D1116069

CONTEMPORARY
NUTRITION
SUPPORT
PRACTICE
A Clinical Guide

www.elsevierhealth.com

Second Edition

CONTEMPORARY
NUTRITION
SUPPORT
PRACTICE

A CLINICAL GUIDE

Laura E. Matarese, MS, RD, LD, FADA, CNSD
Director, Nutrition Intestinal Rehabilitation
The Cleveland Clinic Foundation
Cleveland, Ohio

Michele M. Gottschlich, PhD, RD, LD, CNSD
Director, Nutrition Services
Shriners Hospitals for Children
Cincinnati, Ohio
and
Adjunct Associate Professor
Department of Dietetics and Nutrition Education
College of Allied Health Sciences
University of Cincinnati
Cincinnati, Ohio

SAUNDERS
An Imprint of Elsevier Science
Philadelphia London New York St. Louis Sydney Tokyo

SAUNDERS
An Imprint of Elsevier Science
11830 Westline Industrial Drive
St. Louis, Missouri 63146

Contemporary Nutrition Support Practice, ed 2   ISBN 0-7216-9357-1

NOTICE

Nutrition is an ever-changing field. Standard safety precautions must be followed, but as new research and clinical experience broaden our knowledge, changes in treatment and drug therapy may become necessary or appropriate. Readers are advised to check the most current product information provided by the manufacturer of each drug to be administered to verify the recommended dose, the method and duration of administration, and contraindications. It is the responsibility of the licensed prescriber, relying on experience and knowledge of the patient, to determine dosages and the best treatment for each individual patient. Neither the publisher nor the author assumes any liability for any injury and/or damage to persons or property arising from this publication.

Previous edition copyrighted, 1998.

Library of Congress Cataloging-in-Publication Data

Contemporary nutrition support practice: a clinical guide / [edited by] Laura E.
Matarese, Michele M. Gottschlich. -- 2nd ed.
    p. cm.
  Includes bibliographical references and index.
  ISBN 0-7216-9357-1
   1. Diet therapy. I. Matarese, Laura E. II. Gottschlich, Michele M.

RM216 .C678 2002
615.8'54--dc21

                                     2002026878

Vice President and Publishing Director, Nursing: Sally Schrefer
Editor: Yvonne Alexopoulos
Associate Developmental Editor: Danielle Frazier
Publishing Services Manager: Catherine Jackson
Project Manager: Anne Gassett
Designer: Amy Buxton

EH/MVY

Printed in the United States of America

Last digit is the print number: 9   8   7   6   5   4   3   2   1

To my dear parents
Ben and Rose,
who sacrificed so much so that I may have an education,
and to my brother,
Ben,
the best guy I know!

LEM

I ask a blessing on this book from my true soul mate,
Bill Barkalow, to whom,
along with my cherished children,
Mark, Melissa, and MaryAnn,
and my dear parents,
Norma and Eugene Morath,
this book is dedicated.

MMG

CONTRIBUTORS

Diane M. Anderson, PhD, RD, CSP, FADA
Associate Professor
Department of Pediatrics
Baylor College of Medicine
Houston, Texas
Neonates

Peter L. Beyer, MS, RD
Associate Professor
Department of Dietetics and Nutrition
University of Kansas Medical Center
Kansas City, Kansas
Complications of Enteral Nutrition

Abby S. Bloch, PhD, RD, FADA
Nutrition Consultant
New York, New York
Cancer

Maria G. Boosalis, PhD, MPH, RD, LD
Associate Professor
Department of Clinical Sciences
University of Kentucky
Lexington, Kentucky
Vitamins

Carmen S. Brunner, RD, LD
Clinical Dietitian
Department of Nutrition
Shriners Hospitals for Children
Cincinnati, Ohio
Neurologic Impairments

Jean C. Burge, PhD, RD, CNSD
Associate Professor and Director of the Didactic
Program in Dietetics
Department of Foods and Nutrition
College of Saint Elizabeth
Morristown, New Jersey
Obesity

Theresa A. Byrne, DSc, RD, CNSD
Director, Research and Clinical Services
Nutritional Restart Centers
Wellesley, Massachusetts
Gastrointestinal and Pancreatic Disease

Pamela Charney, MS, RD, CNSD
PhD Student
University of Medicine and Dentistry
    of New Jersey (UMDNJ)
Consultant
Private Practice
Dayton, Ohio
Diabetes Mellitus

Ronni Chernoff, PhD, RD, FADA
Associate Director
Geriatric Research Education and Clinical Center
Central Arkansas Veterans Healthcare System
Director
Arkansas Geriatric Education Center
Professor
Department of Nutrition and Dietetics
University of Arkansas for Medical Sciences
Little Rock, Arkansas
Geriatrics

Tina Colaizzo-Anas, PhD, RD, CDN
Assistant Professor
Department of Dietetics and Nutrition
Buffalo State College
Buffalo, New York
*The Evolution of Nutrition Support Services; Future
Directions*

Charlene W. Compher, PhD, RD, FADA, CNSD
Senior Clinical Specialist
Department of Clinical Nutrition Support Service
University of Pennsylvania Health System
Philadelphia, Pennsylvania
Economics of Nutrition Support

Ann M. Coulston, MS, RD
Nutrition Consultant
Hattner/Coulston Nutrition Associates, LLC
Palo Alto, California
Understanding and Conducting Clinical Research

Gail A. Cresci, MS, RD, CNSD, LD
Assistant Clinical Professor
Department of Surgery
Co-Director, Surgical Nutrition Service
Medical College of Georgia
Augusta, Georgia
Metabolic Stress

Anne M. Davis, MS, RD, CNSD
Senior Clinical Scientist
Department of Clinical Nutrition
Wyeth-Ayerst Global Pharmaceuticals
Philadelphia, Pennsylvania
Pediatrics

Michele A. DeBiasse-Fortin, MS, RD, LDN, CNSD
Chief Clinical Dietitian
Nutrition Support Dietitian
Department of Food and Nutrition Services
Quincy Medical Center
Quincy, Massachusetts
Minerals and Trace Elements

Robert S. DeChicco, MS, RD, LD, CNSD
Manager, Nutrition Support Dietetics
Department of Nutrition Support and Vascular Access
The Cleveland Clinic Foundation
Cleveland, Ohio
Determining the Nutrition Support Regimen

Cade Fields-Gardner, MS, RD, LD, CD
Director of Services
The Cutting Edge
Cary, Illinois
Human Immunodeficiency Virus Infection

David Frankenfield, MS, RD
Chief Clinical Dietitian
Department of Clinical Nutrition
Penn State's Milton S. Hershey Medical Center
Hershey, Pennsylvania
Energy Dynamics

Sue Fredstrom, MS, RD, CNSD
Clinical Nutritionist
Department of Medicine
University of Minnesota
Minneapolis, Minnesota
Carbohydrates

M. Patricia Fuhrman, MS, RD, LD, FADA, CNSD
Chair of Dietetics
Jewish Hospital College of Nursing and Allied Health
Saint Louis, Missouri
Complication Management in Parenteral Nutrition

Susan T. Fussell, PhD, RD, CNSD
Pediatric Dietitian
Duke University
Durham, North Carolina
Enteral Formulations

D. Jordi Goldstein-Fuchs, DSc, RD
Associate Research Professor
Nutrition Education and Research Program
School of Medicine
University of Nevada, Reno
Reno, Nevada
Renal Failure

Michele M. Gottschlich, PhD, RD, LD, CNSD
Director, Nutrition Services
Shriners Hospitals for Children
Cincinnati, Ohio
and
Adjunct Associate Professor
Department of Dietetics and Nutrition Education
College of Allied Health Sciences
University of Cincinnati
Cincinnati, Ohio
Early and Perioperative Nutrition Support; Burns and Wound Healing

Kathy Hammond, MS, RN, RD, LD, CNSN, CNSD
Coordinator, Continuing Education
Clinical Nutrition Specialist
Professional Services
Chartwell Diversified Services, Inc.
Lilburn, Georgia
Adjunct Assistant Professor
University of Georgia
Department of Foods and Nutrition
Athens, Georgia
History and Physical Examination

Jeanette M. Hasse, PhD, RD, LD, FADA, CNSD
Transplant Nutrition Specialist
Baylor Institute of Transplantation Services
Baylor University Medical Center
Dallas, Texas
Solid Organ Transplantation

Ann-Marie Hedberg, DrPh, RD, LD
Assistant Director
Department of Nutrition Services
St. Luke's Episcopal Hospital
Houston, Texas
Quality and Performance Improvement

Wanda Hain Howell, PhD, RD, CNSD
Associate Professor
Department of Nutritional Sciences
University of Arizona
Tucson, Arizona
Anthropometry and Body Composition Analysis

Carol Ireton-Jones, PhD, RD, LD, CNSD, FACN
Director
Department of Nutrition Services
Coram Healthcare
Carrollton, Texas
Home Care

Ruth E. Johnston, MS, RD, LD, CDE
Geriatric Dietitian
Department of Nutrition and Food Service
Central Arkansas Veteran Healthcare System
Little Rock, Arkansas
Geriatrics

Peggy Kaproth, MS, MBA, RPh, RD
Clinical Manager, Aligned Promotions
Department Client Support Services
Advance PCS
Minneapolis, Minnesota
Hepatic Failure

Michael J. Kelley, PhD, RD, CNSD
Senior Project Leader
Ross Products Division
Abbott Laboratories
Columbus, Ohio
Lipids

Bobbi Langkamp-Henken, PhD, RD
Associate Professor
Department of Food, Science, and Human Nutrition
University of Florida
Gainesville, Florida
Evaluating Immunocompetence

Polly Lenssen, MS, RD, CD, FADA
Clinical Nutrition Manager
Department of Clinical Nutrition
Children's Hospital and Regional Medical Center
Seattle, Washington
Hematopoietic Cell Transplantation

Lucinda K. Lysen, RD, LD, RN, BSN
Owner/Director
Private Practice in Nutrition
Chicago, Illinois and Stuart, Florida
Enteral Equipment

Maureen MacBurney, MBA, MS, RD, LD
Manager, Thoracic Surgery Team
Department of Care Coordination
Brigham and Women's Hospital
Boston, Massachusetts
Pregnancy

Julie O'Sullivan Maillet, PhD, RD, FADA
Associate Dean for Academic Affairs and Research
Dean's Office
University of Medicine and Dentistry of New Jersey
Newark, New Jersey
Ethical Considerations

Laura E. Matarese, MS, RD, LD, FADA, CNSD
Director, Nutrition Intestinal Rehabilitation
The Cleveland Clinic Foundation
Cleveland, Ohio
Determining the Nutrition Support Regimen; Rationale and Efficacy of Specialized Enteral and Parenteral Formulas; Pregnancy; Future Directions

Theresa Mayes, RD, LD
Clinical Dietitian
Department of Nutrition Services
Shriners Hospitals for Children
Cincinnati, Ohio
Burns and Wound Healing

Beth McQuiston, MS, RD, LD
Clinical Consultant
Chicago, Illinois
Renal Failure

Elaine R. Monsen, PhD, RD
Professor
Department of Nutrition and Medicine
University of Washington
Seattle, Washington
Understanding and Conducting Clinical Research

Charles M. Mueller, PhD, RD, CNSD, CDN
General Clinical Research Center
Weill Cornell Medical College
New York Presbyterian Hospital
Adjunct Assistant Clinical Professor
Department of Nutrition and Food Studies
New York University
New York, New York
Inflammatory Response and Sepsis

Jennifer Kay Nelson, MS, RD, LD, CNSD
Director
Department of Clinical Dietetics
Mayo Clinic
Rochester, Minnesota
Economics of Nutrition Support

Reneé Piazza-Barnett, MEd, RD, CNSD
Clinical Dietitian Specialist
Department of Nutrition Services
Loma Linda University Medical Center
Loma Linda, California
Combined and Transitional Feeding Modalities

Sandra M. Raup, RD, CNSD
Student
The George Washington University School of Law
Washington, DC
Hepatic Failure

Carol J. Rollins, MS, RD, CNSD, Pharm D, BCNSP
Coordinator, Nutrition Support Team
Arizona Health Sciences Center
Clinical Associate Professor
Department of Pharmacy Practice & Science
University of Arizona
Tucson, Arizona
General Pharmacologic Issues

Mary Krystofiak Russell, MS, RD, LDN, CNSD
Dietitian Clinician
Department of Nutrition Services
Duke University Hospital
Durham, North Carolina
Laboratory Monitoring

Denise Baird Schwartz, MS, RD, FADA, CNSD
Nutrition Support Coordinator
Department of Nutrition Service
Providence Health System
Burbank, California
Pulmonary and Cardiac Failure

Annalynn Skipper, MS, RD, FADA, CNSD
Co-Director, Nutrition Support Service
Assistant Professor
Department of Clinical Nutrition
Rush Presbyterian-St. Luke's Medical Center
Chicago, Illinois
Parenteral Nutrition

Joanne L. Slavin, PhD, RD
Professor
Department of Food, Science, and Nutrition
University of Minnesota
St. Paul, Minnesota
Dietary Fiber

Randi Stanko-Kline, RD, CNSD
Senior Clinical Scientist
Department of Clinical Nutrition
Wyeth-Ayerst Global Pharmaceuticals
Philadelphia, Pennsylvania
Pediatrics

Susan Stoll, MS, RD, CNSD
Nutrition Consultant
Brookline, Massachusetts
Proteins and Amino Acids

Mary M. Sullivan, MPH, RD
Regulatory Affairs Associate
Pharmaceutical Products Division
Abbott Laboratories
Abbott Park, Illinois
Gastrointestinal and Pancreatic Disease

Elizabeth Wall-Alonso, MS, RD, CNSD
Nutrition Support Specialist
Department of Nutrition Services
The University of Chicago Hospital
Chicago, Illinois
Gastrointestinal and Pancreatic Disease

Susan J. Whitmire, RD, CNSD
Nutrition Support Dietitian
Department of Gastroenterology and Nutrition
Geisinger Medical Center
Danville, Pennsylvania
Fluid, Electrolytes, and Acid-Base Balance

Marion F. Winkler, MS, RD, LDN, CNSD
Surgical Nutrition Specialist
Department of Surgery and Nutrition Support
Rhode Island Hospital
Providence, Rhode Island
Quality and Performance Improvement

Steven M. Wood, PhD, RD
Clinical Research Scientist
Department of Medical Nutrition Research and Development
Ross Products Division
Abbott Laboratories
Columbus, Ohio
Evaluating Immunocompetence

Lorraine See Young, RD, MS, LDN, CNSD
Clinical Nutrition Manager for Home Care and Research
Boston Medical Center
Boston, Massachusetts
Proteins and Amino Acids

REVIEWERS

Diana Fullen Bowers, PhD, RD, LD
Adjunct Professor
Columbus State Community College
Columbus, Ohio
Nutrition Support Dietitian
HomeReach, Inc.
Worthington, Ohio
Lecturer
PRN Continuing Education
Westerville, Ohio

Margaret M. Cicirella, MS, MA, RD, LD
Instructor
Department of Nutrition
Case Western Reserve University
Cleveland, Ohio

Gail A. Cresci, MS, RD, CNSD, LD
Assistant Clinical Professor
Department of Surgery
Co-Director, Surgical Nutrition Service
Medical College of Georgia
Augusta, Georgia

Michele A. DeBiasse-Fortin, MS, RD, LDN, CNSD
Chief Clinical Dietitian
Nutrition Support Dietitian
Department of Food and Nutrition Services
Quincy Medical Center
Quincy, Massachusetts

Marianne Duda, MS, RD, LD, CNSD
Nutrition Support Dietitian
Coram Healthcare
Tampa, Florida

Barbara Eldridge, RD, LD
Clinical Trials Coordinator
Cancer Treatment Center
Saint Alphonsus Regional Medical Center
Boise, Idaho

Susan Ettinger, PhD, RD
Chair
Associate Professor
Department of Clinical Nutrition
New York Institute of Technology
Old Westbury, New York

Judith Fish, MMSc, RD, CNSD
Nutrition Consultant
Asheville, North Carolina

Kathy Hammond, MS, RN, RD, LD, CNSN, CNSD
Coordinator, Continuing Education
Clinical Nutrition Specialist
Professional Services
Chartwell Diversified Services, Inc.
Lilburn, Georgia
Adjunct Assistant Professor
University of Georgia
Department of Foods and Nutrition
Athens, Georgia

Mary Jacob, PhD
Professor, Nutritional Sciences
Department of Family and Consumer Sciences
Graduate Coordinator
California State University
Long Beach, California

Betty Kenyon, BS, RD, LMNT
Consultant Dietitian
Panhandle Community Services
Gering, Nebraska
Nutrition Instructor
Western Nebraska Community College
Scottsbluff, Nebraska

Bridget Klawitter, PhD, RD, CD, FADA
Manager
Medical Nutrition Therapy and Diabetes Services
All Saints Healthcare, Inc.
Racine, Wisconsin

Diane T. Kupensky, RN, MSN, CNS
Clinical Resource Coordinator
St. Elizabeth Health Center
Youngstown, Ohio

Joseph Lacy, MS, RD
Assistant Director
Department of Parenteral and Enteral Nutrition
The University Hospital
Cincinnati, Ohio

Polly Lenssen, MS, RD, CD, FADA
Clinical Nutrition Manager
Department of Clinical Nutrition
Children's Hospital and Regional Medical Center
Seattle, Washington

Edith Lerner, PhD
Associate Professor and Vice-Chair
Department of Nutrition
Case Western Reserve University
Cleveland, Ohio

Barbara J. Main, RD, CNSD
Compliance Manager
Department of Dietetics
William Beaumont Hospital
Royal Oak, Michigan

Mary Marian, MS, RD
Clinical Nutrition Research Specialist
Department of Family and Community Medicine
University of Arizona
Tucson, Arizona

Dena McDowell, RD
Clinical Dietitian
Froedtert and Medical College
Milwaukee, Wisconsin

Marlene J. Neville, MMSc, RD, LD, CNSD
Nutrition Support Dietitian
Coram Healthcare
Marietta, Georgia
Nutrition Support Dietitian
Department of Pharmacy
Northside Hospital
Atlanta, Georgia
Clinical Preceptor, Graduate Nutrition Program
University of Georgia
Atlanta, Georgia

Marsha E. Orr, RN, MS
Principal
CreativEnergy, LLC Healthcare Consultants
Mesa, Arizona

Tracey Ryan, RD, CNSD
Chief Clinical Dietitian
Froedtert and Medical College
Milwaukee, Wisconsin

M. Rosita Schiller, PhD, RD, FADA
Professor and Director
Medical Dietetics Division
School of Allied Medical Professions
The Ohio State University
Columbus, Ohio

Carolyn T. Spencer, BS, RD, CNSD
Clinical Dietitian
Department of Clinical Nutrition Support Service
Hospital of the University of Pennsylvania
University of Pennsylvania School of Medicine
Philadelphia, Pennsylvania

FOREWORD TO FIRST EDITION

Although nutrition support is only about 30 years old, nutrition support practice has gone through many changes during those years. The evolution of nutrition support has lead to transformations in the art and science of specialized nutrition, in the methods used to deliver it, and in the roles of the personnel who are responsible for prescribing and evaluating its effectiveness. After many years of experimentation, trial, and failure by outstanding scientists, successful parenteral nutrition in an infant was reported in the late 1960s by Wilmore and Dudrick.[1] Despite this published report, many health professionals were unimpressed with the technique and dubious about any future for this intervention. Although nutrients had been delivered into the gastrointestinal tract by tube for many years, the concept of safely feeding a patient using the circulatory system, accessed by catheter, did not seem reasonable to many physicians and other health professionals. Nutrition support is now accepted practice.

Nutrition support with enteral (tube) feedings traditionally had been the responsibility of dietitians; when parenteral nutrition became an acceptable intervention, responsibility for its management was shifted to the nutrition support team that established the practice standards. The knowledge and skills needed to practice in the area of nutrition support have grown considerably, and this book serves as a source of the most valuable, updated, and current information for the nutrition support practitioner.

The editors and chapter authors are among the most knowledgeable experts in the field of nutrition support. They have included state-of-the-art information on a broad range of topics that are essential to practice for the nutrition support or clinical dietitian. These topics range from understanding the dynamics of the nutrition support team to conducting research in the area of nutrition support. The domain of knowledge required to practice successfully includes comprehensive information on body composition; nutrition assessment; metabolic processes in normal, chronically ill, or acutely ill individuals; the basic principles and techniques of enteral and parenteral nutrition; normal growth, development, and aging; and organ systems disorders. Other key issues involved in nutrition support are quality assurance, ethics, economics, and management policies.

As the health care delivery system changes, shifting the provision of care from the tertiary care setting to community and home-based primary care, the role that specialized nutrition support will have in health care intervention and therapy will change, as will the methods that may have to be implemented. With these changes, dietitians and nutrition support professionals will have the responsibility for ensuring their own positions and responsibilities in nutrition care, whether in hospital, institutional, home, or out-patient settings.

As dietetics professionals, nutrition support practitioners have made a commitment to lifelong education and mandatory continuing education. The responsibility resides with each individual to pursue information that will ensure his or her competency in this area of practice. For nutrition support clinicians, using a book such as this fulfills the ongoing commitment to increase knowledge and apply it in the daily performance of delivering safe, comprehensive, valuable nutrition support. The editors have done a splendid job in compiling a comprehensive, well-organized text written by recognized experts and leaders in the field. They are to be congratulated for adding a valuable reference to the literature of nutrition support.

Ronni Chernoff, PhD, RD, FADA
Associate Director
Geriatric Research Education and Clinical Center
Central Arkansas Veterans Healthcare System
Director
Arkansas Geriatric Education Center
Professor
Department of Nutrition and Dietetics
University of Arkansas for Medical Sciences
Little Rock, Arkansas

REFERENCE

1. Wilmore DW, Dudrick SJ: Growth and development of an infant receiving all nutrients exclusively by vein, *JAMA* 1968; 203:860.

FOREWORD TO SECOND EDITION

The concept of parenteral nutrition and nutrition support practice originated in the late 1960s at the Hospital of the University of Pennsylvania through the pioneering work of Drs. Stanley Dudrick, Douglas Wilmore, Harry Vars, and Jonathan Rhoads. These surgical pioneers would not accept the inevitable progression of malnutrition and death that would often accompany some postoperative complications or complicated diseases. Their concerns for their patients spurred them on to critically acclaimed work in the laboratory followed by its application to critically ill surgical and medical patients. The application of the techniques of parenteral nutrition, or intravenous hyperalimentation as it was called at that time, required the expertise of a multidisciplinary team including a dietitian, nurse, pharmacist, and physician. The combined knowledge of these four fields led to a team that could skillfully and safely support the patient's nutrition needs in a way that the four independent disciplines working alone could not. Although the field is over 30 years old, it is still growing, developing, and redefining itself. Different enteral devices and formulations as well as scientific research in optimizing enteral diets for various disease states continue to evolve. Similarly, parenteral nutrition solutions and additives are evoking great interest in the research lab. The role of glutamine, carnitine, and choline remains to be fully defined. Intestinal rehabilitation programs to maximize intestinal absorption in patients with diseased or shortened intestinal tracts through the use of diet, medication, and trophic hormones are of great current interest.

The etiology of metabolic bone disease and liver disease that can complicate prolonged home parenteral nutrition are being actively investigated. We have learned a lot in the last 35 years, but an increasing number of questions still need to be answered.

The editors of this second edition of *Contemporary Nutrition Support Practice: A Clinical Guide* are well-known, established, expert clinicians who have made significant contributions to the development of the science and art of nutrition support. They both continue to engage in an active clinical practice in nutrition support and have assembled a very knowledgeable group of contributors to update and make this second edition even more useful than the very popular first edition. This text will prove to be of great value to all members of a nutrition support team in helping to provide clinically relevant information related to the care of their patients.

Ezra Steiger, MD, FACS, CNSP
Consultant in General Surgery
Co-Director, Nutrition Support
Director, Intestinal Rehabilitation Program
The Cleveland Clinic Foundation
Cleveland, Ohio

PREFACE

Since 1968 when techniques for intravenous nutrition were introduced, the field of nutrition support has evolved to encompass a very broad and sophisticated knowledge base. There has been a rapid accumulation of scientific information and technical advances. The growing complexity of providing highly specialized nonvolitional feedings has presented the clinician with many new challenges. The nutrition support practitioner must have an astute knowledge of nutrition, physiology, pharmacology, research, and management. All of these elements form the solid foundation for assessment, planning, implementation, and monitoring of the nutrition support regimen.

Numerous changes have occurred in our knowledge of nutrition and our methods of delivery since the first edition. The health care environment continues to change. Over the past several decades, the role of the nutrition support dietitian has expanded and broadened to include added responsibilities, more independence, and greater accountability. The purpose of this book is to provide a comprehensive reference on the principles and practices of nutrition support, with an emphasis on safety, efficacy, and science-based medicine. It is our hope that this book will become a useful reference and tool to the practicing clinician as well as a text for students studying nutrition.

This text is organized in a logical progressive manner addressing basic principles and then progressing to more advanced concepts. It begins with an account of the evolution of nutrition support, followed by assessment of nutritional status, and nutrients for nutrition support. The text then provides a series of chapters on the principles of nutrition support, nutrition support throughout the life cycle, nutrition support in specific system disorders and general systemic disorders, and continuing through nutrition support in physiologic stress. The final section addresses management and professional issues and includes a chapter on future directions. An exhaustive list of references for more in-depth review has also been included.

Progress is made by those who are brave enough to dream and strong enough to persevere. Our dedication to the care of patients and the advancement of practice is evident throughout this book. The thread of collaborative and interdisciplinary management is interwoven throughout the text. This resource will benefit not only dietitians but also any practitioner or educator involved in the area of specialized nutrition support.

The chapters have been written by a distinguished group of authors who have devoted their careers to nutrition support. With the publication of the first edition, it was our hope and intention that this book become the "gold standard" for contemporary nutrition support practice and that it be used to guide and enhance the care of the patients and clients we serve. Thanks to the dedication of the authors and publisher, our vision is becoming a reality.

Laura E. Matarese
Michele Morath Gottschlich

ACKNOWLEDGMENTS

No achievement, great or small, is effectively accomplished in isolation. Listing the entire "team" (e.g., Cincinnati Burns Institute, Shriners Hospitals for Children, The Cleveland Clinic Foundation, Elsevier Science, the American Dietetic Association, Dietitians in Nutrition Support, the American Society for Parenteral and Enteral Nutrition, the American Burn Association, patients, colleagues, relatives, and friends), so many of whom have contributed either directly or indirectly to the development of each of us and thus to this book – would indeed be an insurmountable task! However, a number of very special people have given so much to this venture that not specifically mentioning them would be unthinkable.

First, we would like to express our sincere gratitude to each of our extraordinary contributors, with many of whom we have enjoyed a wonderful professional relationship as well as friendship for years. A very special thanks is extended to our talented medical illustrator, Tamela Grandjean. This book also would not have been possible without the excellent assistance from Yvonne Alexopoulos, Editor, Danielle Frazier, Associate Developmental Editor, and Anne Gassett, Project Manager—all at Elsevier Science.

We would like to acknowledge a number of physicians who have influenced us over the course of our careers. In particular, we recognize and appreciate the opportunities and insights afforded to us by Drs. Josef Fischer, J. Wesley Alexander, Richard E. Miller, Sidney F. Miller, Robert K. Finley, Jr., and Richard J. Kagan, during our formative years. We consider ourselves currently blessed to have exceptional medical directors (Drs. Glenn D. Warden, Ezra Steiger, and Douglas Seidner) and appreciate the continued encouragement, generous moral support, and overwhelming wisdom we gain from them daily.

We appreciate the enthusiasm, assistance, and nurturing we have received over the years from our colleagues, who we feel have influenced and facilitated countless of our professional endeavors, including the development of this book. Lastly, the heartfelt encouragement, exceptional capacity for understanding, and sustenance that we received from our personal friends and family throughout the periods of doubt and exhaustion have culminated in our indebtedness to each of them—we can only recognize and likely never be able to adequately repay this debt.

Michele Morath Gottschlich
Laura E. Matarese

CONTENTS

The Evolution of Nutrition Support Services

1

Tina Colaizzo-Anas, PhD, RD, CDN

I N this chapter we examine the evolution of the team approach to nutrition support, the economic pressures that challenge this specialty service, the transformation of nutrition support as a vehicle for the delivery of functional foods,* and the opportunities that the future may hold for this specialty service.

The Emergence of the Nutrition Support Team

Methods of providing optimal nutrition care for hospitalized patients have changed dramatically since the development and refinement of techniques for parenteral and enteral nutrition. Initially, the ability to provide nutrition to any patient, regardless of disease state, presented many challenges to health care professionals. Parenteral nutrition (PN) was associated with serious metabolic, infectious, and access sites complications.[1,2] Similarly, forced enteral feeding was associated with potential complications, including aspiration,[3-5] pneumothorax,[6] diarrhea,[7] and formula contamination.[8] The need to provide parenteral and enteral nutrition safely and effectively was the catalyst for a new approach to the delivery of nutrition in the hospital: a multidisciplinary team approach to nutrition support.

To ensure appropriate care for patients receiving specialized nutrition therapy, nutrition support teams (NSTs) were formed. The NST provides consultation services for the primary care physician whose patients require parenteral or enteral nutrition (PEN) and any other specialized nutrition support intervention. The team typically includes a physician, a registered dietitian, a nurse, and a pharmacist. Each professional brings to the team unique clinical skills and nutrition knowledge.

Each team member assesses and monitors the patient from the standpoint of his or her respective discipline. By sharing data, expertise, and perspectives, the team members define the patient's nutrition problems and formulate a comprehensive treatment plan. As a result, patient care decisions are products of the team process and not of just one discipline. Monitoring the patient throughout the course of treatment, the NST ensures that the goals of nutrition therapy are met and that morbidity and mortality secondary to misapplication of nutrition support techniques are prevented. By working together, NST clinicians acquire a common core of nutrition support knowledge and refine the clinical and technical skills they need to provide safe and effective nutrition support.

An examination of the results of two surveys performed in 1983 revealed the following facts about early NSTs.[9,10] Team directors were typically physicians with backgrounds in surgery or gastroenterology. Many team members were educated at the graduate level: 17% of the nurses, 35% of the dietitians, and 42% of the pharmacists reported having advanced degrees.[9] Many practitioners had previous clinical experience. The advanced education and clinical background suggested that NST members required skills consistent with an advanced level of practice.

Only a few teams existed before 1975.[11] Some 95% of the teams surveyed were formed after 1975, and 60% of those were formed after 1980 and at the time of the survey could be considered newly formed.[9] It was estimated that, in 1983, 8.3% of all United States hospitals had NSTs.[10] While the primary focus was on inpatient care, more than 50% of the teams surveyed reported outpatient involvement with home parenteral and enteral nutrition patients.[9]

National Nutrition Support Organizations/Certification

By 1975, the growing interest in nutrition support led to the chartering of the American Society for Parenteral and Enteral Nutrition (ASPEN), "a multidisciplinary, professional and scientific organization committed to promoting quality patient care, education and research in the field of nutrition and metabolic support in all health care settings."[12] Since its inception, ASPEN has led the way in developing standards of practice for nutrition support professionals,[13-16] standards of care for patients receiving this complex therapy,[17-20] and guidelines for the use of parenteral and enteral nutrition (Box 1-1). ASPEN has also been instrumental in developing a certification process for nutrition support practitioners. The National Board of Nutrition Support Certification, which was established in 1984, administers certification programs, offering credentials to dietitians, nurses, and physicians. Pharmacists receive nutrition support certification from the Board of Pharmaceutical Specialties. Eligibility criteria for dietitians are the Registered Dietitian credential with a recommended 2 years of experience in specialized nutrition support. Candidates for certification must pass a written examination designed to test the knowledge needed to deliver parenteral and enteral support. Certification extends for 5 years, after which reexamination is required. The application for certification may be found online at http://www.nutritioncare.org/profdev/nbnsc.html.

Paralleling the formation of ASPEN, Dietitians in Critical Care, a dietetics practice group (DPG) of the American Dietetic

*Functional foods refers to foods or ingredients that potentially provide a health benefit beyond traditional nutrition.

Acknowledgment: A special thank you is extended to Karen Buzby, RD, who contributed to the first edition chapter.

Standards and Guidelines for Nutrition Support*

ASPEN Standards for Nutrition Support Pharmacists[13]
ASPEN Standards for Nutrition Support Dietitians[14]
ASPEN Standards for Nutrition Support Nurses[15]
ASPEN Standards for Nutrition Support Physicians[16]
ASPEN Standards for Home Nutrition Support[17]
ASPEN Standards for Nutrition Support: Hospitalized Patients[18]
ASPEN Standards for Nutrition Support of Adult Residents of Long-Term Care Facilities[19]
ASPEN Standards for Nutrition Support: Hospitalized Pediatric Patients[20]
ASPEN Safe Practices for Parenteral Feeding Formulations[21]
Role of the Dietitians in Enteral and Parenteral Nutrition Support, position statement of the American Dietetic Association[22]
Nutrition Intervention in the Care of Persons with Human Immnodeficiency Virus Infection, position statement of the American Dietetic Association[23]

*Standards and guidelines are available from the American Society for Parenteral and Enteral Nutrition, 8605 Cameron Street, Silver Spring, MD 20910.

Association (ADA), was established in 1978. The initial focus of the practice group was patients in the intensive care unit; however, the need for parenteral and enteral nutrition extended beyond the acute stage of illness, frequently to the rehabilitation and outpatient settings. To reflect the expanding scope of practice, the name of the organization was changed to Dietitians in Nutrition Support (DNS). Immediately following the name change in 1987, DNS experienced its greatest increase in membership to approximately 3200 today.

DNS has promoted and advanced the practice of nutrition support by contributing to several ADA position statements of the dietitian's role in nutrition support;[22,23] publishing guidelines for nutrition support; providing continuing education via a monthly newsletter, workshops, and lectures; and providing representation on legislative issues facing nutrition support dietitians. Although specialty and fellow credentials for registered dietitians are available from the ADA, these credentials do not focus solely on nutrition support.

Evolution and Growth of the Nutrition Support Team

Coinciding with advances in parenteral and enteral nutrition were reports of malnutrition in hospitalized patients in the United States.[24,25] Several early studies documented the prevalence of malnutrition in hospitalized patients to be 30% to 50%.[26-29] Despite differences in hospital populations, types of hospitals, diseases studied, and the socioeconomic status of the patients, the prevalence of malnutrition appeared to be relatively predictable. The incidence of malnutrition in hospitalized patients further substantiated the need for a new approach to the delivery of nutrition care to hospitalized patients.

Systematic clinical and experimental studies were undertaken to define the effects of malnutrition on hospital course, risk of complications, and chance of survival. Numerous studies documented the negative impact of malnutrition on clinical outcome.[29-33] Data have been generated that identify specific measures of nutritional status as predictors of increased hospital morbidity and mortality secondary to protein-calorie malnutrition (PCM).[28,30-32,34] Increased awareness of the preva-

lence and consequences of untreated PCM provided a strong incentive for the rapid growth in the use of specialized nutrition support for malnourished patients.

The Early Usage of Nutrition Support

Results from a 1984 marketing survey[35] show that 15% of all patients in U.S. hospitals (5.5 million) received nutrition therapy beyond the standard hospital diet, and that 3.6% of these patients (1.32 million) received PN or enteral nutrition (EN). The average duration of PN was 20.6 days and of EN, 18.5 days.[35] Therefore, parenteral and enteral nutrition services were provided for more than 25 million inpatient days. The cost of PN and EN was more than $3 billion. In recent years, nutrition support professionals have influenced a significant shift toward enteral nutrition whenever possible. Additionally, the average duration of PN and EN likely has decreased, given the current health care financing pressures that are subsequently described. Unfortunately, current data collection reflecting the prevalence of PEN usage is lacking.

Impact of Prospective Payment and Diagnosis-Related Groups

Escalation of costs of medical care led to legislation aimed at controlling and reducing them. In 1982, Congress passed the Tax Equity and Fiscal Responsibility Act, which changed Medicare reimbursement for inpatient hospital services from a cost-based retrospective reimbursement system to a fixed-price prospective payment system (PPS). Diagnosis-related groups (DRGs)* caused hospitals to reevaluate the services they provide. Some institutions decentralized their NSTs, making them informal committees or consultation services only.[36]

Changes in nutrition support staffing were observed between a 1986 and a 1989 survey of dietitians. A decrease in full-time-equivalent nutrition support dietitians was observed.[37] Daily use of nutrition support for inpatients was 3.5% for parenteral and 4.9% for enteral tube feeding and 9.6% for oral supplements.[37]

PPS provided the incentive for NSTs to evaluate the cost-effectiveness of nutrition support therapies. Because parenteral and enteral nutrition therapies are costly and are associated with certain risks, it became clear that procedures were needed that would ensure judicious and appropriate use of nutrition support. Nutrition screening programs were established in hospitals across the country to identify earlier and more precisely patients at risk for malnutrition who need a comprehensive nutrition assessment to determine if nutrition support is needed. In 1993, 90% of hospitals had policies for screening.[38] Today virtually all hospitals have nutrition screening programs to comply with standards issued by the Joint Commission on Accreditation of Healthcare Organizations (JCAHO).

Initially, NSTs focused on becoming a revenue-generating service. Under the current arrangements for health care reim-

*Diagnosis-related groups are categories for reimbursing hospitals for care to Medicare patients based on diagnosis. For example, if a patient were admitted to the hospital for gallbladder removal, Medicare would reimburse the hospital for the preset amount for cholecystectomies regardless of actual costs.

bursement, the focus has shifted to demonstrating how NSTs can significantly save on costs and influence outcome. NSTs can easily reduce costs by guiding discriminate use of the more than 200 formulas on the market, controlling duration of nutrition support, setting policy for indications for nutrition support, reducing waste, and "vetoing" unnecessary laboratory tests. Literally thousands of dollars per patient can be saved when the NST advises against parenteral nutrition because other adequate and less expensive means of nutrition support are available.

The Nutrition Support Team in the 1990s

The unprecedented scrutiny of health care services that started with PPS continued into the 1990s. Health care reform, managed care, case management, and home care are just several issues NSTs faced in the 1990s. Examining team prevalence, structure, services, and responsibilities helps elucidate how NSTs have faced these challenges.

Prevalence

In 1991, ASPEN conducted a survey of all hospitals larger than 150 beds in the United States to determine the prevalence of NSTs and to obtain information about current and planned teams.[39] The results revealed that 484 of the 1680 hospitals (29%) that participated in the survey had an NST. More than half of these teams had been active for 5 years or more, and 21% were well established and had been active longer than 10 years. Twenty-seven percent of the NSTs could be considered recently formed (i.e., active for 5 or fewer years). This indicates that hospital administrators were still receptive to starting NSTs. Well-established teams were more likely to have larger numbers of PEN patients and to have team members who devote more time to nutrition support activities. The longer-standing teams also had more team members financed by the NST department. Of the 1196 hospitals without NSTs, 12% had previously *had* a team and 17% had plans to start a team within the next 2 years.[39]

Organizational Structure

There are two basic models for the organization of a nutrition support service: the nutrition support committee and the nutrition support team or department.[36] Factors that influence how a nutrition support service is organized include institution size; profit versus nonprofit status; university affiliation; level of patient care (case mix); the overall clinical, educational, and research objectives of the hospital; staff availability; and internal politics. Separate cost centers for NSTs may be housed within existing departments, for example, department of dietetics, pharmacy, surgery, or medicine.

Team leadership is important to the overall success of the NST. Leadership needs to be addressed on two levels: patient care and team administration. The physician on the NST must assume leadership in the medical aspects of the patient's nutrition care. Depending on the size of the NST, a team coordinator may be required to assume the responsibility for supervising the administrative and clinical functions of the team. ASPEN standards of practice recommend that the NST director be a physician;[16] however, it is not unusual for the team director to be from another discipline.[39] In teams reporting nonphysician directors, dietitians were more likely to assume the director's position.[39]

Services Provided

The actual number of professionals and support staff on an NST varies from institution to institution, but certain services are common to all teams. The general services provided by NSTs include inpatient consultation, provision of home nutrition support, patient and professional educational programs, research and quality management.

INPATIENT CONSULTATION: ASSESSMENT, THERAPY, MONITORING, AND STANDARDIZATION OF PRACTICE. Depending on the arrangement in a given hospital, the team may provide care to patients only when consulted or may provide care to all patients on PEN. Some teams write the orders for PEN and patient monitoring, whereas others write only the *recommendations* for new orders. One of the factors distinguishing successful NSTs from less successful ones or nonteam arrangements is close coordination among team members to deliver comprehensive, cost-effective patient care. Good coordination is achieved through clear and timely communication among members. To optimize the timeliness of team communication, NST rounds may be scheduled at times when the most data are available. For example, team rounds may be scheduled daily after the results of laboratory values are obtained and patients are seen; after at least 12 hours of the previous day's formula has been infused; after that day's data from the patient, bedside chart, and medical record have been obtained; after team members have communicated with primary physicians, consultants, primary nurses, and other caregivers; and before the order for the PN is due in the pharmacy (Fig. 1-1).

During NST rounds, with the initial presentation of patient data, the dietitian may report to the team the results of nutrition assessment (including fluid and electrolyte status, extraordinary losses, and constraints to nutrient delivery), an opinion on the indication for PEN, results of indirect calorimetry (if available), and initial and final formula goal. The nurse may report on the presence and integrity of nutrient access sites; the pharmacist may report on potential drug interactions; and the physician may report on the anticipated medical or surgical plan. When team members are cross-trained, one team member may assume the responsibility for communicating all of the information about an individual patient.

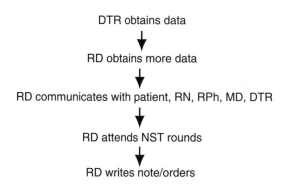

FIGURE 1-1 Model for team communication. *DTR,* registered dietetic technician; *MD,* medical doctor; *NST,* nutrition support team; *RD,* registered dietitian; *RPh,* registered pharmacist; *RN,* registered nurse.

After the initial plan is implemented, team members monitor the patient to prevent complications, including fluid and electrolyte abnormalities, failure to meet nutrition goal targets, nutrient access site problems, and so forth. Intake and output data, laboratory values, medical progress, patient acceptance, and relevant physical examination data are evaluated daily. A deliberate effort must be made to ensure that proper PEN infusions are running, and on schedule; that is, that the actual formula ordered is the one that is being infused. Often, PEN infusions are interrupted for tests and procedures. For this reason, delays in the delivery of the most recently ordered formula may occur. Unless team members monitor to determine that the appropriate formula is being infused, monitoring the patient's tolerance to PEN becomes problematic. Finally, the team members identify targets for discontinuation of PEN and the PEN monitoring protocols.

Generally, the NST devises standardized forms and protocols for ordering and monitoring PEN. Standardization helps streamline communication, reduce ordering errors, and expedite the development of a complete order. While the team promotes consistent use of standardized forms and protocols, it also educates on the use of forms and protocols for implementing individualized PEN regimens and monitoring plans that optimize the potential for meeting medical and nutritional goals.

HOME NUTRITION SUPPORT PROGRAM. A growing trend has been the shift in the use of PEN from the hospital to the home. Data collected from 1988 estimated that 48,000 patients received enteral nutrition and 17,000 patients received PN at home.[40] Data from 1992 revealed a significant increase in home nutrition support, with an estimated 152,000 enteral and 40,000 parenteral nutrition patients.[41]

The NST must ensure that the patient meets eligibility criteria for either enteral or parenteral nutrition at home.[20] As in inpatient care, the team must identify the goals of home nutrition support and devise a comprehensive care plan, including selection of route of nutrient delivery, feeding formula, feeding schedule, and equipment needs.[17] As soon as a patient is identified as a home nutrition support candidate the team should begin assessing the patient's discharge needs and educating patient and family in formula administration and care of the access site. One report of home parenteral nutrition services by a university hospital-affiliated home infusion company indicated that inpatient training had decreased from an average of 12 hours to an average of 4 to 5 hours, with training continued by the home health practitioner.[42] During this time the number of postdischarge educational interventions increased from 0.4 per patient in 1993 to 5.1 in 1997. Home care practitioners often have a major role in patient education and monitoring. Accordingly, responsibility for investigating third-party reimbursement may vary among the NST, the primary physician, and the home care practitioner. The goal is to document the medical necessity of home nutrition support so the patient can obtain financial assistance. Referrals to a home care company for supplies and services are often made by the NST.

Patients should return to the nutrition support outpatient clinic regularly for monitoring. The development of protocols for home nutrition support monitoring ensures the delivery of efficient and cost-effective care. Good communication among the home care company, primary care physician, NST physician, and hospital-based team is essential to achieving a positive patient outcome.

An established NST can be a valuable resource in providing regional home PN and EN programs for other hospitals and institutions that lack their own nutrition support expertise. Some NSTs have expanded the scope of their services and formed home infusion therapy programs to provide antibiotics, chemotherapy, anticoagulation medication, blood products, and fluid and electrolyte replacement at home.[43]

EDUCATIONAL PROGRAMS. The educational efforts of the NST are directed toward patient training and continuing education of health professionals. Of primary importance is the development of easy-to-use patient education materials for home nutrition support. In addition, team members may supervise or directly teach techniques of home nutrition support to patients who require it. Patient support groups can also be organized by the NST as part of the patient education program. These groups address the concerns and needs of long-term home nutrition support patients.

Team members are nutrition support education resources for their discipline. Promoting timely NST consultation requests by providing in-service programs on the detection and prevention of malnutrition should be an objective of the team's professional education efforts. To keep abreast of changes in this and related areas of practice, team members should routinely conduct in-service workshops on new developments in and protocols for nutrition support, organize journal clubs to review and analyze recently published research, and apply new scientific principles to clinical practice.

Many NSTs offer clinical rotations for medical and surgical residents as well as medical, nursing, dietetics, and pharmacy students. Advanced nutrition support training programs and fellowships are also offered by the larger teams to graduate students or health professionals who have previous clinical experience.[44]

RESEARCH. Paralleling NST growth was the expansion of nutrition support research. Many of the larger NSTs have conducted or participated in research. Clinical and laboratory research require a significant commitment in terms of personnel, money, time, and space. These resources may not be available to small NSTs; however, teams in nonteaching hospitals can and often do participate in clinical research. Smaller institutions can evaluate and publish data on selected aspects of their practice (e.g., evaluate catheter infection rate or enteral tube complications to determine the safety and efficacy of the care provided). Both ASPEN and DNS foster and fund nutrition support research.[45] Research grants are awarded annually to members of these organizations.

Current areas of heightened interest in nutrition support research include (1) investigating disease-specific nutrient solutions and enteral formulas, (2) conducting controlled clinical trials to examine the effects on clinical outcome of parenteral and enteral nutrition for specific diseases, (3) identifying the actual cost of resources consumed in the provision of parenteral and enteral nutrition, (4) performing clinical efficacy and cost-effectiveness studies in tandem, (5) performing cost-effectiveness analysis as new and better data become available, (6) documenting patterns of use of parenteral and enteral nutrition services in a variety of patient care settings, and (7) "translating" new findings in molecular and cell biology to clinical trials.

Two areas for which an increasing amount of outcome data have been generated are in the use of immune-enhancing enteral formulas[46] and perioperative nutrition support.[47] In some instances, immune-enhancing enteral formulas have been shown to improve host defense, improve clinical outcome, and reduce resource utilization and costs.[46] Consensus recommendations from the U.S. Summit on Immune-Enhancing Enteral Therapy were derived using an evidence-based medicine approach for determining the types of patients who should receive these formulas, when immune-enhancing medical nutrition therapy should begin, optimal dose and length of therapy, and expected outcomes.[48]

In 1997, the National Institutes of Health, ASPEN, and the American Society for Clinical Nutrition convened an advisory committee to review the current medical literature evaluating the clinical use of nutrition support.[49] The committee identified research priorities with regard to five areas: nutrition assessment, nutrition support in patients with gastrointestinal diseases, nutrition support in wasting diseases, nutrition support in critically ill patients, and perioperative nutrition support. One specific area that is likely to receive increasing attention is the use of anabolic hormones such as insulin and growth hormone to improve nitrogen metabolism in metabolically stressed patients.[50] The objective of using anabolic adjunctive therapy would be to improve clinical outcomes by making protein accretion better, a goal that in many circumstances has remained elusive.

QUALITY MANAGEMENT. JCAHO has refocused and redefined quality assurance in health care. Many NSTs have established quality assessment and improvement programs whose goals are to improve the level of care and examine how care is managed to have a positive fiscal impact in the institution.[52,53] More information on quality assessment and improvement can be found in Chapter 43.

Roles and Responsibilities of Team Members

The NST remains an interdisciplinary group of professionals who share the common goal of providing care to patients who require special nutrition support. Most NSTs continue, typically, to include at least one physician, a registered dietitian, a nurse, and a pharmacist.[39] Collaboration requires a great deal of effort on the part of all team members. Each professional must gain appreciation for and learn to depend on the others' expertise. Because NST professionals serve as resources on all aspects of nutrition support, including assessment of the patient, development of a nutrition care plan, and implementation and monitoring of nutrition support, roles may potentially overlap. To ensure the team's success and efficient functioning, the roles and responsibilities of each professional must be clearly defined.

Although the scope of each professional's practice varies according to that person's position, education, and place of practice, each practitioner should demonstrate competency in nutrition support.[13-16] Certification by the National Board of Nutrition Support Certification is one way practitioners can demonstrate a minimal level of competency in nutrition support.

The roles and responsibilities of the dietitian, nurse, pharmacist, physician, and ancillary professional staff and support personnel are described in the following sections.

NUTRITION SUPPORT DIETITIAN. Often, the responsibility of the nutrition support dietitian (NSRD) begins after a patient identified through nutrition screening is referred to the NST for PEN. The NSRD's first objective is to determine if PEN is indicated. Limiting the use of PEN to those patients who clearly need it is one of the best ways to control costs and prevent complications. In general, parenteral nutrition is indicated when patients cannot be adequately nourished via the gastrointestinal tract. The NSRD reads the patient's medical record and confers with the patient's physicians to seek evidence of (1) gut failure or poor gastrointestinal function, (2) an anticipated prolonged period of bowel rest, (3) preoperative malnutrition, and (4) severity of postoperative complications.

Results of the Veterans Affairs Cooperative Study Group[54] underscore the importance of determining precisely who should receive parenteral nutrition. This multicenter, prospective, randomized trial was conducted to test the hypothesis that perioperative PN decreases the incidence of serious complications after major abdominal or thoracic surgery in malnourished patients. Patients ($n = 395$) were randomly assigned to receive parenteral nutrition for 7 to 15 days before surgery and 3 days afterward *or* no PN. They were monitored for complications for 90 days. Patients were stratified by nutritional status, according to the nutrition risk index or subjective global assessment.* Their malnutrition was classified as borderline, mild, or severe. Two of the most important results of this study were that preoperative patients who were *severely* malnourished and received PN had fewer noninfectious complications than did patients who did not receive PN; and, conversely, the rate of infectious complications was *higher* for borderline or mildly malnourished patients who received PN than for those who did not receive PN. This indicates that PN can do more harm than good when given to the "wrong" patients.

Sometimes, the NSRD is consulted after PEN is initiated. In this situation, the most important responsibility is to ascertain whether the current regimen is an appropriate one. The NSRD must address several important questions: Is the patient at risk for refeeding syndrome? Have the appropriate laboratory tests been ordered and evaluated? Do any critical laboratory values need to be corrected? Do any medical or metabolic constraints on nutrient delivery need to be controlled immediately (e.g., fluid, protein, potassium)? Are medications being administered that critically alter mineral requirements (e.g., large doses of potassium-wasting diuretics) or impose constraints on nutrient delivery (e.g., potassium-sparing medications)? Are any nutrient needs extraordinary (e.g., fluid, potassium, magnesium)? Is the patient being overfed (high-dose dextrose load in a chronic obstructive pulmonary disease patient with elevated P_{CO_2})? After these questions are answered, the identified issues are addressed, and the formula is deemed safe, the NSRD may proceed from the nutrition assessment to designing an individualized parenteral or enteral regimen.

---

*The *nutrition risk index* is a regression equation that uses serum albumin and percentage of usual body weight. *Subjective global assessment* is a nutrition assessment technique that uses patient history and physical signs of malnutrition to classify nutritional status.

After implementing the PEN plan in conjunction with the NST, medical and nursing staff, and the patient, the NSRD monitors the patient daily for tolerance to the PEN regimen. Often, a dietetic technician helps with daily data collection, which may include laboratory values, oral and PEN nutrient intake, intake and output data, changes in medications, information on gastrointestinal tolerance (if enteral nutrition is infused), and information on the patient's acceptance of PEN.

The NSRD records his or her assessment of daily monitoring data in the medical record. In some institutions, a standardized sticker is used to condense the daily notes. These condensed formats facilitate speedy review by medical and nursing staffs. Generally, the daily note includes recommendations for adjusting the PEN regimen. When the dietitian has PEN order-writing privileges, the recommendations are implemented immediately after coordinating with medical staff. If the primary medical service writes the order, it is extremely helpful in getting the recommendations accepted if the rationale for the recommendation is communicated *verbally* to the medical staff.

In this era of critical pathway–guided* patient care, it is important to include the results of ongoing nutrition assessment in the medical record progress notes. In some institutions progress toward nutritional goals is reported weekly. When medically indicated, the NSRD initiates a plan to help patients make the transition from PEN to oral intake or home PEN (HPEN). The objective during transitional feeding is to ensure that the patient achieves nutrient intake goals while PEN is being tapered and oral intake is increasing. The NSRD consults with the clinical dietitian or registered dietetic technician (DTR) to monitor success of dietary interventions, which can include between-meal feedings, oral supplements, and special diets. The objectives in preparing a patient for HPEN are to coordinate the plan fully with the patient, the medical and nursing staff, the NST, and the home nutrition company, to verify that the patient is receiving complete instruction on infusion and monitoring of HPEN, and that the HPEN prescription has been communicated accurately.

NURSE. The nutrition support nurse is the principal resource on implementation of nutrition support, especially administration of feeding formulations and management of access devices.[15] As the primary liaison with the floor nursing staff, the nutrition support nurse conducts educational and quality assurance programs on administration of parenteral and enteral formulas and central venous catheter or feeding tube care. Other nursing responsibilities include (1) facilitating discharge planning, (2) educating patient and family in techniques of home nutrition support, and (3) helping patients and families acquire and maintain an appropriate level of independent care.

PHARMACIST. The NST pharmacist is the expert on compounding feeding formulations. Ensuring the stability of parenteral products, the pharmacist evaluates parenteral solutions for possible incompatibility with admixed drugs and other additives. The pharmacist provides expertise on nutrient-nutrient, drug-nutrient, and drug-disease interactions; drug dosages; and

drug-induced feeding intolerance. The pharmacist helps teach home nutrition support techniques to patients and their families and to other members of the health care team.

PHYSICIAN. The NST physician may be responsible for the medical direction of the team, overseeing patient care activities. The physician may review the nutrition assessment form and approve the therapeutic nutrition plan. Evaluating the pathophysiology and expected clinical course, the physician ensures that the goals of nutrition support, the route of delivery, and the formula selected are clinically appropriate. The physician also monitors the patient throughout therapy by evaluating the impact of changes in clinical status on the nutrition support regimen. In some institutions the NST physician is responsible for placement of the central venous catheter and feeding tubes.

The NST physician may also participate in the administrative responsibilities ensuring that (1) the team has the appropriate multidisciplinary focus, (2) the policies and procedures for the provisions of nutrition support are in place, and (3) educational programs on nutrition support are implemented. In addition, the physician acts as liaison between the team and the hospital administration and medical staff.

ANCILLARY PROFESSIONAL STAFF AND SUPPORT PERSONNEL. The NST may include as few as two persons or as many as 30, depending on the size of the institution and the types of patients. Sometimes people assume multiple roles. A list of professional and administrative ancillary staff appears in Box 1-2.

Nutrition Support Dietitian: Expanding Roles in the New Millennium

Current data on the prevalence of NSTs are scant. However, numerous anecdotal reports suggest that the traditional structure of NSTs is changing. In some instances, NSTs have been dis-

---

BOX 1-2

Functions of Nutrition Support Team Ancillary Personnel

Dietetic technician	Assists in data collection and oral feeding
Medical specialist	Provides support and specialty knowledge on patient care (e.g., infectious disease physician may be involved in caring for patients with catheter infections)
Metabolic technician	Performs indirect calorimetry
Physical therapist	Develops an exercise program to increase patient's general well-being and to increase muscle mass
Reimbursement specialist	Facilitates obtaining third-party reimbursement for home nutrition support and documents medical necessity
Respiratory therapist	Coordinates performance of indirect calorimetry with ventilator-dependent patients
Social worker	Provides psychologic support and addresses social issues and financial concerns related to nutrition support
Data coordinator	Coordinates daily distribution of patient census, laboratory values, and graphic data
Secretary	Keeps records, processes charges, writes reports, does word processing, and carries out miscellaneous secretarial activities
Students	Medicine, dietetics, nursing, and pharmacy

---

*A critical pathway is a preplanned, multidisciplinary, process-based prescription for providing patient care that is designed to produce positive patient outcomes using specific resources.

banded. While the impact of disbanding NSTs is only starting to be studied, dietitians are reportedly assuming many of the activities previously accomplished by the NST. For this reason, the term nutrition support team (NST) is replaced by nutrition support services (NSS) for the remainder of this chapter.

One area in which dietitians are assuming leadership responsibility is in writing orders for parenteral nutrition. According to the ASPEN Standards for Nutrition Support Dietitians, the NSRD may "recommend, write orders, or obtain verbal orders for enteral and parenteral formulations (as guided by professional licensure or delineated by clinical privileges of an institution).[14] The Dietitians in Nutrition Support survey of dietitians writing orders for PEN found that many of them have PN order-writing responsibilities. Thirty-seven percent of the survey sample reported that they "sometimes or always write" parenteral orders. Twenty-three percent signed the parenteral order, and, of those who knew their institutional verbal order-writing policy, slightly more than half took verbal orders. Generally, a physician must cosign dietitian orders. Thirty-three percent of respondents write orders for monitoring parenteral nutrition (e.g., laboratory tests, weight measurements, intake and output). Sixty-two percent of respondents reported having a primary role in setting policy on indications for parenteral nutrition. Much expertise and institutional responsibility are required for writing parenteral nutrition orders. Accordingly, respondents indicated that extended supervised instruction is needed to develop parenteral nutrition order-writing skills. Respondents ranked clinical experience, continuing education, and clinical rotation as part of undergraduate training as the most important forms of training for developing nutrition order-writing skills.[55]

Dietitians who indicated that they write PN orders were no more likely than nonwriters to hold an advanced degree and therefore did not fit the criteria established by the ADA for advanced-level practice. ASPEN's certified nutrition support dietitian (CNSD) credential does not include skills for PN order-writing. It is possible that current dietetics' credentials do not adequately address the competencies required for PN order-writing. Perhaps a new credential is needed for advanced practice in nutrition support.

Expanded roles of NSRDs in the new millenium may include nutrition-focused physical assessment. Additionally, NSRDs are increasingly in the position to place nasoenteric tubes. This practice must be preceded by "specialized training, demonstrated competency, and delineated clinical privileges."[14]

The role of the NSS dietitian in the new millenium needs the support that Congress recently granted to dietitians providing medical nutrition therapy (MNT)* to Medicare beneficiaries with diabetes and renal disease. In 2000, Congress approved coverage for MNT by registered dietitians to these groups under Medicare Part B. Expansion of this legislation to provide coverage for MNT to Medicare beneficiaries on home PN or PEN is needed. Additionally, the recent inclusion of MNT current procedural terminology (CPT) codes† in the American

Medical Association Current Procedural Terminology should support NSRD efforts to secure reimbursement for their services by third-party payers. It is likely that NSRDs will expand their practice as reimbursement improves using CPT codes relevant to services provided to patients under their care.

In addition to expanded roles in clinical practice, NSRDs have expanded their roles in the administrative structure of NSSs. Dietitians are the most frequent nonphysician NSS leaders. According to the ASPEN Standards of Practice for Nutrition Support Dietitians, the scope of practice of the NSRD may include "management of nutrition support services including developing polices and procedures and supervising personnel and budgets; recommending and maintaining enteral and parenteral formularies; evaluating equipment for enteral feeding delivery; participating in nutrition support committees; and assuring optimal reimbursement for nutrition support activities."[14] Additionally, NSRDs are involved in patient education and research. The administrative roles of the NSRD should extend to ensuring that "enteral formulations are prepared according to established guidelines (Hazard Analysis Critical Control Point) for safe, aseptic, and effective nutrition therapy."[14,57] Box 1-3 lists the job responsibilities of an NST RD administrator. This position includes responsibilities for conducting NST rounds; delegating tasks to team members; hiring, training, and evaluating personnel; supervising fee-for-service charge systems and budgets; writing grant proposals; setting policy; writing reports; establishing faculty responsibilities; and overseeing research and development of critical pathways and guidelines for clinical practice and strategic planning.

In addition to expanded roles, the NSRD of the new millenium is likely to expand practice in alternative care settings. For example, home care is the fastest-growing segment of the health care industry and is likely to employ more dietitians.[58] Home health administrators have indicated that they value dietitian involvement in parenteral and enteral nutrition.

Educational Background of Nutrition Support Dietitians

The ASPEN Standards for Nutrition Support Dietitians specifies the minimal qualifications for practice in nutrition support. Three of the following must be documented:[14]

1. Certification by the National Board of Nutrition Support Certification, Inc. as a Certified Nutrition Support Dietitian (CNSD)
2. Formal education, training, or continuing professional education in nutrition support
3. A minimum of 30% to 50% professional practice time devoted to the practice of nutrition support
4. Participation in the health care institution's nutrition support activities
5. Membership in professional societies devoted to nutrition support

A survey by Olree and Skipper[59] indicated that 79% of NSRDs believe that experiences beyond those required for becoming a registered dietitian are needed to provide NSRDs with specialized skills. Currently, most of these experiences are obtained through on-the-job training. A need exists for advanced-level clinical training programs to prepare NSRDs.

---

*Medical nutrition therapy refers to the comprehensive nutrition services provided by registered dietitians as part of the health care team.
†The MNT CPT codes: 97802—MNT individual initial assessment, 15 minutes; 97803—individual reassessment, 15 minutes; 97804—group (2 or more), 30 minutes.[56]

BOX 1-3

Job Responsibilities of Nutrition Support Team Registered Dietitian Administrator

1. Serves as a consultant on advanced concepts of nutrition support to NST personnel and other health care professionals
2. Provides advanced-level nutrition care to NST patients:
   a. Performs comprehensive initial and serial nutrition assessments
   b. Develops and implements specialized nutrition support care plans
   c. Monitors/evaluates/modifies nutrition support management through serial nutrition support and evaluation of the medical record
   d. Counsels patients and families on principles of home nutrition support
   e. Completes discharge planning for patients who will receive home nutrition support
   f. In conjunction with medical staff, orders PN, tube feeding, and monitoring tests
   g. Develops and/or implements guidelines for the practice of nutrition support of inpatients and outpatients
   h. Monitors patients on home nutrition support
3. Conducts NST rounds to review patient management and facilitate achievement of nutrition support goals
4. Delegates responsibilities to support personnel, including the NST administrative assistant and dietetic technician
5. Interviews, hires, trains, evaluates, and counsels NST professional and support staff
6. Supervises fee-for-service charge system and determines recommended fee structure
7. Prepares an annual budget and allocates resources based on the budget
8. Writes grant proposals for revenue generation
9. Advises on NST policy
10. Promotes and maintains effective communication with all members of the NST, dietetics department, and all relevant departments
11. Writes and presents NST reports
12. Develops policies and procedures
13. Carries out faculty responsibilities:
    a. Serves as a clinical preceptor for PEN and critical care nutrition rotations for dietetics students
    b. Develops and/or contributes to the development of learning modules for nutrition assessment, nutrient requirements, PEN, and critical care nutrition
    c. Coordinates educational experiences with discipline representatives for allied health, nursing, and medical students
    d. Assists in the supervision of master's degree/students' research projects
14. Attends and makes presentations at local, regional, and national professional meetings
15. Participates in research activities:
    a. Evaluates scientific literature
    b. Plans and executes research projects and protocols
    c. Collects, analyzes, and evaluates research data
    d. Publishes manuscripts
16. Coordinates quality improvement activities of the NST
    a. Interprets and implements JCAHO standards
    b. Develops and implements continuous quality improvement programs
    c. Develops and implements critical pathways in conjunction with other health care professionals
17. Markets the NST
18. Participates in external professional activities
19. Participates in strategic planning
20. Serves on departmental and interdepartmental committees

Reprinted with permission from Rush-Presbyterian St. Luke's Medical Center, Chicago, Illinois. The NST Coordinator list of responsibilities was developed at Rush-Presbyterian St. Luke's Medical Center and does not reflect current practice.

Future of Nutrition Support Services

In 1994 the DNS practice group of the ADA administered a survey to its membership to identify trends that affect the practice of nutrition.[60] Fifty trends were grouped into categories: cost and outcomes, survival skills, technologic advances, consumer issues, and work environment. As a basis for a discussion of the future of NSSs, we borrowed a few of these categories and added sections on strategies for success (meeting unmet needs, politics, image, and marketing) and professional challenges (clinical privileges and cross-training).

Cost and Outcome

It is likely that the most important NSS priorities will be controlling costs and providing evidence of improvement in patient outcome as a result of NSS interventions. Historically, NSTs have attempted to become revenue-generating centers, but with today's health care reimbursement arrangements (e.g.,

managed care), true worth must be justified by demonstrating good evidence of cost control and decreased incidence of patient complications. When calculating cost savings, it is important to remember that costs rather than charges are considered: when reimbursement was cost based, patient charges were an important economic consideration of nutrition support. With managed care reimbursement arrangements, charges become irrelevant.

Because PEN is expensive and consumes a wide variety of resources, it affords many opportunities for clinicians to control costs. One of the best ways to control costs is to accurately determine which patients are appropriate PEN candidates because feeding a patient enterally rather than parenterally saves thousands of dollars.

Through NSS intervention, significant cost savings can be realized by reducing the number of laboratory tests for monitoring PEN, controlling the amount of PEN solutions to prevent overfeeding, decreasing the average duration of parenteral nutrition therapy, reducing the use of expensive nonstandard PN formulations, standardizing protocols, performing cost analysis of supplies and solutions to determine which products offer the most value, and preventing waste.

It has also been argued that, if NSS interventions result in the ordering of fewer laboratory tests, true cost savings are not likely to be realized unless fewer laboratory technicians are used; that is, many laboratory costs are fixed and do not change with volume.[61] This argument fails to consider the opportunity cost of ordering laboratory tests. *Opportunity cost* is an established economic concept that considers the uncaptured value of other activities that could be performed if fewer laboratory tests were ordered. For example, laboratory tests involve a nurse's time to check the order; a unit clerk's time to transfer the order; a physician's, nurse's, and the NST's time to evaluate the result; a nurse's time to troubleshoot when for some reason the order is not carried out; and an NST's time to troubleshoot when a laboratory value is potentially unreliable (e.g., determining if the blood sample was hemolyzed in a patient who has a high serum potassium value). Although it may be difficult to calculate, when identifying the costs associated with utilization of PEN, it is important to consider opportunity costs. The uncaptured value of these health care workers' time may be higher-quality patient care, which may be more easily realized if fewer laboratory tests were needed as a result of simplified protocols for monitoring PEN.

There are many examples of cost savings by NSTs.[62,63] For example, in our experience, one simple intervention resulted in annual savings to the hospital of $40,000 by determining that one of the more expensive parenteral formulas was not more beneficial therapeutically than the standard formula. Recently, Dodds et al.[64] published reference standards to assess care at institutions where NSTs have been eliminated in cost-saving efforts. These authors documented a symptomatic metabolic complication rate for PN of 0.4%. If the symptomatic complication rate is higher than 0.4%, a strong argument can be made for reinstatement of the NST. Chapter 45 contains a more comprehensive discussion of the cost-effectiveness of nutrition support.

While NSSs have many opportunities to control costs in day-to-day practice, practitioners' responsibilities will be increasingly broadened to include development of guidelines for applying diagnostic, monitoring, and therapeutic procedures designed to control costs and patient complications.[65] Because PEN is expensive and carries serious risks for the patient if administered improperly, NSS expertise is needed to provide accurate information for the development of protocols.

Emphasis on cost control has increased utilization of PEN in the home care setting. This trend is expected to result in the employment of more nutrition support practitioners. Cost controls on reimbursement for home health care services have changed the patterns of nutrition support practice in home care. Critical pathways that optimize the potential for positive patient outcomes have been introduced to home care. Many activities of practitioners working in home infusion companies are being shared by the various nutrition support disciplines, in efforts to increase efficiency. These may include material management, administrative responsibilities, reimbursement management, marketing and sales, and clinical care functions that do not require licensure.[66] Changes in practice are expected to continue.

A recent Institute of Medicine study indicated that nutrition services can commonly be provided through a team approach to care, but the roles of team members are not well defined.[67] The problem with this lack of definition is that it presents a barrier to the development of data on the cost effectiveness of MNT.[68] A proposed model for nutritional care has recently been developed to help dissolve the barriers to collecting cost-effectiveness data.[68] The proposed model includes three components: (1) the trigger event that identifies patients who are candidates for MNT; (2) the nutrition care process, which includes assessment, planning, implementation, documentation, and evaluation; and (3) nutrition-related outcomes that focus on goals that can be disease specific or reflective of clinical pathways or care maps, MNT protocols, or clinical practice guidelines.[68]

Technologic Advances

"New technologies will reshape how, when, and where we practice."[69] Computers are automating many procedures formerly supervised by NSTs.[53] For example, software that is available for PN compounding performs calcium phosphate solubility calculations based on amino acid concentration and type of amino acid solution; offers order entry functions by component, total calories, and distribution of calories between amino acids, dextrose, and lipids; implements controls on electrolytes based on the patient's weight and clinical status; introduces safety features, including limits on osmolality for peripherally infused solutions and warnings of potential overdoses or potential order entry errors; and a variety of labeling options.

Computers have drastically changed the work environment for many health care practitioners. Physical location no longer imposes constraints on the practice setting. Practitioners have computer access to patient records in distant hospitals to provide consultation to primary care providers and supervision for their students. Expanded computerized information systems continue to greatly enhance the NST's ability to provide services within multihospital corporations.

As predicted by the DNS trend analysis, the variety of available specialized food products, medical foods, and disease-specific formulas has continued to increase.[60] Growth factors such as transforming growth factor (TGF-β) have recently been introduced to enteral formulas. In the future, nutrients aimed at modulating immune response or manipulating the stress response in critically ill patients are likely to be included in parenteral nutrition formulas.[70] The ultimate therapeutic objective for some formula additives will be alteration of gene expression.

It is anticipated that advances in genomics and molecular biology will change the practice of clinical nutrition directly and indirectly by using nutrients to regulate gene expression. Nutrient requirements may be altered when hormones produced by recombinant deoxyribonucleic acid (DNA) technology (e.g., growth hormone) are administered. A highly specialized therapy using growth hormone in combination with glutamine and a modified oral diet is already being offered to patients with short-bowel syndrome to improve intestinal morphology and function and reduce dependence on home PN.[71] Likewise, advances in molecular genetics are likely to show that genetic variation may influence dietary responsiveness.

The development of MNT based on advances in genomics and molecular biology dictate expanded responsibility for practitioners of nutrition support. Because the technology of molecular biology brings new products and analytic methods to the field of clinical nutrition, practitioners and educators of practitioners need to acquire an understanding of the fundamental concepts of molecular biology in order to follow progress in biomedical and nutrition research and to determine the implications of molecular research findings for the practice of clinical nutrition.[72] In addition to graphs and tables, nutrition support literature will be intensively laced with data from experiments using molecular biologic techniques such as Northern analysis,[73] Southern analysis, and Western blots.

Advances in technology will require NSRDs to use solid paradigms for decision making with regard to clinical practice. Evidence-based medicine offers one such paradigm. Evidence-based medicine is the practice of identifying the best data on which to base clinical decisions.[74] The process of identifying the best data is laborious and time consuming. Reliance on prospective, randomized, controlled clinical trials along with meta-analyses should be the basis of clinical decision making. Reading medical literature requires practice, which can be fostered through participation in journal clubs and by confirming that clinical decisions are consistent with the patient's values and preferences.

Strategies for Success: Meeting Needs, Politics, Nutrition Support Service Image, and Marketing

The most critical task for NSS survival is to demonstrate reduced health care costs, reduced patient complications, and improved patient outcomes as a result of NSS intervention. Several other initiatives may be taken by NSSs to reduce the threat of cutbacks and increase the potential for expanded administrative support. One effective strategy is to document the benefits of maintaining nutritional status in terms of outcome. It has recently been demonstrated that patients who decline nutritionally have higher hospital charges compared with those who do not ($28,631 vs. $5762).[75] Trujillo et al. recently documented the worth of a metabolic support service by showing that inappropriate use of PN resulted in one half million dollars in patient charges (not including the charges related to treatment of potentially avoidable parenteral nutrition complications.) In this study, PN was determined to be appropriate in 82% of the patients with a metabolic support service consultation compared with 56% without a consultation. Likewise, the metabolic complication rate with consultation was 34% versus 66% without consultation.[76]

By becoming attuned to the hospital's needs and priorities, many NSSs have increased the number of services they provide to add value to their role and fill unmet needs. For example, many NSSs perform venipuncture, offer placement of central venous catheters and surgically placed enteral feeding tubes, provide fluoroscopy and endoscopy for placement of enteral feeding tubes, provide TPN and EN order-writing, and offer home nutrition support and indirect calorimetry.[61,77,78] Meeting a hospital's needs may mean expanding the NSS's practice to include services that are not directly related to providing parenteral and enteral nutrition.[77] These include provision of various home infusion therapies, nutrition counseling for the community, and hospital-wide nutrition screening. One California NSS provides preadmission nutrition screening to

comply with critical pathways for specific diagnosis-related groups.[79]

Although the principal focus of the NSS's efforts to support its financial viability is to demonstrate cost control, opportunities for revenue generation may continue to arise. For example, NSSs may subcontract services to other hospitals in the community where nutrition support resources are not available.

Potential miscommunication, both within the team and between the NSS and other hospital departments, must be dealt with in a proactive way. Conflict can arise among team members because of different views of the scope of practice for specific disciplines. Interdepartmental conflicts can arise when procedures and protocols are not acceptable to all parties involved or are not followed.

Good communication skills based on mutual respect, a nonjudgmental tone, and a commitment to collaborative practice are critical for averting and resolving team conflicts. Firm knowledge of data relevant to the conflict, whether it be quality improvement data or data from the literature, goes a long way toward supporting the NSS's position and credibility. Efforts to market the team and to boost its image must be planned and practiced every day. For example, all NSS members should make it known that they are available and accessible any time. On-call schedules should be distributed to page operators and nursing units.

The NSS should develop a track record of "getting things done," even if these things are only peripherally related to PEN. For example, primary registered nurses should be able to rely on NSS to get the correct bag of PN when needed if problems in delivery arise. The NSS dietetic technician should solve the problem of providing the correct oral snack to a hard-to-please patient. The NSS should take responsibility for guiding the intensive treatment needed when control of blood sugar is difficult to achieve. When the NST goes the extra mile and, in the end, saves time for those in other disciplines while improving the quality of patient care, this contribution, in and of itself, markets the team well. The NSS needs to be vocal about its accomplishments, especially when the team accomplishments enhance the hospital's image. Box 1-4 summarizes strategies for NSS success.

Professional Challenges: Clinical Privileges and Cross-Training

As has been true for many sectors of the U.S. economy, such as industry, universities, and government, today hospitals are the targets of industrial reengineering, as economic pressures force downsizing and restructuring. For those multidisciplinary NSTs that remain, role delineation may have to change if they are to flourish. Developing expanded clinical privileges and cross-training within NST disciplines may be two proactive measures that can enhance the competitive posture of team members.

Expanded clinical privileges have been obtained by using the 1995 JCAHO nutrition standard that requires authorized persons to prescribe or order food and nutrition products in a timely manner.[80] The nutrition order may be written by a nonphysician designee who has been granted clinical privileges to write such orders.[81] Objectives of obtaining expanded clinical privileges include facilitating timely delivery of nutrition care

---

BOX 1-4

Strategies for Nutrition Support Team Success

1. Take the pulse of the environment.
   Continually assess your hospital's situation, needs, and resources.
   Be attuned to emerging consumer demands.
   Stay abreast of evolving health care trends.
2. Think "value-added" and expand your horizons.
   Focus on ways to add value to your hospital.
   Be willing to expand your traditional role.
   Find new niches that fill a void.
3. Collect, analyze, and disseminate data.
   Perform outcome studies on topical issues.
   Use data to demonstrate the team's clinical and nonclinical benefits.
   Emphasize cost savings of NST policies and procedures.
4. Build up your revenue and cost savings.
   Document fees for services and other sources of revenue.
   Document costs saved from NST services.
   Explore new and creative sources of revenue.
5. Practice good politics.
   Be tactful when dealing with opposing views.
   Foster open communication and work toward agreement.
   Use data to gain cooperation.
6. Stay in the spotlight.
   Be accessible to your colleagues.
   Toot your own horn about your achievements.
   Use public relations vehicles to keep your team visible.
7. Nurture vital allies and advocates.
   Communicate regularly with administrators.
   Work with clinicians to build and maintain their support.
   Maintain good relations with the nursing staff.

Reprinted with permission from Martin AL: The nutrition support team: surviving and thriving in an era of reform, *Nutr Clin Pract* 10(suppl):17s, 1995.

---

orders and increasing professional credibility, visibility, and effectiveness.[80] The expanded clinical privileges include taking verbal orders and writing orders in the medical record with physician cosignature for diets, oral and parenteral nutrient solutions, tube feedings, transitional feedings, balance studies, blood glucose monitoring, and HPEN.

Cross-training among NST disciplines historically has been a controversial and sometimes very emotional issue. Examples of cross-training include dietitians performing physical assessments, placing enteral feeding tubes, and performing catheter care and nurses performing nutrition assessment. NST members who have opposed cross-training often believe that it decreases the quality of care and threatens their loyalty to their respective disciplines. When economic pressures limit the size of NSTs, the choice may be to have an NST whose members are cross-trained or no NST at all. The challenge to the NST then is to train individuals from other disciplines well and to establish continuous quality improvement programs to monitor quality. To increase the likelihood that cross-training will be a success, a high degree of respect for the unique contributions of each NST discipline is essential. All NST members should have completed at least one college course in nutrition. All NSTs should have at least one dietitian team member.

The relationship of cross-training to licensure has not been studied. It is possible that cross-training will receive official status in the health care system by virtue of disciplines obtaining expanded clinical privileges.

Summary

Establishing priorities for the allocation of health care resources will continue to be difficult. The NST, like many hospital services, will be confronted with downsizing in order to survive. Reducing team size necessitates maximizing team productivity. Overlap in responsibilities must be eliminated, and changes in roles must be clearly defined. Because trends predict a rapidly changing environment, future leaders will need to be "direction setters, change agents, spokespersons, and mentors."[69] Their challenge will be to convince others of the need for change.

The future will not wait while we close gaps in the literature on the costs and efficacy of nutrition support. More information is urgently needed to help justify the allocation of health care resources for the detection, prevention, and treatment of malnutrition in hospitalized patients. Priority research must be directed toward identifying the best methods of providing cost-effective nutrition support.

Today's practitioners must collate and distribute available information on the cost-effectiveness of nutrition support from the literature and from continuous quality-improvement programs. Critical pathways and quality indicators that generate institution-specific evidence of the cost-effectiveness of nutrition support must be marketed both internally and externally. With this information, hospital administrators, medical staff, boards of trustees, and health professional staff will agree that hospitals cannot afford to be without organized nutrition support services.

REFERENCES

1. Dudrick SJ, Long JM: Applications and hazards of intravenous hyperalimentation, *Annu Rev Med* 28:517-528, 1977.
2. Ryan JA Jr, Abel RM, Abbott WM, et al: Catheter complications in total parenteral nutrition. A prospective study of 200 consecutive patients, *N Engl J Med* 290:757-761, 1974.
3. Boscoe MJ, Rosin MD: Fine bore enteral feeding and pulmonary aspiration, *Br Med J* 289:1421-1422, 1984.
4. Olivares L, Segovia A, Revuelta R: Tube feeding and lethal aspiration in neurological patients: a review of 720 autopsy cases, *Stroke* 5:654-657, 1974.
5. Wynne JW, Modell JH: Respiratory aspiration of stomach contents, *Ann Intern Med* 87:466-474, 1977.
6. Olbrantz KR, Gelfand D, Choplin R, et al: Pneumothorax complicating enteral feeding tube placement, *J Parenter Enteral Nutr* 9:210-211, 1985.
7. Niemiec PW, Vanderveen TW, Morrison JI, et al: Gastrointestinal disorders caused by medication and electrolyte solution osmolality during enteral nutrition, *J Parenter Enteral Nutr* 7:387-389, 1983.
8. Schreiner RL, Eitzen H, Gfell MA, et al: Environmental contamination of continuous drip feeding, *Pediatrics* 63:232-237, 1979.
9. McShane CM, Fox HM: Nutrition support teams—a 1983 survey, *J Parenter Enteral Nutr* 9:263-268, 1985.
10. Sheridan J, Calvert S: *Nutrition support team directory*, Columbus, OH, 1983, Ross Laboratories.
11. NSS Teams: *Nutritional support services* 3(11):35-68, 1983.
12. American Society for Parenteral and Enteral Nutrition: Definition of terms used in A.S.P.E.N. guidelines and standards, *Nutr Clin Pract* 10(1):1-3, 1995.
13. American Society for Parenteral and Enteral Nutrition: Standards of practice for nutrition support pharmacists, *Nutr Clin Pract* 14:275-281, 1999.
14. American Society for Parenteral and Enteral Nutrition: Standards for nutrition support dietitians, *Nutr Clin Pract* 15:53-59, 2000.
15. American Society for Parenteral and Enteral Nutrition: Standards for nutrition support nurses, *Nutr Clin Pract* 16:56-62, 2001.

16. American Society for Parenteral and Enteral Nutrition: Standards for nutrition support physicians, *Nutr Clin Pract* 11(6):235-240, 1996.
17. American Society for Parenteral and Enteral Nutrition: Standards for home nutrition support, *Nutr Clin Pract* 14:151-162, 1999.
18. American Society for Parenteral and Enteral Nutrition: Standards for nutrition support: hospitalized patients, *Nutr Clin Pract* 10(6):208-217, 1995.
19. American Society for Parenteral and Enteral Nutrition: Standards for nutrition support for adult residents of long-term care facilities, *Nutr Clin Pract* 12:284-293, 1997.
20. American Society for Parenteral and Enteral Nutrition: Standards for nutrition support: hospitalized pediatric patients, *Nutr Clin Pract* 11:217-228, 1996.
21. National Advisory Group on Standards and Practice Guidelines for Parenteral Nutrition. Safe practices for parenteral feeding formulations, *J Parenter Enteral Nutr* 22(suppl), 49-66,1998.
22. American Dietetic Association: The role of the registered dietitian in enteral and parenteral nutrition support, *J Am Diet Assoc* 97(3):302-304, 1997.
23. American Dietetic Association: Nutrition intervention in the care of persons with human immunodeficiency virus infection, *J Am Diet Assoc* 100:708-717, 2000.
24. Butterworth CE: The skeleton on the hospital closet, *Nutr Today* March/April:4-8, 1974.
25. Bistrian BR, Blackburn GL, Hallowell E, et al: Protein status of general surgical patients, *JAMA* 230:858-860, 1976.
26. Bistrian BR, Blackburn GL, Vitale J, et al: Prevalence of malnutrition in general medical patients, *JAMA* 235:1567-1570, 1976.
27. Lundvick JL: Evaluation of a nutritional screen when used in oncology, *J Parenter Enteral Nutr* 3:521, 1979 (abstract).
28. Mullen JL, Gertner MH, Buzby GP, et al: Implications of malnutrition in the surgical patient, *Arch Surg* 114:121-125, 1979.
29. Willicuts HD: Nutritional assessment of 1,000 surgical patients in an affluent suburban community hospital, *J Parenter Enteral Nutr* 1:25, 1977.
30. Meakins JL, Pietsch JB, Bubenick O, et al: Delayed hypersensitivity: indicators of acquired failure of host defenses in sepsis and trauma, *Ann Surg* 186:241-250, 1977.
31. Buzby GP, Mullen JL, Matthews DC, et al: Prognostic nutritional index in gastrointestinal surgery, *Am J Surg* 139:160-167, 1980.
32. Mullen JL, Buzby GP, Matthews DC, et al: Reduction of operative mortality and morbidity by combined preoperative and postoperative nutritional support, *Ann Surg* 192:604-613, 1980.
33. Blackburn GL, Bistrian BR, Harvey K: Indices of protein calorie malnutrition as predictors of survival. In Levenson SM (ed): *Nutrition assessment—present status, future directions and prospects,* Columbus, OH, 1981, Ross Laboratories, pp 131-136.
34. Kaminski MV, Fitzgerald MJ, Murphy RJ, et al: Correlation of mortality with serum transferrin and anergy, *J Parenter Enteral Nutr* 1:27, 1977.
35. Steinberg EP, Anderson GF: Implications of medicare prospective payment system for specialized nutrition services, *Nutr Clin Pract* 1:12-28, 1986.
36. American Society for Parenteral and Enteral Nutrition: *Nutrition support team resource kit,* Silver Spring, MD, 1990, ASPEN, pp 1-23.
37. Compher C, Colaizzo T: Staffing patterns in hospital clinical dietetics and nutrition support: a survey conducted by the Dietitians in Nutrition Support dietetics practice group, *J Am Diet Assoc* 92:807-812, 1992.
38. Foltz MB, Schillar MR, Ryan AS: Nutrition screening and assessment: current practices and dietitians' leadership roles, *J Am Diet Assoc* 93:1388-1395, 1993.
39. Regenstein M: Nutrition support teams—alive, well and still growing, *Nutr Clin Pract* 7:296-301, 1992.
40. OASIS Annual Report: *1988 data,* Albany, NY, 1990, The Oley Foundation.
41. North American Home Parenteral and Enteral Nutrition Patient Registry: *Annual report with outcome profiles 1985-1992. 1992 data,* Albany, NY, 1994, The Oley Foundation, pp 1-23.
42. Jones KR, Kovacevish DS, Teitelbaum DH: Establishing a comprehensive database for home parenteral nutrition: six years of data, *Nutr Clin Pract* 15:279-286, 2000.
43. Crocker KS: Current status of home infusion therapy, *Nutr Clin Pract* 7(6):256-263, 1992.
44. Shronts EP, Silverman DW: Impetus for change in educational preparation, *Nutr Clin Pract* 7(suppl 3):9-14, 1992.
45. Schiller MR: Research development, progress and expansion, *Nutr Clin Pract* 7(suppl 3):15-17, 1992.
46. Kudsk KA: Introduction: proceedings from summit on immune-enhancing enteral therapy, *J Parenter Enteral Nutr* 25(2S):S1-S2, 2001.
47. Maxfield D, Geehan D, Van Way CW: Perioperative nutrition support, *Nutr Clin Pract* 16:69-73, 2001.
48. Consensus recommendations from the U.S. Summit on Immune-Enhancing Enteral Therapy, *J Parenter Enteral Nutr* 25(2S):S61-S63, 2001.
49. Klein S, Kinney J, Jeejeebhoy K, et al: Nutrition support in clinical practice: review of published data and recommendations for future research directions, *Am J Clin Nutr* 66:683-706, 1997.
50. Daly JM: The evolution of surgical nutrition: nutrient and anabolic interventions, *Ann Surg* 229:19-20, 1999.
51. Srp F, Ayello EA, Andujar E, et al: Quality of care concepts and nutrition support, *Nutr Clin Pract* 6:131-141, 1991.
52. Powers T, Deckard M, Stark N, et al: A nutrition support team quality assurance plan, *Nutr Clin Pract* 6:151-155, 1991.
53. Geibig CB, Mirtallo JM, Owens J: Quality assurance for a nutrition support service, *Nutr Clin Pract* 6:147-150, 1991.
54. The Veterans Affairs Total Parenteral Nutrition Cooperative Study Group: Perioperative total parenteral nutrition in surgical patients, *N Engl J Med* 325:525-532, 1991.
55. Mueller CM, Colaizzo-Anas T, Shronts E, et al: Order-writing for parenteral nutrition by registered dietitians, *J Am Diet Assoc* 96:764-768, 1996.
56. Current Procedural Terminology (CPT 2001): Chicago, IL, 2001, American Medical Association Press.
57. Loken JK: *The HACCP food safety manual,* New York, 1995, John Wiley & Sons.
58. Schiller MR, Arensberg MB, Kantor B: Administrators' perceptions of nutrition services in home health care agencies, *J Am Diet Assoc* 98:56-61, 1998.
59. Olree K, Skipper A: The role of nutrition support dietitians as viewed by chief clinical and nutrition support dietitians: implications for training, *J Am Diet Assoc* 97:1255-1260, 1997.
60. Williams DM: Top trends affecting nutrition support according to DNS members, *Statline* II(1):2-3, 1995.
61. Clemmer TP: The role of the team in the new health care environment, *Nutr Clin Pract* 10(suppl 2):24S-27S, 1995.
62. Gales BJ, Riley DG: Improved total parenteral nutrition therapy management by a nutrition support team, *Hosp Pharm* 29:469-470, 1994.
63. Goldstein M, Braitman LE, Levine GM: The medical and financial costs associated with termination of a nutrition support team, *J Parenter Enteral Nutr* 24:323-327, 2000.
64. Dodds ES, Murray JD, Trexler KM, et al: Metabolic occurrences in total parenteral nutrition patients managed by a nutrition support team, *Nutr Clin Pract* 16:78-84, 2001.
65. Eddy DM: Broadening the responsibilities of practitioners, *JAMA* 269:1849-1855, 1993.
66. Viall CD, Crocker KS, Hennessy K, et al: High tech home care: surviving and prospering in a changing environment, *Nutr Clin Pract* 10(suppl 2):49S-54S, 1995.
67. Committee on Nutrition Services for MedicareBeneficiaries, Food and Nutrition Board: *The role of nutrition in maintaining health in the nation's elderly,* Washington, DC, 2000, National Academy Press.
68. Splett P, Myers EF: A proposed model for effective nutrition care, *J Am Diet Assoc* 101:357-363, 2001.
69. Parks SC: What does the future hold? *Nutr Clin Pract* 10(suppl 2):38S-40S, 1995.
70. Grant JP: Nutrition support in critically ill patients, *Ann Surg* 220:610-616, 1994.
71. Byrne TA, Morrissey TB, Nattakom TV, et al: Growth hormone, glutamine, and a modified diet enhance nutrient absorption in patients with severe short bowel syndrome, *J Parenter Enteral Nutr* 19:296-302, 1995.
72. Smith RJ: Molecular biology in nutrition support, *Nutr Clin Pract* 7:5-15, 1992.
73. Avissar NE, Ziegler TR, Wang HT, et al: Growth factors regulation of rabbit sodium-dependent neutral amino acid transporter ATB and oligopeptide transporter 1 mRNAs expression after enterectomy, *J Parenter Enteral Nutr* 25:65-72, 2001.
74. Koretz RL. Doing the right thing: the utilization of evidence-based medicine, *Nutr Clin Pract* 15:213-217, 2000.
75. Braunschweig C, Gomez S, Sheenan PM: Impact of declines in nutritional status on outcomes in adult patients hospitalized for more than 7 days, *J Am Diet Assoc* 100:1316-1322, 2000.
76. Trujillo EB, Young LS, Chertow GM, et al. Metabolic and monetary costs of avoidable parenteral nutrition use, *J Parenter Enteral Nutr* 23:109-113, 1999.

77. Martin AL: The nutrition support team: surviving and thriving in an era of reform, *Nutr Clin Pract* 10(suppl):17S-23S, 1995.
78. Bothe A, Steiger E: Worksheet for nutrition support services, *Nutr Clin Pract* 10(suppl):74S, 1995.
79. Schwartz DB, Gudzin D: Preadmission nutrition screening: expanding hospital-based nutrition services implementing earlier nutrition intervention, *J Am Diet Assoc* 100:81-87, 2000.

80. Davis AM, Baker SS, Leary RA: Advancing clinical privileges for nutrition support practitioners: the dietitian as a model, *Nutr Clin Pract* 10:98-103, 1995.
81. Nutrition care. In *The Joint Commission 1995 accreditation manual for hospitals,* vol II, Oakbrook Terrace, IL, 1994, Joint Commission on Accreditation of Healthcare Organizations, p 88.

History and Physical Examination

2

Kathy Hammond, MS, RN, RD, LD, CNSN, CNSD

THE history and physical examination are part of a comprehensive approach to the assessment of nutritional status, along with anthropometric measurements and laboratory data (Fig. 2-1).[1,2] A tactful, investigative approach to the nutrition history and physical examination through interviewing, keen observation, examination techniques, and measurements allows the practitioner to gather key information in the assessment process to formulate an effective plan of nutrition care. In many instances, essential information that might be overlooked in other data and in written reports is picked up through the nutrition history or physical examination.

The relationship between nutritional status and physical examination is evident when a thorough assessment reveals nutritional deficiencies not identified by other assessment approaches. Nutritional deficiencies can be readily apparent in underweight individuals, while being more obscure in those who are overweight. Excessive ingestion of calories and protein does not necessarily mean that micronutrient requirements are met. One must keep in mind that, in general, signs of malnutrition or of clinical disorders that result from various degrees of protein or calorie deficiency are nonspecific. When physical findings are correlated with other assessment data, such as medical and nutrition histories, dietary intake, biochemical markers, and anthropometric measurements, evaluation of nutritional status can be completed.[3] This chapter concentrates on the history and physical examination only as they pertain to the nutritional status of the adult patient. This chapter is geared toward the beginner in physical assessment

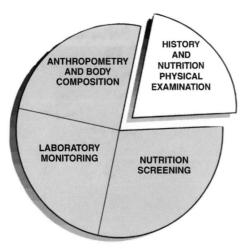

FIGURE 2-1 Assessment of nutritional status.

skills. Other, more detailed texts are available for more advanced clinicians.

Application to Practice

The nutrition history and physical assessment have many applications to clinical practice for today's dietitians. An accurate history investigates physiologic, psychologic, psychosocial, and cultural information about a patient's health. The physical examination provides an objective interpretation of the person as a whole and allows the use of all of the examiner's senses to distinguish variations from "usual wellness." As a result, appropriate planning and implementation of nutrition care can take place, along with effective evaluation of the response to nutrition therapy.

Before beginning any patient contact or care, the clinician must be aware of safety precautions and protective guidelines. Universal precautions guidelines, published by the Centers for Disease Control (CDC), address the prevention of bloodborne diseases. Clinicians must follow proper handwashing techniques, barrier precautions, and other infection control measures.

Nutrition Health History

The nutrition component of the overall health history provides information useful for identifying nutrition-related problems. The nutritional health history provides subjective findings from the patient or a significant other about the past and present nutritional state of health, nutritional health promotion, and other activities that affect nutritional status. Approximately 80% of information on nutritional status comes from the nutritional health history. A thorough history results in a focused physical examination.[4]

The nutritional health history is conducted in a systematic, accurate, and thorough interview session. A successful interview requires effective communication and interpersonal skills. Verbal and nonverbal approaches need to be used appropriately to ensure effective communication. Establishing rapport, along with being empathetic and accepting, are important for establishing a relationship with the patient. Awareness of cultural differences is important to recognize and respect. Components of one's cultural values include religious beliefs, rituals, symbols, language, dietary practices, communication style, education, and race. It is important for the health professional to be aware of differences in culture because how one views health, wellness, and illness can affect the outcome of care.

The interview should take approximately 30 minutes to complete. Controlling and pacing the interview are important for completing it within an appropriate interval. Providing privacy and minimizing interruptions can help. The examiner should establish a "bill of rights" and confidentiality with the patient and should let that person know how long the interview will take. Complicated technical and medical terminology is avoided, and therapeutic techniques of communication are used, such as acceptance, recognition, restating, reflecting, and paraphrasing. The examiner avoids stereotyped comments such as "It's for your own good" and does not reject, approve, disagree, or advise.[5-7]

The nutritional health history is collected in a fairly standard format of the following components: demographic data, chief complaint, present and past illnesses, current health, family history, dietary history, socioeconomic status, personal stress, coping mechanisms, and a review of systems (Table 2-1). The review-of-systems component of the nutritional health interview allows patients to explain their health status to the clinician and enables systematic collection of specific information about present and past problems and health promotion, along with a general overview of health status, including a review of vision and hearing and the integumentary, respiratory, hematologic, cardiovascular, peripheral vascular, gastrointestinal and hepatobiliary, genitourinary, endocrine, neurologic, and musculoskeletal systems (Box 2-1).[5-7] Facts uncovered during the interview process may reveal previous or current nutrition-related concerns. These findings allow a more focused physical examination to follow.[8] The examiner is alert for nonspecific signs and symptoms such as fatigue, cold intolerance, flaky dermatitis, and any other sign that could indicate a nutrition-related problem and requires further investigation.[5] More direct clues in the history that can prompt further investigation of the possibility of malnutrition include recent, unintentional loss of 10% or more of usual body weight in an adult, restricted food intake, a chronic disease, malabsorption, or use of drugs that interact with nutrients.[9] Other questions to focus on include How is the appetite? Is there a history of nausea, vomiting, or early satiety? Is diarrhea or

---

TABLE 2-1

Nutritional Health History

Item	Components
Demographic data	Name, date, age, sex, date of birth, address, occupation, workplace, insurance
Chief complaint	Client's subjective statement of health problem, including onset and duration
	Reason for seeking health care
Present illness and current health	Detailed data about chief complaint as it relates to nutritional status
	Recent diet changes and reasons
	Recent weight loss or gain and over what period of time
	Usual body weight; 20% above or below desirable weight?
	Change in appetite
	Unusual stress/trauma (surgery, job, family)
	Medications, prescriptions
	Alcohol, nicotine, caffeine consumption
Health history	Previous illnesses, trauma, major dental problem that could interfere with ability to shop, prepare food, chew, or swallow
	Allergies—environmental, foods, drugs
	Eating disorders
	Chronic disease or surgery that affects gastrointestinal tract
	Substance abuse
	Nutrition programs
Family health history	Genetic/familial disorders that could affect nutritional status: cardiovascular or gastrointestinal disorders, Crohn's, diabetes, cancer, sickle cell anemia, allergies, food intolerance, obesity
Dietary history	Current food intake pattern using one of the following methods: 24-hour or 7-day recall, as appropriate, food frequency, comparison to dietary guidelines and RDAs
	Special dietary considerations, restrictions
	Fad diets
	Vitamin and mineral supplements
	Commercial dietary supplements
	Nonconventional dietary supplements
	Food preferences, dislikes
	Dietary influences from ethnic, cultural, religious practices
	Counseling needs (based on food knowledge)
Medication history	Recent use of steroids, immunosuppressants, chemotherapy, anticonvulsants, or oral contraceptives
Socioeconomic	Adequate food storage, refrigeration, food preparation
	Payments: SSI, food stamps, WIC
	Who shops, prepares, and cooks food?
Personal	Stress/coping mechanisms, self-concept, social support
	Daily activity level and exercise regimen
Review of systems	Systematic collection of specific information about present and past problems
	Health promotion and maintenance practices
	Includes general overview, vision/hearing, integumentary, respiratory, cardiovascular, hematologic, peripheral vascular, gastrointestinal, genitourinary, endocrine, neurologic, and musculoskeletal systems (see Box 2-1)

BOX 2-1

Review of Systems Related to Nutritional Status

GENERAL

Present weight	Fever
Weakness	Headache
Fatigue	Dizziness
Malaise	Sleep patterns

EYES AND EARS

Nutritional significance: Problems with the eyes can affect ability to shop, prepare food, and read instructions or work home therapy equipment properly without modifications. Ear problems such as pain or infection can affect ability to chew food or hear equipment alarms for home therapy.

Eyes	Ears
Pain	Pain
Vision impairments	Infection
Glasses/contacts	Mastoiditis
Spots/floaters	Vertigo
Recent change in acuity	
Infection	
Glaucoma	
Cataract	

SKIN AND NAILS

Nutritional significance: Problems may indicate particular vitamin, mineral, or protein deficiency.

Itching	Excessive dryness
Tendency to bruising	Pigmentary and other color changes
Texture and moisture	Lesions or rashes
Changes in hair and nails	Use of hair dyes or other agents

RESPIRATORY TRACT

Nutritional significance: Nasal obstruction may affect delivery of nutrition support; lung problems that pose energy restrictions can influence the ability to consume enough food. Substrate composition of feeding can also be influenced.

Nose	Lungs
Injury	Chronic obstructive pulmonary disease
Sinus pain or infection	Cystic fibrosis
Nasal obstruction	Bronchodysplasia
Rhinorrhea or discharge	Sputum production
Dyspnea	Oxygen therapy

BLOOD AND LYMPH NODES

Nutritional significance: Problems may indicate vitamin or protein deficiencies.

Bleeding tendencies	Anemia and treatment
Lymph node enlargement	

CARDIOVASCULAR SYSTEM

Nutritional significance: May affect fluid or substrate composition of feeding regimen

Hypertension
Dyspnea/cyanosis
Coronary artery disease
Edema

GASTROINTESTINAL AND HEPATOBILIARY SYSTEMS

Nutritional significance: Factors related to indigestion, digestion, or absorption of nutrients

Mouth or throat soreness or pain	Hoarseness
Difficulty chewing or swallowing	Bleeding gums

Continued.

constipation present? Are there neuromuscular changes such as tingling or numbness of the fingers? Is there a history of glossitis, stomatitis, or conjunctivitis that might suggest vitamin deficiency? Is there a history of skin rashes or chronic infections suggestive of zinc deficiency? Complementary and alternative medicine (CAM) should also be addressed (herbs, homeopathic remedies, acupuncture, magnets, vitamin, amino acid, and mineral supplements).[10]

Review of Systems Related to Nutritional Status—cont'd

GASTROINTESTINAL AND HEPATOBILIARY SYSTEMS—cont'd

Condition of teeth
Appetite/food intolerances
Nausea or vomiting
Dysphagia
Heartburn
Indigestion
Postprandial pain
Use of antacids
Other abdominal pain or tenderness
Belching
Abdominal masses
Hematemesis
Distention
Flatulence

Expectoration
Use of laxatives
Character of stool
Melena
Change in bowel habits (constipation/diarrhea)
Rectal conditions (pruritus, hemorrhoids, fissures)
Gallbladder disease
Hepatitis
Jaundice
Appendicitis
Abdominal surgery
Colitis
Parasites
Hernia

URINARY TRACT

Nutritional significance: Problems affect substrate composition and calorie and protein requirements of feeding regimens.

Renal colic or stones
Kidney disease (failure, nephrotic syndrome)
Dialysis
Nocturia

Albuminuria
Infections
Polyuria
Oliguria

ENDOCRINE SYSTEM

Nutritional significance: Problems affect substrate composition and calorie and protein requirements of feeding regimens.

Nutritional and growth history
Thyroid function (tolerance to heat, cold, changes in skin; relationship between appetite and weight, nervousness, tremors, drowsiness
Hair distribution and hirsutism

Goiter
Diabetes or symptoms (polyuria, polydipsia, polyphagia)
Sugar in blood or urine
Excessive sweating
Hormone therapy

NERVOUS SYSTEM

Nutritional significance: Problems affect ability to coordinate feeding and requirements for adaptive equipment.

Headache
Nervousness
Sleep disturbances
Paresthesias
Convulsions
Loss of consciousness

Stroke
Sensory or motor disturbances (speech, tremors, weakness)
Vertigo or syncope
Disorientation
Memory loss

MUSCULOSKELETAL SYSTEM

Nutritional significance: Affects ability to self-feed and need for adaptive equipment. Also may reflect some vitamin or mineral imbalances.

Muscles	Joints
Weakness	Pain
Pain or trauma	Stiffness
Cramps	Swelling
Spasms	Rheumatoid arthritis or osteoarthritis
Aches	Bursitis
Atrophy	Gout
Dislocation	Osteomyelitis
Fractures	Osteoporosis
Back (pain, stiffness, limitation, disk disease)	

Adapted with permission from Cecere C, McCash K: Health history and physical examination. In Lewis SM, Collier IC (eds): *Medical-surgical nursing*, St Louis, 1992, Mosby.

Physical Examination

The physical assessment, part of the patient's evaluation, takes a problem-oriented approach to provide and prioritize nutrition care. Findings of the nutritional health history and physical examination constitute the initial database from which a problem list is then constructed, and a plan of care is written for each problem. The plan is then implemented, monitored, and evaluated for effectiveness.[6,7]

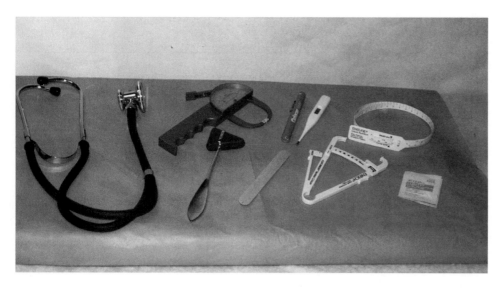

FIGURE 2-2 Equipment for assessment. Stethoscope, Lange skinfold caliper, reflex hammer, tongue blade (*forefront*), penlight, thermometer, Ross skinfold caliper, tape measure, alcohol wipe. (Courtesy of Louis and Vera Pesce.)

Physical assessment is defined as an interpretation of the whole person. It is a collection of data about an individual's state of health. The physical examination reveals objective information related to nutritional status.[6,7,11-14] How well nutrients meet the body's needs can be evaluated through physical examination of body systems. Nutritional and metabolic dysfunction can be assessed by physical examination.[15] Tissues that rapidly proliferate, such as hair, skin, eyes, lips, and tongue papillae, are likely to reveal nutritional deficiencies sooner than other tissues do.[16,17] One must be able to distinguish between nonnutritional causes for similar findings. For example, changes in hair color or texture may be related to chemical alterations such as bleaching, coloring, or other processing. Information can also be gathered regarding the choice of appropriate feeding regimens, such as calorie and protein requirements for a patient with a fever, a healing wound, or an amputation; states that require modification of formula selection, such as fluid limitations; route of feeding, which may be affected by surgical procedures, wounds, or drainage; and the possibility of additional nutrient requirements in the presence of delayed wound healing or an essential fatty acid deficiency.[18]

The nutritional physical examination takes a systems approach, which proceeds from head to toe to assess the state of the patient's nutritional health. It should corroborate with the nutrition health history.[19] A systems approach allows the examiner to concentrate on areas of concern. The process is systematic to ensure an organized and efficient approach to care.[2,6,7] Physical examination for nutrient deficiencies should be done weekly during an acute illness.[18]

A few basic pieces of equipment are necessary to perform a physical examination with a nutrition focus: thermometer, stethoscope, sphygmomanometer, penlight or flashlight, wooden tongue depressor, tape measure, scales, skin calipers, reflex hammer, and nasoscope (Fig. 2-2). To successfully perform a comprehensive physical examination, four basic techniques are used: inspection, palpation, percussion, and auscultation. A nutrition-focused physical examination concentrates on the techniques of inspection, palpation, and auscultation.

Inspection is the examination technique used most frequently. Inspection entails critical observation by smell, sight,

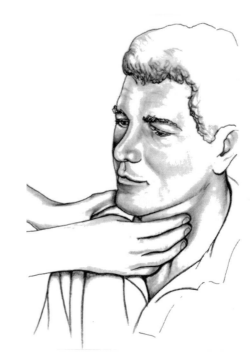

FIGURE 2-3 Light palpation.

and hearing. Inspection should not be hurried, lest important observations be missed. Initially, the area of interest is assessed generally. This broad observation is followed by a closer, more detailed look at that area including critical observation of its color, texture, size, and shape. Good lighting is essential for adequate assessment.[6,7,15,16]

Palpation follows inspection. Palpation—examining body structures, pulsations, and vibrations by touch—also allows assessment of the texture, size, warmth, tenderness, and mobility of the body. Palpation can be either light or deep as controlled by the pressure of the fingers or hand. Light palpation involves gently pressing in to a depth of 1 cm (Fig. 2-3), while deep palpation involves pressing in to a depth of approximately 4 cm (Fig. 2-4). Light palpation is usually adequate for nutrition examination.

Percussion follows palpation and involves tapping fingers and hands quickly and sharply against body surfaces such as the chest and abdomen. The goal of percussion is to produce sounds to locate organ borders and assess organ shape and position. It also determines if the organ is solid or filled with fluid or gas.[7,16] There are two methods of percussion, direct and indirect. Direct percussion is performed by tapping the fingertips or hand directly against the body structure (Fig. 2-5). Indirect percussion is performed by using the nondominant hand as the stationary hand. The middle finger or pleximeter is hyperextended and the distal portion is placed firmly against the patient's skin. The middle finger of the dominant hand strikes the pleximeter with the fingertip, not the finger pad. It should hit at a right angle to the stationary finger. The finger strikes twice and is

withdrawn immediately, to avoid interfering with vibrations (Fig. 2-6). This procedure continues symmetrically, first on one side of the body, then on the other, as in percussion of the posterior thorax.[7,15,16] Different tissues produce different sounds (Table 2-2).

Auscultation uses a stethoscope to listen to sounds produced by organs and viscera, such as the lungs, heart, blood vessels, stomach, and intestines. These sounds reflect movement of air or fluid through different parts of the body. Auscultation is usually the final technique used in physical assessment, except in the abdomen, where it is used second, after inspection. Bowel sounds may be disrupted by palpation. Sounds should be described in terms of pitch (high or low), amplitude (loudness), duration (length), and frequency (how often).[7,15]

The examiner must respect the patient's dignity and provide privacy. Only the body area being examined is uncovered and the patient must not be overexposed. When examination of the particular body part is completed, that part is covered again. The purpose of the examination and each part of it is explained

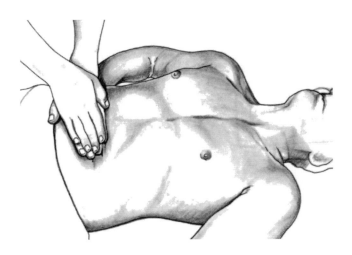

FIGURE 2-4 Deep palpation.

TABLE 2-2
Percussion Sounds[7,10]

Sound	Structure of Origin	Pitch	Amplitude	Quality
Tympany	Stomach, intestine	High	Loud	Drumlike
Dullness	Dense structures (liver, spleen, diaphragm)	High	Soft	Thudlike
Flatness	Muscle, bone	High	Soft	Dull
Resonance	Lungs	Low	Loud	

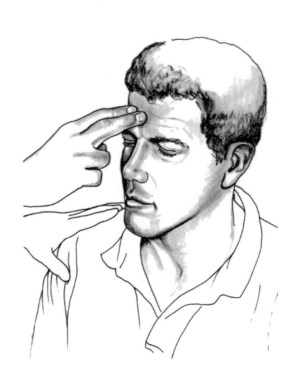

FIGURE 2-5 Direct percussion.

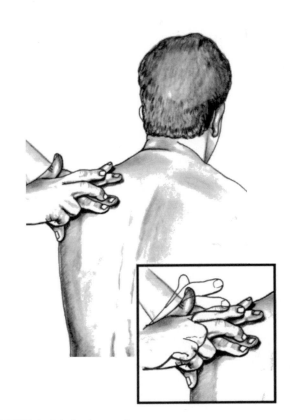

FIGURE 2-6 Indirect percussion.

as the examination proceeds, to decrease anxiety and fear, even if the patient is comatose.

The physical examination consists of a head-to-toe progression to assess nutritional status. The examination includes a general survey, vital signs, anthropometrics, and assessment of the head and neck and of the respiratory, cardiovascular, gastrointestinal, musculoskeletal, nervous, and integumentary systems.[4,5,7,10,11] Box 2-2 provides the screening format for a nutrition-focused physical examination, and Table 2-3 describes signs and symptoms that may indicate nutritional deficiencies.

General Survey

The general survey reveals much information at initial contact with the patient because it reflects his or her overall nutritional

---

BOX 2-2
Outline for Screening Physical Examination

1. General Survey
Observe general state of health (patient is seated)
  Body features
  State of consciousness and arousal
  Speech
  Body movements
  Physical signs
  Nutritional status
  Stature

2. Vital Signs
Record vital signs:
  Blood pressure
  Radial pulse
  Respiration
Record height and weight

3. Integument
Inspect and palpate skin for the following:
  Color
  Lesions
  Scars
  Bruises
  Edema
  Moisture
  Texture
  Temperature
  Turgor
  Vascularity
Inspect and palpate nails for the following:
  Color
  Lesions
  Size
  Flexibility
  Shape
  Angle

4. Head and Neck
Inspect and palpate head for the following:
  Shape and symmetry of skull
  Masses
  Tenderness
  Hair
  Scalp
  Skin
  Temporal arteries
  Temporomandibular joint
  Sensory (CN V, light touch, pain)
  Motor (CN VII, shows teeth, purses lips, raises eyebrows)
  Looks up, wrinkles forehead (CN VII)
  Raises shoulders against resistance (CN XI)

Inspect and palpate (occasionally auscultate) neck for the following:
  Skin (vascularity and visible pulsations)
  Symmetry
  Postural alignment
  Range of motion
  Pulses and bruits (carotid)
  Midline structure (trachea, thyroid gland, cartilage)
  Lymph nodes (preauricular, postauricular, occipital, mandibular, tonsillar, submental, anterior and posterior cervical, infraclavicular, supraclavicular)
Inspect and palpate eyes for the following:
  Visual acuity
  Eyebrows
  Position and movement of eyelids
  Visual fields
  Extraocular movements (CN III, IV, VI)
  Cornea, sclera, conjunctiva
  Pupillary response
  Red reflex
  Eyeball tension
Inspect and palpate ears for the following:
  Placement
  Pinna
  Auditory acuity (Weber's or Rinne, whispered voice, ticking watch)
  Mastoid process
  Auditory canal
  Tympanic membrane
Inspect and palpate nose and sinuses for the following:
  External nose
    Shape
    Blockage
  Internal nose
    Patency of nasal passages
    Shape
    Turbinates or polyps
    Discharge
  Frontal and maxillary sinuses
Inspect and palpate mouth for the following:
  Lips (symmetry, lesions, color)
  Buccal mucosa (Stensen's and Wharton's ducts)
  Teeth (absence, state of repair, color)
  Gums
  Tongue for strength (asymmetry, ability to stick out tongue, side to side, fasciculations)
  Palates
  Tonsils and pillars
  Uvular elevation (CN IX)
  Posterior pharynx
  Gag reflex (CN X)
  Jaw strength (CN XI)
  Moisture
  Color
  Floor of mouth

Continued.

status.[4] The general state of health is observed, including orientation, speech, body type, mobility, and signs of nutritional depletion such as wasting of skeletal muscle or subcutaneous fat and weight loss. Loss of muscle mass over quadriceps and deltoids is seen with nutritional depletion. The examiner must keep in mind that muscle mass varies with activity level and with nutritional status. Activities such as weight lifting and

running increase muscle mass, whereas unused muscles, especially in the arms and legs, undergo atrophy, as seen in prolonged bed rest. Loss of subcutaneous fat is usually noticeable in the face (hollow cheeks), triceps, thighs (quadriceps),[19] and waist. Profound weight loss is also noted on general inspection. Findings noted in the general survey usually reflect long-term nutritional depletion rather than early depletion.[15,20]

BOX 2-2
Outline for Screening Physical Examination—cont'd

5. Extremities
Observe size and shape, symmetry and deformity, involuntary movements
Inspect and palpate arms, fingers, wrists, elbows, shoulders for the following:
  Strength
  Range of motion
  Crepitus
  Joint pain
  Swelling
  Fluid
Test reflexes:
  Biceps
  Triceps
  Brachioradialis
  Patellar
  Achilles
  Plantar
Inspect and palpate legs for the following:
  Strength of hips
  Edema
  Hair distribution
  Pulses (dorsalis pedis, posterior tibialis)

6. Posterior Thorax
Inspect for muscular development, respiratory movement, approximation of AP diameter
  Palpate for symmetry of respiratory movement, tenderness of CVA, spinous processes, tumors or swelling, tactile fremitus
  Percuss for pulmonary resonance
  Auscultate for breath sounds

7. Anterior Thorax
  Assess breasts for configuration, symmetry, dimpling of skin
  Assess nipples for rash, direction, inversion, retraction
  Initiate teaching or review of breast self-exam
  Inspect for PMI, other precordial pulsations
  Palpate for thrills, lifts, heaves, tenderness over precordium
  Inspect neck for venous distention, pulsations, waves
  Palpate axillae
  Palpate breasts
  Auscultate for rate and rhythm, character of S_1 and S_2 in the aortic, pulmonic, Erb's point, tricuspid, mitral areas; bruits at carotid, epigastrium; breath sounds at RML

8. Abdomen
  Inspect for scars, shape, symmetry, bulging, muscular position and condition of umbilicus, movements (respiratory, pulsations, presence of peristaltic waves)
  Auscultate for peristalsis, bruits
  Percuss border of liver, four abdominal quadrants
  Palpate to confirm positive findings; check liver (size, surface contour, tenderness); spleen; kidney (size, contour, consistency, tenderness, mobility); urinary bladder (distention); femoral pulses; inguinofemoral nodes

9. Completion of Examinations of Extremities
Observe the following:
  Range of motion of hips, knees, ankles, feet
  Crepitus
  Joint pain
  Swelling
  Fluid
  Muscle development
  Coordination (heel to shin)
  Homan's sign
  Proprioception (position sense of great toe)

10. Neurologic
  Motor status observations
    Gait
    Toe walk
    Heel walk
    Drift
  Coordination
    Finger to nose
    Romberg's sign
  Spine (scoliosis)

11. Genitalia*
Male external genitalia
  Inspect penis, noting hair distribution, prepuce, glans, urethral meatus, scars, ulcers, eruptions, structural alterations
  Inspect epidermis of perineum, rectum
  Inspect skin of scrotum; palpate for descended testes, masses, pain
Female external genitalia
  Inspect hair distribution; mons pubis; labia (minora and majora); urethral meatus; Bartholin's, urethral, Skene's glands (may also be palpated, if indicated); introitus
  Assess for presence of cystocele, rectocele, prolapse
  Inspect perineum, rectum

From McCash K. Health history and physical examination. In Lewis SM, Heitkemper MM, Dietsen SR (eds): *Medical-surgical nursing*, St Louis, 2000, Mosby, p 74.
AP, anteroposterior; *CVA*, costovertebral angle; *PMI*, point of maximal impulse; *RML*, right middle lobe.
*If the nurse has the appropriate training, the speculum and bimanual examination of women and the prostate gland examination of men should be performed after this inspection.

TABLE 2-3

Nutrition Deficiencies Revealed by Physical Examination[3,8,9,12,18]

Deficient Nutrient	Findings
GENERAL SURVEY	
Protein, calories	Loss of weight, muscle mass, or fat stores; growth retardation, infection
Protein, thiamine	Edema (ankles and feet) (rule out sodium and water retention, pregnancy, protein-losing enteropathy)
Obesity	Excessive fat stores
Vitamin A	Poor growth
Iron	Anemia, fatigue
SKIN	
Protein, vitamin C, zinc	Poor wound healing, pressure ulcers
Fat, vitamin A	Xerosis (rule out environmental, lack of hygiene, aging, uremia, hypothyroidism)
	Follicular hyperkeratosis
	Mosaic dermatitis (plaques of skin in center, peeling at periphery on shins)
Vitamin C	Slow wound healing
Niacin	Red, swollen skin lesions
Zinc	Delayed wound healing, acneiform rash, skin lesions, hair loss
Vitamin K or C	Excessive bleeding, petechiae, ecchymoses; small red, purple, black or blue, hemorrhagic spots
Dehydration (fluid)	Poor skin turgor
NAILS	
Iron	Koilonychia (rule out cardiopulmonary disease)
Protein deficiency	Dull, lusterless with transverse ridging across nail plate
Vitamin A, C	Pale, poor blanching, irregular, mottled
Protein, calories	Bruising, bleeding
Vitamin C	Splinter hemorrhages
HAIR	
Protein	Hair lacks shine, luster (cause may be environmental or chemical)
	Thin, sparse (fine, silky, and sparse with wide gaps between hairs)
Protein, copper	Dyspigmentation (lightening of normal hair color; consider if hair is bleached or dyed)
	Flag sign (alternating bands of light and dark hair in young children): rare
	Easily plucked
Copper	Corkscrew hair (Menkes syndrome)
FACE	
Protein	Diffuse depigmentation, swelling
	Moon face (rounded cheeks with pursed mouth, seen in preschoolers)
Calcium	Facial paresthesias
EYES	
Iron, folate, or vitamin B_{12}	Pale conjunctivae (anemia)
Vitamin A	Bitot's spots (more common in children)
	Conjunctival xerosis (rule out chemical or environmental irritation)
	Corneal xerosis
	Keratomalacia
Pyridoxine, niacin, riboflavin	Angular palpebritis
Hyperlipidemia	Corneal arcus, xanthelasma
NOSE	
Riboflavin, niacin, pyridoxine	Seborrhea on nasolabial area, nose bridge, eyebrows, and backs of ears (rule out poor hygiene)
LIPS AND MOUTH	
Niacin, riboflavin	Cheilosis
	Angular scars
Riboflavin, pyridoxine, niacin, iron	Angular stomatitis

Continued.

Vital Signs

Measurements of temperature, pulse, respiration, and blood pressure are also significant sources of data. These measures, referred to as *vital signs*, help monitor essential body functions and afford insight into the functional capacity of specific organs, especially heart and lungs. Vital signs establish base-line measurements, identify physiologic disorders and changes over time, and monitor response to therapy.[7]

TABLE 2-3

TABLE 2-3
Nutrition Deficiencies Revealed by Physical Examination—cont'd

Deficient Nutrient	Findings
TONGUE	
Niacin, riboflavin, folic acid, iron, B_{12}	Atrophic filiform papillae
	Glossitis
Zinc	Taste atrophy
Riboflavin	Magenta tongue
TEETH	
Excess sugar, vitamin C	Edentia, caries
Fluorosis	Mottled
GUMS	
Vitamin C	Spongy, bleeding, receding
NECK	
Iodine	Enlarged thyroid
Protein, bulimia	Enlarged parotids (bilateral)
Excess fluid	Venous distention, pulsations
THORAX	
Protein, calories	Decreased muscle mass and strength, shortness of breath, fatigue; decreased pulmonary function
CARDIAC SYSTEM	
Thiamine	Heart failure
GASTROINTESTINAL SYSTEM	
Protein, calories, zinc, vitamin C	Poor wound healing
Protein	Hepatomegaly
URINARY TRACT	
Dehydration	Dark, concentrated urine
Overhydration	Light, dilute urine
MUSCULOSKELETAL SYSTEM	
Vitamin D, calcium	Rickets, osteomalacia
Vitamin D	Persistently open anterior fontanel (after age 18 months), craniotabes (softening of skull across back and sides before age 1 year)
	Epiphyseal enlargement (painless) at wrist, knees, and ankles
	Pigeon chest and Harrison's sulcus (horizontal depression on lower chest border)
Protein	Emaciation, muscle wasting, swelling, pain, pale hair patches
Vitamin C	Swollen, painful joints
Thiamine	Pain in thighs, calves
NERVOUS SYSTEM	
Protein	Psychomotor changes (listless, apathetic)
	Mental confusion
Thiamin, B_6	Weakness, confusion, depressed reflexes, paresthesias, sensory loss, calf tenderness
Niacin, vitamin B_{12}	Dementia
Calcium, magnesium	Tetany

Anthropometric Measurements

Measurements of triceps skinfold and arm muscle circumference provide more accurate means of assessing somatic fat and protein stores. Height and weight are also measured to assess weight for height, usual body weight, ideal body weight, and percent weight change. These values, discussed in Chapter 3, should be compared to previous recordings.[19]

Skin and Nails

The skin is observed while assessing each body system because it can provide pertinent information on nutritional status. The skin is inspected for color, pigmentation, abnormal color, bruising, lesions, and edema. Any changes in skin color, texture, temperature, pigmentation, or moisture should be noted and further examined.[21] Skin color varies with genetic makeup. Generally, it ranges from ivory to pinkish to ruddy tan to light to dark brown, and it may have yellow or olive overtones. Hygiene of the skin should also be noted. Next, the skin should be palpated for temperature, moisture, turgor, and texture.[15,16,21,22] Temperature is checked using the backs of the hands and palpating the skin bilaterally. Healthy skin is warm and dry. Any moisture should be noted. Diaphoresis is associated with elevated temperature or fever, and it increases the metabolic rate. Moisture also reflects the state of hydration as evidenced by assessing skin turgor. Skin turgor is assessed by pinching a fold of skin (usually on the anterior chest under the clavicle) and noting its ability to spring back promptly. If skin remains pinched up or "tents" and assumes its normal position slowly skin turgor is poor; this probably reflects dehydration or extreme weight loss.[15,16] On the other hand, edema may be present if the skin looks puffy and tight. Edema, not normally present, is the accumulation of fluid in the intercellular spaces.[16] Edema is most notable in dependent parts of the body such as the sacrum and lower extremities. Accumulation of excess fluid in the tissues can be caused by increased hydrostatic pressure such as that associated with heart failure and renal failure. On the other hand, protein deficits can cause decreased capillary oncotic pressure and resultant fluid accumulation in the tissues. Edematous skin is palpated gently with the thumb or forefinger, and the indentations are observed. If edema (commonly known as *pitting edema*) is present, it may range from 1+ for slight indentation (about 2 mm) to 4+ for deep indentation (about 8 mm).[15]

Unexposed areas of the skin normally feel smooth and firm, whereas exposed areas of skin have a slightly rougher texture. Follicular hyperkeratosis, which feels like sandpaper, consists of spinelike plaques on the buttocks, thighs, elbows, and knees. Xerosis is indicated by general dryness and shedding of the skin. Skin is thinner on eyelids and ears and thicker on the palms of the hands and soles of the feet. Bleeding, petechiae, ecchymoses, and hemorrhagic areas should be noted.[9,15,16]

The skin should be assessed for wounds and ulcers. Pressure ulcers develop in immobile patients and with prolonged bed rest. These ulcers, most notable on bony prominences, result from prolonged pressure in areas such as the back of the neck, scapulas, wrists, elbows, hips sacrum, and heels, and in other tender areas such as the ears. Pressure ulcers are staged on a scale of 1 to 4, according to the extent of damage to skin layers and underlying structures such as muscle, bone, fascia, or connective tissue.[6,15] Several skin assessment scales are available for predicting risk of developing pressure sores. One scale in particular, the Braden Scale,[23] includes a subscale to measure usual food intake patterns ranging from very poor to excellent. A second layer of potential responses is listed for those receiving enteral or parenteral nutrition. Because in some instances these regimens are not prescribed or managed to the fullest benefit of the patient, the rating of excellent is not listed.

Wounds are an important part of skin assessment because poor nutritional status is reflected in poor wound healing. Wounds need to be accurately described and monitored in order to adjust nutritional parameters as necessary. Wounds are inspected for size, color, depth, drainage, swelling, and stage of healing. Accurate assessment of these parameters is important to determine nutritional outcomes. Wounds can be easily described using basic descriptions or measurements (e.g., the wound is about the size of a quarter or dime) to more sophisticated methods. Special disposable rulers are available along with tracers (plastic sheets and grids), photography, and even ultrasonic surface scanners; however, the most important fact to remember is to track the data collected to evaluate progress. Upon inspection, normal findings include some redness and swelling of the wound in the early stages of healing. Any swelling that causes separation of the suture line or is associated with pus formation is abnormal. As healing progresses, swelling and redness decrease, and the wound edges should have fused when the sutures are removed. The wound bed should be bright red and moisture should be evident. Any dryness, dehiscence, evisceration, or fistula formation requires immediate attention.[15]

Along with skin, nails are inspected and palpated for shape and contour, angle, and any lesions.[15,22] Normally, nail surfaces are slightly curved or flat and the edges are smooth and rounded. The nail surface should be smooth and regular. The nail plate is translucent, giving way to the pinkish nail bed color in whites and a bluish hue in dark-skinned peoples. To assess circulation, the nails should be gently squeezed between the thumb and forefinger. The nail blanches white when squeezed and when released should again turn pink. How long the blanched nail takes to return to its normal color is the capillary refill time, usually less than 3 seconds. Any bleeding or bruising should be noted because it could indicate malnutrition. Concave nails can indicate iron-deficiency anemia. *Koilonychia* describes spoon-shaped, brittle, and thin nails.[8] Nails that blanch poorly or are irregular and mottled in appearance may reflect vitamin deficiencies.[8,14,20]

Head and Neck

Physical examination of the head by inspection and palpation includes the scalp, hair, face, eyes, nose, mouth, and neck. The scalp is inspected and palpated for shape and symmetry and for masses and tenderness of the skull. General hygiene is noted for sores, drainage, flakiness, and rashes. Hair is inspected for color, pigmentation, distribution pattern, shine, texture, and quantity. Gently pulling hair away from the scalp between the fingers assesses ease of hair loss and degree of pluckability, which may be associated with protein or zinc deficiency.

The face is inspected and palpated for skin color, lesions, texture, depth, and moisture. Wasting may be evident in hollowing of the temporalis and cheeks. Cranial nerves may also be part of the examination. Cranial nerve V (trigeminal) is tested by asking the patient to clench the teeth and noting the strength of muscle contraction. Cranial nerve VII (facial) is tested by having the patient show both upper and lower teeth.[5] These nerves can affect the ability to eat properly.

Next, the eyes are inspected and palpated. The skin around the eyes should be noted for scaling, redness, and other discoloration. Angular palpebritis is manifested when corners of the eyes are cracked and red. The color of the conjunctivae, sclerae, and corneas should be assessed. The conjunctivae can be checked by gently pulling down the skin below the lower lid and having the patient look upward.[22] The conjunctivae should be pink and without drainage. If the conjunctiva is pale, investigation for anemia may be warranted. Xerosis can produce dryness of the conjunctivae and corneas. The sclerae are normally white. Yellowing is usually associated with jaundice, whereas thin sclerae may look bluish; however, both tinges are normal variations in black persons. The cornea is inspected with a flashlight, examining from the side of the eye. Corneal xerosis is evidenced by a dull, milky, hazy, opaque appearance on the lower central area of the eye.[24] Keratomalacia may also be detected as bilateral softening of the entire cornea, or part of it and a gelatinous white or yellow appearance.[3,8,9,24] Arcus senilis—a grayish white ring or arc around the cornea—is due to lipid deposition that occurs with normal aging, but in young persons it can signal hyperlipoproteinemia.[16] Soft, raised, yellow plaques on the eyelids at the inner canthus, called *xanthelasma*, develop around the fifth decade of life, mostly in women. These plaques are seen with high and normal cholesterol levels.[11] Also, the whites of the eyes should be inspected for Bitot's spots, which are dry, gray, yellowish or white, foamy spots.[3,8,9,24] If the practitioner is trained in using an ophthalmoscope, further examination of the eye may be conducted by inspecting the interior of the eye for evidence of certain diseases such as diabetes mellitus, hypertension, and atherosclerosis.

After completion of the eye examination, the external and internal aspects of the nose are inspected. The shape and symmetry of the external nose is noted, along with any discharge. Color and consistency of the discharge may indicate bleeding, trauma, or infection.[15,16] Nasolabial seborrhea appears as scaly, dry, greasy skin and yellowish or salmon-colored material around the nostrils.[3,8,924] Inspection of the internal aspects of the nose follows the external examination. Patency of each nostril is checked by obstructing one nostril, having the patient exhale with mouth closed, and feeling for the puff of air with the fingertips. Further examination follows, using a nasal speculum or penlight or the light on an ophthalmoscope. The head is tilted back slightly, if the patient is able, and patency of the nasal passage is examined, especially if there is the possibility that a feeding tube may be placed. Any blockage, polyps, or deviation of the septum that could affect tube placement should be noted.[15] Any feeding device already in place should be noted, along with condition of mucous membranes, to make sure a sinus tract or infection has not developed from the tube. The mucous membranes should be pinkish red. Enlarged, boggy, and bluish nasal turbinates may indicate allergy.

The oral cavity—jaws, lips, teeth, tongue, gums, and buccal mucosa—follows next in the examination. The jaws are inspected and palpated by having the patient open and close them while exposing the teeth. The upper and lower front teeth should align with a slight overbite. Malocclusion is significant when it interferes with effective chewing. Jaw movements from side to side should also be noted.[15] The parotid glands can be inspected and palpated at this time. The parotid glands, located anterior to the ear lobes, may become enlarged secondary to bulimia and other states of starvation or to infections

such as mumps and isolated parotitis.[17] The lips are inspected and palpated for symmetry, lesions, and color. Cheilosis is noted when lips are red and swollen, with vertical cracks noted at the center of the lower lip. Cracks, redness, and flakiness at the corners of the mouth indicate angular stomatitis.[8,9,24]

The tongue is inspected and palpated for color, fissures, cuts, moisture, texture, and symmetry. Inspection is performed by having the patient stick the tongue out as far as possible. The examiner should note symmetry at this time. The tongue should protrude in midline without tremors. Abnormalities of strength and symmetry may indicate a problem with cranial nerve XII (hypoglossal), which can affect the ability of a patient to chew certain foods properly.[15,16] The tongue should be pink and moist, without fissures or cuts, and its texture should appear slightly rough because of the taste buds. Atrophic filiform papillae (taste buds) appear shrunken, and the tongue is smooth and slick. With glossitis the tongue is beefy red, appears atrophic, and is painful.[8,9,17,24] Any other tongue color (e.g., magenta) could indicate a nutrition-related disorder. One must also distinguish the protective white coating the tongue forms during inflammatory processes from white plaques that may adhere to the tongue as exudates during infective states. Next, the inner mouth is inspected with a tongue blade for the color of the buccal mucosa, which may vary depending on race. The mucosa of blacks may have a slightly blue undertone, whereas in whites the mucosa usually has pink or red undertones. The remainder of the oral mucosa in all races should be some shade of pink, depending on mucosal thickness.[4,15] The mucosa should appear moist if saliva secretion is adequate, and no lesions or cuts should be present. The gag reflex can also be assessed at this time by gently touching the posterior wall of the pharynx with a tongue blade to elicit a response. Assessment of the gag reflex tests cranial nerves IX (glossopharyngeal) and X (vagus).[15,16]

The teeth and gums are also inspected and palpated at this time. The teeth are assessed for the state of repair, tooth loss, and inflammatory processes. White or brownish patches or mottling should be noted. Gums are inspected for color, texture, and cuts. Spongy, receding, pale, and bleeding gums indicate a nutrition-related disorder.[15,16] Feeding devices should be noted at this time, as well as the condition of the device and surrounding anatomy.

Proceeding from head to toe, the neck is inspected and palpated next. The neck veins should be inspected to assess for distention, which may give an indication of fluid status. The neck is inspected to assess the thyroid gland for midline structure, including enlargement (e.g., a goiter).[15] The examination is usually performed while standing behind the patient, who sits up straight and bends the head slightly forward and to the right to help relax the muscles. The examiner places the right-hand fingers between the trachea and sternomastoid muscle, retracting the muscle slightly and asking the patient to swallow. The thyroid should move slightly upward. This is repeated on the left side (Fig. 2-7). Normally, the thyroid is not palpable. Hardened nodules or masses are abnormal, and palpation should not elicit any tenderness. Although this is more awkward, the thyroid can be assessed while standing in front of the patient. With the patient's head tipped slightly forward and to the right, the right thumb displaces the trachea slightly to the patient's right, and the

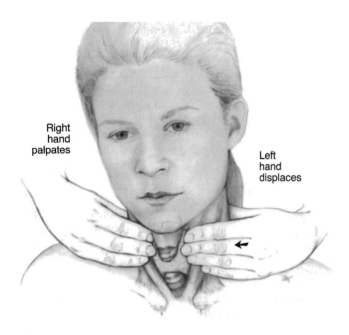

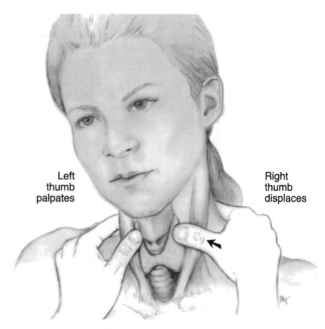

FIGURE 2-7 Examination of thyroid from behind. (From Jarvis C: *Physical examination and health assessment,* Philadelphia, 1992, WB Saunders, p 283.)

FIGURE 2-8 Examination of thyroid from front. (From Jarvis C: *Physical examination and health assessment,* Philadelphia, 1992, WB Saunders, p 284.)

left thumb and fingers are placed around the sternomastoid muscle, palpating for lobe enlargement as the patient swallows (Fig. 2-8).[16] The examiner also notes any feeding devices.

Thorax

The anterior and posterior thorax are inspected for shape, muscle and lung development, and symmetry.[22,25] Muscle mass and fat stores in the anterior and posterior thorax should be noted, along with respiratory rate, depth, and rhythm. Hypertrophied muscles may indicate the use of accessory muscles to breath.[25] Malnutrition is usually an indirect result of underlying respiratory problems. In states of malnutrition, respiratory muscle mass, strength, and efficiency decrease. Respiratory muscle mass is thought to decline in proportion to body weight.[3] Energy needs (and calorie requirements) are generally increased in patients with respiratory disease because much energy is used just to breathe. Many times, the patient with chronic respiratory disease cannot consume enough food because of fatigue caused by increased work of breathing, shortness of breath, and decreased oxygen saturation.[3] A vicious cycle develops, beginning with a decline in pulmonary function and increased energy needs that exceed food intake capability and progressing to nutritional depletion. In normal adults, resting rate of respirations ranges from 16 to 20 breaths per minute, and they are even in depth and regular in rhythm. With respiratory disease, respiratory rate increases, the breathing pattern is deep or shallow, depending on the cause of the disease, and the rhythm irregular. The lungs may also be auscultated with a stethoscope for presence and quality of breath sounds. The flat diaphragm of the stethoscope is held firmly against the patient's anterior chest wall and the examiner listens throughout the thorax, from side to side, comparing breath sounds. Auscultation is reliable to determine the presence of fluid, mucus, or obstruction within the respiratory tract.[25,26] Breath sounds also should be auscultated posteriorly for more

detailed assessment. Breath sounds should be clear on auscultation. Abnormal sounds—muffled ones, crackling, popping, wheezing, or gurgling—indicate abnormalities and should be further evaluated for underlying causes.[5]

Heart

Physical examination of the heart, with a view to nutrition, previously began with assessment of blood pressure for hypertension or hypotension. Cardiac status affects nutrition management when fluid volume or substrate alterations such as lipid disorders are a concern. In patients with known cardiac failure, signs and symptoms of cardiac cachexia (see Chapter 30) should be assessed carefully. Cardiac cachexia results from moderate to severe heart failure. The temporal and supraclavicular areas should be inspected for both fat and muscle wasting. Also, with cardiac decompensation, inadequate circulation results in shortness of breath.[3] With practice and expertise, the clinician can learn to auscultate the heart for rate and rhythm.[22] With skill, the clinician can evaluate heart sounds (S_1 and S_2/lub-dub) along with the presence of S_3 or S_4. Inspection of any central venous access devices should be completed at this time and the appearance of the exit site noted. The catheter exit site should be free of excessive redness, swelling, and drainage.

Abdomen

The abdomen is next examined using the following sequence: inspection, auscultation, percussion, and palpation. The abdomen should be inspected for skin color, contour, scars, shape, symmetry, bulging, muscle development, position and condition of the umbilicus, and movements. For examination, the abdomen is divided into four quadrants. The examiner should be familiar with the normal anatomy of each quadrant in order to be able to identify deviations from the norm (Fig. 2-9).[27]

To inspect the contour of the abdomen, the examiner stands to the right of the patient's exposed abdomen and looks down

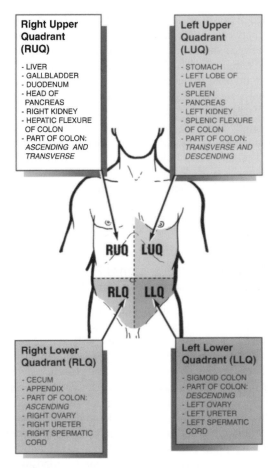

Right Upper Quadrant (RUQ)

- LIVER
- GALLBLADDER
- DUODENUM
- HEAD OF PANCREAS
- RIGHT KIDNEY
- HEPATIC FLEXURE OF COLON
- PART OF COLON: *ASCENDING AND TRANSVERSE*

Left Upper Quadrant (LUQ)

- STOMACH
- LEFT LOBE OF LIVER
- SPLEEN
- PANCREAS
- LEFT KIDNEY
- SPLENIC FLEXURE OF COLON
- PART OF COLON: *TRANSVERSE AND DESCENDING*

Right Lower Quadrant (RLQ)

- CECUM
- APPENDIX
- PART OF COLON: *ASCENDING*
- RIGHT OVARY
- RIGHT URETER
- RIGHT SPERMATIC CORD

Left Lower Quadrant (LLQ)

- SIGMOID COLON
- PART OF COLON: *DESCENDING*
- LEFT OVARY
- LEFT URETER
- LEFT SPERMATIC CORD

FIGURE 2-9 Quadrants of the abdomen.

at the abdomen; then, stooping or sitting, the examiner notes the profile from the rib margin to the pubic bone. The contour of the abdomen normally ranges from flat to rounded and assists in determining nutritional status.[5,15,16] Loss of subcutaneous fat, as with nutritional depletion, reveals a scaphoid abdomen. Gas distention and obesity make the abdomen round to protuberant with an inverted umbilicus; whereas, ascites is associated with generalized enlargement of the abdomen and

an everted umbilicus and tight, glistening skin (Fig. 2-10).[15,16] Next, the symmetry of the abdomen is noted. It should be bilaterally symmetric, without masses or bulging. The umbilicus should lie at the midline and be inverted and without signs of inflammation or discoloration. The skin is also inspected for color, warmth, and texture. The skin should be warm and dry, with good turgor.

After inspection, bowel sounds are auscultated using a stethoscope to assess peristalsis.[4] Auscultation is done second in assessing the abdomen, so as not to stimulate pressure on the bowel, which can alter motility and bowel sounds.[27,28] Using the diaphragm of the stethoscope, the examiner listens, starting at the lower right quadrant where the ileocecal valve is located, because bowel sounds are normally always present in this area. Bowel sounds are the result of the movement of air and fluid through the small intestine. If sounds are hypoactive or absent, the examiner listens for 1 or 2 minutes in each quadrant. Normal bowel sounds are high pitched and gurgling, occurring at irregular intervals anywhere from 5 to 34 times per minute. Hyperactive bowel sounds are loud and high pitched rushing or splashing.[5,22,27,28] Increased bowel sounds indicate increased motility as seen with laxatives, gastroenteritis, or a resolved ileus. Diminished bowel sounds, soft and spaced apart, are present with slowed motility, inflamed bowel or surrounding tissue, electrolyte imbalances (hypokalemia, hyponatremia), and postoperatively. The absence of bowel sounds may be indicative of possible ileus or peritonitis. High-pitched "tinkling" bowel sounds alert the examiner to fluid or air under tension and possible "early" bowel obstruction.[5,27] Light percussion can be used to assess tympany, dullness, or density of abdominal contents and liver span. Dullness is heard over solid organs and masses.[5,15,16] Tympany is usually predominant and heard over air-filled areas such as the stomach and even small bowel and colon when air is present. The gastric air bubble can be percussed at the left anterior lower rib cage. The size of the gastric air bubble depends on the time lapsed since the last feeding. Palpation is performed last, to determine the size and location of specific organs and any masses or tenderness. The examiner lightly palpates all four abdominal quadrants systematically, using circular motions of the fingertips. Deep palpation

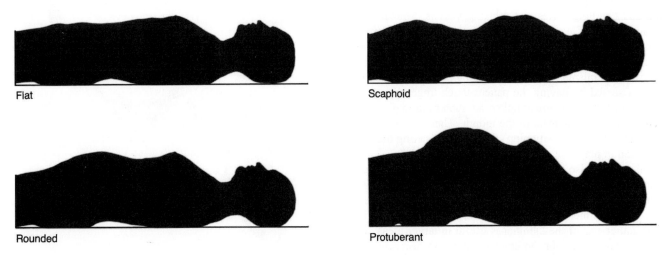

Flat

Scaphoid

Rounded

Protuberant

FIGURE 2-10 Inspection of the abdomen: contour. (From Jarvis C: *Physical examination and health assessment,* Philadelphia, 1992, WB Saunders.)

may follow. The abdomen should be free of palpable masses and tenderness. The liver can be palpated at this time if that is deemed necessary. During the abdominal assessment, ostomies and feeding devices are noted and inspected for appearance, position, and the presence of drainage, inflammation, or tenderness. Of course, if the patient complains of pain, clinical judgment should be used in performing these techniques.

Renal

With advanced practice, assessment of the renal and urinary system can be completed in conjunction with assessment of the abdomen. The flank regions are assessed for symmetry, color, pain, or discomfort. The kidneys are not usually palpable.[5] For metabolic and nutritional assessment, it is important to note urine color and turbidity, which reflects the patient's fluid status. Normal urine is amber-yellow and clear. In states of dehydration, urine output is small and the urine can be dark and concentrated.

Musculoskeletal

The musculoskeletal system is inspected and palpated next. General inspection of the arms and legs assesses fat stores and muscle mass. In states of nutritional depletion, fat stores are notably depleted, as is muscle mass. Prolonged bed rest also causes muscle mass wasting, evidenced in the gastrocnemius muscle in the lower leg and the deltoid muscle in the upper arm. Skinfold measurements are useful for assessing fat and muscle stores. Inspection and palpation of the arms, fingers, wrists, elbows, and shoulders are done to assess the patient's motor skills and ability to eat and manipulate eating utensils. Adaptive equipment may be needed. Inspection seeks range-of-motion impairments, swelling, arthritis, and other joint changes and deformities. Palpation for swelling, pain, and tenderness should also be completed.[5,15,16,25]

Neurologic

Neurologic assessment is important to further assess the patient's ability to perform independent eating tasks such as hand-mouth coordination, use of eating utensils to pick up food, and handling plates and drinking vessels. Mental alertness and signs of dementia or behavior disturbances can be noted during general conversation and by the patient's appropriate answers to questions. Motor status can be assessed by gait. Any generalized weakness should be noted. Coordination can be assessed by having the patient touch finger to nose or having him or her perform simple tasks such as preparing food and raising eating utensils to the mouth. These are important considerations for "transitioning" the patient to taking foods by mouth and in preparing him or her for discharge.[15,16]

Reflexes are also tested to seek central nervous system disturbances. A reflex hammer is used to assess reflexes. The pointed end of the hammer is used to strike small areas, as when the examiner's finger overlies the biceps tendon. The larger, flatter end of the hammer is useful in larger areas such as the patellar tendon or the brachioradialis, to decrease pain. To elicit a deep tendon response, the limb must be relaxed and

positioned properly and symmetrically. The examiner holds the hammer between thumb and index finger, allowing it to swing freely between the palm and other fingers. Moving from the wrist, the hammer is struck briskly on the tendon.

Reflexes tested include the biceps, triceps, brachioradialis, abdominal, patellar, ankle, and plantar responses.[5] The patellar tendon is usually easily accessible for testing. The lower legs should dangle freely to flex the knee and stretch the tendons. Next, the tendon is struck below the patella. The knee should extend. The reflexes should be compared symmetrically. The reflex response is graded on a scale from 0 to 4, where 0 indicates no reflex, 2+ indicates average to normal response, and 4+ indicates hyperactivity (Figs. 2-11 to 2-15).[16] See Table 2-3 for specific nutrient deficiencies revealed by the physical examination.

Considerations for Nutritional Physical Assessment of Elderly Persons

Physical examination of elderly patients may require special adaptations because of associated changes in physiologic function, nutritional status, and dietary intake.[30] Age-related changes in the gastrointestinal tract include altered swallowing coordination, a reduction in the capacity to secrete hydrochloric acid in the stomach (results in a decreased absorption of vitamin B_{12} and folic acid), reduction in motility, and a reduction in hepatic blood flow. Caution should be used when examining the abdomen because the liver is easily palpated with increased size, and pain reception within the abdominal wall may also be diminished.[6] Changes in body composition compartments between fat and muscle occur (see Chapter 3). Age-related changes affect kidney function and endocrine function (see Chapter 28). Changes in musculoskeletal system affect functional status on a daily basis. Changes in mental capacity

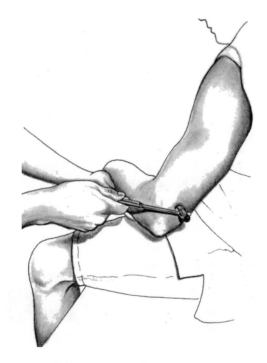

FIGURE 2-11 Eliciting the triceps reflex.

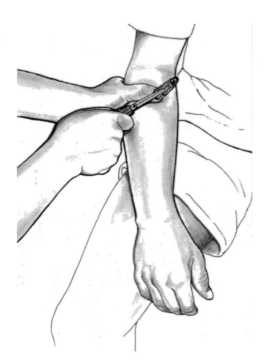

FIGURE 2-12 Eliciting the brachioradialis reflex.

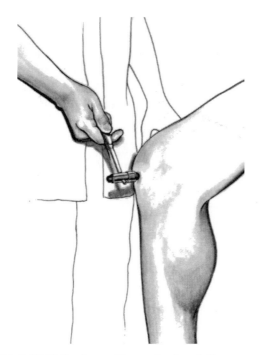

FIGURE 2-13 Eliciting the quadriceps reflex (knee jerk).

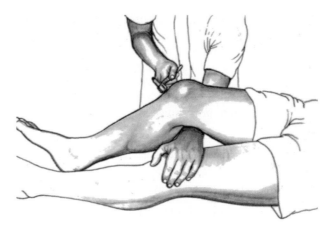

FIGURE 2-14 Eliciting the quadriceps reflex (supine position).

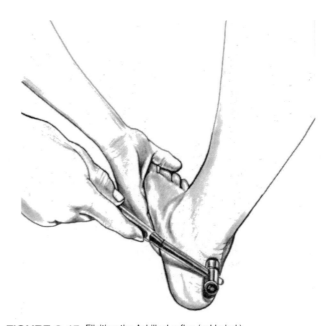

FIGURE 2-15 Eliciting the Achilles' reflex (ankle jerk).

may also be evident.[31] In conducting the nutrition history, the accuracy is of concern because of declining memory or the reluctance to provide information.[32] In general, a quiet environment should be provided.

The patient must be kept warm because subcutaneous fat decreases with age. Because the elderly patient often lacks fat and muscle reserves, careful examination for any underlying chronic disease or injury must take place. As much of the examination as possible should be performed with the patient in one position because physical limitations such as limited range of motion of the extremities, decreased reflexes, and decreased sense of balance can make it difficult for the patient to assume different positions. An elderly person's skin should be handled with much care because fragile skin and loss of subcutaneous tissue place him or her at risk for skin breakdown.[6] The anteroposterior diameter of the chest wall may be increased indicating chronic obstructive lung disease. In many cases, this condition causes a tendency to tire out easily with large meals.[32] Digestive functions such as intestinal motility can also diminish with inactivity, decreased fluid intake, or limited intake of a wide variety of foods.[6, 32]

Summary

The nutrition history and physical examination provides much valuable information when assessing nutritional status. The initial interview and physical examination call for hands-on skills and contact with the patient that cannot be reproduced in figures from laboratory tests. One must remember that it takes much skill and practice to become proficient in physical examination techniques. The more practice one receives, the more comfortable and proficient he or she becomes. Reviewing competency standards along with standards of practice can assist the nutrition practitioner performing various skill sets.[34,35]

REFERENCES

1. American Dietetic Association: ADA's definitions for nutrition screening and nutritional assessment, *J Am Diet Assoc* 94(8):838-839, 1994.
2. Butterworth CE, Blackburn GL: Hospital malnutrition, *Nutr Today* March/April:8-18, 1975.
3. Hammond KA: Dietary and clinical assessment. In Mahan LK, Stump-Escott S (eds): *Krause's food, nutrition and diet therapy,* ed 10, Philadelphia, 2000, WB Saunders, pp 353-379.
4. Poncar PJ: Who has time for a head to toe assessment? *Nursing* 25(3):59, 1995.
5. Bates B, Bickley LS, Hoekelman RA (eds): *A guide to physical examination and history taking,* ed 6, Philadelphia, 1995, JB Lippincott.
6. McCash K: Health history and physical examination. In Lewis SM, Collier IC, Heitkemper MM (eds): *Medical-surgical nursing,* ed 5, St Louis, 1999, Mosby, pp 66-78.
7. Herbert J: Health history and physical assessment. In Bauxbaum BS, Mauro E, Norris CG (eds): *Illustrated manual of nursing practice,* ed 2, Springhouse, PA, 1994, Springhouse.
8. Hammond KA: Physical assessment: a nutritional perspective, *Nurs Clin North Am* 32(4):779-790, 1997.
9. Owen G: Physical examination as an assessment tool. In Simko MD, Cowell C, Gilbride JA (eds): *Nutrition assessment,* ed 2, Gaithersburg, MD, 1995, ASPEN.
10. Hodge P, Ullrich S: Does your assessment include alternative therapies? *RN* 62(6):47-49, 1999.
11. ASPEN Board of Directors: Standards for home nutrition support, *Nutrition in Clinical Practice* 14(3):151-161, 1999.
12. ASPEN Board of Directors: Guidelines for the use of parenteral and enteral nutrition in adult and pediatric patients, *J Parenter Enteral Nutr* 26(11): 1SA-138SA, 2002.
13. ASPEN Board of Directors: *Clinical pathways and algorithms for delivery of parenteral and enteral nutrition support in adults,* Silver Spring, MD, 1998, American Society for Parenteral and Enteral Nutrition.
14. Shopbell JM, Hopkins B, Shronts E: Nutrition screening and assessment. In Gottschlich MM (chief ed): *The science and practice of nutrition support: a case based core curriculum,* 2001, American Society for Parenteral and Enteral Nutrition, Dubuque, IA Kendall/Hunt Publishing, pp 107-140.
15. Fuller J, Schaller-Ayers J (eds): *Health assessment: a nursing approach,* ed 2, Philadelphia, 1994, JB Lippincott, pp 115-184.
16. Jarvis C: *Physical examination and health assessment,* Philadelphia, 1992, WB Saunders.
17. Weinsier RI, Morgan SL (eds): *Fundamentals of clinical nutrition,* St Louis, 1993, Mosby.
18. Hammond KA: The nutritional dimension of physical assessment, *Nutrition* 15(5):411-419, 1999.
19. Jeejeebhoy KN: Nutritional assessment, *Gastroenterol Clin North Am* 27(2):348-369, 1998.
20. Konstantinides NN: Nutritional care. In Bauxbaum BS, Mauro E, Norris CG (eds): *Illustrated manual of nursing practice,* ed 2, Springhouse, PA, 1994, Springhouse.
21. Talbot L, Curtis L: The challenges of assessing skin indicators in people of color, *Home Healthcare Nurse* 14(3):167-173, 1996.
22. Hargrove-Huttel RA: Nursing health assessment. In *Lippincott's medical-surgical nursing,* ed 3, Philadelphia, 2001, Lippincott.
23. Braden B: Using the Braden scale for predicting pressure sore risk, *Support Line* 18(4):14-17, 1996.
24. Grant A, DeHoog S: *Nutrition assessment and support,* Seattle, WA, 1991, Northgate Station.
25. O'Hanlon-Nichols T: The adult pulmonary system, *Am J Nurs* 98(2):39-45, 1998.
26. Murphy LM, Bickford V: Physical assessment of the cardiopulmonary system: nutritional implications, *Support Line* 19(2):8-11, 1997.
27. Goff K: Assessment of the gastrointestinal tract, *Support Line* 19(2):3-7, 1997.
28. Langan JC: Abdominal assessment in the home: from A to Z, *Home Health Care Nurse* 16(1):50-57, 1998.
29. Neal L: Basic musculoskeletal assessment, *Home Health Care Nurse* 15(4):227-233, 1997.
30. Rush D: Nutrition screening in old people: its place in a coherent practice of preventive health care, *Annu Rev Nutr* 17:101-125, 1997.
31. Simon LJ, Russell C: Impact of the physiologic changes associated with aging on nutrition assessment, *Support Line* 20(3):3-7, 1998.
32. Barrocas A, Belcher D, Champagne C, et al: Nutrition assessment: practical approaches, *Clin Geriatric Med* 11(4):675-713, 1995.
33. Plummer E: Trauma in the elderly, *Advance for Nurses* 2(21):22-23, 2000.
34. ASPEN Board of Directors: Interdisciplinary nutrition support core competencies, *Nutrition in Clinical Practice* 14(6):331-333, 1999.
35. ASPEN Board of Directors: Standards of practice for nutrition support dietitians, *Nutrition in Clinical Practice* 15(1):53, 2000.

Anthropometry and Body Composition Analysis

3

Wanda Hain Howell, PhD, RD, CNSD

Body Composition and Nutrition Care

The provision of nutrition care requires the integration of data on diet and/or nutrient intake, clinical and metabolic status, and body weight and composition. Several approaches are necessary because alterations in nutritional status occur through a series of successive steps.[1] Inadequate or excessive intake, possibly combined with increased needs, leads to metabolic alterations reflected in biochemical changes, which in turn are expressed in altered body composition parameters. Eventually, clinical signs and symptoms develop that are associated with increased risk of morbidity and mortality.

The evaluation of nutrient intake and clinical and metabolic status are described elsewhere in this volume. The focus of this chapter is the application of body weight and composition to the assessment, planning, implementation, and monitoring of nutrition care. Specifically, body composition analysis aids nutrition care by enabling the nutrition support team:

- To identify nutrition risk associated with inadequate or excessive levels of total or regional body composition compartments (fat, protein, bone, and water)
- To design care plans based on appropriate levels of body weight and body compartment size
- To monitor changes in body weight and composition that are associated with alterations in physiologic states
- To monitor growth, development, and age-related changes in body composition
- To evaluate the effectiveness of nutrition interventions in improving body composition

Principles of Body Composition in Health and Disease

The term *body composition* refers to the distribution and size of the components of total body weight. Traditionally, research in this area has been based on the two-compartment model of body composition defined as

$$Bwt = FM + FFM$$

where *Bwt* is total body weight, *FM* is fat mass, and *FFM* is fat-free body mass.[2-4] More recently, as a result of new techniques (e.g., dual-energy x-ray absorptiometry and neutron activation analysis), investigators have favored multicompartment models because of their improved accuracy and wider applicability. The most general of these models, outlined in Table 3-1, partitions FFM into total body water (*TBW*), osseous mineral (*Mo*),

TABLE 3-1

General Multicompartment Body Composition Model*

Compartment	Amount (kg)	% Body Weight
Water	42	60
Extracellular	18	26
Intracellular	24	34
Fat (nonessential)	12	17
Protein	10.6	15
Bone mineral (osseous)	3.7	5.3

Adapted from Wang ZM, Pierson RN Jr, Heymsfield SB: The five-level model: a new approach to organizing body-composition research, *Am J Clin Nutr* 56:20, 1992.
*Reference man, 70 kg, 20-30 years old.

and protein (*P*) compartments. Total body weight is thus defined as

$$Bwt = FM + TBW + Mo + P$$

In healthy adults, body composition is relatively stable, which allows for the extrapolation of certain body compartment measurements from the direct measurement of others. For example, the hydrodensitometric two-compartment model of body composition defines body weight as the sum of FM and FFM and is based on the assumption that the density of FFM is constant and universal. These assumptions, however, may not be valid in certain states of health and disease. Research suggests that blacks and Hispanics have higher bone mineral mass and bone density than whites.[5-7] The result of using the two-compartment model in these groups would be to underestimate body fat. In contrast, children have relatively little mineral and more body water than adults.[8] The body density of elderly persons is also less than that of "reference man" owing to lower bone mineral content.[9] Thus, the relative body fat of children and elders is overestimated by the traditional two-compartment model.

Multicompartment models accommodate differences in the water, mineral, and protein content of FFM that are associated with ethnicity, gender, age, and pathologic states. The choice among various multicompartment models is based on which compartments are of primary interest. Nutrition care professionals are often concerned about metabolically active compartments and fluid status. Fluid status can be addressed by further subdividing total body water into extracellular and intracellular compartments. The partitioning of FFM into inactive extracellular mass (ECM), which is composed of extracellular solids (ECS) and extracellular fluid (ECF), and metabolically active body cell mass (BCM) allows a focus on BCM. This multicompartment model can be presented as:

$$Bwt = FM + BCM + ECS + ECF$$

The relative size and distribution of these compartments vary in states of disease compared with states of health. In a healthy person, BCM and ECM are roughly equivalent in size, each accounting for some 35% to 40% of total body weight.[10] The FM contributes the residual 20% to 25% of total body weight. Comparatively, obese individuals have increased FM and ECM (including extracellular water [ECW]), and reduced BCM, intracellular water (ICW), and TBW. Catabolic, malnourished patients commonly have reduced total body weight, FM, BCM, and ICW and an expanded ECM compartment (including ECW). Volume-expanded patients present with increased ECW that is reflected in increased TBW and total body weight. These patients' cardiac, renal, and pulmonary systems are stressed by the circulatory overload. Conversely, volume-depleted patients present with reductions in body weight and in all fluid compartments (TBW, ICW, and ECW). Organ systems may be threatened by reduced blood flow.

Use of appropriate techniques to assess these alterations in body composition, to design intervention strategies to correct them, and to evaluate improved response to therapy is desirable for provision of optimal nutrition care. The following review of available techniques for assessing body composition focuses on their indications for use, their limitations, and their applicability in the clinical setting.

Laboratory Methods of Determining Body Composition

Hydrodensitometry

Hydrodensitometry (underwater weighing) is the foundation of the traditional two-compartment model of body composition. This method measures body volume (density) and relies on the assumption that the density of FM and the components of FFM (water, mineral, and protein) are constant and universal and that individuals differ from the reference values only in their amount of fat, while their FFM is assumed to be 73.8% water, 19.4% protein, and 6.8% mineral.[3]

Using these assumptions, two equations are commonly employed to convert body density (Db) from hydrostatic weighing into percentage of body fat (%BF):

Siri[11]   %BF = (4.95/Db) − 4.50
Brozek[3]   %BF = (4.57/Db) − 4.142

The %BF can then be expressed as FM (kg) divided by total body weight (kg). Based on the two-compartment model, FFM (kg) is the difference between total body weight and FM.

The procedure used most widely to determine body density involves measurements of mass with the body submersed in water and in air. The difference between the two values is the *apparent body volume* or density. Correction must be made, however, for residual lung volume, which can be as high as 1 to 2 L. This may be accomplished by the open-circuit approach with a spirometer and a nitrogen analyzer, allowing for the measurement of nitrogen washout of the lungs simultaneously with the underwater weighing.[12] Alternatively the closed-circuit oxygen dilution technique involves having the subject breathe in and out of a spirometer filled with a known volume and concentration of oxygen until the nitrogen concentration in the lungs and in the spirometer has equilibrated.[13] This approach has the advantage of more rapid measurements. A small correction (100 ml) for gastrointestinal gas volume is also made.

Hydrodensitometry can be adapted for field use, but it has obvious limitations in the clinical setting. Because the typical procedure requires total submersion of the subject, it is not useful for sick persons or for some children and older people. Despite its limitations, hydrostatic weighing is the most widely accepted criterion or reference method by which other methods for measuring body FM are validated. The goal of much of the current research in body composition is to develop alternative methods that are as precise but more broadly applicable. One of the new techniques, dual-energy x-ray absorptiometry (DXA), shows much promise as an alternative to hydrodensitometry.

Imaging Techniques

DUAL-ENERGY X-RAY ABSORPTIOMETRY. The development of DXA proceeded from two early techniques used to measure bone mineral content and density. The principle of absorptiometry for studying bone composition is that bone mineral content is assumed to be directly proportional to the amount of photon energy absorbed by the bone.[14] The first of the traditional techniques, single-photon absorptiometry (SPA), uses iodine-125 as the photon source and measures bone mineral in the radius and ulna only.[15,16] Dual-photon absorptiometry (DPA) is a modification of SPA and uses gadolinium-153, which emits photons at two energy levels. Two energy levels eliminate the need for assuming a constant thickness of soft tissue in the scan path and allow measurement of total body bone mineral content. Refinements of the DPA technique ultimately allowed estimates of soft tissue (FM and FFM) and total body bone mineral content.[17-20]

The need for an alternative energy source (owing to the instability of gadolinium-153 over time) was a primary factor that led to the development of DXA. The use of x-rays as the photon source improved the resolution of images obtained and reduced scan time. In both the DXA and DPA systems, the photon source is mounted beneath a table on which the subject lies and is opposite a detector above the table. The source and detector are connected and thus pass across the body simultaneously.

Total and regional body composition analysis by DXA is based on the principle that when a beam of x-rays passes through the body, the beam is attenuated (reduced in intensity) in proportion to the size and composition of the individual tissue components.[21] Soft tissues (fat and bone-free, fat-free tissue) restrict the flux of x-rays less than bone. The ratio of the restriction at the low and high x-ray levels employed in DXA is a function of the proportion of fat and lean tissue.[22]

The use of x-rays as the radiation source results in lower radiation exposure (0.05 to 1.5 mrem) for DXA than for DPA (10 to 15 mrem).[22] Such low levels of radiation compare very favorably with those for conventional radiography (chest films and computed tomography [CT]), which range from 25 to 270 mrem. This feature promotes the general applicability of DXA for estimating total body composition in healthy subjects of all ages, except for pregnant women and obese or very tall persons.[23-25] Those larger than the scan area (>193 cm × 58 to 65 cm) may not be measured accurately. A novel approach to this problem that has been investigated involves scanning the right half of the body and, assuming bilateral symmetry, doubling the values to estimate total body composition.[26]

The applicability of DXA for assessing body composition in disease states has not been extensively investigated. Studies of the sensitivity of DXA to small changes in hydration levels (1 to 3 kg) support the accuracy of this technique in detecting dehydration.[27,28] Similarly, DXA was found to measure accurately the effect of removing 1 to 4 kg of fluid during hemodialysis.[29] Investigations of the sensitivity of DXA in reflecting body composition changes with weight loss have yielded conflicting results.[30-33] These inconsistent results are due, at least in part, to the use of equipment and body composition soft tissue analysis software from different manufacturers. Three types of DXA hardware are currently available: Hologic QDR, Lunar DPX, and Norland XR. Each manufacturer has developed several versions of body composition software that can yield different results.[34] Because of this disparity among software products, assessment of the validity or the accuracy of DXA estimates of soft tissue is confounded.

The most obvious limitation to routine use of DXA for soft tissue analysis is that it is not currently approved for that purpose in the United States except in research protocols. DXA is, however, used extensively for clinical evaluation and monitoring of bone mineral content and density. DXA-derived estimates of total body bone mass are also useful in the multicompartment approach to body composition assessment. With further research, it holds great promise of becoming a reference method for body composition analysis.

COMPUTED TOMOGRAPHY. The most common application of CT to body composition analysis is measurement of regional adipose tissue content. Although both DXA and CT relate differences in x-ray attenuation to differences in the density of body components, the two methods produce several differences in results. CT produces three-dimensional cross-sectional tissue analyses of targeted sites, whereas DXA produces two-dimensional regional and total body compartment analyses. Therefore, CT allows for measurement of absolute volumes rather than the proportional tissue composition produced by DXA. One reported advantage of DXA as compared with CT for body composition analysis is that DXA measures the proportion of *fat* in the scan area rather than the volume of *adipose tissue* that CT measures.[22]

The value of CT in evaluating changes in muscle and adipose tissue in malnourished persons has been demonstrated.[35] Cross-sectional differences in abdominal fat distribution during aging have also been identified with CT.[37,38] The most current area of research using CT as a criterion or reference method evaluates the role of visceral adipose tissue, specifically the mesenteric and omental adipose stores, in increasing morbidity and mortality from cardiovascular diseases and type 2 diabetes mellitus.[39]

MAGNETIC RESONANCE IMAGING. Because, in contrast to DXA and CT, magnetic resonance imaging (MRI) does not employ ionizing radiation, it has potential as one of the few noninvasive available methods for directly assessing body composition. This approach is based on the principle that body elements with isotopes containing an odd number of protons or neutrons possess magnetic properties that allow them to align with an external magnetic field applied across part of the body. In the presence of this magnetic field a radiofrequency signal is directed into the body target site, causing some nuclei to go from a low-energy state to a high-energy one and to "flip" out of alignment with the magnetic field. When the radiofrequency signal is removed, some nuclei flip back into alignment and emit the radiofrequency they had acquired. This emitted energy is characteristic of specific organic compounds that define a specific type of body tissue.[40]

Currently, for body composition purposes, MRI can image protons (hydrogen) and phosphorus-31. Consequently, it has been used to differentiate fat from tissue containing water (bone-free, fat-free body mass).[41] The principal limitation of the technique is its poor ability to detect and measure other important elements of organic compounds such as carbon and nitrogen.[25] Efforts are underway to refine the technique for this purpose.

Elemental Analysis Techniques

TOTAL BODY POTASSIUM COUNTING. Total body potassium-40 counting is a traditional method of measuring elemental potassium in the body. The procedure used most is similar to that described for DXA, except that it involves the administration of cesium-137 as the energy source and a whole-body count of the gamma rays emitted, from which attenuation factors are determined.[42]

Measured potassium values have been used to estimate FFM and FM in the traditional two-compartment model of body composition.[2,14] These estimations assume constant potassium content in FFM. This assumption reduces the applicability of this technique for estimating FFM in various states of disease. The high cost and limited availability of the equipment needed to perform total body potassium counting generally restrict its use to research.

NEUTRON ACTIVATION ANALYSIS. Direct in vivo measurement of most of the elemental composition of the body became possible with the development of neutron activation analysis (NAA). Several types of NAA systems have been designed for specific elemental analyses: inelastic neutron scattering for carbon analysis;[43] prompt-gamma-ray NAA for nitrogen;[44] and delayed-gamma-ray NAA for sodium, chlorine, calcium, and phosphorus analyses.[45] All of these systems operate using the same general principle. A moderated beam of fast neutrons is delivered to the subject. Capture of these neutrons creates unstable isotopes of the target elements. As these isotopes stabilize, they emit gamma-ray energy levels that are characteristic of the target elements. The gamma-ray energy is analyzed by standard gamma spectrographic techniques, which identify and quantify the elements.[14]

The use of NAA combined with potassium-40 analysis allows direct measurement of more than 98% of the elemental composition of the body.[46] Elemental compositions measured by these techniques are also used to validate other body composition methods. For example, NAA of elemental calcium has been used as the reference measure in studies to evaluate the accuracy of DXA in determining bone mineral content.[9]

Several factors, however, preclude the routine clinical use of these NAA methods. The high cost and limited availability of the necessary instrumentation, the need for skilled professionals to operate the equipment, and the significant levels of ionizing radiation associated with these methods limit their use to research.

Isotope Dilution Techniques

Investigators have traditionally used the isotopes of hydrogen, deuterium, and tritium, to measure TBW by isotope dilution in healthy and diseased persons. Isotope dilution is generally considered the criterion or reference method for quantifying TBW. Because tritium is a radioactive tracer, more recent studies have favored use of the stable isotope deuterium (also referred to as *heavy water* or D_2O). The refinement of infrared absorption and isotope ratio mass spectrometry assay techniques has facilitated analysis of deuterium in biologic fluids (blood, urine, saliva, and respiratory tract water).[47,48] Although use of the stable isotope tracer, oxygen-18, is reported to give the most accurate estimates of TBW, its cost is prohibitive for routine use (minimum $500 per dose versus about $7 per dose for deuterium).[14]

The basic assumptions of the method are that the isotope is distributed evenly in body water and is exchanged by the body in a manner similar to water.[49] The typical procedure for using stable isotopes for this purpose involves drinking a predetermined quantity of the tracer mixed in a known volume of water, waiting between 2 to 4 hours for the tracer to equilibrate in body fluids, and giving a sample of blood, urine, or saliva for analysis of isotope concentration. The calculation of TBW is based on the relationship:

$$C_1 V_1 = C_2 V_2$$

where C_1 is the initial concentration of the tracer in a known volume (V_1) of water, C_2 is the final concentration of the tracer in the biologic sample, with V_2 calculated as the volume of TBW.[14]

Estimation of ECW is based on the same relationship. In this case, however, sodium bromide, rather than a stable isotope, is most often used as the tracer. Sodium bromide is a water-soluble compound that enters cells in very limited amounts and so is distributed almost entirely in ECW and excreted in the urine. After the dose equilibration period, serum sodium bromide concentration is used to quantify ECW.[50,51] ICW is estimated as the difference between measured TBW and ECW.

The isotope dilution technique using deuterium as the tracer and urine sampling is clinically applicable for estimating TBW because of its noninvasive character. Analysis of isotopes in biologic fluids is, however, expensive enough to rule out routine use of the technique. In addition, the equilibration period may need to be extended to 6 to 10 hours if the patient is fluid overloaded or has reduced renal perfusion or reduced urine output. Correction for fluid taken in from enteral tube or parenteral feeding before and during the equilibration period has also been recommended.[46]

Estimating FFM and FM using the two-compartment model and direct measurement of TBW is not appropriate for patients whose hydration status is altered. This model is based on the assumption of a constant hydration factor of the FFM. This assumption is invalid for malnourished catabolic patients who have reduced FM and increased ECW. TBW measurements can appropriately be incorporated into multicompartment models in which other body and water compartments are assessed.

Field Methods for Measuring Body Composition
Anthropometric Techniques

BODY WEIGHT AND BODY MASS INDEX. Body weight alone and body weight standardized for height or body mass index (BMI) are the two nutrition assessment variables reported most frequently. Errors in the measurement and use of body weight as a clinical variable are common. Clinical decisions are often based on patients' self-reports rather than on measured weight and height. Furthermore, instruments used to measure these indices are seldom routinely calibrated. Finally, a variety of standards have been used to interpret these measurements.

Traditional reference standards include those from the World Health Organization (WHO) and the Metropolitan Life Insurance Company. The limitations associated with using these standards have been reviewed. An important one is the fact that they do not include data representative of the U.S. population.[52] In addition, the classification categories used in these standards assume the same (normal) distribution of total body weight across all age groups. This assumption is not valid for two reasons: body weight is not normally distributed within *any* age group, and the shape of the distribution of body weight varies across age groups.[36]

For these reasons and to encourage uniform use, body weight reference tables compiled by Frisancho from the first and second samples of the National Health and Nutrition Examination Surveys (NHANES), conducted during 1971 to 1974 and 1976 to 1980, are provided in the appendices at the end of this text. These tables contain the most current anthropometric data available for the noninstitutionalized U.S. population derived from a sample of 43,774 subjects (35,931 whites; 7125 blacks; and 718 others), aged 1 to 74 years. All tables report data in percentiles to appropriately accommodate "nonnormative" distributions of indices. Data from the third NHANES survey (1988 to1994) are currently being analyzed and will be used to update reference standards in the near future.[53]

Limitations associated with the use of statistically derived (population-based) desirable body weights were discussed during the recent American Health Foundation Roundtable on Healthy Weight.[54] Low reported correlations between BMI (except at the extremes) and morbidity or mortality rates were cited as a primary limitation. Acknowledging the morbidity and mortality associated with significant overweight and underweight, the participants supported the use of statistically derived standards in population screening for nutritional risk.

The outcome of this roundtable discussion was the publication of public health recommendations for a healthy-weight target, which was defined as "a reasonable upper limit for body weight that would offer a reduction in disease risk and be within reach for most overweight adults."[55] The Expert Panel on Healthy Weight arrived at a healthy weight target of a BMI below 25 for adults, which was converted to a height-weight ratio (in inches and pounds) for easy use by the general public.

Healthy-weight guidelines were not issued for children and adolescents or for persons older than 65 years. The National Center for Health Statistics (NCHS) has, however, published revised growth charts that use BMI as an indicator of over-weight in children 2 to18 years old.[56]

In addition to a healthy-weight target, a healthier-weight goal was recommended by the expert panel for those adults whose weight already exceeded the target. This healthier-weight goal defines successful weight loss as an amount that reduces disease risk rather than the amount necessary to achieve ideal body weight. The goal is equivalent to 2 BMI units, or weight loss of about 4.5 to 7.3 kg (10 to 16 lb).[55] This level of weight loss was considered achievable and maintainable. Incremental weight loss at this level was recommended only after a maintenance period of at least 6 months. Professional and public responses to these recommendations are likely to be mixed. Future research will reveal the extent to which the public and nutrition care community have embraced these new reference values for body weight and weight loss.

Faulty estimates of body weight and use of inappropriate reference standards can introduce errors throughout the nutrition care process and have promoted the use of body weight change, rather than weight alone, as the key variable in assessing nutritional risk. BMI or body weight alone lacks sensitivity in classifying nutritional risk.[57,58] Variations in one or more of the components of FFM can lead to errors in interpretation of total body weight. Dynamic changes in fluid status, muscle mass, and bone mass may not be reflected in changes in total body weight. Likewise, nutritional repletion of catabolic patients cannot be evaluated solely by monitoring changes in body weight because of altered use of nutrients during physiologic stress.

Estimates of the composition of body weight are, therefore, necessary to accurately assess and monitor nutritional status. Without direct laboratory measures of body composition, alternative indirect field methods that have been validated using laboratory techniques can be used for this purpose. It is important to remember, however, that no single type of data can be used as the sole basis for assessing or monitoring nutritional status. This is best accomplished by integrating body composition data with those from evaluation of nutrient intake, clinical and medical status, family, social and medical history, and biochemical profiles. The anthropometric methods used most widely to assess the composition of total body weight are described in the following sections.

SKINFOLD MEASUREMENTS. Skinfold measurements, particularly of the triceps area, have been used in the clinical setting to estimate energy reserves in subcutaneous tissue. The use of the skinfold technique can appropriately be applied in nutrition screening protocols to assign patients to categories of relative risk on this variable. Combined measurements of triceps skinfold and mid-upper arm circumference have also been applied successfully to classify patients according to relative estimates of arm muscle and fat areas (Box 3-1). Classification of nutritional risk based on these parameters requires reference data that are not available for elders or ethnic minorities. This use of skinfold measurements and arm circumferences in these population groups is problematic. In addition, the validity of these measurements for estimating body composition in very obese

and heavily muscled subjects is questionable because of the technical difficulties of performing the measurements.[59]

Skinfold measurements may be useful for assessing long-term change in subcutaneous adipose tissue stores and derived muscle area in patients who have chronic conditions or are being renourished by enteral or parenteral support over months or years (e.g., patients with acquired immunodeficiency syndrome [AIDS] or short-bowel syndrome). The assessment of short-term changes in body composition, particularly in acutely stressed patients, cannot, however, be made with confidence. This limitation in the skinfold method is related to basic assumptions implicit in its application, which are violated in both healthy and diseased persons. All persons exhibit short-term hydration-related body tissue variations. These fluid shifts are pronounced with medical conditions such as congestive heart failure and liver or kidney disease. In addition, errors in estimating muscle area from triceps skinfold and arm circumference measurements can be introduced by rapid changes in muscle glycogen stores or variations in the level of fat or the presence of edema in muscle tissue.[35]

A related limitation of the skinfold method is its inability to assess absolute amounts of adipose tissue or body protein stores. Equations used to predict FM (or %BF) and FFM from skinfold measurements in healthy populations are not valid in diseased populations.[60] In theory, disease-specific equations could be developed using a reference method such as DXA, but it would be difficult to obtain large enough study samples whose duration and severity of disease and treatment modality are comparable.

Another factor that may compromise the accuracy of skinfold measurements is observer error. This error can be introduced when all measurements are taken by the same person or when different observers take measurements. Intraobserver error can be reduced by extensive training and practice. Interobserver error depends on what site is being measured (the triceps site has about 3.0% interobserver error)[61] and what procedure is followed to perform the measurement. The Anthropometric Standardization Reference Manual was developed from the Arlie Consensus Conference to provide detailed, standardized descriptions for the identification and measurement of sites commonly used in anthropometry.[62] The ultimate goal in producing this manual was to encourage use of uniform procedures in body composition studies. These procedures have, appropriately, been adopted for use in the third NHANES survey.

Differences in the type of calipers used and their calibration can also introduce intraobserver and interobserver error. Both metal and plastic calipers should be calibrated routinely using Vermier calipers or calibration blocks.[63] Metal calipers should be recalibrated according to manufacturer's instructions, or the calipers should be returned for recalibration. Differences between brands of calipers have been documented. Harpenden calipers routinely produce significantly smaller values than do Lange calipers, probably because their greater jaw force increases compression at the site.[64] In the hands of well-trained and experienced observers, no significant differences have been shown between measurements made with plastic and with metal calipers.[61,65,66] It is important to emphasize that observers in these studies were very well-trained and experienced anthropometrists. An extensive list of sources for body composition equipment and contact information has been published.[63]

BOX 3-1

Clinical Insight: Anthropometric Parameters

MEASUREMENT PROCEDURES

Mid-Upper Arm Circumference (AC)

1. Keeping the subject's right arm parallel to the body, bend the elbow 90 degrees.
2. Using either a metallic tape or an insert tape, measure the distance between the acromion (the bony protrusion on the back of the upper shoulder) and the olecranon process (tip) of the elbow. If an insert tape is used, the same number should appear at the top of the shoulder and the elbow, and the midpoint is given by the mark on the tape.
3. Mark the midpoint between these two landmarks.
4. Ask the subject to relax the arm, so it hangs loose and parallel to the body.
5. Position the metric tape around the upper arm at the marked midpoint. Make sure that the tape is snug but not so tight as to indent or pinch the skin.
6. Record the AC to the nearest 0.1 cm.

Triceps Skinfold Thickness (TSF)

1. Locate the previously marked midpoint on the posterior or back side of the right upper arm.
2. With the subject's arm hanging loosely at the side, palpate the measurement site at the midpoint to become familiar with distinguishing muscle from adipose soft tissue.
3. From 1 cm above the midpoint, grasp a vertical pinch of skin and only the subcutaneous fat layer between the thumb and index finger. The skinfold should be gently pulled away from the underlying muscle.
4. Place the skinfold calipers at the midpoint and release the jaw pressure slowly while maintaining a grasp of the skinfold. Three readings should be taken in quick succession, and the average of the three recorded to the nearest 0.1 mm. Each reading should be taken as soon as the jaws of the caliper come into contact with the skin after the pressure is completely released and the dial reading has stabilized (about 4 seconds).

COMPUTATION OF DERIVED ANTHROPOMETRIC PARAMETERS

Calculations of mid-upper arm fat area (AFA) and arm muscle area (AMA) are based on measurements of AC and TSF. Equations for estimating AMA corrected for bone area are presented because they provide more accurate assessments of bone-free muscle area.[35] The computational steps are outlined below. These examples assume that AC is 30 cm and TSF is 25 mm (2.5 cm). (It is essential to convert TSF to centimeters for the following computations.)

1. Determine total upper arm area (TAA):

$$TAA\ (cm^2) = AC^2/4 \times \pi$$

$$TAA = 30^2/12.57 = 71.6\ cm^2$$

2. Determine uncorrected AMA:

$$AMA\ (cm^2) = [AC-(TSF \times \pi)]^2/4 \times \pi$$

$$AMA = [30-(2.5 \times 3.1416)]^2/12.57$$

$$AMA = 490.44/12.57$$

$$AMA = 39\ cm^2$$

3. Determine corrected AMA (AMA_c):

$$Males = AMA_c - 10\ cm^2 = 29.0\ cm^2$$

$$Females = AMA_c - 6.5\ cm^2 = 32.5\ cm^2$$

4. Determine AFA as the difference between TAA and *uncorrected* AMA:

$$AFA\ (cm^2) = TAA - AMA$$

$$AFA = 71.6 - 39.0 = 32.6\ cm^2$$

Note: Arm fat index (AFI) or percent fat area (%FA) can be determined as follows:

$$AFI\ or\ \%FA = (AFA/TAA) \times 100$$

$$AFI\ or\ \%FA = (32.6/71.6) \times 100 = 45.5\%$$

INTERPRETATION OF ANTHROPOMETRIC PARAMETERS

Comparing the percentile ranking of a specific individual on the various anthropometric measurements with a classification scheme is the basis for interpreting these values. Reference data in percentiles for TSF, AMA, and AFA appear in the appendices. Because the reference data are those compiled by Frisancho from the NHANES I and II data, it is appropriate to use the classification categories derived statistically from these data.[36] The table below displays the percentile categories and their interpretation for arm muscle and arm fat areas as well as total body weight.

Percentile Rank	AMA	AFA	Total Body Weight
<5	Muscle deficit	Fat deficit	Total body wasting
5.1-15	Below average	Below average	Below average
15.1-85	Average	Average	Average
>85	Above average musculature	Excess fat	Excess total body weight

To reduce these errors, it is recommended that repeated skinfold measurements be performed by a single, well-trained observer who always uses the same equipment and standardized methods. Furthermore to reduce errors associated with fluctuations in ECW, it is recommended that measurements be taken in the morning on fasted subjects after they have voided and that no measurements be taken in women the week before or during a menstrual period.[67]

The standardized procedures developed at the Arlie Consensus Conference are recommended because they are the procedures used to collect reference data for the NHANES surveys. The procedures for measuring standing mid-upper arm circumference and triceps skinfold thickness are outlined in Box 3-1. Reference data for comparison appear in the appendices.

Measurements for recumbent bedridden or wheelchair-bound subjects follow the same general procedure but require the subject to lie on the left side. Reference data for interpretation of recumbent anthropometric measurements are limited to a small nonrepresentative sample of white men and women aged 65 to 90 years.[68]

BODY BREADTHS AND CIRCUMFERENCES. Total body weight varies not only with gender and age, but also with body dimensions. Body lengths are determined by measuring recumbent length in infants and children up to 3 years and stature in those older than 3 years. Skeletal dimensions provide information on frame size, which is necessary for accurate interpretation of weight and muscle area measurements.

Elbow breadth and wrist circumference have been used to determine frame size because these measurements are affected less by adipose tissue than are shoulder and hip measurements.[69,70] Elbow breadth is generally considered more accurate and is the variable used to determine frame size in the NHANES surveys. Box 3-2 explains procedures for frame size measurement and interpretation.

Abdominal circumference is preferred to skinfold thicknesses in obese subjects because of the technical problems associated with taking skinfold measurements for them. Percentage of body fat-prediction equations developed for women use abdominal circumference, height, and weight as predictors, and those for men use abdominal circumference and body weight as predictors.[71,72]

The waist-hip circumference ratio (WHR) has been used to assess distribution of adipose tissue. Determination of this ratio is problematic in very obese persons because they lack a definable waist and the iliac crest landmarks are inaccessible.

BOX 3-2

Clinical Insight: Frame Size

MEASUREMENT PROCEDURE

Elbow breadth is most accurately measured using either sliding or spreading calipers and the following procedure:[36]
1. Raise the subject's right arm so that the forearm is parallel to the body and flexed to a 90-degree angle.
2. Facing the subject, palpate the lateral and medial epicondyles of the humerus (the two prominent bones on either side of the elbow) and place the caliper jaws parallel or slightly at a slant to these two sites.
3. Measure the greatest bony width across the elbow joint twice to the nearest 0.1 cm; take the average of the two measurements.

Note: If sliding calipers are not available, elbow breadth can be estimated by placing the thumb and index finger of one hand parallel to the body on the epicondyles. The distance between the tips of the thumb and index finger is measured as the elbow breadth.

MEASUREMENT INTERPRETATION

The National Health and Nutrition Examination Survey (NHANES) classification of frame size as small, medium, or large is based on the Frame Index 2 value, which is derived thus:

$$\text{Frame index 2} = \text{elbow breadth (mm)/stature (cm)} \times 100$$

This index accommodates age-related changes in weight and stature. The computation is made after converting the units of elbow breadth from centimeters to millimeters (by multiplying by 10). The derived Frame Index 2 is compared with the reference values for small, medium, and large frames, as defined below for the appropriate age and gender of the subject.

Age (yrs)	Male			Female		
	Small	**Medium**	**Large**	**Small**	**Medium**	**Large**
18.0-24.9	<38.4	38.4 to 41.6	>41.6	<35.2	35.2 to 38.6	>38.6
25.0-29.9	<38.6	38.6 to 41.8	>41.8	<35.7	35.7 to 38.7	>38.7
30.0-34.9	<38.6	38.6 to 42.1	>42.1	<35.7	35.7 to 39.0	>39.0
35.0-39.9	<39.1	39.1 to 42.4	>42.4	<36.2	36.2 to 39.8	>39.8
40.0-44.9	<39.3	39.3 to 42.5	>42.5	<36.7	36.7 to 40.2	>40.2
45.0-49.9	<39.6	39.6 to 43.0	>43.0	<37.2	37.2 to 40.7	>40.7
50.0-54.9	<39.9	39.9 to 43.3	>43.3	<37.2	37.2 to 41.6	>41.6
55.0-59.9	<40.2	40.2 to 43.8	>43.8	<37.8	37.8 to 41.9	>41.9
60.0-64.9	<40.2	40.2 to 43.6	>43.6	<38.2	38.2 to 41.8	>41.8
65.0-69.9	<40.2	40.2 to 43.6	>43.6	<38.2	38.2 to 41.8	>41.8
70.0-74.9	<40.2	40.2 to 43.6	>43.6	<38.2	38.2 to 41.8	>41.8

Adapted from Frisancho AR: *Anthropometric standards for the assessment of growth and nutritional status,* Ann Arbor, MI, 1990, The University of Michigan Press, p 28.

The WHR has been reported to be strongly associated with visceral fat, although waist circumference alone may be a better predictor of visceral fat deposition than WHR.[73-75] The significance of level of visceral (omental and mesenteric) adipose tissue is its reported relationship to higher risk for chronic diseases. In response to the evidence supporting waist circumference as a predictor of morbidity and mortality from chronic disease, WHO has published a waist circumference scale to classify overweight and obesity.[76] This association is hypothesized to be secondary to the mobilization of large amounts of free fatty acids from these adipose depots directly into the liver, thus promoting the altered metabolism often associated with coronary artery disease and type 2 diabetes mellitus.[77]

SPECIAL ANTHROPOMETRIC CONSIDERATIONS

Height or Stature. When stature cannot be measured because of the patients' inability to stand or to excessive spinal curvature, knee height is an appropriate alternative parameter.[68] Knee height is measured most accurately on the left side with large sliding calipers while the subject lies supine with the knee and ankle flexed to 90 degrees. The fixed blade of the caliper is placed under the heel and the other blade on the anterior surface of the thigh just proximal to the patella. The shaft of the calipers is held parallel to the shaft of the tibia, and pressure is applied to compress the tissue.[36] Two measurements are recorded to the nearest 0.1 cm. The average of the two measurements is converted to full stature using the following equations:[78]

Males	64.19–(0.04 × age) + (0.02 × knee ht)
Females	84.88–(0.24 × age) + (1.83 × knee ht)

An alternative measure of stature for persons with spine anomalies is arm span.[79] Arm span can be measured with the subject standing or lying supine and requires free extension of the arms. Anthropometers provide the most accurate measurements, although a nonflexible tape estimate can be made. For bedridden patients, the fixed end of the anthropometer or tape is placed at the tip of one middle finger (not the fingernail) and the moveable end at the other, passing over the clavicles.[80] In young middle-aged adults, arm span is equivalent to stature. For elderly persons it provides an estimate of maximum stature at maturity, before age-related bone loss occurred.

Weight. Adjustments in total body weight for amputations are generally estimated using figures published for percentage of total body weight of individual body parts. The percentage adjustments for the most common amputations are listed below:[81]

Hand	0.8%	Foot	1.8%
Forearm and hand	3.1%	Lower leg and foot	7.1%
Entire arm	6.5%	Entire leg	18.6%

Weight measurements of nonambulatory subjects require a wheelchair balance beam or electronic scale or a bed scale. Detailed procedures for the use of the Scale-Tronix Lift Bed Scale have been published.[82] All institutional healthcare facilities should be equipped with portable wheelchair and bed scales.

Bioelectrical Impedance Analysis

Bioelectrical impedance analysis (BIA) is considered a precise, rapid, safe, noninvasive, and portable method of assessing body composition. As such, it warrants increased consideration for use in the clinical setting. Compared with skinfold measurements as a field method, it has a similar level (less than 1% difference) of relative predictive accuracy in estimating FFM but has the advantage of requiring less training and experience to take accurate measurements.[83] Bioimpedance analyzers are, however, more expensive than skinfold calipers (ranging from about $4000 to $7000), but considerably less so than equipment used in the laboratory methods to assess body composition.

One advantage of the skinfold technique is the availability of reference data from large population studies that provide standards for interpreting measurements. Although many research studies have employed BIA technology to assess body composition, there is considerable diversity in characteristics of the study samples, in equipment, in measurement procedures, and in equations used to predict body composition parameters. The lack of comparability of currently available research data is a serious limitation to establishing the general validity of the technique.

The limitation of scarce BIA reference data will be alleviated, in part, when the NHANES III BIA data become available. This survey was the first of the NHANES to incorporate BIA in the data collection protocol. Organization and analysis of these data have been ongoing since collection ended in 1994. More extensive information than ever before will be available on body composition of a large, representative sample, using standardized BIA procedures and equipment.

BASIC PRINCIPLES. Single-frequency total body BIA involves the introduction of a small (less than 1 mA) alternating electrical current to the body at a frequency of 50 kHz and measurement of the differential opposition (impedance) of body tissues to its flow. Tissues that contain little water and electrolytes, such as fat and bone, are poor conductors and have great resistance to the flow of the current. Biologic tissues such as blood, viscera, organs, and muscle are good conductors because of their high fluid and electrolyte content. Heavily muscled persons have lower impedance measurements than persons with much adipose tissue. Impedance to the flow of electrical current is a function of resistance (opposition of the extracellular body mass to the current flow) and reactance (the additional opposition due to the capacitance of cell membranes and tissue interfaces or of intracellular mass [BCM]).

Estimates of body composition using BIA are based on the principle that impedance to current flow through the body is directly related to the length of the body (stature) and inversely related to its cross-sectional area. Mathematically expressed in terms of body volume rather than cross-sectional area, the equation $V = \rho S^2/Z$ is derived, where V is volume of conductive tissues (TBW or FFM), ρ is the resistance to the flow of current per unit of length of the conductor (assumed to be constant), S is stature, and Z is impedance. Thus, the volume of TBW or FFM is related directly to body stature and inversely to impedance. The contribution of resistance to impedance is much greater than that of reactance, so the previous equation can be rewritten as $V = \rho S^2 R$, where R is whole body resistance.[14]

This equation is based on the assumptions that the conductor has a homogeneous composition, a fixed cross-sectional area, and a uniform density distribution. These assumptions are not valid in the human body, particularly in association with disease. The cross-sectional area of the body is not constant, stature is not the actual length of the conductor, and the specific resistivity (ρ) varies with the amounts and distribution of body tissues and fluids. Nevertheless, statistical associations have been established between S^2/R and TBW or FFM in diverse samples of children and adults.

Bioelectrical Impedance Analysis Prediction Equations

Population-specific and generalized equations have been derived for the prediction of body composition parameters from BIA data. Most of the population-specific equations predict TBW or FFM from S^2/R alone, S^2/R plus body weight or S plus R plus weight. These equations can be applied only to subjects whose characteristics are similar to those of the population subgroup for which they were validated. Age-specific,[84] race-specific,[85,86] weight-specific,[87,88] and physical activity-specific[89] equations have been validated. Generalized BIA prediction equations commonly include factors such as age, weight, and gender as predictors and have been validated on more diverse populations.[90-94] These generalized equations are therefore often less accurate in their prediction of TBW or FFM than are the population-specific equations. A comprehensive list of BIA equations was recently published.[95]

Like skinfold equations, BIA equations must be validated using a direct measure of TBW (usually by isotope dilution) and FM (usually by hydrodensitometry or DXA). Most of the published equations have been validated using the two-compartment model of body composition. As discussed previously, this model is based on the faulty assumption that FFM always consists of 73.82% water. Estimates of FFM are based on this ratio and on direct measurement of TBW by isotope dilution. The extent to which a person's FFM does not consist of 73.82% water is directly related to the size of errors in the estimation of that person's FM and FFM. Only a few BIA equations have been validated using a multicomponent model to derive more accurate estimates of FFM or FM.[84,86,96-98]

Assessment of the ability of BIA to determine changes in body composition is particularly important in judging its applicability for clinical use. The accuracy of BIA for determining changes in TBW before and after dialysis has been evaluated. BIA-derived TBW change was found to be correlated very highly with volume of fluid removed during dialysis,[99] but less strongly with changes in total body weight before and after dialysis.[100] Compared with hydrodensitometry, BIA was found to underestimate short-term changes in FFM resulting from 2 days of hypocaloric feeding.[101] In contrast, BIA accurately predicted TBW change after a 2-week fast, and after 7 to 19 weeks of a hypocaloric diet when compared with TBW change derived from isotope dilution.[91,102] Thus, it appears that whole-body BIA predicts large changes more accurately than it does small changes (less than 1 to 2 kg) in TBW or FFM.

NEW DEVELOPMENTS IN BIOELECTRICAL IMPEDANCE ANALYSIS. A review of the role of BIA in nutrition assessment of hospitalized patients emphasized the potential of the technique to distinguish regional and total body ICW from ECW and to estimate TBW volume. Two recent developments have enhanced the capability of the BIA technology to provide these features desired for clinical use.

Segmental bioelectrical impedance analysis. The assumption on which BIA was originally based—that the human body is a conductor of uniform length and cross-sectional area—creates errors in its estimates of TBW and FFM. The human body (excluding the head) is more appropriately conceptualized as five separate cylinders: the two arms, the two legs, and the trunk. A procedure for segmental bioelectrical impedance analysis (SBIA) was recently described.[103] The procedure involves placing two additional voltage-sensing electrodes on the left wrist and left ankle, in addition to those on the right wrist and ankle (see Box 3-3). An impedance index produced by data from cross-body electrode pairs was shown to reflect accurately both segmental and total body fat. The potential of this modified BIA technique to estimate regional body fat has obvious public health implications. In addition, the potential for SBIA to monitor segmental body water changes could have valuable clinical applications. Further research in SBIA will provide insight into its expanded utility as compared with whole-body BIA.

Multiple-frequency bioelectrical impedance analysis. A second new development in BIA technology is the use of multiple electrical current frequencies rather than the traditional single 50-kHz frequency. Estimates of TBW from BIA are related to total body resistance measures. The other component of impedance, reactance, is theoretically a measure of the quantity of cell membrane and, as such, is an index of BCM. The level of impedance is a function of the level of current frequency. At low frequencies (5 to 15 kHz) the capacitive effect of cells is sufficient to block the flow of current through the cells, and the resistance measured reflects ECW volume. At frequencies higher than 100 kHz, current penetrates the cell membranes, allowing estimates of combined ECW and ICW. For validation purposes, these estimates are compared with direct measures of ECW and TBW by isotope dilution (e.g., sodium bromide and deuterium, respectively).

Studies of dialysis patients and those receiving intravenous infusions have demonstrated that fluid volume changes during hemodialysis or intravenous infusion could be detected more accurately by measuring the change in impedance at two

---

BOX 3-3

Procedure for Measuring Bioimpedance

The standard measurement protocol for whole-body, single-frequency BIA, regardless of equipment, is outlined below.[83]

1. Perform measurements on fasted subjects (at least 2 hours postprandial) who have abstained from alcohol and strenuous exercise for at least 12 hours and who are not dehydrated. Subjects should remove jewelry (except plain rings) before the measurement.
2. Place the subject supine on a nonconducting surface in a room of normal temperature. Remove the right shoe and sock or stocking.
3. Abduct the limbs from the body to approximately 45 degrees.
4. Prepare skin surfaces for electrode placement with isopropyl alcohol.
5. Accurately place electrodes at anatomic sites.
6. Repeat the measurement in triplicate.

frequencies (1.5 and 150 kHz) as compared with using the 50-kHz single frequency.[104-107] In a study of 53 general surgical patients, however, no difference was seen between TBW and ECW estimates in single-frequency and multifrequency bioimpedance analysis (MFBIA).[108] Recent reports support the accuracy of MFBIA (compared with isotope dilution) for estimating TBW and ECW in hemodialysis patients.[109,110] Similar results were obtained in studies of patients with blunt trauma and sepsis.[111]

Bioimpedance spectroscopy. Bioimpedance spectroscopy (BIS) (Xitron Technologies, San Diego, California) is a variation of MFBIA in which impedance is generally measured over a wide spectrum of frequencies (5 to about 1000 kHz), with TBW and ECW volumes calculated through the application of Cole-Cole curve-fitting modeling procedures and equations derived from mixture theory. Several studies reported positive results using this technology in healthy individuals.[112-117] Recent studies report the use of BIS to measure changes in the body fluid components of clinical populations with emphasis on ICW volume as an indicator of BCM.[118] The sensitivity of several impedance methods for measuring ICW change was studied over an average of 20 weeks in patients with human immunodeficiency virus (HIV) infection who were receiving anabolic steroid therapy.[118] ICW was determined before and after therapy using five impedance methods (BIS, 50-kHz impedance, 50-kHz parallel reactance, difference between 200-kHz impedance and 5-kHz impedance, and difference between 500-kHz impedance and 5-kHz impedance) and compared with ICW derived by difference from TBW and ECW measurements by dilution methods (deuterium and sodium bromide, respectively). The multiple-frequency modeling approach of BIS was the only method that predicted ICW changes that were not statistically different from the isotope dilution-derived measurements of ICW change. In addition, the BIS method predicted FFM change accurately compared with the accretion of lean tissue estimated from nitrogen balance measured daily for 21 days by 24-hour urine and fecal collections following gonadal hormone replacement therapy in HIV-positive men.[119] It was also reported that the BIS method predicted FFM change more accurately than DXA or deuterium dilution. Because the cellular compartment would have retained most of the increased nitrogen,[120] the results of this study strongly suggest that the BIS method is sensitive to changes in BCM. This remains an exciting area of investigation with significant potential for clinical application.

NATIONAL INSTITUTES OF HEALTH TECHNOLOGY ASSESSMENT CONFERENCE ON BIOELECTRICAL IMPEDANCE ANALYSIS. A Technology Assessment Conference entitled, "Bioelectrical Impedance Analysis in Body Composition Measurement" was held December 12 to 14, 1994. At the close of this conference, during which leading experts in the field presented evidence related to BIA methods, the National Institutes of Health (NIH) Technology Assessment Panel published the following conclusions (abridged):[121]

- BIA provides a reliable estimate of TBW under most conditions. Subsequent estimation of FFM and %BF vary in validity, depending on the population or individual studied and on the applicability of the prediction equation used to estimate these parameters of body composition.

- BIA can be a useful technique for body composition analysis in healthy persons and in those with chronic conditions such as mild-to-moderate obesity, diabetes mellitus, and other medical conditions in which major disturbances of water distribution are not prominent.

- The ability of BIA to predict adiposity accurately in severely obese persons is limited. In addition, BIA is not useful in measuring short-term changes in body composition (e.g., in response to diet or exercise) among individuals.

- Although there may be instances in critical illness for which TBW assessment by BIA may be useful (e.g., dialysis patients), there does not appear to be an established role for the technique in the critical care setting.

- Further research is recommended in BIA technology, the basic science of impedance measurements, determinations of ICW and ECW, correlations with clinical outcome in specific patient populations, and longitudinal clinical follow-up of the NHANES III subjects.

- No specific, well-defined procedure for routine BIA measurements is practiced. Therefore, the panel recommends that a committee of appropriate expert scientists and instrument manufacturers be formed who are charged with setting instrument standards and methods.

- Calculations of body composition parameters from the basic electrical measurements should include population-specific equations and report the standard errors of the estimate for the individual.

Its high cost and limited availability preclude use of BIA for routine clinical assessment of body composition.

Ultrasound

The use of ultrasound for body composition analysis was developed as an alternative to skinfold measurements for estimating body fat.[122] This technique uses high-frequency sound waves that are produced by a piezoelectric crystal in a transducer (probe). These sound waves are introduced through the skin by the probe and reflected from interfaces between tissues (mainly deep fascia) that have different acoustic properties. The reflected acoustic energy is transformed to an electrical energy signal. This "echo" produces cross-sectional images of the target tissues that are visualized on an oscilloscope.[60] The beta-mode ultrasound instrument can measure subcutaneous adipose and muscle tissue thickness, muscle cross-sectional area, and abdominal depth.

The precision of ultrasound measurement of adipose tissue is high: reported coefficients of reliability are 91% to 98%.[123,124] Beta-mode ultrasound and skinfold measurements of subcutaneous adipose tissue have been compared[123,125] and found to be similar in accuracy for prediction of body density. Skinfold measurements have the advantage of lower cost and portability. Ultrasound measurements, however, can be made in obese subjects and at some sites (e.g., sacral and paraspinal) where calipers cannot be applied.[60]

Near-Infrared Interactance

A relatively new commercial near-infrared (NIR) analyzer (Futurex-5000) has gained popularity in fitness centers as a field method of estimating %BF. The infrared interactance technique was originally developed to predict the starch, oil, water, and protein content of grains.[126] This technology was applied to the study of body composition using a sophisticated, very precise computerized spectrophotometer.[127] Because of the results of this single, small-sample, unreplicated study, and a computer simulator to predict the accuracy of a low-cost, portable, wide-slit spectrophotometer, the Futurex-5000 was marketed.[128] The technique is based on the principles of light absorption and reflection using NIR spectroscopy.[14] An electromagnetic energy signal is generated by a monochronator and transmitted by a fiberoptic probe to a depth of up to 4 cm into the biceps area, where it is scattered and reflected off the bone back to the conductor. Theoretically, the degree of scattered and reflected energy, interactance energy, is linearly related to the water, fat, and protein composition of the target site (the biceps). The Futurex-5000 uses derived optical density measures (level of interactance energy) and those from a Teflon block as the optical standard, along with weight, height, gender, and exercise level in equations to predict %BF.[63]

Several investigators have reported unacceptable prediction errors for the Futurex-5000 equations used to estimate %BF.[129-133] The manufacturer's equations are reported to underestimate systematically average %BF,[134-136] the degree of underestimation being directly related to the level of adiposity.

Conclusion

A summary of the characteristics of the various methods described in this chapter is provided in Table 3-2. Laboratory methods provide the most precise, accurate, and direct measures of body composition, but their expense and limited availability preclude routine clinical use. Of the field methods described that provide indirect measures of body composition, the various bioelectrical impedance techniques appear to hold the greatest promise for routine clinical use. These techniques

are very precise, safe, noninvasive, and relatively inexpensive. Investigations on the clinical application of this technology using multicompartment criterion models are a priority research area in the field of body composition determination.

REFERENCES

1. Young VR, Marchini JS, Cortiella J: Assessment of protein nutritional status, *J Nutr* 120(suppl 11):1496-1502, 1990.
2. Behnke AR, Wilmore JH: *Evaluation and regulation of body build and composition,* Englewood Cliffs, NJ, 1974, Prentice-Hall, pp 2, 22, 32-34.
3. Brozek J, Grande F, Anderson JT, et al: Densitometric analysis of body composition: revision of some quantitative assumptions, *Ann NY Acad Sci* 110(Pt 1):113-140, 1963.
4. Siri WE: Body composition from fluid spaces and density: analysis of methods, *University of California Radiation Laboratory Report,* 3349, Berkely, CA, Printed for the U.S. Atomic Energy Commission 1956.
5. Côté K, Adams WC: Effect of bone density on body composition estimates in young adult black and white women, *Med Sci Sports Exerc* 25(2):290-296, 1993.
6. Ortiz O, Russell M, Daley TL, et al: Differences in skeletal muscle and bone mineral mass between black and white females and their relevance to estimates of body composition, *Am J Clin Nutr* 55(1):8-13, 1992.
7. Schutte JE, Townsend EJ, Hugg J, et al: Density of lean body mass is greater in blacks than in whites, *J Appl Physiol* 56(6):1647-1649, 1984.
8. Lohman TG, Boileau RA, Slaughter MH: Body composition in children and youth. In Boileau RA (ed): *Advances in pediatric sport sciences,* vol 1, Biological Issues, Champaign, IL, 1984, Human Kinetics, pp 29-57.
9. Heymsfield SB, Wang J, Lichtman S, et al: Body composition in elderly subjects: a critical appraisal of clinical methodology, *Am J Clin Nutr* 50(suppl 5):1167-1175, 1989.
10. Shizgal HM: Nutritional assessment with body composition measurements by multiple isotope dilution, *Infusionstherapie* 17(suppl 3):9-17, 1990.
11. Siri WE: Body composition from fluid spaces and density: analysis of methods. In Brozek J, Henschel A (eds): *Techniques for measuring body composition: proceedings of a conference, Quartermaster Research and Engineering Center, Natick, MA, January 22-23, 1959,* Washington, DC, 1961, National Academy of Sciences National Research Council, pp 223-244.
12. Akers R, Buskirk ER: An underwater weighing system utilizing "force cube" transducers, *J Appl Physiol* 26(5):649-652, 1969.
13. Wilmore JH: A simplified method for determination of residual lung volumes, *J Appl Physiol* 27(1):96-100, 1969.
14. Lukaski, HC: Methods for the assessment of human body composition: traditional and new, *Am J Clin Nutr* 46(4):537-556, 1987.
15. Cameron JR, Sorenson J: Measurement of bone mineral in vivo: an improved method, *Science* 142(3589):230-232, 1963.
16. Mazess RB, Cameron JR: Direct readout of bone mineral content using radionuclide absorptiometry, *Int J Appl Radiat Isotopes* 23(10):471-479, 1972.
17. Gotfredsen A, Jensen J, Borg J, et al: Measurement of lean body mass and total body fat using dual photon absorptiometry, *Metabolism* 35(1):88-93, 1986.
18. Mazess RB, Peppler WW, Gibbons M: Total body composition by dual-photon (153Gd) absorptiometry, *Am J Clin Nutr* 40(4):834-839, 1984.
19. Heymsfield SB, Wang J, Heshka S, et al: Dual-photon absorptiometry: comparison of bone mineral and soft tissue mass measurements in vivo with established methods, *Am J Clin Nutr* 49(6):1283-1289, 1989.
20. Going SB, Pamenter RW, Lohman TG, et al: Estimation of total body composition by regional dual photon absorptiometry, *Am J Hum Biol* 2(6):703-710, 1990.
21. Lang P, Steiger P, Faulkner K, et al: Osteoporosis. Current techniques and recent developments in quantitative bone densitometry, *Radiol Clin North Am* 29(1):49-76, 1991.
22. Lohman, TG: Dual energy x-ray absorptiometry. In Roche AF, Heymsfield SB, Lohman TG (eds): *Human body composition,* Champaign, IL, 1996, Human Kinetics, pp 63-78.
23. Mazess R, Collick B, Trempe J, et al: Performance evaluation of a dual-energy x-ray bone densitometer, *Calcif Tiss Int* 44(3):228-232, 1989.
24. Mazess RB, Barden HS, Bisek JP, et al: Dual-energy x-ray absorptiometry for total-body and regional bone-mineral and soft-tissue composition, *Am J Clin Nutr* 51(6):1106-1112, 1990.

TABLE 3-2

Comparison of Methods to Determine Human Body Composition*

Method	Cost	Precision Technical Difficulty	Precision Fat-Free Mass	Precision % Fat
Isotope dilution (TBW)				
Deuterium	2	3	3	3
Oxygen-18	5	5	4	4
Total body potassium counting (^{40}K)	4	4	4	3
Densitometry	3	4	5	5
Skinfold thickness	1	3	2	2
Arm circumference	1	2	2	2
Neutron activation analysis (NAA)	5	5	5	5
Dual-energy x-ray absorptiometry (DXA)	4	4	5	5
Dual-photon absorptiometry (DPA)	4	4	4	4
Ultrasound	3	3	3	3
Bioelectrical impedance analysis (BIA)	2	1	4	4
Computed tomography (CT)	5	5	?	?
Magnetic resonance imaging (MRI)	5	5	?	?

Adapted from Lukaski HC: Methods for the assessment of human body composition: traditional and new, *Am J Clin Nutr* 46:551, 1987.
*Ranking system: 1 = least; 5 = greatest; ? = unknown at this time.

25. Heymsfield SB, Wang Z, Wang J, et al: Theoretical foundation of dual energy x-ray absorptiometry (DEXA) soft tissue estimates: validation in situ and in vivo, *FASEB J* 8(4-5):A278, 1994 (abstract 1603).
26. Tataranni PA, Ravussin E: Use of dual-energy x-ray absorptiometry in obese individuals, *Am J Clin Nutr* 62(4):730-734, 1995.
27. Going SB, Massett MP, Hall MC, et al: Detection of small changes in body composition by dual-energy x-ray absorptiometry, *Am J Clin Nutr* 57(6):845-850, 1993.
28. Nord RH, Payne RK: DXA vs underwater weighing: comparison of strengths and weaknesses, *Asia Pacific J Clin Nutr* 4:173-175, 1995.
29. Horber FF, Thomi F, Casez JP, et al: Impact of hydration status on body composition as measured by dual energy x-ray absorptiometry in normal volunteers and patients on haemodialysis, *Br J Radiol* 65(778):895-900, 1992.
30. Jensen LB, Quaade F, Sorensen OH: Bone loss accompanying voluntary weight loss in obese humans, *J Bone Miner Res* 9(4):459-463, 1994.
31. Lukaski HC, Siders WA, Gallagher SK: Decreased bone mineral status assessed by dual-energy x-ray absorptiometry (DXA) in obese women during weight loss, *Am J Clin Nutr* 56(4):768, 1992 (abstract 82).
32. Svendsen OL, Haarbo J, Hassager C, et al: Accuracy of measurements of body composition by dual-energy x-ray absorptiometry in vivo, *Am J Clin Nutr* 57(5):605-608, 1993.
33. Svendsen OL, Haarbo J, Hassager C, et al: Accuracy of measurements of total-body soft-tissue composition by DXA in vivo. In Ellis KJ, Eastman JD (eds): *Human body composition: in vivo methods, models, and assessment,* New York, 1993, Plenum, pp 381-383.
34. Van Loan MD, Thompson J, Butterfield G, et al: Comparison of bone mineral content (BMC), bone mineral density (BMD), lean and fat measurements from two different bone densitometers, *Med Sci Sports Exerc* 26(suppl 5):S40, 1994 (abstract 231).
35. Heymsfield SB, McManus C, Smith J, et al: Anthropometric measurement of muscle mass: revised equations for calculating bone-free arm muscle area, *Am J Clin Nutr* 36(4):680-690, 1982.
36. Frisancho AR: *Anthropometric standards for the assessment of growth and nutritional status,* Ann Arbor, Michigan, 1990, The University of Michigan Press, pp 28, 41-42, 51-52, 54, 60-63.
37. Borkan GA, Gerzof SG, Robbins AH, et al: Assessment of abdominal fat content by computed tomography, *Am J Clin Nutr* 36(1):172-177, 1982.
38. Borkan GA, Hults DE, Gerzof SG, et al: Comparison of body composition in middle-aged and elderly males using computed tomography, *Am J Phys Anthropol* 66(3):289-295, 1985.
39. Seidell JC: Relationships of total and regional body composition to morbidity and mortality. In Roche AF, Heymsfield SB, Lohman TG (eds): *Human body composition,* Champaign, IL, 1996, Human Kinetics, pp 345-353.
40. Baumgartner RN, Rhyne RL, Garry PJ, et al: Imaging techniques and anatomical body composition in aging, *J Nutr* 123(suppl 2):444-448, 1993.
41. Alger JR, Frank JA: The utilization of magnetic resonance imaging in physiology, *Annu Rev Physiol* 54:827-846, 1992.
42. Cohn SH, Dombrowski CS, Pate HR, et al: A whole-body counter with an invariant response to radionuclide distribution and body size, *Phys Med Biol* 14(4):645-658, 1969.
43. Kehayias JJ, Heymsfield SB, Dilmanian FA, et al: Measurement of body fat by neutron inelastic scattering: comments on installation, operation, and error analysis. In Yasumura S, Harrison JE, McNeill KG, et al (eds): *In vivo body composition studies: recent advances,* New York, 1990, Plenum, pp 339-346.
44. Heymsfield SB, Wang Z, Baumgartner RN, et al: Body composition and aging: a study by in vivo neutron activation analysis, *J Nutr* 123(suppl 2):432-437, 1993.
45. Cohn SH, Dombrowski CS: Measurement of total-body calcium, sodium, choline, nitrogen, and phosphorus in man by in vivo neutron activation analysis, *J Nucl Med* 12(7):499-505, 1971.
46. Heymsfield SB, Matthews D: Body composition: research and clinical advances—1993 A.S.P.E.N. research workshop, *J Parenteral Enteral Nutr* 18(2):91-103, 1994.
47. Halliday D, Miller AG: Precise measurement of total body water using trace quantities of deuterium oxide, *Biomed Mass Spectrom* 4(2):82-87, 1977.
48. Lukaski HC, Johnson PE: A simple, inexpensive method of determining total body water using a tracer dose of D_2O and infrared absorption of biological fluids, *Am J Clin Nutr* 41(2):363-370, 1985.
49. Pinson EA: Water exchanges and barriers as studied by the use of hydrogen isotopes, *Physiol Rev* 32(2):123-134, 1952.
50. Forbes GB: *Human body composition: growth, aging, nutrition, and activity,* New York, 1987, Springer-Verlag, pp 6-19.
51. McCullough AJ, Mullen KD, Kalhan SC: Measurements of total body and extracellular water in cirrhotic patients with and without ascites, *Hepatology* 14(6):1102-1111, 1991.
52. Grant A, DeHoog S: *Nutritional assessment and support,* ed 4, revised, expanded. Seattle, 1991, Anne Grant/Susan DeHoog, pp 9-85.
53. Kuczmarski RJ, Flegal KM, Campbell SM, et al: Increasing prevalence of overweight among US adults. The National Health and Nutrition Examination Surveys, 1960-1991, *JAMA* 272(3):205-211, 1994.
54. Abernathy RP, Black DR: Healthy body weights: an alternative perspective, *Am J Clin Nutr* 63(suppl 3):448S-451S, 1996.
55. Meisler JG, St Jeor S: Summary and recommendations from the American Health Foundation's expert panel on healthy weight, *Am J Clin Nutr* 63(suppl 3):474S-477S, 1996.
56. Kuczmarski RJ, Ogden CL, Grummer-Strawn LM, et al: *CDC growth charts: United States. Advance data from vital and health statistics, No. 314,* Hyattsville, MD, 2000. National Center for Health Statistics.
57. Smalley KJ, Knerr AN, Kendrick ZV, et al: Reassessment of body mass indices, *Am J Clin Nutr* 52(3):405-408, 1990.
58. Garn SM, Leonard WR, Hawthorne VM: Three limitations of the body mass index, *Am J Clin Nutr* 44(6):996-997, 1986.
59. Gray DS, Bray GA, Bauer M, et al: Skinfold thickness measurements in obese subjects, *Am J Clin Nutr* 51(4):571-577, 1990.
60. Roche AR: Anthropometry and ultrasound. In Roche AF, Heymsfield SB, Lohman TG (eds): *Human body composition,* Champaign, IL, 1996, Human Kinetics, pp 167-189.
61. Lohman TG, Pollock ML, Slaughter MH, et al: Methodological factors and the prediction of body fat in female athletes, *Med Sci Sports Exerc* 16(1):92-96, 1984.
62. Harrison GG, Buskirk ER, Carter JE, et al: Skinfold thicknesses and measurement technique. In Lohman TG, Roche AF, Martorell R (eds): *Anthropometric standardization reference manual,* Champaign, IL, 1988, Human Kinetics, pp 55-70.
63. Heyward VH, Stolarczyk LM: *Applied body composition assessment,* Champaign, IL, 1996, Human Kinetics, pp 29, 56-65, 186-189.
64. Gruber JJ, Pollock ML, Graves JE, et al: Comparison of Harpenden and Lange calipers in predicting body composition, *Res Q Exerc Sport* 61(2):184-190, 1990.
65. Hawkins JD: Analysis of selected skinfold measuring instruments, *J Phys Ed Recreat Dance* 54(1):25-27, 1983.
66. Leger LA, Lambert J, Martin P: Validity of plastic skinfold caliper measurements, *Hum Biol* 54(4):667-675, 1982.
67. Bunt JC, Lohman TG, Boileau RA: Impact of total body water fluctuations on estimation of body fat from body density, *Med Sci Sports Exerc* 21(1):96-100, 1989.
68. Chumlea WC, Roche AF, Steinbaugh ML: Estimating stature from knee height for persons 60 to 90 years of age, *J Am Geriatr Soc* 33(2):116-120, 1985.
69. Grant JP: *Handbook of total parental nutrition,* Philadelphia, 1980, WB Saunders.
70. Frisancho AR, Flegel PN: Elbow breadth as a measure of frame size for US males and females, *Am J Clin Nutr* 37(2):311-314, 1983.
71. Weltman A, Seip RL, Tran ZV: Practical assessment of body composition in adult obese males, *Hum Biol* 59(3):523-555, 1987.
72. Weltman A, Levine S, Seip RL, et al: Accurate assessment of body composition in obese females, *Am J Clin Nutr* 48(5):1179-1183, 1988.
73. Seidell JC, Oosterlee A, Thijssen MA, et al: Assessment of intra-abdominal and subcutaneous abdominal fat: relation between anthropometry and computed tomography, *Am J Clin Nutr* 45(1):7-13, 1987.
74. Busetto L, Baggio MB, Zurlo F, et al: Assessment of abdominal fat distribution in obese patients: anthropometry versus computerized tomography, *Int J Obes* 16(10):731-736, 1992.
75. Weits T, van der Beek EJ, Wedel M, et al: Computed tomography measurement of abdominal fat deposition in relation to anthropometry, *Int J Obes* 12(3):217-225, 1988.
76. World Health Organization: Obesity: preventing and managing the global epidemic of obesity. Report of WHO Consultation of Obesity, Geneva, June 3-5, 1997.
77. Bjorntorp P: "Portal" adipose tissue as a generator of risk factors for cardiovascular disease and diabetes, *Arteriosclerosis* 10(4):493-496, 1990.
78. Chumlea WC: Methods of nutritional anthropometric assessment for special groups. In Lohman TG, Roche AF, Martorell R (eds): *Anthropometric standardization reference manual,* Champaign, IL, 1988, Human Kinetics, pp 93-95.
79. Kwok T, Whitelaw MN: The use of armspan in nutritional assessment of the elderly, *J Am Geriatr Soc* 39(5):492-496, 1991.

80. Lohman TG: Anthropometry and body composition. In Lohman TG, Roche AF, Martorell R (eds): *Anthropometric standardization reference manual,* Champaign, IL, 1988, Human Kinetics, pp 125-129.

81. Brunnstrom S: *Clinical kinesiology,* ed 2, Philadelphia, 1966, FA Davis, p 269.

82. Jensen TG, Englert DM, Dudrick SJ: *Nutritional assessment: a manual for practitioners,* Norwalk, CT, 1983, Appelton-Century-Crofts, p 53-64.

83. Kushner RF: Bioelectrical impedance analysis: a review of principles and applications. *J Am Coll Nutr* 11(2):199-209, 1992.

84. Houtkooper LB, Going SB, Lohman TG, et al: Bioelectrical impedance estimation of fat-free body mass in children and youth: a cross-validation study, *J Appl Physiol* 72(1):366-373, 1992.

85. Rising R, Swinburn B, Larson K, et al: Body composition in Pima Indians: validation of bioelectrical resistance, *Am J Clin Nutr* 53(3):594-598, 1991.

86. Stolarczyk LM, Heyward VH, Hicks VL, et al: Predictive accuracy of bioelectrical impedance in estimating body composition of Native American women, *Am J Clin Nutr* 59(5):964-970, 1994.

87. Gray DS, Bray GA, Gemayel N, et al: Effect of obesity on bioelectrical impedance, *Am J Clin Nutr* 50(2):255-260, 1989.

88. Segal KR, Van Loan M, Fitzgerald PI, et al: Lean body mass estimation by bioelectrical impedance analysis: a four-site cross-validation study, *Am J Clin Nutr* 47(1):7-14, 1988.

89. Houtkooper LB, Going SB, Westfall CH, et al: Prediction of fat-free body corrected for bone mass from impedance and anthropometry in adult females, *Med Sci Sports Exerc* 21(suppl 2):S39, 1989 (abstract 229).

90. Deurenberg P, van der Kooij K, Evers P, et al: Assessment of body composition by bioelectrical impedance in a population aged greater than 60 y, *Am J Clin Nutr* 51(1):3-6, 1990.

91. Gray DS: Changes in bioelectrical impedance during fasting, *Am J Clin Nutr* 48(5):1184-1187, 1988.

92. Kushner RF, Schoeller DA: Estimation of total body water by bioelectrical impedance analysis, *Am J Clin Nutr* 44(3):417-424, 1986.

93. Lukaski HC, Bolonchuk WW: Estimation of body fluid volumes using tetrapolar bioelectrical impedance measurements, *Aviat Space Environ Med* 59(12):1163-1169, 1988.

94. Van Loan M, Mayclin P: Bioelectrical impedance analysis: is it a reliable estimator of lean body mass and total body water? *Hum Biol* 59(2):299-309, 1987.

95. Houtkooper LB, Lohman T, Going SB, et al: Why bioelectrical impedance analysis should be used for estimating adiposity, *Am J Clin Nutr* 64(suppl 3):436S-448S, 1996.

96. Guo S, Roche AF, Houtkooper L: Fat-free mass in children and young adults predicted from bioelectric impedance and anthropometric variables, *Am J Clin Nutr* 50(3):435-443, 1989.

97. Lohman TG: *Advances in body composition assessment, Current Issues In Exercise Science Monograph Number 3,* Champaign, IL, 1992, Human Kinetics, pp 53, 124.

98. Van Loan MD, Boileau RA, Slaughter MH et al: Association of bioelectrical resistance with estimates of fat-free mass determined by densitometry and hydrometry, *Am J Hum Biol* 2(3):219-226, 1990.

99. Böhm D, Odaischi M, Beyerlein C, et al: Total body water: changes during dialysis estimated by bioimpedance analysis, *Infusionstherapie* 17(suppl 3):75-78, 1990.

100. Kurtin PS, Shapiro AC, Tomita H, et al: Volume status and body composition of chronic dialysis patients: utility of bioelectric impedance plethysmography, *Am J Nephrol* 10(5):363-367, 1990.

101. Deurenberg P, Weststrate JA, van der Kooij K: Body composition changes assessed by bioelectrical impedance measurements, *Am J Clin Nutr* 49(3):401-403, 1989.

102. Kushner RF, Kunigk A, Alspaugh M, et al: Validation of bioelectrical-impedance analysis as a measurement of change in body composition in obesity, *Am J Clin Nutr* 52(2):219-223, 1990.

103. Organ LW, Bradham GB, Gore DT, et al: Segmental bioelectrical impedance analysis: theory and application of a new technique, *J Appl Physiol* 77(1):98-112, 1994.

104. Tedner B: Equipment using an impedance technique for automatic recording of fluid-volume changes during haemodialysis, *Med Biol Eng Comput* 21(3):285-290, 1983.

105. Tedner B, Lins LE: Fluid volume monitoring with electrical impedance technique during hemodialysis, *Artif Organs* 8(1):66-71, 1984.

106. Tedner BT, Jacobson HS, Linnarsson D, et al: Impedance fluid volume monitoring during intravenous infusion in healthy subjects, *Acute Care* 10(3-4):200-206, 1984.

107. Tedner B, Lins LE: Fluid volume changes during hemodialysis monitored with the impedance technique, *Artif Organs* 9(4):416-420, 1985.

108. Hannan WJ, Cowen SJ, Fearon KC, et al: Evaluation of multi-frequency bio-impedance analysis for the assessment of extracellular and total body water in surgical patients, *Clin Sci (Colch)* 86(4):479-485, 1994.

109. Ho LT, Kushner RF, Schoeller DA, et al: Bioimpedance analysis of total body water in hemodialysis patients, *Kidney Int* 46(5):1438-1442, 1994.

110. Cha K, Chertow GM, Gonzalez J, et al: Multifrequency bioelectrical impedance estimates the distribution of body water, *J Appl Physiol* 79(4):1316-1319, 1995.

111. Finn PJ, Plank LD, Clark MA, et al: Progressive cellular dehydration and proteolysis in critically ill patients, *Lancet* 347(9002):654-656, 1996.

112. Chumlea WC, Guo SS, Baumgartner RN, et al: Determination of body fluid compartments with multiple frequency bioelectric impedance. In Ellis KJ, Eastman JD (eds): *Human body composition: in vivo methods, models, and assessment,* New York, 1993, Plenum, pp 23-26.

113. Azcue M, Wesson D, Neuman M, et al: What does bioelectrical impedance spectroscopy (BIS) measure? In Ellis KJ, Eastman JD (eds): *Human body composition: in vivo methods, models, and assessment,* New York, 1993, Plenum, pp 121-123.

114. Deurenberg P, Schouten FJM, Andreoli A, et al: Assessment of changes in extracellular water and total body water using multifrequency bioelectrical impedance. In Ellis KJ, Eastman JD (eds): *Human body composition: in vivo methods, models, and assessment,* New York, 1993, Plenum, pp 129-132.

115. Van Loan MD, Withers P, Matthie J, et al: Use of bioimpedance spectroscopy to determine extracellular fluid, intracellular fluid, total body water, and fat-free mass. In Ellis KJ, Eastman JD (eds): *Human body composition: in vivo methods, models, and assessment,* New York, 1993, Plenum, pp 67-70.

116. Mitchell CO, Rose J, Familoni B, et al: The use of multifrequency bioelectrical impedance analysis to estimate fluid volume changes as a function of the menstrual cycle. In Ellis KJ, Eastman JD (eds): *Human body composition: in vivo methods, models, and assessment,* New York, 1993, Plenum, pp 189-191.

117. van Marken Lichtenbelt WD, Westerterp KR, Wouters L, et al: Validation of bioelectrical-impedance measurements as a method to estimate body-water compartments, *Am J Clin Nutr* 60(2):159-166, 1994.

118. Earthman CP, Matthie JR, Reid PM, et al: A comparison of bioimpedance methods for detection of body cell mass change in HIV infection, *J Appl Physiol* 88(3):944-956, 2000.

119. Van Loan MD, Strawford A, Jacob M, et al: Monitoring changes in fat-free mass in HIV-positive men with hypotestosteronemia and AIDS wasting syndrome treated with gonadal hormone replacement therapy, *AIDS* 13(2):241-248, 1999.

120. James HM, Dabek JT, Chettle DR, et al: Whole body cellular and collagen nitrogen in healthy and wasted man, *Clin Sci (Colch)* 67(1):73-82, 1984.

121. National Institutes of Health: *Bioelectrical impedance analysis in body composition measurement,* National Institutes of Health Technology Assessment Statement, Dec 12-14, 1994, Bethesda, MD, 1994, NIH Office of Medical Applications of Research, pp 3-28. http://text.nlm.nih.gov

122. Booth RA, Goddard BA, Paton A: Measurement of fat thickness in man: a comparison of ultrasound, Harpenden calipers, and electrical conductivity, *Br J Nutr* 20(4):719-725, 1966.

123. Abe T, Kondo M, Kawakami Y, et al: Prediction equations for body composition of Japanese adults by B-mode ultrasound, *Am J Hum Biol* 6(2):161-170, 1994.

124. Bellisari A, Roche AF, Siervogel RM: Reliability of B-mode ultrasonic measurements of subcutaneous adipose tissue and intra-abdominal depth: comparisons with skinfold thicknesses, *Int J Obes Relat Metab Disord* 17(8):475-480, 1993.

125. Fanelli MT, Kuczmarski RJ: Ultrasound as an approach to assessing body composition, *Am J Clin Nutr* 39(5):703-709, 1984.

126. Norris KH: Extracting information from spectrophotometric curves. Predicting chemical composition from visible and near-infrared spectra. In Martens H, Russwurm H, Jr (eds): Food Research and Data Analysis: *Proceedings from the IUFoST Symposium, September 20-23, 1982,* Oslo, Norway, London, 1983, Applied Science Publishers, p 95-113.

127. Conway JM, Norris KH, Bodwell CE: A new approach for the estimation of body composition: infrared interactance, *Am J Clin Nutr* 40(6):1123-1130, 1984.

128. Conway JM, Norris KH: Noninvasive body composition in humans by near infrared interactance. In Ellis KJ, Yasumura S, Morgan WD (eds): *In vivo body composition studies.* Proceedings of an International Symposium held at Brookhaven National Laboratory, New York, on September 28-October 1, 1986. London, 1987, The Institute of Physical Sciences in Medicine, pp 163-170.

129. Heyward VH, Jenkins KA, Cook KL, et al: Validity of single-site and multi-site models of estimating body composition of women using near-infrared interactance, *Am J Hum Biol* 4(5):579-593, 1992.

130. Eaton AW, Israel RG, O'Brien KF, et al: Comparison of four methods to assess body composition in women, *Eur J Clin Nutr* 47(5):353-360, 1993.

131. Elia M, Parkinson SA, Diaz E: Evaluation of near infra-red interactance as a method for predicting body composition, *Eur J Clin Nutr* 44(2):113-121, 1990.

132. Hortobagyi T, Israel RG, Houmard JA, et al: Comparison of body composition assessment by hydrodensitometry, skinfolds, and multiple site near-infrared spectrophotometry, *Eur J Clin Nutr* 46(3):205-211, 1992.

133. McLean KP, Skinner JS: Validity of Futrex-5000 for body composition determination, *Med Sci Sports Exerc* 24(2):253-258, 1992.

134. Davis PG, Van Loan M, Holly RG, et al: Near infrared interactance vs. hydrostatic weighing to measure body composition in lean, normal, and obese women, *Med Sci Sports Exerc* 21(suppl 2): S100, 1989 (abstract 595).

135. Hicks V, Heyward V, Flores A, et al: Validation of near-infrared interactance (NIR) and skinfold (SKF) methods for estimating body composition of American Indian women, *Med Sci Sports Exerc* 25(suppl 5):S152, 1993 (abstract 848).

136. Houmard JA, Israel RG, McCammon MR, et al: Validity of a near-infrared device for estimating body composition in a college football team, *J Appl Sport Sci Res* 2(5):53-59, 1991.

Mary Krystofiak Russell, MS, RD, LDN, CNSD

Assessment of Protein Status Using Hepatic Transport Proteins

Biochemical assessment of nutritional status provides information on both somatic and visceral (nonmuscle) compartments of the body. The somatic compartment is composed of skeletal muscle and adipose tissue. Creatinine-height index (CHI) and urinary 3-methylhistidine (3-MH) are biochemical methods, used in addition to anthropometry, to estimate somatic protein stores. The visceral compartment includes the organs and structural components of the body; serum albumin, transferrin, transthyretin (TTR, or prealbumin), and retinol-binding protein (RBP) are laboratory indices commonly used to assess protein status. Nitrogen balance studies monitor nutrition intervention and provide an assessment of stress level and an estimate of protein requirements. C-reactive protein (CRP) measures the degree of the inflammatory response and can be helpful in determining when to maximize nutrition support of the stressed patient. Fibronectin (FN) and insulin-like growth factor I (IGF-I, or somatomedin C) have potential as markers of the efficacy of nutrition support therapy.

Determinants such as synthesis, degradation, and distribution all should be considered when evaluating transport protein concentrations. Table 4-1 provides a summary of important data used in assessment of transport protein levels. Transport proteins used in nutrition assessment are designated "negative acute-phase reactants" because levels of these proteins drop significantly during an acute phase response, such as that to inflammation. The magnitude of the drop is related to (1) downregulation of gene expression and translation, (2) increased catabolism, (3) transfer to extravascular pools, and (4) reduced synthesis related to reduced availability of dietary amino acids.[1-3] Analysis of trends in protein concentrations, with attention to the direction of change, is more important than assessment of a single level because there is no single indicator of nutritional status or effectiveness of therapy. Sound clinical recommendations are derived from evaluating biochemical results in conjunction with diet history, physical assessment, anthropometry, the clinical status of the patient, and experience/clinical judgment.

Albumin

PHYSIOLOGY. Albumin was first recognized in 1837 as a protein necessary for vascular transport of molecules, maintenance of the vascular system, and prevention of edema.[4]

Synthesized in the liver, albumin has a half-life of 20 days and is the most abundant plasma protein. The normal total body pool of albumin is 3 to 4 g/kg for females and 4 to 5 g/kg for males.[4] Most albumin (60%) is contained in the extravascular space, with 30% to 40% of that in the skin. The remaining extravascular albumin is distributed throughout the muscles and viscera. Intravascular albumin (40%) is primarily responsible for plasma colloid oncotic pressure.

Serum albumin is most useful as a prognostic screening tool for hospitalized patients because it is easily measured and inexpensive, and it has been identified as a key marker of nutritional risk.[5-7] Low serum albumin levels have been associated with increased morbidity, mortality, and increased length of stay in several patient populations.[3,8-18] Chlebowski and colleagues observed that patients with the acquired immunodeficiency syndrome (AIDS) whose initial serum albumin level was less than 2.5 g/dl had a median survival time of 17 days. Patients with a normal serum albumin value (greater than 3.5 g/dl) had a median survival of more than 960 days.[13] Biochemical alterations consistent with kwashiorkor occur when the serum albumin level falls below 3.0 g/dl.[14] An albumin level of less than 4.0 g/dl is a powerful predictor of death in patients with end-stage renal disease.[15,16] Development of pressure ulcers has been associated with hypoalbuminemia and, consequently, with increased in-hospital mortality and increased mortality in long-term care settiings.[17-19] The increase in interstitial edema associated with low serum albumin is thought to be responsible for accelerated tissue damage, interference with respiration, and delayed wound healing.[17]

CLINICAL UTILITY AND LIMITATIONS. As an indicator of protein-energy balance in the acute-care setting, albumin is limited by its long half-life, large body pool, and poor sensitivity and specificity.[2,3,20-21] Serum albumin levels more often reflect the acute response to hypermetabolism and insult than they do depletion of body mass.[1-3] Cytokines, such as interleukin-1 (IL-1), interleukin-6 (IL-6), and tumor necrosis factor released from phagocytic cells, reorient hepatic synthesis of plasma proteins and increase muscle protein breakdown to provide needed energy and protein.[1,2] A sharp drop in albumin is frequently seen after trauma, surgery, or stress. An average decrease of 0.5 g/dl in serum albumin has been seen in 70% of patients who undergo surgery.[22] Vanek notes that serum albumin levels in severely ill patients may decrease by 1 to 1.5 g/dl over a few days.[3] I have frequently noted drops in serum albumin of up to 2 g/dl after acute stress or surgery. Further decreases can occur, despite apparently adequate nutrition support.[3,21] The acute fall in serum albumin associated

Acknowledgment: A special thank you is extended to M. Patricia McAdams, MS, RD, LDN, who contributed to the first edition chapter.

TABLE 4-1

Quick Reference for Hepatic Transport Proteins

Transport Protein	Clinical Significance	Half-Life	Nonnutritional Factors that Increase Value	Nonnutritional Factors that Reduce Value
Albumin	Vascular transport Maintenance of colloid oncotic pressure Prognostic screening tool Key marker of nutrition risk Marker of inflammatory response to hypermetabolism and insult Poor marker of protein-energy balance in acute care Negative acute-phase reactant	21 days	Dehydration Reduced plasma volume Exogenous administration	Overhydration Insufficient protein intake Increased catabolism Increased excretion Alteration in synthesis due to acute stress Acute or chronic inflammation Age Liver failure
Transferrin	Iron transport Poor marker of protein-energy balance in acute care May correlate with nitrogen balance Negative acute-phase reactant	8-10 days	Iron-deficiency anemia Oral contraceptives Acute hepatitis Chronic blood loss Dehydration	Liver failure Increased excretion Alteration in synthesis due to acute stress Acute or chronic inflammation
Transthyretin (prealbumin)	Thyroxine transport Rapid response to malnutrition Rapid increase with adequate protein intake Negative acute-phase reactant	2-3 days	Dehydration Renal failure Glucocorticosteroid therapy	Liver failure Alteration in synthesis due to acute stress Acute or chronic inflammation Overhydration
Retinol-binding protein	Retinol transport Sensitive indicator of protein or energy restriction Negative acute-phase reactant	12 hr	Renal failure	Hyperthyroidism Chronic liver disease Cystic fibrosis Vitamin A deficiency Alteration in synthesis due to acute stress
Fibronectin	Function in cell adhesion, cell and tissue differentiation, wound healing, opsonization Correlates with nitrogen balance and energy intake Negative acute-phase reactant	15 hr	FN-rich cryoprecipitate or blood products	Malnutrition Burns Trauma Sepsis Fasting Binding to actin, fibrin, DNA, *Staphylococcus aureus*
Somatomedin-C	Growth peptide Regulates anabolic activity Positive correlation with nitrogen balance in stress and infection	2-4 hr	Renal failure, liver disease, autoimmune disease (due to interference with assay of binding proteins)	

DNA, deoxyribonucleic acid; *FN*, fibronectin.

with critical illness is part of the inflammatory response to injury and is related to increased microvascular permeability and to the shift in albumin distribution from the vascular to the interstitial space.[2,3,22-23]

INTERPRETATION OF SERUM LEVELS. Hypoalbuminemia occurs in approximately 25% of hospitalized patients[9] and can be classified by severity (Table 4-2). Low albumin levels may result from insufficient protein intake; increased losses; and alterations in fluid status, synthesis, and degradation. During stress, synthesis of albumin is depressed as the liver prioritizes its function to the production of positive acute-phase reactants, which include C-reactive protein, fibrinogen, haptoglobin, and ceruloplasmin.[22,24] In addition, during the acute-phase response to injury, increased degradation of albumin occurs; the degraded amino acids become part of the amino acid pool to be used for protein synthesis. Significant losses of albumin occur with thermal injury, nephrotic syndrome, protein-losing enteropathy, cirrhosis, and chronic bronchitis.[2,22,23] Other causes of hypoalbuminemia, possibly independent of or codependent with nutritional status,

TABLE 4-2

Normal and Deficiency States As Defined by Serum Protein Markers

	Normal	Mild	Moderate	Severe
Albumin (g/dl)	3.5-5.0	2.8-3.5	2.1-2.7	<2.1
TFN (mg/dl)	200-400	150-200	100-150	<100
TTR (mg/dl)	15.7-29.6	10-15	5-10	<5
RBP (mg/dl)	2.7-7.6			

Data from Shopbell J, Hopkins B, Shronts E: Nutrition screening and assessment. In Gottschlich M (ed): *The science and practice of nutrition support: a case-based core curriculum*, Dubuque, IA, 2001, ASPEN/Kendall Hunt, pp 107-140.

RBP, Retinol-binding protein; *TFN*, transferrin; *TTR*, transthyretin.

include liver disease, infection, multiple myeloma, acute or chronic inflammation, and rheumatoid arthritis.[23] Age may also contribute to altered albumin metabolism. Hypoalbuminemia in elderly patients may be related to a reduced albumin pool and increased fractional catabolic rate of albumin.[25]

Increased levels of albumin, independent of nutritional status, are seen with dehydration, decreased plasma volume, and during the administration of exogenous albumin to maintain fluid volume in the vascular space. Anabolic hormones and corticosteroids can increase albumin levels. Albumin levels measured under these conditions are not, contrary to common reference, "falsely" elevated but rather are higher because of nonnutritional factors, and therefore are not very useful as nutrition assessment or monitoring tools.

Transferrin

PHYSIOLOGY. Transferrin, a β-globulin synthesized in the liver, is primarily responsible for iron absorption and transport. Transferrin binds with ferric iron and transports it to the bone marrow to be used for hemoglobin synthesis, to storage sites in the liver reticuloendothelial cells, and to gastrointestinal mucosal cells for incorporation into some enzymes. Transferrin regulates the rate at which iron is released from the mucosal cells into general circulation. Transferrin is normally saturated to about one third of its total iron-binding capacity (TIBC). In iron deficiency, transferrin levels rise in proportion to the deficiency of iron stores in bone marrow and liver. After correction of iron-deficiency anemia, serum transferrin is the last hematologic index to return to normal.

CLINICAL UTILITY AND LIMITATIONS. Transferrin has a half-life of 8 to 10 days and equilibrates more rapidly with the extravascular space than does albumin.[2,20] Although more valuable than albumin in monitoring protein-energy balance, transferrin has been criticized for its lack of specificity and sensitivity;[20,26] however, other investigators have found transferrin concentration to correlate closely with transthyretin concentration and to changes in nitrogen balance.[27] Church and Hill found rising transferrin levels to indicate positive nitrogen balance, although falling levels did not reflect the reverse.[28] Transferrin was superior to other serum proteins, as well as to sepsis incidence and fistula output, in predicting spontaneous gastrointestinal fistula closure, in a study by Kuvshinoff and colleagues.[29]

Serum transferrin can be measured directly through radial immunodiffusion or calculated from TIBC by various formulas (Box 4-1).[2,30-31] Calculating transferrin from TIBC can underestimate levels in iron-deficient persons.[30] In addition, the relationship between TIBC and transferrin varies among laboratories. The relationship should be validated in each institution rather than relying on published formulas.[2,32]

INTERPRETATION OF SERUM LEVELS. Elevated transferrin levels are associated with iron-deficiency anemia, use of oral contraceptives, acute hepatitis, chronic blood loss, and dehydration.

BOX 4-1

Calculation of Transferrin from Total Iron-Binding Capacity*[30,31]

Miller	(0.68 × TIBC)	+ 21	=	157 mg/dl
Danzinger	(0.76 × TIBC)	+ 18	=	170 mg/dl
Blackburn	(0.80 × TIBC)	− 43	=	117 mg/dl
Grant	(0.87 × TIBC)	+ 10	=	184 mg/dl
Heymsfield	(0.90 × TIBC)	− 4.5	=	175.5 mg/dl

*Calculations assume TIBC value of 200.

Depressed transferrin levels, independent of nutritional status, are seen in end-stage liver disease; in protein-losing conditions; and after surgery, trauma, or infection. Transferrin may be unreliable as a nutrition parameter during administration of antibiotics.[33]

Transthyretin (Thyroxine-Binding Prealbumin)

PHYSIOLOGY. Transthyretin (TTR) carries thyroxine and facilitates the transport of RBP.[20,34] TTR has a high concentration of tryptophan, which exerts a key role in protein synthesis. The half-life of TTR is 2 days.[33] The short half-life and high tryptophan content make TTR a sensitive marker of protein deficiency.[20,34]

CLINICAL UTILITY AND LIMITATIONS. Use of TTR to monitor the efficacy of nutrition support is well documented in the literature.[28,33-38] TTR responds quickly to the onset of malnutrition and rises rapidly with adequate protein intake.[28,33,35] In patients who receive and tolerate optimal nutrition support, the TTR level may increase 4 mg/dl per week.[33] However, persistent sepsis, acute respiratory distress syndrome (ARDS), purulent abscesses, and similar clinical situations may blunt or prevent this increase.[2] Winkler and coworkers reported that plasma concentrations of TTR and RBP improved within the first week of nutrition support therapy and persisted throughout its administration.[36] Serum transferrin did not respond until the end of therapy. No significant difference was observed in serum albumin levels. Tuten and associates observed a significant increase in TTR levels in the presence of positive nitrogen balance in patients receiving nutrition support.[37] Others noted TTR to be a sensitive nutrition indicator and a valuable prognostic index for oncology patients.[39,40] Milano and colleagues observed a rapid drop in TTR 2 to 3 months before death.[40]

Boosalis' group found TTR to be more sensitive than albumin as a marker of nutrition support therapy in patients with head injuries;[21] however, these authors felt that the interval between initiation of therapy and change in TTR level diminished its clinical utility in this population. Despite their healthy premorbid state, these patients had depressed TTR and albumin levels on admission. TTR, like other plasma proteins, is a negative acute phase reactant and in these circumstances has limited value as a nutrition assessment tool.

Transthyretin is more expensive to measure than albumin, which is part of a multichemistry panel. However, Mears reports that screening using serum TTR may actually improve reimbursement well beyond the laboratory cost. With colleagues, she found that inclusion of TTR in an admission screening panel identified 44% of patients at nutritional risk, who would have been missed if evaluated by serum albumin alone.[38] After patient admission and during a proscribed nutrition repletion regimen, the investigators monitored TTR every 3 days until a goal of 25 mg/dl was reached. By identifying protein-calorie malnutrition and including it as part of the discharge diagnosis, the institution was able to obtain an additional $20,000 from Medicare reimbursement for 2 consecutive years.

INTERPRETATION OF SERUM LEVELS. Decreased levels of TTR are associated, in addition to stress, with hepatitis, liver failure, zinc deficiency, cirrhosis, and inflammation.[36] Some authors recommend following TTR and CRP levels to monitor the acuity of the inflammatory response. When CRP is at its height, TTR is likely to be at its nadir. As CRP falls, TTR should increase if nutrition support is adequate. The increase in TTR may correlate with positive nitrogen balance.[1] Higher levels of TTR are seen with dehydration and in renal failure because of altered degradation and excretion by the kidneys.[2,41,42] Decreased RBP breakdown may be indirectly responsible for the increase in serum TTR seen in renal failure;[41] however, in patients with stable renal function, a trend analysis of serum TTR levels may be appropriate for nutrition monitoring. Corticosteroid therapy stimulates TTR synthesis, raising serum concentrations independent of nutrition therapy.[2,33]

Retinol-Binding Protein

PHYSIOLOGY. RBP is a single polypeptide chain that circulates in plasma, with a half-life of 12 hours, as a TTR-RBP complex. RBP, synthesized in the liver, transports the alcohol form of vitamin A from the liver to peripheral tissues.[33]

CLINICAL UTILITY AND LIMITATIONS. Because of its short half-life and small body pool, RBP is considered a sensitive indicator of protein or calorie restriction and a marker of nutrition support adequacy.[35,36] The TTR-RBP complex responds in parallel with protein deficiency, and measurement of either TTR or RBP has been proposed as an early marker of prekwashiorkor and marasmus.[20] However, in clinical practice, measurement of TTR is preferred over RBP because its half-life is longer, and TTR is not as significantly affected by end-stage liver or chronic renal disease.[33]

INTERPRETATION OF SERUM LEVELS. Serum levels of RBP are decreased in hyperthyroidism, chronic liver disorders, cystic fibrosis, vitamin A deficiency, and stress.[31] A sharp elevation of RBP is also seen with renal disease because of reduced catabolism by the kidneys.[2,33,41,42] Figure 4-1 describes sequential protein markers tested in a 58-year-old man with renal disease.[43] Of note is the more dramatic rise in RBP, as compared with TTR ("prealbumin" in the figure). This figure also illustrates the importance of serial measurements and evaluation of the directional change in prealbumin and RBP, rather than interpretation of an isolated value.

C-Reactive Protein

PHYSIOLOGY. The exact function of CRP is not clear. What is known is that levels of this protein rise very early in acute stress (within 4 to 6 hours of surgery or trauma) and in heart disease and may increase up to 1000-fold.[24]

CLINICAL UTILITY AND LIMITATIONS. CRP rises until the catabolic phase of the stress response is over and falls rapidly with anabolism. Use of CRP in conjunction with TTR may "pinpoint" the optimal timing of aggressive nutrition support.

INTERPRETATION OF SERUM LEVELS. CRP has a wide reference range, 60 to 8000 µg/L, with the median value 500 µg/L. In mild inflammation and viral infections, the concentration increases to 10 to 40 mg/L; in acute inflammation and bacterial infections the concentration may rise quickly to 40 to 200 mg/L. In severe sepsis or trauma, serum concentration may exceed 300 mg/L.[24] CRP is elevated in rheumatoid arthritis and other connective tissue disorders. Slightly elevated levels may predict coronary events.[44]

Fibronectin

PHYSIOLOGY. Fibronectin (FN) is a glycoprotein in lymph, amniotic fluid, cerebrospinal fluid, interstitial matrix, and plasma.[45] Of the serum protein markers, FN is unique in that it is not synthesized exclusively in the liver.[33] Active synthesis of FN takes place in endothelial cells, peritoneal macrophages, hepatocytes, and fibroblasts. Plasma FN has multiple ligand-binding sites that facilitate its role in cell adhesion, cell and tissue differentiation, wound healing, microvascular integrity, and opsonization of particulate matter. Deposition in tissues, especially at sites of injury and inflammation, is characteristic of FN. Such deposition is very important to wound healing and maintenance of vascular permeability.[45] The large molecular weight of FN prevents its leakage from plasma during the capillary leak syndrome associated with acute

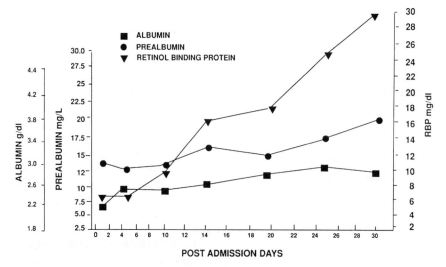

FIGURE 4-1 Serial levels of albumin, prealbumin (TTR), and retinol-binding protein (RBP). (From Spiekerman AM: Proteins used in nutritional assessment, *Clin Lab Med* 13[2]:359, 1993.)

inflammation. Its small extravascular pool means it does not readily return to plasma when blood concentrations decrease, as does serum albumin;[1] this makes interpretation of serum levels less subject to the effects of acute stress.

CLINICAL UTILITY AND LIMITATIONS. With a half-life of 12 hours, FN responds quickly to nutrition support and has been correlated with nitrogen balance and also with cumulative calorie and nitrogen intake.[46] Decreased levels of FN have been observed in malnutrition, burns, trauma, and sepsis as a result of decreased synthesis and deposition of FN in sites of injury and inflammation.[46] Studies in healthy volunteers have demonstrated decreases in plasma FN concentrations after fasting, which subsequently return to normal after refeeding.[47,48]

Mattox and colleagues evaluated use of serum FN and somatomedin C (SMC) as nutritional markers during enteral nutrition support in critically ill patients.[49] By day 7 of nutrition support, both FN and SMC concentrations increased significantly from baseline. SMC continued to rise and peaked by day 14; concentrations declined by day 21. Peak levels of FN were seen at day 7. Serum concentrations of FN on days 14 and 21 were not significantly different than the baseline value.

This response of FN has been reported by others.[50] Kirby and colleagues studied plasma FN in 27 patients receiving both parenteral and enteral nutrition support.[50] Plasma FN concentration significantly increased in all patients after 1 week of therapy; however, no significant changes were observed in subsequent weeks. In this study, plasma FN did not correlate with nitrogen balance, serum albumin, or total lymphocyte count. A correlation was observed between FN and transferrin. FN levels lack specificity and can be affected by the caloric and dextrose-lipid composition of the nutrition support regimen.[46]

INTERPRETATION OF SERUM LEVELS. Normal levels of plasma FN are shown in Table 4-3. As with other negative acute phase reactants, FN is not a reliable indicator of nutritional status in the presence of acute stress and inflammation. Low levels of FN, independent of nutritional status, may be the result of FN binding to actin, fibrin, deoxyribonucleic acid (DNA), or *Staphylococcus aureus*. Higher levels may be seen during administration of FN-rich cryoprecipitate or blood products;[46] a patient's coagulation status also affects FN levels.[49]

Somatomedin C

PHYSIOLOGY. SMC is a growth hormone–dependent growth peptide, synthesized in the liver, with a proinsulin-like structure and anabolic properties.[46] Levels of SMC are influenced by both hormone secretion and nutrient intake.[33,51] SMC in its bound form has a half-life of 2 to 4 hours and is not affected by circadian variation, acute stress, inflammatory response, or exercise.[33]

SMC mediates the growth-promoting effects of growth hormone and regulates biologic growth and anabolic activity. Biologic activities are related to the progression of cells from resting phase to active cell division. Anabolic activity is concerned with synthesis of protein and DNA precursors.[33,51]

CLINICAL UTILITY AND LIMITATIONS. SMC has been proposed as a sensitive marker of malnutrition and of the response to nutrition support.[52-54] Low levels of SMC are observed in malnourished patients and in fasted obese subjects, and significant increases are seen with refeeding.[52,53] Dietary fat, carbohydrate, and protein have varying effects on somatomedin activity. Unterman studied the utility of SMC and traditional nutrition indices (transferrin, albumin, lymphocytes) in the assessment of hospitalized, malnourished patients receiving nutrition support.[54] SMC was the only index that correlated with intake of protein and calories. SMC has been shown to positively correlate with nitrogen balance during stress and infections.[55]

INTERPRETATION OF SERUM LEVELS. The reference range for SMC is listed in Table 4-3. As with other indices of nutritional status, interpretation of serum SMC levels in nutrition support monitoring may be difficult in patients with liver, kidney, and autoimmune diseases.[33] Laboratory values are affected by the SMC-binding proteins and the extraction method used in testing.[2,33] Cost and available analytic methods limit use of SMC at present.[2]

Summary

In clinical practice, albumin appears most useful in screening, and TTR and transferrin are most useful for serial monitoring of patients receiving nutrition support. CRP measures the extent of the inflammatory response, while FN and SMC are potential measures of nutritional status and adequacy of therapy. Figure 4-2 shows serial changes in four visceral protein markers.[33] Nutrition intervention was initiated on day 2. Albumin remains unchanged while TTR (prealbumin), FN, and SMC increase during therapy.

Use of hepatic transport proteins and nitrogen balance in nutrition support monitoring requires concomitant evaluation of other factors that may affect interpretation. There is no single definitive marker of nutritional status or response to intervention. Formulate recommendations for nutrition therapy from a review of all available objective and subjective information and with sound clinical judgment.

Somatic Protein Assessment

Serum levels of albumin, transferrin, and other proteins reflect visceral protein status and physiologic stress level. Urinary creatinine excretion (and derived CHI) and urinary 3-MH excretion are indices of somatic (muscle) protein status. Unfortunately, both measures have limited application; neither is commonly used for determining lean body mass, for reasons detailed below.

Creatinine-Height Index

PHYSIOLOGY. Creatinine (Cr), formed at a constant daily rate of 1.7% from muscle creatine, is not retained by muscle but is distributed in total body water and cleared unaltered by the kidneys. Daily urine output of Cr can (under conditions of relatively constant muscle creatine) be used as a measure of total

TABLE 4-3

Reference Range of Potential Measures of Protein Status

Protein	Reference Range (mg/L)	Half-Life (hr)
Fibronectin	220-400	15
Somatomedin C	0.10-0.40	2

Data from Spiekerman AM: Nutritional assessment (protein nutriture), *Anal Chem* 67: 429R-436R, 1995.

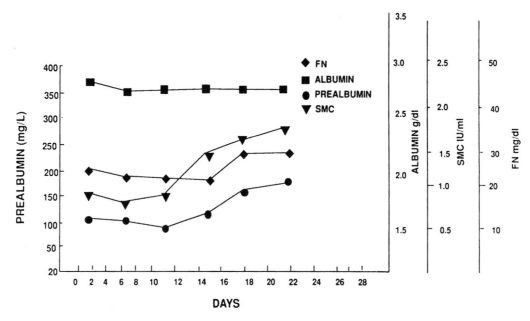

FIGURE 4-2 Serial changes in visceral proteins. Note that albumin remained unchanged, while prealbumin, fibronectin (FN), and somatomedin C (SMC) increased during the course of nutritional therapy. Nutritional intervention began on day 2. (Spiekerman AM: Proteins used in nutritional assessment, *Clin Lab Med* 13[2]:362, 1993).

body muscle mass. Population studies have demonstrated a good correlation between Cr output and lean body mass[56] One gram of excreted Cr is equivalent to approximately 17 to 20 kg of muscle.[57] On average, fat-free skeletal muscle comprises 49% of total fat-free weight (data from animal and human studies).[58] For persons on an unrestricted diet, lean body mass (LBM) in kilograms is 3.288 mmol per day Cr (0.0291 mg per day Cr) plus 7.38.[56] For persons on a meat-free diet, LBM (kg) is 2.723 mmol per day Cr (0.024 mg per day Cr) plus 20.7.[59]

These equations apply to young and middle-aged adults in good health but cannot be applied directly to children, the elderly, or ill persons of any age. Correlation coefficients for the two equations suggest that 97% and 91%, respectively, of intersubject variability in LBM can be accounted for by differences in urinary Cr excretion. Significant variations in Cr output can occur in individuals within a given population. Because muscle creatine concentration is the sum of creatine synthesized and dietary creatine (principally from meat), persons with different eating habits may have significantly different body creatine pools.[60] Use of urinary Cr excretion to assess muscle mass can thus produce significant errors. In addition, urine Cr can be affected by age and gender, and it is also subject to circadian variations[59] that can range from 1.4% to 36% over a 5-day collection period.[56] For this reason, abbreviated collections (i.e., 4 hours) are not indicated;[56] consecutive daily collections over 3 days are best to increase test accuracy.

EXPECTED VALUES. Creatinine excretion can be expressed in terms of height or body weight.[61] Expression in terms of height is considered more reliable because variations in body weight arise from different proportions of adipose tissue, or fluid imbalance.[61,62] Height is minimally affected by adult malnutrition, and Cr excretion continues to correlate with body cell mass, even with weight loss.[63] Average daily Cr excretion for men is 23 mg/kg ideal body weight; for women it is 17 to

18 mg/kg ideal body weight.[64] Imbembo and Walser[65] combined data from several studies (some of healthy persons, some hospitalized but without renal or hepatic dysfunction) conducted between 1963 and 1971 to derive an average regression equation for Cr excretion in milligrams per kilogram (y) as it varies with age (A) and gender.

Men: $y = 28.2 - 0.172A$
Women: $y = 21.9 - 0.115A$

Decreased Cr excretion with age results from three factors: decreased muscle mass per kilogram of body weight, decreased muscle creatine concentration, and possibly decreased meat consumption.[65] From the regression equations and ideal weight for height and frame size (based on the 1983 Metropolitan Life Insurance Company tables) expected urinary Cr excretion can be calculated for women and for men (Table 4-4).

EQUATION. The CHI compares measured Cr excretion for the subject to the expected excretion for persons of similar height and gender and is a laboratory method for assessing skeletal muscle (and, thus, somatic protein stores).[66]

$$CHI = \frac{\text{actual 24-hour urinary Cr excretion}}{\text{expected 24-hour urinary Cr excretion}} \times 100$$

INTERPRETATION. The CHI is expressed as a percentage of a standard, with a value of 90% to 100% considered to reflect normal muscle mass.[62] A CHI less than 80% suggests skeletal muscle depletion; 60% to 80%, moderate deficit in muscle mass; and less than 60%, severe deficit in muscle mass.[67]

LIMITATIONS. By far the most common source of error is incomplete urine collection, which occurs in metabolic general medical-surgical wards and in intensive care units.[68] An error as small as 15 minutes in a urine collection period may represent an error of 1% in urine Cr excretion; longer discrepancies in collection times could cause even more significant errors.[56]

Expected Creatinine Excretion (mg/day) in Men and Women of Ideal Weight

Height (cm)	Age (yr)						
	20-29	30-39	40-49	50-59	60-69	70-79	80-89
MEN							
146	1258	1169	1079	985	896	807	716
148	1284	1193	1102	1005	915	824	733
150	1308	1215	1123	1025	932	839	747
152	1334	1240	1145	1045	951	856	762
154	1358	1262	1166	1064	968	872	775
156	1390	1291	1193	1089	990	892	793
158	1423	1322	1222	1115	1014	913	812
160	1452	1349	1240	1132	1035	932	829
162	1481	1376	1271	1160	1055	950	845
164	1510	1403	1296	1183	1076	969	862
166	1536	1427	1318	1203	1094	986	877
168	1565	1454	1343	1226	1115	1004	893
170	1598	1485	1372	1252	1139	1026	912
172	1632	1516	1401	1278	1163	1047	932
174	1666	1548	1430	1305	1167	1069	951
176	1699	1579	1458	1331	1211	1090	970
178	1738	1615	1491	1361	1238	1115	992
180	1781	1655	1529	1395	1269	1143	1017
182	1819	1690	1561	1425	1296	1167	1038
184	1855	1724	1592	1450	1322	1190	1059
186	1894	1759	1625	1483	1349	1215	1081
188	1932	1795	1658	1513	1377	1240	1103
190	1968	1829	1689	1542	1402	1263	1123
WOMEN							
140	858	804	754	700	651	597	548
142	877	822	771	716	666	610	560
144	898	841	790	733	682	625	573
146	917	859	806	749	696	638	586
148	940	881	827	768	713	654	600
150	964	903	848	787	732	671	615
152	984	922	865	803	747	685	628
154	1003	940	882	819	761	698	640
156	1026	961	902	838	779	714	655
158	1049	983	922	856	796	730	670
160	1073	1006	944	877	815	747	686
162	1100	1031	966	899	835	766	703
164	1125	1064	990	919	854	783	719
166	1148	1076	1010	938	871	799	733
168	1173	1099	1032	958	890	817	749
170	1199	1124	1055	980	911	835	766
172	1224	1147	1077	1000	929	853	782
174	1253	1174	1102	1023	951	872	800
176	1280	1199	1126	1045	972	891	817
178	1304	1223	1147	1065	990	908	833
180	1331	1248	1171	1087	1011	927	850

Adapted from Walser M, Imbembo AL, Margolis S, Elfert G (eds): *Nutritional management: the Johns Hopkins handbook*, Philadelphia, 1984, WB Saunders, p 24.

Creatinine excretion declines with age, presumably because of decreasing muscle mass, but standard values for excretion in persons older than 55 years have not been developed,[63] in part because of the variable decrease in height in elders secondary to spinal changes and narrowing of cartilage that bears weight.[69] Even if standards for the elderly were available, their application would be difficult because of problems in measur-ing height of elders who are bedridden or unable to stand up straight.[70] In fact, obtaining an accurate height is a problem in nearly all hospitalized patients, not only the elderly. Without an accurate height, the CHI is useless.[70]

Emotional stress, catabolism, rhabdomyolysis, bed rest, strenuous exercise, and the second half of the menstrual cycle can cause increases in urinary Cr, as can addition of meat to a previously meat-free diet, or after starvation.[70] Sepsis, trauma, and fever can significantly increase urinary Cr: elevations of 20% to 100% over normal values are seen in patients in the initial posttrauma stage.[71] Compromised renal function, low urine output for any reason, and muscle atrophy unrelated to malnutrition can decrease measured urinary Cr, resulting in an unreliable CHI value.

CLINICAL UTILITY. CHI was proposed in 1970 as a method for assessment of recovery of malnourished children or for detection of marginal malnutrition.[72] Unfortunately, little research has been done over the last 25 years to support recommendation of this assessment tool today. The reasons include the following: (1) difficulties inherent in accurate 24-hour urine collection (particularly the recommended 3-day collection); (2) inability of standard tables to account for Cr excretion changes associated with age, disease, physical training, drug therapy, or metabolic state;[73] (3) use of medium-frame, ideal-weight tables for calculation of standard Cr excretion values (failing to consider the wide range of body habitus in both healthy and ill adults);[54] and (4) unavailability of sufficient data in the literature from which to calculate percentiles.[63]

There is no valid, reasonably priced, and readily available method for measuring muscle mass as a means of validating the CHI, so its reliability in humans is difficult to assess.[74,75] Initial weight gain during nutrition therapy (no matter how appropriate) may be principally water and fat, rather than lean body mass, with very little resultant change in CHI.[76] Bedridden patients will not develop much lean body mass because of the absence of weight-bearing activity. An increase in CHI is not seen in these patients even with adequate nutrition support.[77] The effect on muscle mass accretion of range of motion activities or other bed-bound types of physical therapy is not known. In the anabolic stage of recovery (not often seen in hospitalized patients who are discharged early to "less acute" facilities) as gluconeogenesis ceases, a modest increase in CHI may occur.[76]

Direct measures of body composition (e.g., neutron activation analysis and total body count of isotopes such as potassium-40) have been validated for longitudinal assessment of body composition. This expensive technology is confined principally to research centers and is impractical for routine clinical use.[78]

3-Methylhistidine

PHYSIOLOGY. Measurement of urine 3-MH excretion is used to assess muscle protein metabolism. Methylhistidine is a modified amino acid found in actin and myosin of muscle. When myofibrillar protein is catabolized, 3-MH is not reused for protein synthesis but is excreted in the urine.[79] The amount of urinary 3-MH serves as a measure of muscle protein turnover or somatic protein reserves.[80]

EXPECTED VALUES. Reported values of urinary 3-MH excretion in healthy adults range from 1.3 ± 0.1 to 7.8 ± 0.4 μmol/kg per day;[81] traumatized or septic adults excrete 6.3 ± 0.7 (females) and 11.8 ± 2.2 μmol/kg per day (males).[82]

CLINICAL UTILITY AND LIMITATIONS. In spite of its theoretic value as a measure of muscle mass, the clinical use of 3-MH is confounded by several factors. The subject must abstain from meat for several days to eliminate 3-MH from dietary sources. The correlation between 3-MH excretion, lean body mass, muscle mass, and total body fat-free mass is high ($r > 0.8$) in normal persons who eat no meat for 3 days.[81,82] This limitation does not affect persons receiving parenteral or most forms of enteral nutrition; however, they would not be considered "normal" as compared with the subjects measured in studies cited above. Some endogenous 3-MH is derived from cardiac and smooth muscle; not all comes from skeletal muscle.[79] Turnover of gastrointestinal tract muscle can exceed that of skeletal muscle by 20%.[83] Methylhistidine is present only in myofibrillar protein, not in the sarcoplasmic protein that is the constituent of approximately one third of skeletal muscle protein.[84] Excretion of 3-MH in nutritional depletion states varies with the type of depletion (protein versus protein and calories). With protein depletion, 3-MH output declines steadily and does not rise until repleted through a protein-rich diet, suggesting muscle conservation.[79] With protein-calorie deficiency, however, 3-MH output initially increases (most likely because carbon is needed for gluconeogenesis), then decreases as fat stores are tapped.[85] Excretion of 3-MH varies with age and hormone status.[79] In laboratory animals insulin therapy decreases output of 3-MH.[86] Thyroxine secretion, corticosteroid secretion under stress,[87] trauma, and infection increase 3-MH output, as does presence of more lean body mass. All of these factors must be considered when evaluating changes in 3-MH excretion.[86]

Clinical use of 3-MH as a measure of protein turnover and somatic muscle stores is limited by lack of standards for interpretation[82] and need for labor-intensive laboratory assay procedures.[1] In addition, the day-to-day variation of 3-MH is thought to be very high,[88] although this observation has not been studied thoroughly.

Estimation of Protein Requirements

Nitrogen Balance

Nitrogen balance is the only biochemical measurement that reflects the status of both the somatic and visceral protein pools.[1] A valid nitrogen balance finding is a sensitive and specific monitor of the adequacy of nutrition support and a marker of physiologic stress.[32] Calculation of nitrogen balance is shown in Box 4-2. Nitrogen balance is equal to nitrogen input (which is calculated by dividing protein intake by the factor 6.25 for most formulations) minus nitrogen output. The percentage of protein as nitrogen in some parenteral and enteral formulations varies; consult product information for specifics. Calculation of nitrogen balance for patients consuming food orally may be challenging outside of a metabolic ward.

INTERPRETATION. Negative nitrogen balance indicates protein catabolism, and positive balance generally correlates with net protein synthesis. A frequently stated goal of nutrition support intervention is a positive nitrogen balance of 2 to 4 g of nitrogen per day. This is very difficult to achieve in critically ill patients.

BOX 4-2

Nitrogen Balance Calculation

Nitrogen balance = Nitrogen intake − Nitrogen output

$$\frac{\text{24-hr protein intake (g)} - (\text{24-hr UUN (g)} + 4\ g^{\dagger})}{6.25^{*}}$$

$$\frac{\text{24-hr protein intake (g)} - (\text{24-hr TUN (g)} + 2\ g^{\dagger})}{6.25^{*}}$$

Adapted from Russell M: Serum proteins and nitrogen balance. Evaluating response to nutrition support, *Support Line*, XVII:3-8, 1995.
TUN, Total urea nitrogen; *UUN*, urinary urea nitrogen.
*Most protein sources contain 16% nitrogen. Check source for exact amount.
†Estimate of fecal, dermal, miscellaneous, and nonurea nitrogen losses.

In these patients, nitrogen losses can exceed 30 g per day as a result of increased catabolism related to cytokine release and the physiologic response to injury, immobilization, and infection.[3] Minimizing nitrogen loss is a more realistic goal, along with physical therapy and/or muscle stimulation as possible and provision of appropriate calories to minimize protein use as an energy source.[3] As the metabolic stress response subsides, positive nitrogen balance may be a feasible goal.

CLINICAL UTILITY AND LIMITATIONS. Many factors can affect nitrogen balance calculations (Box 4-3).[89,90] A true nitrogen output determination would require measurement of the nitrogen content of urine, feces, sweat, and wounds, as well as sloughed skin, hair, and nails. In clinical practice, urine is the sample most often collected. Urinary urea nitrogen (UUN) is assumed to represent 80% to 90% of total urea nitrogen (TUN) in healthy, nonstressed persons.[91] Investigators have proposed several different factors for estimating nonurea losses and nitrogen losses from stool, skin, and miscellaneous sources. A factor of 2 to 4 g added to UUN, as reported by Blackburn and coworkers, is commonly used to estimate nonmeasured nitrogen losses.[66] Konstantinides recommended that a factor of 25% be added to UUN to account for the nonurea component of the urine and another factor for nitrogen losses from stool and

---

BOX 4-3

Factors That Influence Nitrogen Balance Determination/Calculations

Incontinence, spills, timing of sample
Losses from skin, sweat, hair, nails, blood draws, menstruation
Body fluid losses from nasogastric tube, paracentesis, peritoneal dialysis, surgical drains
Gastrointestinal losses
Draining wounds and fistulas
Thermal injury or exfoliative disease
Renal disease
Immobility
Hormone or steroid therapy
Nutrient composition of feedings
Equilibration after change in protein intake or provision

Data from Shopbell J, Hopkins B, Shronts E: Nutrition screening and assessment. In Gottschlich M (ed): *The science and practice of nutrition support: a case-based core curriculum*, Dubuque, IA, 2001, ASPEN/Kendall Hunt, pp 107-140; Murray RL: Protein and energy requirements. In Krey SH, Murray RL (eds): Dynamics of nutrition support, Norwalk, CT, 1986, Appleton-Century-Crofts, pp 188-192.

skin.[91] Burge proposed that UUN plus measurement of urinary ammonia provides a more reliable estimate of TUN than does UUN alone.[92] In that study of patients receiving nutrition support, UUN alone accounted for 90% and the combination of UUN plus ammonia for 96% of TUN. To estimate nitrogen losses in pediatric patients, Maldonado and coworkers suggested the following formula:[93]

[UUN (g/L)/2 × urine volume (L)] + 0.8 g

A significant amount of nitrogen may be lost (and unaccounted for) in patients with draining wounds. Nitrogen losses can be estimated using the following factors:[94]

<10% open wound = 0.02 g nitrogen per kilogram per day

11% to 30% open wound = 0.05 g nitrogen per kilogram per day

>31% open wound = 0.12 g nitrogen per kilogram per day

Measurement of TUN is not available in many hospital laboratories; UUN is most commonly used to determine nitrogen balance. Loder and coworkers studied the relationship between UUN and TUN in three groups: (1) nutritionally depleted preoperative, (2) nonseptic postoperative, and (3) stressed intensive care patients.[95] UUN accurately approximated TUN in only the first group. Patients in the other two groups excreted much more nonurea nitrogen, so UUN was less useful in these patients as an index of total nitrogen excretion. Helms and colleagues concluded from a study of postsurgical, preterm neonates receiving parenteral nutrition support that actual measurements are required for accurate nitrogen balance assessments.[96] UUN measurement showed wide intrapatient and interpatient variability; this resulted in significant underestimation of nitrogen loss. In a retrospective study by Konstantinides and colleagues, nitrogen balance values calculated with UUN were compared with direct measurement of TUN.[97] In this surgical and trauma population, the UUN-TUN ratio for the entire population was 80.0% ± 12.0% (range, 12% to 112%). Based on these numbers, if UUN values are substituted for TUN in nitrogen balance equations, an error of as much as 12 g per day could result. Grimble and colleagues also reported variances in the UUN-TUN ratio in adult surgical patients fed enterally or parenterally.[98] Patients receiving enteral nutrition had UUN-TUN ratios from 57% to 109% and those fed parenterally had ratios from 25% to 95%; in healthy and fasted subjects the UUN-TUN ratios were 87% and 84%, respectively. As the degree of stress increased, the variability in UUN-TUN ratio became progressively larger.[91,95,98] Actual measurement of TUN is more accurate and is preferred over UUN for use in balance studies.

Clinicians now have the opportunity to measure nitrogen via pyrochemiluminescence (PCL), which is safer and more cost effective than the traditional Kjeldahl procedure.[91,98] The availability of TUN assessment, however, remains a limiting factor for many, although some national laboratories do offer the test and a quick turnaround time. The clinician must be aware of the inherent drawbacks and disadvantages of using UUN to estimate TUN in nitrogen balance calculations. As with all potential indicators of nutrition status, evaluate nitrogen balance results in conjunction with other nutrition parameters and the clinical status of the patient.

Urea Kinetics

Determination of nitrogen balance in the absence of renal failure is relatively straightforward, if a complete urine sample is obtained. It is more complex in patients with compromised renal function, but it is still valuable for monitoring and evaluating nutrition support of patients with kidney disease.[99]

DEFINITION. Urea kinetic modeling is a single-pool pharmacokinetic model originally developed for use in hemodialysis patients.[100,101] Its use for determining nitrogen balance in acutely ill patients with varying degrees of renal function was first proposed in the early 1980s.[102,103] Current applications include determination of optimal daily protein intake; management of nutrition therapy in chronic renal failure;[99,102,104,105] and, less commonly, monitoring of nutrition support in critically ill patients.

BACKGROUND. The urea kinetic model relates the principles of mass balance to blood urea nitrogen (BUN), net urea nitrogen generation, and renal function. The model proposed by Sargent and colleagues[106] is based on the direct relationship of protein catabolic rate (PCR), in grams per 24 hours, to rate of urea nitrogen generation (GUN) in milligrams per minute. This relationship is expressed as:

$$\text{PCR (g/24 hr)} = [\text{GUN (mg/min)} + 1.2] \times 9.35$$

Comparison of PCR to total protein intake can be used to determine nitrogen balance.[90] Calculation of nitrogen balance via GUN and PCR requires extensive data collection using a flowsheet or personal digital assistant and software to facilitate the calculations. GUN is expressed as the amount of serum urea nitrogen multiplied by the volume of serum cleared by the kidney (or total body water), to which is added UUN.[90] A fundamental assumption of this model is that urea is equally distributed in total body water (TBW).[105] TBW of normal adults can be estimated from a nomogram,[107] using the subject's dry weight.[90] The weight of accumulated fluid associated with edema or ascites is added to the value determined from the nomogram. A less precise method for estimating TBW is to multiply body weight in kilograms by 0.58 for males and by 0.55 for females.[106] This method, however, fails to account for changes in TBW that occur with age and changes in body fat.[90] Whitmire reports a wide variation in TBW, relative to age, gender, and relative proportion of lean body mass to adipose tissue.[108] TBW as a percentage of body weight varies from 80% in premature infants to 42% in an obese adult female; average values for adult males and females are 60% and 50%, respectively.[109]

Determination of PCR allows the clinician to assess the amount of protein needed to obtain neutral, or slightly positive, nitrogen balance. Each gram of protein catabolized (and not used for anabolism) results in the production of 0.154 of urea nitrogen, which either remains in body water or is excreted.[102,103] This degree of urea production occurs only when net protein catabolism exceeds 11 g per day. The catabolized protein makes up for fecal nitrogen losses and for production of nitrogenous compounds such as Cr, uric acid, and ammonia.[101,102]

EQUATIONS. The following list describes the terms used to calculate GUN.[90] (Note the respective units of measure.)

KrUN   Residual urea clearance by the kidney (ml/min)

UUN   Urine urea nitrogen concentration (mg/ml)

BUN	Serum urea nitrogen (mg/ml)
U_v	Volume of urine collection (ml)
t	Time interval of urine collection (min)
V_u	Estimated urea volume of body water (ml)
θ	Time interval between blood samples (min)
BUN_1	Postdialysis BUN (mg/ml)
BUN_2	Predialysis BUN (mg/ml)
V_{u1}	Urea volume of dry body weight (ml)
V_{u2}	V_{u1} + interdialysis weight gain (ml)
$\overline{BUN}$	Mean BUN

$$\frac{BUN_1 + BUN_2}{2} \text{ (mg/ml)}$$

As Murray suggested in her classic description,[90] four different clinical situations can lend themselves to application of the principles of urea kinetics.

1. Nondialyzed, nutritionally stable patients with progressive renal failure but relatively stable BUN
   a. Calculate KrUN

   $$KrUN = \frac{UUN}{\overline{BUN}} \times \frac{Uv}{t}$$

   b. Calculate GUN

   $$GUN = BUN \times KrUN$$

   c. Calculate PCR

   $$PCR = (GUN + 1.2) \times 9.35$$

2. Nondialyzed, catabolic (nutritionally unstable) patient, with rapidly rising BUN
   a. Calculate KrUN

   $$KrUN = \frac{UUN}{\overline{BUN}} \times \frac{Uv}{t}$$

   b. Calculate GUN

   $$GUN = \frac{(BUN_2 - BUN_1)(V_u) + (\overline{BUN} \times KrUN)}{\theta}$$

   c. Calculate PCR

   $$PCR = (GUN + 1.2) \times 9.35$$

3. Dialyzed patient without urea nitrogen loss in urine (anuric patient)
   a. Calculate GUN

   $$GUN = \frac{(V_{u2} \times BUN_2) - (V_{u1} \times BUN_1)}{\theta}$$

   b. Calculate PCR

   $$PCR = (GUN + 1.2) \times 9.35$$

4. Dialyzed patient with urea nitrogen losses in urine
   a. Calculate KrUN

   $$KrUN = \frac{UUN}{\overline{BUN}} \times \frac{Uv}{t}$$

b. Calculate GUN

$$GUN = \frac{(BUN_2 + V_{u2}) - (BUN_1 \times V_{u1})}{\theta} + (\overline{BUN} \times KrUN)$$

c. Calculate PCR

$$PCR = (GUN + 1.2) \times 9.35$$

INTERPRETATION. Protein balance equals protein intake minus PCR minus losses.[104] Converting this equation to one for nitrogen balance requires dividing all components by 6.25, the average amount of protein to yield 1 g of nitrogen.[101] Determination of PCR by way of urea kinetic modeling can help identify hemodialysis patients with suboptimal protein intake. Repeat PCR values below 1 g/kg body weight per day generally indicate inadequate protein intake;[110] however, PCR is not a measure of protein catabolism because protein degradation in humans far exceeds protein intake. Isotope dilution studies have shown that protein synthesis and catabolism may each equal 45 to 55 of nitrogen daily (equivalent to the protein in 1 to 1.5 kg of muscle).[111] In situations where hypercatabolism of protein exists, provision of protein in amounts greater than 1.5 g/kg does not reduce the catabolism but rather contributes to increased excretion of nitrogenous waste.[112]

In the acutely ill patient with normal renal function, nitrogen balance determined via urea kinetics correlates closely[99,113] with balance determined by conventional methods.[66] As renal function declines, the correlation between the two methods decreases because the conventional nitrogen balance technique does not account for renal insufficiency or changes in the urea pool.

Leblanc and colleagues proposed a method using urea nitrogen appearance (UnA) and normalized protein catabolic rate (nPCR) to quantify the protein catabolic response in ICU patients. They observed a positive correlation between UnA and Cr production rate, a poor correlation between serum albumin and lean body mass/body weight, a weak relation to clinical outcome of UnA and nPCR, and a wide variance in UnA in critically ill patients with acute renal failure.[114]

Kosanovich and colleagues showed that progressive increases in energy intake with constant protein intake resulted in improved nitrogen balance; however, these studies were not performed in a steady state of protein balance and urea metabolism.[99] Particularly in critically ill patients, provision of energy in excess of needs may result in CO_2 retention, hepatic steatosis, or other undesirable consequences.

Nutritional Anemias

A complete nutrition assessment includes screening for nutritional anemia (one of the most common medical problems worldwide). Deficiencies of iron, folic acid, or vitamin B_{12} can be caused by malnutrition, alcoholism, growth, or pregnancy, and by various chronic diseases. The nutrition support dietitian should have a working knowledge of the manifestations of these anemias and an excellent reference for quick access when specific questions arise.[115]

Background

Anemia is a condition in which a deficiency in the size or number of erythrocytes or their hemoglobin content limits oxygen and carbon dioxide exchange between blood and tissue cells.[115] Anemias are classified, on the basis of hemoglobin content and cell size, as macrocytic, hypochromic-microcytic, or normochromic-normocytic (Table 4-5). Causes of these anemias include chronic disease, drug therapy, hemorrhage, genetic abnormalities, and nutritional deficiencies. Nutritional anemias are caused by a lack of one or more nutrients required for normal erythrocyte synthesis.[115] A deficiency can arise from inadequate consumption, absorption, or utilization of a nutrient or increased utilization, excretion, or destruction.[116] To characterize an anemia as *nutritional* requires both of the following features: (1) lack of a specific nutrient must produce the anemia, and (2) provision of the nutrient must correct it. By this definition there are only three simple nutritional anemias: those due to lack of iron, vitamin B_{12}, or folic acid.[117] These, along with the anemia of chronic disease, are reviewed. Other nutrition-related anemias include copper deficiency anemia (seen in infants fed cow's milk, or adults with malabsorption or receiving copper-free parenteral nutrition) and sideroblastic (pyridoxine-responsive) anemia, caused by an inherited defect in an enzyme involved in heme synthesis.[115]

To help differentiate the nutritional causes of anemia, the complete blood count (CBC) is useful. Microcytic anemia is most often associated with iron deficiency, while deficiencies of folate or B_{12} result in macrocytic anemia. However, because the CBC is not specific, additional data are needed. Leukocyte and platelet counts, if low, suggest bone marrow failure; if high, anemia or infection. The reticulocyte count increases anytime red blood cell production increases. When this value is high, look for bleeding or hemolysis as possible causes of anemia.[1]

Rarely, if ever, are the nutritional anemias a compelling concern in the nutrition support of critically ill patients. Nonetheless, an understanding of the basic biochemical and hematologic background and the nutritional implications and treatment of these anemias is important. Nutrition support dietitians should be able to help differentiate nutritional anemias from those due to other causes.[1] Anemias complicate many diseases, and more than one type can be present simultaneously.[118] They may be identified in the initial nutrition assessment or discovered while monitoring results of nutrition support in a long-term care facility or in the home. Progress in

TABLE 4-5

Morphologic Classification of Anemia

Morphologic Type	Underlying Abnormality	Clinical Syndromes	Treatment
Macrocytic (MCV >94, MCHC >31)			
Megaloblastic	Vitamin B_{12} deficiency	Pernicious anemia	Vitamin B_{12}
	Folic acid deficiency	Nutritional megaloblastic anemias, sprue, and other malabsorption syndromes	Folic acid
	Inherited disorders of DNA synthesis	Orotic aciduria	According to nature of disorder
	Drug-induced disorders of DNA synthesis	Chemotherapeutic agents, anticonvulsants, oral contraceptives	Stop offending drug and administer folic acid
Nonmegaloblastic	Accelerated erythropoiesis	Hemolytic anemia	Treatment of underlying disease
	Increased membrane surface area		
	Obscure		
Hypochromic-microcytic (MCV <80, MCHC <31)			
	Iron deficiency	Chronic loss of blood, inadequate diet, impaired absorption, increased demands	Ferrous sulfate and correction of underlying cause
	Disorders of globin synthesis	Thalassemia	Nonspecific
	Disorders of porphyrin and heme synthesis	Pyridoxine-responsive anemia	Pyridoxine
	Other disorders of iron metabolism		
Normochromic-normocytic (MCV 82-92, MCHC >30)			
	Recent blood loss	Various	Transfusion, iron
			Correct underlying condition
	Overexpansion of plasma volume	Pregnancy	Restore homeostasis
		Overhydration	
	Hemolytic diseases		According to nature of disorder
	Hypoplastic bone marrow	Aplastic anemia	Transfusions
		Pure red blood cell aplasia	Androgens
	Infiltrated bone marrow	Leukemia, multiple myeloma, myelofibrosis	Chemotherapy
	Endocrine abnormality	Hypothyroidism, adrenal insufficiency	
	Chronic disorders		Treatment of underlying disease
	Renal disease	Renal disease	
	Liver disease	Cirrhosis	

From Mahan LK, Escott-Stump S (eds): *Krause's food, nutrition, and diet therapy*, ed 10, Philadelphia, 2000, WB Saunders, p 782; as adapted from Wintrobe MM, et al: *Clinical hematology*, ed 8, Philadelphia, 1981, Lea & Febiger.
MCV (mean corpuscular volume), volume of one red blood cell expressed in femtoliters (fl): *MCHC* (mean corpuscular hemoglobin concentration), concentration of hemoglobin expressed in grams per deciliter (dl).

treatment of existing anemias can be monitored with greater understanding if the pathophysiology of the underlying disease is understood.

Iron-Deficiency Anemia (Hypochromic, Microcytic)

PREVALENCE. Iron deficiency, the most prevalent nutrition deficiency in the world,[119] is a condition in which the total body iron is inadequate for the formation of hemoglobin, iron enzymes, and other iron-containing compounds. This condition responds to iron therapy, in contrast to conditions in which the iron supply to the developing red blood cell is insufficient (such as the anemia of chronic disease).[1,120] Dietary iron deficiency is most common in infants and small children, who grow fast,[119] and in menstruating females. In adults, iron deficiency can result from a diet inadequate in heme iron (such as vegetarian); increased losses (menses or chronic bleeding from hemorrhoids, ulcer, cancer, or parasitic infection); increased requirements (pregnancy, lactation);[119,120] or defective release of iron stores because of chronic inflammation or other disorders, drug interference, or impaired absorption (diarrhea, achlorhydria, celiac disease).[115] Iron deficiency can develop after gastric bypass surgery for morbid obesity, gastrectomy, vagotomy with gastroenterostomy, or Billroth II procedure[119] because of reduced gastric acidity, rapid intestinal transit, and loss of the gastric secretions essential for absorption. Iron deficiency, regardless of the cause, develops from a disturbance in an essentially closed, carefully conserved system of iron metabolism.

STAGES OF DEVELOPMENT. The sequential stages of iron status, from normal to overload on the positive side and from normal to deficient on the negative side, were eloquently described by Herbert (Fig. 4-3).[121] Iron deficiency, the end result of a long period of negative iron balance, develops in three stages: depletion of stores (ferritin and hemosiderin), deficiency of erythropoiesis, and anemia.

DIAGNOSIS. Several laboratory tests are available to help diagnose iron deficiency. *Hemoglobin* alone is not an appropriate tool for the diagnosis of iron deficiency because of its delayed response to iron deficiency, nonspecificity for the type of anemia, and wide variations among normal subjects; however, it may be a useful screening tool. Reduction in hemoglobin synthesis rate results in the production of smaller (microcytic), less hemoglobin-dense (hypochromic) cells (see Table 4-5).

Serum iron is insensitive to the early stages of iron depletion and may even be normal in mild anemia. A level below 60 g/dl indicates severe depletion. Pregnancy, menstruation, recent ingestion of iron, hepatitis, time of day, or iron contamination of needles or glassware may affect the level.[121] Serum iron significantly varies day-to-day even in healthy people.[1] *Percent*

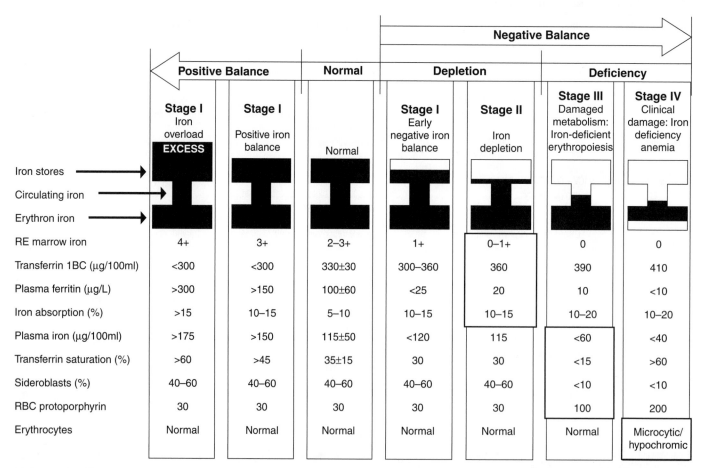

	Positive Balance		Normal	Depletion		Deficiency	
	Stage I Iron overload EXCESS	Stage I Positive iron balance	Normal	Stage I Early negative iron balance	Stage II Iron depletion	Stage III Damaged metabolism: Iron-deficient erythropoiesis	Stage IV Clinical damage: Iron deficiency anemia
RE marrow iron	4+	3+	2–3+	1+	0–1+	0	0
Transferrin 1BC (µg/100ml)	<300	<300	330±30	300–360	360	390	410
Plasma ferritin (µg/L)	>300	>150	100±60	<25	20	10	<10
Iron absorption (%)	>15	10–15	5–10	10–15	10–15	10–20	10–20
Plasma iron (µg/100ml)	>175	>150	115±50	<120	115	<60	<40
Transferrin saturation (%)	>60	>45	35±15	30	30	<15	>60
Sideroblasts (%)	40–60	40–60	40–60	40–60	40–60	<10	<10
RBC protoporphyrin	30	30	30	30	30	100	200
Erythrocytes	Normal	Normal	Normal	Normal	Normal	Normal	Microcytic/ hypochromic

FIGURE 4-3 Sequential stages of iron status. *RE,* Reticuloendothelial cells; *TIBC,* total iron-binding capacity; *RBC,* red blood cell. (From Herbert V, et al: Vitamin C-driven free radical generation from iron, *J Nutr* 126:1214S, 1996. Copyright 1990, 1995 by Victor Herbert.)

iron absorption increases with development of deficiency (as well as overload) but is not specific for the individual stages. *Total iron binding capacity (TIBC)* depends on the number of free binding sites on the transferring molecule.[1] TIBC increases in iron deficiency, hepatitis, hypoxemia, pregnancy, and in the presence of therapy with oral contraceptive agents or estrogen replacement therapy. The normal range reportedly varies, 47 to 70 µmol/L[119] or 28 to 56 µg/L.[1] TIBC falls in malignant disease, nephrosis, inflammatory disease, and megaloblastic or hemolytic anemia.[1]

Transferrin saturation (serum iron divided by total iron-binding capacity) measures iron supply to tissues. This indicator falls when the amount of stored iron available for release to transferrin drops and when dietary iron intake is low.[1] Levels below 16% are insufficient for red cell production. Transferrin saturation is more specific for iron status than hemoglobin or hematocrit, but as with many of the others is not a "perfect" indicator of iron status.[1] *Ferritin* is a storage protein for iron.[1] Its concentration is directly proportional to body iron stores. Serum ferritin levels below 10 ng/ml specifically indicate prelatent iron deficiency[119] in the absence of chronic infection, nonspecific inflammatory bowel disease, cancer, or chronic liver disease. Because ferritin is an acute-phase reactant, its level increases in the presence of inflammation. *Zinc (or erythrocyte) protoporphyrin-heme ratio (ZnPP/heme)* measures iron supply to developing red blood cells. When iron available for incorporation into porphyrin is insufficient, zinc is substituted. This molecule does not bind oxygen.[115] Iron deficiency results in an increased ZnPP-heme ratio, but the test cannot distinguish between anemia due to iron deficiency and that caused by lead poisoning or chronic inflammation.[1] *Serum transferrin receptor (sTfR)* is a relatively new test for iron deficiency that is not affected by presence of inflammation.[1] This protein binds holotransferrin (transferrin plus Fe(III)) during cellular iron uptake, resulting in a drop in cellular iron levels as sTfR increases.[1] Serum transferrin receptor monitors iron status effectively in normal individuals and in patients with iron overload or inflammation and/or infection;[1,122] it may replace ferritin as a sensitive, specific, and reliable indicator of iron status.[122]

Bone marrow aspirate (fixed and stained with Prussian blue) can be evaluated for the presence of hemosiderin, a dense aggregate of ferritin and a storage form of iron. Marrow hemosiderin stores are graded from 0 to 6+, and a good correlation is observed between this grading and the marrow iron content (which is normally 4+ to 5+) in iron deficiency and the anemia of chronic disease.[123] Because this procedure is quite invasive, its use in routine diagnosis of iron deficiency should be limited.[1]

Megaloblastic Anemias Caused by Folic Acid or Vitamin B$_{12}$ Deficiency

DESCRIPTION. Megaloblastic anemia is characterized, on a blood film, by macroovalocytosis (large, oval shape) of erythrocytes and hypersegmentation (presence of multiple nuclear lobes) of granulocytes, particularly neutrophils. These distinctive cells, the morphologic expression of retarded DNA synthesis, are caused most often by deficiency of folic acid (pteroylglutamic acid) or vitamin B$_{12}$ (cyanocobalamin), or both.[117] Folic acid deficiency appears within 2 to 4 months of

cessation of folate ingestion and/or absorption.[115] In contrast, B$_{12}$ deficiency does not occur for 3 to 6 years after cessation of B$_{12}$ absorption, and not until 20 to 30 years after cessation of B$_{12}$ ingestion (Box 4-4).[117]

ETIOLOGY. Causes of megaloblastic anemias are summarized in Box 4-5 and are reviewed in more detail elsewhere.[115,117] Folic acid deficiency anemia, most common in pregnant women (nearly a third of them, worldwide), also affects infants of deficient mothers, alcoholics, narcotics addicts, and patients with tropical sprue.[115,117] It is most often caused by inadequate absorption and utilization of folic acid, prolonged dietary deficiency, or increased demands of growth.[115] B$_{12}$ deficiency (pernicious anemia) is most often observed in patients with gastric disorders, owing to insufficient or absent secretion of intrinsic factor, a glycoprotein in gastric juice that is required for B$_{12}$ absorption, or with small bowel disorders such as gluten-sensitive enteropathy or regional enteritis.[117] It is also seen, though rarely, in strict vegetarians.[115,117]

DIAGNOSIS. Plasma homocysteine rises with B$_{12}$, folate, and B$_6$ deficiencies, so this indicator is not useful for differentiation among the anemias. Measurements of serum B$_{12}$, serum folate, and red blood cell folate are needed to attribute an anemia to folic acid deficiency. Folic acid deficiency anemia is diagnosed on blood film by large (macrocytic), immature (megaloblastic) red blood cells and decreased platelet and leukocyte counts and is characterized by very low levels of both serum folate (less than 3 ng/ml) and red cell folate (less than 140 ng/ml). Red blood cell folate is the superior measure of folate nutrition because it reflects folate status at the time the red cells were formed.[115] Serum B$_{12}$ is normal, and formiminoglutamate (FIGlu) excretion is significantly increased[115,124] in megaloblastic anemia.

FIGlu is an intermediate in the conversion of histidine to glutamate. The final step in this pathway is the formation of glutamate from FIGlu by transfer of the formimino group to tetrahydrofolate (which plays an important role in the synthesis of guanine, adenine, and thymine, which are used for formation of DNA and RNA). In folate deficiency, this step is impaired; FIGlu is excreted in the urine. In the FIGlu excretion test, a loading dose of histidine (15 g) is given. Urine is then collected for 8 hours; urinary FIGlu is measured at the end of the collection. Normal FIGlu excretion is 1 to 17 mg per 24 hours; persons with folate deficiency may excrete 185 to 2047 mg per 24 hours.[124] Some 50% of patients with B$_{12}$ deficiency also exhibit increased (though less) FIGlu excretion, in the range of 23 to 260 mg per 24 hours.

In vitamin B$_{12}$-deficiency anemia (also macrocytic, megaloblastic), serum B$_{12}$ levels are decreased moderately (below 100 pg/ml), in the presence of normal serum and red cell folate levels.[117] If B$_{12}$ deficiency is suspected to be the result of malabsorption, the Schilling test, the most popular test for B$_{12}$ absorption, is recommended.[125] A 1000-µg intramuscular dose of nonradioactive B$_{12}$ is administered, along with a 0.5- to 2.0-µg oral dose of radiolabeled vitamin. The radioactivity in urine collected 24 to 72 hours after this dose is measured. The injection partially saturates the B$_{12}$-binding sites, thus allowing urinary excretion of vitamin that would otherwise be retained. Approximately 18% of the vitamin is excreted under these conditions. In pernicious anemia or other disorders caused by lack

---

BOX 4-4

Causes of Vitamin B₁₂ and Folate Deficiency

I. *Vitamin B₁₂ deficiency*
  A. Inadequate ingestion
  B. Inadequate absorption
    1. Gastric disorder
      a. Addisonian pernicious anemia
      b. Autoimmune-associated gastric atrophy
    2. Gastrectomy, total or subtotal
    3. Antibody to intrinsic factor
    4. Small intestinal disorder
      a. Gluten-induced enteropathy
      b. Tropical sprue
      c. Regional enteritis
      d. Strictures or anastomoses
      e. Intestinal resection
      f. Cancer
      g. Drug-induced malabsorption (colchicine, neomycin, para-aminosalicylic acid, ethanol)
      h. Long-term ingestion of calcium-chelating agents
      i. Inadequately alkaline pH in the ileum
      j. Competition for absorption by parasites or bacteria
      k. HIV
      l. Pancreatic disease
  C. Inadequate utilization
    1. B₁₂ antagonists (experimental agents)
    2. Congenital or acquired enzyme deficiency or deletion
    3. Abnormal B₁₂ binding in serum
    4. Inadequate serum B₁₂ binding protein
  D. Increased requirements
    1. Hyperthyroidism
    2. Increased hematopoiesis?
    3. Infancy
    4. Parasitization by fetus or by malignant tissue?
  E. Increased excretion
    1. Inadequate serum B₁₂ binding protein
    2. Liver disease; possibly renal disease
  F. Increased destruction by antioxidants
    1. Pharmacologic doses of ascorbic acid
II. *Folate deficiency*
  A. Inadequate Ingestion
    1. Poor diet
    2. Chronic alcoholism

  B. Inadequate absorption, upper one-third of the small intestine
    1. Malabsorption syndromes
      a. Gluten-sensitive enteropathy
      b. Tropical sprue
      c. Associated with certain liver and skin disorders
    2. Drugs
      a. Anticonvulsants, such as phenytoin
      b. Barbiturates
      c. Ethanol
      d. Excess glycine or methionine
      e. Cholestyramine
      f. Sulfasalazine
    3. Specific malabsorption of folate
      a. Congenital or acquired nonconjugase defects
      b. Inadequate intestinal or biliary nonconjugases
      c. Conjugase inhibitors
    4. Blind loop syndrome
  C. Inadequate utilization
    1. Folic acid antagonists
      a. 4-amino-4 deoxyfolate (i.e., methotrexate)
      b. 2,4-diaminopyrimidine (i.e., trimethoprim)
      c. Triamterene
      d. Diamidine compounds (i.e., pentamidine)
    2. Enzyme deficiency, congenital or acquired
    3. Vitamin B₁₂ deficiency
    4. Alcohol
    5. Ascorbic acid deficiency
    6. Excess glycine, methionine
  D. Increased requirements
    1. Extra tissue demand by fetus, nursing infant, or malignant tissue
    2. Infancy
    3. Increased hematopoiesis
    4. Increased metabolic activity
    5. Drugs (L-dopa?)
  E. Increased excretion
    1. Vitamin B₁₂ deficiency
    2. Liver disease?
    3. Kidney dialysis
    4. Chronic exfoliative dermatitis
  F. Increased destruction
    1. Oxidant in diet?

From Mahan LK, Escott-Stump S (eds): *Krause's food, nutrition, and diet therapy,* ed 10, Philadelphia, 2000, WB Saunders, pp 780-790, 794. From Shils M, Olson J, Shike M (eds). *Modern nutrition in health and disease,* ed 9, Lippincott Williams & Wilkins, 1998.
? = possible unproven cause

---

of intrinsic factor (total or partial gastrectomy, gastric bypass, functional absence of intrinsic factor), absorption decreases significantly to 0.5% of the radiolabeled dose but is corrected to nearly normal values (13%) by oral ingestion of intrinsic factor plus vitamin B₁₂. With deficiency of vitamin B₁₂ caused by malabsorption (sprue, small bowel overgrowth, selective B₁₂ malabsorption, chronic pancreatitis), the decrease in B₁₂ absorption is not altered by administration of intrinsic factor (3.6% and 3.3%).[124] Incomplete urine collection and renal disease, which can delay excretion of the vitamin by as much as 72 hours, affect test results.

Vitamin B₁₂ deficiency can result in folic acid deficiency by causing entrapment of folate as 5-methyltetrahydrofolate. Without B₁₂, methyltetrahydrofolate cannot release its methyl group to tetrahydrofolate, which is the optimal substrate for cellular folate polyglutamate synthesis.[115] Synthesis of other folate coenzymes is thus blocked, and folic acid deficiency is the result. Deficiency of methyltetrahydrofolate leads to megaloblastic anemia as a result of restricted DNA synthesis.[124]

Anemia of Chronic Disease

Although not a nutritional anemia, the anemia of chronic disease,[1,119] also known as *the anemia of chronic disorders,*[120] is one of the most common anemias and the one most nutrition support practitioners will likely observe. Defined as a mild to moderate anemia that frequently accompanies inflammation, infection, trauma, or neoplastic disease (see Box 4-4) and persists longer than 1 to 2 months,[125] the disease is characterized by hypoferremia (measured by serum ferritin) in spite of abundant iron stores.

Conditions Associated with the Anemia of Chronic Disorders

Chronic infections
   Pulmonary infections: abscesses, emphysema, tuberculosis, pneumonia
   Subacute bacterial endocarditis
   Pelvic inflammatory disease
   Osteomyelitis
   Chronic urinary tract infections
   Chronic fungal disease
   Meningitis
Chronic, noninfectious inflammations
   Rheumatoid arthritis
   Rheumatic fever
   Systemic lupus erythematosus
   Severe trauma
   Thermal injury
   Adjuvant disease in rats
   Sterile abscesses
Malignant diseases
   Carcinoma
   Hodgkin's disease
   Lymphosarcoma
   Leukemia
   Multiple myeloma
Miscellaneous
   Alcoholic liver disease
   Congestive heart failure
   Thrombophlebitis
   Ischemic heart disease
   "Idiopathic"

From Lee GR, Bithell TC, Foerster J, et al. (eds): *Wintrobe's clinical hematology*, ed 9, Philadelphia, 1993, Lippincott Williams & Wilkins.

Anemia of chronic disease is generally a normocytic, normochromic anemia that develops in the first 1 or 2 months of illness and remains stable, with severity correlated with that of the underlying disease. Often, it arises from shortened red cell survival time, impaired marrow response, and disturbance in iron metabolism. It is likely one manifestation of the metabolic response resulting from cellular immune system stimulation, involving macrophage activity and cytokine elaboration (particularly IL-1 and tumor necrosis factor). Therapy for the anemia of chronic disorders focuses on the underlying disorder. Because the anemia is an adaptive response to the disease, it often should not be treated.[126]

Conclusion

Albumin, transferrin, transthyretin, and nitrogen balance studies (both UUN and TUN) remain the best-researched measures of protein status and those likely to yield reproducible results in common clinical settings. Albumin is beneficial as a screening parameter for large populations; transthyretin and transferrin may be part of the monitoring process for patients receiving nutrition support. Other laboratory indicators of protein status such as 3-MH, CHI, and urea kinetics are complicated to measure and in some cases lack appropriate standards; seasoned practitioners in very controlled settings may use them in challenging situations. Because no single labora-

tory test can provide definitive assessment of nutrition status and response to intervention, the clinician must develop recommendations using objective and subjective data, common sense, and finely honed clinical judgment.

Basic hematologic data are usually available for every patient. Review of these data, combined with an understanding of the clinical condition of the patient, allows the dietitian to screen for anemias and to suggest management and treatment options, adding value to the nutrition assessment.

The need for laboratory data to assess nutritional status and to monitor nutrition support must be justified in the managed care environment. Including specific laboratory tests in clinical paths designed for management of specific diseases or diagnoses may minimize criticism of test utility and may maximize the availability of appropriate nutrition outcome data.

REFERENCES

1. Carlson T: Laboratory data in nutrition assessment. In Mahan K, Escott-Stump S (eds): *Krause's food, nutrition, and diet therapy,* ed 10, Philadelphia, 2000, WB Saunders, pp 380-398.
2. Veldee M: Nutrition assessment, therapy, and monitoring. In Burtis C, Ashwood E (eds): *Tietz textbook of clinical chemistry,* Philadelphia, 1999, WB Saunders, pp 1359-1394.
3. Vanek V: The use of serum albumin as a prognostic or nutritional marker and the pros and cons of IV albumin therapy, *Nutr Clin Prac* 13(2):110-122, 1998.
4. Rothschild MA, Oratz M, Schreiber SS: Albumin synthesis, *N Engl J Med* 286(14):748-757, 1972.
5. Buzby GP, Mullen JL, Matthews DC, et al: Prognostic nutritional index in gastrointestinal surgery, *Am J Surg* 139(1):160-167, 1980.
6. Harvey KB, Moldawer LL, Bistrian BR, Blackburn GL: Biologic measures for the formulation of a hospital prognostic index, *Am J Clin Nutr* 34(10):2013-2022, 1981.
7. Mullen JL, Gerther MH, Buzby GP, et al: Implications of malnutrition in the surgical patient, *Arch Surg* 114(2):121-125, 1979.
8. Seltzer MH, Fletcher HS, Slocum BA, Ensler PE: Instant nutritional assessment in the intensive care unit, *J Parenter Enteral Nutr* 5(1):70-72, 1981.
9. Reinhardt GF, Mysocofski JW, Wilkens DB, et al: Incidence and mortality of hypoalbumic patients in hospitalized veterans, *J Parenter Enteral Nutr* 4(4):357-359, 1980.
10. Harvey KB, Ruggier JA, Regan CS, et al: Hospital morbidity-mortality risk factors using nutritional assessment, *Am J Clin Nutr* 31(4):703, 1978 (abstract).
11. Rich MW, Keller AJ, Schechtman KB, et al: Increased complications and prolonged hospital stay in elderly cardiac surgical patients with low serum albumin, *Am J Cardiol* 63(11):714-718, 1989.
12. Yamanaka H, Nishi M, Kanemaki T, et al: Preoperative nutritional assessment to predict postoperative complication in gastric cancer patients, *J Parenter Enteral Nutr* 13(3):286-291, 1989.
13. Chlebowski RT, Grosvenor MB, Bernhard NH, et al: Nutritional status, gastrointestinal dysfunction, and survival in patients with AIDS, *Am J Gastroenterol* 84(10):1288-1293, 1989.
14. Whitehead RG, Coward WA, Lunn PG: Serum albumin concentration and the onset of kwashiorkor, *Lancet* 1(794):63-66, 1973.
15. Owen WF, Lew NL, Liu Y, et al: The urea reduction ratio and serum albumin concentration as predictors of mortality in patients undergoing hemodialysis, *N Engl J Med* 329(14):1001-1006, 1993.
16. Lowrie EG, Lew NL: Death risk in hemodialysis patients: the predictive value of commonly measured variables and an evaluation of death rate differences between facilities, *Am J Kidney Dis* 15(5):458-482, 1990.
17. Allman RM, Laprade CA, Noel LB, et al: Pressure sores among hospitalized patients, *Ann Intern Med* 105(3):337-342, 1986.
18. Hanan K, Scheele L: Albumin vs. weight as a predictor of nutritional status and pressure ulcer development, *Ostomy Wound Management* 33:22-27, 1991.
19. Gilmore S, Robinson G, Posthauer M, Raymond J. Clinical indicators associated with unintentional weight loss and pressure ulcers in elderly residents of nursing facilities, *J Am Diet Assoc* 95:984-992, 1995.

20. Igenbleek Y, Van Den Schrieck HG, De Nayer P, De Visscher M: Albumin, transferrin and the thyroxine-binding prealbumin/retinol binding protein (TBPA-RBP) complex in assessment of malnutrition, *Clin Chim Acta* 63(1):61-67, 1975.
21. Boosalis MG, Ott L, Levine AS, et al: Relationship of visceral proteins to nutritional status in chronic and acute stress, *Crit Care Med* 17(8):741-747, 1989.
22. Doweiko JP, Nompleggi DJ: The role of albumin in human physiology and pathophysiology. Part III. Albumin and disease states, *J Parenter Enteral Nutr* 15(4):476-483, 1991.
23. Fleck A, Raines G, Hawker F, et al: Increased vascular permeability: a major cause of hypoalbuminemia in disease and injury, *Lancet* 1(8432):781-784, 1985.
24. Thompson D, Milton-Ward A, Whicker J: The value of acute-phase protein measurements in clinical practice, *Ann Clin Biochem* 29 (Pt 2):123-131, 1992.
25. Misra DP, Loudon JM, Staddon GE: Albumin metabolism in elderly patients, *J Gerontol* 30(3):304-306, 1975.
26. Roza AM, Tuitt D, Shizgal HM: Transferrin: a poor measure of nutritional status, *J Parenter Enteral Nutr* 8(5):523-528, 1984.
27. Fletcher JP, Little JM, Gust PK: A comparison of serum transferrin and serum prealbumin as nutritional parameters, *J Parenter Enteral Nutr* 11(2):144-147, 1987.
28. Church JM, Hill GL: Assessing the efficacy of intravenous nutrition in general surgical patients: Dynamic nutritional assessment with plasma proteins, *J Parenter Enteral Nutr* 11(2):135-139, 1987.
29. Kuvshinoff B, Brodish R, McFadden D, Fischer J: Serum transferrin as a prognostic indicator of spontaneous closure and mortality in gastrointestinal cutaneous fistulas, *Ann Surg* 217(6):615-622, 1993.
30. Miller SF, Morath MA, Finley RR: Comparison of derived and actual transferrin: a potential source of error in clinical nutrition assessment, *J Trauma* 21(7):548-550, 1981.
31. Russell M: Serum proteins and nitrogen balance: evaluating response to nutrition support, *Support Line* XVII:3-8, 1995.
32. Crosby LO, Giandomenico A, Forster J, Mullen JL: Relationships between serum total iron-binding capacity and transferring, *J Parenter Enteral Nutr* 8(3):274-278, 1983.
33. Spiekerman AM: Nutritional assessment (protein nutriture), *Anal Chem* 67(12):429R-436R, 1995.
34. Ingenbleek Y, Young V: Transthyretin (prealbumin) in health and disease: nutritional implications, *Ann Rev Nutr* 14:495-533, 1994.
35. Shetty PS, Watrasiewicz KE, Jung RT, James WP: Rapid-turnover proteins: an index of subclinical protein-energy malnutrition, *Lancet* 2(8136):230-232, 1979.
36. Winkler MF, Gerrior SA, Pomp A, Albina JE: Use of retinol-binding protein and prealbumin as indicators of the response to nutrition therapy, *J Am Diet Assoc* 89(5):684-687, 1989.
37. Tuten MB, Wogt S, Dasse F, Leider Z: Utilization of prealbumin as a nutritional parameter, *J Parenter Enteral Nutr* 9(6):709-711, 1985.
38. Mears E: Outcomes of continuous process improvement of a nutritional care program incorporating serum prealbumin measurements, *Nutrition* 12(7-8):479-484, 1996.
39. Bourry J, Milano G, Caldani C, Schneider M: Assessment of nutritional proteins during parenteral nutrition of cancer patients, *Ann Clin Lab Sci* 12(3):158-162, 1982.
40. Milano G, Cooper EH, Goligher JC, et al: Serum prealbumin, retinol-binding protein, transferrin, and albumin levels in patients with large bowel cancer, *J Natl Cancer Inst* 61(3):687-691, 1978.
41. Cano N, DiConstanxo-Dufetel J, Calaf R, et al: Prealbumin-retinol-binding protein complex in hemodialysis patients, *Am J Clin Nutr* 47(4):664-667, 1988.
42. Smith FR, Goodman DS, Zaklama M, et al: Serum vitamin A, retinol-binding protein, and prealbumin concentrations in protein-calorie malnutrition: 1. A functional defect in hepatic retinol release, *Am J Clin Nutr* 26(9):973-981, 1973.
43. Hopkins B: Assessment of nutritional status. In Gottschlich M, Matarese L, Shronts E (eds): *Nutrition support dietetics core curriculum,* ed 2, Silver Spring, MD, 1993, ASPEN.
44. Gabay C, Kushner I: Acute phase proteins and other systemic responses to inflammation, *N Engl J Med* 340(6):448-454, 1999.
45. Saba TM, Kiener JL, Holman JM Jr: Fibronectin and the critically ill patients: current status, *Intensive Care Med* 12(5):350-358, 1986.
46. Bounpane EA, Brown RO, Boucher BA, et al: Use of fibronectin and somatomedin-C as nutritional markers in the enteral nutrition support of traumatized patients, *Crit Care Med* 17(2):126-132, 1989.
47. Howard L, Dillon B, Saba TM, et al: Decreased plasma fibronectin during starvation in man, *J Parenter Enteral Nutr* 8(3):237-244, 1984.
48. Horowitz GD, Groege JS, Legaspi A, Lowry SF: The response of fibronectin to differing parenteral caloric sources in normal man, *J Parenter Enteral Nutr* 9(4):435-438, 1985.
49. Mattox TW, Brown RO, Boucher BA, et al: Use of fibronectin and somatomedin C as markers of enteral nutrition support in traumatized patients using a modified amino acid formula, *J Parenter Enteral Nutr* 12(6):592-596, 1988.
50. Kirby DF, Marder RJ, Craig RM, et al: The clinical evaluation of plasma fibronectin as a marker for nutritional depletion and repletion and as a measure of nitrogen balance, *J Parenter Enteral Nutr* 9(6):705-708, 1985.
51. Minuto F, Barreca A, Adami GF, et al: Insulin-like growth factor-1 in human malnutrition: Relationship with some body composition and nutritional parameters, *J Parenter Enteral Nutr* 13(4):392-396, 1989.
52. Clemmons DR, Underwood LE, Dickerson RN, et al: Use of plasma somatomedin C/insulin-like growth factor 1 measurements to monitor the response to nutritional repletion in malnourished patients, *Am J Clin Nutr* 41(2):191-198, 1985.
53. Clemmons DR, Klibanski A, Underwood LE, et al: Reduction of plasma immunoreactive somatomedin C during fasting in humans, *J Clin Endocrinol Metab* 53(6):1247-1250, 1981.
54. Unterman TG, Vasquez RM, Slas AJ, et al: Nutrition and somatomedin. X111. Usefulness of somatomedin C in nutritional assessment, *Am J Med* 78(2):228-234, 1985.
55. Burgess E. Insulin-like growth factor 1: a valid nutritional index during parenteral feeding of patients suffering an acute phase response, *Ann Clin Biochem* 29(Pt 2):137-144, 1992.
56. Forbes GB, Bruining GJ: Urinary creatinine excretion and lean body mass, *Am J Clin Nutr* 29(12):1359-1366, 1976.
57. Heymsfield SB, Arteaga C, McManus C, et al: Measure of muscle mass in humans: validity of the 24-hour urinary creatinine method, *Am J Clin Nutr* 37(3):478-494, 1983.
58. Forbes GB: Body composition: Influence of nutrition, physical activity, growth, and aging. In Shils M, Olsen J, Shike M, Ross A (eds): *Modern nutrition in health and disease,* ed 9, Baltimore, 1999, Williams & Wilkins, pp 789-809.
59. Lewis JS, Bunker ML, Getts SS, Essien R: Variability of creatinine excretion of normal, phenylketonuric, and galactosemic children and children treated with anticonvulsant drugs, *Am J Clin Nutr* 28(4):310-315, 1975.
60. Crim MC, Calloway DH, Margen S: Creatine metabolism in men: creatine pool size and turnover rate in relation to creatine intake, *J Nutr* 106(4):371-381, 1976.
61. Sauberlich HE: *Laboratory tests for the assessment of nutritional status,* Boca Raton, 1999, CRC Press, p 454.
62. Bistrian BR, Blackburn G, Sherman M, Scrimshaw NS: Therapeutic index of nutritional depletion in hospitalized patients, *Surg Gynecol Obstet* 141(4):512-516, 1975.
63. Bistrian BR, Blackburn GL: Assessment of protein-calorie malnutrition in the hospitalized patient. In Schneider HA, Anderson CE, Coursin DB: *Nutritional support of medical practice,* ed 2, Philadelphia, 1983, Harper and Row, pp 128-139.
64. Phinney SD: The assessment of protein nutriture in the hospitalized patient, *Clin Lab Med* 1(4):767-774, 1981.
65. Imbembo AL, Walser W: Nutritional assessment. In Walser M, Imbembo AL, Margolis S, Elfert G (ed): *Nutritional management: the Johns Hopkins handbook,* Philadelphia, 1984, WB Saunders, pp 9-30.
66. Blackburn GL, Bistrian BR, Maini BS, et al: Nutritional and metabolic assessment of the hospitalized patient, *J Parenter Enteral Nutr* 1(1):11-22, 1977.
67. Murray RL: Interpreting the nutritional assessment. In Krey SH, Murray RL (eds): *Dynamics of nutrition support: assessment, implementation, evaluation,* Norwalk, CT, 1986, Appleton-Century-Crofts, pp 155-181.
68. Grant JP: Nutritional assessment in clinical practice, *Nutr Clin Pract* 1:3-11, 1986.
69. Trotter M, Gleser GC: The effect of aging on stature, *Am J Phys Anthropol* 9:311, 1951.
70. Williams CS: Laboratory values and their interpretation. In Krey SH, Murray RL (eds): *Dynamics of nutrition support: assessment, implementation, evaluation,* Norwalk, CT, 1986, Appleton-Century-Crofts, pp 83-97.
71. Schiller WR, Long CL, Blakemore WS: Creatinine and nitrogen excretion in seriously ill and injured patients, *Surg Gynecol Obstet* 149(4):561-566, 1979.

72. Arroyave G, Dining J, Freuk S, Gopalan C et al: Assessment of protein nutritional status: a committee report, *Am J Clin Nutr* 23(6):807-819, 1970.

73. Boileau RB, Hortsman DH, Buskirk ER, et al: The usefulness of urinary creatinine excretion in estimating body composition, *Med Sci Sports* 4:85-90, 1972.

74. Cohn SH, Vaswani AN, Vartsky D, et al: In vivo quantitation of body nitrogen for nutritional assessment, *Am J Clin Nutr* 35(suppl 5):1186-1191, 1982.

75. Heymsfield SB, McManus C, Stevens V, Smith J: Muscle mass: reliable indicator of protein-energy malnutrition severity and outcome, *Am J Clin Nutr* 35(suppl 5):1192-1199, 1982.

76. Matarese LE: Reassessment and determining an end point of therapy. In Krey SH, Murray RL (eds): *Dynamics of nutrition support: assessment, implementation, evaluation,* Norwalk, CT, 1986, Appleton-Century-Crofts, pp 479-487.

77. Umapathy KP, Mavk PB, Dozier EA: Effect of immobilization on urinary excretion of creatine and creatinine with certain possible ameliorating measures applied, *Ind J Nutr Dietet* 10:292, 1973.

78. Lipkin EW, Bell S: Assessment of nutritional status: the clinician's perspective, *Clin Lab Med* 13(2):329-352, 1993.

79. Matthews D: Protein and amino acids. In Shils M, Olsen J, Shike M, Ross A (eds): *Modern nutrition in health and disease,* ed 9, Baltimore, 1999, Williams & Wilkins, pp 11-48.

80. Young VR, Munro HN: N-tau-methylhistidine (3-methylhistidine) and muscle protein turnover: an overview, *Fed Proc* 37(9):2291-3000, 1978.

81. Lukaski HC, Mendez J, Buskrik ER, Cohn SH: Relationship between endogenous 3-methylhistidine excretion and body composition, *Am J Physiol* 240(3):E302-E307, 1981.

82. Long CL, Birkhan RH, Geiger RN, et al: Urinary excretion of 3-methylhistidine: an assessment of muscle protein catabolism in adult normal subjects and during malnutrition, sepsis, and trauma, *Metabolism* 30: 765-776, 1981.

83. Wassner JJ, Li JB: N-tau-methylhistidine release: contributions of rat skeletal muscle, GI tract, and skin, *Am J Physiol* 243(2):E293-E297, 1982.

84. Dwyer J, Kenler S: Assessment of nutritional status in renal disease. In Mitch WE, Klahr S (eds): *Nutrition and the kidney,* Boston, 1993, Little, Brown, pp 61-95.

85. Haverberg LN, Deckelbaum L, Bilzanes C, et al: Myofibrillar protein turnover and urinary N-tau-methylhistidine output. Response to dietary supply of protein and energy, *Biochem J* 152:503-510, 1975.

86. Nakhooda F, Wei CN, Marliss EB: Muscle protein catabolism in diabetes: 3-methylhistidine excretion in the spontaneously diabetic "BB" rat, *Meta Clin Exp* 29(12):1272-1277, 1980.

87. Tomas FM, Munro HN, Young VR: Effect of glucocorticoid administration on the rate of muscle protein breakdown in vivo in rats, as measured by urinary excretion of N-tau-methylhistidine, *Biochem J* 178(1):139-146, 1979.

88. Forbes GB: *Human body composition: growth, aging, nutrition, and activity,* New York, 1987, Springer-Verlag.

89. Shopbell J, Hopkins B, Shronts E: Nutrition screening and assessment. In Gottschlich M (ed): *The science and practice of nutrition support: a case-based core curriculum,* Dubuque, IA, 2001, ASPEN/Kendall Hunt, pp107-140.

90. Murray RL: Protein and energy requirements. In Krey SH, Murray RL (eds): *Dynamics of nutrition support,* Norwalk, CT, 1986, Appleton-Century-Crofts, pp 188-192.

91. Konstantinides FN: Nitrogen balance studies in clinical nutrition, *Nutr Clin Pract* 7(5):231-238, 1992.

92. Burge JC, Choban P, McKnight T, et al: Urinary ammonia plus urinary urea nitrogen as an estimate of total urinary nitrogen in patients receiving parenteral nutrition support, *J Parenter Enteral Nutr* 17(6):529-531, 1993.

93. Maldonado J, Faus MJ, Bayes R, et al: Apparent nitrogen balance and 3-methyl histidine urinary excretion in intravenously fed children with trauma and infections, *Eur J Clin Nutr* 42(2):93-100, 1988.

94. Gottschlich M. Burns. In Gottschlich M, Matarese L, Shronts E (eds): *Nutrition support dietetics core curriculum,* ed 2, Silver Spring, MD, 1993, ASPEN.

95. Loder PB, Kee AJ, Horsburgh R, et al: Validity of urinary urea nitrogen as a measure of total urinary nitrogen in adult patients requiring parenteral nutrition, *Crit Care Med* 17(4):309-312, 1989.

96. Helms RA, Alvarado-Hughes M, Fernandes ET, Storm MC: Nitrogen balance determinations in preterm neonates, *J Parenter Enteral Nutr* 13(1):19S, 1989 (abstract).

97. Konstantinides FN, Konstantinides NN, Li JC, et al: Urinary urea nitrogen: too insensitive for calculating nitrogen balance studies in surgical clinical nutrition, *J Parenter Enteral Nutr* 15(2):189-193, 1991.

98. Grimble GK, West MF, Acuti A, et al: Assessment of an automated chemiluminescence nitrogen analyzer for routine use in clinical nutrition, *J Parenter Enteral Nutr* 12(1):100-106, 1988.

99. Kosanovich JM, Dumler F, Horst M, et al: Use of urea kinetics in the nutritional care of the acutely ill patient, *J Parenter Enteral Nutr* 9(12):165-169, 1985.

100. Sargent JA, Gotch FA: Mathematical modeling of dialysis therapy, *Kidney Int* 18(suppl 10):S2-S10, 1980.

101. Sargent JA: Control of dialysis by a single-pool urea model. The National Cooperative Dialysis Study, *Kidney Int* (suppl 13):S19-S25, 1983.

102. Sargent JA, Gotch FA: Nutrition and treatment of the acutely ill patient using urea kinetics, *Dial Transplant* 10:314-322, 1981.

103. Sargent JA: Urea mass balance: nutrition and treatment of the acutely ill patient, *Nutr Supp Serv* 2:32-39, 1982.

104. Goldstein DJ, Frederico CB: The effect of urea kinetic modeling on the nutrition management of hemodialysis patients, *J Am Diet Assoc* 87(4):474-479, 1987.

105. O'Donnell L: Nutritional applications of urea kinetics, *Support Line* XIII(2):6-9, 1991.

106. Sargent J, Gotch F, Borah M, et al: Urea kinetics: a guide to nutritional management of renal failure, *Am J Clin Nutr* 31(9):1696-1702, 1978.

107. Moore FD, Oleson KH, McMurray JD, et al: *The body cell mass and its supporting environment: body composition in health and disease,* Philadelphia, 1963, WB Saunders.

108. Whitmire S: Fluid and electrolytes. In Matarese L, Gottschlich M (eds). *Contemporary nutrition support practice,* Philadelphia, 1995, WB Saunders, p 134.

109. Whitmire S: Fluid and electrolytes. In Gottschlich M (ed): *The science and practice of nutrition support: a case-based core curriculum,* Dubuque, IA, 2001, ASPEN/Kendall Hunt, pp 53-83.

110. Bergstrom J: Nutritional requirements of hemodialysis patients. In Mitch WE, Klahr S (eds): *Nutrition and the kidney,* ed 2, Boston, 1993, Little, Brown, pp 263-289.

111. Mitch WE: Restricted diets and slowing the progression of chronic renal insufficiency. In Mitch WE, Klahr S (eds): *Nutrition and the kidney,* ed 2, Boston, 1993, Little, Brown, pp 243-262.

112. Druml W: Nutritional support in acute renal failure. In Mitch WE, Klahr S (eds): *Nutrition and the kidney,* ed 2, Boston, 1993, Little, Brown, pp 314-345.

113. Shronts EP, Teasley KM: Clinical utility of urea kinetics for calculating nitrogen balance in acutely ill patients, *Nutr Supp Serv* 8(6):12-15, 1988.

114. Leblanc M, Garred L, Cardinal J, et al: Catabolism in critical illness: estimation from urea nitrogen appearance and creatinine production during continuous renal replacement therapy, *Am J Kid Dis* 32(3):444-453, 1998.

115. Kasdan T. Medical nutrition therapy for anemia. In Mahan LK, Escott-Stump S (eds): *Krause's food, nutrition, and diet therapy,* ed 10, Philadelphia, 2000, WB Saunders, pp 781-800.

116. Herbert V, Das K: Folic acid and vitamin B_{12}. In Shils ME, Olson JA, Shike M (eds): *Modern nutrition in health and disease,* ed 8, vol 1, Philadelphia, 1994, Lea & Febiger, pp 402-425.

117. Herbert V: Hematology and the anemias. In Schneider HA, Anderson CE, Coursin DB (eds): *Nutritional support of medical practice,* ed 2, Philadelphia, 1983, Harper and Row, pp 386-409.

118. Lang CE, Cashman MD: Nutritional status. In Skipper A (ed): *Dietitian's handbook of enteral and parenteral nutrition,* Rockville, MD, 1989, Aspen Publishers, pp 5-18.

119. Chanarin I: Nutritional aspects of hematologic disorders. In Shils M, Olsen J, Shike M, Ross A (eds): *Modern nutrition in health and disease,* ed 9, Baltimore, 1999, Williams & Wilkins, pp 1419-1437.

120. Beutler E: The common anemias, *JAMA* 259(16):2433-2437, 1988.

121. Herbert J: Everyone should be tested for iron disorders, *J Am Diet Assoc* 92(12):1502-1509, 1992.

122. Ahluwalia N: Diagnostic utility of serum transferring receptors measurement in assessing iron status, *Nutr Rev* 1(5 Pt 1):133-141, 1998.

123. Lee GR: Microcytosis and the anemias associated with impaired hemoglobin synthesis. In Lee GR, Bithell TC, Foerster J, et al. (eds): *Wintrobe's clinical hematology,* ed 9, vol 1, Philadelphia, 1993, Lea & Febiger, pp 791-807.

124. Lee GR: Megaloblastic and nonmegaloblastic macrocytic anemias. In Lee GR, Bithell TC, Foerster J, et al. (eds): *Wintrobe's clinical hematology,* ed 9, vol 1, Philadelphia, 1993, Lea & Febiger, pp 745-790.

125. Carmel R: Pernicious anemia: The expected findings of very low serum cobalamine levels, anemia and macrocytosis are often lacking, *Arch Intern Med* 148(8):1712-1714, 1988.

126. Lee GR: The anemia of chronic disorders. In Lee GR, Bithell TC, Foerster J, et al. (eds): *Wintrobe's clinical hematology,* ed 9, vol 1, Philadelphia, 1993, Lea & Febiger, pp 840-851.

Evaluating Immunocompetence

5

Bobbi Langkamp-Henken, PhD, RD

Steven M. Wood, PhD, RD

THROUGHOUT history, links between nutrition and function of the immune system have been demonstrated repeatedly by the simultaneous occurrence of famine and devastating, contagious infectious diseases. During times of war or natural disaster, sources of adequate nutrition may be limited; consequently, nutritional depletion and subsequent immune-mediated changes occur that threaten survival. Malnutrition and nutrient deficiencies affect the immune system in a number of ways. Malnutrition impairs the ability of immune cells to recognize foreign stimuli, alters proliferative responses of various immune cells, impairs antigen presentation, reduces phagocytic and cytolytic cellular capacity, alters membrane or enzyme function, and perturbs the cooperative interactions and communication between the various types of immune system cells.[1-12] There is also evidence that pharmacologic levels of nutrients (i.e., levels above which deficiencies are prevented) and nonnutritive dietary components improve immune function.[13-24] Recently, researchers demonstrated that the nutritional status of a host can influence the genomic structure of viruses.[25] Therefore, nutritional status affects the ability of the host to ward off disease and infection and influences the pathogenic virulence of organisms and viruses.

Over the years, the sciences of immunology and nutrition have progressed from using simple tests of immune function to predict the degree of malnutrition to using complex techniques to identify the roles nutrients play in immune function, infection, and clinical outcome.[14,17-20,26-29] Although most of the laboratory tests discussed in this chapter are not available in house to clinicians practicing in community hospitals, practitioners must understand immune function tests and the limitations associated with each test in order to critically evaluate the literature and provide "state of the art" nutrition support. The purpose of this chapter is to provide a basic understanding of the immune system, the laboratory tests used to assess the impact of nutrient intake on immune function, the limitations associated with these tests, and the value of the tests in predicting clinical outcome. To this end, the chapter presents the two arms of the immune system (i.e., the innate and acquired immune systems) and selected tests used to assess immune response (Table 5-1). Although the two systems are separated for illustrative purposes, typically they work in concert to eliminate pathogens and malignant cells or to respond to physiologic processes.

Innate (Natural) Immunity

The immune system consists of a network of tissues, organs, cells, and molecules that protect the body from encroachments by foreign substances and organisms and from malignant and autoimmune cells. Immune mechanisms are of two types—innate and acquired. Innate immunity is inborn and does not rely on prior exposure to infectious microbes or foreign macromolecules. Physiochemical barriers, such as skin and gastric or mucous secretions (including pH and enzymes), are the first line of defense against the invasion of pathogens. In addition to these physiochemical barriers, macrophages, granulocytes, natural killer cells, and complement participate in innate immunity.

Evaluating Granulocyte Function

Granulocytes, which consist of neutrophils, eosinophils, and basophils, are white blood cells (leukocytes) that attack and eliminate microbes and dead tissue. Neutrophils, also called *polymorphonuclear leukocytes* (PMNs) because of their multilobed nuclei, are the most abundant (50% to 70%) of the white blood cells. The principal function of neutrophils is to destroy foreign microbes during an acute inflammatory response. Eosinophils and basophils constitute approximately 1% to 3% and less than 1%, respectively, of the white blood cells. Eosinophils play an important role in the defense against parasitic organisms. Basophils' functions are not based on phagocytic (engulfment) functions but rather their ability to release potent biologic mediators into the cellular microenvironment.

Bacterial cell walls (endotoxin) or secreted toxins (exotoxin) stimulate macrophages and other cells such as the vascular endothelium to secrete cytokines. These cytokines induce inflammation by promoting neutrophil adhesion to vascular endothelium and neutrophil migration into infected tissue (chemotaxis). The recruited neutrophils eliminate microbes by phagocytic processes. Microbes that are opsonized or "coated" with antibody or complement are more readily engulfed by neutrophils. This enhanced phagocytosis occurs because neutrophils have receptors for antibodies and complement. After being ingested, the microbes within the neutrophil are killed by the discharge (degranulation) of the contents of cytoplasmic granules into the phagocytic vacuoles. Killing is accomplished during the degranulation process by the release of cytotoxic proteins, destructive enzymes, and newly generated toxic oxidants—reactive oxygen and nitrogen molecules (respiratory burst).

Defects in neutrophil function can be attributed to reduced numbers of normal neutrophils or altered neutrophil function. Typically, a complete blood cell count (CBC) and a differential white blood cell count are performed to determine the number

TABLE 5-1

Selected Tests Used to Assess Components of the Innate and Acquired Immune System

Immune System Component	Functions in Innate Immunity	Functions in Acquired Immunity	Function	Selected Tests to Assess Immune Status	Purpose of Test
Neutrophil	X		Destroy foreign microbes during acute inflammatory response	WBC with differential	Determine total number of circulating cells
				MPO	Estimate neutrophil infiltration into tissues
				NBT, Ferricytochrome c reduction	Assess intracellular killing, specifically, respiratory burst
				Microbicidal assays	Measure bacteria-killing capacity
Macrophage	X		Destroy foreign microbes	Microbicidal assays	Measure bacteria-killing capacity
	X	X	Cytokine secretion	ELISA	Measure cytokines in body fluids or cell culture supernatants
				Bioassays	Measure cytokines in body fluids or cell culture supernatants
				ELISPOT	Detect individual cytokine-secreting cells
Complement	X		Lysis of cells, bacteria, or viruses	AH_{50}	Measure complement associated hemolytic activity
	X		Opsonize foreign microbes	Microbicidal assays	Estimate serum complement opsonic activity
				ELISA	Estimate complement component and protein levels
		X	Lysis of cells, bacteria, or viruses	CH_{50}	Measure complement associated hemolytic activity
Large granular lymphocytes (NK cells)	X		Nonspecific killing of abnormal cells	^{51}Cr- or fluorochrome-release assay	Measure cytotoxic activity in vitro
				Intravenous injection of radiolabeled target cells	Measure cytotoxic activity in vivo
T Lymphocytes		X	Cell-mediated immunity	Flow cytometry	Characterize cell subtypes or surface receptor expression
				Proliferation assays	Measure the ability of lymphocytes to proliferate in vitro to various mitogens
				MLR	Characterize the cellular basis of rejection of transplanted tissue
				DTH	Measure cell-mediated immunity in vivo

Continued.

of circulating neutrophils. The extent of neutrophil infiltration into tissue or organs in animals can be evaluated by assaying the tissue or organ for the granular enzyme myeloperoxidase (MPO).[30] The MPO assay is a relatively easy and reproducible procedure for estimating neutrophils; however, it does not distinguish between neutrophil and monocyte MPO and eosinophil peroxidase activity. Additionally, the location of the neutrophils—circulating, marginating, or infiltrating—cannot be determined with the assay.[31] Stained histologic sections or immunohistochemical analysis with fluorescence-labeled anti-neutrophil antibodies can be used to localize neutrophils. In humans, neutrophil MPO or lipocalin (a neutrophil-specific protein) can be measured in lung lavage fluid or expectorated sputum as an indication of neutrophil activity.[32,33]

Tests are available to evaluate chemotaxis, recognition and adhesion, ingestion, degranulation, and intracellular killing. Because neutrophils are terminally differentiated cells they cannot be propagated in tissue culture. Assays used to determine neutrophil function must be done the same day the neutrophils are isolated. Common tests for assessing neutrophil function include respiratory burst as well as phagocytosis and microbial killing assays. To determine the functional capacity of neutrophils to generate toxic oxidants during a respiratory burst, stimulated neutrophils are incubated with nitroblue tetrazolium (NBT). Neutrophils that function normally chemically reduce NBT, which produces a detectable color change in the dye. The reduced NBT can be measured spectrophotometrically to quantitate the "respiratory burst." The generation of a respiratory burst and the subsequent reduction of NBT require that the phagocytic processes that occur before oxidative killing be intact.[34] The rate of formation of superoxide can be quantitated by stimulating neutrophils in the presence of ferricytochrome c. As the ferricytochrome c is reduced, a color change is produced that can be measured spectrophotometrically.[34]

TABLE 5-1					
Selected Tests Used to Assess Components of the Innate and Acquired Immune System—cont'd					
Immune System Component	Functions in Innate Immunity	Functions in Acquired Immunity	Function	Selected Tests to Assess Immune Status	Purpose of Test
Helper T Th1 Th2		X	Overall orchestration of specific immunity via cytokine secretion (secreted cytokines also used to identify Th1 and Th2 subclasses)	ELISA	Measure cytokines in body fluids or cell culture supernatants
				Bioassays	Measure cytokines in body fluids or cell culture supernatants
				ELISPOT	Detect individual cytokine-secreting cells
CTL		X	Lysis of virus-infected cells, tumor cells, or allografted cells	^{51}Cr-release assay	Measure the ability of CTL to lyse target cells
B Lymphocytes		X	Antibody production	Flow cytometry	Characterize cell class and isotype
				ELISA	Determine serum immunoglobulin concentrations
				Nephelometry	Determine serum immunoglobulin concentrations
				RIA	Determine serum immunoglobulin concentrations
				RID	Determine serum immunoglobulin concentrations
				PFC	Determine serum immunoglobulin concentrations
				ELISPOT	Detect individual antibody-secreting cells
		X	Antibody production in vaccination response	HI	Detect vaccine-specific antibodies

AH$_{50}$, Alternate pathway hemolytic activity; *CH$_{50}$*, classical pathway hemolytic activity; *CTL*, cytotoxic T lymphocytes; *DTH*, delayed-type hypersensitivity; *ELISA*, enzyme-linked immunosorbent assay; *ELISPOT*, enzyme-linked immunospot assay; *HI*, hemagglutination inhibition; *MLR*, mixed leukocyte reaction; *MPO*, myeloperoxidase; *NBT*, nitroblue tetrazolium dye reduction test; *PFC*, plaque-forming cell assay; *RIA*, radioimmunoassay; *RID*, radial immunodiffusion assay; *WBC*, white blood count.

Phagocytosis should be determined whenever measuring microbial killing. If the neutrophils are unable to ingest the microbe, "normal" killing will be mistakenly assumed. Traditionally, microbial killing was evaluated by incubating neutrophils with serum (a source of antibodies and complement for opsonization of bacteria) and a known bacterium. The opsonized bacteria are ingested and killed by the neutrophils. Uningested bacteria are destroyed with the addition of an antibiotic. Neutrophils are lysed, and the viable intracellular bacteria are quantitated by mounting the lysed neutrophil solution on culture plates. The killing capacity is determined by counting the colonies of bacteria that grow on the culture plates. Fewer colonies equates to more killing. The normal percent killing capacity is 93% to 98% in 60 to 90 minutes; however, this can vary, depending on assay conditions.[34] Newer techniques assess microbial killing and phagocytosis using fluorescein-labeled, viable bacteria.[35]

Neutrophil dysfunction has been observed in seniors, patients with human immunodeficiency virus (HIV), patients with cirrhosis, and infants receiving long-term parenteral nutrition.[36-39] Trauma, surgery, chemical exposure, and environmental factors also alter neutrophil function and render patients more susceptible to infection.[40-43] In 2202 surgical patients, Christou demonstrated a statistically significant correlation between sepsis and preoperative neutrophil adherence and chemotaxis.[44] Preoperative neutrophil chemotaxis was found to be lower in patients who became septic, whereas neutrophil adherence was increased. Neutrophil phagocytosis and bacterial killing were not different in septic and nonseptic patients, and neutrophil function did not correlate with mortality.[44]

Although neutrophils protect against invading microbes, they have little intrinsic ability to differentiate between the pathogen and host tissue, and therefore, must rely on antibodies, complement, and cytokines to identify appropriate targets. Loss of the contents of the neutrophil granules into the extracellular fluid results in tissue injury and additional inflammation. Consequently, activated neutrophils have been implicated as mediators of ischemia-reperfusion injury, adult respiratory distress syndrome (ARDS), and the onset of sepsis.[36,45] Because neutrophils play an integral role in host defense and host injury, functional tests must be interpreted in the context of patient diagnosis.

Several limitations are associated with neutrophil function assays. For example, neutrophil function is typically evaluated in vitro on neutrophils obtained from the circulating blood pool; however, the majority of neutrophil function in vivo is carried out by marginating or extravascular neutrophils and not by circulating neutrophils. Additionally, the half-life of circulating neutrophils is approximately 7 hours.[46] Therefore, when tests of neutrophil function are repeated on blood samples drawn at 14-hour intervals, the blood could contain entirely different cell populations.

Evaluating Macrophage Function

Monocytes circulate in the blood and lymph and then migrate through blood vessel walls into tissues and organs, at which time they become macrophages (through the process of differentiation). Like neutrophils, macrophages are capable of ingesting and destroying antigens but also play a role in presenting foreign antigens and activating T and B lymphocytes, whereas neutrophils do not have this function. Activated macrophages secrete cytokines and factors important in the inflammatory process. For example, liver macrophages (Kupffer cells) remove matter and microbes from the systemic circulation and in the process release interleukin-1 (IL-1), interleukin-6 (IL-6), and tumor necrosis factor (TNF) (cytokines responsible for the acute-phase response), and complement proteins (discussed in the following section). Methods used for assessing macrophage phagocytosis and microbial killing are similar to those discussed for neutrophils. However, macrophage function can be discriminated from neutrophil function by altering the incubation time in the microbial killing assays or by measuring cell size, granularity, or cytokine production (i.e., TNF-α, or IL-1; see Cytokine Production). It is also important to note that macrophages play a role in many immune responses and that there are assay techniques to evaluate particular functions separately.

Murine (mouse) models have demonstrated that activating macrophages in some cases and inhibiting macrophage function in others can be protective, depending on the conditions.[5,47] Following septic challenge, excessive macrophage function may actually be detrimental. Antibodies against interferon gamma (IFN-γ, a cytokine that enhances macrophage function) block IFN-γ activity, thereby decreasing macrophage respiratory burst and TNF release, and increasing the survival rate from acute sepsis.[47] In protein-energy malnutrition (PEM), the host response to infective challenge is significantly depressed, and macrophage respiratory burst, phagocytosis, and *C. albicans* killing are significantly impaired.[4] In this case, treatment with IFN-γ enhances macrophage function and ultimately *C. albicans* killing.[5] These studies demonstrate that enhancing immune function is not always advantageous and that immune function tests must be interpreted in the context of

the patient's diagnosis. Furthermore, macrophages have a number of functions in the natural immune system and additional functions in the acquired immune system (i.e., antigen presentation and cytokine production; see Acquired Immune System). Because of the large number of diverse functions of macrophages, it is important to keep in mind that the demonstration of an adequate function from a single immunity test (e.g., microbial killing or TNF release) does not guarantee uncompromised immune function.

Evaluating Complement Function

Complement is a collective term for a functionally linked system of proteins that react in a cascadelike sequence. Three major functions of the complement system include lysis of cells, bacteria, or enveloped viruses; opsonization of foreign organisms or particles; and mediation of the inflammatory response. Patients with a complement deficiency have increased susceptibility to pyogenic infections (e.g., *Neisseria meningitidis, Hemophilus influenzae, Streptococcus pneumoniae*) and to illnesses characterized by autoantibodies and immune complexes.[48] The complement cascade can be activated in various sequences and by numerous agents. The classical, alternative, or lectin pathways are used to describe three routes for complement activation (Fig. 5-1). Within acquired immunity, activation of complement occurs by the binding of the first complement protein, C1, to antigen-antibody complexes (the classical pathway). The alternative and lectin pathways do not require antibodies to initiate the activation cascade; hence, they are considered to be a part of innate

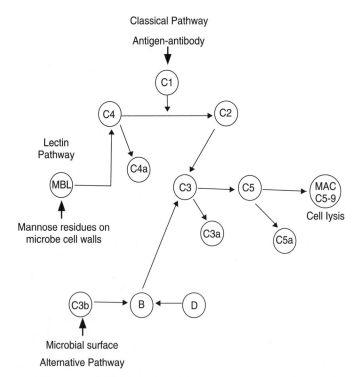

FIGURE 5-1 Simplified overview of the complement system. The complement cascade can be activated by three routes: Classical, Lectin, and Alternative Pathways. All three pathways generate C3 and ultimately membrane attack complexes (MAC). The anaphylatoxins, C3a, C4a, and C5a are generated during the cascade. *MBL,* Mannan-binding lectin.

immunity. The alternative pathway is activated by the binding of C3b complement protein to microbial surfaces. The lectin pathway is activated by the binding of an acute phase protein, mannan-binding lectin (MBL), to mannose residues on glycoproteins or carbohydrates present on microbes.[49] Activation of complement via all pathways results in sequential activation of a series of proteins that leads to the formation of the membrane attack complex (MAC). The MAC consists of several soluble complement components (C5 through C9) that organize into a pore structure on the target cell surface and induce osmotic lysis.

C3b is a complement component that participates in the complement cascade and acts as an opsonin to enhance the phagocytic processes of neutrophils and macrophages. Phagocytosis of C3b-coated microorganisms is most likely the major defense against systemic bacterial and fungal infections. C3a, C4a, and C5a are called *anaphylatoxins* because they mediate inflammatory processes. For example, the anaphylatoxins bind to mast cells and basophils and release vasoactive mediators such as histamine, thus increasing vascular permeability and smooth muscle contraction. C5a is principally responsible for these effects and for promoting neutrophil adhesion and chemotaxis.[50]

The activation of the complement system involves many sequential steps of proteolytic enzyme activation, which acquire activity through the action of other proteases; thus, amplification is immense in this system. An enzyme activated at one step generates many activated components at the next step. To keep such a system under control, soluble and membrane-bound proteins act as inhibitors at different steps in the cascade.[51]

Well-known studies have correlated reduced plasma concentrations of complement components and complement function with malnutrition and increased morbidity and mortality.[52-56] For example, in 1980 Alexander and colleagues showed that despite higher caloric intake, severely burned children with lower protein intakes (16.5% of desired caloric intake from protein) had a diminished C3 level and opsonic index, which translated into more bacteremic days and a worse survival compared to children with similar injuries receiving an aggressive protein feeding (23% of caloric intake from protein).[52] While maintaining both plasma concentrations of complement and complement function are important, inappropriate or excessive activation of complement can lead to the pathogenesis of ischemia/reperfusion injury following cardiovascular accidents, tissue transplantation, cardiopulmonary bypass, or septic shock.[45,57-60] Therapeutic inhibition of complement using soluble complement receptors or antibodies against key complement proteins or receptors appears to minimize ischemia/reperfusion injury and inflammatory diseases.[50,51,58-61]

Complement function via the classical (antibody-activated) pathway is determined in vitro by measuring hemolytic activity. A titration curve is generated by incubating sheep erythrocytes and rabbit antisheep cell antibodies with diluted human serum samples. Complement proteins in the serum are activated when the rabbit antisheep cell antibodies bind to the sheep erythrocytes (antibody-antigen complexes formation). Complement MAC lyse the erythrocytes and hemoglobin is released. The amount of released hemoglobin is measured spectrophotometrically. The inverse of the concentration of sample serum required to lyse 50% of the sheep erythrocytes is called the CH_{50}. For example, if a 1/80 dilution of serum lyses 50% of the sheep erythrocytes, the CH_{50} is 80 U/ml. Functional assessment of the alternative pathway of complement is done in a similar manner, except that rabbit erythrocytes are used as the target cells and as inducers of complement activity. Results are reported as AH_{50}. The CH_{50} and AH_{50} assays are bioassays (using viable sheep and rabbit erythrocytes) and therefore measure complement function but are subject to variability associated with reaction conditions. Calibrated human serum standards or pooled normal human serum should be included in every assay to standardize results and minimize interassay variability. Individual complement components in serum can be quantitated using antibodies specific for a given component in enzyme-linked immunosorbent assays (ELISA) or radioimmunoassays (RIA) (see Cytokine Production for method descriptions). The individual complement component C3, which functions as an opsonin, is central to all complement pathways and is frequently measured.[44,62-64] A reduction of as much as 60% in C3 must occur before opsonization is altered.[64]

Evaluating Natural Killer Cell Activity

Natural killer (NK) cells are cytotoxic lymphocytes capable of rapid, nonspecific killing of abnormal cells, regardless of prior sensitization, antigen presentation, major histocompatibility complex (MHC) restriction, or clonal expansion.[65,66] NK cells also produce cytokines such as IFN-γ, a cytokine that influences T- and B-lymphocyte functions.[67]

NK lymphocytes, also known as *null cells, non-T, non-B lymphocytes*, and *large granular lymphocytes* (LGL), make up approximately 5% to 10% of the entire lymphocyte population.[68,69] NK cells contain less nuclear material and more cytoplasm than small lymphocytes and are important in the surveillance and killing of various tumors,[70,71] viruses,[72,73] and pathogenic microbes.[74-78] Decreased NK cell cytotoxicity has been noted in association with solid neoplasms or untreated leukemias as well as increased risk of infection in the elderly.[79,80] Moreover, NK cell cytotoxicity is inversely correlated with tumor growth and metastasis.[81,82] NK cell activity is also reduced in AIDS patients but appears to be normal in asymptomatic carriers of HIV-1.[83] Unlike other cytotoxic responses that require days or weeks to achieve full potency, NK cells react within minutes of target cell exposure. NK cell function does not require interactions with other cells such as macrophages or helper T lymphocytes (although cytokines such as IL-2, IL-7, IL-12 or prostaglandins such as prostaglandin E_2 [PGE_2] can influence NK activity). Activation of NK cells more than likely requires target cell contact; however, the nature of the NK receptor molecule remains unclear.

Cytotoxic activity of NK cells is assessed in vitro using target tumor cells (K562 or Daudi cells). K562 cells, derived from a patient in blastic crisis with leukemia,[84] and Daudi cells, derived from a Burkitt's lymphoma cell line, are susceptible to the cytotoxic effects of NK cells. To assess cytotoxicity, target cells are prelabeled with a radioisotope such as chromium-51 (^{51}Cr), or a fluorochrome such as 2'7'-bis(carboxyethyl)-5,6-carboxyfluorescein (BCECF-AM) or Calcien AM (Molecular Probes, Inc., Eugene, Oregon). The target cells and the peripheral blood mononuclear lymphocytes, which include NK cells, are then mixed in various ratios and incubated. During the incubation, the NK cells destroy the target cells and release the radioisotope or fluorochrome.[85,86] The amount of radioisotope released from the cells into the culture medium or the fluorochrome retained by the target cells is determined by counting radioactivity or by measuring fluorescence with a flow cytometer or fluorescence concentration analyzer. Target cell uptake and spontaneous release of ^{51}Cr vary from assay to assay. Fluorochrome labeling of target cells seems to be more consistent than radiolabeling, yet BCECF-AM is affected by the pH of culture media during labeling. Calcein AM is not sensitive to pH and is retained much longer than ^{51}Cr,[87] thus allowing longer incubation.

Controls are used to assess the two extremes of cytotoxicity–no NK-mediated target cell lysis (target cells incubated without NK cells) and complete cytotoxicity (addition of detergent to lyse all target cells). It is important to match experimental controls for gender and age. NK-cell activity tends to vary with age and to be greater in males. Tilden and coworkers reported an increase in NK-cell cytotoxicity,[88] whereas Facchini and colleagues reported a decrease with age.[89] Target and NK cells must be properly prepared. Contaminating monocytes or PMNs can suppress NK-cell cytotoxic activity, while contaminating erythrocytes can enhance activity.

An alternate method (single cell suspension assay) for assessing NK-cell cytotoxicity is described by Bonavida and associates.[90] K562 cells are incubated with NK embedded in agarose. After an incubation period, the cells bound to the K562 cells and those destroyed are counted.

Evaluation of NK-cell cytotoxicity is fairly easy to perform; however, a substantial number of cells is required. The ^{51}Cr- or fluorochrome-release assay (discussed above) measures lytic function of a cell suspension of NK and target cells. One NK cell can lyse many target cells. The single cell suspension assay is more tedious to perform but provides specific information on binding and lytic capacity of a single NK cell.

Several investigators report enhancement of in vivo NK cytotoxicity.[91-94] Radiolabeled target cells were injected intravenously into animals whose NK activity was manipulated. At different points after injection of the target cells, the animals were killed and organ (spleen, liver, lungs) radioactivity was measured. Enhanced cytotoxicity, decreased tumor growth, and increased survival time were noted in the animals whose NK cells were manipulated for enhanced activity.[93-95] Major limitations of most in vivo NK cell studies are the associated high variability and low reproducibility.[94] A portion of the variability may be attributed to other cells such as macrophages and lymphocyte-activated killer cells that can lyse the radiolabeled target cells.

NK cell cytotoxicity is frequently assessed in nutrition intervention studies designed to evaluate the effects of nutrient deficiency and supplementation on immune function.[6,8,96,97] In healthy seniors, decreased serum selenium and zinc appear to correlate with a decreased percentage of NK cells.[8] Decreased serum vitamin E concentrations are associated with depressed NK cell cytotoxicity.[6,8] For example, depressed NK function was observed in a 16-month-old patient with Shwachman syndrome (an autosomal recessive syndrome characterized in part by pancreatic insufficiency, fat malabsorption, severe vitamin E

deficiency). Supplementation with vitamin E normalized NK cell activity and cessation of supplementation decreased activity, demonstrating a nutritional effect on NK cell activity.[6] Increased NK cytotoxicity is interpreted as a beneficial outcome. As our understanding of NK cells increases, we will be better able to interpret changes in NK function in relation to patient outcomes.

Summary
Physiochemical barriers, phagocytic cells, complement, and NK cells function within innate immunity, nonspecifically providing the first line of defense against invading organisms. While innate immune mechanisms function independently from acquired ones, the two also work in concert. For example, macrophages present antigen and secrete cytokines to activate T lymphocytes. Activated T lymphocytes and NK cells secrete IFN-γ, which enhances macrophage phagocytic activity. Additionally, acquired immune responses, such as antibody-induced complement activation, augment the innate immune response by directing phagocytes into infected areas and enhancing phagocytosis. The role of acquired immunity in host defense is discussed in the following section.

Acquired Immunity
Acquired immunity is also called "specific" or "adaptive" immunity. Like innate immune responses, acquired immune mechanisms also function to eliminate invading microbes; however, two additional features of acquired immunity—antigen-specific amplification and memory—are important in host defense. Once a lymphocyte recognizes an antigen, the lymphocyte is induced to proliferate until sufficient lymphocytes are available to mount an adequate immune response. During the amplification process, memory cells are generated. These lymphocytes "remember" the inciting antigen and are available to respond to subsequent exposures. Because of the presence of memory cells, subsequent exposures to the same antigen generate an immune response that is more rapid in onset and more intense.

Acquired immune responses are mediated by substances such as antibodies in body fluids (humoral immunity) or by immune cells (cell-mediated immunity). Efficient removal of inciting antigens by the acquired immune system depends on a coordinated effort and communication between the different components of the humoral and cell-mediated immune responses. Communication is brought about by direct cell-to-cell contact and secreted cytokines or immune regulatory molecules. Assessment of acquired immune responses focuses not only on the cells and antibodies involved in cell-mediated and humoral immunity but also on the secreted cytokines and molecules involved in the intercellular communication process.

Evaluating T-Lymphocyte Function
Cell-mediated immunity is carried out by T lymphocytes, which originate from the bone marrow and mature in the thymus. T lymphocytes are of two functionally distinct populations, T helper lymphocytes and cytotoxic T lymphocytes (CTLs). At this time, there is controversy in the literature regarding whether a third population of "suppressor T lympho-

cytes" exists or whether T helper lymphocytes and CTLs perform suppressor functions under certain conditions.

Monoclonal antibodies have been developed to identify or react with selected cell surface molecules on T helper lymphocytes and CTLs. The identified cell surface molecules that have been defined are given a *cluster of differentiation* (CD) designation. Antibodies that recognize the CD are termed *anti-CD*.... T helper lymphocytes are generally referred to as CD4+ lymphocytes, whereas CTLs are generally referred to as CD8+ lymphocytes. T helper lymphocytes of a single phenotype (i.e., the same cell surface molecules) can be subclassified as Th1 or Th2, based on their function and the cytokines they secrete. The Th1 cytokines, which are predominantly IL-2 and IFN-γ, activate T lymphocytes and macrophages. The Th1 subset is responsible for cell-mediated immune functions, such as delayed-type hypersensitivity and activation of cytotoxic T lymphocytes. Th2 cytokines, which are predominantly IL-4 and IL-10, help with B-lymphocyte functions. Recent studies suggest that dietary nucleic acids may promote a shift in Th1 to Th2 balance toward Th1 responses.[13,98] When mice were fed a nucleic acid supplemented diet versus a nucleic acid free diet, there was an increase in Th1 cytokines and a decrease in Th2 cytokines and associated antibodies.[13,98] Zinc deficiency adversely affects Th1 lymphocyte function and cell-mediated immunity, while zinc supplementation seems to improve Th1 responses.[99] On the other hand, high-level dietary vitamin A appears to enhance Th2-mediated immune responses.[16]

CD4+ T lymphocytes use their T-cell receptors to recognize antigens in conjunction with the MHC class II molecules on antigen-presenting cells (APC). Macrophages, dendritic cells, and B lymphocytes are examples of APCs. Once receptor binding occurs between the T lymphocyte and APC, production of IL-2 and IL-2 receptor is induced. IL-2 serves as a growth factor responsible for the initiation of cell cycling in the particular T lymphocyte that is secreting the IL-2, as well as nearby T lymphocytes.

CTLs are a subset of T lymphocytes whose proliferation and differentiation depend on IL-2. The function of CTLs is to lyse target cells such as virus-infected cells, tumor cells, or organ or tissue allografts (transplanted tissue). Like T-helper-lymphocyte activation, CTL killing is antigen specific. CTLs that recognize antigen bind to the antigen-expressing target cell and release pore-forming proteins and cell toxins to kill the target cell.

Activated T lymphocytes mediate many functions, including induction and suppression of cell activity, destruction of infected cells, and the overall orchestration of the immune response. Therefore, evaluation of T-lymphocyte response requires phenotypic quantitation and functional assessment. Methods used to assess T-lymphocyte number, phenotype, and function are discussed in the following sections. T lymphocytes are often evaluated in vitro on peripheral blood samples, but keep in mind that the phenotypes and functions of lymphocytes may vary depending on their location (e.g., peripheral blood, systemic lymph nodes, gut-associated lymphoid tissues, spleen, and various body fluids).

CELL ENUMERATION. The number and percentage of circulating lymphocytes are routinely evaluated in clinical settings by obtaining a WBC and differential count. The total lymphocyte count (TLC), which represents both T- and B- and NK-cell populations, is calculated by multiplying the white blood cell count by the percentage of lymphocytes. Typically, lymphocyte counts of 1500 to 1800 mm³ are associated with mild nutritional depletion, while TLCs of 900 to 1500 mm³ and less than 900 mm³ are associated with moderate and severe depletion, respectively.[100] This is a readily available immune parameter that correlates with malnutrition[10,63] and increased morbidity and mortality in hospitalized patients.[101-104] TLC is not a specific indicator of nutrition status because it decreases with aging, acquired immunodeficiency syndrome, and radiotherapy. Additionally, TLC is depressed with the administration of immunosuppressive medications, such as corticosteroids and chemotherapeutic agents, and is increased with infection and lymphoma.[63,105,106]

With advanced technology, subpopulations of lymphocytes, instead of just TLC, can now be assessed. Flow cytometry technology, also known as flow microfluorometry or flow cytofluorometry, is used to count cell populations. Additionally, flow cytometry is used to characterize cell-surface antigens and phenotypes (T lymphocytes versus B lymphocytes or CD4+ T lymphocytes versus CD8+ T lymphocytes). To characterize the CD4+ lymphocyte population of a blood sample, whole blood samples are drawn and red blood cells are removed. The remaining cells are incubated with antibodies against CD4 (anti-CD4 antibodies) that are labeled with a fluorochrome such as fluorescein isothiocyanate (FITC) or phycoerythrin (PE). The fluorochrome-labeled, anti-CD4 antibodies bind to cells with the CD4 surface molecules (i.e., T helper lymphocytes). Labeled and unlabeled cells are injected into the flow cytometer and individually illuminated by a laser. Lymphoid cell populations are initially separated by size and granularity (internal structure). Cell size is determined by measuring forward light scatter, and granularity by measuring 90-degree sideways light scatter. Cells that are larger, smaller, or more granular than lymphocytes (i.e., neutrophils) are "gated" out, so that the analysis focuses on lymphocytes. The CD4+ subpopulation is identified by exciting the fluorochrome-labeled, anti-CD4 antibody bound to these cells. The fluorochrome absorbs light at a specific wavelength and emits light at a different wavelength. By measuring the intensity of the fluorescence, the frequency of CD4+ cells and the relative amount of the cellular antigenic determinants can be ascertained. Because fluorescence intensity is an arbitrary measure, data must be compared with known standards or controls. Histograms are used to plot data.

Studies have used flow cytometry to examine the effect of nutrition or nutrients on lymphocyte subpopulations, such as T lymphocytes (CD3+ cells), helper T lymphocytes (CD4+ cells), cytotoxic T lymphocytes (CD8+ cells), naive T lymphocytes (CD45RA+ cells), memory T lymphocytes (CD45RO+ cells) and activated T lymphocytes (CD25 or CD69).[10,17,28,63] In a recent in vitro study Granato and others showed that an olive oil-based emulsion could preserve IL-2 receptor (CD25) expression on CD4+ and CD8+ cells compared with soybean oil lipid emulsion typically used in parenteral nutrition solutions.[28] Other studies have attempted to characterize lymphocyte populations in the severely malnourished to identify the cause of starvation-induced impairment of immune function.[10] CD4+

T-lymphocyte populations are routinely measured in the diagnosis and treatment of human immunodeficiency virus (HIV) and acquired immunodeficiency syndrome (AIDS). Flow cytometric techniques can also be used to differentiate B lymphocyte populations from T lymphocytes using fluorescent-labeled antibodies to CD19 or CD20.[107,108]

ASSAYS OF PROLIFERATION (LYMPHOCYTE BLASTOGENESIS). Stimulation of lymphocytes by certain agents (typically mitogens) results in cellular events that culminate in cellular division (DNA synthesis). Whole-blood samples are drawn and the lymphocytes are isolated by density gradient centrifugation. This is done by layering blood on a polysucrose medium. Red blood cells and granulocytes are aggregated by the polysucrose and centrifuged through the medium. Lymphocytes remain at the plasma-medium interface. The lymphocytes are removed, washed, and incubated in triplicate in 96-well plates containing culture medium and autologous serum, pooled human serum, or fetal calf serum. A mitogen is added at time zero, and DNA synthesis is measured 72 hours later by assessing the incorporation of a radioactive nucleoside precursor such as tritiated thymidine (^{3}H-thymidine) into newly synthesized DNA. The incorporation of ^{3}H-thymidine is related to the ability of the cell to respond to the mitogen (cellular activation and division—lymphocyte proliferation).

DNA synthesis is reported as counts per minute of ^{3}H. Some researchers normalize data by subtracting the background count per minute (unstimulated cultures) from the stimulated count per minute (stimulated cultures) or by dividing the stimulated count per minute by the background value (stimulation index). These data manipulations can obscure significant differences in the background count per minute, which may account for all measurable differences among experimental groups. When data are presented in this manner, it is important to present the range of background count per minute. High background counts may be due to contamination of cultures or to cross-contamination between culture wells.

Mitogens used to activate T lymphocytes include anti-CD3, concanavalin A (Con A), or phytohemagglutinin (PHA), whereas T and B lymphocytes can be stimulated by phorbol esters (phorbol-12-myristate-13-acetate [PMA]) plus ionomycin or pokeweed mitogen (PWM).[10,28,109,110] Mitogen-induced proliferation is also useful in estimating signal transduction or assessing growth factor requirements for lymphocytes. Mitogens such as PHA and Con A nonspecifically stimulate 80% to 90% of the T lymphocytes and are thus convenient to use. Mitogens, however, do not physiologically activate T lymphocytes.[111] In vivo, stimulation of T lymphocytes occurs when the T-cell receptor binds antigen presented in the MHC class II molecule on the APC. Less than 0.0001% to 0.01% of resting T lymphocytes respond to a conventional antigen.[112] Using an antigen to stimulate T lymphocytes in vitro would require a prohibitive number of cells to measure proliferative responses and biochemical changes. Superantigens or allogeneic stimulator cells (see One-Way Mixed Leukocyte Reaction) stimulate a reasonable number of cells and are therefore used as a physiologic means of T-lymphocyte activation.[111]

The lymphocyte proliferative response in vitro is frequently used as an indicator of immunocompetence in nutrient depletion or nutrient supplementation studies.[10,26,28,29,63,113] Cells taken from the study and control populations are cultured in medium for 3 to 7 days. While the nutrient intake of study patients may have been quite different from that of the control patients (e.g., added arginine) the nutrient composition of the incubation medium is identical for both groups. Therefore, culture conditions do not reflect conditions in vivo. Cells that are not responsive in vivo because of nutrient deprivation may now respond in vitro. Conversely, cells that respond in vivo may not respond in vitro after being removed from their normal environment. Frequently, autologous serum (serum and cells taken from the same individual) is used in proliferation assays. Inhibitory or stimulatory factors formed in vivo and secreted into the serum under the experimental conditions may alter the proliferative response in vitro.

Malnutrition, aging, major burns, and long-chain polyunsaturated fatty acid intravenous lipid emulsions are a few conditions or interventions that depress lymphocyte proliferation.[7,9,10,27,28,63,114] Nutrition research frequently tries to manipulate the proliferative response by nutrient supplementation; however, only a few studies to date have correlated an improved proliferative response with an improved clinical outcome.[20,113,115]

ONE-WAY MIXED LEUKOCYTE REACTION. Another method of measuring T-lymphocyte activation and proliferation is the one-way mixed leukocyte reaction (MLR). The MLR is used to assess histocompatibility for tissue transplant. An MLR is induced by culturing mononuclear leukocytes (stimulator cells) from a "normal" donor with mononuclear leukocytes from a test subject (responder cells). The stimulator cells are pretreated with mitomycin C or gamma irradiation to prevent proliferation without killing the cells. The cells are cultured for 4 to 7 days. If the stimulator and responder cells contain different alleles of the MHC genes, the responder T lymphocytes become activated and proliferate. Proliferation is measured by the incorporation of ^{3}H-thymidine into DNA (see Assays of Proliferation). When the MLR is used in research as a physiologic means for T-lymphocyte activation, intersubject variability is great. This is because the proliferative response depends on the degree of genetic disparity between stimulating and responding cells. To minimize variability, pooled human allogeneic cells can be frozen in aliquots and used as stimulator cells.[116]

CYTOTOXIC T-LYMPHOCYTE ASSAYS. CTL and NK function are assessed in much the same way. Target cells such as Epstein-Barr virus-transformed B lymphoblasts are radiolabeled with ^{51}Cr and incubated with different dilutions of CTLs and anti-CD3 to stimulate the cells. When CTLs kill the target cells, ^{51}Cr is released. To control for spontaneous release of ^{51}Cr from the target cells, radiolabeled target cells are incubated without CTLs. Maximum release of ^{51}Cr is determined by lysing the labeled target cells. At the end of the incubation period, the ^{51}Cr released into the cell-free supernatant is counted in a gamma counter. The percentage of specific lysis is determined by subtracting the spontaneous release from the experimental release and dividing this quantity by the maximum release minus the spontaneous release. If mononuclear cell populations are used as the source of CTLs, additional controls must be added to the assay to account for NK lysis of the target cells.

CYTOKINE PRODUCTION. Cytokines play an integral role in immune response, cell differentiation, and proliferation. The term *cytokine* is a universal term for lymphokines, monokines, and interleukins. Cytokines are hormone-like peptides or glycopeptides of low molecular weight that mediate intercellular communication. Typically, cytokines are produced by more than one cell type and have a diverse effect on many target cells. This nonspecificity has led to much confusion because cytokines were originally identified and described according to the cells that produced them and the actions they induced in the target cells. Once cytokines are produced, they interact with specific cell-surface receptors. Cellular activation can upregulate receptor expression. Receptors can be shed from cells and act as inhibitory molecules by binding to secreted cytokines. The relatively short half-life of cytokines allows tight regulation of their actions.

Cytokines can be measured by several means. The sensitivity and precision required to quantitate cytokine levels dictate which assay should be used. The ELISA is a reproducible, nonradioactive technique for detecting or measuring cytokines in body fluids and cell culture supernatants. Because antibodies stick to the plastic surface of ELISA plates, the plates can be coated with antibodies (typically monoclonal antibodies) that recognize the cytokine being assayed. Supernatants or fluids that contain the cytokine are added to the wells of the ELISA plate and incubated. The antibodies "capture" the cytokine. The wells are then washed to remove unbound cytokines, and a second antibody (typically a polyclonal antibody) that also recognizes the cytokine being assayed is added to the wells. After an incubation period and subsequent washing, a third antibody that recognizes the second antibody and that is also conjugated with an enzyme is added to each well. Finally, the substrate for the enzyme is added to each well. As the enzyme metabolizes the substrate, a color change is produced. The degree of color change depends on the amount of cytokine present. The color change is quantitated, and the concentration of the test sample is calculated from a standard curve. While the second antibody could be conjugated with the enzyme, a third antibody typically is used to amplify the signal (i.e., increase the degree of color change). To prevent nonspecific binding of the second or third antibodies to the ELISA plate, a protein such as albumin can be added to the wells. This technique can be modified to include radiolabeled ligands or antibodies in the amplification step (RIA). Cytokines present in dilute concentrations (nanograms to picograms per milliliter) can be measured with a high degree of accuracy using these methods.

Bioassays are another way of measuring cytokine levels. Cell lines that cannot propagate without a certain cytokine added to the culture medium are used as a "bioassay" for that particular cytokine.[117] Cell supernatants or body fluids containing the cytokine to be assayed and the cytokine-dependent cells are added to wells in a microtiter plate. Known quantities of recombinant cytokine are added to other wells that contain the cytokine-dependent cells. The cells are then incubated. After a period of time, cell division is measured in the cells (see Assays of Proliferation). The amount of cell division depends on the amount of cytokine in the supernatant or fluid: the higher the concentration of the cytokine, the more the cells proliferate. To determine the concentration of cytokine, the proliferation in each well of the microtiter plate is compared to a standard curve generated from the proliferation that occurred in the wells containing known concentrations of the recombinant cytokine. Bioassays are valuable for determining whether the secreted cytokines are biologically active; however, ELISA determinations are used more often.

Frequently measured cytokines include the proinflammatory cytokines—IL-1, IL-6, and TNF—that modulate immune responses and orchestrate metabolic changes during an acute inflammatory response. Functions of these cytokines are discussed in detail in Chapter 35. Recently, Th1 cytokines (IL-2, IFN-γ) and Th2 cytokines (IL-4, IL-5, IL-6, IL-10) have been measured to ascertain the mechanism by which nutrition or nutritional supplementation affects immune function.[13,16,98,99,118,119]

DELAYED-TYPE HYPERSENSITIVITY. Although the majority of immune reactions occur locally within tissues, immune function is typically evaluated in vitro on cellular or humoral components of the immune system taken from the peripheral blood. Consequently, immune function in vitro may not correlate with actual responses in tissues. The DTH test, also known as *delayed cutaneous hypersensitivity* or *cell-mediated immunity skin test*, is one of the few immune function tests performed in vivo. A panel of antigens such as *Mycobacterium tuberculosis*, tetanus toxoid, diphtheria toxoid, and *C. albicans* are injected intradermally (usually in the forearm) to assess T-lymphocyte function. Antigen-induced reactivity, measured by millimeters in diameter of induration (swelling) and erythema (redness) at 24 and 48 hours, is characterized by an infiltrate consisting predominantly of T lymphocytes. The inability to react to any of the injected antigens is termed *anergy*. The term *relative anergy* is commonly used to define the ability to react to only one skin-test antigen from a battery of antigens;[120,121] however, this designation is arbitrary.

For a subject to respond to the antigen, the subject must have been previously exposed to or immunized against the antigen. In addition to no previous exposure to an antigen, malnutrition, advanced age, immunosuppressive diseases, immunosuppressive therapy, and technical errors in administering skin test antigens are associated with anergy.[19,106,122-126] Thus, caution is warranted in interpreting results or comparing outcomes from studies of different patient populations.

More recently, the antigenic response from a battery of skin test antigens has been evaluated. By using a battery of skin test antigens, the likelihood of previous exposure to at least one antigen increases. The DTH test score is then reported as the number of positive antigen test sites and/or the sum of average diameters for all skin test antigens.[14,19,20,119] Because of the risk of an anaphylactic reaction, medical supervision is essential during delayed-type hypersensitivity (DTH) testing.

Epidemiologic and clinical studies have confirmed that malnourished children suffer more frequent and severe infections. DTH testing has been used as a tool to predict morbidity risk in pediatric populations.[127] Shell-Duncan and Wood noted that immunologic status in children, as measured by DTH anergy, predicted gastrointestinal and respiratory infections and that nutritional status also was a factor in immunocompetence.[128] DTH has been used to document the adverse effect of age and stress on immune function, predict risk of infection, and determine the immunologic influence of specific nutrients (i.e., vitamin E).[14,19,20,119]

Evaluating B-Lymphocyte Function

B lymphocytes, which make up 5% to 10% of the total lymphocyte population, are the precursors of antibody-secreting cells (plasma cells). Antibodies or immunoglobulins are glycoproteins produced by plasma cells and B lymphocytes that neutralize antigen or mark it for elimination. There are five major classes of immunoglobulins, which are described in Table 5-2. Major classes can be further divided into subclasses based on structure (e.g., IgA_1 and IgA_2). Methods for determining serum immunoglobulin concentrations include ELISA, nephelometry, RIA, radial immunodiffusion (RID), plaque-forming cell assay (PFC), and enzyme-linked immunospot assay (ELISPOT).

QUANTITATION OF IMMUNOGLOBULINS. ELISA, which is frequently used to measure immunoglobulins, is a very versatile, sensitive, and quantitative technique that requires little equipment, and many of the reagents are available commercially (see Cytokine Production). Currently, many diagnostic laboratories use an automated nephelometric system to measure immunoglobulins. While instrumental costs are high compared to those of methods such as ELISA, nephelometric measurements are quick and easy to perform.

Nephelometry is the measurement of light scatter produced by the reflection of transmitted light rays. Antibody concentration can be determined by measuring the amount of light scatter produced when the antibody-antigen complexes are formed. Typically, a known concentration of antigen is assayed to generate a standard curve. The degree of light scatter depends on the size of the antibody-antigen complexes and the rate of the precipitation reaction between the complexes. Other conditions that can influence the determinations include sample condition, temperature, and mixing of the reagents. It is important to control as much as possible for these factors, as for any of the immunoassays described here.

RID, a method historically used to quantitate immunoglobulin concentrations, was based on the principle that when antigens and antibodies diffuse through agarose gel they form immune complexes. These complexes become visible as a precipitation ring.[129] More advanced techniques, such as the ELISA, have replaced RID.

The PFC assay is an effective in vitro method that is frequently used in animal models to measure the number of antibody-secreting cells in a cell population (e.g., peripheral blood, spleen, lymph nodes, tonsils). The PFC assay measures antibody formation in response to a primary or secondary immune challenge. To measure a secondary immune response, animals must first be "primed" in vivo. Typically this is accomplished by injecting erythrocytes from another animal species (e.g., sheep red blood cells) into the experimental animal. Antibody production is then measured by plating B lymphocytes from the primed animal with complement and antiimmunoglobulin on culture plates layered with red blood cells from the species used to prime the animal. If the B lymphocytes are secreting antibodies that recognize the plated red blood cells, the antibody binds to the target cell. MACs are formed (see Evaluating Complement Function), producing a clear circular area of lysed red blood cells (plaque) around the antibody-producing cell. The plaque surrounds the antibody-producing lymphocyte. Each plaque reflects one antibody-secreting lymphocyte. This assay can be modified to measure all classes of immunoglobulins or to determine the number of antibody-secreting cells. While the PFC assay is very useful for determining effective B-lymphocyte responses, it is used mainly in animal studies because priming includes injection of heterologous erythrocytes.

The ELISPOT assay, developed to detect individual antibody-secreting cells, became an alternate method to the PFC assay.[130-132] In the ELISPOT assay, tissue culture plates are coated with antigen. Antibody-secreting cells are added, and the cells are incubated. If the cells are secreting antibody that recognizes the antigen, antibody-antigen complexes are formed. The plates are washed to remove any antibody that is not bound to the antigen. An antiimmunoglobulin antibody conjugated to an enzyme (e.g., horseradish peroxidase or alkaline phosphatase) is added to the culture plate. The antiimmunoglobulin enzyme binds the secreted antibody. Substrate for the enzyme is added to the culture plates. As the substrate is metabolized by the enzyme, a color change (a spot) is observed. The spots are counted to determine how many cells are secreting antibody particular to the antigen coated on the plate.[131] Antigens used in this assay are those typically used to vaccinate humans. An advantage of the ELISPOT assay is that the antibody-secreting potential of individual cells taken from tissue biopsies of lung or intestine can be assessed.[133,134] The ELISPOT assay can also be modified to assess cytokine production.[135]

The evaluation of antibodies can provide valuable information on how well the acquired immune system is functioning. Nutritional studies have examined antibody concentrations, classes, and subclasses as an indication of systemic and mucosal immune responses, immunoglobulin response to vaccination, and Th1 versus Th2 balance.[98,115,118,136,137] For example, Sudo and associates measured serum antibodies in mice maintained on a nucleic acid–free or nucleic-acid supplemented diet.[98] Total IgM, IgG, IgG1, and IgE were reduced and IgG2a did not change in the nucleic acid supplemented mice compared with mice fed the nucleic acid–free diet. This pattern of antibody expression suggests a shift in the Th1/Th2 balance toward Th1-mediated immune function or cell mediated immune function.[98] Studies from the laboratory of Kudsk routinely measure IgA as an indication of mucosal immune function in studies examining the effect of route of feeding on mucosal immunity.[118,138,139]

TABLE 5-2

Major Classes of Immunoglobulin (Antibody) and Defining Characteristics

Immunoglobulin	Characteristic
IgG	Most abundant immunoglobulin in normal serum
IgA	Predominant immunoglobulin in external secretions: breast milk; tears; and digestive, bronchial, and genitourinary secretions
IgM	First immunoglobulin produced in a primary antibody response
IgD	Found on the membrane of mature B cells, biologic effector function yet to be determined
IgE	Immunoglobulin responsible for allergic reactions

VACCINE RESPONSE. Another in vivo measurement of immune function is the quantitation of a vaccine response (specific antibody production). The purpose of a vaccine is to expose the immune system to noninfectious antigens so that the immune system recognizes and rapidly responds to the infectious agent on subsequent encounters. The response requires cooperation between antigen-presenting T and B lymphocytes and can be quantitated to provide an index of how well the immune system is functioning. Any cellular dysfunction can potentially cause a decrease in antibody production.

Vaccine response can be evaluated by ELISA (to measure vaccine-specific antibodies) or ELISPOT (to detect individual cells secreting vaccine-specific antibodies). Recently, there has been interest in the nutrition arena in measuring vaccine response. It is well known that seniors frequently receive influenza vaccines but don't respond as well as a younger population.[140] Several studies examining the effect of nutrition or age on the immune system of seniors have measured the antibody response to influenza vaccines using the hemmagglutination inhibition (HI) method to quantitate antibody levels in blood or serum.[141] This tests detects antibodies that prevent influenza virus hemmagglutination (clumping of red blood cells). When influenza virus and red blood cells are mixed at optimal concentrations there is a distinct pattern of agglutination. When antibodies specific for influenza are present, the agglutination is blocked. Therefore, one measures the relative concentration based on standardized dilutions of test and references samples. The HI titer is reported as the reciprocal of the highest dilution that caused complete inhibition of agglutination. An antibody titer equal to or above 40 is generally believed to provide significant protection against influenza, while a fourfold increase in HI antibody titer indicates a specific immune response to the vaccine.

Vaccine response is decreased with nutrient deficiencies, stress, and advanced age.[136,137] When studying the effectiveness of vaccination, for example in the seniors, nutritional aspects are rarely taken into consideration, yet nutrition plays a large and influential role in vaccination response. In 1992, Chandra demonstrated that vitamin and mineral supplementation significantly increased the influenza vaccine response in seniors above the placebo group.[113] In 1997, Meydani and others showed that supplemental vitamin E (200 to 800 mg α-tocopherol) increased antibody response to the hepatitis B vaccine but did not enhance antibody response to tetanus toxoid or diphtheria vaccinations in seniors.[19]

There is added confidence when evaluating the effects of nutrients if several indices of immune function indicate that a formula or compound provides benefit to the immune system. For example, a recently completed study examined immune responses (including antibody response and lymphocyte proliferation to influenza vaccine components) and the incidence of upper respiratory tract infections (URTI) in seniors who consumed a balanced nutritional formula containing 360 kcal and 13 g of protein plus vitamins, minerals, antioxidants, fructooligosaccharides, and structured lipids or an isocaloric, isonitrogenous control product.[115] Seniors are at increased risk of URTI and age-associated immune senescence; however, the researchers noted a decrease in the average days of symptoms of URTI in the group who received the nutritional supplement.

There was also a higher percentage of subjects in the treatment versus control groups (87% versus 41%) who achieved a fourfold increase in serum antibody titer to the influenza vaccine. And lastly, the specific lymphocyte proliferation to influenza components was greater in the treatment versus the control group. In conclusion, the unique formula improved immune function, enhanced influenza vaccine effectiveness, and reduced the days of symptoms of URTI in seniors. This study also provides a good example of a nutritional study that used laboratory and clinical-based outcomes to evaluate immune function.

Summary

Acquired immune responses are critical for host defense. Lymphocytes interact with other cells and recognize antigen. Activated lymphocytes proliferate until sufficient cells are available to mount an adequate immune response. Cytokines, secreted during the activation process, aid in the regulation of cell differentiation and proliferation, antibody generation and secretion, and cell-cell communication. Ultimately, the inciting antigen is cleared by opsonin-enhanced phagocytosis or cytolysis. Laboratory tests used to evaluate immunocompetence focus on every aspect of an immune response, ranging from antigen recognition to antigen elimination.

Conclusion

The complexity of an immune response and the many factors that affect immune function make it difficult to define an "optimal" response. Complexity is reduced by analyzing individual components of the integrated response and by combining laboratory-based measurements with clinical outcomes. Laboratory tests used successfully to evaluate immunocompetence must be informative, discriminating, and clinically relevant. Typically, this has required the characterization of a normal immune response with the deviation from normal being indicative of an unfavorable outcome. Unfortunately, normal immune function is difficult to assess in humans because so many factors—age, sex, active disease or infection, medication, nutritional status—affect immune function.

Laboratory tests routinely used to evaluate immunocompetence must be both available to the clinician and clinically relevant. Most of the laboratory tests discussed in this chapter are not available "in house" to clinicians practicing in community hospitals. Patient samples can be sent to outside laboratories, but this involves delay and extra expense. Many of the functional assays described in this chapter require 3 to 7 days to perform. Because of short hospital stays and dramatically changing conditions of acutely ill patients, the clinical relevance of such studies is questionable. Currently, clinical and basic scientists use immune function testing. Nutrients are being manipulated in an attempt to modulate the immune system and favorably affect patient outcomes. Because it is the responsibility of the nutrition practitioner to interpret the results of these studies and apply them, a basic understanding of the immune system, immune function assays, and the limitations associated with each assay is a necessity. The nutrition practitioner must also recognize the implications associated with enhancing or inhibiting immune function in specific patient populations.

REFERENCES

1. Wu G, Flynn NE, Flynn SP, et al: Dietary protein or arginine deficiency impairs constitutive and inducible nitric oxide synthesis by young rats, *J Nutr* 129(7):1347-1354, 1999.
2. Hildebrandt M, Rose M, Mayr C, et al: Alterations in expression and in serum activity of dipeptidyl peptidase IV (DPP IV, CD26) in patients with hyporectic eating disorders, *Scand J Immunol* 50(5):536-541, 1999.
3. Conzen SD, Janeway CA: Defective antigen presentation in chronically protein-deprived mice, *Immunology* 63(4):683-689, 1988.
4. Redmond HP, Leon P, Lieberman MD, et al: Impaired macrophage function in severe protein-energy malnutrition, *Arch Surg* 126(2):192-196, 1991.
5. Redmond HP, Shou J, Kelly CJ, et al: Protein-calorie malnutrition impairs host defense against *Candida albicans, J Surg Res* 50(6):552-559, 1991.
6. Adachi N, Migita M, Ohta T, et al: Depressed natural killer cell activity due to decreased natural killer cell population in a vitamin E-deficient patient with Shwachman syndrome: reversible natural killer cell abnormality by alpha-tocopherol supplementation, *Eur J Pediatr* 156(6):444-448, 1997.
7. Fulop T, Wagner JR, Khalil A, et al: Relationship between the response to influenza vaccination and the nutritional status in institutionalized elderly subjects, *J Gerontol A Biol Sci Med Sci* 54(2):M59-M64, 1999.
8. Ravaglia G, Forti P, Maioli F, et al: Effect of micronutrient status on natural killer cell immune function in healthy free-living subjects aged ≥90 y, *Am J Clin Nutr* 71(2):590-598, 2000.
9. Kawakami K, Kadota J, Iida K, et al: Reduced immune function and malnutrition in the elderly, *Tohoku J Exp Med* 187(2):157-171, 1999.
10. Allende LM, Corell A, Manzanares J, et al: Immunodeficiency associated with anorexia nervosa is secondary and improves after refeeding, *Immunology* 94(4):543-551, 1998.
11. Kyzer S, Binyamini J, Chaimoff C, et al: The effect of surgically induced weight reduction on the serum levels of the cytokines: interleukin-3 and tumor necrosis factor, *Obes Surg* 9(3):229-234, 1999.
12. Herselman M, Moosa MR, Kotze TJ, et al: Protein-energy malnutrition as a risk factor for increased morbidity in long-term hemodialysis patients, *J Ren Nutr* 10(1):7-15, 2000.
13. Nagafuchi S, Hachimura S, Totsuka M, et al: Dietary nucleotides can up-regulate antigen-specific Th1 immune responses and suppress antigen-specific IgE responses in mice, *Int Arch Allergy Immunol* 122(1):33-41, 2000.
14. Gianotti L, Braga M, Fortis C, et al: A prospective, randomized clinical trial on perioperative feeding with an arginine-, omega-3 fatty acid-, and RNA-enriched enteral diet: effect on host response and nutritional status, *J Parenter Enteral Nutr* 23(6):314-320, 1999.
15. Lewis B, Langkamp-Henken B: Arginine enhances in vivo immune responses in young, adult and aged mice, *J Nutr* 130(7):1827-1830, 2000.
16. Cui D, Moldoveanu Z, Stephensen CB: High-level dietary vitamin A enhances T-helper type 2 cytokine production and secretory immunoglobulin A response to influenza A virus infection in BALB/c mice, *J Nutr* 130(5):1132-1139, 2000.
17. Fortes C, Forastiere F, Agabiti N, et al: The effect of zinc and vitamin A supplementation on immune response in an older population, *J Am Geriatr Soc* 46(1):19-26, 1998.
18. Santos MS, Gaziano JM, Leka LS, et al: Beta-carotene-induced enhancement of natural killer cell activity in elderly men: an investigation of the role of cytokines, *Am J Clin Nutr* 68(1):164-170, 1998.
19. Meydani SN, Meydani M, Blumberg JB, et al: Vitamin E supplementation and in vivo immune response in healthy elderly subjects. A randomized controlled trial, *JAMA* 277(17):1380-1386, 1997.
20. Girodon F, Galan P, Monget AL, et al: Impact of trace elements and vitamin supplementation on immunity and infections in institutionalized elderly patients: a randomized controlled trial. MIN. VIT. AOX. Geriatric Network, *Arch Intern Med* 159(7):748-754, 1999.
21. Del Rio M, Ruedas G, Medina S, et al: Improvement by several antioxidants of macrophage function in vitro, *Life Sci* 63(10):871-881, 1998.
22. Matsuzaki T, Chin J: Modulating immune responses with probiotic bacteria, *Immunol Cell Biol* 78(1):67-73, 2000.
23. Yu R, Park JW, Kurata T, et al: Modulation of select immune responses by dietary capsaicin, *Int J Vitam Nutr Res* 68(2):114-119, 1998.
24. Estrada A, Yun CH, Van Kessel A, et al: Immunomodulatory activities of oat beta-glucan in vitro and in vivo, *Microbiol Immunol* 41(12):991-998, 1997.
25. Levander OA, Beck MA: Selenium and viral virulence, *Br Med Bull* 55(3):528-533, 1999.
26. de Beaux AC, O'Riordain MG, Ross JA, et al: Glutamine-supplemented total parenteral nutrition reduces blood mononuclear cell interleukin-8 release in severe acute pancreatitis, *Nutrition* 14(3):261-265, 1998.
27. Berger MM, Spertini F, Shenkin A, et al: Trace element supplementation modulates pulmonary infection rates after major burns: a double-blind, placebo-controlled trial, *Am J Clin Nutr* 68(2):365-371, 1998.
28. Granato D, Blum S, Rossle C, et al: Effects of parenteral lipid emulsions with different fatty acid composition on immune cell functions in vitro, *J Parenter Enteral Nutr* 24(2):113-118, 2000.
29. Langkamp-Henken B, Herrlinger-Garcia KA, Stechmiller JK, et al: Arginine supplementation is well tolerated but does not enhance mitogen-induced lymphocyte proliferation in elderly nursing home residents with pressure ulcers, *J Parenter Enteral Nutr* 24(5):280-287, 2000.
30. Karimbakas J, Langkamp-Henken B, Percival SS: Arrested maturation of granulocytes in copper deficient mice, *J Nutr* 128(11):1855-1860, 1998.
31. Grisham MB, Benoit JN, Granger DN: Assessment of leukocyte involvement during ischemia and reperfusion of intestine, *Methods Enzymol* 186:729-742, 1990.
32. Schmekel B, Seveus L, Xu SY, et al: Human neutrophil lipocalin (HNL) and myeloperoxidase (MPO). Studies of lung lavage fluid and lung tissue, *Respir Med* 94(6):564-568, 2000.
33. Bresser P, Out TA, van Alphen L, et al: Airway inflammation in nonobstructive and obstructive chronic bronchitis with chronic *Haemophilus influenzae* airway infection. Comparison with noninfected patients with chronic obstructive pulmonary disease, *Am J Respir Crit Care Med* 162(3 Pt 1):947-952, 2000.
34. Clark RA, Nauseef WM: Isolation and functional analysis of neutrophils. In Coligan JE, Kruisbeek AM, Margulies DH, et al. (eds): *Current protocols in immunology,* New York, 1996, Wiley, pp 7.23.21-27.23.17.
35. Martin E, Bhakdi S: Flow cytometric assay for quantifying opsonophagocytosis and killing of *Staphylococcus aureus* by peripheral blood leukocytes, *J Clin Microbiol* 30(9):2246-2255, 1992.
36. Okada Y, Klein NJ, van Saene HK, et al: Bactericidal activity against coagulase-negative staphylococci is impaired in infants receiving long-term parenteral nutrition, *Ann Surg* 231(2):276-281, 2000.
37. Mastroianni CM, d'Ettorre G, Forcina G, et al: Interleukin-15 enhances neutrophil functional activity in patients with human immunodeficiency virus infection, *Blood* 96(5):1979-1984, 2000.
38. Fiuza C, Salcedo M, Clemente G, et al: In vivo neutrophil dysfunction in cirrhotic patients with advanced liver disease, *J Infect Dis* 182(2):526-533, 2000.
39. Corberand J, Ngyen F, Laharrague P, et al: Polymorphonuclear functions and aging in humans, *J Am Geriatr Soc* 29(9):391-397, 1981.
40. Azuma Y, Shinohara M, Wang PL, et al: Comparison of inhibitory effects of local anesthetics on immune functions of neutrophils, *Int J Immunopharmacol* 22(10):789-796, 2000.
41. Hitzfeld B, Friedrichs KH, Ring J, et al: Airborne particulate matter modulates the production of reactive oxygen species in human polymorphonuclear granulocytes, *Toxicology* 120(3):185-195, 1997.
42. Pelletier M, Savoie A, Girard D: Activation of human neutrophils by the air pollutant sodium sulfite (Na(2)SO(3)): comparison with immature promyelocytic HL-60 and DMSO-differentiated HL-60 cells reveals that Na(2)SO(3) is a neutrophil but not a HL-60 cell agonist, *Clin Immunol* 96(2):131-139, 2000.
43. Solomkin JS: Neutrophil disorders in burn injury: complement, cytokines, and organ injury, *J Trauma* 30(12 suppl):S80-85, 1990.
44. Christou NV: Host-defense mechanisms in surgical patients: a correlative study of the delayed hypersensitivity skin-test response, granulocyte function and sepsis, *Can J Surg* 28(1):39-46, 49, 1985.
45. Xiao F, Eppihimer MJ, Willis BH, et al: Complement-mediated lung injury and neutrophil retention after intestinal ischemia-reperfusion, *J Appl Physiol* 82(5):1459-1465, 1997.
46. Kozol RA: Neutrophil recruitment to the gastrointestinal tract, *J Surg Res* 53(3):310-315, 1992.
47. Redmond HP, Chavin KD, Bromberg JS, et al: Inhibition of macrophage-activating cytokines is beneficial in the acute septic response, *Ann Surg* 214(4):502-508; discussion 508-509, 1991.
48. Leitao MF, Vilela MM, Rutz R, et al: Complement factor I deficiency in a family with recurrent infections, *Immunopharmacology* 38(1-2):207-213, 1997.
49. Suankratay C, Mold C, Zhang Y, et al: Mechanism of complement-dependent haemolysis via the lectin pathway: role of the complement regulatory proteins, *Clin Exp Immunol* 117(3):442-448, 1999.

50. Haynes DR, Harkin DG, Bignold LP, et al: Inhibition of C5a-induced neutrophil chemotaxis and macrophage cytokine production in vitro by a new C5a receptor antagonist, *Biochem Pharmacol* 60(5):729-733, 2000.

51. Kirschfink M: Controlling the complement system in inflammation, *Immunopharmacology* 38(1-2):51-62, 1997.

52. Alexander JW, MacMillan BG, Stinnett JD, et al: Beneficial effects of aggressive protein feeding in severely burned children, *Ann Surg* 192(4):505-517, 1980.

53. Suskind R, Edelman R, Kulapongs P, et al: Complement activity in children with protein-calorie malnutrition, *Am J Clin Nutr* 29(10):1089-1092, 1976.

54. Haller L, Zubler RH, Lambert PH: Plasma levels of complement components and complement haemolytic activity in protein-energy malnutrition, *Clin Exp Immunol* 34(2):248-252, 1978.

55. Chandra RK: Immunocompetence in undernutrition, *J Pediatr* 81(6):1194-1200, 1972.

56. Chandra RK: Serum complement and immunoconglutinin in malnutrition, *Arch Dis Child* 50(3):225-229, 1975.

57. Hazelzet JA, de Groot R, van Mierlo G, et al: Complement activation in relation to capillary leakage in children with septic shock and purpura, *Infect Immun* 66(11):5350-5356, 1998.

58. Zamora MR, Davis RD, Keshavjee SH, et al: Complement inhibition attenuates human lung transplant reperfusion injury: a multicenter trial, *Chest* 116(1 suppl):46S, 1999.

59. Fitch JC, Rollins S, Matis L, et al: Pharmacology and biological efficacy of a recombinant, humanized, single-chain antibody C5 complement inhibitor in patients undergoing coronary artery bypass graft surgery with cardiopulmonary bypass, *Circulation* 100(25):2499-2506, 1999.

60. Collard CD, Vakeva A, Morrissey MA, et al: Complement activation after oxidative stress: role of the lectin complement pathway, *Am J Pathol* 156(5):1549-1556, 2000.

61. Zimmerman JL, Dellinger RP, Straube RC, et al: Phase I trial of the recombinant soluble complement receptor 1 in acute lung injury and acute respiratory distress syndrome, *Crit Care Med* 28(9):3149-3154, 2000.

62. Houdijk AP, Nijveldt RJ, van Leeuwen PA: Glutamine-enriched enteral feeding in trauma patients: reduced infectious morbidity is not related to changes in endocrine and metabolic responses, *J Parenter Enteral Nutr* 23(5 suppl):S52-S58, 1999.

63. Gelas P, Cotte L, Poitevin-Later F, et al: Effect of parenteral medium- and long-chain triglycerides on lymphocytes subpopulations and functions in patients with acquired immunodeficiency syndrome: a prospective study, *J Parenter Enteral Nutr* 22(2):67-71, 1998.

64. Chandra RK: Immunodeficiency in undernutrition and overnutrition, *Nutr Rev* 39(6):225-231, 1981.

65. Seeley JK, Golub SH: Studies on cytotoxicity generated in human mixed lymphocyte cultures. I. Time course and target spectrum of several distinct concomitant cytotoxic activities, *J Immunol* 120(4):1415-1422, 1978.

66. Ortaldo JR, Bonnard GD, Kind PD, et al: Cytotoxicity by cultured human lymphocytes: characteristics of effector cells and specificity of cytotoxicity, *J Immunol* 122(4):1489-1494, 1979.

67. Trinchieri G: Biology of natural killer cells, *Adv Immunol* 47:187-376, 1989.

68. Robertson MJ, Ritz J: Biology and clinical relevance of human natural killer cells, *Blood* 76(12):2421-2438, 1990.

69. Lotzova E: Natural killer cells: immunobiology and clinical prospects, *Cancer Invest* 9(2):173-184, 1991.

70. Talmadge JE, Meyers KM, Prieur DJ, et al: Role of NK cells in tumour growth and metastasis in beige mice, *Nature* 284(5757):622-624, 1980.

71. Hanna N: Role of natural killer cells in control of cancer metastasis, *Cancer Metastasis Rev* 1(1):45-64, 1982.

72. Bukowski JF, Woda BA, Welsh RM: Pathogenesis of murine cytomegalovirus infection in natural killer cell-depleted mice, *J Virol* 52(1):119-128, 1984.

73. Ebihara K, Minamishima Y: Protective effect of biological response modifiers on murine cytomegalovirus infection, *J Virol* 51(1):117-122, 1984.

74. Clark IA, Allison AC: *Babesia microti* and *Plasmodium berghei yoelii* infections in nude mice, *Nature* 252(5481):328-329, 1974.

75. Eugui EM, Allison AC: Differences in susceptibility of various mouse strains to haemoprotozoan infections: possible correlation with natural killer activity, *Parasite Immunol* 2(4):277-292, 1980.

76. Hunter KW, Folks TM, Sayler PC, et al: Early enhancement followed by suppression of natural killer cell activity during murine malarial infection, *Immun Lett* 1(2):209-212, 1981.

77. Murphy JW, McDaniel DO: In vitro reactivity of natural killer (NK) cells against *Cryptococcus neoformans, J Immunol* 128(4):1577-1583, 1982.

78. Hidore MR, Murphy JW: Correlation of natural killer cell activity and clearance of *Cryptococcus neoformans* from mice after adoptive transfer of splenic nylon wool-nonadherent cells, *Infect Immun* 51(2):547-555, 1986.

79. Ogata K, Yokose N, Tamura H, et al: Natural killer cells in the late decades of human life, *Clin Immunol Immunopathol* 84(3):269-275, 1997.

80. Vaquer S, Jorda J, Lopez de la Osa E, et al: Clinical implications of natural killer (NK) cytotoxicity in patients with squamous cell carcinoma of the uterine cervix, *Gynecol Oncol* 36(1):90-92, 1990.

81. Kadish AS, Doyle AT, Steinhauer EH, et al: Natural cytotoxicity and interferon production in human cancer: deficient natural killer activity and normal interferon production in patients with advanced disease, *J Immunol* 127(5):1817-1822, 1981.

82. Alvarez de Mon M, Casas J, Laguna R, et al: Lymphokine induction of NK-like cytotoxicity in T cells from B-CLL, *Blood* 67(1):228-232, 1986.

83. Scott-Algara D, Vuillier F, Cayota A, et al: Natural killer (NK) cell activity during HIV infection: a decrease in NK activity is observed at the clonal level and is not restored after in vitro long-term culture of NK cells, *Clin Exp Immunol* 90(2):181-187, 1992.

84. Lozzio CB, Lozzio BB: Human chronic myelogenous leukemia cell-line with positive Philadelphia chromosome, *Blood* 45(3):321-334, 1975.

85. Chen G, Wood S, Watson RR: Modulation by drugs and measurement of natural killer cell activity. In Watson RR (ed): *In vitro methods of toxicology,* Boca Raton, FL, 1992, CRC Press, pp 53-65.

86. Wood SM, Beckham C, Yosioka A, et al: Beta-carotene and selenium supplementation enhances immune reponse in aged humans, *Integr Med* 21(2):85-92, 2000.

87. Wierda WG, Mehr DS, Kim YB: Comparison of fluorochrome-labeled and ^{51}Cr-labeled targets for natural killer cytotoxicity assay, *J Immunol Methods* 122(1):15-24, 1989.

88. Tilden AB, Grossi CE, Itoh K, et al: Subpopulation analysis of human granular lymphocytes: associations with age, gender and cytotoxic activity, *Nat Immun Cell Growth Regul* 5(2):90-99, 1986.

89. Facchini A, Mariani E, Mariani AR, et al: Increased number of circulating Leu 11+ (CD 16) large granular lymphocytes and decreased NK activity during human ageing, *Clin Exp Immunol* 68(2):340-347, 1987.

90. Bonavida B, Bradley TP, Grimm EA: Frequency determination of killer cells by a single-cell cytotoxic assay, *Methods Enzymol* 93:270-280, 1983.

91. Riccardi C, Puccetti P, Santoni A, et al: Rapid in vivo assay of mouse natural killer cell activity, *J Natl Cancer Inst* 63(4):1041-1045, 1979.

92. Djeu JY, Huang KY, Herberman RB: Augmentation of mouse natural killer activity and induction of interferon by tumor cells in vivo, *J Exp Med* 151(4):781-789, 1980.

93. Riccardi C, Santoni A, Barlozzari T, et al: In vivo natural reactivity of mice against tumor cells, *Int J Cancer* 25(4):475-486, 1980.

94. Riccardi C, Santoni A, Barlozzari T, et al: Role of NK cells in rapid in vivo clearance of radiolabeled tumor cells. In Herberman RB (ed): *Natural cell-mediated immunity against tumor,* New York, 1980, Academic, pp 1121-1139.

95. Gorelik E, Wiltrout RH, Okumura K, et al: Role of NK cells in the control of metastatic spread and growth of tumor cells in mice, *Int J Cancer* 30(1):107-112, 1982.

96. Bogden JD: Studies on micronutrient supplements and immunity in older people, *Nutr Rev* 53(4 Pt 2):S59-S64; discussion S64-S55, 1995.

97. Corbeel LM, Ceuppens JL: Natural killer cell activity and hypovitaminosis E, *Eur J Pediatr* 156(6):449-450, 1997.

98. Sudo N, Aiba Y, Takaki A, et al: Dietary nucleic acids promote a shift in Th1/Th2 balance toward Th1-dominant immunity, *Clin Exp Allergy* 30(7):979-987, 2000.

99. Prasad AS: Effects of zinc deficiency on Th1 and Th2 cytokine shifts, *J Infect Dis* 182(suppl 1):S62-S68, 2000.

100. Shopbell JM, Hopkins B, Shronts EP: Nutrition screening and assessment. In Gottschlich MM (ed): *The science and practice of nutrition support: a case-based core curriculum,* Dubuque IA, 2001, Kendall/Hunt Publishing Company, pp 107-140.

101. Lewis RT, Klein H: Risk factors in postoperative sepsis: significance of preoperative lymphocytopenia, *J Surg Res* 26(4):365-371, 1979.

102. Morath MA, Miller SF, Finley RK Jr: Nutritional indicators of postburn bacteremic sepsis, *J Parenter Enteral Nutr* 5(6):488-491, 1981.

103. Harvey KB, Bothe A Jr, Blackburn GL: Nutritional assessment and patient outcome during oncological therapy, *Cancer* 43(5 suppl):2065-2069, 1979.

104. Seltzer MH, Fletcher HS, Slocum BA, et al: Instant nutritional assessment in the intensive care unit, *J Parenter Enteral Nutr* 5(1):70-72, 1981.

105. Wikby A, Johansson B, Ferguson F, et al: Age-related changes in immune parameters in a very old population of Swedish people: a longitudinal study, *Exp Gerontol* 29(5):531-541, 1994.
106. Cosimi AB, Brunstetter FH, Kemmerer WT, et al: Cellular immune competence of breast cancer patients receiving radiotherapy, *Arch Surg* 107(4):531-535, 1973.
107. Shearer WT, Easley KA, Goldfarb J, et al: Prospective 5-year study of peripheral blood CD4, CD8, and CD19/CD20 lymphocytes and serum Igs in children born to HIV-1 women. The P(2)C(2) HIV Study Group, *J Allergy Clin Immunol* 106(3):559-566, 2000.
108. Terzakis JA: Distinguishing B and T lymphocytes by scanning electron microscopy, *Ultrastruct Pathol* 24(4):205-209, 2000.
109. Son NH, Murray S, Yanovski J, et al: Lineage-specific telomere shortening and unaltered capacity for telomerase expression in human T and B lymphocytes with age, *J Immunol* 165(3):1191-1196, 2000.
110. De AK, Kodys KM, Pellegrini J, et al: Induction of global anergy rather than inhibitory Th2 lymphokines mediates posttrauma T cell immunodepression, *Clin Immunol* 96(1):52-66, 2000.
111. Langkamp-Henken B, Johnson LR, Viar MJ, et al: Differential effect on polyamine metabolism in mitogen- and superantigen-activated human T-cells, *Biochim Biophys Acta* 1425(2):337-347, 1998.
112. Kotb M: Role of superantigens in the pathogenesis of infectious diseases and their sequelae, *Curr Opin Infect Dis* 5:364-374, 1992.
113. Chandra RK: Effect of vitamin and trace-element supplementation on immune responses and infection in elderly subjects [see comments], *Lancet* 340(8828):1124-1127, 1992.
114. Lesourd BM: Nutrition and immunity in the elderly: modification of immune responses with nutritional treatments, *Am J Clin Nutr* 66(2):478S-484S, 1997.
115. Langkamp-Henken B, Bender BS, Gardner EM, et al: Nutritional formula enhanced immune function and reduced upper respiratory tract infection (URTI) in a randomized, double-blind, controlled trial in older adults, *Faseb J* 15(4):A63, 2001.
116. Kirk SJ, Hurson M, Regan MC, et al: Arginine stimulates wound healing and immune function in elderly human beings, *Surgery* 114(2):155-159; discussion 160, 1993.
117. Gillis S, Ferm MM, Ou W, et al: T cell growth factor: parameters of production and a quantitative microassay for activity, *J Immunol* 120(6):2027-2032, 1978.
118. Wu Y, Kudsk KA, DeWitt RC, et al: Route and type of nutrition influence IgA-mediating intestinal cytokines, *Ann Surg* 229(5):662-667; discussion 667-668, 1999.
119. Pallast EG, Schouten EG, de Waart FG, et al: Effect of 50- and 100-mg vitamin E supplements on cellular immune function in noninstitutionalized elderly persons, *Am J Clin Nutr* 69(6):1273-1281, 1999.
120. Meakins JL, Pietsch JB, Bubenick O, et al: Delayed hypersensitivity: indicator of acquired failure of host defenses in sepsis and trauma, *Ann Surg* 186(3):241-250, 1977.
121. Christou NV, McLean AP, Meakins JL: Host defense in blunt trauma: interrelationships of kinetics of anergy and depressed neutrophil function, nutritional status, and sepsis, *J Trauma* 20(10):833-841, 1980.
122. Moulias R, Devillechabrolle A, Lesourd B, et al: Respective roles of immune and nutritional factors in the priming of the immune response in the elderly, *Mech Ageing Dev* 31(2):123-137, 1985.
123. Gordin FM, Hartigan PM, Klimas NG, et al: Delayed-type hypersensitivity skin tests are an independent predictor of human immunodeficiency virus disease progression. Department of Veterans Affairs Cooperative Study Group, *J Infect Dis* 169(4):893-897, 1994.
124. Copeland EM, Fadyen BV Jr, Dudrick SJ: Effect of intravenous hyperalimentation on established delayed hypersensitivity in the cancer patient, *Ann Surg* 184(1):60-64, 1976.
125. Hersh EM, Gutterman JU, Mavligit G, et al: Host defense, chemical immunosuppression, and the transplant recipient. Relative effects of intermittent versus continuous immunosuppressive therapy with reference to the objectives of treatment, *Transplant Proc* 5(3):1191-1195, 1973.
126. Law DK, Dudrick SJ, Abdou NI: Immunocompetence of patients with protein-calorie malnutrition. The effects of nutritional repletion, *Ann Intern Med* 79(4):545-550, 1973.
127. Zaman K, Baqui AH, Yunus M, et al: Malnutrition, cell-mediated immune deficiency and acute upper respiratory infections in rural Bangladeshi children, *Acta Paediatr* 86(9):923-927, 1997.
128. Shell-Duncan B, Wood JW: The evaluation of delayed-type hypersensitivity responsiveness and nutritional status as predictors of gastro-intestinal and acute respiratory infection: a prospective field study among traditional nomadic Kenyan children, *J Trop Pediatr* 43(1):25-32, 1997.
129. Mancini GA, Carbonara O, Heremans JF: Immunochemical quantitation of antigens by single radial immunodiffusion, *Immunochemistry* 2:235-254, 1965.
130. Johnson CW, Williams WC, Copeland CB, et al: Sensitivity of the SRBC PFC assay versus ELISA for detection of immunosuppression by TCDD and TCDD-like congeners, *Toxicology* 156(1):1-11, 2000.
131. Czerkinsky CC, Nilsson LA, Nygren H, et al: A solid-phase enzyme-linked immunospot (ELISPOT) assay for enumeration of specific antibody-secreting cells, *J Immunol Methods* 65(1-2):109-121, 1983.
132. Sedgwick JD, Holt PG: A solid-phase immunoenzymatic technique for the enumeration of specific antibody-secreting cells, *J Immunol Methods* 57(1-3):301-309, 1983.
133. Flo J, Elias F, Benedetti R, et al: Reversible effects on B and T cells of the gut-associated lymphoid tissues in rats malnourished during suckling: impaired induction of the immune response to intra-Peyer patches immunization with cholera toxin, *Clin Immunol Immunopathol* 80(2):147-154, 1996.
134. Lycke N: A sensitive method for the detection of specific antibody production in different isotypes from single lamina propria plasma cells, *Scand J Immunol* 24(4):393-403, 1986.
135. Vazquez E, Gil A, Garcia-Olivares E, et al: Weaning induces an increase in the number of specific cytokine- secreting intestinal lymphocytes in mice, *Cytokine* 12(8):1267-1270, 2000.
136. Vedhara K, Cox NK, Wilcock GK, et al: Chronic stress in elderly carers of dementia patients and antibody response to influenza vaccination, *Lancet* 353(9153):627-631, 1999.
137. Kiecolt-Glaser JK, Glaser R, Gravenstein S, et al: Chronic stress alters the immune response to influenza virus vaccine in older adults, *Proc Natl Acad Sci USA* 93(7):3043-3047, 1996.
138. Li J, Kudsk KA, Gocinski B, et al: Effects of parenteral and enteral nutrition on gut-associated lymphoid tissue, *J Trauma* 39(1):44-51; discussion 51-42, 1995.
139. Renegar KB, Johnson CD, Dewitt RC, et al: Impairment of mucosal immunity by total parenteral nutrition: requirement for IgA in murine nasotracheal anti-influenza immunity, *J Immunol* 166(2):819-825, 2001.
140. Nicholson KG, Kent J, Hammersley V, et al: Acute viral infections of upper respiratory tract in elderly people living in the community: comparative, prospective, population based study of disease burden, *Br Med J* 315(7115):1060-1064, 1997.
141. Salk JE: Simplified procedure for titrating hemagglutinating capacity of influenza virus and the corresponding antibody, *J Immunol* 49:87-98, 1944.

Energy Dynamics 6

David Frankenfield, MS, RD

MODERN nonvolitional nutrition support has allowed clinicians to nourish the most critically ill patients in the hospital, patients with metabolic derangements who are unable to self-feed. The challenge is that, without the patient's internal cues for guidance and with considerable interpatient variability, we must provide adequate energy substrate without overfeeding. This chapter focuses on normal energy dynamics and the changes observed in hospital patients, the measurement and prediction of energy expenditure, and the consequences of providing energy substrate.

The History of Energy Dynamics

A good starting point for a discussion of the history of energy dynamics is the seventeenth century, with the experiments of William Boyle. While developing a device to create a vacuum, Boyle discovered that air was necessary to sustain both a flame and the life of small animals.[1,2] What component of air sustains both processes was not discovered until the eighteenth century, when Joseph Priestley discovered oxygen and Antoine Lavoisier named it and recognized it as the element that sustains combustion and life. Lavoisier went on to relate the uptake of oxygen by an animal to the release of carbon dioxide and heat by that animal. This was a seminal discovery in the science of calorimetry.[2]

In the nineteenth century, it was discovered that gas exchange (oxygen consumption and carbon dioxide production) is proportional to the amount of heat given off when a substrate is burned (oxidized) in a bomb calorimeter. The latter part of the nineteenth century saw many advances in the science of calorimetry and energy metabolism in both Europe and the United States. During this time, the relationship between gas exchange and heat production in vitro was found to hold true in vivo in animals and humans.[2,3] Such whole-body experiments were made possible by the development of direct calorimeters (chambers in which the subject resided while heat release into the environment was measured) and then the discovery that direct calorimetry measurements were proportional to indirect calorimetry measurements (the measurement of gas exchange of a living being). Many classic experiments of normal and altered metabolism were conducted in the early part of the twentieth century by investigators such as Atwater, Benedict, DuBois, and others.[2,4-6] In 1919, Harris and Benedict related basal metabolic rate to sex, age, and body size.[5] The Harris-Benedict equations for basal energy expenditure (BEE) remain to this day basic calculations in the workup of patients for nutrition support.

Calorimetry chambers were common in hospitals until the 1950s, being the primary tool for diagnosing and monitoring thyroid dysfunction.[2] As biochemical markers of thyroid function became available, most of the calorimetry chambers were dismantled, so that measurement of energy expenditure generally became unavailable in the hospital setting. Calorimetry chambers remained and still remain in use for research into the role of activity, genetics, and other factors in determining metabolic rate.

With the advent and widespread use of parenteral and tube feeding in the late 1960s and 1970s came a strong stimulus for the development of portable, bedside methods of measuring energy expenditure. In the 1980s several types of portable indirect calorimeters were made commercially available for clinical care and clinical research use. Much data on metabolic rates of various patient groups has since been published, some of it contradictory. Even with the reintroduction of calorimetry into the clinical arena, the use of predictive equations remains the most often used method of assigning an energy requirement to patients.

Energy Metabolism
Overview

The body requires a constant supply of energy to maintain homeostasis (i.e., life). The form this life-sustaining energy takes is the nucleotide adenosine triphosphate (ATP). As critical as it is to life, only enough ATP is present in the body at any given time, to last a few seconds to minutes. Thus, mechanisms have evolved to constantly convert more complex forms of chemical energy (the macronutrients carbohydrate, protein, lipid, and sometimes ethanol) into ATP, and to interconvert the macronutrients, depending on needs.[2,7]

Cellular Metabolism, Gas Exchange, and Heat Production

The basic method of energy conversion in animals is to oxidize complex macronutrients in a controlled manner by cleaving carbon bonds (a process called *decarboxylation*) and hydrogen bonds (*dehydrogenation*), capturing the resulting free energy by coupling the decarboxylation and dehydrogenation (oxidation) reactions to a reduction reaction ($NAD^+ + H_2 = NADH + H^+$).[8] Carbon dioxide and heat are released in the decarboxylation reaction. The carbon dioxide is transported to the lungs and expired; the heat is dissipated mainly through the skin. The $NADH + H^+$ enters the electron transport chain, which consists of a series of reduction-oxidation reactions of progressively lower redox potential. At each redox step, energy is released and captured by the phosphorylation of adenosine diphosphate ($ADP + P_1 = ATP$).[8] The terminal reaction of the electron transport chain is the reduction of oxygen to water. The ATP is used immediately for cellular chemical reactions. The chemical energy released by ATP dephosphorylation during cellular chemical reactions is converted to heat, and the heat is dissipated. Thus, in cellular metabolism of macronutrients, carbon dioxide is produced, oxygen is consumed, and heat is generated in proportion to the amount of substrate being oxidized (Fig. 6-1). All current methods of determining energy expenditure and substrate utilization rely on the relationship between cell metabolism, gas exchange, and heat release.

The relationships among oxidation of substrate, oxygen consumption, carbon dioxide production, and release of heat are constant. Each substrate produces a particular amount of heat for a given amount of oxygen consumption and a unique ratio of carbon dioxide production (Vco_2) to oxygen consumption (Vo_2) (respiratory quotient or RQ) (Table 6-1). The relationships among substrate oxidation, Vo_2, Vco_2, and heat release were elucidated in the late nineteenth and early twentieth centuries from bomb calorimetry studies and subsequent empiric balancing of chemical equations.[3,9-12] For fat and carbohydrate, combustion in a bomb calorimeter yields the same end products as enzymatic oxidation in the body (carbon

dioxide, water, and heat), so bomb calorimetry data are directly applicable to animal metabolism. Protein, however, is burned more completely in the bomb calorimeter (carbon dioxide, water, sulfate, nitrogen) than in the body (carbon dioxide, water, sulfate, urea). Thus, a correction factor must be used to account for incomplete combustion of protein in the body when applying bomb calorimetric constants to animal metabolism.

In 1988, Livesey and Elia published two landmark papers listing corrected constants for a large number of whole foods; medical foods; and individual fatty acids, carbohydrates, and amino acids (see Table 6-1).[13,14] Instead of stoichiometry, an algebraic approach was taken to validate the constants and equations used for gas exchange correlations with cellular metabolism.

Patterns of Cellular Substrate Metabolism

In healthy persons the pattern of substrate utilization is determined mainly by the amount and types of food consumed, mediated mostly by the central nervous system (CNS) and hormones whose serum levels are tuned to the feeding state. In ill patients energy expenditure and substrate utilization are mediated by complex interactions of many factors: CNS input, hormones, growth factors, certain peptides and amino acids, cytokines, and eicosanoids, whose levels are tuned more so to the disease state than the feeding state.[15] A detailed description of the mediators of energy expenditure is beyond the scope of this chapter.

STARVATION. If no food is consumed, insulin levels fall while glucagon and other counterregulatory hormone levels rise, creating a mildly catabolic state. Free fatty acids are readily available in this low insulin state, and the body develops a lipid and protein substrate economy; however, there is an obligatory

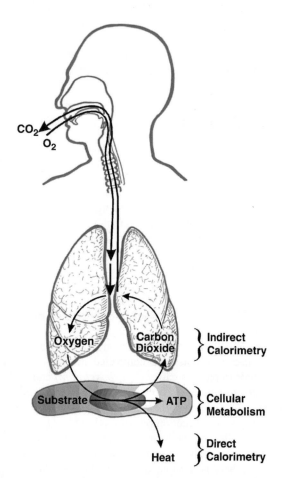

FIGURE 6-1 The relationship between cellular metabolism, heat production, and gas exchange.

TABLE 6-1

Examples of Constants for Heat Release and Gas Exchange for Carbohydrate, Fat, and Protein

Substrate/Investigator	−ΔHc (kcal/g)	CeO₂ (kcal/L)	RQ
CARBOHYDRATE			
Livesey, Elia[13]			
Glucose	3.72	4.98	1.0
Starch	4.18	5.05	1.0
Glycogen	4.19	5.05	1.0
Schumburg,[9] Zuntz	—	5.05	1.0
FAT			
Livesey, Elia[13]			
Palmitic acid	9.30	4.65	0.696
Safflower oil	9.42	4.70	0.722
Adipose tissue	9.45-9.54	4.68-4.70	0.709-0.722
Cathcart[10]	—	4.74	0.72
PROTEIN			
Livesey, Elia[13]			
Glutamine	3.61	4.59	0.89
Leucine	6.89	4.64	0.73
Food protein	4.17-5.06	4.63-4.68	0.814-0.874*
Lusk[3]	—	4.46	0.80

CeO₂, Caloric equivalent of oxygen; *ΔHc*, heat of combustion; *RQ*, respiratory quotient.
*Recommended RQ for protein, 0.835.

requirement for carbohydrate in CNS tissue and immune cells. In a starved state, when no exogenous or stored form of carbohydrate is available, protein must be converted to carbohydrate (through a process called *gluconeogenesis*) to satisfy obligatory needs. Unfortunately, there is no "storage form" of protein, so for every catabolized molecule of protein there is some loss of body function. In fact, death from starvation is often related to immune system and organ dysfunction secondary to protein depletion rather than exhaustion of available metabolic fuel. To spare protein the body musters several adaptations during starvation.[16] These include incomplete oxidation and recycling of available carbohydrate, reduction of metabolic rate, increased oxidation of body lipid, and ketone production from body lipids. In fully adapted starvation, ketone bodies can substitute for a large portion of the carbohydrate needed by the CNS and immune cells and can be used by skeletal and heart muscle.

FEEDING. When food is consumed, insulin levels rise, glucagon and other counterregulatory hormone levels fall, and the organism becomes anabolic. Insulin inhibits lipolysis (reducing free fatty acid availability) and enhances glucose uptake by cells. Gluconeogenesis is suppressed; exogenous carbohydrate is oxidized; and glycogen stores, body protein, and body lipid are repleted. Excess carbohydrate is disposed of by oxidation and glycogenesis. De novo lipogenesis is not significant, except in the most extreme conditions of carbohydrate overfeeding.[17,18] Excess carbohydrate intake leads to weight gain by suppressing lipid oxidation.

CRITICAL ILLNESS. In critically ill patients, substrate metabolism is markedly different from either normal starvation or fed states. Levels of glucagon (and other counterregulatory hormones) are elevated, but so is insulin. The glucagon increase is of a greater magnitude than that of insulin, so the glucagons-insulin ratio is increased. Other biochemical mediators such as cytokines are elevated while some growth factors are suppressed. High insulin levels suppress ketogenesis but do not suppress gluconeogenesis. Furthermore, dietary glucose loses the ability to completely suppress gluconeogenesis. Both free fatty acids and glucose are available for oxidation, whereas in normal metabolism only one would predominate in a given metabolic state (fatty acids in fasting and glucose in fed states). Glucose uptake is lower than would be expected based on the serum insulin level (i.e., insulin resistance), but total daily glucose uptake is increased. Glucose and lipid recycling rates are accelerated.[19,20] Critically ill patients have higher than normal energy expenditure and catabolic rates. Patients remain catabolic, gluconeogenic, and in negative nitrogen balance despite adequate calorie and high protein intake.[21] Body fat is capable of sparing protein from oxidation to cover calorie deficits during feeding of mixed-fuel nutrition support, although not to the point of achieving nitrogen equilibrium.[21]

Methods of Assessing Energy Expenditure

Four methods are available for determining energy expenditure: indirect calorimetry (portable cart and respiration chamber), Fick equation, direct calorimetry, and doubly labeled water. None measures cellular metabolic rates directly: all rely on correlations between cellular metabolism, gas exchange, and heat production to determine energy expenditure indirectly.

Indirect Calorimetry

Indirect calorimetry is the most used technique for measuring energy expenditure in both clinical and research settings. All indirect calorimetry methods have in common the measurement of inspired and expired gas volumes and concentrations. These data are used to calculate Vo_2 and Vco_2, the quantities being proportional to substrate utilization and energy expenditure (see Figs. 6-1 and 6-2). Indirect calorimeters are of two basic types: respiration chamber calorimeters, in which the subject resides and breathes freely inside a chamber, and portable devices, in which expired air is collected via face mask, canopy, or from a mechanical ventilator and is funneled into the instrument for analysis (Fig. 6-3). (At the time of this writing, new hand-held calorimeters are becoming available.) Indirect calorimeters can be further classified by whether they are open or closed circuit. In open-circuit indirect calorimeters, the patient's inspired air source is room air or comes from a mechanical ventilator. In closed-circuit indirect calorimeters, the inspired air source is an air or oxygen tank in the calorimeter.

Respiration chambers are most often employed in research settings, where they contribute important information on familial/genetic determinants of resting metabolic rate, the partitioning of total metabolic rate into its component parts, and the effect of various activities on total metabolic rate. The portable, open-circuit indirect calorimeter is the type most often used in

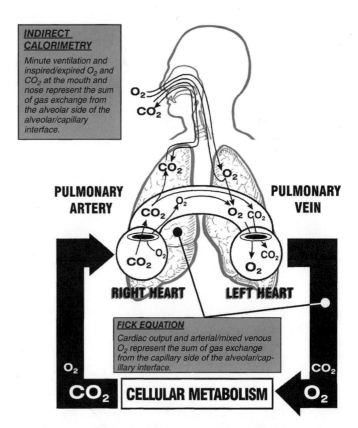

FIGURE 6-2 The relationship between cellular metabolism, blood gas content, and gas exchange, demonstrating the points of measurement for indirect calorimetry and the Fick equation. Cellular metabolism consumes inspired oxygen and produces carbon dioxide, which is excreted by the lungs. Indirect calorimetry measures gas exchange across the alveoli, whereas the Fick equation measures exchange across the pulmonary vasculature.

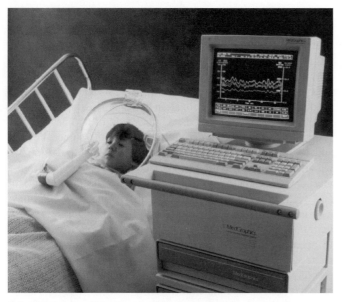

FIGURE 6-3 A typical modern portable indirect calorimeter with canopy set up to measure gas exchange in a subject breathing room air. (Courtesy of Medical Graphics Corporation, St. Paul, Minnesota.)

hospitals, although closed-circuit, portable indirect calorimeters are available.

INSTRUMENTATION. An indirect calorimeter has four basic components: a carbon dioxide analyzer, an oxygen analyzer, a volume-measuring device, and a microprocessor for calculation and data management. Gas analyzers and volume-measuring devices work in any of several ways, but the results generally are similarly accurate. To convert gas measurements to standard conditions, indirect calorimeters must also be able to measure

air temperature and pressure and to dry or otherwise account for the water content of air.

CALCULATIONS. To perform gas exchange analysis, six quantities must be measured or calculated: fraction of inspired and expired oxygen and carbon dioxide concentrations (F_{IO_2}, F_{EO_2}, F_{ICO_2}, and F_{ECO_2}), and inspired and expired minute gas volume (V_I, V_E). From these quantities, V_{O_2} and V_{CO_2} can be calculated:

$$V_{O_2} \text{ (ml/min)} = (F_{IO_2} \times V_I) - (F_{EO_2} \times V_E)$$

$$V_{CO_2} \text{ (ml/min)} = (F_{ECO_2} \times V_E) - (F_{ICO_2} \times V_I)$$

Most indirect calorimeters measure gas concentrations and V_E. However, inspired minute gas volume must be calculated in open-circuit indirect calorimetry, since the opportunity to divert the entire inspired volume into the indirect calorimeter does not exist (this limitation does not exist for closed-circuit indirect calorimeters, which can measure V_I). Open-circuit indirect calorimeters use the Haldane transformation to calculate inspired volume from expired volume, F_{IO_2}, F_{EO_2}, and F_{ECO_2}:

$$V_I = (1 - F_{EO_2} - F_{ECO_2}/1 - F_{IO_2}) \times V_E$$

One significant consequence of relying on the Haldane transformation is that an upper limit of F_{IO_2} is set (60% to 85%, depending on the particular indirect calorimeter). Above a certain F_{IO_2} limit, the denominator of the Haldane equation approaches 0, small errors in F_{IO_2} are amplified, and the calculation of V_I becomes unreliable (Fig. 6-4).[22,23]

DERIVATION OF ENERGY EXPENDITURE FROM GAS EXCHANGE DATA.
Under proper conditions, gas exchange (V_{O_2} and V_{CO_2}) is proportional to cellular metabolism (substrate utilization and energy expenditure). Energy expenditure (EE) is calculated from V_{O_2} and V_{CO_2} (along with nitrogen excretion as a measure of protein oxidation), by multiplication by various constants for

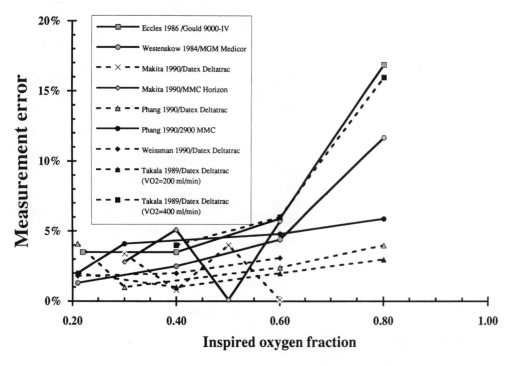

FIGURE 6-4 Measurement error in gas exchange at various fractions of inspired oxygen, for several indirect calorimeters. (From Chiolero RL, Bracco D, Revelly JP: Does indirect calorimetry reflect energy expenditure in the critically ill patient? In Wilmore DW, Carpentier YA (eds): *Metabolic support of the critically ill patient*, Berlin, 1993, Springer-Verlag, p 95.)

caloric equivalents of oxygen (constants obtained from bomb calorimetry, stoichiometric analysis, and nutrient balance studies). Several sets of constants are available;[3,9-14,24,25] most results agree within 2% of one another.[26]

The original method for calculating energy expenditure was quite cumbersome, involving the measurement of gas exchange and urinary nitrogen loss, calculation of nonprotein RQ, and consultation of a table to compute heat equivalent of oxygen at the measured nonprotein RQ. In 1949, Weir, noting that the cumbersome nature of the energy expenditure calculations had led to improper use of the method, published a simplified set of energy expenditure calculations.[27] Using constant values of calorie equivalents of oxygen for carbohydrate, fat, and protein, Weir derived the following energy expenditure equation:

$$EE \text{ (kcal/d)} = V_{O_2} (3.94) + V_{CO_2} (1.11) - \text{urea nitrogen excretion } (2.17)$$

V_{O_2} and V_{CO_2} are expressed in liters per day, urea nitrogen in grams per day. The urea nitrogen factor is a correction for incomplete protein oxidation in vivo. Weir noted that the error in ignoring the protein correction to energy expenditure was only 1% for every 12.3% protein contribution to total energy expenditure. Thus, the energy expenditure calculation could be further simplified:

$$EE \text{ (kcal/d)} = V_{O_2} (3.9) + V_{CO_2} (1.1)$$

(Some calorimeters express V_{O_2} and V_{CO_2} in ml/min instead of l/d. In such cases, a multiplier of 1.44 is included in the equation.)

Because a larger than normal portion of energy expenditure is accounted for by protein in critically ill patients, it was thought to be inappropriate to ignore the protein correction. Thus, Bursztein and coworkers calculated energy expenditure in critically ill patients from V_{O_2} and V_{CO_2}, with and without correcting for urea nitrogen excretion.[28] As with Weir's data in healthy persons, Bursztein found that only small errors were introduced into the calculation by ignoring the correction for incomplete protein oxidation, even though protein oxidation was higher than normal.

ACCURACY AND LIMITATIONS OF INDIRECT CALORIMETRY. Accuracy of properly calibrated indirect calorimeters is generally high, with errors of less than 4%. Accuracy of gas concentration and volume measurements is reduced by increasing or fluctuating F_{IO_2} and by high expired minute volume.[23,29-31] A safe upper limit of F_{IO_2} is 60%, although some indirect calorimeter manufacturers claim accuracy up to F_{IO_2} of 80% (see Fig. 6-4). Excessive fluctuation of F_{IO_2} might be corrected by replacing the ventilator's air-oxygen blender, if it is insufficiently accurate for metabolic monitoring. The air-oxygen blender is a device on the ventilator that mixes hospital air and pure oxygen to achieve an oxygen-enriched air mixture for the patient to breathe. The acceptable degree of accurate mixing by this blender for clinical purposes is less than that required for calorimetry measurements, so it may be difficult to get the blender changed for the sake of the metabolic measurement (i.e., the blender is providing adequate clinical service and thus there is no great incentive to switch out the blender). An alternative to replacing the air-oxygen blender is to place another blender in line for additional blending (a simple 1- to 3-L steel canister placed in the expired air collection line of the calorimeter may suffice). Finally, the indirect calorimeter gas analyzers

and volume-measuring devices must be calibrated before each test and tested regularly in vitro.

The fundamental concept of indirect calorimetry to bear in mind is that a respiratory measurement (gas exchange) is being used to assess a cellular process (substrate utilization and metabolic rate). Under steady state conditions these processes are aligned and indirect calorimetry is in fact a measurement of energy expenditure. In nonsteady state conditions, even if the indirect calorimeter is accurately measuring gas exchange, the gas exchange does not reflect cellular energy expenditure. A strong link between gas exchange and cell metabolism depends on numerous factors. The patient must have a stable breathing pattern and expired minute volume or be measured over an extended time (see Indirect Calorimetry Protocols). The body pool of carbon dioxide must be in a steady state. If not, the carbon dioxide measured at the point of respiration will not equal that produced at the point of cell metabolism. For example, a person who purposely hyperventilates (breathes faster than normal) to excrete more carbon dioxide will appear by indirect calorimetry to have increased his V_{CO_2} when in fact what he has done is to briefly reduce his whole-body pool of carbon dioxide. On the other hand, an actual change in V_{CO_2} at the cellular level does not appear immediately as a change in gas exchange because the carbon dioxide pool is quite large (200 to 240 ml/kg), as compared with the typical V_{CO_2} (3 to 4 ml/min per kilogram).[32,33] Note that it is possible to get an accurate indirect calorimetry measurement of energy expenditure in a person with high or low carbon dioxide pool, as long as the size of the pool does not change during the measurement. Compared to V_{CO_2}, V_{O_2} is a robust measurement because the total body pool of oxygen is less than 1 L (i.e., the oxygen pool is about 15 ml/kg body weight versus a typical V_{O_2} of 3 to 5 ml/min per kilogram).[22] A change in V_{O_2} at the cellular level is quickly reflected in the gas exchange measurement.

An obvious problem affecting the link between gas exchange measurement and cellular metabolism is the presence of air leaks. Patient air can leak from chest tubes, through bronchopleural fistulae, around endotracheal or tracheostomy cuffs, facemasks or head canopies, or at any tubing connection in the mechanical ventilator or indirect calorimeter circuits. Air leak represents gas that has participated in cellular metabolism and gas exchange but is not presented to the indirect calorimeter for analysis. Underestimation of cellular metabolic rate will result from an air leak. A special type of "air leak" is the use of extracorporeal oxygenation or carbon dioxide removal, in which gas exchange occurs across a medical device rather than the lung. The indirect calorimeter could be connected to such devices and the gas exchange measured, but the validity of such measurements is not known.

FICK EQUATION. Oxygen consumption and carbon dioxide production can be calculated from blood measurements across the heart, in a method analogous to measurement of gas exchange across the lung (see Fig. 6-2). The required quantities are whole-body blood flow (cardiac output), whole-body venous oxygen and carbon dioxide concentrations (mixed venous blood from the pulmonary artery), and whole-body arterial oxygen and carbon dioxide concentrations (arterial blood from any site). *Mixed venous blood* refers to blood from all tissues of the body, fully mixed together. A mixed venous blood sample is necessary for Fick equations (more accurately called reverse Fick equations) because it blends regional differences in oxygen utilization into a whole-body value. Mixed venous blood occurs only in the pulmonary artery. Because of the need for mixed venous blood and cardiac output measurements, a pulmonary artery catheter (e.g., Swan-Ganz catheter) is necessary for Fick-calculated Vo_2 and Vco_2. Therefore, the Fick equation is calculated only for critically ill patients who require a pulmonary artery catheter for aggressive hemodynamic monitoring. (A pulmonary artery catheter would never be placed solely for nutrition assessment.)

The data and equations required to calculate Vo_2 by the Fick equation are as follows:

1. Cao_2 (ml/dl) = 1.39 (Hgb) × Sao_2/100 + 0.0031 (Pao_2)

2. Cvo_2 (ml/dl) = 1.39 (Hgb) × Svo_2/100 + 0.0031 (Pvo_2)

3. Vo_2 (ml/min) = Cardiac output × 10 Cao_2 – Cvo_2

Hgb is hemoglobin in g/dl, Sao_2 is arterial oxygen saturation, Pao_2 is partial pressure of oxygen in arterial blood (in mm Hg), Svo_2 is venous oxygen saturation, and Pvo_2 is partial pressure of oxygen in venous blood (in mm Hg). Carbon dioxide production can be calculated using the same principle as for Vo_2, except that carbon dioxide is substituted for oxygen and carbon dioxide content analysis is more involved, requiring adjustment for temperature and blood pH using the Henderson-Hasselbalch equation.[34] Oxygen consumption by the Fick method is much more accurate than Vco_2 by the Fick method. Brandi and coworkers[35] calculated Vo_2 and Vco_2 by the Fick method and compared the results to those of indirect calorimetry. The coefficient of determination (R^2) for Vo_2 between the methods was 0.92, whereas for Vco_2 the R^2 was only 0.26. In fact, Vco_2 is generally not calculated by the Fick method because of the unreliability of the results. Energy expenditure is predominantly a function of Vo_2, and can be calculated ignoring Vco_2, if RQ is assumed:

EE (kcal/d) = (Vo_2 × Heo_2) × 1440 min/d

At RQ 0.86, the heat equivalent of O_2 (Heo_2) = 0.00486 kcal/ml, so the equation multiplies out to:

EE (kcal/d) = Vo_2 × 7

Many studies have compared energy expenditure and Vo_2 by the Fick method and indirect calorimetry. Strengths of association vary (R^2 = 0.49 to 0.92).[35-41] Strongest associations are found in the most stable patients. For example, Brandi noted an R^2 of 0.92 between Fick and indirect calorimetry measurements of energy expenditure in a group of postoperative patients who were hemodynamically stable, were not receiving inotropes, and were not mechanically ventilated.[35] In contrast, Gerold and colleagues[36] measured energy expenditure in unstable patients with hyperdynamic trauma and multiple organ failure, all of whom were mechanically ventilated and most of whom were receiving inotropes. The R^2 between Fick and indirect calorimetry for these patients was only 0.49. In addition to this potential random error, there is a systematic error (underestimation) in the Fick calculation of Vo_2 and energy expenditure because of "contamination" of oxygenated blood in the

pulmonary vein by bronchial venous return, causing oxygen dilution and carbon dioxide enrichment.[42] Because of the limitations of the Fick method in unstable patients, indirect calorimetry is the preferred way of determining energy expenditure. If indirect calorimetry is not available, good clinical judgment is probably more accurate than Fick equations in determining energy expenditure.

DIRECT CALORIMETRY. Direct calorimetry measures heat release from an organism and was the original technique for measuring energy expenditure in humans. Direct calorimeters rely on the correlation between heat loss and cellular metabolism to calculate energy expenditure (see Fig. 6-1). Specially designed chambers or restrictive water-cooled body suits are required to measure heat loss. The impracticality (often impossibility) of placing hospitalized patients into special rooms or body suits makes direct calorimetry inappropriate for hospitalized patients, but direct calorimeters are still used in research settings.

DOUBLY LABELED WATER. The doubly labeled water technique of energy expenditure measurement is not widely used in hospitalized patients; however, a short review of the method is in order. The technique of doubly labeled water was developed in the 1950s for use in laboratory animals,[42] and was first used in humans in 1982.[43] The technique involves administration of a stable isotope of water ($^2H_2^{18}O$) and measurement of the disappearance rate of the isotope over several days. Hydrogen-2 disappearance is proportional to water turnover, while ^{18}O disappearance is proportional to water turnover plus Vco_2. Therefore, the difference between ^2H and ^{18}O disappearance gives Vco_2. Oxygen consumption is not measured. Rather, the food quotient (FQ) must be calculated (FQ = sum of Vco_2/sum of Vo_2 for all foods consumed in the diet, calculation of which necessitates accurate food records). From FQ and measured Vco_2, Vo_2 can be calculated. Alternatively, if FQ is not known, an RQ can be assumed, allowing calculation of Vo_2 and thus energy expenditure.

The advantages of the doubly labeled water technique are that total rather than resting energy expenditure (REE) is measured, and the measurement is repeatable over several days. One disadvantage of the doubly labeled water technique is the reliance on FQ to calculate Vo_2. The doubly labeled water technique is especially useful in field studies of free-living humans because it measures energy expenditure associated with activity without the subject having to wear measurement equipment or remain confined in the space of a direct or indirect calorimeter chamber. Validation studies have been performed in healthy humans[44,45] but not in ill humans who have altered substrate metabolism that might interfere with the Vo_2 calculation from FQ.

Methods of Assessing Substrate Utilization
Indirect Calorimetry

Net substrate utilization can be calculated from Vo_2, Vco_2, and metabolized protein (traditionally represented by urea nitrogen excretion). Numerous calculation systems exist for net substrate utilization, using constant values for RQ, heat of combustion, and heat equivalent of oxygen for the various fuel substrates (see Table 6-1). Westenskow and coworkers[26] showed that the various calculation methods agree with one another within approximately 2%, probably because all the systems have in common similar assumptions of chemical composition and calorie equivalent of the substrates being used. Livesey and Elia[13,14] have pointed out that these general assumptions are reasonably true for most typical carbohydrate and lipid substrates but probably are not true for proteins (see Table 6-1). Proteins are composed of many amino acids in varying concentrations, and individual amino acids have strikingly different Vo_2 and Vco_2 values. Some atypical protein sources (e.g., high branched-chain amino acid, glutamine, or other parenteral amino acid solutions, some disease-specific enteral feedings) can therefore introduce significant errors into substrate utilization calculations, which assume a standard protein as the basis for calculations. Compounding this problem, endogenous protein oxidation contributes to total protein oxidation and so should be considered a protein source. Another problem with protein utilization calculations is that most bomb calorimetry constants assume that urea is the end product of protein oxidation; however, protein can be oxidized to end products besides urea (mostly ammonia and creatinine), and the extent to which this occurs can introduce further error into substrate utilization calculations. Finally, gluconeogenesis can affect substrate utilization calculations if the new glucose is not metabolized but is added to the body pool and excreted in the urine (excreted glucose is included as metabolized carbohydrate in the standard calculations).

Isotope Method

For purposes of research, a large number of stable and radioactive isotopes are available to assess substrate utilization. Isotope studies take the general method of infusing a particular isotope, then measuring the incorporation of that isotope into various tissues, body fluids, expired air, or intermediary metabolites.[19-21] Isotope studies allow researchers to trace the intermediary metabolism of the nutrient of interest; indirect calorimetry provides only net substrate utilization rates.

Like indirect calorimetry, isotope methods have associated errors (loss of isotope to body pools, reutilization of isotope).[13,14] Jeevanandam, in a study of lipid metabolism in young and elderly trauma patients, used both indirect calorimetry and isotope methods and obtained similar results with the two methods.[46]

Determinants of Energy Expenditure

Total daily energy expenditure in healthy, well-nourished adults is composed of basal requirements, requirements for activity, and requirements associated with substrate metabolism (thermogenic effect of feeding). Children have an additional requirement for growth, and sick persons may have additional energy requirements associated with the illness.

Basal Energy Expenditure

Basal energy expenditure (BEE) is the energy expenditure of a healthy person at full repose, before or immediately upon awakening, before eating or engaging in any activity. BEE is the minimum amount of energy the body needs to maintain homeostasis. In some research studies, the terms REE and BEE are used interchangeably, although it is incorrect and confusing to do so. (REE has less strict activity restrictions than BEE.)

BEE for adults is principally a function of body size, or more specifically fat-free mass.[47,48] The organs that comprise fat-free mass contribute disproportionately to BEE given their mass (Table 6-2).[49] Gender and age have been associated with BEE.[5] Many of the age and gender effects on BEE are due to covariations among BEE, gender, age, and fat-free mass. (Elderly people and females tend to have smaller fat-free mass than younger people and males, and in turn have lower BEEs). Several investigators, however, after controlling for fat-free mass[50-52] still found attenuated BEE in elderly as compared with young subjects and in females versus males,[50,51,53-55] indicating age and gender effects independent of their effects on fat-free mass.

Ambient temperature can affect BEE. If ambient temperature lies outside the *zone of thermoneutrality,*[56] the ambient temperature range outside of which the nude body must change its energy expenditure rate to maintain core body temperature. In normal humans, the zone of thermoneutrality is 27° to 29° C. In ill humans, the zone is higher (e.g., 32° C in burn patients).

BEE accounts for 60% to 70% of the total daily energy expenditure. Even in very active persons or hypermetabolic critically ill ones, BEE accounts for no less than 50% of total energy expenditure. Because BEE accounts for such a large portion of the total energy expenditure, numerous attempts have been made to construct predictive standards for BEE.[3-6,57] Perhaps the most famous reference standard for BEE is that published by Harris and Benedict in 1919.[5] Despite criticism, even by the original authors of the standards,[57] that the Harris and Benedict data are 5% to 10% too high, and despite more recent and often larger studies of BEE,[58-63] the Harris-Benedict regression equations for predicting BEE remain the most often quoted and used reference for BEE in clinical settings and in research. Because of their historic significance and continued common use, the data of Harris and Benedict deserve close attention.

Three indirect calorimetry techniques were used by Harris and Benedict in data collection: the majority of tests were performed using a portable closed-circuit "universal respiration apparatus" (Fig. 6-5).[64] Other tests were performed using an indirect calorimetry chamber or the Tissot gasometer.[2] Energy

TABLE 6-2

Contribution to Basal Energy Expenditure of Body Tissues

Body Tissue	% of Total Body Weight	% of Basal Energy Expenditure	Daily Energy Expenditure (kcal/kg tissue)
Adipose	21–33*	5	4.5
Muscle	30–40*	15–20*	13
Organs†	5–6*	60	200–440‡
Other§	33	15–20*	12

From Elia M: Organ and tissue contribution to metabolic rate. In Kinney JM, Tucker HN (eds): *Energy metabolism: tissue determinants and cellular corollaries,* New York, 1992, Raven Press, p 63.
*Range is reference female (low) and reference male (high) from Snyder WS, Cook MJ, Nasset ES, et al. Report of the Task Group on Reference Man. International Commission on Radiological Protection, No. 23, Oxford, 1975, Pergamon Press.
‡Brain, kidney, liver, heart.
†Range is liver (200), brain (240), kidney, and heart (440).
§Bone, skin, intestine, glands.

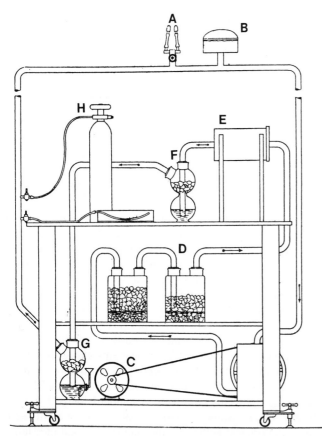

FIGURE 6-5 Diagram of the portable, closed-circuit indirect calorimeter used by Harris and Benedict in their experiments with BEE. *(A)* Tubes inserted into subject's nose; *(B)* "tension equalizer" to equalize air pressure inside the system; *(C)* rotary blower for circulating expired air through the system; *(D)* sulfuric acid bottles to dry expired air; *(E)* canister of soda lime to remove carbon dioxide from expired air; *(F)* repeat air drying by sulfuric acid; *(G)* rehydration of air in preparation for rebreathing; *(H)* oxygen tank to replenish expired air before rebreathing. (From Benedict FG: An apparatus for studying the respiratory exchange, *Am J Physiol* 24[3]:345, 1909.)

expenditure was calculated from V_{O_2} and V_{CO_2}, ignoring protein oxidation. If either V_{O_2} or V_{CO_2} were unavailable, an RQ of 0.85 was assumed, and the missing value was calculated algebraically. Subjects were tested on the morning after a 12-hour fast and were often tested several times per day over several days; however, subjects were required to journey to the test site, which could increase their metabolic rate. Muscle movement during testing was detected objectively by attaching motion detection devices to the bed or directly to the patient. Mean data are displayed in Table 6-3. Note in particular the low mean and range of ages and body sizes. Multiple regression analysis of the data (one of the first applications of this statistical method to human physiology) yielded the following predictive equations for BEE:

Males: BEE = 66.4730 + 13.7516 (w) + 5.0033 (s) − 6.7550 (a)

Females: BEE = 655.0955 + 9.5634 (w) + 1.8496 (s) − 4.6756 (a)

where *w* is weight in kg, *s* is stature (height) in cm, *a* is age in years. The R^2 between predicted and measured BEEs for males was 0.75, for females 0.53 (Fig. 6-6).

TABLE 6-3

Summary of Data from Harris and Benedict's Basal Energy Expenditure Series

Variable	Original Series, 1919 (mean ± SD/range)	Subsequent Series 1928, 1935 (mean ± SD/range)
MALES		
Subjects	136	33
Age (yr)	27 ± 9 (16-63)	43 ± 24 (21-91)
Height (cm)	173 ± 8 (148-198)	173 ± 8 (154-188)
Weight (kg)	64 ± 10 (33-109)	70 ± 19 (52-157)
BMI*	21 ± 3 (15-33)	24 ± 7 (17-56)
Measured BEE	1632 ± 205 (997-2559)	1591 ± 323 (910-2821)
Predicted BEE	1631 ± 178 (1101-2426)	1607 ± 331 (1041-2870)
FEMALES		
Subjects	103	66
Age (yr)	31 ± 14 (15-74)	54 ± 24 (18-88)
Height (cm)	162 ± 5 (151-176)	158 ± 7 (138-180)
Weight (kg)	56 ± 11 (36-94)	59 ± 13 (32-97)
BMI*	22 ± 4 (12-35)	24 ± 5 (16-40)
Measured BEE	1349 ± 156 (985-1765)	1230 ± 194 (799-1619)
Predicted BEE	1349 ± 112 (1056-1723)	1260 ± 188 (854-1664)

BEE, Basal energy expenditure; *BMI*, body mass index.
*Body mass index calculated as wt/ht^2 (kg/cm^2).

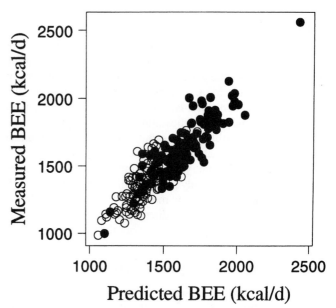

FIGURE 6-6 Plot of predicted and measured BEE from the original data of Harris and Benedict.[5] *Closed circles,* men ($R^2 = 0.75$, $p < .0001$); *open circles,* women ($R^2 = 0.53$, $p < .0001$).

The original Harris-Benedict data have been criticized for insufficient numbers of obese and elderly patients. In 1928 and 1935 Benedict published supplemental series of subjects (32 males, 66 females),[57,65] increasing the range of age and body sizes reported in the original series (see Table 6-3). In the combined series, BEE predicted by the Harris-Benedict equations for males varied from measured BEE by 5% ± 4%, 15% of the predictions deviating from measured BEE by more than 10%.

For females, the mean difference was 6% ± 5%, and 19% of predicted values deviated from measured values by more than 10%.

Development of predictive standards for BEE remains a relevant and ongoing topic of research because a very reliable standard has yet to be found. Recent attempts to construct standards have concentrated on the effects on BEE of body composition, gender, and age.[58] Other important factors to consider are genetics, physical fitness, and nutritional status.[66]

Activity Energy Expenditure

Physical activity is the component of energy expenditure under conscious control of the healthy individual. Various activities require different amounts of muscle work and associated energy expenditure.[67,68] For hospitalized patients, however, physical activity is usually limited by fatigue, pain, depression, or confinement. Long suggested a simple adjustment for activity: 120% of BEE for bedridden patients and 130% for ambulatory patients.[69]

The metabolic rate of critically ill patients has been measured during various intensive care unit activities—bathing, chest physiotherapy, measurement of body weight, chest radiography, and dressing changes.[70,71] Although such activities can increase energy expenditure 20% to 35%, the duration of the activity is usually brief, so effect on 24-hour total energy expenditure is minor (i.e., the activity factor for most intensive care unit patients is approximately 5%).

Another factor to be considered in critically ill patients is pharmacologic inhibition of activity.[72,73] Weissman has shown that morphine decreases energy expenditure.[72] Paralyzing agents minimize or eliminate muscle activity as a contributor to energy expenditure.[73] However, in at least one study, the dose of morphine and the use of medical paralytics was actually associated with increased energy expenditure.[74] This observation probably is explained by the fact that the more critically ill patients have greater inflammatory injury (a more severe hypermetabolism) and also tend to require heavier sedation and are more likely to need medical paralytics. Thus, it may be true that the sedated or paralyzed patient has a lower metabolic rate than if he or she were not sedated or paralyzed, but it is not necessarily true that sedation and/or medical paralysis lead to a normometabolic state. This is understandable from Table 6-2, which indicates that only 20% of REE is derived from skeletal muscle. Sedation and medical paralysis would have their effects on metabolic rate mainly by reducing this small portion of the total REE.

Thermogenic Effect of Feeding

Thermogenic effect of feeding refers to the phenomenon of increased energy expenditure in response to eating. This phenomenon has been known for more than 100 years, although its causes, mediation, and purpose remain ill-defined.[75] Thermogenic effect of feeding has an obligatory and a facultative component.[76] The obligatory component is associated with digestion, absorption, and disposition of the feeding. The facultative component is associated with sympathetic input and thus can be blocked by inhibiting the sympathetic nervous system. The thermogenic effect of feeding has two phases: the postprandial phase and a chronic response to prolonged overfeeding.[75,76]

Rubner first described the thermogenic effect of food as "specific dynamic action," believing the increased energy expenditure to be "specific" to protein ingestion.[77] Others, however, demonstrated that thermogenesis occurred with ingestion of carbohydrate and fat, as well as with protein.[78] The term *specific dynamic action* thus gave way to *diet-induced thermogenesis.*

Studies in animals during the 1930s and 1940s demonstrated that diet-induced thermogenesis was more pronounced when nutrients were fed individually than when they were fed in a mixed meal. Additionally, diet-induced thermogenesis was found to be more pronounced during overfeeding than under-feeding.[79,80] More recently, other factors have been found to affect the degree of thermogenesis associated with feeding, including the ratio of protein, fat, and carbohydrate in the diet; fiber content of the meal; nutritional status of the subject; time when the diet is consumed; psychological stress; and factors that modulate sympathetic nervous system function, such as age, coffee consumption, smoking, and the spiciness of the food in the diet.[75,81] Parenteral and enteral feeding have thermogenic effects.[82]

The modern concept of diet-induced thermogenesis (now called the *thermogenic effect of feeding*) includes the following elements: (1) it is not specific to protein; (2) mixed diet has less effect than a single nutrient; (3) a small meal has less effect than a large meal; (4) a meal eaten in the evening has less effect than a meal eaten in the afternoon, which has less effect than a meal eaten in the morning; and (5) malnourished people have an attenuated thermogenic response as compared with well-nourished ones.[75,81] Because intraindividual differences in thermogenic response are pronounced and because many physiologic factors modify the extent of the thermogenic effect of feeding, it is difficult to predict the extent of the thermogenic response in an individual hospital patient. Rather, if a patient's energy expenditure is going to be measured to guide nutrition support, the measurement should be performed during feeding, especially in patients who are fed continuously, thus eliminating the need to predict thermogenic effect of feeding.

Energy Dynamics During Illness

Many hospitalized patients are hypermetabolic, and the degree varies much from patient to patient and from day to day.[74,83]

A plethora of published papers describe the level of hypermetabolism in various disease states (blunt trauma and burns, major and elective surgery, medical diseases, inflammatory states such as sepsis and pancreatitis). Some of the earliest work on altered energy expenditure in illness was published by DuBois, who determined that energy expenditure increased 13% per degree centigrade and 7% per degree Fahrenheit of body temperature.[6] These predictive factors remain in use today.

In the 1960s, Kinney and colleagues began to study energy expenditure in critically ill patients, using a nonportable head canopy, indirect calorimetry system installed permanently into a four-bed intensive care unit.[84] Among Kinney's early observations was that the relationship between fever and energy expenditure was more complex than that delineated by DuBois (some patients were hypermetabolic but not febrile, some were febrile but not hypermetabolic, some conformed to DuBois's prediction).[85] An accumulation of over 200 studies by Kinney's group led to the following recommended modifications to BEE for hospitalized patients: major tissue depletion 60% to 80% of BEE, major elective surgery 110% of BEE, multiple injury 110% to 125% of BEE, major sepsis 120% to 150% of BEE, major burns 150% to 200% of BEE.[86]

As a direct continuation of Kinney's work, Calvin Long published in 1979 a series of stress factors for hospitalized patients.[69] Subjects in Long's paper were classified by conditions such as elective surgery, "skeletal" (motor vehicle) and "blunt" (gunshot) trauma, sepsis, or burns. A total of 39 spontaneously breathing patients were studied. Elevation of energy expenditure above BEE was 120% for uncomplicated elective surgery patients, 135% for trauma, 160% for severe sepsis (what would today be described as systemic inflammatory response syndrome), and 210% for severe burns. Although published 18 years ago, Long's stress factors are still widely used to calculate energy expenditure in modern intensive care units. Some or all of these ranges for hypermetabolism may be dated because of advances in patient care (better wound care, nutrition support, mechanical ventilation to reduce work of breathing and to allow deeper sedation). Kinney pointed out that, from the 1960s to the 1980s, the range in measured metabolic rates dropped from 60% to 200% of BEE to 80% to 160% of BEE.

Beginning in the 1980s, accurate, portable indirect calorimeters capable of measuring mechanically ventilated and spontaneously breathing patients have been available, leading to a large number of publications of resting energy expenditure in hospitalized patients. Along with the associated explosion of published reports of energy expenditure in hospitalized patients came contradictory results. Most studies in elective surgery postoperative intensive care unit patients are consistent with Kinney's data showing a 10% increase in REE.[69,70,86-91] For trauma, some investigators suggest that Long's standards are too high (115% to 124% versus Long's standard of 135%); other papers suggest that REE in trauma patients is much higher than that reported by Long or Kinney (150% to 160%).[21,82,92-95]

Early studies of burn patients showed marked hypermetabolism, up to 200% of BEE.[69] Later reports have demonstrated that a portion of burn hypermetabolism was related to ambient temperature. Burn patients allowed to control ambient room temperature who had occlusive dressings had significant reductions in hypermetabolism (from 178% to 121% of calculated basal expenditure).[96]

Studies of medical patients indicate that conditions such as cirrhosis, pancreatitis, and Crohn's disease have negligible effects on energy expenditure, if the patient is not critically ill.[97-100] Critical medical illness is associated with hypermetabolism.[100] Guillain-Barré syndrome, a condition of complete body paralysis but of activated inflammatory response, causes a hypermetabolic response on the order of 150% to 168% of BEE.[101] Similarly, medical intensive care unit patients with sepsis (infection, fever, tachycardia, tachypnea) can have REE on the order of 155% of BEE,[102] similar to that seen with post-trauma sepsis.[93]

Given the apparent discrepancies in REE among published studies, the question arises, Why? It is possible that care practices that affect energy expenditure vary from institution to institution, such as sedation practices, levels of hemodynamic

"push" (inotropes, volume resuscitation), and use of antipyretics and cooling blankets. Such practices may or may not be reported in the published papers. The physiologic state of the patient at the time of the measurement can have a significant effect on energy expenditure.[102] Description or stratification of patients by reason for admission (trauma, surgery, medicine) may obscure or inappropriately mix physiologic states and create discrepancies. For example, data from our own institution show similar degrees of hypermetabolism (mean 140% of BEE) in trauma, major surgery, and medical intensive care unit patients when fever is present. Afebrile patients had REEs of approximately 125% of BEE, whether they were trauma, major surgery, or medical patients.[103]

Assessment of Energy Dynamics in Clinical Practice

Indirect Calorimetry Protocols

The ideal indirect calorimetry apparatus and measurement protocol would allow for continuous measurement of all mechanically ventilated patients in the intensive care unit to assess the effects of feeding, clinical condition, physical activity, and day-to-day variations on energy expenditure. Although such indirect calorimetry systems exist and provide vast amounts of metabolic and pulmonary function data, they are very expensive, labor intensive, and difficult to maintain.[104] The more common indirect calorimetry apparatus is the portable unit that measures one patient at a time. A rather severe limitation is therefore placed on the number of indirect calorimetry tests that can be performed. Several compromises from the ideal 24-hour indirect calorimetry measurement must be made to increase the total number of measurements that can be performed.

Weissman and colleagues[70] have shown that, although intensive care unit activities (e.g., bathing, dressing changes, chest physiotherapy) can increase energy expenditure significantly, these increases are usually transient and thus add little more than 5% to overall REE. Other investigators have confirmed this observation (Fig. 6-7).[71-74] Therefore, unless indirect calorimetry is being attempted in an agitated, physically active patient, a short measurement under resting conditions, with an assumed increase of 5% for activity, will suffice.

The resting state is usually defined as a period of time when the patient is undisturbed by hospital personnel and is lying quietly in bed. It is desirable to begin the state of rest at least 15 minutes before the calorimetry measurement is initiated and to maintain the state to the end of the measurement. Nutrient intake does not have to be interrupted for a measurement of REE in the setting of nutrition support practice (which usually involves continuous infusion of feeding), although it should be interrupted for 12 hours in clinical situations where the subject is taking intermittent meals in order for the results to be comparable to published standards). In mechanically ventilated patients, ventilator settings that will change expired minute volume should not be made within the hour preceding a metabolic measurement.

Measurement duration is another important aspect in designing a protocol.[23] To reduce the effect of respiratory artifacts and to detect changes in V_{CO_2} (which take longer to manifest than changes in V_{O_2}), a common indirect calorimetry

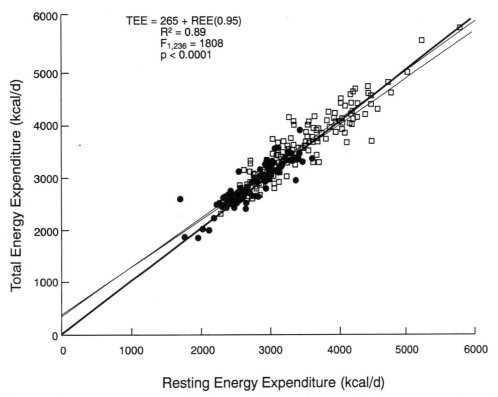

TEE = 265 + REE(0.95)
$R^2 = 0.89$
$F_{1,236} = 1808$
$p < 0.0001$

FIGURE 6-7 Relationship between resting and total energy expenditure in critically ill, sedated, mechanically ventilated trauma patients *(closed circles)* and patients with multiple organ failure *(open squares)*. (From Frankenfield DC, Wiles CE, Bagley S, et al: Relationship between resting and total energy expenditure in injured and septic patients, *Crit Care Med* 22:1796, 1994.)

protocol for resting patients is a 30-minute measurement during which the coefficients of variation (standard deviation/mean) of Vo_2, Vco_2, and V_E are not more than 10%. Such a protocol allows a dedicated indirect calorimetry technician to measure a maximum of 12 patients in an 8-hour period (optimistically assuming that all 12 patients are found in a resting state and that it takes 10 minutes to set up each 30-minute test). Frankenfield and coworkers[105] have found in mechanically ventilated patients that a 5-minute protocol that accepts coefficients of variation of not more than 5% for Vo_2, Vco_2, and V_E provides data comparable to those from the 30-minute protocol, especially if the patient is sedated (Fig. 6-8). Using the 5-minute protocol and making the same optimistic assumptions that all patients are found in a resting state and that setup time is 10 minutes, a maximum of 32 patients can be measured in an 8-hour workday. The abbreviated protocol thus affords more comprehensive surveillance of energy expenditure than the 30-minute one.

For an agitated, mechanically ventilated patient, measurement over several hours is probably justified because physical activity increases energy expenditure by more than 5% and the correct increment would be almost impossible to predict.

Lucid, spontaneously breathing patients being measured with a canopy system (see Fig. 6-3) should be measured longer than mechanically ventilated patients. A longer measurement period is necessary because the patient is more aware of the indirect calorimetry equipment and the operator and therefore needs time to relax and achieve a steady state.

Uncooperative, spontaneously breathing patients are not candidates for indirect calorimetry because they cannot be asked to relax and probably will not tolerate being under the canopy long enough. Patients who are breathing on their own but require supplemental oxygen cannot be measured with open-circuit indirect calorimeters because an accurate sample of inspired air cannot be obtained for analysis.

Calculation Protocols

In many hospitals no equipment for measuring energy expenditure is available. Even when indirect calorimetry is available, the demand for measurements can exceed the number of measurements that can be performed. Therefore, calculation of energy expenditure remains a large part of nutrition assessment in the hospital. Energy expenditure can be calculated in many ways, but most have in common some assessment of BEE plus an allowance for activity and injury.

Probably the most common equations for BEE are the Harris-Benedict equations,[5] which are based on body size with age and gender modifiers. The equations of Mifflin are similar in form to the Harris-Benedict equations,[58] are more recent, and are based on a larger database, but they have not found widespread usage. Comparison of calculated BEE using the two sets of equations demonstrates similarity between standards, with a tendency for Mifflin to give a slightly lower value for BEE (Table 6-4) (consistent with other observations that the Harris-Benedict equations overestimate BEE).[57] The variables in the Harris-Benedict and Mifflin equations are those known to

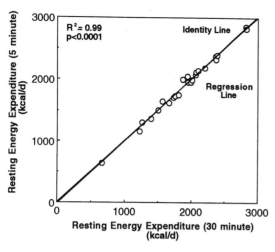
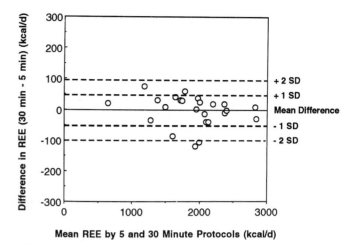

FIGURE 6-8 Relationship between a standard 30-minute protocol for resting energy expenditure and 5-minute measurement.[109] *Left:* Regression of 5- and 30-minute data showing the degree of linearity between methods. *Right:* Plot of residuals (difference between 5- and 30-minute data) versus mean of the 5- and 30-minute data, demonstrating the accuracy of the 5-minute protocol. (From Frankenfield DC, Sarson GY, Smith JS, et al: Validation of an abbreviated indirect calorimetry protocol in critically ill patients, *J Am Coll Nutr* 15[4]:397-402, 1996.)

TABLE 6-4

Differences in Calculated Basal Energy Expenditure Using the Harris-Benedict and Mifflin Equations*†

	Height (cm)	Weight (kg)‡	Percent Ideal Weight (%)	Harris-Benedict (kcal)	Mifflin (kcal)	Difference (kcal)§	Percent Difference (%)
Male	160	56	100	1395	1390	5	0.4
	160	75	135	1656	1580	76	5.0
	170	67	100	1596	1563	33	2.1
	170	100	150	2048	1893	155	7.6
	180	78	100	1797	1735	62	3.5
	180	120	155	2372	2155	217	9.1
	180	137	175	2605	2325	280	10.7
Female	160	52	100	1321	1224	97	7.3
	160	70	135	1506	1414	92	6.1
	170	61	100	1446	1397	49	3.4
	170	90	150	1766	1727	39	2.3
	180	70	100	1571	1569	2	0.1
	180	109	155	1872	1879	7	0.4
	180	123	175	2007	2029	22	1.1

* See text for the Harris-Benedict equations for basal metabolism.[5] Mifflin equations for resting energy expenditure: Men = 5 + (10 × wt) + (6.25 × ht) − (5 × age); Women = −161 + (10 × wt) + (6.25 × ht) − (5 × age).[58]
†Age set at 35 years.
‡Actual weight used in all calculations.
§Percent difference is the difference between the methods/Harris-Benedict.

affect or predict fat-free mass, the energy-consuming tissue in the body.

A common misconception is that Harris and Benedict did not measure obese people to develop their standards. Therefore it is assumed that use of actual weight in the Harris-Benedict equations will overestimate BEE in people with body weight greater than about 125% of ideal or body mass index (BMI) greater than about 28 kg/m[2].[57] These assumptions have led to the widespread clinical practice of calculating an adjusted, or metabolically active body weight for overweight people; for example, (1) (actual weight–ideal weight) × 0.25 + ideal weight; (2) ideal weight × 1.3; and (3) actual weight[0.75]. In fact, Harris and Benedict included subjects with BMI up to 35 kg/m[2] in their study, so the use of adjusted body weight, at least up to this limit of BMI,[106] might not be justified.[107] The Mifflin equations avoid controversy over the need for adjustments to body weight because many obese people were measured in the development of the standard, and actual weight was used in the computation.

Once BEE has been calculated, allowance must be made for activity, diet-induced thermogenesis, and injury. Each allowance introduces further error into the overall calculation of energy expenditure. It is in the assignment of the modifier to BEE that conflicting published reports of energy expenditure in hospitalized patients can cause uncertainty. Many practitioners use Long's or Kinney's multipliers, others use any one of the more recent reports, and still others with access to indirect calorimeters in their facility use multipliers developed in house. Although no set of multipliers is preferred, the reference used in a particular hospital should be based on data obtained in that hospital or on carefully reviewed studies of patients similar (e.g., in injury severity, level of sedation) to those being cared for in that hospital.

More recent methods for predicting energy expenditure in ill patients are based on physiologic and anthropometric variables in multiple regression equations. The appeal of this approach is that a continuum of calculated energy expenditure is created (as opposed to the strict categorization of the stress multipliers) and that the predicted energy expenditure can be recalculated daily from clinical data. Swinamer was one of the first to develop one of these equations:[95]

$$REE = BSA(941) - age(6.3) + T_{max}(104) + RR(24) + V_T(804) - 4243$$

where *BSA* is body surface area, T_{max} is maximum body temperature (centigrade), *RR* is respiratory rate (breaths/min), and V_T is tidal volume (L). The R^2 for this multiple regression equation versus measured REE was 0.77 ($p < .001$).

Later, Ireton-Jones formulated an equation as follows:[108]

$$REE = wt(5) - age(10) + sex(281) + trauma(292) + burns(851) + 1925$$

where sex was male = 1 and female = 0, trauma and burns were yes = 1, no = 0.

Frankenfield and colleagues developed a multiple regression equation for trauma or posttrauma patients with multiple organ failure:[94]

$$REE = BEE(1.5) + body\ temp(250) + V_E(100) + dobut(40) + MOF(300) - 11000$$

where *body temp* is body temperature during study (degrees centigrade), V_E is expired minute volume (L/min), *dobut* is dobutamine dose(μg/kg per minute), and *MOF* is presence of multiple organ failure.

The R^2 of the equation versus measured REE was 0.77 ($p < .0001$) (compared with an R^2 of 0.30 for calculated BEE versus measured REE, and 0.45 for Long-modified BEE versus measured REE).

We have developed a regression equation for our institution (the *Penn State equation*) from a retrospective review of 169 indirect calorimetry tests on trauma, surgical, and medical intensive care patients:

$$REE = BEE(1.1) + V_E(32) + T_{max}(140) - 5340$$

with abbreviations and units as above. The R^2 of the multiple regression equation versus measured REE was 0.70 ($p < .0001$) as compared with 0.50 for BEE versus measured REE, and 0.55 for Long-modified BEE versus measured REE.[69]

A limited number of validation studies have been performed on some of these equations. Flancbaum[109] compared the Ireton-Jones and Frankenfield equations to Fick-derived REE and calorimetric REE in 36 patients in an intensive care unit (ICU). None of the calculation methods performed well. There was only limited correlation between the calculated and measured REE (ranging from 0.26 for Ireton-Jones to 0.39 for Frankenfield). The Ireton-Jones equation had a smaller average and range of difference from measured REE (150 kcal/day with a range of –67 to 368 kcal/day). An informal validation (unpublished) of the Swinamer, Ireton-Jones, and Penn State equations performed on 13 ICU patients revealed high correlations with measured REE (R^2 0.90 for Swinamer, 0.94 for Penn State, and 0.73 for Ireton-Jones). For the Swinamer equation, only 31% of the calculations were within 10% of measured REE (greatest error = 36% from measured), compared with 69% for the Ireton-Jones equation (greatest error = 28% from measured), and 85% for the Penn State equation (greatest error = 17% from measured).

Energy Substrates Available for Use in Nutrition Support

Four types of macronutrients are available: carbohydrate, lipid, protein, and alcohol. Alcohol (ethanol) generally is not used as a calorie substrate in nutrition support because of its toxicity, although experiments have been conducted to that end. Some institutions treat or prevent delirium tremens by providing ethanol to patients with significant history of ethanol abuse. Ethanol is metabolized and yields ATP and so must be considered in the nutrition support plans of patients receiving it. In a bomb calorimeter, ethanol produces 7.1 kcal/g of fuel;[13] however, subjects given isocaloric substitution of ethanol as a major portion of their calorie intake lose weight, suggesting that less than 7.1 kcal/g is available in vivo.[107] Ethanol may provide fewer calories in vivo than in vitro because of the way it is metabolized. Experienced drinkers use not only the acetaldehyde system to metabolize ethanol but also the inducible microsomal ethanol oxidase system (MEOS). MEOS must be primed with NADPH (the reduced form of nicotinamide-adenine dinucleotide), so less NADPH is available for ATP production.[110] Alternatively, weight loss during ethanol consumption may be due to altered hormone release or some other factor that leads to increased protein breakdown.[111]

Carbohydrate is most often provided as glucose of varying polymer sizes (glucose, maltodextrin, hydrolyzed starch; calorie density 3.4 to 4.0 kcal/g). Some tube feedings contain fructose (as a monosaccharide or as sucrose) and dietary fiber (indigestible polysaccharide). Dietary fiber and other indigestible carbohydrates are extensively fermented to short-chain fatty acids by bacteria in the colon. A variable portion of the short-chain fatty acids (calorie density 3.5 to 5.9 kcal/g)[13] is absorbed from the colon and thus provides fuel for the patient.[112]

Lipids are available as long-chain triglycerides (parenterally and enterally) and increasingly as medium-chain triglycerides (currently only available in enteral form). Soybean and safflower oils are the only long-chain fat sources in parenteral use in the United States. A wider variety of long-chain fats (e.g., canola, soybean, menhaden, rapeseed oils) incorporating a greater range of free fatty acids is used in enteral products. Long-chain lipids provide 9 kcal/g and medium-chain lipids 8 kcal/g.

Amino acid solutions for parenteral administration are synthetically produced, and the amino acid profile is based on the physiologic requirement for nitrogen balance in healthy adults. In enteral formulas, food sources of protein are used, most commonly casein, whey, or soy protein.

An important and very basic controversy exists in regard to whether protein should be considered a calorie substrate. When nutrition support became a clinical reality in the 1960s, nutrient prescriptions were typically calculated in nonprotein calories (carbohydrate plus lipid intake equal to predicted or measured energy expenditure). Today, no standardization exists for the inclusion or exclusion of protein energy into the calculation of calorie intake. Shea and Topalian found that 51% of nutrition support teams apply the nonprotein calorie standard and 49% the total calorie standard.[113]

The concept of nonprotein calories apparently is based on the rationale that infused protein is intended for protein synthesis and not for oxidation for ATP production. Basic biochemistry, however, offers no foundation for this, since protein is metabolized extensively and used for energy and for synthetic processes.[114] For example, the branched-chain amino acids are major oxidative fuels for muscle tissue.[115] The glutamine that results from branched-chain amino acid deamination in the muscle is used as oxidative fuel in the gut and in the cells of the immune system.[116-118] In the liver, amino acids are oxidized directly and are also converted to glucose, which is subsequently oxidized.[119] Garlik and others found that unfed healthy humans derive 11% of their metabolic rate from protein oxidation.[120] Upon feeding, the proportion of metabolic rate derived from protein increases to 18%. In injured patients, urea nitrogen excretion data suggest that 25% or more of the metabolic rate is derived from protein (either direct oxidation or via gluconeogenesis).[86] Young and coworkers suggested that oxidative amino acid utilization is a significant determinant of protein requirement.[114]

The choice of the nonprotein versus the total calorie standard is not simply an academic one. Provision of too much carbohydrate and lipid is associated with a variety of deleterious effects in the lungs, liver, and immune system. If total calories is the proper standard, carbohydrate and lipid intake can be decreased by an amount equal to the protein content of the nutrient infusion (calorie density of protein or amino acid solutions ranges from 4 to 6 kcal/g).[13]

Effect of Substrate Provision on Gas Exchange

There is a link between nutrient intake and respiratory requirements. Nutrient consumption increases both V_{O_2} and V_{CO_2}. The increased carbon dioxide load increases the arterial partial pressure of carbon dioxide (Pa_{CO_2}). The body responds to the increase in Pa_{CO_2} by increasing expired minute volume to expel the accumulating carbon dioxide.[2] An increase in expired minute volume is of minor consequence to someone with normal pulmonary function, but in a patient with impaired pulmonary function it can precipitate the need for mechanical ventilation or prevent successful weaning from mechanical ventilation.

A series of papers (summarized in reference 121) published in the early 1980s examined the effects of carbohydrate, lipid, and amino acid intake on V_{O_2} and V_{CO_2} in depleted and in injured patients. Carbohydrate and amino acids were both found

to increase V_{CO_2} and respiratory drive. Substitution of a portion of the carbohydrate with lipid led to decreased V_{CO_2}. From these studies came the notion that critically ill patients should be fed high-fat diets. It must be pointed out, however, that calorie intake in these studies was 135% to 200% of measured REE. Whether the effect of feeding on V_{CO_2} was due to high carbohydrate intake per se or to overfeeding in general could not be determined in these studies.

More recently, Talpers and colleagues[122] designed a two-part study in which mechanically ventilated patients were fed total calories at a rate of 130% of calculated BEE, with varying amounts of carbohydrate (40%, 60%, and 75% of total calorie intake). Carbon dioxide production did not change significantly as carbohydrate intake changed (Fig. 6-9). In part two of the

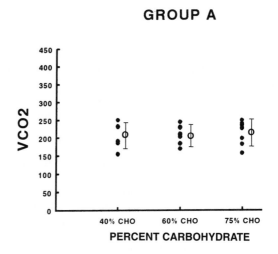

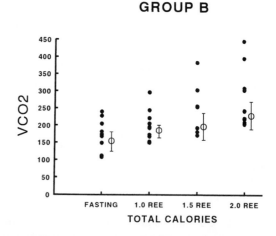

FIGURE 6-9 Effect on carbon dioxide production of increasing carbohydrate intake without increasing total calorie intake (130% of BEE, *top*) and increasing total calorie intake at constant percent of calories as carbohydrate (60% of total calories, *bottom*). Subjects are stable intensive care unit patients failing to wean from mechanical ventilation. (From Talpers SS, Romberger DJ, Bunce SB, Pingleton SK: Nutritionally associated increased carbon dioxide production: excess total calories versus high proportion of carbohydrate calories, *Chest* 102[2]:551-555, 1992.)

experiment, carbohydrate was held constant at 60% of total calorie intake, but total calorie intake was increased (fasting, 100%, 150%, and 200% of calculated BEE). As calorie intake increased, so did V_{CO_2}. Part two of the study was limited by the fact that as total calorie intake increased so did total carbohydrate intake, so the question of the relative effects of carbohydrate versus total calorie overfeeding on V_{CO_2} was not answered. Talpers clearly showed that if patients are not overfed, increasing carbohydrate does not greatly increase V_{CO_2}.

Conclusion

Energy expenditure is crucial to the maintenance of life. In the process of energy metabolism, organic substrates and oxygen are consumed and carbon dioxide and heat are produced. The relationships between substrate and oxygen consumption and carbon dioxide and heat production can be exploited to calculate the energy expenditure and substrate utilization of the patient. Hospitalized patients have altered substrate utilization and energy expenditure that must be considered when designing a nutrition support regimen.

There is significant variability in basal and total energy expenditure of healthy persons and hospitalized patients. Accurate prediction of energy requirements is important but difficult. Measurement of energy expenditure by indirect calorimetry is the preferred method of determining energy requirements. If indirect calorimetry is not available, predictive equations become necessary. Regression equations based on physiologic variables seem to be more accurate than multiplication of BEE based on disease category, although regression-derived predictions do not approach the accuracy of indirect calorimetry. Accurate provision of calorie substrate is necessary to prevent the complications associated with overfeeding and underfeeding. The practice of providing nonprotein calories equal to measured energy expenditure has the effect of overfeeding. Protein is an oxidative fuel and should be counted in the daily calorie prescription, reducing the need for carbohydrate and lipid and the attendant complications of overfeeding these substrates.

REFERENCES

1. Kleiber M: *The fire of life,* New York, 1961, John Wiley.
2. Burstein S, Elwyn DH, Askanazi J, Kinney JM: *Energy metabolism, indirect calorimetry, and nutrition,* Baltimore, 1989, Williams & Wilkins.
3. Lusk G: *The elements of the science of nutrition,* ed 4, Philadelphia, 1928, WB Saunders.
4. Atwater WO, Benedict FG: *A respiration calorimeter with appliances for the direct determination of oxygen,* Publication No. 42, Washington, DC, 1905, Carnegie Institute.
5. Harris JA, Benedict FG: *A biometric study of basal metabolism in man,* Publication No. 279, Washington, DC, 1919, Carnegie Institute.
6. DuBois EF: The basal metabolism in fever, *JAMA* 77(5):352-357, 1921.
7. Newsholme EA, Start C: *Regulation in metabolism,* London, 1973, John Wiley.
8. Becker WM: Aerobic production of ATP: electron transport. In Zubay G (ed): *Biochemistry,* Reading, MA, 1984, Addison-Wesley, pp 363-407.
9. Zuntz N, Schumburg GH: *Studien zur einer Physiologie des Marsches,* Berlin, 1901, Berlin Publishers.
10. Cathcart EP, Cuthbertson DP: The composition and distribution of the fatty substances of the human subject, *J Physiol* 72(3):349-360, 1931.
11. Rubner M: Calorimetrische Untersuchungen, I. Einleitung, *Z Biol* 21:250, 1885.
12. Michaelis AM: A graphic method of determining certain numerical factors in metabolism, *J Biol Chem* 59(1):51-58, 1924.
13. Livesey G, Elia M: Estimation of energy expenditure, net carbohydrate utilization, and net fat oxidation and synthesis by indirect calorimetry: evaluation of errors with special reference to the detailed composition of fuels, *Am J Clin Nutr* 47(4):608-628, 1988.
14. Elia M, Livesey G: Theory and validity of indirect calorimetry during net lipid synthesis, *Am J Clin Nutr* 47(4):591-607, 1988.
15. Rothwell NJ: Hypothalamus and thermogenesis. In Kinney JM, Tucker HN (eds): *Energy metabolism: tissue determinants and cellular corollaries,* New York, 1992, Raven Press, pp 229-245.
16. Cahill GF: Starvation in man, *N Engl J Med* 282(12):668-675, 1970.
17. Acheson KJ, Flatt JP, Jequier E: Glycogen synthesis versus lipogenesis after a 500 g carbohydrate meal in man, *Metabolism* 31(12):1234-1240, 1982.
18. Acheson KJ, Schutz Y, Bessard T, et al: Glycogen storage capacity and de novo lipogenesis during massive carbohydrate overfeeding in man, *Am J Clin Nutr* 48(2):240-247, 1988.
19. Jeevanandam M, Young DH, Schiller WR: Nutritional impact on the energy cost of fat fuel mobilization in polytrauma victims, *J Trauma* 30(2):147-154, 1990.
20. Shaw JH, Wolfe RR: An integrated analysis of glucose, fat, and protein metabolism in severely traumatized patients, *Ann Surg* 209(1):63-72, 1989.
21. Frankenfield DC, Smith JS, Cooney RN: Accelerated nitrogen loss after traumatic injury is not attenuated by achievement of energy balance, *J Parent Ent Nutr* 48(6):324-329, 1997.
22. Chiolero RL, Bracco D, Revelly JP: Does indirect calorimetry reflect energy expenditure in the critically ill patient? In Wilmore DW, Carpentier YA (eds): *Metabolic support of the critically ill patient,* Berlin, 1993, Springer-Verlag, p 95.
23. Ultman JS, Bursztein S: Analysis of error in the determination of respiratory gas exchange at varying F_{IO_2}, *J Appl Physiol* 50(1):210-216, 1981.
24. Ben Porat M, Sideman S, Bursztein S: Energy metabolism rate equation for fasting and postabsorptive subjects, *Am J Physiol* 244(2):R764-R769, 1983.
25. Lusk G: Analysis of the oxidation of mixtures of carbohydrate and fat. A correction, *J Biol Chem* 59(1):41-42, 1924.
26. Westenskow DR, Schipke CA, Raymond JL, et al: Calculation of metabolic expenditure and substrate utilization from gas exchange measurements, *J Parenter Enteral Nutr* 12(1):20-24, 1988.
27. Weir JB DeV: New methods for calculating metabolic rate with special reference to protein metabolism, *J Physiol* 109(1):1-9, 1949.
28. Bursztein S, Sapher P, Singer P, Elwyn DH: A mathematical analysis of indirect calorimetry measurements in acutely ill patients, *Am J Clin Nutr* 50(2):227-230, 1989.
29. Makita K, Nunn J, Royston B: Evaluation of metabolic measuring instruments for use in critically ill patients, *Crit Care Med* 18(6):638-644, 1990.
30. Phang PT, Rich T, Ronco J: A validation and comparison study of two metabolic monitors, *J Parenter Enteral Nutr* 14(3):259-264, 1990.
31. Takala J, Keinanen O, Vaisanen P, Kari A: Measurement of gas exchange in intensive care: laboratory and clinical validation of a new device, *Crit Care Med* 17(10):1041-1047, 1989.
32. Barstow TJ, Cooper DM, Sobel E, et al: Influence of increased metabolic rate on ^{13}C bicarbonate washout kinetics, *Am J Physiol* 259(1):R163-R171, 1990.
33. Armon Y, Cooper DM, Springer C, et al: Oral [^{13}C] bicarbonate measurement of CO_2 stores and dynamics in children and adults, *J Appl Physiol* 69(5):1754-1760, 1990.
34. Douglas AR, Jones NL, Reed JW: Calculation of whole blood CO_2 content, *J Appl Physiol* 65(1):473-477, 1988.
35. Brandi LS, Gvana M, Mazzanti T, et al: Energy expenditure and gas exchange measurements in post-operative patients: thermodilution versus indirect calorimetry, *Crit Care Med* 20(9):1273-1283, 1992.
36. Gerold K, Stoklosa J, Frankenfield DC: Oxygen consumption calculated by Fick equation poorly predicts oxygen consumption measured by indirect calorimetry, *Chest* 100(2):125S, 1991.
37. Liggett SB, St. John RE, Lefrank SS: Determination of resting energy expenditure utilizing the thermodilution pulmonary artery catheters, *Chest* 91(4):562-566, 1987.
38. Myburgh JA, Webb RK, Worthley LI: Ventilation/perfusion indicies do not correlate with the difference between oxygen consumption measured by the Fick principle and metabolic monitoring systems in critically ill patients, *Crit Care Med* 20(4):479-482, 1992.

39. Cobean RA, Gentilello LM, Parker A, et al: Nutritional assessment using a pulmonary artery catheter, *J Trauma* 33(3):452-456, 1992.

40. Williams RR, Fuenning CR: Circulatory indirect calorimetry in the critically ill, *J Parenter Enteral Nutr* 15(5):509-512, 1991.

41. Blasi A: Bronchial circulation: anatomical viewpoint. In Cumming G, Bonsignore G (eds): *Pulmonary circulation in health and disease,* New York, 1980, Plenum Press, pp 19-26.

42. Lifson N, Gordon GB, McClintock R: Measurement of total carbon production by means of $D_2{}^{18}O$, *J Appl Physiol* 7(7):704-710, 1955.

43. Schoeller DA, Van Santen E: Measurement of energy expenditure in free-living humans by using doubly labeled water, *J Nutr* 118(10):1278-1289, 1988.

44. Schoeller DA, Ravussin E, Schutz Y, et al: Energy expenditure by doubly labeled water: validation in humans and proposed calculation, *Am J Physiol* 250(5):R823-R830, 1986.

45. Westerterp KR, Brouns F, Saris WH, ten Hoor F: Comparison of doubly labeled water with respiratory low- and high-activity levels, *J Appl Physiol* 65(1):53-56, 1988.

46. Jeevanandam M, Young DH, Schiller WR: Energy cost of fat-fuel mobilization in geriatric trauma, *Metabolism* 39:144-149, 1990.

47. Ravussin E, Lillioja S, Anderson TE, et al: Determinants of 24-hour energy expenditure in man, *J Clin Invest* 78(6):1568-1578, 1986.

48. Webb P: Energy expenditure and fat-free mass in men and women, *Am J Clin Nutr* 34(3):1816-1826, 1981.

49. Elia M: Organ and tissue contribution to metabolic rate. In Kinney JM, Tucker HN (eds): *Energy metabolism: tissue determinants and cellular corollaries,* New York, 1992, Raven Press, p 63.

50. Poehlman ET, Toth MJ: Mathematical ratios lead to spurious conclusions regarding age- and sex-related differences in resting metabolic rate, *Am J Clin Nutr* 61(3):482-485, 1995.

51. Poehlman ET, Goran MI, Gardner AW, et al: Determinants of decline in resting metabolic rate in aging females, *Am J Physiol* 264(3):E450-E455, 1993.

52. Tanner JM: Fallacy of per-weight and per-surface area standards and their relation to spurious correlations, *J Appl Physiol* 2(1):1-15, 1949.

53. Poehlman ET, Melby CL, Badylak SF: Relation of age and physical exercise status on metabolic rate in younger and healthy older men, *J Gerontol* 46(2):B54-B58, 1991.

54. Fukagawa NK, Bandini LG, Young JB: Effect of age on body composition and resting metabolic rate, *Am J Physiol* 259(2):E233-E238, 1990.

55. Arciero PJ, Goran MI, Poehlman ET: Resting metabolic rate is lower in women than in men, *J Appl Physiol* 75(6):2514-2520, 1993.

56. Elwyn DH, Kinney JM, Askanazi J: Energy expenditure in surgical patients, *Surg Clin North Am* 61:545-556, 1981.

57. Benedict FG: Basal metabolism data on normal men and women (series II) with some considerations on the use of prediction standards, *Am J Physiol* 85(3):607-620, 1928.

58. Mifflin MD, St. Jeor ST, Hill LA, et al: A new predictive equation for resting energy expenditure in healthy individuals, *Am J Clin Nutr* 51(2):241-247, 1990.

59. Owen OE, Karle E, Owen RS, et al: A reappraisal of the caloric requirements of healthy women, *Am J Clin Nutr* 44(1):1-19, 1986.

60. Owen OE, Holup JL, D'Alessio DA, et al: A reappraisal of the caloric requirement of men, *Am J Clin Nutr* 46(6):875-885, 1987.

61. Boothby WM, Berkson J, Dunn HL: Studies of the energy metabolism of normal individuals: a standard for basal metabolism, with a nomogram for clinical application, *Am J Physiol* 116(3):468-484, 1936.

62. Robertson JD, Reid DD: Standards for the basal metabolism of normal people in Britain, *Lancet* 1(6715):940-943, 1952.

63. Schofield WN: Predicting basal metabolic rate, new standards and review of previous work, *Hum Nutr Clin Nutr* 39(suppl):5-41, 1985.

64. Benedict FG: An apparatus for studying the respiratory exchange, *Am J Physiol* 24(3):345-374, 1909.

65. Benedict FG: Old age and basal metabolism, *N Eng J Med* 212(24):1111-1122, 1935.

66. Ravussin E, Bogardus C: Relationship of genetics, age, and physical fitness to daily energy expenditure and fuel utilization, *Am J Clin Nutr* 49:968-975, 1989.

67. Consolazio CF, Johnson RE, Pecora LJ: The computation of metabolic balances. In *Physiologic measurements of metabolic functions in man,* New York, 1963, McGraw-Hill, p 313.

68. Altman PL, Dittmer DS: *Metabolism,* Washington, DC, 1968, Federation of American Societies for Experimental Biology.

69. Long CL, Schaffel N, Geiger JW, et al: Metabolic response to injury and illness: estimation of energy and protein needs from indirect calorimetry and nitrogen balance, *J Parenter Enteral Nutr* 3(6):452-456, 1979.

70. Weissman C, Kemper M, Damask MC, et al: Effect of routine intensive care interactions on metabolic rate, *Chest* 86(6):815-818, 1984.

71. Swinamer DL, Phang PT, Jones RL, et al: Twenty-four hour energy expenditure in critically ill patients, *Crit Care Med* 15(7):637-643, 1987.

72. Rodriguez JL, Weissman C, Damask MC, et al: Morphine and postoperative rewarming in critically ill patients, *Circulation* 68(6):1283-1346, 1983.

73. Robertson CL, Clifton GL, Grossman RG: Oxygen utilization and cardiovascular function in head-injured patients, *Neurosurgery* 15(3):307-314, 1984.

74. Frankenfield DC, Wiles CE III, Bagley S, Siegel JH: Relationships between resting and total energy expenditure in injured and septic patients, *Crit Care Med* 22(11):1796-1804, 1994.

75. James WPT: From SDA to DIT to TEF. In Kinney JM, Tucker HN (eds): *Energy metabolism. Tissue determinants and cellular corollaries,* New York, 1992, Raven Press, pp 163-186.

76. Jequier E, Schutz Y: Energy expenditure in obesity and diabetes, *Diabetes Metab Rev* 4(6):583-593, 1988.

77. Rubner M: *Die Gesetze des Energieverbrauchs bei der Ernahrung,* Lepizig, 1902, Franz Deuticke.

78. Lusk G: Metabolism after ingestion of dextrose and fat, including the behavior of water, urea, and sodium chloride solutions, *J Biol Chem* 13(1):27-47, 1912.

79. Forbes EB, Swift RW: Associative dynamic effects of protein, carbohydrate, and fat, *J Nutr* 27(6):453-468, 1944.

80. Blaxter KL: *Energy metabolism in animals and man,* Cambridge, 1989, Cambridge University Press.

81. Romon M, Edme JL, Boulenguez C, et al. Circadian variation of diet induced thermogenesis, *Am J Clin Nutr* 57(4):476-480, 1993.

82. Askanazi J, Carpentier YA, Elwyn DH, et al: Influence of total parenteral nutrition in fuel utilization in injury and sepsis, *Ann Surg* 191(1):40-46, 1980.

83. Vermeij CG, Feenstra BW, van Lanschot J, Bruining HA: Day-to-day variability of energy expenditure in critically ill surgical patients, *Crit Care Med* 17(7):623-626, 1989.

84. Kinney JM, Morgan AP, Domingues FJ, Gildner KJ: A method for continuous measurement of gas exchange and expired radioactivity in acutely ill patients, *Metabolism* 13(3):205-211, 1964.

85. Kinney JM, Roe F: Caloric equivalent of fever, *Ann Surg* 156(4):610-622, 1962.

86. Kinney JM, Duke JH, Long CL, et al: Tissue fuel and weight loss after injury, *J Clin Pathol* 23(suppl 4):65-72, 1968.

87. Baker JP, Detsky AS, Stewart S, et al: Randomized trial of total parenteral nutrition in critically ill patients: metabolic effects of varying glucose-lipid ratios as an energy source, *Gastroenterology* 87(1):53-59, 1984.

88. Savino JA, Dawson JA, Agarwall N, et al: The metabolic cost of breathing in critical surgical patients, *J Trauma* 25(12):1126-1133, 1985.

89. Mann S, Westenskow DR, Houtchens BA: Measured and predicted caloric expenditure in the acutely ill, *Crit Care Med* 13(3):173-177, 1985.

90. Fredrix EW, Soeters PB, von Meyenfeldt MF, Saris WH: Resting energy expenditure in cancer patients before and after gastrointestinal surgery, *J Parenter Enteral Nutr* 15(6):604-607, 1991.

91. Quebbeman EJ, Ausman RK, Schneider TC: A re-evaluation of energy expenditure during parenteral nutrition, *Ann Surg* 195(3):282-286, 1982.

92. Boulanger BR, Nayman R, McClean RF, et al: What are the clinical determinants of early energy expenditure in critically injured adults? *J Trauma* 37(6):969-974, 1994.

93. Hwang TL, Huang SL, Chen MF: The use of indirect calorimetry in critically ill patients—the relationship of measured energy expenditure to Injury Severity Score, Septic Severity Score, and APACHE II score, *J Trauma* 34(2):247-251, 1993.

94. Frankenfield DC, Omert LA, Badellino MM, et al: Prediction of energy expenditure from clinically obtainable variables in trauma and septic patients, *J Parenter Enteral Nutr* 18(5):398-403, 1994.

95. Swinamer DL, Grace MG, Hamilton SM, et al: Predictive equation for assessing energy expenditure in mechanically ventilated critically ill patients, *Crit Care Med* 18(6):657-661, 1990.

96. Caldwell FT, Wallace BH, Cone JB, Manuel L: Control of the hypermetabolic response to burn injury using environmental factors, *Ann Surg* 215(5):485-490, 1992.

97. Stokes MA, Hill GL: Total energy expenditure in patients with Crohn's disease: measurement by combined body scan technique, *J Parenter Enteral Nutr* 17(1):3-7, 1993.

98. Vermeij CG, Feenstra BW, Oomen AMFA, et al: Assessment of energy expenditure by indirect calorimetry in healthy subjects and patients with liver cirrhosis, *J Parenter Enteral Nutr* 15(4):421-425, 1991.

99. Dickerson RN, Vehe KL, Mullen JL, Feurer ID: Resting energy expenditure in patients with pancreatitis, *Crit Care Med* 19(4):484-490, 1991.
100. Liggett SB, Renfro AD: Energy expenditures of mechanically ventilated nonsurgical patients, *Chest* 98(3):682-686, 1990.
101. Roubenoff RA, Borel CO, Hanley DF: Hypermetabolism and hypercatabolism in Guillain-Barré syndrome, *J Parenter Enteral Nutr* 16(5):464-472, 1992.
102. Kreymann G, Grosser S, Buggisch P, et al: Oxygen consumption and resting metabolic rate in sepsis, sepsis syndrome, and septic shock, *Crit Care Med* 21(7):1012-1019, 1993.
103. Frankenfield DC, Smith JS, Cooney RN, et al: Relative association of fever and injury with hypermetabolism in critically ill patients, *Injury* 28(9-10):617-621, 1997.
104. Turney SZ, McAslan TC, Cowley RA: The continuous measurement of pulmonary gas exchange and mechanics, *Ann Thorac Surg* 13(3):229-242, 1972.
105. Frankenfield DC, Sarson GY, Smith JS, et al: Validation of an abbreviated indirect calorimetry protocol in critically ill patients, *J Am Coll Nutr* 15(4):397-402, 1996.
106. Feurer ID, Crosby LO, Buzby GP, et al: Resting energy expenditure in morbid obesity, *Ann Surg* 197:17-21, 1983.
107. Frankenfield DC, Muth ER, Rowe WA: The Harris-Benedict studies of human basal metabolism: history and limitations, *J Am Diet Assoc* 98(4):439-445, 1998.
108. Ireton-Jones CS, Turner WW, Liepa GW, et al: Equations for estimating energy expenditure in burn patients with special reference to ventilatory status, *J Burn Care Rehabil* 13:330-333, 1992.
109. Flancbaum L, Choban PS, Sambucco S, et al: Comparison of indirect calorimetry, the Fick method, and prediction equations in estimating the energy requirements of critically ill patients, *Am J Clin Nutr* 69:461-466, 1999.
110. Reinus JF, Heymsfield, SB, Wiskind R, et al: Ethanol: relative fuel value and metabolic effects in vivo, *Metabolism* 38(2):125-135, 1989.
111. Pirola RC, Lieber CS: The energy cost of the metabolism of drugs, including alcohol, *Pharmacology* 7(3):185-196, 1972.
112. Southgate DAT, Durin JV: Calorie conversion factors. An experimental reassessment of the factors used in the calculation of the energy value of human diets, *Br J Nutr* 24(2):517-535, 2001.
113. Shea R, Topalian J: Use of nonprotein calories vs. total calories when estimating nutritional plans: results of a practitioner survey. Presented at ASPEN 17th Clinical Congress, 1993.
114. Young VR, Meredith C, Hoerr R, et al: Amino acid kinetics in relation to protein and amino acid requirements: the primary importance of amino acid oxidation. In Garrow JS, Halliday D (eds): *Substrate and energy metabolism in man,* London, 1985 John Libbey, pp 119-133.
115. Elia M, Livesay G: Effects of ingested steak and infused leucine on forelimb metabolism in man and the fate of the carbon skeletons and amino groups of branched chain amino acids, *Clin Sci* 64(5):517-526, 1983.
116. Newsholme EA, Newsholme P, Curi R, et al: A role for muscle in the immune system and its importance in surgery, trauma, sepsis, and burns, *Nutrition* 4(4):261-288, 1988.
117. Ashy AA, Ardawi MSM: Glucose, glutamine, and ketone body metabolism in human enterocytes, *Metabolism* 37(6):602-609, 1988.
118. Ardawi MSM: Glutamine and glucose metabolism in human peripheral lymphocytes, *Metabolism* 37(1):99-103, 1988.
119. Shaw JHF, Klein S, Wolfe RR: Assessment of alanine, urea, and glucose interrelationships in normal subjects and in patients with sepsis with stable isotopic tracers, *Surgery* 97(5):557-568, 1985.
120. Garlick PJ, McNurlan, McHardy, et al: Rates of nutrient utilization in man measured by combined respiratory gas analysis and stable isotope labelling: effect of food intake, *Hum Nutr Clin Nutr* 41C:177-191, 1987.
121. Robin AP, Askanazi J, Cooperman A, et al: Influence of hypercaloric glucose infusions on fuel economy in surgical patients: a review, *Crit Care Med* 9(9):680-686, 1981.
122. Talpers SS, Romberger DJ, Bunce SB, Pingleton SK: Nutritionally associated increased carbon dioxide production: Excess total calories versus high proportion of carbohydrate calories, *Chest* 102(2):551-555, 1992.

Proteins and Amino Acids

7

Lorraine See Young, RD, MS, LDN, CNSD

Susan Stoll, MS, RD, CNSD

PROTEIN is an essential component of all living things. A knowledge of how proteins are utilized by the healthy body and how protein metabolism changes with disease to support body systems needed for fighting infection and for tissue repair is essential in nutrition support. Proteins are required as catalysts or enzymes for metabolic reactions, as antibodies, as chemical messengers (hormones), and as important structural components of cells. Dietary proteins are important principally as sources of amino acids, some of which are *essential* (indispensable); that is our bodies cannot manufacture them, so they are an essential part of the diet. There are also nonessential (dispensable) amino acids, which are synthesized from available carbon and nitrogen precursors in the body. In addition, there are a few amino acids that under normal circumstances can be manufactured by the body but with certain clinical conditions become "conditionally essential" (Table 7-1). Moreover, any larger, newly identified protein compounds (casomorphins, lactoferrin, glutathione) are proving to have vital roles in nutrition and metabolism.

The distinction between essential and nonessential amino acids is not always clear cut. Certain amino acids that adult animals can synthesize may need to be provided to an immature animal.[1] In addition, when protein metabolism is altered because of trauma, infection, or specific organ dysfunction, synthesis of a particular amino acid may be insufficient, and then that amino acid becomes conditionally essential. This area is currently under intensive scientific investigation. New evidence is emerging not only on how the metabolism and requirements of specific amino acids change during disease but also on how nutrition support professionals may be able to utilize certain amino acids as part of new therapeutic strategies to enhance the efficacy of enteral and parenteral nutrition.

Before reviewing the applicability of specific amino acids as part of the newer nutrition therapies, we first review amino acid requirements at various stages of life. We review the newest ways to assess human protein status and to define the optimal amounts of protein and energy required during illness and stress to modify the metabolic response and to achieve nitrogen retention. Finally, we discuss how we can use the newer concepts of amino acids metabolism to provide a well-balanced amino acid–dipeptide parenteral solution that best supports critically ill patients.

Amino Acid Requirements

The requirements for the 11 essential amino acids were first established in 1957 by Rose, who performed now classic nitrogen balance studies.[2] Historically these requirements have served as the standards for designing enteral and parenteral nutrition formulas. As scientific methods became more sophisticated, balance studies were supplemented with plasma amino acid response curves; growth rates, when evaluating requirements in infants and children; and, most recently, kinetic studies using noninvasive stable isotope tracer techniques to evaluate protein turnover. Because of the results of these newer methods, there has been renewed debate regarding the definition of optimal levels of certain amino acids in normal adults, specifically leucine, threonine, valine, and lysine. One scientific group proposes that the minimum requirements of the indispensable amino acids need major revisions upward; the other group contends that the Food and Agriculture Organization, World Health Organization of the United Nations (FAO/WHO/UN) 1985 recommendations of indispensable amino acid requirements remain 11% of the total protein requirements.[3,4] Young[3] suggests a new revised estimate (Table 7-2).

TABLE 7-1

Amino Acid Classification

Indispensable	Dispensable	"Conditionally Essential"
Phenylalanine	Alanine	Cysteine
Isoleucine	Aspartic acid	Glutamine
Leucine	Asparagine	Arginine
Lysine	Glutamic acid	Taurine
Methionine	Glycine	Tyrosine
Histidine	Proline	
Threonine	Serine	
Tryptophan		
Valine		

TABLE 7-2

Tentative Revised Estimates of Amino Acid Requirements of Healthy Adult Humans

Amino Acid	Requirement (mg/kg/day)	Pattern* (mg/g protein)
Isoleucine	23	35
Leucine	40	65
Lysine	30	50
Methionine and cystine	13	25
Phenylalanine and tyrosine	39	65
Threonine	15	25
Tryptophan	6	10
Valine	20	35

Adapted from Young VR: Adult amino acid requirements: the case for a major revision in current recommendations, *J Nutr* 124:1517S-1523S, 1994.
*Values rounded to nearest 5.

This new proposed amino acid pattern is essentially the same as that for 2- to 5-year-old children (FAO/WHO/UN, 1985) Thus, Young's group maintains that the amino acid requirement pattern does not change substantially between early childhood and adult life.[3]

To define the optimal requirement for protein requires judgment about the benefit of any particular level of intake and associated oxidative losses. The minimum intakes of specific indispensable amino acids required to meet the body's physiologic needs are defined as the smallest amounts that achieve equilibrium amino acid balance in the body (i.e., daily intake ~ daily oxidation = 0).[5] Millward[4] believes that the 1985 FAO/WHO/UNU recommendations are appropriate for minimal requirement standards and that a definition of optimal needs requires value judgments to be made about the beneficial metabolic effects of intakes in excess of minimal (the *anabolic drive*). This anabolic drive has yet to be identified in humans. In addition, Millward contends that stable isotope balance studies of specific amino acids do not provide unequivocal support for increasing minimum requirements.[4]

Historically, amino acid requirements focused on two processes: growth (in the sense of protein [nitrogen] deposition) and maintenance (more difficult to define). The pattern of amino acids required for protein deposition is determined largely by the amino acid composition of the proteins deposited, as determined by nitrogen balance studies.[6] They define optimal amino acids patterns for efficient amino acid deposition. In other words, they are minimal requirements for maximum growth or optimal health.[3,6]

Although the debate surrounding amino acid requirements has focused on normal requirements, these results and the methods used to determine the requirements must be know to nutrition support dietitians. Clinicians must be able to adapt and modify normal requirements to seriously ill patients whose end-organ dysfunction may necessitate modifications in protein intake. As scientists debate the definition of normal metabolism and more clearly define what amino acids or protein substances are needed to "maintain" the body in condition and in what amounts, the clinical dietitian needs to be prepared to translate the newest research findings into guidelines for practice.

Protein quality and quantity are the key factors that determine how protein requirements are met. Effective protein utilization also depends on an adequate energy supply. Protein synthesis requires a full supply of amino acids; if one of the essential amino acids is lacking, a new protein cannot be made because the metabolic pathway for protein synthesis allows no substitutions.[7] For the most part, high-quality proteins (i.e., those that contain all of the amino acids in the proper portions) come from animal sources such as eggs, milk, meat, and fish. Measurements of protein quality include biologic value and chemical score. The *biologic* value is a measure of the nitrogen retained for growth or maintenance and is expressed as nitrogen retained divided by nitrogen absorbed. The *chemical* score compares the amino acid composition of food with that of a high-quality protein such as egg. For hospitalized patients the goal is to give high-quality proteins so as not to overburden the body with the task of metabolizing extra, unneeded amino acids. All commercially available enteral formulas contain high-quality protein.

Amino acid imbalances, antagonisms, and toxicities are also major concerns. The lack of one essential amino acid can produce an imbalance that can result in growth failure or negative nitrogen balance. Amino acid antagonism can occur among amino acids that are structurally related; that is, an excessive amount of one of the branched-chain amino acids (leucine, isoleucine, valine) can depress utilization of the other two. Toxicity can also result when disproportionate amounts of amino acids are administered. Although this effect usually manifests in children as poor growth, it can be cause of concern with injudicious use of specialized adult formulas designed for "stress" or organ dysfunction.[8]

Methods of Protein Assessment Turnover

Loss of body protein or lean body mass (LBM) is associated with many conditions (acute, chronic illness and starvation) seen in the hospital setting and is a major contributor to mortality. Loss of LBM or specifically of muscle mass is also associated with advanced age. Glucocorticoids are also involved in accelerating protein degradation. The primary objective of nutrition therapy in the critically ill is to attenuate losses and maintain LBM and the size of the protein pool to optimize the body's ability to repair itself (i.e., wound healing and fighting infection). Methods for assessing protein nutrition in hospitals and clinics have historically given information about the degree of malnutrition and the effectiveness of nutrition support. These data are only estimates because the techniques are based on various assumptions that are usually not valid in the clinical setting. In the future, the ability to accurately measure protein stores and protein metabolism may give us more information about disease states and ultimately facilitate the design of more rational nutrition therapies. The methods for assessing protein nutrition are traditional methods: nitrogen balance, protein turnover, 3-methylhistidine (3-MH), and urinary creatinine excretion. Newer techniques are bioelectrical impedance assay (BIA) and dual-energy x-ray absorptiometry (DXA). These methods are discussed in more detail in the chapters on assessment of nutritional status (see Chapter 3).

Protein Turnover

The measurement of whole body protein turnover in humans was a significant advancement in nitrogen balance studies. Nitrogen balance reflects the overall balance between protein synthesis and protein breakdown. A given nitrogen balance can be achieved within a wide range of protein synthesis and breakdown rates. *Protein turnover*, the measurement of protein synthesis and degradation, provides information about protein metabolism.

The body proteins are constantly in flux, and in healthy persons equilibrium is maintained by the sum of ongoing anabolic and catabolic processes over a 24-hour period. In normal individuals, whole-body protein turnover cycles throughout the day between periods of feeding, when protein synthesis exceeds protein breakdown, and periods of fasting, when breakdown exceeds synthesis. This process is altered by various diseases and physiologic states and by changes in nutrient intake (e.g., parenteral and enteral nutrition infusion).

By giving the patient a stable, isotope-labeled amino acid, protein turnover can be followed. The labeled amino acid enters the free amino acid pool and is incorporated into newly synthesized protein. Over time, the labeled amino acid is lost as protein is broken down. The rate at which a label is lost from a particular protein depends on the rate at which that protein is broken down or resynthesized. Using these principles, Stein,[9] in a thorough review of protein turnover, described two methods for measuring protein turnover: the flux method and the end-product method. The flux method measures the incorporation of isotope into the free amino acid pool. The end-product method measures the rate and proportion of isotope excreted in the urine.

Newer methods of stable isotope tracer methodology, mass spectrometry, and effective purification techniques enable the measurement of protein synthesis at the tissue (liver, gut, muscle) level, individual protein level, and specific protein fraction.[10] Today, assessment of protein turnover is used only in research studies, but the findings help in the development of optimal nutrition support methods. Protein turnover assessment can determine if muscle wasting is due to reduced synthesis, increased breakdown, or a combination of the two.

Protein turnover studies can help define optimal amounts of protein and particular proteins or amino acids needed to attenuate protein losses in normal and abnormal physiologic states. Also, protein turnover methods can monitor and quantify metabolic changes in response to modifications of nutrient intake and evaluate the effects of nutrition support. Protein gain is related not only to protein intake but also to energy intake; thus, protein-energy relationships are significant. Protein and energy must be supplied concurrently. Also, there is an optimal range of calorie and protein intake that optimizes nitrogen retention and substrate utilization.

Optimizing Nitrogen-Energy Relationships

In healthy persons, nitrogen equilibrium is related to adequacy of calorie intake. Calloway and Spector noted that when calories are supplied without protein, nitrogen sparing occurs.[11] The maximum protein sparing occurs at almost 700 nonprotein calories per day. Increasing calories over this amount does not improve nitrogen balance; only adding protein will do that. Then, nitrogen balance improves further with the addition of protein and energy to the diet. Calloway and Spector concluded that with fixed but adequate protein intake, the energy level is the deciding factor in nitrogen balance, and with fixed and adequate calorie intake, nitrogen intake determines nitrogen balance (Fig. 7-1).

In normal and depleted "nonstressed" persons, nitrogen balance is achieved as long as adequate calories are provided and protein accounts for about 8% of calories (calorie-nitrogen ratio 300:1). Once nitrogen balance is achieved in normal persons, further increases in calories or protein do not promote positive nitrogen balance (nitrogen balance stays at zero); however, in starved or depleted persons, without the hypermetabolism associated with stress, the addition of more protein promotes positive nitrogen balance, and lost protein is replenished. The hypermetabolism associated with various diseases (i.e. burns, multiple trauma) is characterized by protein catabo-

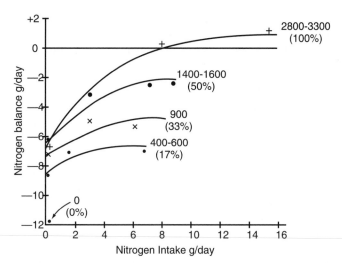

FIGURE 7-1 At any level of nitrogen intake, increasing calorie intake improves nitrogen balance, and at any level of calorie intake, increasing nitrogen intake improves balance. The range of calorie intake in these active young men is listed to the right of each isobar. The number in parentheses below each calorie intake expresses total calorie intake as a percentage of total daily metabolic expenditure, as measured or estimated in the enteral feeding studies. (From Wilmore DW: Energy requirements for maximum nitrogen retention. In Green HL, Holliday MA, Munro HN: *Proceedings of a symposium on amino acids*, American Medical Association, Philadelphia, 1977, pp 47-57. Adapted from Calloway DH, Spector H: Nitrogen balance as related to calorie and protein intake in active young men, *Am J Clin Nutr* 2:405-412, 1954.)

lism and negative balance. This increase in metabolic activity causes calorie needs to increase and protein requirements to double to approach nitrogen equilibrium. The optimal calorie-nitrogen ratio is 150:1, about 15% to 20% of energy being derived from protein.[9] Current clinical practice includes providing calories to meet metabolic demands and providing 1.5 g of protein/kg per day. There is evidence that providing protein in excess of this amount affords no additional advantage in improving nitrogen balance.[12] The exception to this general rule is the patient with a large burn injury who loses large amounts of protein through the burn wound. For these patients it is reasonable to provide up to 2 g of protein per kilogram per day.[13] Nutrition support for a critically ill person improves nitrogen retention by increasing synthesis but has minimal effect on decreasing catabolism; thus, positive nitrogen balance may not be a realistic goal in critically ill persons. Anabolic hormones or growth factors may improve nitrogen balance in some populations. The efficacy of these anabolic agents is being evaluated. Several studies have shown that glucose-based and lipid-based parenteral solutions have similar effects on nitrogen balance. In current practice, the majority of nonprotein calories provided are carbohydrates and less than 30% of calories are lipids, to avoid potential complications associated with high linoleic acid intake in critical illness (i.e., adult respiratory distress syndrome [ARDS], sepsis).

Functions of Amino Acids in Critical Care

Amino acid requirements of critically ill persons have recently received a tremendous amount of attention. Methods of feeding the critically ill have changed drastically since the inception of special enteral and parenteral feedings. Amino acids, protein, and other major nutrients were once provided principally with the goal of preventing nutrient deficiencies and maintaining energy and protein balance until the patient was "cured" by the surgeon's hand or by drug therapy. Little thought was given to how specific nutrients might affect the body's response to stress, infection, or trauma. Our current approach to feeding critically ill persons focuses more on the use of specific nutrients as therapeutic modulators of the metabolic response. In addition to nourishing the human body, specific nutrients, including certain amino acids, may actually enhance the body's own curative powers. Two main functions of amino acids—maintenance of host defenses and of neuromuscular function (i.e., maintenance of both higher neural function and mobility)—are critically important.[6]

Protein Substances and Immune Function

In terms of host immune defense, protein and some individual amino acids play key roles in two important areas. It is well established that protein depletion is associated with impaired immune function, partly because of the limited availability of amino acids to support synthesis of cell proteins and hepatic acute-phase protein response.[14,15] Proteins are also essential as structural components to help maintain a barrier in the skin, lungs, and gastrointestinal tract to prevent invasion of pathogenic organisms.

The end products of the metabolism of some amino acids are crucial intermediates in the maintenance of various physiologic functions that are not directly related to protein metabolism. Table 7-3 lists some of these substances.[6] One of the compounds, essential for host defense, is glutathione (GHS), a tripeptide and a key free radical scavenger. It is essential for lymphocyte activation and is synthesized from glutamate, glycine, and cysteine.[16] Plasma and tissue GSH levels are low with protein malnutrition and clinical conditions such as cirrhosis, sepsis, trauma, shock, and HIV infection.[17-20]

TABLE 7-3
A Partial List of Physiologically Important End Products of Amino Acid Metabolism

Product	Precursor	Function
Glutathione	Cysteine, glutamate, glycine	Oxidant defense
Creatine	Glycine, arginine	Muscle function
Taurine	Cysteine	Neural function Muscle function? Osmoregulation? Oxidant defense?
Nitric acid	Arginine	Immune function Neural function Blood vessel tone
Carnitine	Lysine	Fat oxidation
Brain glutamate	Glutamate	Neurotransmitter
Brain glycine	Glycine	Neurotransmitter

Adapted from Reeds PJ, Hutchens TW: Protein requirements: from nitrogen balance to functional impact, *J Nutr* 124:1754S-1764S, 1994.
? = possible role

Glutathione

Cysteine is known to be one of the limiting amino acids for GSH synthesis. It has been shown that GSH levels can be restored by providing cysteine in the diet.[21] Welbourne, however, has demonstrated that glutamine (GLN) is the rate-limiting amino acid for GSH synthesis in the kidney in vitro.[22] There is also evidence in experimental animals that the provision of exogenous GLN improves survival after massive hepatic necrosis because of a variety of oxidant stresses, by preserving hepatic GSH levels.[23] Klimberg and colleagues demonstrated in vivo that supplemental GLN could prevent cyclophosphamide-induced depletion of intracellular cardiac GSH, resulting in decreasing cardiotoxicity and improved survival.[24]

There is also more recent evidence, in rats and again from Klimberg's laboratory, that oral GLN supplementation enhances selectivity of antitumor drugs by protecting normal tissues from (and possibly sensitizing tumor cells to) chemotherapy-related injury.[25] Rats that received 1 g/kg per day of GLN and subsequently underwent methotrexate chemotherapy had decreased levels of tumor GSH, but they increased or maintained host GSH stores. The lower levels of GSH in tumor cells correlated with greater tumor volume loss.[25]

Deficiency of GSH stores, readily seen during serious illness, can predispose patients to ongoing tissue damage from oxygen free radicals. And although it has yet to be proven in human studies, these data suggest that patients who require nutrition support and who do not receive this GSH precursor amino acid or an alternative supplement may have limited ability to maintain their antioxidant stores when they most need them.[26] GSH deficiency in patients may lead to increased morbidity and mortality, not only because this tripeptide is vital for defense against oxidants but also because it is essential for the leukocyte function and proliferation required for metabolism of many cellular compounds and for wound repair.[27]

Arginine is an amino acid that can be valuable when the immune system is compromised. In postoperative surgical patients, arginine supplementation enhances T-lymphocyte response and increases helper T-cell numbers, and T-cell function rapidly returns to normal as compared with control patients.[28] Arginine is discussed in greater detail in later sections.

The Concept of Conditionally Indispensable Amino Acids

The current focus in the development of amino acid preparations is to provide solutions specific to critically ill patients or those who have certain metabolic disorders. Provision of certain amino acids as single nutrients can improve the tolerance to nitrogen load in the presence of illness or organ dysfunction. In essence, some classic "nonessential" amino acids have to be relabeled as "conditionally indispensable" substrates.[29] Administering required substrates can facilitate the anabolic response to a life-threatening disease.[30] Some of the amino acids considered in this category are arginine, histidine, serine, taurine, cysteine, tyrosine, and glutamine (see Table 7-1).

Arginine

Arginine, originally classified by Rose as a conditionally essential amino acid, is an intermediary metabolite in the urea cycle, where it is hydrolyzed to urea and ornithine by the enzyme arginase.[2] As a component of the urea cycle, arginine is indirectly linked to the citric acid cycle and to oxidation of fuel molecules for energy. Conversion to ornithine explains arginine's role in the production of polyamines, which are key molecules in cell growth and differentiation.[31] Arginine is also a critical substrate for production in vivo and in vitro of nitric oxide (NO) via conversion to citrulline. Arginine's role in NO production is apparently critical to the body's homeostatic mechanisms, because NO appeared to be a major regulator of the vascular endothelium (vasodilator) and is involved in macrophage physiology, among other cell functions.

Arginine has received renewed attention in the context of critical illness because of its potential role in immunomodulation.[32] It is hypothesized that arginine enhances the depressed immune responses associated with trauma, sepsis, or malnutrition. In experimental animal and human studies, arginine supplementation improved cellular response, decreased trauma-induced reduction in T-cell function, and accelerated phagocytosis.[33] Interestingly, glutamine increases the production of arginine via citrulline produced from glutamine metabolism in the gut. This may account for some of the immunostimulating and beneficial clinical effects observed with glutamine supplementation.[34] It is important to note that arginine competes with lysine for tubular reabsorption.[35] Thus, parenteral administration of excessive amounts of arginine can result in lysine deprivation.

Glutamine

The amino acid glutamine has received considerable scientific attention in the past decade because of evidence (initially generated in animal models but now also in humans) of its metabolic importance in health and during critical illness. Glutamine performs numerous unique physiologic and biochemical functions in addition to being a structural unit of protein.[36,37] It is the most abundant amino acid in plasma (600 to 900 µm/l) and in skeletal muscle (~20 mM/l), and thus represents more than 50% of the total free amino acid pool in the body.[38] One of the more important functions of glutamine is that, together with alanine, it transports more than half of the circulating amino acid nitrogen, being the principal carrier because of its two amino moieties.[39,40] It is a major substrate for renal ammoniagenesis and is thus essential for maintaining acid-base balance.[41] It is a major precursor of nucleotides and other macromolecules and a regulator of protein synthesis. Moreover, glutamine is the principal respiratory fuel for cells of the intestinal tract and is essential for many other rapidly proliferating cells, such as stimulated lymphocytes, endothelial cells, fibroblasts, and malignant cells, which suggests that glutamine may play a role in certain clinical conditions.[5,42-44] Sir Hans Krebs, a prominent biochemist, remarked in a special lecture on glutamine metabolism in the animal body, "Most amino acids have multiple functions, but glutamine appears to be the most versatile" (Box 7-1).[45]

Dietary GLN requirements appear to increase markedly during certain catabolic states because cellular requirements of the primary GLN-utilizing tissues (intestinal and immune cells, kidney, and perhaps other tissues such as wounds) are increased, GLN utilization by body tissues apparently exceeds endogenous GLN production from skeletal muscle and liver

---

BOX 7-1

Important Metabolic Functions of Glutamine

Major substrate for gluconeogenesis
Interorgan nitrogen and carbon transport
Essential precursor for nucleotide synthesis
Essential amino acid in synthesis of body proteins
Substrate for renal ammoniagenesis
Stimulation of glycogen synthesis
Regulator of protein synthesis and breakdown rates
Important metabolic fuel source for rapidly replicating cells

Adapted from Ziegler T, Young LS: Therapeutic effects of specific nutrients. In Rombeau J, Caldwell MC (eds): *Enteral and tube feeding,* ed 3, Philadelphia, 1996, WB Saunders.

---

during catabolic illness, even during provision of standard enteral and parenteral feeding.[46] GLN deficiency may develop if the increased GLN requirements of GLN-utilizing tissues are not met by adequate dietary provision of GLN; however, standard parenteral feedings do not contain GLN, and only a few enteral products are enriched in this amino acid. Reduced GLN concentrations in intracellular and plasma pools appear to be coupled with altered structure and function of the key tissues that synthesize or utilize GLN (e.g., skeletal muscle breakdown and weakness, gut mucosal atrophy, and immune cell dysfunction can develop).[45,46]

As the key role of glutamine in health and disease came into focus over the past 10 years, it became clear to scientists and nutritionists that its ubiquitous nature and its physiologic and metabolic importance justified reclassification. GLN has historically been considered a nonessential amino acid because it can be synthesized by almost all body tissues in adequate amounts during health. Under certain pathophysiologic conditions, however, the need for nonessential or dispensable amino acid can exceed the amount the body synthesizes. This is the case with glutamine. Amino acids that need to be supplied exogenously in certain cases, such as glutamine, are called *conditionally essential*.[29,45]

It is well established that GLN deficiency develops after injury or infection. In the animal model, supplying GLN enterally or parenterally not only prevents GLN deficiency but also improves overall outcome. Although an exhaustive review of the literature is not possible here, the safety and stability of parenteral and enteral GLN have been well established. GLN-enriched enteral formulas are now commercially available. They offer a theoretic advantage over parenteral diets containing GLN because they provide GLN directly to the gut mucosa and splanchnic tissue and in animal models exert similar metabolic and clinical effects. However, because only 60% to 70% of enteral glutamine is extracted by the splanchnic tissue, it will take longer to reverse the glutamine deficiency state seen in critical illness and raise plasma levels.[47] It may be prudent to supply glutamine intravenously during the first few days of injury as glutamine-containing tube feedings are advanced to goal. This may be especially important because the function of glutamine as an antioxidant precursor and immunostimulant may be time dependent.[34]

More recently, Houdijk and associates[48] from the Netherlands evaluated the infectious morbidity in multiple trauma patients who were randomly fed either a glutamine-containing enteral formula (Alitraq) or a control formula that was isocaloric and isonitrogenous. The patients were fed the formulas for a minimum of 5 days. The glutamine-containing group had significantly lower incidence of pneumonia, sepsis, and bacteremia at the end of a 15-day study period. The glutamine-fed group also had higher GLN and arginine levels and lower tumor necrosis factor receptor p55 and p75 levels. There was no difference in mortality.[48]

Jensen and associates recently published a preliminary report on the metabolic effects of a commercially available GLN-enriched tube feeding formula in critically ill patients.[49] Arterial and venous amino acids and lymphocyte subsets in peripheral blood were assessed in 28 intensive care unit patients randomized to receive 10 days of isocaloric, isonitrogenous tube feedings that differed sixfold in GLN content. The GLN-supplemented group had a better phenylalanine-tyrosine ratio (an indicator of the protein catabolic response) and a significantly greater rise in the helper T cell (CD4+)–suppressor T cell (CD8+) ratio (an indication of improved immune function).

An increasing number of studies have documented benefits of parenteral nutrient solutions enriched with free GLN or various GLN dipeptides, which are available in Europe. Both intravenous forms of GLN have pros and cons; both are somewhat more expensive to manufacture than standard amino acid solutions. The solutions that contain GLN require special procedures that require additional personnel and there is an added cost if they are made with solutions that contain essential amino acid predominantly, because these are generally more expensive than standard amino acid solutions. In the future large-scale production of these solutions may reduce costs of manufacturing.

The original clinical trials of GLN-enriched nutrition focused primarily on nitrogen and amino acid metabolism. Improved nitrogen retention and maintenance of plasma GLN concentrations were first observed by Furst, Stehle, and associates, who studied patients receiving ALA-GLN dipeptide-enriched parenteral nutrition (PN) following major abdominal operations or trauma.[50,51] Vinnars, Wernerman, and Hammarqvist and colleagues evaluated nitrogen balance and blood and intracellular muscle amino acid concentrations in patients receiving several experimental amino acids in balanced PN solutions after elective cholecystectomy.[52-54] A standard amino acid solution was compared with an isonitrogenous and isocaloric solution containing either ALA-GLN dipeptides or free GLN. The GLN solutions resulted in significantly improved nitrogen balance, smaller skeletal muscle intracellular GLN losses, and preserved muscle protein synthesis as compared with the GLN-free solutions. The available human data suggest that as patients become more critically ill, it takes greater amounts of exogenous glutamine to improve nitrogen economy and maintain muscle GLN concentrations. This may be due to increased GLN utilization and requirements in tissues such as the gut mucosa and immune cells.[7] Recent human studies have demonstrated the gut trophic effects of GLN dipeptides.[55, 56] Van der Hulst and colleagues[55] studied the effects of glycyl-L-GLN dipeptide-enriched parenteral feeding given for 10 to 14 days to patients who require PN for stable intestinal disease. Patients who received the GLN-enriched solution exhibited slightly greater intestinal villus height and significantly less intestinal permeability than

control patients who received standard PN. Similarly, Tremel and others demonstrated that critically ill patients who received L-alanyl-GLN dipeptides had significantly enhanced absorption of oral D-xylose as compared with controls who received standard PN, both after 8 days.[56]

Two randomized double-blind controlled trials were recently performed in catabolic bone marrow-transplant patients.[57,58] In the first trial, 45 adult recipients of allogeneic transplants for hematopoietic malignancies were randomized to receive either standard or GLN-supplemented parenteral nutrition starting on day 1 after marrow transplantation. The patients had received intensive chemotherapy and total body irradiation 1 week before. The parenteral nutrition the patients received was isocaloric and isonitrogenous; however, one group received 0.57 g per kilogram GLN per day (about 40 g), the other received no GLN. The patients were allowed to eat, but because of severe mouth ulcers, nausea, vomiting, and profuse diarrhea, their oral intake was minimal. Metabolic monitoring included nitrogen balance, evaluation of laboratory indices, monitoring for clinical infection and microbial colonization, time until marrow engraftment, length of hospital stay, and other data related to hospital morbidity.

The patients were clinically similar and had similar nutrient intakes. The group who received GLN, however, had less microbial colonization, developed fewer clinical infections, and were discharged from the hospital 7 days sooner than those who received standard parenteral nutrition. Nitrogen balance was also improved in the group of patients who received GLN. The reduction in hospital stay in the bone marrow transplantation (BMT) study significantly reduced hospital costs (by about $21,000/patient), principally charges for room and board.[59] There were no differences between the groups in incidence of fever, antibiotic requirements, or time to neutrophil engraftment.

In the second study, Schloerb and colleagues[58] duplicated the earlier study design and also showed reduced length of stay in bone marrow-transplant patients. These findings strengthened the evidence that GLN is in fact efficacious and cost-effective in humans.[58] Box 7-2 summarizes the beneficial effects of intravenous glutamine in the clinical setting.

BOX 7-2

Beneficial Effects of Dietary Supplementation with Intravenous GLN or GLN Dipeptide in Clinical Settings

---

Sustained plasma GLN levels in catabolic stress (GLN and GLN dipeptide)
Sustained skeletal muscle intracellular GLN levels after trauma or operation (GLN dipeptide)
Improved nitrogen balance in catabolic states (GLN and GLN dipeptide)
Attenuated 3-MH excretion after BMT (GLN)
Enhanced skeletal muscle protein synthesis rates (GLN dipeptide)
Attenuated extracellular fluid expansion after BMT (GLN)
Increased D-xylose absorption in critical illness (GLN dipeptide)
Improved intestinal nutrient absorption in severe short-bowel syndrome combined with a modified diet and growth hormone (GLN)
Reduced microbial colonization and clinical infection after BMT (GLN)
Enhanced lymphocyte recovery after BMT (GLN)
Shortened hospital length of stay after allogenic or autologous BMT (GLN)

Adapted from Ziegler T, Young LS: Therapeutic effects of specific nutrients. In Rombeau J, Caldwell MC (eds): *Enteral and tube feeding*, ed 3, Philadelphia, 1996, WB Saunders. *BMT,* Bone marrow transplantation; *GLN,* glutamine.

More recently, Griffiths and colleagues[60] designed a randomized blinded trial to evaluate glutamine-containing PN on morbidity and mortality in trauma patients. The study population of 84 parenterally fed patients was chosen from a cohort of 156 severely ill patients based on the patients intolerance to enteral feedings over 48 hours or intraabdominal processes precluding enteral nutrition. In the glutamine recipients, there was improved survival at 6 months postinjury and reduced hospital costs per survivor ($46,403 versus $94,077), despite the fact they received the GLN-PN for only 5 days while in the ICU.

A recent review of the glutamine literature by Buchman suggests using a more cautious approach when extrapolating animal data to humans.[61] He readily acknowledges that the reduced length of hospitalization seen in many clinical trials evaluating GLN is an important finding, but feels it may be a too simplistic explanation to suggest this outcome is attributable to GLN supplementation alone. In addition, many clinical trials with GLN use glycine as the control amino acid. There is new evidence to suggest glycine may be immune-enhancing in its own right.[62,63] Moreover, there is still a paucity of data regarding glutamine's mechanisms of action during critical illness, which Buchman[61] considers ample reason to be prudent with GLN supplementation in the clinical setting.

Based on data available to date, GLN should be considered an important dietary amino acid in a number of clinical settings (see Box 7-2); however, additional randomized, blinded, and controlled trials are needed to define further which patient subgroups might benefit from GLN supplementation.

Branched-Chained Amino Acids

Branched-chain amino acid (BCAA) solutions have been proposed as a treatment for catabolic or stressed patients, especially those with sepsis, trauma, or severe burns. Special BCAA-enriched solutions have also been developed for patients with liver failure, principally to treat portal-systemic encephalopathy (PSE).

BCAAs account for about 35% of all essential amino acids and 14% of skeletal muscle amino acids in humans. In the postabsorptive state, a significant proportion of skeletal muscle amino acids uptake is accounted for by BCAAs.[64] Initially, interest in the BCAAs derived from studies performed in vitro or in animal models that suggested BCAAs (especially leucine) or their ketoacids have a regulatory and anabolic role in protein metabolism by increasing rates of skeletal muscle protein synthesis or decreasing rates of protein degradation. Also, patients with hepatic failure demonstrate decreased circulating BCAA and accumulation of aromatic amino acids (phenylalanine, tyrosine, tryptophan) and methionine in the blood.[65,66] The theory is that an increased aromatic amino acid–BCAA ratio may increase tryptophan uptake across the blood-brain barrier and contribute to increased cerebral serotonin levels and to precipitation or exacerbation of encephalopathy. Thus, provision of amino acid transport across the blood-brain barrier was suggested as a method for improving hepatic encephalopathy and enhancing nitrogen balance.[1]

BCAA-enriched parenteral and enteral nutrition have been investigated fairly extensively both as a way to improve nitrogen balance in critically ill persons and as therapy for hepatic encephalopathy. To summarize, the results of meta-analysis of randomized clinical trials of BCAA-enriched parenteral nutrition in hepatic encephalopathy were published in 1989.[67] The authors concluded that slight but significant improvement in hepatic encephalopathy may occur when cirrhosis patients are given parenteral BCAA-enriched solutions (which may thus allow larger amounts of protein to be administered), but their effects on mortality seem to be inconsistent. The recently published clinical guidelines of the American Society for Parenteral and Enteral Nutrition suggest that BCAA-enriched enteral or parenteral nutrition should be used for hepatic encephalopathy only when, in spite of standard medical care (lactulose/neomycin), the encephalopathy makes it impossible to provide adequate protein to the patient.

Recent randomized trials in catabolic and critically ill patients without hepatic disease that compared BCAA-enriched parenteral nutrition with standard parenteral formulas showed no significant clinical outcome or metabolic differences.[68,69] The American Society for Parenteral and Enteral Nutrition clinical guidelines state that, because proven effects on clinical outcomes are lacking, BCAA-supplemented diets cannot be routinely advocated for critically ill patients.[70]

Histidine

It is well established that infants have a specific requirement for dietary histiine.[71] There is also evidence that histidine is required during uremia, and including it in diets for uremic patients improves nitrogen economy.[64] Plasma histidine levels drop when even normal, healthy men consume a histidine-deficient diet for a long time. This suggests that patients who require long-term PN might benefit from histidine supplementation.

Serine

Serine, another nonessential amino acid, may become conditionally essential in kidney disease because endogenous synthesis may not cover the body's requirement.[72] Serine depletion may be another limiting factor for protein synthesis in patients with impaired kidney function.

Taurine

Taurine is beginning to receive more attention as a potentially important amino acid for nutrition support. Although taurine is the most abundant intracellular free amino acid in the human body, it is not incorporated into body protein.[73] Taurine is important in bile acid conjugation, cell volume regulation, neural and retinal function, platelet aggregation, antioxidation, membrane stabilization, detoxification, calcium homeostasis, and neuromodulation.[74,75] Several studies have reported low plasma and urinary taurine levels in adults with catabolic illnesses such as cancer[75] or after operative injury, burns, and chemotherapy or irradiation, and inflammatory processes suggesting total body taurine depletion in these conditions.[75-77] Taurine has also been shown to be effective in the treatment of congestive heart failure. It is thought to have cardioprotective effects against calcium-mediated cell damage.[78] The rate-limiting enzyme for synthesis of taurine from methionine or cysteine, cysteine sulfinic acid decarboxylase, may be inhibited during catabolic illness.[79] Taurine is clearly important in infants, but to date, no studies have identified any beneficial effects of taurine supplementation for adult patients.[31]

Cysteine

In healthy adults, the sulfur-containing amino acid cysteine can be synthesized from methionine via the liver-specific trans-sulfuration pathway. The activity of cystathionase, the key enzyme in the transsulfuration pathway, is low or undetectable in the liver tissue of fetuses and preterm and term infants.[80] In persons with liver disease, body cysteine requirements are not covered because of diminished transsulfuration capacity. Cysteine needs to be administered in such cases. Stegink demonstrated that healthy men given intravenous methionine solutions that contained no cysteine had depressed levels of all three forms of circulating cysteine—free cysteine and free and protein-bound cystine.[81] Parenteral solutions may need to contain cysteine and adequate methionine. During heat sterilization and storage, parenteral cysteine is oxidized rapidly to cystine, which is very poorly soluble and thus precipitates in solution.

Tyrosine

Another traditionally nonessential amino acid for adult humans is tyrosine, which is synthesized from phenylalanine by hydroxylation. Tyrosine is considered conditionally indispensable for premature infants and for persons who have liver or kidney disease or phenylketonuria. It has been reported that administration of standard PN to patients with cirrhosis resulted in low plasma tyrosine, cysteine, and taurine levels because of impaired liver synthetic capabilities.[82] Tyrosine is also unstable in solution when its concentration exceeds 0.4 to 0.5 g/L. Thus, it may be difficult to provide sufficient amounts to cover increased tyrosine requirements for the clinical conditions previously described.

Protein (Amino Acid) Balance

To our knowledge, alteration of clinical outcome by enteral or parenteral repletion of these amino acids has not been reported to date. Some of the amino acids mentioned are either totally lacking in standard parenteral amino acid formulations (taurine, cysteine, glutamine) or are present in very small amounts (tyrosine). Current intravenous amino acid formulas may provide limiting or excessive amounts of certain amino acids and thus may be unbalanced for patients with certain medical conditions; however, as stated earlier, it is difficult to determine amino acid requirements or to diagnose amino acid "deficiency" as measured by plasma levels or free amino acid levels in tissues. Amino acid levels are in a state of flux and are affected by previous nutritional status, amino acid and energy intakes, underlying disease, severity of illness, and the patient's age and sex.[31,33]

Gazzaniga and colleagues studied the effects on plasma amino acids and nitrogen balance of a pediatric amino acid formula administered as part of balanced PN to stable adult patients.[83] The formula contained 33% BCAA (a proportion intermediate between adult standard and BCAA-enriched solutions) and increased amounts (as compared with standard adult amino acid solutions) of histidine, tyrosine, and arginine, and it included taurine. Patients received the solution with or without added cysteine HCl (0.5 mmol/kg per day) and a total protein dose of 1.5 g/kg per day for at least 6 days. Positive nitrogen balance was achieved in each group of adult patients (cysteine supplemented, +3.21 0.70 g per day versus no cysteine, +1.75 0.70 g per day; not significant (NS)) and plasma tyrosine levels normalized in each group. A significant positive correlation was observed between the increase in taurine levels in plasma and improved nitrogen balance, but only in the group who received cysteine supplementation. Positive correlation was also noted between improved nitrogen balance and plasma levels of cysteine, total cysteine plus cystine, tyrosine, and ornithine. Although a control group who received standard adult solutions was not studied, these findings suggest possible benefits for adults from amino acid solutions that initially were tailored for infants and children.

Other Proteins in Parenteral and Enteral Nutrition: Ornithine α-Ketoglutarate and α-Ketoglutarate

Ornithine α-ketoglutarate (OKG) and α-ketoglutarate (AKG) have been studied extensively in Europe.[84] OKG is a salt formed of one AKG molecule and two ornithine molecules. After intravenous or enteral administration, OKG dissociates into ornithine and AKG.[84-86] Both are GLN biosynthetic precursors: They are converted to glutamate in the body and then synthesized to GLN by the enzyme GLN synthetase.[84] AKG is also a key intermediary in the Krebs cycle, and ornithine is a central amino acid in the urea cycle. OKG has been shown to stimulate release of growth hormone and insulin, and ornithine is important in polyamine synthesis.[84]

Administration of enteral OKG in amounts from 16 to 20 g per day improved nitrogen retention and protein synthesis in postsurgical, burn and sepsis patients.[84-86] Enteral OKG enhanced nitrogen balance in association with increased GLN, growth hormone (GH), and insulin-like growth factor I (IGF-I) levels, as compared with matched patients who received OKG-free isonitrogenous tube feedings.[87] In postoperative and critically ill patients, intravenous OKG and AKG induce metabolic and protein-sparing effects very similar to those produced by GLN and GLN dipeptide. In a study of children with growth retardation secondary to short-bowel syndrome, OKG (15 g per day) added to PN was associated with accelerated growth and increased GLN and IGF-I levels.[88] Further research is needed to identify other potential outcomes of this therapy.

Carnitine

The incidence of serious liver complications associated with long-term parenteral nutrition is reported to vary between 15% to 40%. Although rare, deaths have occurred.[89] Typically, liver histology shows steatosis, steatonecrosis, intrahepatic cholestasis, and cholelithiasis. Although the causes of these liver abnormalities are multifactorial, carnitine deficiency has been implicated as one possible cause of fatty liver. Carnitine is essential for the transport of long chain fatty acids and is necessary for β-oxidation. Carnitine is not normally added to PN and low plasma levels have been reported in patients on long-term PN. Although parenteral administration of L-carnitine has been shown to improve skeletal muscle weakness, hypoglycemia, and impaired liver function,[90] it was not effective in reducing hepatic fat accumulation after 1 month of supplementation.[91]

Choline

Although choline is not considered an essential nutrient in human health because it is synthesized endogenously from phosphatidylethanolamine, it may become conditionally essential in patients not receiving choline from their diets, such as those on long-term PN. Choline is required for synthesis of phospholipids and is essential for all membranes and is an important donor of methyl groups. It has been shown that malnourished patients with preexisting liver dysfunction may not be able to synthesize sufficient choline because of defective methyl transfer reactions.[92] Buchman and coworkers, in two separate studies,[93,94] supplemented long-term PN patients with low plasma choline levels and liver steatosis with 1 to 4 g parenteral choline chloride for 6 weeks and 24 weeks, respectively. Choline concentrations were increased to the normal range, liver function tests improved, and assessment of liver steatosis based on liver-spleen computed tomography (CT) scan showed significant improvement, suggesting that choline may be a required nutrient in long-term PN patients.

Dipeptides in Nutrition Support

The amino acids tyrosine and cysteine are poorly soluble, and GLN, although unstable if heat sterilized, can be added to standard PN as a single amino acid under certain conditions. In Europe, where PN solutions must be heat sterilized, GLN has gained wider acceptance for use as a dipeptide than as a single amino acid as in the United States. The dipeptides are highly soluble in water and sufficiently stable during sterilization procedures to be approved by the authorities as constituents of parenteral solutions.[33] Synthetic dipeptides made with GLN, tyrosine, and cysteine have been shown to clear rapidly from plasma after parenteral administration without accumulating in tissues, and little is lost in the urine.[33]

Patients who underwent elective major surgery were infused with L-alanyl-L-glutamine (ALA-GLN)-supplemented PN over 5 days. Nitrogen balance improved on each postoperative day as compared with values for control subjects who received isonitrogenous and isoenergetic PN without the peptides.[95] The improvement in nitrogen balance was also associated with maintenance of intracellular GLN levels, whereas patients who received the peptide-free solution exhibited a significant decrease in GLN levels as compared with their preoperative values. Short-term infusions of ALA-GLN have positive effects on muscle protein synthesis as assessed by ^{13}C leucine incorporation in postsurgical patients receiving GLN-free parenteral nutrition. Moreover, ALA-GLN-supplemented PN was shown in ICU patients to prevent the PN-related intestinal atrophy so common with GLN-free PN.[56] Box 7-2 summarizes the beneficial effects of glutamine dipeptides in the clinical setting.

Dipeptides Versus Single Amino Acids in Enteral Nutrition

Controversy persists about the use of intact protein as peptides of varying chain lengths versus single amino acids in enteral nutrition. Many claims are made about the absorption properties of amino acids versus those of dipeptide, tripeptide, and oligopeptide in the compromised gastrointestinal tract. Early studies of the digestion and absorption of enteral formulas suggested that proteins needed to be hydrolyzed to amino acids if absorption was to occur.[96] More recent research in this area has identified dipeptide and tripeptide carrier systems, whereby the peptide form of certain amino acids is absorbed more rapidly than the single amino acid. Proponents of peptide-containing enteral formulas contend that these formulas are tolerated better than elemental diets. They claim that protein hydrolysate formulas produce less stool output, fewer symptoms of nausea and vomiting from high osmolar elemental diets, greater nitrogen utilization, and greater insulin secretion, and peptide absorption is affected less by pathologic states than is free amino acid absorption.[97] The problem with many of these studies that compare enteral formulas is that often they did not control for other factors that can affect amino acid and protein absorption (e.g., sodium content, peptide chain lengths, and fat and carbohydrate sources). In fact, when these factors are controlled for, nitrogen balance and body weight are no different with enzymatic hydrolysate or a free amino acid formula in patients with a normal gastrointestinal tract.[98] It seems that further research is needed in this area, specifically in patients with disorders of gastrointestinal function.

Conclusion

Protein is an essential macronutrient of all living things. Knowledge of the function of protein and its component amino acids is important in determining the amount and type required in health and disease. Consideration of the route of administration may have clinical consequences. It is apparent that appropriate use of protein alters outcome in some circumstances.

REFERENCES

1. Jackson AA: Amino acids: essentials and nonessential? *Lancet* (1):1034-1037, May, 1983.
2. Rose WC: The amino acid requirements of adult man, *Nutr Abstr Rev* 27:631-647, 1957.
3. Young VR: Adult amino acid requirements: the case for a major revision in current recommendations, *J Nutr* 124:1517S-1523S, 1994.
4. Millward J: Can we define indispensable amino acid requirements and assess protein in adults? *J Nutr* 124:1509S-1516S, 1994.
5. Young VR, Bier DM: Amino acid requirements in the adult human: how well do we know them? *J Nutr* 117:1484-1487, 1987.
6. Reeds PJ, Hutchens TW: Protein requirements: from nitrogen balance to functional impact, *J Nutr* 124:1754S-1764S, 1994.
7. Stein TP, Levine GM: Human macronutrient requirements. In Rombeau JL, Caldwell MD (eds): *Enteral and tube feeding,* Philadelphia, 1984, WB Saunders, pp 73-83.
8. Harper AE, Benevenga NJ, Wohlhueter RM: Effects of ingestion of disproportionate amounts of amino acids, *Physiol Rev* 50:428-558, 1970.
9. Stein TP: Nutrition and protein turnover: a review, *J Parenter Enter Nutr* 6:444-454, 1982.
10. Balagopal P: In vivo measurement of protein synthesis in humans, *Curr Opin Clin Nutr Metab Care* 1(5):467-473, 1998.
11. Calloway DH, Spector H: Nitrogen balance related to calorie and protein intake in active young men, *Am J Clin Nutr* 2:405-412, 1954.
12. Shaw JH, Wildbore M, Wolfe RR: Whole body protein kinetics in severely septic patients: the response to glucose infusion and total parenteral nutrition, *Ann Surg* 205(3):288-294, 1987.
13. Alexander, JW, MacMillen, BG, et al: Beneficial effects of aggressive protein feeding in severely burned children, *Ann Surg* (4):192:505-517, 1980.
14. Chandra RK: Nutrition and immunity: lessons from the past and new insights into the future, *Am J Clin Nutr* 53:1087-1101, 1991.

15. Colley CM, Fleck A, Goode AW, et al: Early time course of the acute phase protein response in man, *J Clin Pathol* 36:203-207, 1983.

16. Droge W, Pottmeyer-Gerber C, Schmidt H, et al: Glutathione augments the activation of cytotoxic T lymphocytes in vivo, *Immunobiology* 172:151-156, 1986.

17. Shi ECP, Fisher R, McEvoy M, et al: Factors influencing hepatic glutathione concentrations: a study in surgical patients, *Clin Sci* 62:279-283, 1982.

18. Stein HJ, Oosthuizen MMJ, Hinder RA, et al: Oxygen free radicals and glutathione in hepatic ischemia/reperfusion injury, *J Surg Res* 50:398-402, 1991.

19. Buhl R, Jaffe HA, Holyroyd KH, et al: Systemic glutathione deficiency in symptom-free HIV-seropositive individuals, *Lancet* Dec 2; 2 (8675): 1294-1298, 1989.

20. Burgunder JM, Lauterburg BH: Decreased production of glutathione in patients with cirrhosis, *Eur J Clin Invest* 17:408-414, 1987.

21. Grimble RF, Jackson AA, Persaud C, et al: Cysteine and glycine supplementation modulate the metabolic response to tumor necrosis factor-alpha in rats fed a low protein diet, *J Nutr* 122:2066-2073, 1992.

22. Welbourne TC: Ammonia production and glutamine incorporation into glutathione in the functioning rat kidney, *Can J Biochem* 57:233-237, 1979.

23. Hong RW, Rounds JD, Helton WS, et al: Glutamine preserves liver glutathione after lethal hepatic injury, *Ann Surg* 215(2):114-119, 1992.

24. Vanderpool D, Schaefer RF, Klimberg VS, et al: Oral glutamine protects against cytoxan induced cardiotoxicity and death. Presented at the Association for Academic Surgery, November 10-13, Hershey, PA, 1993.

25. Rouse K, Nwokedi E, Woodliff JE, et al: Glutamine enhances selectivity of chemotherapy through changes in glutathione metabolism, *Ann Surg* 221:420-426, 1995.

26. Robinson MK, Ahn MS, Rounds JD, et al: Parenteral glutathione monoester enhances tissues antioxidant stores, *J Parenter Enter Nutr* 16:413-418, 1992.

27. Hamilos DL, Zelarney P, Mascali JJ: Lymphocyte proliferation in glutathione-depleted lymphocytes: direct relationship between glutathione availability and the proliferative response, *Immunopharmacology* 18:223-235, 1989.

28. Daly JM, Reynolds J, Thom A, et al: Immune and metabolic effects of arginine in the surgical patient, *Ann Surg* 208(4):512-523, 1988.

29. Chipponi JX, Bleier JC, Santi MT, et al: Deficiencies of essential and conditionally essential nutrients, *Am J Clin Nutr* 35:1112-1116, 1982.

30. Wilmore DW: Catabolic illness: strategies for enhancing recovery, *N Engl J Med* 325:695-702, 1991.

31. Ziegler TR, Young LS: Therapeutic effects of specific nutrients. In Rombeau J, Caldwell MD (eds): *Enteral and tube feeding,* ed 3, Philadelphia, 1996, WB Saunders.

32. Kirk SJ, Barbul A: Role of arginine in trauma, sepsis, and immunity, *J Parenter Enter Nutr* 14:226S-229S, 1990.

33. Furst P, Stehle P: Are we giving unbalanced amino acid solutions? From protein hydrolysates to tailored solutions. In Wilmore DW, Carpentier YA (eds): *Metabolic support of the critically ill patient,* New York, 1993, Springer-Verlag.

34. Wilmore DW, Shapert JK: Role of glutamine in immunologic responses, *Nutrition* 14:618-626, 1998.

35. Vinnars E, Furst P, Hallgren B, et al: The nutritive value in man of non-essential amino acids infused intravenously (together with the essential ones). Individual non-essential amino acids, *Acta Anaesth Scand* 14: 147-172, 1970.

36. Smith RJ: Glutamine metabolism and its physiologic importance, *J Parenter Enter Nutr* 14(4):40S-44S, 1990.

37. Smith RJ, Wilmore DW: Glutamine nutrition and requirements, *J Parenter Enter Nutr* 14(4):94S-99S, 1990.

38. Bergstrom J, Furst P, Noree LO, et al: Intracellular free amino acid concentration in human muscle tissue, *Appl Physiol* 36:693-697, 1974.

39. Marliss EB, Aoki TT, Pozefsky T, et al: Muscle and splanchnic glutamine and glutamate metabolism in postabsorptive and starved man, *J Clin Invest* 50:814-817, 1971.

40. Souba WW, Herskowitz K, Austgen TR: Glutamine nutrition: theoretical considerations and therapeutic impacts, *J Parenter Enter Nutr* 14S: 237S-243S, 1990.

41. Pitts RF: Renal production and excretion of ammonia, *Am J Med* 36: 720-742, 1964.

42. Windmueller HG, Spaeth AE: Identification of ketone bodies and glutamine as the major respiratory fuels in vivo for postabsorptive rat small intestine, *J Biol Chem* 253:69-76, 1985.

43. Newsholme EA, Crabtree B, Ardawi MS: Glutamine metabolism in lymphocytes: its biochemical, physiological and clinical importance, *Q J Exp Physiol* 70:473-489, 1985.

44. Kovacevic Z, Morris HP: The role of glutamine in the oxidative metabolism of malignant cells, *Cancer Res* 32:326-333, 1972.

45. Lacey JM, Wilmore DW: Is glutamine a conditionally essentially amino acid? *Nutr Rev* 48:297-309, 1990.

46. Ziegler TR, Smith RJ, Byrne TA, et al: Potential role of glutamine supplementation in nutrition support, *Clin Nutr* 12(suppl 1):S82-S90, 1993.

47. Hankard RG, Darmon D, Sager BK, et al: Response of glutamine metabolism to exogenous glutamine in humans, *Am J Physiol* (4 Pt 1), 269:E663-670, 1995.

48. Hodijk APJ, Rijnsburger ER, Jansen J, et al: Randomized trial of glutamine-enriched enteral nutrition on infectious morbidity in patients with multiple trauma, *Lancet* 352:772-776, 1998.

49. Jensen GL, Miller RH, Talabiska D, et al: A double-blind, prospective, randomized study of glutamine-enriched versus standard peptide-based feeding in the critically ill, *Am J Clin Nutr* 64(4):615-621, 1993 (abstract).

50. Stehle P, Mertes N, Puchstein CH, et al: Effect of parenteral glutamine peptide supplements on muscle glutamine loss and nitrogen balance after major surgery, *Lancet* 1(8632):231-233, Feb 4,1989.

51. Furst P, Albers S, Stehle P: Glutamine-containing dipeptides in parenteral nutrition, *J Parenter Enter Nutr* 14(suppl 4):118S-124S, 1990.

52. Vinnars E, Hammarqvist F, von der Decken A, et al: Role of glutamine and its analogs in posttraumatic muscle protein and amino acid metabolism, *J Parenter Enter Nutr* 14:125S-129S, 1990.

53. Hammarqvist F, Wernerman J, Ali R, et al: Addition of glutamine to total parenteral nutrition after elective abdominal surgery spares free glutamine in muscle, counteracts the fall in muscle protein synthesis, and improves nitrogen balance, *Ann Surg* 209:455-461, 1989.

54. Wernerman J, Hammarqvist F, Ali MR: Glutamine and ornithine-alpha-ketoglutarate but not branched chain amino acids reduce the loss of muscle glutamine after surgical trauma, *Metabolism* 38:63-66, 1989.

55. Van der Hulst RRW, Van Kreel BK, et al: Glutamine and the preservation of gut integrity, *Lancet* 341(8857):1363-1365, May 29,1993.

56. Tremel H, Kienle B, Weileman LS, et al: Glutamine dipeptide supplemented TPN maintains intestinal function in the critically ill, *Gastroenterology* 107:1595-1601, 1994.

57. Ziegler TR, Young LS, Benfell K, et al: Clinical and metabolic efficacy of glutamine- supplemented parenteral nutrition after bone marrow transplantation: a randomized, double-blind, controlled study, *Ann Intern Med* 116:821-828, 1992.

58. Schloerb PR, Amare M: Total parenteral nutrition with glutamine in bone marrow transplantation and other clinical applications (a randomized, double-blind study), *J Parenter Enter Nutr* 17:407-413, 1993.

59. MacBurney M, Young LS, Ziegler TR, et al: A cost-evaluation of glutamine-supplemented parenteral nutrition in adult bone marrow transplantation, *J Am Diet Assoc* 94:1263-1266, 1994.

60. Griffiths, RD, Jones, C, Palmer, TEA: Six-month outcome of critically ill patients given glutamine supplemented parenteral nutrition, *Nutrition* 13:295-302, 1997.

61. Buchman, AL: Glutamine: commercially essential or conditionally essential? A critical appraisal of the human data, *Am J Clin Nutr* 74:25-32, 2001.

62. Hall JC: Glycine, *J Parenter Enter Nutr* 22:393-398, 1998.

63. Ascher E, Hanson JN, Cheng W, et al: Glycine preserves function and decreases necrosis in skeletal muscle undergoing ischemia and reperfusion injury, *Surgery* 129:231-235, 2001.

64. Furst P: 15N-studies in severe renal failure. II. Evidence for the essentiality of histidine, *Scand J Clin Lab Invest* 30:307-312, 1972.

65. Freund H, Dienstag J, Lehrich J, et al: Infusion of branched-chain amino acid solution in patients with hepatic encephalopathy, *Ann Surg* 196(2):209-220, 1982.

66. Cerra FB, Chung NK, Fischer JE, et al: Disease-specific amino acid infusion (F080) in hepatic encephalopathy: a prospect randomized, double-blind controlled trial, *J Parenter Enter Nutr* 9:288-295, 1985.

67. Naylor CD, O'Rourke K, Detsky AS, et al: Parenteral nutrition with branched chain amino acids in hepatic encephalopathy: a meta-analysis, *Gastroenterology* 97:1033-1042, 1989.

68. Lenssen P, Cheney CL, Aker SN, et al: Intravenous branched chain amino acid trial in bone marrow transplant recipients, *J Parenter Enter Nutr* 11:112-118, 1987.

69. Jimenez FJ, Ortiz LC, Morales MS, et al: Prospective study on the efficacy of branched-chain amino acids in septic patients, *J Parenter Enter Nutr* 15:252-261, 1991.

70. American Society for Parenteral and Enteral Nutrition Board of Directors: Guidelines for the use of parenteral and enteral nutrition in adult and pediatric patients, *J Parenter Enter Nutr* 17(suppl 4):1SA-52SA, 1993.

71. Snyderman SE: The protein and amino acid requirements of the premature infant. In Janxix JHP, Visser HKA, Troelstra JA (eds): *Metabolic processes in the fetus and newborn infant,* Leiden, 1970, Stenfert Kroese, pp 128-141.

72. Bergstrom J, Alvestrand A, Furst P: Plasma and muscle free amino acids in maintenance hemodialysis patients without protein malnutrition, *Kidney Int* 38:108-114, 1990.

73. Laidlaw SA, Kopple JD: Newer concepts of the indispensible amino acids, *Am J Clin Nutr* 46:593-605, 1987.

74. Wright CE, Tallan HH, Lin YY, et al: Taurine: biological update, *Annu Rev Biochem* 55:427-453, 1986.

75. Gray GE, Landel AM, Mequid MM: Taurine-supplemented total parenteral nutrition and taurine status of malnourished cancer patients, *Nutrition* 10:11-15, 1994.

76. Paauw JD, Davis AT: Taurine concentrations in serum of critically injured patients and age- and sex-matched healthy control subjects, *Am J Clin Nutr* 52:657-660, 1990.

77. Desai TK, Maliakkal J, Kinzie JL, et al: Taurine deficiency after intensive chemotherapy and/or radiation, *Am J Clin Nutr* 55:708-711, 1992.

78. Stapleton PP, O'Flaherty L, Redmond P, et al: Host defense—a role for the amino acid taurine, *J Parenter Enteral Nutr* 22:42-48, 1998.

79. Martensson J, Larson J, Schildt BO: Metabolic effects of amino acid solutions in burned patients: with emphasis on sulfur amino acid metabolism and protein breakdown, *J Trauma* 25:427-432, 1985.

80. Sturman JA, Gaull G, Raiha NCR: Absence of cystathionase in human fetal liver. Is cystine essential? *Science* 169:74-76, 1970.

81. Steginck LD, Den Besten L: Synthesis of cysteine from methionine in normal adult subjects: effect of route of alimentation, *Science* 178:514-516, 1972.

82. Rudman D, Williams PJ: Nutrient deficiencies during total parenteral nutrition, *Nutr Rev* 43:1-13, 1985.

83. Gazzaniga AB, Waxman K, Day AT, et al: Nitrogen balance in adult hospitalized patients with the use of a pediatric amino acid model, *Arch Surg* 123:1275-1279, 1988.

84. Cynober L: Ornithine alpha-ketoglutarate in nutritional support, *Nutrition* 7:313-322, 1991.

85. Leander U, Furst P, Vesterberg K, et al: Nitrogen sparing effect of Ornicetil in the immediate postoperative state: clinical biochemistry and nitrogen balance, *Clin Nutr* 4:43-51, 1985.

86. Cynober L, Lioret N, Coudray-Lucas C, et al: Action of ornithine alpha-ketoglutarate on protein metabolism in burn patients, *Nutrition* 3:187-191, 1987.

87. Jeevanandam M, Ali MR, Peterson SR: Substrate and hormonal changes due to dietary supplementation with ornithine alpha ketoglutarate in critically ill trauma victims, *Clin Nutr* 11(suppl):26, 1992 (abstract).

88. Moukarzel A, Gorski AM, Boya I, et al: Growth retardation in children on long term total parenteral nutrition (TPN): effects of ornithine alpha-ketoglutarate, *Clin Nutr* 7(suppl):13, 1988 (abstract).

89. Cavicchi M, Beau P, Crenn P, et al: Prevalence of liver disease and contributing factors in patients receiving home parenteral nutrition for permanent intestinal failure, *Ann Intern Med* 132:525-532, 2000.

90. Krahenbuhl S: Carnitine metabolism in chronic liver disease, *Life Sciences* 59(19):1579-1599, 1996.

91. Bowyer BA, Miles JM, Haymond MW, Fleming CR: L-carnitine therapy in home parenteral nutrition patients with abnormal liver tests and low plasma carnitine concentrations, *Gastroenterology* 94:434-438, 1988.

92. Shronts E: Essential nature of choline with implications for total parenteral nutrition, *J Am Diet Assoc* 96:639-649, 1997.

93. Buchman AL, Dubin MD, Moukarzel AA, et al: Choline deficiency: a cause of hepatic steatosis during parenteral nutrition that can be reversed with intravenous choline supplementation, *Hepatology* 22:1399-1403, 1995.

94. Buchman AL, Ament ME, Sohel M, et al: Choline deficiency causes reversible hepatic abnormalities in patients receiving parenteral nutrition: proof of a human choline requirement: a placebo-controlled trial, *J Parenter Enteral Nutr* 25:260-268, 2001.

95. Stehle P, Zander J, Mertes N, et al: Effect of parenteral glutamine peptide supplements on muscle glutamine loss and nitrogen balance after major surgery, *Lancet* 1(8632):231-233, Feb 4, 1989.

96. Brinson RR, Hanumanthu SK, Pitts WM: a reappraisal of the peptide-based enteral formulas: clinical applications, *Nutr Clin Pract* 4:211-217, 1989.

97. Silk DBA: Peptide enteral formulas, *Crit Care Med* 17:708-709, 1989 (letter).

98. Moriarty KJ, Hegarty JE, Fairclough PD, et al: Relative nutritional value of whole protein, hydrolysed protein and free amino acid in man, *Gut* 26:694-699, 1985.

Carbohydrates

8

Sue Fredstrom, MS, RD, CNSD

CARBOHYDRATE (CHO) is a paradoxical nutrient. Current recommendations call for it to contribute about 55% of the total daily calorie intake, although it is not always considered "essential."[1] Carbohydrate thus constitutes the major energy source of all feedings—oral, enteral, and parenteral. To cells, glucose provides most of the usable energy, but free glucose rarely exists in foods. Generally carbohydrate is easily absorbed, yet malabsorption of one CHO, lactose, afflicts the majority of the world's population to at least some degree.

After a brief review of definitions used with CHO, the functions, digestion, absorption, and metabolism of CHO and the requirements for CHO and their alterations in health and disease are discussed. Sources of CHO currently used in enteral and parenteral nutrition support are surveyed.

Definitions

CHOs are compounds of carbon, hydrogen, and oxygen in the form $C_n(H_2O)_n$, where n is 3, 4, 5, 6, or 7.[2,3] They are commonly referred to as *sugars* or *saccharides*, but chemically, CHOs are aldehydes or ketones with hydroxyl groups on the nonterminal carbons. The stochiometric position of a hydroxyl group and of the aldehyde group and the presence of a ketone or alcohol determine some of the properties of a specific sugar: its "absorbability" and its function in the body. The most common sugars have 3, 5, or 6 carbons and are termed *tri*oses, *pent*oses, and *hex*oses, respectively. Alcohols of sugars occur naturally and are used therapeutically (e.g., sorbitol) and as sweeteners in food processing.

A single sugar unit, or monosaccharide, can be linked to another through a glycoside bond, forming a disaccharide. (The term *glucosidic* is used in some texts.) A chain with more sugar units is an oligosaccharide (3 to 10 units) or a polysaccharide (more than 10 units).[2,4] When the bonds are such that branches are formed, the polysaccharide is called a *starch*. Glycoside bonds are referred to as α- or β-bonds, depending on their orientation. Humans can digest only the α-bonds, with the exception of lactose, a β-glycoside. Dietary fiber CHOs are linked by β-bonds indigestible to humans (see Chapter 13). CHOs important in nutrition support include the monosaccharides, glucose and fructose; disaccharides, sucrose and lactose; maltodextrins (the oligosaccharide product of starch hydrolysis); starch; and dextrose (an anhydrous form of glucose used parenterally). Galactose is found in fermented milk products. Legumes usually contain large amounts of raffinose oligosaccharides, which, although they have α-linkages, are not well digested in the small intestine. See Table 8-1 for the monosaccharide composition of disaccharides and some oligosaccharides.

TABLE 8-1
Intestinal Membrane Digestion of Major Dietary Saccharides*

Saccharide	Monosaccharide Components	Enzymes	Extent of Digestion (%)
Sucrose	Glucose Fructose	Sucrase	100
Maltose	Glucose	Isomaltase	50
		Maltase	25
		Sucrase	25
Isomaltose	Glucose	Isomaltase	95
		Maltase	5
Lactose	Galactose Glucose	Lactase	100
Raffinose	Galactose Glucose Fructose	Bacterial fermentation	

*Starches are digested in the lumen by salivary and pancreatic amylases.[5,6]

Carbohydrate Function
Functions as Food

As a food source, most CHOs are plant derived. In the United States, 60% of CHO is consumed in the form of starch; much of the rest is sucrose and fructose.[1,2] Lactose, the sugar in milk, provides up to 10% of CHO to adults and much more to infants. Average daily total CHO intake is 287 g for adult males and 177 g for females, or roughly 50% of total energy.[1]

Principally, CHO foods provide energy. Naturally occurring CHO in food or added CHO can act as a sweetener, improving palatability. As a general rule the smaller the molecule the sweeter the taste and the higher the osmolality. In large enough quantities sugar acts as a preservative. CHO can improve the appearance of baked goods and other products, increase the viscosity of foods, or stabilize emulsions. Some CHOs used for these purposes are indigestible to humans and provide energy only when fermented by bacteria.

Functions in the Body

Because glucose can be synthesized from amino acids and the intermediates pyruvate and lactate, CHO is not absolutely essential. However, only CHO can produce energy in anaerobic conditions.[7] Brain and nerve tissue use glucose exclusively except in times of prolonged starvation. Other tissues—erythrocytes,

105

leukocytes, the lens of the eye, and the renal medulla—use glucose preferentially but do not metabolize it completely.[8] When glucose is otherwise unavailable, gluconeogenesis is increased to provide it to the tissues that require it. Inclusion of CHO in the diet thus spares protein and reduces nitrogen excretion. In fact, it has been observed that for each extra kilocalorie in the diet, nitrogen excretion is reduced 1.5 mg.[9] Although this applies to both CHO and fat, CHO is more efficient.[10]

A primary function of CHO (shared with protein) is the enhancement of insulin secretion, thus initiating anabolism.[11] Carbohydrates differ in their ability to increase blood glucose, and therefore stimulate insulin. This ability is measured as *glycemic index*: the concentration of blood glucose observed by consumption of a food relative to that of white bread.[12] Simple CHOs have a high glycemic index, and therefore result in greater insulin secretion than the more slowly assimilated complex CHO.

CHO has numerous other physiologic effects in the body. Although its effect is controversial, CHO may increase satiety.[13,14] When present in the gut lumen, CHO, fat, and protein stimulate hormonelike substances secreted by the gut, notably gastric inhibitory peptide, which alters gastric and intestinal secretions.[5,9] Carbohydrate improves sodium absorption and increases excretion of calcium, magnesium, and possibly chromium.[5] On the other hand, lactose may improve calcium uptake. Glucose metabolism generates adenosine triphosphate (ATP), a source of energy in many reactions; NADH, an electron source in redox reactions; and, through the pentose pathway, NADPH. One of the functions of NADPH is participation in the recycling of oxidized glutathione.[3,7] Sugars are components of compounds that have a variety of functions in the body. The pentoses deoxyribose and ribose form part of the structure of ribonucleic acid (RNA) and deoxyribonucleic acid (DNA). Other CHOs are integral to certain proteins, notably those that form collagen and certain hormones, and still others form mucopolysaccharides with lipids. CHO may also play a role in cell-to-cell "messaging" and transport.[3]

Digestion and Absorption

Digestion

Ingested CHO must be hydrolyzed to monosaccharides before being absorbed. The enzymes involved, collectively called the α-glycosidases, act only on α-bonds between saccharide units. Some of the oligosaccharides and those CHOs with β-bonds (except lactose) escape digestion and, therefore, absorption in the small intestine. They pass into the colon, where they are fermented by bacteria.

Amylase is present in saliva and in the gut lumen from pancreatic secretions. It begins the hydrolysis of starch. Salivary amylase is inhibited by gastric acid, but its action is likely preserved to some extent by the buffering of foods in the stomach.[2,6] Pancreatic amylase does have some brush border activity.[2,5,15] Its end products are oligosaccharides, also called *α-limit dextrins*.[2] Enzymes responsible for further hydrolysis are synthesized in the brush border of the enterocytes. They are found principally, but not exclusively, in the upper and middle jejunum, very close to the site of absorption. Table 8-1 lists sugars that are substrates for specific enzymes. Although their names imply specificity to maltose and sucrose, maltase and sucrase act on most disaccharides and on the α-limit dextrins.[2,5] Digestion is very rapid and rarely rate limiting to absorption of CHO. Again lactase is the exception. It is specific to lactose, is secreted in the duodenum, and because it has a slower rate of action, it can limit the rate of absorption of the sugar.

Disaccharidase enzyme activity is stimulated by the presence of fructose and of CHO and fat.[2,16] Sucrose and fructose (but not glucose) increase sucrase and maltase activity. The presence of food increases the number of enterocytes, thus enhancing enzyme synthesis as well. Whether disaccharide enzyme regulation is translational or transcriptional is controversial, and in some cases it may involve both processes.[15] Lactase is probably controlled translationally because messenger RNA (mRNA) for the enzyme can be found in persons who express little of the enzyme.[2,17] Initially, lactase is synthesized as a "prolactase" and the "pro" sequence may control posttranslational modification.

Absorption and Malabsorption

Absorption of the monosaccharides occurs by active transport, carrier-mediated diffusion, and simple diffusion. Glucose and fructose are the most abundant sugars presented for absorption. An estimated 95% of glucose is absorbed actively.[15] Active transport of glucose and galactose involves a family of sodium-dependent carrier known as *SGLTs*.[2,18] When sodium is in its receptor site on the carrier, its affinity for glucose is increased. Sodium-potassium ATPase acts as a cotransporter by providing energy for this carrier.[2] Interestingly, glucose from disaccharides is absorbed more quickly than free glucose, likely because of the brush border site of the disaccharidases and the use of nonsodium-dependent transporters.[6] Absorption of maltodextrins is slower, limited by the rate of hydrolysis, which is in turn determined by chain length.[6] SGLTs are also present in the kidney to facilitate resorption of glucose from urine.

Fructose absorption uses facilitated diffusion, the rate of which may depend on the concentration of the sugar. A carrier known as *GLUT 5* is necessary for fructose absorption.[2] Sugar alcohols and L-isomers of glucose and galactose are absorbed by diffusion, a relatively slow process. Flow of water into the lumen is enhanced by these sugars to decrease their concentration. Consuming more than 50 g of sugar alcohol can cause cramping and diarrhea.

At the basolateral membrane, hexoses enter the blood by facilitated diffusion.[2,15] The carriers involved exist in five isoforms, referred to as *GLUT 1-5*. Each isoform is specific to the tissue in which it is expressed, or as mentioned above in the case of GLUT 5, to the sugar it carries. Basal, noninsulin-mediated glucose uptake depends on GLUT 1, found in many tissues and highest in brain and placenta.[2,19] GLUT 2 is found in liver, pancreas, kidney, and small intestine and may be involved in hepatic release of glucose and in insulin secretion. GLUT 4, found in skeletal muscle and fat, is sensitive to insulin and thus has a role in glucose control.[2,19]

Malabsorption of most CHOs is rare, and tolerance to a CHO load is generally limited by absorptive capacity.[4] There are rare inborn errors of metabolism in which necessary digestive enzymes or carrier proteins are missing.[2] In most instances, however, CHO malabsorption is secondary to a gastrointestinal disease such as celiac sprue or gastric infection. With small bowel atrophy, as with starvation, parenteral nutrition for bowel rest, or in a critically ill patient, disaccharidase levels and activity also decrease, causing a secondary deficiency of enzymes.[15,20] Maldigestion of lactose and sucrose in children with human immunodeficiency virus (HIV) was recently reported.[21] Symptoms of malabsorption are bloating; cramping; flatulence; borborygmus; and watery, osmotic diarrhea with pH less than 6.[11,22] When colonic pH is less than 5, fermentation is inhibited, so CHO, usually in the form of glucose, appears in the stool.[22] When villus repair is possible, the presence of food in the lumen stimulates enzyme synthesis by the enterocytes. This process takes about 5 days.[23]

Food properties and processing can alter digestibility and absorption.[6,24] Heating of foods containing disaccharides can hydrolyze the sugars, making them more available for enzyme action. Particularly in the case of starch, particle size, physical form, and degree of processing alter accessibility to amylase. Raw starch is relatively indigestible, but when cooked, starch is partially hydrolyzed or gelatinized and is less resistant to amylase. Cooling once again renders the starch difficult to hydrolyze, and it may escape digestion and absorption in the small intestine. Such CHO, termed *resistant starch*, is fermented in the cecum. Nonabsorbable sugars such as raffinose are fermented as well.

Metabolism

Metabolic Control

Of primary importance in the metabolism of food by all organisms is provision of a continuous supply of needed fuels, even though they are consumed sporadically. Metabolic pathways have developed to extract energy during the fed state and to provide needed energy during short-term and long-term deprivation. When the macronutrient composition of the diet changes, metabolism is "fine-tuned" to adjust to those changes.

Hormones—notably insulin and the counterregulatory hormones glucagon, cortisol, growth hormone, epinephrine—and substrates closely control CHO metabolism.[8] Their expression depends on the physiologic state of the body. Insulin is also influenced by the composition of the diet. Control may be exerted by allosterically inhibiting or activating enzymes, by modifying an enzyme, or by altering protein synthesis.[3,8] These paths are further altered by disease, exercise, and stress. In the case of stress or injury, the inherent control mechanisms are largely ineffective but may serve to ensure adequate glucose availability to the immune system or to healing wounds.[25] The metabolism of CHO was discussed in detail by Welborn and Moldower and by Elwyn and Bursztein and is reviewed briefly here.[8,25-27]

Fed State

Once absorbed, CHO is delivered to the liver and other tissues, notably skeletal muscle and brain. The liver extracts some of the glucose and much of the fructose for glycogen storage. The amount, however, is somewhat controversial. It has been estimated that the liver takes as much as 40% to 50% of the glucose from an oral meal.[28] Others have estimated that most

glucose (73%) is taken up by muscle for oxidation and storage there.[29] Gerard and colleagues, using nuclear magnetic resonance spectroscopy (NMR), found that 19% of a glucose load is stored in the liver.[30] Differences in technique may explain the differences in results; most recent studies, however, indicate that most glucose is taken up peripherally.[8]

Glucose is first metabolized to pyruvate and lactate by glycolysis and then oxidized through the Krebs cycle in liver, muscle, and adipose tissue. About 40% of glucose infused at 5 to 6 mg/kg per minute is oxidized.[31] The actual oxidation rate varies with intake, degree of exercise, and the tissue under study.[8,26] Several micronutrients are required for CHO oxidation, notably thiamine, niacin, riboflavin, phosphorus, and magnesium. Most unoxidized glucose is stored as glycogen.

When CHO is supplied in sufficiently large quantities, its oxidation predominates, even in the postprandial state, and fat oxidation is suppressed.[32] De novo lipogenesis eventually ensues, and the CHO is stored as fat. Under normal conditions in healthy persons who consume a self-selected diet, lipogenesis from CHO rarely happens.[8,32,33] With overfeeding of CHO, as in metabolic studies and in parenteral hyperalimentation, fat is synthesized from CHO after maximal glycogen storage.[34,35] After 7 days of excess feeding in one study, CHO was used only for oxidation and lipogenesis; glycogenesis had stopped.[34]

Insulin secretion increases with a glucose load. The absolute glucose concentration and its rate of change are the principal regulators of the hormone, but other CHOs, certain amino acids and fatty acids, metabolites, and ketones also affect insulin concentration.[28] Insulin improves transport of glucose into all tissues except the liver, but has no direct effect on oxidation.[8] The increase in CHO oxidation observed with insulin is mediated by the decrease in free fatty acid concentration caused by insulin.[8,26] Known as an *anabolic hormone*, insulin enhances protein, glycogen, and fat synthesis while decreasing protein breakdown in muscle and lipolysis in adipose tissue.[25]

Futile cycles, or substrate cycles, converting glucose to glucose-6-phosphate, alanine, or lactate and back, are more active after a meal.[26,36] These cycles may allow the body to amplify the metabolic pathway if needed; they also generate some heat.

Responses to CHO feeding—insulin secretion, oxidation rate, glycogen synthesis, and lipogenesis—are altered as intake changes. With sudden decreases or increases, these changes may take several days as the body adapts and reaches a new steady state. In the previously cited experiment,[34] excessive amounts of CHO required 1 day for oxidation to "plateau" and 7 days for lipogenesis to stabilize. When the overfeeding ceased, neither oxidation nor lipogenesis returned to normal for 2 days. In another example, McDevitt and associates[37] performed 96-hour continuous whole-body calorimetry while feeding five diets in random order to lean and obese women. The experimental diets provided 50% more calories than needed for energy balance as fat or as glucose, fructose or sucrose, with the energy balance diet serving as the control. All of the CHO diets induced glycogen synthesis on the first day and increased CHO oxidation in the following days, with a steady state reached by day 3 or 4. In all of the overfeeding diets, 88% of excess calories were stored as fat. No differences were seen between body types. These alterations in glucose disposal have implications for clinical practice. Studies of energy expenditure in patients who are given a large CHO load may not reflect the steady state if the studies are performed early in the course of feeding.

Fructose can enter the glycolysis pathway as fructose 1-phosphate in the liver or as fructose 6-phosphate in adipose tissue. The liver metabolizes most of the fructose. While serum glucose concentrations are decreased, higher triglyceride, lactate, and uric acid levels have been associated with fructose than with glucose feeding.[3] In the liver, galactose is converted to glucose, a necessary step, since galactose and its alcohol are toxic.[3]

Postabsorptive State

In the postabsorptive state, defined by some to be 8 hours after a meal, the hormonal status of the body and the metabolic pathways change to ensure a continual supply of glucose.[25,27] Glucagon is the dominant hormone, driving hepatic glycogenolysis and gluconeogenesis to increase liver glucose output. Epinephrine promotes glycogenolysis in muscle, and glucocorticoids enhance gluconeogenesis. Glycogenolysis predominates in the first hours. Some researchers have found gluconeogenesis to plateau 4 hours after a meal and to remain at that level for 60 more hours of fasting.[38] In this study, glycogenolysis was constant from hours 4 to 22, then decreased through 46 hours, and was minimal until the study's end.

With prolonged starvation, the body gradually adapts by decreasing basal energy expenditure and protein turnover, thus sparing protein stores.[9] Oxidation of fat by muscle and liver provides more energy. The brain adapts through alteration of the blood brain barrier to increase passage of ketones and use them as fuel.

Metabolic Alterations in Stress and Disease

In postoperative stress, trauma, and sepsis, hormonal control of metabolism is affected by increased cytokines, notably interleukin-1 (IL-1) and tumor necrosis factor (TNF), and actions of the sympathetic nervous system.[19,25,27] Insulin, glucagon, epinephrine, and cortisol are all increased. Energy expenditure rises with increases in body temperature and oxygen consumption; protein turnover is greater; and despite ongoing protein synthesis, there is net catabolism.[39] These metabolic changes are difficult to modify with hormonal or dietary interventions. For example, it has been demonstrated in injured persons that glucose intake in excess of 600 g per day suppresses gluconeogenesis.[40] The same process is retarded by 125 g of glucose in healthy subjects.[25] A recent study by Tappy and colleagues demonstrated that neither a high CHO or high-lipid, low-CHO continuous enteral feeding decreased gluconeogenesis or enhanced splanchnic uptake of glucose in two groups of seven patients.[41]

Alterations in CHO metabolism are manifested as increased serum glucose and insulin, increased protein breakdown, and enhanced futile cycling. Hyperglycemia and hyperinsulinemia vary directly with the severity of injury or degree of stress.[42,43] Insulin secretion in response to CHO infusion is exaggerated in patients. The liver, however, does not respond to insulin and glucose concentrations that normally decrease gluconeogenesis, and hepatic glucose output is enhanced.[29] Glucose uptake is enhanced in peripheral tissues, especially tissues involved in the immune response. Glucose uptake in this case likely involves a GLUT carrier not responsive to insulin, probably GLUT 1, and appears to be mediated by TNF, IL-1, and possibly other cytokines.[19] Oxidation of preformed glucose during trauma, sepsis, and burns is decreased, but when measured by isotope techniques to include all sources, it is metabolized to a greater degree than normal. It is thought that the hyperglycemia of illness or injury may be driven by an increased need for glucose.[26,27] Because of the high concentrations of available insulin and glucose, glycogen synthesis does occur, sometimes to an exaggerated degree.[27] Lipolysis and fat oxidation also increase with stress, but ketone production is minimal, because mitochondrial uptake of long-chain fatty acids is suppressed by insulin.

Rossi-Fanelli and colleagues reported that more than 60% of cancer patients studied had abnormal glucose tolerance tests and that glucose intolerance is an early manifestation of the disease.[44] Rapid glucose turnover and decreased peripheral disposal are thought to be the major factors in this problem. Tumors prefer glucose for fuel, metabolizing it through glycolysis. A number of measures for inhibiting glycolysis have been studied, but results have been equivocal.[44]

Carbohydrate Requirements

Requirements in Health

For healthy persons, current recommendations for CHO intake are based on the requirements and recommendations for protein and fat and have been determined largely by the difference between total caloric need and the calories supplied by the other macronutrients.[1] More recently, the relative ratio of CHO and fat in the diet has been studied and discussed. Increased insulin secretion accompanied by decreased insulin sensitivity found with high CHO diets lead to increased triglyceride synthesis, especially in persons who are not active.[45] This appears to be especially true for CHO with a high glycemic index. Diets emphasizing these foods are thought to lead to obesity and type 2 diabetes but this hypothesis is controversial.[46] While total calorie intake remains the most important factor in determining body weight, 45% to 55% of calories as CHO, with the caveat that complex CHO be stressed, has been suggested.[45]

To provide the brain with necessary glucose and maintain nitrogen balance, a CHO-free diet must provide 155 g of protein per day. Under these conditions, the brain was also considered to be using ketones for energy, but that fuel provided only 20% of the total requirement.[8] Complete fat oxidation requires glucose. Fifty grams of exogenous CHO per day is considered sufficient to meet this need under conditions of maximal gluconeogenesis and adaptation.[1]

Requirements in Disease

A discussion of specific requirements for CHO in specific disease states is beyond the scope of this chapter. More information can be found in the chapters of this book regarding the disease of interest. In general, for diagnoses in which protein or fat may be limited, the CHO requirement is increased, as dictated by those restrictions. Two examples are end-stage renal and hepatic disease. In both cases, increased intake of CHO spares protein and replaces energy lost through protein restriction.

Current recommendations for type 1 diabetes patients (see Chapter 37) encourage a consistent daily intake of CHO based on the patient's diet history.[47] For type 2 diabetics, goals of dietary treatment include normalizing serum glucose and lipids and attaining ideal weight. A recent multicenter study compared a diet of 55% CHO and 30% fat to one of 40% CHO and 45% fat with a large percentage of monounsaturates in patients with type 2 diabetes. Improved glucose control and decreased plasma insulin, triglyceride, and cholesterol were associated with the higher-fat diet.[48]

Care must be exercised in feeding patients with respiratory disease. When respiratory function is limited, disposal of increased carbon dioxide from CHO oxidation may be difficult and may cause ventilator dependence.[49] Nutrition support must be optimized to prevent undernutrition and overnutrition. Recently, it was suggested that nitrogen balance be monitored to determine whether calories are sufficient, rather than relying on energy expenditure estimates.[50] It may be difficult to predict whether a patient will be able to tolerate a high calorie or CHO load.[51]

It has been recommended that stressed patients receive at least 50% of their resting energy requirement (REE) as CHO and that the energy provided should total 125% of the REE.[27] Generally 5 mg/kg per minute is the upper limit for CHO. This level approaches an excessive calorie load for most adults.[29] As much as 80% of energy needs can be provided as CHO.[27] In persons with diabetes or respiratory failure or stressed patients whose disease is resistant to insulin, CHO may have to be decreased. Ultimately, the final concentration of CHO to be given also depends on the patient's protein and fat requirements.

Carbohydrate in Nutrition Support
Metabolism in Enteral Nutrition

Changes in CHO metabolism in a person taking enteral feedings can be seen when intake is significantly different from usual amounts, as previously noted. Most other alterations in CHO metabolism from enteral feeding are associated with the feeding schedule. Intermittent feedings are similar to meals and allow for the normal ebb and flow of metabolism. Continuous feedings, on the other hand, cause the rates of CHO oxidation and deposition to be constant throughout the day.[8] Whether these rates are greater than those with interrupted feedings is not clear. Campbell and associates compared bolus feedings given every 2 hours or night feedings to continuous feeding and found oxygen consumption to be significantly greater in the groups fed continuously.[52,53] Patients in these experiments were fed 1.7 to 1.8 times their REE and may have been overfed. Using 1.4 times REE in healthy volunteers, lower energy expenditure was observed with continuous than with intermittent feeding in another study.[54]

Chen and coworkers[55] determined uptake of glucose increases in the liver, but not muscle, when continuous enteral feedings were given to dogs. In contrast, dogs supported by PN had greater than normal glucose uptake in both liver and muscle. Plasma insulin and glucagon concentrations were higher in the dogs given enteral nutrition. It was concluded that

continuous enteral nutrition may lead to greater insulin requirements than PN because of poor muscle glucose uptake and that this may be a disadvantage of enteral feeding. Comparison between continuous and intermittent feeding schedules was not done.

Metabolism in Parenteral Nutrition

Parenteral glucose has a "metabolic fate" similar to that of ingested CHO. According to Wolfe, 73% of glucose, either oral or intravenous, is disposed of in skeletal muscle.[29] Hyperglycemia associated with parenteral nutrition in nonstressed, nondiabetic patients can be simply the result of a higher than normal glucose load. A recent study found that 18 of 37 nondiabetic patients who received CHO in parenteral nutrition at a rate of more than 5.0 mg/kg per minute exhibited hyperglycemia, whereas 5 patients were hyperglycemic while being infused CHO at 4.1 to 5.0 mg/kg per minute, and patients fed at rates no greater than 4 mg/kg per minute were euglycemic.[56] In addition to possible or frank diabetes, steroids and other medications can also contribute to hyperglycemia of parenteral nutrition.[57]

It is generally recommended that parenteral nutrition be tapered at the start and end of infusions to prevent hyperglycemia and (especially) hypoglycemia. Krzywda and coworkers found in a group of 18 patients, including 6 with diabetes, that glucose rose at the start of infusion and returned to preinfusion concentrations within an hour of discontinuing parenteral nutrition without problems.[58] On the other hand, sudden drops in plasma glucose have been noted within 30 minutes of cessation of parenteral nutrition.[57] Abnormal serum glucose level is perhaps the most common metabolic complication of parenteral nutrition. Because of the possibility of inducing nonketotic hyperosmolar coma, on the one extreme, or severe hypoglycemia, on the other, glucose levels must be monitored frequently and treated if necessary. Hyperosmolar, nonketotic coma, which has a 50% mortality rate, is preventable not only by monitoring but with appropriate hydration because many cases are the result of dehydration. Hyperglycemia can also be a risk factor for development of infection. Treatment of hyperglycemia includes removal of excessive CHO calories and administration of insulin.

Patients fed parenterally are more susceptible to fatty infiltration of the liver when fed excessive CHO calories. Increased alkaline phosphatase and transaminase concentrations and jaundice are also observed.[35] In most cases, 150% of REE and 80% of total calories as CHO is considered to be the upper limit for parenteral nutrition.

Sources of Carbohydrate in Nutrition Support Formulas
Enteral Formulas

CHOs for enteral formulas must be easily soluble; easily digested; and, in most cases, of lowest possible osmolality. A product marketed for oral consumption must be palatable as well. The CHOs that meet these criteria are corn syrup solids, hydrolyzed cornstarch, maltodextrins, and other glucose polymers, and all are commonly used in formulas.[59] Corn syrup solids, hydrolyzed cornstarch, and maltodextrins are similar but differ in the degree of hydrolysis: maltodextrins are the least hydrolyzed and therefore the lowest in osmolality.[60] Hydrolysis of corn syrup solids and hydrolyzed cornstarch varies in extent but produces the simple CHOs glucose, maltose, isomaltose, and triose. Some longer chains are also available. Generally, the lower the osmolality, the more complex the CHO. Glucose polymers vary less in chain length, ranging from 2 to 10 glucose units.[4] Some sucrose is used in products intended to be taken orally. Very few, if any, enteral products contain lactose at this time, so lactose content is of little concern. Fruits and vegetables are currently being used in a few products.

Modular tube feedings can be "designed" to meet needs of patients for whom commercial products are inappropriate. Intravenous dextrose (70%) has been used in this type of feeding.[61] Glucose polymers are also available for this purpose.

Parenteral Nutrition

The CHO in parenteral nutrition formulas is most often dextrose monohydrate. It is available in 5% to 70% solutions, supplying 3.4 kcal/g dextrose. The pH ranges from 3.7 to 4.0 and osmolarity is 50 mOsm per percent of dextrose.[62] Because of the sometimes adverse effects of large glucose loads, alternative CHO sources have been investigated. One, glycerol, is available as ProCalAmine, a premixed product that also contains amino acids and is designed for peripheral infusion. It provides 250 kcal/L and 735 mOsm/L and has proved safe for adults.[62,63]

Conclusion

CHO, while not strictly speaking, essential, is very important for metabolism, energy balance, and viability of the body. Consideration of using CHO as a fuel or a foodstuff must also take into account other macronutrients and micronutrients. Given enterally or parenterally, its "metabolic fate" appears to be about the same. Use or misuse of CHO can have profound effects on the body, especially in disease. Monitoring for abnormalities and attending to any that arise are important activities of nutrition support.

REFERENCES

1. Food and Nutrition Board: *Recommended daily allowances,* ed 10, Washington, DC, 1989, National Academy Press, pp 39-43.
2. Levin RI: Carbohydrates. In Shils ME, Olson JA, Shike M (eds): *Modern nutrition in health and disease,* ed 9, Philadelphia, 1999, Lea & Febiger, pp 49-65.
3. Stryer L: Carbohydrates. In *Biochemistry,* ed 3, New York, 1988, WH Freeman, pp 315-348.
4. Gottschlich MM, Shronts EP, Hutchins AM: Defined formula diets. In Rombeau JL, Rolandelli RH (eds): *Clinical nutrition. Enteral and tube feeding,* ed 3, Philadelphia, 1997, WB Saunders, pp 207-239.
5. Johnson LR (ed): Regulation: peptides of the gastrointestinal tract. In *Gastrointestinal physiology,* St Louis, 1985, Mosby, pp 1-14.
6. Southgate DAT: Digestion and metabolism of sugars, *Am J Clin Nutr* 62(suppl):203S-211S, 1995.
7. Brosnan JT: Comments on metabolic needs for glucose and the role of gluconeogenesis, *Eur J Clin Nutr* 53(1):S107-111, 1999.
8. Elwyn DH, Bursztein S: Carbohydrate metabolism and requirements for nutritional support. Part I, *Nutrition* 9:50-67, 1993.
9. Waterlow JC: Metabolic adaptation to low intakes of energy and protein, *Ann Rev Nutr* 6:495-526, 1986.
10. Munro HN: Carbohydrate and fat as factors in protein utilization and metabolism, *Physiol Rev* 31:449-488, 1951.
11. Moran JR, Greene HL: Digestion and absorption. In Rombeau JL, Caldwell MD (eds): *Clinical nutrition. Enteral and tube feeding,* Philadelphia, 1990, WB Saunders, pp 10-33.
12. Wolever TMS, Jenkins DJA, Jenkins AL, Josse JG: The glycemic index: methodology and clinical implications, *Am J Clin Nutr* 54:846-854, 1991.
13. Rolls BJ, Hammer VA: Fat, carbohydrate, and the regulation of energy intake, *Am J Clin Nutr* 62(suppl):1086S-1095S, 1995.
14. Marmonier C, Chapelot D, Louis-Sylvestre J: Effects of macronutrient content and energy density of snacks consumed in a satiety state on the onset of the next meal, *Appetite* 34:161-168, 2000.
15. Levin RJ: Digestion and absorption of carbohydrates—from molecules and membranes to humans, *Am J Clin Nutr* 59(suppl):690S-698S, 1994.
16. Goda T, Takase S: Dietary carbohydrate and fat independently modulate disaccharidase activities in rat jejunum, *J Nutr* 124:2233-2239, 1994.
17. Sebastio G, Villa M, Sartorio R, et al: Control of lactase in human adult-type hypolactasia and in weaning rabbits and rats, *Am J Hum Genet* 45:489-497, 1989.
18. Hediger MA, Coady MJ, Ikeda TS, et al: Expression cloning and cDNA sequencing of the Na+/glucose cotransporter, *Nature* 330:379-381, 1987.
19. Mizock BA: Alterations in carbohydrate metabolism during stress: a review of the literature, *Am J Med* 98:75-84, 1995.
20. Gudmand-Hoyer E: The clinical significance of disaccharide maldigestion, *Am J Clin Nutr* 59(suppl):735S-741S, 1994.
21. Yolken RH, Hart W, Oung I, et al: Gastrointestinal dysfunction and disaccharide intolerance in children infected with human immunodeficiency virus, *Pediatrics* 118(3):359-363, 1991.
22. Holtug K, Clausen MR, Hove H, et al: The colon in carbohydrate malabsorption: short-chain fatty acids, pH, and osmotic diarrhoea, *Scand J Gastroenterol* 27:545-552, 1992.
23. Potten CS, Loeffler M: Stem cells: attributes, cycles, spirals, pitfalls and uncertainties. Lessons from the crypt, *Development* 110:1001-1020, 1990.
24. Bjork I, Granfeldt Y, Liljeberg H, et al: Food properties affecting the digestion and absorption of carbohydrates, *Am J Clin Nutr* 59(suppl):699S-705S, 1994.
25. Welborn MB, Moldawer LL: Glucose metabolism. In Rombeau JL, Rolandelli RH (eds): *Clinical Nutrition. Enteral and Tube Feeding,* ed 3, Philadelphia, 1997, WB Saunders, pp 61-80.
26. Elwyn D H, Bursztein S: Carbohydrate metabolism and requirements for nutritional support. Part II, *Nutrition* 9:164-177, 1993.
27. Elwyn DH, Bursztein S: Carbohydrate metabolism and requirements for nutritional support. Part III, *Nutrition* 9:255-267, 1993.
28. Wilmore DW: *The metabolic management of the critically ill,* New York, 1977, Plenum.
29. Wolfe RR: Carbohydrate, *ASPEN Clinical Congress* 18:422-426, 1994.
30. Gerard DP, Rothman DL, Magnusson I, et al: Net liver glycogen synthesis and pathways in humans following an oral glucose load measured using 13C NMR spectroscopy, *Clin Res* 41:130A, 1993.
31. Katz J, McGarry JD: The glucose paradox. Is glucose a substrate for liver metabolism? *J Clin Invest* 74:1901-1909, 1984.
32. Hellerstein MK: De novo lipogenesis in humans: metabolic and regulatory aspects, *European J Cl Nutr* 53S 1:S53-65, 1999.
33. Jequier E: Carbohydrates as a source of energy, *Am J Clin Nutr* 59(suppl):682S-685S, 1994.
34. Acheson KJ, Schutz Y, Bessard T, et al: Glycogen storage capacity and de novo synthesis during massive carbohydrate overfeeding in man, *Am J Clin Nutr* 48:240-247, 1988.
35. Quigley EM, Marsh MN, Shaffer JL, et al: Hepatobiliary complications of total parenteral nutrition, *Gastroenterology* 104:286-301, 1993.
36. Katz J: Energy balance and futile cycling. In *Assessment of energy balance in health and disease,* Evansville, IL, 1980, Ross Labs, pp 63-66.
37. McDevitt RM, Poppitt SD, Murgatroyd PR, Prentice AM: Macronutrient disposal during controlled overfeeding with glucose, fructose, sucrose or fat in lean and obese women, *Am J Clin Nutr* 72:369-377, 2000.
38. Rothman DL, Magnusson I, Katz LD, et al: Quantitation of hepatic glycogenolysis and gluconeogenesis in fasting humans with 13C NMR, *Science* 254:573-576, 1991.
39. Cerra FB: Metabolic response to injury. In Cerra FB (ed): *Manual of critical care,* St Louis, 1987, Mosby, pp 117-145.
40. Elwyn DH, Kinney JM, Jeevanandam M, et al: Influence of increasing carbohydrate intake on glucose kinetics in injured patients, *Ann Surg* 190:117-127, 1979.

41. Tappy L, Berger M, Schwarz JM, McCamish M, Revelly JP, Schneiter P, Jequier E, Chiolero R: Hepatic and peripheral glucose metabolism in intensive care patients receiving continuous high- or low-carbohydrate enteral nutrition, *J Parenter Enteral Nutr* 23:260-267, 1999.

42. Stoner HB, Frayn K, Barton R, et al: The relationships between plasma substrates and hormones and the severity of injury in 277 recently injured patients, *Clin Sci* 56:563-573, 1979.

43. Jeevanandam M, Grote-Holman AE, Chikenji T, et al: Effects of glucose on fuel utilization and glycerol turnover in normal and injured man, *Crit Care Med* 18:125-135, 1990.

44. Rossi-Fanelli F, Cascino A, Muscaritoli M: Abnormal substrate metabolism and nutritional strategies in cancer management, *J Parenter Enteral Nutr* 15:680-683, 1991.

45. Grimm JJ: Interaction of physical activity and diet: implications for insulin-glucose dynamics, *Pub Health Nutr* 2:363-368, 1999.

46. Bessesen DH: The role of carbohydrate in insulin resistance, *J Nutr* 131:2782S-2786S, 2001.

47. Nutrition recommendations and principles for people with diabetes mellitus, position paper approved by the Executive Committee of the American Diabetes Association, *J Am Diet Assoc* 94:504-506, 1994.

48. Garg A, Bantle JP, Henry RR, et al: Effects of varying carbohydrate content of diet in patients with non-insulin-dependent diabetes mellitus, *JAMA* 271:1421-1428, 1994.

49. Ireton-Jones CS, Borman KR, Turner WW Jr: Nutrition considerations in the management of ventilator-dependent patients, *Nutr Clin Pract* 8(2):60-64, 1993.

50. Christman JW, McClain RW: A sensible approach to the nutritional support of mechanically ventilated critically ill patients, *Intens Care Med* 19:129-136, 1993.

51. Fogle P, Fredstrom S, Rios M: Superior mesentery artery syndrome impeded enteral nutrition support in a lung transplant candidate, *ASPEN Clinical Congress* 19:190A, 1995.

52. Campbell IT, Morton RP, Cole RA, et al: A comparison of the effects of intermittent and continuous nasogastric feeding on the oxygen consumption and nitrogen balance of patients after major head and neck surgery, *Am J Clin Nutr* 38:870-878, 1983.

53. Campbell IT, Morton RP, MacDonald IA, et al: Comparison of the metabolic effects of continuous postoperative enteral feeding and feeding at night only, *Am J Clin Nutr* 52:1107-1112, 1990.

54. Heymsfield SB, Casper K, Grossman GD: Bioenergetic metabolic response to continuous v intermittent nasoenteric feeding, *Metab Clin Exp* 1987;36:570-575, 1987.

55. Chen SS, Donmeyer C, Zhang Y, Hande SA, Lacy DB, McGuinness OP: Impact of enteral and parenteral nutrition on hepatic and muscle glucose metabolism, *J Parenter Enter Nutr* 24:255-260, 2000.

56. Rosmarin DK, Wardlaw GM, Mirtallo J: Hyperglycemia associated with high, continuous infusion rates of total parenteral nutrition dextrose, *Nutr Clin Pract* 11:151-156, 1996.

57. Warner B, Bower R: Complications of therapy. In Lang C (ed): *Nutritional support in critical care,* Rockville, MD, 1987, Aspen Publishers.

58. Krzywda EA, Andris DA, Whipple JK, et al: Glucose response to abrupt initiation and discontinuation of total parenteral nutrition, *J Parenter Enteral Nutr* 17:64-67, 1993.

59. Shronts EP, Havala TI: Formulas. In Teasley-Strausberg KM (ed): *Nutrition support handbook. A compendium of products with guidelines for usage,* Cincinnati, OH, 1992, Harvey Whitney, pp 147-186.

60. Storm HM, Lin P: Forms of carbohydrate in enteral nutrition formulas, *Support Line* 18:7-9, 1996.

61. Bernard DKH, Mandt J, Shronts EP: Creation of a unique modular enteral feeding system, *Support Line* 15:10-14, 1993.

62. Teasley-Strausberg KM (ed): II. Carbohydrate solutions. In *Nutrition support handbook. A compendium of products with guidelines for usage,* Cincinnati, OH, 1992, Harvey Whitney, pp 73-79.

63. Tao RC, Kelley RE, Yoshimura NN, et al: Glycerol: its metabolism and use as an intravenous energy source, *J Parenter Enteral Nutr* 7:479-488; 1983.

Lipids

Michael J. Kelley, PhD, RD, CNSD

HISTORICALLY, fat has been regarded as a calorie-dense energy source. In this century, the presence of fat in the diet has assumed added importance with the realization that a source of linoleic and linolenic acids is necessary for health. New information suggests that certain fats are metabolically active beyond their ability to provide kilocalories (kcal). The differences in fuel utilization and requirements associated with stress have become clearer. Furthermore, potentially detrimental effects have recently been ascribed to ingestion of excessive fat and to the more subtle effects of ω-3 as compared with ω-6 fatty acid imbalances in critical care.

The topics covered in this chapter include lipid metabolism during digestion and absorption and in fed, fasted, and stressed states. Experimental support for the inclusion of lipid in feedings for critically ill patients, how much lipid, and what type(s) are also explored. The amount of lipid used is addressed by a review of data on the body's utilization of lipid during critical illness; however, the full scope of the debate over whether glucose kilocalories or lipid kilocalories should predominate in the nonprotein energy component is not covered in this chapter. Cohen[1] and Long and Long[2] have specifically addressed this topic and their conclusions are discussed.

Lipid Metabolism

Digestion and Absorption

Digestion and absorption of dietary lipids involve complex interactions between the lipid components; however, major components of the process are known and they are summarized here. A recent and excellent detailed review has been presented by Linscheer and Vergroesen.[3] The surface area of ingested triglyceride (TG) is much increased by the mechanical and emulsification mechanisms of chewing and gastric action. Lingual lipase is secreted by the serous glands on the back of the tongue. Lingual lipase and gastric lipase both cleave preferentially at the sn-3 position, which produces diglycerides (DGs) and fatty acids (FAs). Both enzymes work optimally at acid pH, so that approximately 30% of ingested TG is hydrolyzed during the 2 to 4 hours of gastric emptying after a meal. The gastric chyme, which contains TG, DG, and FA in small, oily droplets, is delivered intermittently in small amounts to the duodenum.

The cells of the intestinal mucosa can absorb only two hydrolytic products of TG digestion, 2-monoglycerides (2-MG) and free FA (FFA). Partial hydrolysis of the TG and DG delivered in chyme is accomplished by pancreatic lipase in the small intestine. The presence of the lipid components of

chyme and the acid pH in the duodenum induce release of cholecystokinin (CCK) and secretin. Secretin stimulates secretion of bicarbonate by the pancreas, whereas CCK produces enzyme secretion by the pancreas and contraction of the gallbladder to release bile into the intestinal lumen. The bicarbonate brings the pH of the acid chyme to approximately 6.5, and bile further emulsifies lipid to the form of micelles. Pancreatic lipase (with the necessary help of the small pancreatic protein colipase) continues the hydrolysis of the remaining TG and DG. Pancreatic lipase has greatest affinity for FAs at the sn-1 and sn-3 positions (i.e., the two outside FAs of the TG). The affinity of the enzyme for FAs at the sn-2 position is much less avid, so the products of this digestion are FA and 2-MGs. These products are incorporated into mixed micelles that contain partial glycerides, FFA, bile acids, and cholesterol. The components of these mixed micelles are then taken up into cells of the lumen by passive diffusion.

Free cholesterol in the diet requires no digestion but rather is emulsified by the components of bile. Cholesteryl esters (cholesterols linked to FAs) are hydrolyzed to cholesterol plus FA by pancreatic cholesterol esterase. Phospholipids undergo hydrolysis of the FA in the sn-2 position by pancreatic phospholipase A_2. The resultant lysophospholipids, cholesterol, and FAs produced by these actions are absorbed by passive diffusion into enterocytes along with the products of TG digestion.

Once inside the enterocyte, FA and MG are reesterified to TGs, which are then incorporated into chylomicrons. The chylomicrons, which also contain cholesterol, cholesteryl ester, phospholipid, and protein, are secreted by the enterocytes into the local lymph vessels and enter the blood stream through the thoracic duct. By virtue of this transport mechanism, TGs are presented to peripheral tissues. Lipoprotein lipase is an endothelial membrane enzyme found in capillaries. This lipase hydrolyzes the TG, releasing FFAs that diffuse into the local adipocytes, where they are reesterified and stored as TG. In muscle, the FAs may be reesterified or used immediately for energy. The chylomicron, now termed a *chylomicron remnant,* is reduced in size and contains proportionally more cholesterol and phospholipid. The remnant is ultimately cleared by the liver. Both cholesterol and phospholipid can be used by the liver immediately, stored for a while, or repackaged as lipoprotein to be exported (cholesterol and phospholipid in very-low-density lipoprotein and phospholipid in high-density lipoprotein).

The process of digestion and absorption of TG is affected by the chain length of the FAs involved. When medium-chain fatty acids (MCFAs) are present as part of medium-chain triglycerides

(MCTs) or structured triglycerides (STGs), the process is somewhat different. MCFAs have a chain length of 6 to 12 carbons. The normal source of MCT for commercial preparations is coconut oil, from which MCTs are produced that contain predominantly C8 and C10 saturated FAs. When palm kernel oil is used, C12 saturated FAs are present in larger amounts than C8 and C10 saturated FAs. MCTs are soluble in water and diffuse into luminal cells as TGs or FAs faster than TGs with long-chain fatty acids (LCFAs).

Shorter-chain FAs are preferentially hydrolyzed by pancreatic lipase. Thus, C8 and C10 FAs are hydrolyzed much more rapidly than C16 to C20, and the rate of hydrolysis for C20 and C22 is so slow that it is likely that some of these FAs from fish oil remain undigested and unabsorbed. The majority of MCFAs are not reesterified by the enterocytes and pass directly into the portal blood supply. (If larger doses of MCTs are fed or if MCFAs are in the 2 position of structured TG, MCFAs will also be found in mixed TGs in lymphatic chylomicrons.) These FAs proceed to the liver, where the majority are taken up and metabolized for energy. If the supply of MCFAs exceeds the liver's capacity to metabolize them, ketones are produced, which are then released into the blood. These properties of MCTs are the basis for their use in cases when normal lipid digestion and absorption are impaired, as with advanced liver disease or cholestasis. MCTs may also be employed when intolerance to lipid is apparent but no impairment to TG digestion and absorption is obvious. Used this way, MCTs are a useful nonprotein, nonglucose form of energy, but it is important to remember that the metabolism of FAs in MCT is different from that of longer-chain FAs. Following absorption, LCFAs are delivered largely to adipose tissue and are mobilized in response to metabolic demands over time. When these FAs are released, they can supply energy to a number of cell types, including liver and muscle. MCFAs, on the other hand, are delivered immediately to the liver, where most are metabolized for energy or ketone production. The ketones are largely metabolized for energy by muscle.

Recent investigations have shown that confirming the absorption of FAs from MCTs in foods absorbed via the portal vein has not been simple. Earlier animal and human studies that used oil alone or suspended FAs alone have supported the idea that MCFAs are absorbed by the portal route. Early data also indicated that MCTs might be largely intact when absorbed, and that the MCTs are subsequently hydrolyzed by intracellular lipase within the cells of the intestinal mucosa.

You and associates[4] infused rats with a commercially available enteral formula that contained 2.5% fat by kilocalories. Fat was added to this diet to bring the fat kilocalories to 25% by adding either commercial sunflower oil (LCT), a standard MCT preparation, an isomolar mixture of 50% LCT and 50% MCT, or an isomolar mixture of 50% LCT/50% 2-monodecanoic acid. The free FA composition of plasma from the portal vein and the FA composition of lymph TGs were determined after 20 hours of continuous feeding. The percent of MCFAs in portal plasma was much lower than might be expected for the MCT fed group and was actually higher in the LCT fed group. The percent of C8 and C10 was not reported, possibly because these FAs were not detected. The mean percent of C12 was 3.76% for the LCT/2-monodecanoin group, 4.65% for the MCT group, 4.87% for the LCT/MCT group, and 5.37% for the LCT group. The percent of C10 in lymph TG was lowest for the LCT-fed group and highest for the MCT group, but was still only 3.89% for the latter group. The authors suggested the following explanations for why their data seemed to differ from other work in the field: The MCT was given continuously, as an emulsion, in a mixture with other nutrients. They reasoned that this would provide a relatively lower dose of MCT per unit of time, compared with other studies that used a bolus injection or a higher dose of infusion. They also suggested that intestinal cells might have used some of the MCFA in the synthesis of longer chain FAs. Sigalet and others[5] dosed rats with a bolus mixture of radiolabeled C12 and C16 in stable emulsion and collected portal blood over 4 hours and lymph over 20 hours. They reported that 51% of the dose of C12 was accounted for in lymph and that less than 1% appeared in the portal and jugular veins. The authors acknowledged that their ability to account for only a portion of the administered label (for which reasonable explanations exist) had been experienced by other investigators in this area and had not yet been explained sufficiently. The results of these studies do not challenge the earlier observations that MCTs are quickly hydrolyzed and absorbed, but do open questions regarding the route of absorption when MCTs are part of mixed nutrient formula.

Fed State

FFA levels in blood are lower or reduced in the fed state as compared with starvation. In the starved state, FFA levels rise within the first week. This reflects the increased mobilization of FAs as an energy source. The data reviewed by Newsholme and Leech illustrate this point:[6] Plasma FA concentrations were 0.3 mM in the fed state, 1.14 mM after 7 days' starvation, and 1.44 mM after 28 days' starvation. The increased concentrations of FFA result in increased delivery of FFA to liver. Delivery of increased FFAs to liver in turn drives ketone synthesis, and ketones are subsequently exported to other tissues (i.e., muscle) for fuel. The total ketone concentrations reviewed by Newsholme and Leech were 0.02 mM in the fed state, 4.53 mM after 7 days' starvation, and 7.32 mM after 28 days' starvation.

Stressed State

Plasma levels of FFA in the stressed state have been observed to vary widely among individuals. Increased plasma FFA concentrations have been reported by some, and others have reported levels near those in the fed or postabsorptive state. The answer may lie in the variability of postinjury hormone levels or oxygen transport. The observed increases in hormone concentrations following injury were reviewed by Wilmore[7] (Table 9-1). While the elevations of epinephrine and glucagon would seem to drive elevation of FFA levels, insulin levels may also increase in response to increased gluconeogenesis and blood glucose concentrations and subsequently attenuate the FFA-elevating effects of these hormones. Like the hormones listed in Table 9-1, postinjury insulin levels have been observed to vary between basal levels and levels four to five times basal values. Elevated insulin levels in critically ill persons are frequently accompanied by insulin resistance to glucose transport by muscle tissue. The insulin resistance is not necessarily active in adipose tissue, and, therefore, lipolysis can still be

TABLE 9-1

Reported Elevation of Circulating Hormone Levels Above Basal Levels During Stress

Hormone	Elevation Above Basal Value (%)
Norepinephrine	2-22
Epinephrine	3-48
Cortisol	1.3-6.5
Glucagon	0-13

inhibited by insulin. In addition, elevated catecholamine levels can overcome the inhibition of lipolysis by higher insulin levels. There are also variations in tissue perfusion after injury, which in turn affect oxygen transport and fuel utilization.[8]

Thus, fat metabolism during critical illness has been widely characterized as featuring FFA levels near postabsorptive levels; however, it appears that fat metabolism may vary among different critical illnesses and between the "ebb" and "flow," or early and later stages, of injury response.

For the nutrition support professional, the more relevant issues are what percentage of energy expenditure is supplied by lipid, and the lipid requirements of the nutrition support regimen. Little and coworkers[9] reported a respiratory quotient (RQ) of 0.78 in 12 postabsorptive, fasting trauma patients; this indicated that a major energy source was FA oxidation.[7] The median time after injury was 2.5 hours, plasma glucose was 8.4 mM, plasma FFA was 1.0 mM, and insulin was 16 mU/L. Therefore, both glucose and FFAs were elevated over postabsorptive values but insulin was not.

In his review, Cohen concluded that fat oxidation normally accounted for 70% to 90% of resting energy expenditure (REE) of a fasting patient in the stressed state.[10] The release of FFA from adipose tissue is increased in the stressed state, but FFA levels in blood may not be increased because liver uptake and reesterification of FFA are also increased in this state. Therefore, in this condition, the utilization of fat for fuel is high, but the levels of FA in blood may not be. The situation is altered somewhat when stressed patients are fed. First, there may be a difference between calculated and actual energy expenditure. Goran and coworkers measured total energy expenditure (TEE) in burned children to determine how closely TEE was related to predicted energy expenditure.[11] TEE was not as high as would be predicted by use of the Harris-Benedict equation (basal energy expenditure [BEE]) with activity and injury factors. Their data indicated that TEE was more closely related to REE than to BEE and that TEE was not as high as would be predicted by BEE with activity and injury factors. These data also suggest that the use of the Harris-Benedict equation together with an activity factor and the injury factor for burns would result in overfeeding, an important point regardless of what feeding regimen is chosen.

As reviewed by Long and Nelson, when glucose was infused at a rate of 5 to 6 mg/kg body weight per minute, 60% of V_{CO_2} was derived from glucose, and the respiratory quotient was greater than 1.0.[12,13] Burke and colleagues[14] reported that glucose oxidation rates increased with increased loads of glucose. The V_{CO_2} derived from glucose plateaued at about 50%, with RQ values near 1.0 at glucose infusion rates of 5 to 6 mg/kg per minute. Glucose infusion rates greater than 5 to 6 mg/kg per minute increased RQ without further increasing the V_{CO_2} derived from glucose. Assuming that daily nitrogen losses reflect the oxidation of amino acids, Long and Nelson estimated the percentage of energy derived from amino acids to be 20%. The remainder, 20%, is therefore assumed to be supplied by FA. Thus, if the substrate mix fed to critically ill patients is to reflect utilization, they suggest its composition be 60% carbohydrate, 20% lipid, and 20% protein. Therefore, it appears that fat continues to be a major energy source in a stressed patient who is fed.

There have been other suggestions in the literature that less than 30% (perhaps 15% to 20%) of energy from fat in formulas may be optimal for the lipid contribution. Mochizuki and coworkers compared isonitrogenous, isocaloric diets in guinea pigs with burns on 30% of their body surface.[15] The diets provided 0%, 5%, 15%, and 30% of kilocalories as fat. Based on differences in postburn body weight, muscle mass, cumulative nitrogen balance, serum albumin, and total liver fat, the authors concluded that the optimal proportion of lipid in this model was between 5% and 15% of kilocalories. Gottschlich and associates developed a modular tube feeding formula (M) that contained 15% kilocalories as fat (50% menhaden fish oil, 50% safflower oil) and compared this regimen with a commercially available critical care formula (C) and a commercial formula enriched with protein and micronutrient modules (CPM) added at the site.[16] The rate of wound infections was significantly lower in the M group, as was length of stay divided by the percentage of the burn. The death rate was lower in both the M and CPM groups, but the results narrowly missed significance. This small study contained only 14 to 19 patients per group. Chi-square analyses (performed by C. Bush, Ross Products Division, Abbott Laboratories) indicate that this distribution of results for death would be significant with a 50% increase in subjects per group (i.e., between 21 and 29 subjects per group). Pneumonia, total number of infectious episodes, and percentage of patients who experienced diarrhea were likewise lower (approaching statistical significance) in the M group as compared with those for the other two groups. These results may reflect differences in the composition of the fat, protein, or micronutrient content of the diets, but the possibility that the optimal percentage of energy from lipid may be between 15% and 20% must be considered.

Garrel and colleagues[17] also studied formulations with more modest dietary fat levels, with and without fish oil, for burn patients. Forty-three severely burned adults who were assigned to three groups received enteral nutrition that contained (1) 35% kilocalories as fat, (2) 15% kilocalories as fat, or (3) 15% kilocalories as fat, in each case with 50% of fat from fish oil (1.3 g/L eicosapentaenoic acid [EPA], 20:5n3 and 0.7 g/L docosahexaenoic acid [DHA], 22:6n3). Total energy needs were estimated using the Curreri formula and were found to approximate 1.3 times the REE. Patients also received parenteral nutrition containing 20% glucose, 10% Intralipid, and amino acids at rates adjusted to match the energy composition of the enteral feeding. Patients on low-fat support (both low-fat groups combined) had fewer cases of pneumonia (3 of 24 versus 7 of 13, $p = .02$), shorter time to healing (1.2 versus 1.8 days divided by the percentage of body surface area burned,

$p = .01$), and better indices of respiratory and nutrition status. There were no differences between the two low-fat groups for these variables. The results to date from studies that used less than 30% fat kilocalories, with or without a source of ω-3 FAs, show promise but must be followed up with more definitive trials.

For the nutrition support professional, an important point has surfaced about nutrition for critically ill persons: a formulation based on standard calculations of basal energy expenditure with stress and activity factors applied may result in overfeeding the critically ill patient. The maximum rate of glucose oxidation is finite, and supplying lipid at a rate that exceeds the body's ability to clear it can have negative consequences (see next section). Thus, it is important to supply adequate energy but not too much.

Lipid Deficiency, Need, and Excess

Recommendations for lipid intake during critical illness are conservative in the face of uncertainty about exact requirements for fat and optimal amounts and types of lipid. To prevent essential FA deficiency, 2% to 4% of the calorie requirement should be supplied by linoleic acid. The average percentage of FAs as linoleic acid is 51% in soy oil, 55% in corn oil, and 75% in safflower oil.[3] When supplied as soy, corn, or safflower oil, approximately 10% of kilocalories as lipid would supply adequate linoleic acid.[18] α-Linolenic acid, also considered to be essential, is found in soybean and canola oils (about 7% of total FAs in both oils) and in trace amounts in corn and safflower oils.[3] Therefore, enteral and parenteral products that use corn or safflower oil as a lipid source can supply adequate linolenic acid by incorporating soy or canola oil.[3,18]

Long's recommendation that energy supplied as fat not exceed 20% of kilocalories appears to be supported by available data, although confirmation by well-designed studies is still needed.[2] Furthermore, this level of lipid appears to apply equally to different critical illnesses, despite differences in metabolic derangements, and to nutrition supplied either enterally or parenterally.

As much as 60% of kilocalories has been supplied as lipid, without discernible ill effects; however, there may be metabolic effects of lipid or its components that argue for a smaller percentage of lipid. One reason for administering large proportions of lipid has been to meet estimated energy requirements without increasing V_{CO_2}. In his review of this area, however, Cohen[1] distinguished between studies in which patients were overfed (i.e., intake exceeded energy expenditure) and others in which kilocalories were matched to energy expenditure. In overfed patients, carbohydrate alone did indeed produce increases in V_{CO_2} as compared with glucose-lipid mixtures; however, when intake matched energy expenditure, Cohen concluded, "There are few if any significant differences in V_{CO_2} between groups." Thus, moderate calorie intake appears to be more important than the fuel source.

The protein-sparing effects of carbohydrate and lipid kilocalories appear to be equal, or perhaps slightly greater for carbohydrate.[19,20] Kolhardt and associates found the protein-sparing effect of high-lipid intravenous nutrition to be less than that of glucose.[21] Postsurgical, "nonseptic" patients

were given either high-lipid intravenous nutrition (75% of nonprotein kilocalories as lipid) or intravenous isocaloric, isonitrogenous glucose nutrition (100% of nonprotein kilocalories as glucose) for 14 days. Lipid nutrition patients experienced significant decreases in fat-free mass (mean, 1.7 kg), body weight (mean, 2.9 kg), and total body nitrogen (mean, 109 g) as compared with those fed glucose. On the basis of these measures, high-lipid intravenous nutrition does not seem to confer benefits beyond those seen when glucose was the nonprotein calorie source.

Additional recommendations pertain to administration of lipid in parenteral nutrition. By this route of administration, no more than 1 g/kg per day is recommended.[16] This recommendation pertains to both the amount administered and the rate of administration. Several studies in animal systems and humans contributed to this recommendation. Seidner and coworkers measured the clearance of radiolabeled technetium-sulfur colloid in 18 patients given parenteral nutrition (PN).[22] Forty-three percent of nonprotein kilocalories were given as a 20% emulsion over a 10-hour period. Clearance of technetium-sulfur colloid was not changed after a single 10-hour infusion of lipid but was reduced by 41% ($p < .05$) at the end of infusion on the third day of lipid infusions. The same group later found that continuous 24-hour administration of the same lipid emulsion in the same daily dose did not reduce clearance of technetium-sulfur colloid.[23] The maximum recommended rate, 1 g/kg per day, corresponds to 30% of total kilocalories. At 60% of total kilocalories, a rate of 2 g/kg per day is reached (at 60% of nonprotein kilocalories, the rate is 1.9 g/kg per day).

ω-3 Fatty Acids

The feeding of ω-3 FAs to critically ill patients has been a subject of great interest in recent years. The FAs receiving the most attention have been eicosapentaenoic acid (EPA; 20:5, ω-3) and docosahexaenoic acid (DHA; 22:6, ω-3), which are derived from fish oil. Following a single meal containing 0.5 g of fish oil per kilogram body weight, these FAs appeared as plasma FFAs in all lipoprotein fractions, reaching peak levels after 5 to 7 hours.[24]

With regular intake, the incorporation of dietary FAs into plasma lipids is rapid, and incorporation into cell membranes occurs over a period of days.[25,26] In the phospholipids of cell membranes, the ω-3 FAs become substrates for the formation of prostaglandins and thromboxanes via the cyclooxygenase pathway and leukotrienes via the lipoxygenase pathway.[25] When the ω-3 FAs enter these two pathways, they compete with arachidonic acid (20:4, ω-6) as a substrate (Fig. 9-1).[25,27]

Some arachidonate-derived (ω-6) products of these pathways such as prostaglandin E_2 (PGE_2) and leukotriene B_4 (LTB_4) are considered mediators of inflammatory events. Eicosanoid products formed by these pathways from ω-3 FAs (e.g., PGE_3 instead of PGE_2 and LTB_5 instead of LTB_4) appear to be less inflammatory. Over time, an increase in ω-3 FA content of the diet can alter the products of these pathways. For example, Turini and coworkers fed a diet supplemented with 13.8 g of either vegetable oil or sardine oil (containing 3.3 g EPA and 1.2 g DHA) to healthy male subjects for 42 days.[28] Stimulated neutrophils from the fish oil group produced 41%

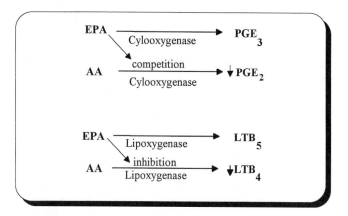

FIGURE 9-1 Conversion of arachidonic acid (AA) and eicosapentaenoic acid (EPA) to prostaglandin and leukotriene eicosanoid metabolites. The eicosanoids in the figure serve as examples (not the full spectrum) of the different series of prostaglandins and leukotrienes generated by each fatty acid. Note the proposed inhibition of AA to PGE_2 by EPA, presumably because of competition for the pathway.

less LTB_4 and 30% less 5-hydroxyeicosatetraenoic acid (5-HETE) than neutrophils from subjects fed vegetable oil. Only dietary fish oil also increased the production of LTB_5 and 5-hydroxyeicosapentaenoic acid (5-HEPE; both derived from EPA), which were not produced by neutrophils before dietary supplementation. All comparisons between pretreatment and posttreatment in the fish oil group were significant at $p < .05$. The difference in production of LTB_4 between posttreatment fish oil and vegetable oil groups was significant at $p < .06$; all other fish oil vs. vegetable oil comparisons were significant at $p < .05$. Li and colleagues found a similar pattern in CD-1 mice that were fed diets of different FA content.[29] When the diets were supplemented with EPA, the EPA content of liver phospholipids rose and the stimulated production of LTE_5 rose, while production of LTE_4, LTB_4 and PGE_2 diminished. In fact, production of LTE_5 was not detectable when diets were supplemented with oleic acid or arachidonic acid instead of EPA. Conversely, only trace amounts of LTB_4 were detected when the diet contained EPA. Production of PGE_2 was also diminished when the diet contained EPA. When compared with the control group that was fed oleic acid, the group fed EPA exhibited 50% less total eicosanoid production (all differences cited were statistically significant).

Severe injury due to trauma or burns can produce immunosuppressive effects in addition to inflammation. The immunosuppressive effects may be mediated, in part, by increased eicosanoid synthesis. Macrophages can carry a large percentage of their total FAs as arachidonic acid and release PGE_2 when stimulated.[30] In fact, the ability of macrophages to release PGE_2 may be enhanced by the conditions produced by injury and possibly also by some of the measures used in critical care. In animal models, increases in PGE_2 have been produced by anesthesia and transfusion, transfusion alone, hemorrhage, and crush-amputation injuries.[31-34] Ertel and colleagues observed that hemorrhage and resuscitation resulted in a rise in circulating PGE_2 levels.[35,36] The effects of PGE_2 observed in studies in vitro include inhibition of mitogen activation, proliferation and migration of lymphocytes, and generation of cytotoxic cells.[37]

Increased PGE_2 isolated from burn patients' serum and commercially prepared PGE_2 have been reported to suppress mixed-lymphocyte cultures.[38,39] Faist and colleagues[40] reported that the response of peripheral blood mononuclear cells to phytohemagglutinin (PHA) was depressed more than 30% below baseline values between 5 and 7 days after surgery in 11 of 19 patients. The response to PHA was improved with the addition of indomethacin, an inhibitor of cyclooxygenase and, therefore, of prostaglandin synthesis. The evidence in this area has led to the idea that injury or infection that contributes to critical illness can induce overproduction of PGE_2 by macrophages, leading to suppression of lymphocyte functions that are essential to fighting infection.

If PGE_2 production by macrophages after injury is key to immunosuppression, postinjury interventions to reduce PGE_2 should decrease immunosuppression and reduce the risk of complications. Faist and colleagues treated 23 postsurgical patients with indomethacin and studied infectious complications and aspects of cell-mediated immunity.[41] Fifty percent of control patients had an infectious episode, compared with 31% of the indomethacin group, but this difference was not statistically significant. Measures of CD3+, CD4+, interleukin-2 (IL-2) receptor lymphocytes, and Leu M3+ mononuclear leukocytes, measured as percentages of preoperative baseline values, were significantly greater for the indomethacin group at points between days 1 and 7 after surgery. Proliferation of peripheral blood mononuclear cells in response to PHA were also greater at points between 1 and 7 days after surgery. Measures of delayed-type hypersensitivity also increased in indomethacin-treated patients as compared with control patients. The clinical evidence from this small, unblinded trial supports the PGE_2-based mechanism proposed on the basis of the animal studies.

Because the immunosuppressant effect of experimental injury appeared to be related to increased PGE_2 secretion by macrophages, the potential of ω-3 FAs to reduce PGE_2 production has also been investigated. Ertel and colleagues fed mice for 3 weeks with diets containing fat from corn, safflower, or fish oils, after which they induced experimental hemorrhage. Release of PGE_2 by peritoneal macrophages was significantly increased, and selected macrophage and splenocyte functions were reduced only in the corn and safflower oil groups.[42]

Both Barton and coworkers and Peck and coworkers reported decreases in mortality in animal models of sepsis when ω-3 FAs were incorporated into animal diets.[43,44] In the former study, the mortality rate was decreased by half, although this did not attain statistical significance, perhaps because of small sample size. PGE_2 secretion by Kupffer cells stimulated with lipopolysaccharide was significantly reduced in fish oil-fed rats. In the study by Peck's group, guinea pigs were fed one of nine diets, whose proportion of fat was 3.5%, 14%, or 56%, and fat composition was 100% Microlipid (rich in linoleic acid), 100% MaxEPA (fish oil containing 35% ω-3 FAs), or a 50:50 mixture of the two. The level of fat did not affect outcome. Survival was 39% for animals fed the 50:50 mixture, 21% for those fed Microlipid, and 9% for those fed 100% fish oil (survival rates were totaled for all three levels of fat).

Johnson and colleagues[45] compared mortality rates for rats with sepsis induced by cecal ligation and puncture (CLP). Rats were fed chow or essential fatty acid-deficient chow supplemented daily with 1 ml of fish oil (MaxEPA), linoleic acid, or normal saline for 2 weeks before the CLP procedure. Survival after CLP in the chow-plus-fish oil group was 80%, for the linoleic acid group 50%, and for the normal saline group 55% (results significant, $p < .05$).

Gogos and associates[46] supplemented the diets of well-nourished and malnourished cancer patients for 40 days with fish oil capsules that supplied approximately 3 g of EPA and 2 g of DHA daily.[43]None of the patients, nor their placebo-fed, well-nourished and malnourished control patients received any additional form of treatment for the cancer. The ratio of helper T cells to suppressor T cells was lower in both groups of malnourished patients at the beginning of the trial and was increased only in the fish oil–fed group. A similar increase in the well-nourished group fed fish oil nearly attained statistical significance ($p = .07$). TNF synthesis by peripheral blood mononuclear cells was lower in the malnourished patients and was increased to a level near those of the well-nourished patients and control subjects after 40 days. The survival of all malnourished patients trailed that of the well-nourished groups, but fish oil supplementation extended the survival of patients in each of those groups compared with their placebo-fed counterparts. In their review of the literature, the authors made reference to studies and reviews that indicated that dietary ω-3 PUFAs reduced metastatic spread of cancer in animal models. Graffini and others[47] studied the effect of fish oil on metastic cancer growth in rats by injecting rats with an established colon carcinoma line (CC531). After 3 weeks on a low-fat (soybean oil) basal diet or basal diet supplemented with safflower or fish oil, animals received an injection of cancer cells into the portal vein. After 3 more weeks, rats fed the safflower oil diet and the fish oil diet were found to have greater numbers of tumors and larger volumes of cancer cells than animals fed the low-fat diet, and the greatest increase was in the animals fed the fish oil diet. These authors were careful to point out that they studied only postmetastatic events. However, this study does indicate that the effect of fish oil FAs should be defined for events throughout the development and spread of cancer cells before putting fish oil to indiscriminate use in cancer treatment.

It may be that some of the injury-related events leading to immunosuppression are related to the generation of PGE_2 and others are not. Tomkins and coworkers reported that a glycopeptide found in the serum of patients with severe burns or multiple trauma inhibited IL-2 synthesis by peripheral blood mononuclear cells.[48] This inhibition was not reversed by indomethacin or antibodies to PGE_2, which indicated an immunosuppressive mechanism independent of the generation of PGE_2.

Kelley and coworkers[49] studied the effect of DHA on immunocompetence by feeding healthy young men a diet that contained 6 g of DHA per day (in place of 6 g of linoleic acid) and supplemented with 20 mg of α-tocopherol for 90 days. Total white blood cells were reduced by 10%, as the result of a 21% decrease in polymorphonuclear leukocytes, after 90 days. Despite these changes, both indices remained within the normal range. Delayed type hypersensitivity response, serum concentrations of IgG, and the proliferative response of peripheral blood mononuclear cells did not differ between the treatment and control groups.

Robinson and Field[50] studied the effect of dietary ω-3 FAs and exercise, alone and in combination, on immune cell activation in sedentary and exercise-trained rats. The cytotoxicity of splenic natural killer cells in sedentary rats was increased by ω-3 FAs, compared with a low ω-3 FA diet, as was the percentage of activated T and B cells and macrophages in spleen after concanavalin A stimulation. When exercise was added to the high ω-3 FA diet, the same indices were not different from those of sedentary rats fed a low ω-3 FA diet. The authors made several excellent points in their discussion: in general, investigations into immune cell numbers and activities have focused on blood-derived lymphocytes and have not made observations on effects in lymphocytes from other tissues. In addition, the diets fed to rats in such studies have frequently contained a much higher percentage of fat and ω-3 FAs than would be found in physiologically relevant human diets. It has been suggested that high levels of fish oil-derived FAs in the diet are inhibitory to natural killer cell activity while more physiologic levels of these FAs may be stimulatory for the same activity.

Specialized enteral formulas have been developed to contain a mixture of nutrients that are thought to be helpful to the recovery of patients. Clinical studies that have used specialized enteral formulas are difficult to interpret when the focus is on a specific class of nutrients such as lipids. Given this limitation, the results of such studies still have value and are often the only examples of the clinical use of specialized lipids in enteral nutrition. Gadek and associates[51] reported the use of an enteral formula (denoted as EPA+GLA) that contained 55.2% of kilocalories as lipid in patients considered at risk for developing acute respiratory distress syndrome (ARDS). The lipid blend included 25% MCT oil, 20% borage oil (a source of ω-linolenic acid [GLA]), and 20% fish oil (sardine oil as a source of EPA), along with canola oil and lecithin. The formula also contained amounts of micronutrients that differed from the isocaloric, isonitrogenous control formula. Gas exchange (P_{AO_2}/F_{IO_2}), the primary variable, was 25% higher in the EPA+GLA group by day 4 and remained higher at day 7. Time on ventilator was 3.6 days less, intensive care unit stay was 3.8 days less, and total new organ failures (10% vs. 25%) were reduced in the EPA+GLA group compared with the control group. Mortality was 16% in the EPA+GLA group versus 25% in the control group (intent to treat), but this difference did not attain statistical significance. Mortality was 12% for the EPA+GLA group and 19% for the control group (not significant). Kenler and colleagues investigated the use of an enteral formula that contained a structured TG made with fish oil and MCT oil compared with control lipid in postsurgical cancer patients.[52] This study is discussed in more detail in the next section. Mortality was low in both groups and was not different between groups. The number of subjects with more than one infection during hospital stay was significantly lower in the structured TG group. The results from these two clinical studies are in line with basic research studies that demonstrated a positive effect of ω-3 FAs in immune function.

Some investigators have begun to question the efficacy benefits of "immune enhancing" enteral formulas. Suchner and coworkers[53] specifically suggested that formulas which contain ω-3 FAs from fish oil may aggravate systemic inflammation and have an adverse effect on outcome. However, studies cited in the section on ω-3 polyunsaturated FAs in that study, including two meta-analyses, did not support that position. In addition, in the work of Gadek and colleagues,[51] Kenler and others,[52] and Gottschlich,[16] the use of diets containing fish oil–derived ω-3 FAs have been associated with improvement across several outcome measures (statistically significant); the studies by Gadek and associates[51] and Gottschlich[16] reported decreased mortality, although not statistically significant.

FAs from the ω-3 family can also enter into the nutrition support of transplant patients. Grimminger and colleagues[54] fed heart transplant recipient rats 9 g/kg body weight of fish oil–derived or soybean oil–derived fat via continuous emulsion. Graft survival for fish oil–infused animals was 12.9 ± 0.4 days (mean ± standard error of the mean) versus 10.4 ± 0.7 for soybean oil–infused animals and 7.6 ± 0.3 for saline-infused controls. Ventura and colleagues[55] administered 3 g per day of ω-3 FAs to orthotopic cardiac transplant recipients with hypertension in a 12-week prospective, randomized, double-blind study. A control group of patients were fed an equal amount of ω-6 FAs. The patients fed ω-3 FAs exhibited significant reductions in mean arterial pressure (120 ± 7 versus 102 ± 7 mm Hg, baseline versus 12 weeks, respectively). Systemic vascular resistance was also significantly reduced only in the ω-3 FA group, a result also observed by others.[56] The authors concluded that ω-3 FAs could be used as an adjuvant for treatment of hypertension in cyclosporine-treated cardiac transplant patients.

The effect of ω-3 FAs on accelerated coronary arteriosclerosis following transplant has also been assessed in a heterotopic heart transplant rat model.[57] Following transplant, animals were fed 2 ml/kg per day of fish oil, an equal amount of safflower oil plus aspirin (1 mg/kg per day), and dipyrimadole (3 mg/kg per day) or an equal amount of safflower oil only. At 110 days after transplantation, animals fed fish oil had significantly less severe allograft coronary arteriosclerosis, as assessed by histologic examination scores, than either of the other two groups. These studies are among the literature that suggests therapeutic use of ω-3 FAs for nutrition support of transplant patients.

These studies are among a body of literature that supports the hypothesis that an increase in dietary (or parenterally administered) ω-3 FAs increases the ω-3 content of membrane phospholipids, which in turn reduces the production of inflammatory eicosanoids, while increasing the production of the less-inflammatory eicosanoids, by competing with arachidonic acid for entry to the eicosanoid synthetic pathways. Some of the data also suggests that some effects of ω-3 FAs are mediated by pathways other than the cyclooxygenase and lipoxygenase pathways. Several important questions remain to be resolved. Is the inclusion or substitution of ω-3 FAs alone in the nutrition regimen sufficient to improve patient outcomes, or must they be combined with other active nutrients? Must they be in a distinct structure (see following section), or is the effect of the ω-3 FAs too subtle to affect patient outcomes such as length of stay? Like much of the data cited in this chapter, those generated with animal models seem very promising, but the human clinical data appear to be less clear cut. Assuming the efficacy of ω-3 FAs,

the optimal mix of FAs and amount of total fat will have to be determined. In addition, the administration of ω-3 FAs that contain 5 or 6 double bonds per molecule may increase the requirement for antioxidants like vitamin E.

Structured Lipids

Structured lipids, or structured TGs, are manufactured by mixing sources of TGs that contain FAs of different lengths. The FAs are hydrolyzed from the glycerol moieties and then reesterified. The process causes the FAs to be redistributed in a random fashion. Figure 9-2 illustrates the concept of hydrolysis followed by reesterification. The most common application has been the production of structured TGs that contain MCFAs and LCFAs for research purposes. The FAs are reesterified randomly (Fig. 9-2). This may be disadvantageous. LCFAs having 20 or 22 carbons are hydrolyzed less efficiently from the 1 or 3 position on glycerol by pancreatic lipase, compared with shorter members of the long-chain family; however, C20 and C22 FAs are absorbed efficiently as monoglycerides when they occupy the 2 position. In fish oils, EPA (C20:5) and DHA (C22:6) can occupy the 1 or 3 position. The hydrolysis and reesterification procedure redistributes some of these FAs to the 2 position (sn-2). Christensen and associates compared the absorption of EPA and DHA from TGs in which EPA and DHA were specifically located at the sn-2 position (and decanoate at the sn-1 and sn-2 positions) with TGs having the same (mol %) of EPA, DHA, and decanoate, but randomly distributed.[58] In gastrostomy-fed rats, both the fate of absorption and the mol % of EPA and DHA were greater for the oil in which the LCFAs were located at the sn-2 position, but the total amount absorbed over 24 hours in response to a single bolus was similar for both oils. This supports earlier work by Jandacek and colleagues that

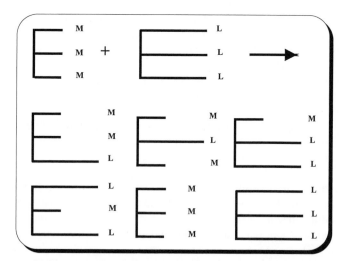

FIGURE 9-2 Synthesis of structured triglycerides from MCFAs *(M)* and LCFAs *(L)*. The starting triglycerides (the two triglycerides at the top of the diagram) are hydrolyzed (i.e., the FAs are detached from the glycerol backbone and then reesterified to the glycerol molecules). The six structures in the lower part of the diagram are the possible products created by the process by which the FAs are randomly reesterified to glycerol molecules. This is the least expensive method of synthesis. Specific products can be produced by using specific enzymes that perform the deesterifications and reesterifications at particular positions on the glycerol backbone.

had shown more rapid absorption of TGs with MCFAs at the 1 and 3 positions and LCFAs at the 2 position versus LCFAs at all three positions.[59] The implication from this work is that, when feeding with LCFAs such as EPA and DHA is beneficial or when absorptive capacity may be reduced, or both, EPA and DHA are delivered better by a structured TG featuring the LCFAs in the 2 position. Hubbard and McKenna found absorption of linoleic acid (18:2) in cystic fibrosis patients to be much more rapid when linoleate was a component of a structured lipid (MCT oil and sunflower oil) rather than safflower oil.[60] Using a rat model, Tso and colleagues reported that STG made with MCT and fish oil was absorbed more quickly through lymph than a physical mix of the components.[61] When intestinal injury was induced by ischemia and reperfusion, lymphatic transport of lipid was reduced as compared with uninjured controls; however, the rate of transport of STG and the amount transported were greater than for the physical mix. Remarkably, the rate and amount of STG transport in rats injured by ischemia and reperfusion was nearly identical to absorption of the physical mix in uninjured rats. The results in cystic fibrosis patients and the rat model of intestinal injury suggest that lipid absorption may also be improved in other conditions where lipid absorption may be impaired, such as Crohn's disease, short bowel syndrome, or a critical illness.

Parenteral use of STGs has also been investigated, although to a lesser extent than for enteral applications. In measuring glycerol kinetics in parenterally fed rats, Drews and coworkers found similar rates of FA oxidation when rats received long-chain TGs, LCT-MCT physical mixture, and structured lipid from LCT-MCT mixture;[62] however, the rate of glycerol production was significantly higher for LCT than for STG, and rates for physical mixture were midway between the two. The glycerol was produced from hydrolysis of endogenous TG, and the results were consistent with higher rates of TG-free FA recycling, which would increase energy expenditure and could account for poorer calorie effectiveness of LCT as compared with STG. Pscheidl and colleagues found greater sequestration of bacteria in liver and spleen and less in lungs of endotoxin-treated rats fed parenterally with structured lipid (LCFAs on sn-2 position) versus the physical mixture, both made with LCT and MCT.[63] The greater sequestration in liver and spleen indicates superior function of the reticuloendothelial system in response to structured lipid. Finally, Sandstrom and coworkers demonstrated the safety and tolerance of a structured lipid (LCT from soy oil plus MCT), administered parenterally, versus a standard LCT emulsion derived from soy oil.[57] The data demonstrated no difference in safety and tolerance between the STG emulsion (73403, Kabi Pharmacia AB) and Intralipid 20%. The same group later reported that this STG emulsion administered parenterally to postoperative patients resulted in significantly higher whole-body fat oxidation than LCT fed at 120% of basal requirement of nonprotein kilocalories.[65] The effect was not seen at 80% of basal requirement of nonprotein kilocalories. No details of the molecular composition of the STGs were given in this report.

The enteral and parenteral use of structured lipids in burn injury models was studied extensively by Bistrian's group. DeMichele and colleagues found a positive and significantly greater nitrogen balance in enterally fed burned rats when modified dairy fat (12% MCT; 7% LCT; and 81% structured lipid made with 50% butter oil, 35% MCT, and 15% safflower oil) and Captex 810B (39% MCT, 2% LCT, 59% STG made with 64% MCT, 36% safflower oil) were compared with MCT or LCT alone.[66] The modified dairy fat group also exhibited less body weight loss and increased muscle and liver fractional and absolute protein synthetic rates than did the other groups. This study was particularly important because it indicated that at least part of the effectiveness of structured lipid is due to the physical rearrangement of LCFAs and MCFAs along the glycerol backbone and not necessarily to the inclusion of ω-3 FAs, which were included in later investigations. DeMichele and colleagues subsequently demonstrated in a similar burn model that structured lipid produced significantly greater nitrogen balance and liver and muscle protein synthetic rates than did a physical mixture of equivalent FA composition.[67] Similar results were reported by the same group for a structured lipid from MCT and fish oil versus safflower oil.[68] The same group later investigated the properties of parenteral administration of an MCT-fish oil-structured TG fed at several levels in rats stressed by burn plus endotoxin.[69] Although some of the previously observed benefits of STG were observed again, others were not. When energy fed was compared with energy needs (determined by indirect calorimetry), it was found that the animals had been overfed. The authors speculated that overfeeding could blunt some of the benefits observed with structured lipid and suggested that STG, fed at relatively low fat intakes (i.e., below 30%) coupled with the prevention of overfeeding, might maximize the benefits provided by this type of lipid.

Sandstrom and colleagues reported the clinical safety and tolerance of parenterally infused STGs.[64,65] Safety, tolerance, and some distinct clinical benefits for postsurgical cancer patients have been reported by Kenler and coworkers.[52] Fifty adult patients with upper gastrointestinal malignancies received Osmolite HN (O-HN; Ross Laboratories) or a fish oil–structured lipid formula (FOSL-HN) fed into the jejunum after abdominal surgery. The two formulas were isonitrogenous and isoenergetic and different only in lipid composition. Lipid provided 30% of kilocalories and was 48.4% MCT, 38.7% corn oil, 9.7% soybean oil, and 3.2% soy lecithin in O-HN and 70.0% STG from fish oil plus MCT, 20.0% canola oil, 6.8% soybean oil, and 3.2% soy lecithin in FOSL-HN. Total patients with gastrointestinal complications, number of days with complications, and the number of actual reported complications were all significantly less in the FOSL-HN group. Although the number of patients with any infection was similar between the groups, five of seven patients had more than one infection in the O-HN group, as compared with one of six in the FOSL-HN group ($p = .037$). The number of days on PN was 29 for the O-HN group versus 11 for the FOSL-HN group ($p = .004$). Serum chemistries, hematology, urinalysis, and tests of liver and renal function were not different between the groups.

On the scientific side, some investigations have been undertaken to compare the efficacy of structured lipids containing ω-3 and MCFAs with that of ω-6 FAs, but no systematic effort to determine the optimal mixture of FAs to be incorporated into the structured lipid has been made. The optimal mixture would

need to be determined largely on the basis of efficacy in critically ill persons, and efficacy may vary with the type of injury
(i.e., trauma versus surgical insult). The efficiency of absorption and, for lipids containing ω-3 FAs, the possible need for
additional a-tocopherol to protect the larger number of double
bonds remain to be determined. The total percentage of lipid
that is optimal may change when a structured lipid is substituted for a physical mixture of lipid, or when structured lipid
and native TGs are combined. Finally, for the purposes of continued research, knowledge of the molecular composition of
structured lipids becomes important. This entails determination
of the identification of the FA at each position in the TG(s)
under study.

Structured lipids have been investigated extensively and
have been incorporated into several enteral products as of this
writing. Several issues associated with the production of
structured lipids can influence how and when these lipids
appear in products. It is more costly to use structured lipids
than common sources of TGs because of the cost of manufacturing the specialty lipid, which is greater than the cost of
obtaining one or more oils that are commodities. The issue of
the costs of royalties or licensing fees will in time affect more
potential ingredients (as they can almost any ingredient).
Managed care plans also have constraints on the prices they
are willing to pay for special purpose enteral or parenteral formulas. At some point, an intersection will be reached between
the function of specialty lipids in nutrition support products
and the cost of those products, where cost-effectiveness "casts
the final vote."

Conclusion

The investigation of lipid sources for nutrition support regimens continues to be an exciting area of investigation.
Nutrition support practice and products are not at the point at
which the practitioner can manipulate the amount and type of
lipid to benefit the patient. The potential uses of specialty lipids
include all critical illnesses and extend to transplantation and to
areas such as cancer and pediatrics. The promise generated by
animal studies must still be confirmed in human clinical trials.
This is rendered difficult in part by the relative uniformity of
conditions and lack of complications available in animal
studies, as compared with human trials. Animal trials are also
typically not confounded by administration of myriad other
therapeutic regimens. Where benefit seems to be apparent, it is
not clear how much benefit is obtained by feeding specialty
lipids *after* injury compared with feeding *before* injury (as
would be possible with some types of surgery, including transplantation). Human clinical trials can also be complicated by
the need to feed test lipids in a matrix of other nutrients. The
expense of varying only one nutrient in a formula across a
broad range and repeating the procedure for all nutrients of
interest is beyond the budgetary means of the largest manufacturers, and probably beyond the means of government
funding agencies. The potential of lipids in nutrition support to
influence outcomes is apparent enough to warrant further
investigation, but it will likely be some time before the specific
formulations that produce optimal effects for each condition
are known.

REFERENCES

1. Cohen FJ: Glucose vs. lipid calories. In Zaloga GP (ed): *Nutrition in critical care,* St Louis, 1994, Mosby, pp 169-182.
2. Long JM III, Long CL: Fuel metabolism. In Zaloga GP (ed): *Nutrition in
critical care,* St Louis, 1994, Mosby, pp 35-54.
3. Linscheer WG, Vergroesen AJ: Lipids. In Shils ME, Olson JA, Shike M
(eds): *Modern nutrition in health and disease,* vol 1, Philadelphia, 1994,
Lea & Febiger, pp 47-88.
4. You YQ, Ling PR, Qu Z et al: Effect of continuous enteral medium-chain
fatty acid infusion on lipid metabolism in rats, *Lipids* 33(3):261-266, 1998.
5. Sigalet DL, Winkelaar GB, Smith LJ: Determination of the route of
medium-chain and long-chain fatty acid absorption by direct measurement
in the rat, *J Parenter Enter Nutr* 21(5):275-278, 1997.
6. Newsholme EA, Leech AR: The integration of metabolism during
starvation, refeeding, and injury. In Newsholme EA, Leech AR (eds):
Biochemistry for the medical sciences, Chichester, 1983, Wiley, pp 536-581.
7. Wilmore DW: Are the metabolic alterations associated with critical illness
related to the hormonal environment? *Clin Nutr* 5:9-19, 1986.
8. Schlichtig R, Ayres SM: Fuel and oxygen metabolism in health and critical
illness. In Schlichtig R, Ayres SM (eds): *Nutrition support of the critically
ill,* Chicago, 1988,Year Book, pp 49-74.
9. Little RA, Stoner HB, Frayn KN: Substrate oxidation shortly after accidental injury in man, *Clin Sci* 61(6):789-791, 1981.
10. Cohen FJ: Glucose vs. lipid calories. In Zaloga GP (ed): *Nutrition in critical care,* St Louis, 1994, Mosby, pp 169-182.
11. Goran MI, Peters EJ, Herndon DN, Wolfe RR: Total energy expenditure in
burned children using the doubly labeled water technique, *Am J Physiol*
259(4 Pt 1):E576-E585, 1990.
12. Long CL, Nelson KM: Nutritional requirements based on substrate fluxes
in trauma, *Nutr Res* 13:1459-1478, 1993.
13. Long CL, Nelson KM, Akin JM Jr, et al: A physiologic basis for the
provision of fuel mixtures in normal and stressed patients, *J Trauma*
30(9):1077-1086, 1990.
14. Burke JF, Wolfe RR, Mullany CJ, et al: Glucose requirements following
burn injury: Parameters of optimal glucose infusion and possible hepatic
and respiratory abnormalities following excessive glucose intake, *Ann
Surg* 190(3):274-285, 1979.
15. Mochizuki H, Trocki O, Dominioni L, et al: Optimal lipid content for enteral
diets following thermal injury, *J Parenter Enter Nutr* 8(6):638-646, 1984.
16. Gottschlich MM, Jenkins M, Warden GD, et al: Differential effects of three
enteral dietary regimens on selected outcome variables in burn patients,
J Parenter Enter Nutr 14(3):225-236, 1990.
17. Garrel DR, Razi M, Lariviere F, et al: Improved clinical status and length
of care with low-fat nutrition support in burn patients, *J Parenter Enter
Nutr* 19(6):482-491, 1995.
18. Skipper A, Marian MJ: Parenteral nutrition. In Gottschlich MM, Matarese
LE, Shronts EP (eds): *Nutrition support dietetics core curriculum,* ed 3,
Silver Spring, MD, 1993, American Society for Parenteral and Enteral
Nutrition, pp 105-123.
19. Van Itallie TB, Moore FD, Geyer RP, Stare FJ: Will fat emulsions given
intravenously promote protein synthesis? Metabolic studies on normal
subjects and surgical patients, *Surgery* 36:720-731, 1954.
20. Bark S, Holm I, Hakansson I, Wretlind A: Nitrogen-sparing effect of fat
emulsion compared with glucose in the postoperative period, *Acta Chir
Scand* 466:40-41, 1976.
21. Kohlhardt SR, Smith RC, Rose A, Allen B: Effect of high-lipid high-nitrogen intravenous nutrition on total body nitrogen, visceral protein synthesis
and nitrogen balance, *Br J Surg* 82(1):64-68, 1995.
22. Seidner DL, Mascioli EA, Istfan NW, et al: Effects of long-chain triglyceride emulsions on reticuloendothelial system function in humans,
J Parenter Enter Nutr 13(6):614-619, 1989.
23. Jensen GL, Mascioli EA, Seidner DL, et al: Parenteral infusion of long-
and medium-chain triglycerides and reticuloendothelial system function in
man, *J Parenter Enter Nutr* 14(5):467-471, 1990.
24. Gibney MJ, Daly E: The incorporation of n-3 polyunsaturated fatty acids
into plasma lipid and lipoprotein fractions in the postprandial phase in
healthy volunteers, *Eur J Clin Nutr* 48(12):866-872, 1994.
25. Palombo JD, DeMichele SJ, Boyce PJ, et al: Metabolism of dietary
ω-linolenic acid vs. eicosapentaenoic acid in rat immune cell phospholipids during endotoxemia, *Lipids* 33(11):1099-1105, 1998.
26. Palombo JD, DeMichele SJ, Boyce PJ, et al: Effect of short-term enteral
feeding with eicosapentaenoic and ω-linolenic acids on alveolar
macrophage eicosanoid synthesis and bactericidal function in rats, *Crit
Care Med* 27(9):1908-1915, 1999.

27. Lindgren JA, Edenius C, Samuelsson B: Eicosanoid metabolism and function—nutritional modulation. In Kinney JM, Borum PR (eds): *Perspectives in clinical nutrition,* Chicago, 1989, American Dietetic Association, pp 379-391.

28. Turini ME, Powell WS, Behr SR, Holub BJ: Effects of fish-oil and vegetable-oil formula on aggregation and ethanolamine-containing lysophospholipid generation in activated human platelets and on leukotriene production in stimulated neutrophils, *Am J Clin Nutr* 60(5):717-724, 1994.

29. Li B, Birdwell C, Whelan J: Antithetic relationship of dietary arachidonic acid and eicosapentaenoic acid on eicosanoid production in vivo, *J Lipid Res* 35(10):1869-1877, 1994.

30. Schultz RM: The role of macrophage-derived arachidonic acid oxygenation products in the modulation of macrophage and lymphocyte function. In Hadden JW, Szentivanyi A (eds): *The reticuloendothelial system,* New York, 1985, Plenum, p 129.

31. Ross WB, Leaver HA, Yap PL, et al: Macrophage prostaglandin E$_2$ and oxidative responses to endotoxin during immunosuppression associated with anaesthesia and transfusion, *Prostaglandins Leukot Essent Fatty Acids* 49(6):945-953, 1993.

32. Ross WB, Leaver HA, Yap PL, et al: Prostaglandin E$_2$ production by rat peritoneal macrophages: role of cellular and humoral factors in vivo in transfusion-associated immunosuppression, *FEMS Microbiol Immunol* 2(5-6):321-325, 1990.

33. Ayala A, Meldrum DR, Perrin MM, Chaudry III: The release of transforming growth factor-beta following haemorrhage: its role as a mediator of host immunosuppression, *Immunology* 79(3):479-484, 1993.

34. Pretus HA, Browder IW, Lucore P, et al: Macrophage activation decreases macrophage prostaglandin E$_2$ release in experimental trauma, *J Trauma* 29:1152-1157, 1989.

35. Ertel W, Morrison MH, Meldrum DR, et al: Ibuprofen restores cellular immunity and decreases susceptibility to sepsis following hemorrhage, *J Surg Res* 53:55-61, 1992.

36. Ertel W, Morrison MH, Ayala A, et al: Blockade of prostaglandin production increases cachectin synthesis and prevents depression of macrophage functions after hemorrhagic shock, *Ann Surg* 213(3):265-271, 1991.

37. Ayala A, Chaudry IH: Dietary n-3 polyunsaturated fatty acid modulation of immune cell function before or after trauma, *Nutrition* 11(1):1-11, 1995.

38. Stephan RN, Conrad PH, Saizawa M, et al: Prostaglandin E$_2$ depresses antigen-presenting cell function of peritoneal macrophages, *J Surg Res* 44(6):733-739, 1988.

39. Ninnemann JL, Stockland AE: Participation of prostaglandin E$_2$ in immunosuppression following thermal injury, *J Trauma* 24(3):201-207, 1984.

40. Faist E, Kupper TS, Baker CC, et al: Depression of cellular immunity after major injury. Its association with posttraumatic complications and its reversal with immunomodulation, *Arch Surg* 121(9):1000-1005, 1986.

41. Faist E, Ertel W, Cohnert T, et al: Immunoprotective effects of cyclooxygenase inhibition in patients with major surgical trauma, *J Trauma* 30(1):8-18, 1990.

42. Ertel W, Morrison MH, Ayala A, Chaudry III: Modulation of macrophage membrane phospholipids by n-3 polyunsaturated fatty acids increases interleukin-1 release and prevents suppression of cellular immunity following hemorrhagic shock, *Arch Surg* 128(1):15-20, 1993.

43. Barton RG, Wills CL, Carlson A, et al: Dietary omega-3 fatty acids decrease mortality and Kupffer cell prostaglandin E$_2$ production in a rat model of chronic sepsis, *J Trauma* 31(6):768-774, 1991.

44. Peck MD, Ogle CK, Alexander JW: Composition of fat in enteral diets can influence outcome in experimental peritonitis, *Ann Surg* 214(1):74-82, 1991.

45. Johnson JA, Griswold JA, Muakkassa FF: Essential fatty acids influence survival in sepsis, *J Trauma* 35(1):128-131, 1993.

46. Gogos CA, Ginopoulos P, Salsa B, et al: Dietary omega-3 polyunsaturated fatty acids plus vitamin E restore immunodeficiency and prolong survival for severely ill patients with generalized malignancy: a randomized control trial, *Cancer* 82(2):395-402, 1998.

47. Griffini P, Fehres O, Klieverik L, Vogels IMC, et al: Dietary omega-3 polyunsaturated fatty acids promote colon carcinoma metastasis in rat liver, *Cancer Res* 58(15):3312-3319, 1998.

48. Tompkins SD, Gregory S, Hoyt DB, Ozkan AN: In vitro inhibition of IL-2 biosynthesis in activated human peripheral blood mononuclear cells by a trauma-induced glycopeptide, *Immunol Lett* 23(3):205-209, 1990.

49. Kelley DS, Taylor PC, Nelson GJ, et al: Dietary docosahexaenoic acid and immunocompetence in young healthy men, *Lipids* 33(6):559-566, 1998.

50. Robinson LE, Field CJ: Dietary long-chain (n-3) fatty acids facilitate immune cell activation in sedentary, but not exercise-trained rats, *J Nutr* 128(3):498-504, 1998.

51. Gadek JE, DeMichele SJ, Karlstad MD, et al: Effect of enteral feeding with eicosapentaenoic acid, gamma-linolenic acid, and antioxidants in patients with acute respiratory distress syndrome, *Crit Care Med* 27(8):1409-1420, 1999.

52. Kenler AS, Swails WS, Driscoll DF, et al: Early enteral feeding in postsurgical cancer patients. Fish oil structured lipid-based polymeric formula versus a standard polymeric formula, *Ann Surg* 223(3):316-333, 1996.

53. Suchner U, Kuhn KS, Furst P: The scientific basis of immunonutrition, *Proc Nutr Soc* 59(4):553-563, 2000.

54. Grimminger G, Grimm H, Fuhrer D, et al: Omega-3 lipid infusion in a heart allotransplant model. Shift in fatty acid and lipid mediator profiles and prolongation of transplant survival, *Circulation* 93(2):365-371, 1996.

55. Ventura HO, Milani RV, Lavie CJ, et al: Cyclosporine-induced hypertension. Efficacy of omega-3 fatty acids in patients after cardiac transplantation, *Circulation* 88(5 Pt 2):II281-285, 1993.

56. Homan-van-der-Heide, JJ, Bilo HJ, Tegzess AM, Donker AJ: The effects of dietary supplementation with fish oil on renal function in cyclosporine-treated renal transplant recipients, *Transplantation* 49(3):523-527, 1990.

57. Sarris GE, Mitchell RS, Billingham ME, et al: Inhibition of accelerated cardiac allograft arteriosclerosis by fish oil, *J Thorac Cardiovasc Surg* 97(6):841-854, 1989.

58. Christensen MS, Hoy CE, Becker CC, Redgrave TG: Intestinal absorption and lymphatic transport of eicosapentaenoic (EPA), docosahexaenoic (DHA), and decanoic acids: dependence on intramolecular triacylglycerol structure, *Am J Clin Nutr* 61(1):56-61, 1995.

59. Jandacek RJ, Whiteside JA, Holcombe BN, et al: The rapid hydrolysis and efficient absorption of triglycerides with octanoic acid in the 1 and 3 positions and long-chain fatty acid in the 2 position, *Am J Clin Nutr* 45(5):940-945, 1987.

60. Hubbard VS, McKenna MC: Absorption of safflower oil and structured lipid preparations in patients with cystic fibrosis, *Lipids* 22(6):424-428, 1987.

61. Tso P, Lee T, Bobik E, et al: Lymphatic absorption of structured triacylglycerols (STG) vs its physical mix (PM) in a rat model of fat malabsorption, *Am J Physiol* 277 (2 Pt 1):G 333-340, 1999.

62. Drews D, Schluter MD, Stein TP: Glycerol kinetics with parenteral lipid emulsions (long-chain triglycerides, medium-chain triglycerides, and structured lipids) in rats, *Metabolism* 42(6):743-748, 1993.

63. Pscheidl E, Hedwig-Geissing M, Winzer C, et al: Effects of chemically defined structured lipid emulsions on reticuloendothelial system function and morphology of liver and lung in a continuous low-dose endotoxin rat model, *J Parenter Enter Nutr* 19(1):33-40, 1995.

64. Sandstrom R, Hyltander A, Korner U, Lundholm K: Structured triglycerides to postoperative patients: a safety and tolerance study, *J Parenter Enter Nutr* 17(2):153-157, 1993.

65. Sandstrom R, Hyltander A, Korner U, Lundholm K: Structured triglycerides were well tolerated and induced increased whole body fat oxidation compared with long-chain triglycerides in postoperative patients, *J Parenter Enter Nutr* 19(5):381-386, 1995.

66. DeMichele SJ, Karlstad MD, Babayan VK, et al: Enhanced skeletal muscle and liver protein synthesis with structured lipid in enterally fed burned rats, *Metabolism* 37(8):787-795, 1988.

67. DeMichele SJ, Karlstad MD, Bistrian BR, et al: Enteral nutrition with structured lipid: effect on protein metabolism in thermal injury, *Am J Clin Nutr* 50(6):1295-1302, 1989.

68. Teo TC, DeMichele SJ, Selleck KM, et al: Administration of structured lipid composed of MCT and fish oil reduces net protein catabolism in enterally fed burned rats, *Ann Surg* 210(1):100-107, 1989.

69. Gollaher CJ, Fechner K, Karlstad M, et al: The effect of increasing levels of fish oil-containing structured triglycerides on protein metabolism in parenterally fed rats stressed by burn plus endotoxin, *J Parenter Enter Nutr* 17(3):247-253, 1993.

Fluid, Electrolytes, and Acid-Base Balance

10

Susan J. Whitmire, RD, CNSD

THE distribution and composition of body fluids have profound effects on cell function. Optimal physiologic functioning relies on a stable internal environment, which the body maintains through a sophisticated network of homeostatic mechanisms. Disease, injury, and operative trauma can disrupt fluid and electrolyte balance, altering cell environment and, ultimately, cell function. Even small changes in pH, electrolyte concentrations, and fluid status can have adverse consequences. A thorough understanding of normal fluid and electrolyte physiology is requisite to anticipating, recognizing, and treating fluid and electrolyte imbalances associated with illness and injury. This chapter reviews the principles of fluid, electrolyte, and acid-base balance as they relate to nutrition support, emphasizing recognition, assessment, and treatment of their various derangements.

Body Fluids

Composition and Distribution

TOTAL BODY WATER. Water is the principal constituent of the human body, comprising nearly 70% to 75% of body weight at birth.[1,2] A physiologic loss of body water occurs during the first few months after birth as infants adjust to their new environment. Total body water (TBW) decreases to 65% by 1 year of age and remains stable until puberty.[1] Further reductions occur with age because of changes in body composition (Table 10-1). Because adipose tissue contains very little water, females and older persons who generally have larger proportions of body fat

compared to lean body mass, have less TBW. Although age and amount of lean body mass affect TBW, its percentage remains fairly constant from day to day in healthy persons.[1]

Distribution of Body Fluids

Body water is divided into two main compartments. Intracellular fluid (ICF) accounts for approximately two thirds of TBW. Extracellular fluid (ECF)—intravascular, interstitial, and transcellular fluid—comprises the remaining third.[1] Intravascular fluid is the noncellular component of blood and is synonymous with plasma. Intravascular fluid accounts for approximately 25% of ECF, corresponding to only 8% of TBW. Interstitial fluid is the fluid surrounding cells in body tissues. It also includes lymph. Transcellular fluids are those that collect in specific locations as a result of transport processes through cells. Transcellular fluids include cerebrospinal, pleural, pericardial, intraocular, and gastrointestinal (GI) fluids. Although they comprise a very small fraction of TBW, the total amount of fluid transported daily across the transcellular spaces is much greater.

COMPOSITION OF BODY FLUIDS. Fluids within each of these compartments contain specific concentrations of solutes, both electrolytes and nonelectrolytes (Fig. 10-1).[4,5] *Nonelectrolytes* are substances that do not dissociate in solution, such as glucose, urea, and creatinine. Electrolytes are substances that dissociate into positively and negatively charged ions, cations and anions, capable of conducting electrical current. Sodium (Na^+) is the principal cation in ECF; potassium (K^+) is the primary cation in ICF. Chloride (Cl^-) is the principal extracellular anion and organic phosphate (PO_4^{3-}) the principal intracellular anion. Nonelectrolytes are generally measured by weight per unit volume (e.g., milligrams per deciliter). Electrolytes are measured in terms of number of particles (millimoles) or combining capacity (milliequivalents) per unit volume.

A *mole* of any substance is simply its gram molecular weight. A millimole (mmol) is that same value expressed in milligrams (mg). For example, a mole of Na^+ is 23 g; a millimole is 23 mg. Similarly, a mole of sodium chloride (NaCl) is 58 g (Na = 23, Cl = 35); a millimole is 58 mg.

An *equivalent* is determined by dividing an ion's gram molecular weight by its valence. A milliequivalent (mEq) is the molecular weight in milligrams divided by the valence. For instance 1 mEq of Na^+ equals 23 mg divided by 1, or 23 mg. Similarly, a mEq of calcium (Ca^{2+}) equals 40 mg divided by 2, or 20 mg.

To convert from milligrams to milliequivalents of a substance, divide its weight (mg) by its molecular weight (mg) and

---

TABLE 10-1

Total Body Water in Relation to Age, Sex, and Lean Body Mass[1-3]

Age	TBW (% Body Weight)
Premature infant	80-85
Term infant	70-75
One year	65
Young adult	♂60 ♀50
Older adult	♂52 ♀47
Obese adult	♂50 ♀42
Lean adult	♂70 ♀60
Emaciated adult	70-75

TBW, total body water.

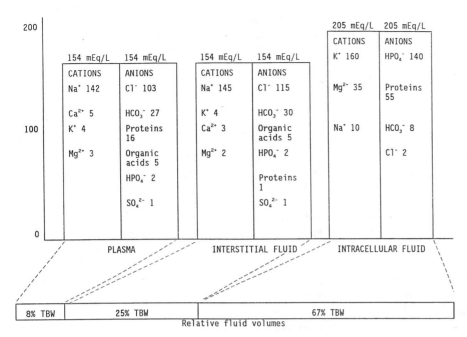

FIGURE 10-1 Composition of body fluids. (Adapted from Gallagher-Allred C: Fluid and electrolyte requirements. In Krey SH, Murray RL [eds]: *Dynamics of nutrition support,* Norwalk, CT, 1986, Appleton-Century-Crofts, p. 253; Lusting JV: Fluid and electrolyte therapy. In Hay WW, Groothuis JR, Hayward AR, Levin MJ [eds]: *Current pediatric diagnosis and treatment,* ed 12, East Norwalk, CT, 1995, Appleton Lange, p. 1180.)

multiply by its valence. To convert from millimoles to milliequivalents, multiply the number of millimoles by the valence. For univalent ions, such as Na^+, a milliequivalent equals a millimole because there is 1 mEq per millimole. With divalent ions such as Ca^{2+} and magnesium (Mg^{2+}) there are 2 mEq per millimole. Thus, 1 mmol Na^+ = 1 mEq; 1 mmol Ca^{2+} = 2 mEq; and 1 mmol Mg^{2+} = 2 mEq. One milliequivalent of any substance combines chemically with 1 mEq of any other substance that has the opposite charge. In any solution, the number of milliequivalents of cations and anions is equal.

Movement of Fluid and Solutes Between Compartments

MEMBRANES. Fluid compartments are separated by semipermeable membranes. Cell membranes separate the ICF from the ECF; capillary membranes separate the intravascular fluid from the interstitial fluid; and epithelial membranes separate both the interstitial and intravascular fluids from transcellular fluids. Very small molecules such as water and urea pass easily through all membranes. However, not all solutes disperse equally in the ICF and ECF. Differences in membrane permeability, transporters, and active pumps regulate solute distribution and account for the unique fluid composition of individual compartments.[2] Large molecules such as proteins are contained primarily in the intravascular space because of the low permeability of capillary membranes. Under certain conditions (e.g., "leaky capillary syndrome") membrane permeability can increase, allowing proteins to pass into the interstitial space. This in turn reduces intravascular colloid pressure and results in increased flux of water from the intravascular to the interstitial space. This process is often referred to as *third spacing.*

TRANSPORT PROCESSES. Movement of substances across a membrane occurs via diffusion, active transport, filtration, and osmosis. In diffusion, particles move along a concentration gradient from an area of high concentration to one of low - concentration. Small particles and those that are lipid soluble pass through the membrane by simple diffusion. Larger,

lipid-insoluble particles such as glucose require a carrier substance in a process termed *facilitated diffusion.* Diffusion also occurs with changes in electrical potential across the membrane such that cations follow anions crossing the membrane and vice versa.

In the absence of an electrical or concentration gradient, *active transport* is required. The movement of a substance from a milieu of low concentration to one of high concentration requires energy and the availability of a carrier substance. Transport ceases when the carrier substance becomes saturated. Active transport is important in the movement of glucose, proteins, Na^+, K^+, and hydrogen (H^+).

When substances move from an area of high hydrostatic pressure to one of low pressure, it is termed *filtration.* Hydrostatic pressure is the pressure contributed by the weight of the fluid. Through this process, the kidneys are able to filter more than 180 L of plasma every day.

Osmosis is the movement of water through a semipermeable membrane from an area of low solute concentration to an area of high solute concentration. Osmotic pressure is the amount of hydrostatic pressure required to halt this flow of water.

INTRAVASCULAR AND INTERSTITIAL FLUID EXCHANGE. There is a constant exchange of fluid across capillary membranes separating the intravascular and interstitial spaces. This fluid, termed "ultrafiltrate," consists of water and small solutes that pass easily through membrane pores.[2] Larger solutes, such as proteins, do not readily cross the capillary membrane. Exchange of fluid between these compartments facilitates delivery of nutrients from the plasma to the cell membrane and removal of substances secreted by the cell. Hydrostatic pressure and colloid osmotic pressure govern movement of ultrafiltrate between the vascular and interstitial spaces. Capillary hydrostatic pressure promotes movement of ultrafiltrate from the intravascular to the interstitial space. Colloid osmotic pressure and lymphatic flow promote return of ultrafiltrate to the vascular space. Colloid osmotic pressure (also called *oncotic pressure*) refers to the osmotic pressure exerted by the proteins contained within a fluid compartment. Plasma proteins consist principally of albumin and globulins. Albumin has a molecular weight of 60,000 and contributes nearly three quarters of the oncotic pressure exerted by plasma proteins.[1] The albumin concentration of interstitial fluid is only 1 g/dl, one quarter that of the intravascular fluid.[2] A reduction in colloid osmotic pressure favors movement of ultrafiltrate from the plasma to the interstium and results in edema.

WATER MOVEMENT ACROSS CELL MEMBRANES. *Osmolality* reflects a solution's ability to create osmotic pressure and thus determine the direction and extent of water movement between fluid compartments. It is measured in terms of the number of osmotically active particles per kilogram of solvent. In clinical practice, osmolality is more easily expressed in terms of osmotically active particles per unit volume—*milliosmoles* per liter (mOsm/L). This value does not reflect the chemical combining capacity of the dissolved substances, but rather the number of particles present when the substance dissociates. For instance, a millimole of NaCl dissociates into a millimole of Na^+ and a millimole of Cl^-, contributing 2 mOsm. A millimole of magnesium sulfate ($MgSO_4$) dissociates similarly to provide 2 mOsm per mmol. However, a millimole of Na_2SO_4 dissociates into 2 mmol of Na^+ and 1 mmol of SO_4^{2-}, contributing a total of 3 mOsm. One mmol of an un-ionized substance (e.g., glucose) equals 1 mOsm.

Cell membranes are completely permeable to water such that water crosses the cell membrane until the osmolalities are equal on both sides of that membrane. Within each compartment, the total number of osmotically active particles is 290 to 310 mOsm/L. The osmolality of a fluid compartment is determined largely by the particles restricted to that compartment. Thus, plasma osmolality is determined primarily by its Na^+ concentration. Plasma osmolality can be calculated as follows:

$$\text{Plasma Osm}_c (\text{mOsm/L}) = 2 \times [Na^+] + [BUN]/2.8 + [glucose]/18$$

Dividing BUN by 2.8 converts from milligrams nitrogen (N) per deciliter to millimoles urea per liter (N has an atomic weight of about 14, a molecule of urea contains 2 atoms of N, and there are 10 dl per L). Similarly, dividing glucose by 18 converts from milligrams per deciliter to millimoles per liter (molecular weight of glucose is approximately 180).[6]

Measured osmolality (Osm_m) is determined directly by some type of osmometer and includes all detectable osmoles. The osmol gap is the difference the between measured and calculated osmolality (Osm_m-Osm_c).[7-11] Although a normal range has not yet been established, positive gaps greater than 10 mOsm/L are considered abnormal.[6] The osmol gap, along with effective osmolality, may be useful in evaluating hyponatremia and assessing risk of cerebral edema.[6]

Effective osmolality is the portion of total osmolality that actually has potential to induce flow of water across cell membranes. Very small particles such as urea and ethanol move easily across cell membranes. As such, they do not induce flow of water and are termed *ineffective osmoles*.[2,6] Effective osmolality is synonymous with tonicity and is determined by subtracting the concentration of ineffective osmoles, in millimoles per liter, from the measured osmolality (to convert ethanol, an ineffective osmole, from milligrams per deciliter to millimoles per liter, divide by 4.6; divide BUN by 2.8 as previously

described). Similarly, deleting the BUN term from the equation for Osm_c yields calculated effective plasma osmolality. Normal effective osmolality is 270 to 285 mOsm/L. Any condition that changes the effective osmolality in either compartment induces flow of water from the compartment with lower effective osmolality to the compartment with higher effective osmolality until the osmolalities reequilibrate. Changes in ICF or ECF volume without concomitant changes in effective osmolality do not result in similar redistribution of water because without creation of an osmotic gradient, there is no inducement of water flow. When the effective osmolality of the ECF is low compared with that of the ICF, the risk of cerebral edema increases.[6]

Fluid Balance

FLUID GAINS. The average adult consumes 2000 to 2500 ml of water daily.[1] Approximately 1500 ml is ingested as fluid.[12] The remainder is extracted from solid food or is produced during oxidative metabolism.[1,5] Approximately 300 ml of water is generated daily from the oxidation of carbohydrates, protein, and fat (Box 10-1).[12,13]

FLUID LOSSES. Fluid losses normally occur via the kidneys, lungs, skin, and GI tract. Other contributors to fluid loss include surgical drains and chest tubes, fistulas, open wounds, and hemorrhage. Additionally, fluids sometimes shift into normally nonequilibrating spaces. Although this *"third-space shift"* does not result in decreased TBW, it reduces the proportion of usable fluids in the intracellular and intravascular compartments.

The kidneys are the primary regulators of fluid and electrolyte status. Of the 180 L of plasma filtered by the kidneys daily, only about 1500 ml is excreted as urine.[13] Average urine output is 40 to 80 ml/hr for adults and 0.5 ml/kg per hour for children. Urine osmolality is determined by the amount of metabolic wastes and urine volume. Healthy kidneys have a maximal concentrating ability of 1400 mOsm/kg water. However, the ability to concentrate urine decreases with advanced age.[14,15] To rid the body of the daily load of metabolic wastes, at least 400 ml of urine must be produced (*obligatory urine output*).

Nearly 500 to 600 ml of fluid are lost through the skin every day.[1,13] Insensible dermal fluid loss is not from sweat, but rather from water vapor formed within the body and lost through the skin.[1] These losses account for approximately 75% of total insensible losses[1] and average 6 ml/kg per day for an adult.[13] This amount increases substantially with burns and fever.

BOX 10-1

Average Daily Fluid Gains and Losses in Adults

Fluid Gains		Fluid Losses	
Sensible		Sensible	
Oral fluids	1100-1400 ml	Urine	1200-1500 ml
Solid foods	800-1000 ml	Intestinal	100-200 ml
Insensible		Insensible	
Oxidative metabolism	300 ml	Lungs	400 ml
		Skin	500-600 ml
Total	2200-2700 ml	Total	2200-2700 ml

Adapted from Horn MM, Swearingen PL (eds): *Pocket guide to fluid, electrolyte, and acid-base balance*, ed 2, St Louis, 1993, Mosby, p 23.

TABLE 10-2

Volume and Electrolyte Content of Gastrointestinal Secretions

Type of Secretion	Volume (ml/24 hr)	Na⁺ (mEq/L)	K⁺ (mEq/L)	Cl⁻ (mEq/L)	HCO₃⁻ (mEq/L)
Saliva	1500 (500-2000)	10 (2-10)	26 (20-30)	10 (8-18)	30 —
Stomach	1500 (100-4000)	60 (9-116)	10 (0–32)	130* (8-154)	—
Duodenum	— (100-2000)	140 —	5 —	80 —	—
Ileum	3000 (100-9000)	140 (80-150)	5 (2-8)	104 (43-137)	30 —
Colon	—	60	30	40	—
Bile	— (50–800)	145 (131-164)	5 (3-12)	100 (89-180)	35 —
Pancreas	— (100-800)	140 (113-185)	5 (3-7)	75 (54-95)	115 —

Adapted from Shires GT, Shires GT III, Lowry SF: Fluid, electrolyte, and nutritional management of the surgical patient. In Schwartz SI (ed): *Principles of surgery*, ed 6, New York, 1994, McGraw Hill, p 65.
* Lower with achlorhydria.

Insensible fluid is essentially void of electrolytes and is generally considered free water loss. Sensible fluid loss via sweat varies with climate and individual activity levels. Under extreme conditions, losses can approach 2 L/hr. Although sweat does contain appreciable amounts of electrolytes (15 to 60 mmol Na⁺/L, 5 to 10 mmol K⁺/L), it is nonetheless hypotonic.[1]

Insensible fluid loss also occurs via the lungs, accounting for approximately 25% of total insensible losses.[1] Amounts vary, depending on humidity and depth of respiration, but are generally on the order of 400 ml/day. With hyperventilation and an unhumidified tracheostomy, losses can reach 1.0 to 1.5 L/day.[1]

Despite large volumes of fluid (6 to 8 L) that traverse the GI tract daily, only 100 to 200 ml are lost. Electrolyte concentrations of GI secretions vary, but are generally isotonic or slightly hypotonic (Table 10-2). During illness, the GI tract can be a site of considerable fluid loss via gastric suctioning, vomiting, diarrhea, and fistula drainage. If losses are not replaced, severe fluid deficits can result.

FLUID REQUIREMENTS. To maintain fluid balance, requirements should be established so that fluid input matches output. Maintenance requirements must take into account insensible water loss as well as water lost in urine, sweat, and feces. Additionally, allowances must be made for alterations in metabolic states that affect fluid requirements. Of these, fever is perhaps the most common. Fluid requirements increase by 12.5% for each degree increase in body temperature above 37° C. Other factors that increase fluid needs are hypermetabolism, hyperventilation, exercise, increased ambient temperature, low humidity, high altitude, and high intake of fiber, caffeine, or alcohol.[1,16] Methods for estimating fluid requirements are shown in Box 10-2.

REGULATION OF FLUID VOLUME, DISTRIBUTION, AND OSMOLALITY. ECF is in a constant state of flux. The body reacts with its surroundings, prompting various homeostatic mechanisms to make

BOX 10-2

Calculation of Daily Fluid Requirements[4,17]

METHOD 1

16-30 yr, active	40 ml/kg
20-55 yr	35 ml/kg
55-75 yr	30 ml/kg
>75 yr	25 ml/kg

METHOD 2

1. 100 ml/kg for the first 10 kg body weight
2. 50 ml/kg for the second 10 kg body weight
3. Age ≤ 50 yr:
   20 ml/kg for each additional kilogram body weight
4. Age >50 years:
   15 ml/kg for each additional kilogram body weight

METHOD 3
1 ml/kcal

adjustments necessary to maintain normal extracellular volume, composition, and osmolality. This in turn ensures a relatively constant cell environment and facilitates normal cell function. The body regulates Na⁺ and water independently, although combined defects in Na⁺ and water homeostasis are common.

Regulation of Water Balance/Osmolality. Despite wide fluctuations in Na⁺ and water intake, normal plasma osmolality is maintained within a narrow range (275 to 290 mOsm/L) by mechanisms capable of detecting a 1% to 2% change in tonicity. Water balance is regulated by the thirst mechanism, along with the renal actions of antidiuretic hormone (ADH), also called *arginine vasopressin (AVP)*. Disorders of water homeostasis result in hyponatremia or hypernatremia. Failure to maintain normal ECF tonicity results in redistribution of water between the ECF and ICF compartments. With increased ECF tonicity, water moves from the ICF to the ECF, causing cells to shrink. Conversely, with decreased ECF tonicity, water moves from the ECF to the ICF, causing cells to swell. The symptoms of osmolality derangements are principally neurologic because of changes in brain cell function.

Thirst is the body's signal to seek fluid and is the primary defender of cell volume. The thirst mechanism is stimulated by an increase in plasma tonicity and to a lesser extent by a decrease in ECF volume. However, because maintenance of adequate effective ECF volume and tissue perfusion takes precedence over maintenance of normal ECF tonicity, a low effective ECF volume stimulates the thirst mechanism even if plasma tonicity is low.[2] The average osmotic threshold for thirst is 290 to 295 mOsm/L.[18] Thirst ceases with ingestion of fluid and restoration of normal plasma tonicity. In persons with impaired thirst perception (e.g., elders) or inability to obtain fluid independently (e.g., neurologically impaired individuals, intubated patients, infants), other methods must be relied on to assess the need for additional fluid.[14-16,19]

ADH, the principle determinant of renal water excretion, is produced by the hypothalamus and released by the posterior pituitary gland. Increased effective plasma osmolality, decreased intravascular volume, and decreased blood pressure stimulate release of ADH. Stress, pain, surgery, and certain medications can also increase ADH release. ADH acts by increasing reabsorption of water in the renal tubule collecting ducts, allowing the kidneys to excrete more concentrated urine.

Regulation of Na⁺ Balance/Extracellular Fluid Volume. The vascular compartment of the ECF must be maintained to ensure adequate tissue perfusion, and thus adequate delivery of nutrients and removal of metabolic wastes. For the most part, total body Na⁺ *content* determines ECF volume. Control over renal Na⁺ excretion is the primary means of preserving intravascular volume. Hormones, neuronal activity, and hemodynamic factors act in concert to influence renal Na⁺ retention and excretion.[2]

Acute changes in intravascular volume are first detected by volume receptors in the carotid sinuses, aortic arch, cardiac atria, and renal vessels. These receptors respond indirectly to volume changes by responding to changes in stretch in the arterial or atrial walls. Such changes ultimately lead to alterations in cardiac output, vascular resistance, thirst, and renal handling of Na⁺ and water. A decrease in stretch, signaling a decrease in intravascular volume, results in increased sympathetic tone, which increases cardiac output and arterial resistance, and ultimately blood pressure.

Increased sympathetic tone and decreased renal perfusion also stimulate the kidneys to release renin, a proteolytic enzyme. Through the action of renin, angiotensin is converted to angiotensin I, which is subsequently converted to angiotensin II, a potent vasoconstrictor. Angiotensin II also stimulates release of aldosterone by the adrenal cortex. Aldosterone exerts its effect in the renal tubules, resulting in increased Na⁺ reabsorption, water retention, and increased K⁺ and H⁺ excretion. Release of aldosterone is also stimulated by increased plasma [K⁺], decreased [Na⁺], and increased adrenocorticotropic hormone (ACTH) levels.

Atrial natriuretic peptide (ANP), a hormone released by the cardiac atria, is also involved in regulation of effective ECF volume. ANP is released in response to elevated atrial pressure and acts to reduce both blood pressure and vascular volume. In addition to direct vasodilation, ANP increases Na⁺ and water excretion by the kidneys, decreases renin synthesis, decreases aldosterone release, and decreases release of ADH.

Volume Disorders

No single laboratory test is adequate for assessing acute volume changes. The amount, composition, and distribution of fluid lost or gained exert varying effects on laboratory indices. Diagnosis of ECF volume deficit or excess relies heavily on clinical examination, but certain laboratory tests are indirect indicators of changes in ECF volume. It is important to note that plasma Na⁺ *concentrations* are *not indicative* of volume status. Normal, high, and low plasma [Na⁺] can occur in states of volume excess or deficit.[1,2]

EXTRACELLULAR FLUID VOLUME DEPLETION (HYPOVOLEMIA) AND DEHYDRATION. Although often used interchangeably, the terms *volume depletion* and *dehydration* describe two distinct entities.[20] Volume depletion, or more appropriately, ECF volume depletion, refers to a fluid deficit within the vascular compartment resulting from a net loss of total body Na⁺. Dehydration refers to intracellular water deficits arising from ECF hypertonicity and altered water metabolism.[20] Volume depletion and dehydration can, and frequently do, occur together. However, they are treated differently and warrant separate discussion.

ECF volume depletion results from a net loss of total body Na⁺ *content*. Etiologies include renal Na⁺ loss (e.g., diuretics, osmotic diuresis, hypoaldosteronism, salt-wasting nephropathies), and extrarenal Na⁺ loss (e.g., hemorrhage, loss of GI fluids from vomiting, gastric suctioning, diarrhea, or fistula drainage).[21-23] Intravascular volume depletion can also occur with ECF redistribution (e.g., hypoalbuminemia, capillary leak).

Diagnosis relies on history, physical examination, and supportive laboratory data. With an ECF deficit sufficient to reduce glomerular filtration rate (GFR), BUN rises. Assuming healthy kidneys, the creatinine usually does not increase proportionately. Thus, an increased ratio of BUN to creatinine (> 20:1) is often used to distinguish between prerenal and renal azotemia.[23] Changes in hematocrit concentration also reflect ECF volume changes and are inversely correlated. The appropriate response to hypovolemia is enhanced renal Na⁺ and water reabsorption. Thus, urine Na⁺ should be less than 20 mmol/L, except in cases of vomiting or acute tubular necrosis.[23] Urine specific gravity and osmolality are generally greater than 1.015 mOsm/L and 450 mOsm/L, respectively.

Signs and symptoms of ECF volume depletion vary according to severity. Central nervous system (CNS) signs range from sleepiness, apathy, and slow responsiveness to decreased tendon reflexes, stupor, and coma. Cardiovascular signs include orthostatic hypotension, tachycardia, collapsed veins and collapsing pulse. Severe ECF depletion is characterized by hypotension, distant heart signs, cold extremities, and absent peripheral pulses. Decreased skin turgor is characteristic, but not diagnostic of ECF volume depletion.[1,23,24] Temperature generally decreases with hypovolemia and normalizes with restoration of ECF volume.

Dehydration results from ECF hypertonicity and altered water metabolism.[20] A diagnosis of dehydration cannot be made without measurement of plasma [Na⁺] or determination of plasma tonicity. ECF hypertonicity reflects an increase in effective osmoles compared to body water as a result of net water loss (e.g., increased insensible losses, loss of hypotonic fluids), or solute gain (e.g., administration of hypertonic saline). Signs and symptoms of acute dehydration include thirst, dry sticky mucous membranes, decreased saliva and tears, tachycardia, hypotension, and fever.[1] CNS signs arise in association with decreased brain cell volume and include altered mental status, weakness, neuromuscular excitability, focal neurologic deficits, and occasionally coma or seizures.[21] CNS signs may be mitigated if development of ECF hypertonicity is gradual in nature. The brain adapts by taking up Na⁺ and K⁺ salts initially, then generating new intracellular solutes (organic osmolytes) to lessen the tonicity gradient between ICF and ECF and minimize loss of water from brain cells.[2,6,16,18,20,25-31]

Treatment. Disorders of ECF volume depletion and dehydration can, of course, occur simultaneously. Conceptualizing them as distinct entities, however, reduces the risk for therapeutic error. Factors to consider include selection of appropriate replacement fluid and rate of correction. In addition to correcting the volume deficit, attention must be given to replacing any ongoing obligatory fluid losses. Electrolyte concentrations and osmolarities of common intravenous fluids are listed in Table 10-3. Formulas commonly used in devising treatment for disorders of water and Na⁺ balance are listed in Box 10-3.

TABLE 10-3

Electrolyte Concentrations and Osmolarities of Common Intravenous Fluids*

	Sodium (mmol/L)	Potassium (mmol/L)	Calcium (mmol/L)	Chloride (mmol/L)	Lactate (mmol/L)	Osmolarity (mOsm/L)
5% dextrose solution	0	0	0	0	0	278
10% dextrose solution	0	0	0	0	0	556
0.9% NaCl (normal saline) solution	154	0	0	154	0	308
Sodium lactate solution	167	0	0	0	167	334
5% dextrose, 0.45% NaCl (half normal saline) solution	77	0	0	77	0	432
5% dextrose, 0.9% NaCl (normal saline) solution	154	0	0	154	0	586
Ringer's solution	147.5	4	2.2	156	0	309
Lactated Ringer's solution	130	4	1.5	109	28	273
5% dextrose in Ringer's solution	147.5	4	2.2	156	0	587
5% dextrose in lactated Ringer's solution	130	4	1.5	109	28	551

* For sodium, potassium, chloride and lactate, one mmol is equal to 1 millequivalent.

BOX 10-3

Formulas used in Implementing Selected Treatment for Water and Na+ Disorders[1,29,30]

FORMULA 1.   **CALCULATION OF WATER DEFICIT**

$$\text{Water deficit} = \text{TBW} \times \left[\frac{\text{current } [Na^+]_p}{140} - 1 \right]$$

Water deficit is in L, TBW is in L (see Table 10–1 for % TBW), and current plasma [Na+] is in mmol/L.

FORMULA 2.   **CALCULATION OF TOTAL NA+ REQUIRED TO INCREASE PLASMA [NA+] TO DESIRED CONCENTRATION**

$$Na^+ \text{ requirement} = \text{TBW} \times (\text{desired}[Na^+]_p - \text{current}[Na^+]_p)$$

Na+ requirement is in mmol, TBW is in L, and desired and current plasma [Na+] are in mmol/L.

FORMULA 3.   **ESTIMATION OF EFFECT OF 1 L RETAINED INFUSATE ON PLASMA [NA+]**

$$\Delta[Na^+]_p = \frac{(\text{infusate } Na^+ + \text{infusate } K^+) - \text{plasma } Na^+}{\text{TBW} + 1}$$

$\Delta[Na^+]_p$ is the change in plasma [Na+] in mmol/L, infusate Na+ and K+ are the amounts (in mmol) of Na+ and K+ contained in 1 L infusate, plasma Na+ is the amount of Na+ in 1 L plasma, TBW is total body water in L, and 1 represents the additional L of fluid contributed by retention of 1 L infusate. From: Adrogué HJ, Madias NE: Aiding fluid prescription for the dysnatremias, *Int Care Med* 23:309–316, 1997.

Treatment of ECF volume depletion centers on restoration of plasma volume and takes precedence over treatment of hyperosmolar disorders. Correction proceeds at a rate faster than that for hyperosmolar disorders because of the importance of maintaining intravascular volume and adequate tissue perfusion. Fluid choices for expansion of ECF include normal saline (NS), blood products, and colloids. NS is more effective than hypotonic saline solutions at restoring ECF because, without an osmotic gradient, there will be no redistribution of water from the ECF to the ICF compartment. In other words, administration of 1 L NS will expand the ECF by 1 L. Administration of 1 L ½ NS (0.45% NaCl) is equivalent to administration of 500 ml NS and 500 ml electrolyte-free water (e.g., 5% dextrose

in water). The 500 ml NS will remain in the ECF. The 500 ml electrolyte-free water will distribute equally between the ICF and ECF according to compartment size: two thirds and one third, respectively. Thus, two thirds of 500 ml, or 335 ml, will redistribute to the ICF and one third of 500 ml, or 165 ml, will remain in the ECF, such that administration of 1 L 0.45% NaCl solution expands the ECF compartment by 665 ml (500 ml + 165 ml). Compartmental redistribution of select intravenous fluids and indications for use are summarized in Table 10-4.

Treatment of dehydration centers on correction of free water deficit and restoration of intracellular volume. Calculation of free water deficit is shown in Box 10-3. Whenever possible water should be given orally or through a nasogastric tube.[32]

TABLE 10-4

Compartmental Distribution of Select Intravenous Solutions and Indications for Use

Intravenous Solution	Compartmental Distribution of 1 L Infusate*			Indication
	ICF	ECF		
		Total	Intravascular	
5% Dextrose in water (D₅W)	667 ml	333 ml	83 ml	Correction of water deficit; replacement of electrolyte-free fluid losses
Normal saline (NS) (0.9% NaCl in water)	0 ml	1000 ml	250 ml	Treatment of ECF volume depletion; isotonic fluid replacement; maintenance IV fluid
½ NS (0.45% NaCl in water)	335 ml	665 ml	166 ml	Treatment of combined ECF volume depletion and dehydration; hypotonic fluid replacement
D₅ ½ NS (5% dextrose and (0.45% NaCl in water)	335 ml	665 ml	166 ml	Treatment of combined ECF volume depletion and dehydration; hypotonic fluid replacement
D₅NS (5% dextrose and 0.9% NaCl in water)	0 ml	1000 ml	250 ml	Treatment of ECF volume depletion; isotonic fluid replacement; maintenance IV fluid
Hypertonic saline (3% NaCl in water)	⇓	⇑	⇑	Treatment of severe symptomatic hyponatremia; change in ICF and ECF volumes dependent on degree of hyponatremia

ECF, extracellular fluid; *ICF*, intracellular fluid; *IV*, intravenous; *TBW*, total body water.
* Assumes ICF = ⅔ TBW, ECF = ⅓ TBW, intravascular (plasma) volume = ¼ ECF, infusion given under conditions of normal ECF tonicity, and glucose homeostasis maintained with infusion of dextrose-containing solutions.

Alternatively, intravenous electrolyte-free or hypotonic saline solutions can be used effectively to correct free water deficits. The intravenous solution selected depends on the desired rate of correction and the presence of concomitant ECF volume depletion or ongoing istonic or hypotonic fluid losses. Because of neurologic complications associated with rapid influx of water into brain cells as ECF osmolality decreases, care should be taken to avoid rapid correction of free water deficits. A general guideline is to replace no more than half the calculated water deficit in the first 24 hours. However, more important than the amount of fluid administered is the change in plasma [Na⁺] observed with treatment. Although there is no consensus for optimal rate of correction, suggested rates are generally on the order of 1.0 mmol/L per hour decrease in plasma [Na⁺] for hypernatremia of rapid (i.e., hours) development and 0.5 mmol/L per hour for hypernatremia of longer or unknown development.[8,28,32] Individuals in whom dehydration developed gradually are thought to be at greater risk of developing neurologic sequelae with rapid correction of hypernatremia.[32] Formula 3 in Box 10-3 predicts the change in plasma [Na⁺] induced by retention of 1 L of any infusate and may be useful as an adjunct in determining appropriate rate of infusion for the selected intravenous fluid.[30,32] Care must be given to providing appropriate maintenance fluids in addition to those required to correct deficits.

HYPERVOLEMIA. Expansion of the ECF volume (hypervolemia) occurs with decreased renal excretion of Na⁺ and water (e.g., with acute or chronic renal failure, nephrotic syndrome, cirrhosis, heart failure), excessive intravenous fluid administration, or interstitial fluid plasma fluid shifts (e.g., mobilization of third-space fluids, overadministration of hypertonic intravenous solutions).

Signs and symptoms of hypervolemia include shortness of breath, orthopnea, edema, increased blood pressure, weight gain, distended neck veins, crackles, rhonchi, wheezes, tachycardia, and moist skin.[1]

Treatment. Treatment of hypervolemia centers on restriction of Na⁺ and water, often in combination with diuretic therapy. Modification of nutrition support regimens should include volume restriction and removal or reduction of Na⁺ from parenteral nutrition formulations. Dialysis or continuous arteriovenous hemofiltration may be necessary when fluid overload is life threatening.

Electrolytes

Electrolyte disorders can occur concurrently with or independent of fluid imbalances. They result from a variety of medical and surgical conditions in which abnormal electrolyte losses or gains persist or in which normal regulatory mechanisms are rendered ineffective. Recognition and correction of these disorders is crucial to preventing a host of potentially life-threatening physiologic sequelae. In many instances parenteral nutrition (PN) formulations can be readily modified to aid in correction of fluid and electrolyte imbalances. Daily electrolyte additions to PN formulations and daily reference intakes (DRIs) are listed in Table 10-5. Electrolyte concentrations and osmolarities of commonly used intravenous solutions are listed in Table 10-3.

Sodium

Na⁺ is the most abundant extracellular cation. Na⁺ gains are realized through diet, medications, and Na⁺-containing intravenous fluids (e.g., saline solutions, PN formulations). Daily

TABLE 10-5

DRIs and Daily Electrolyte Additions to Adult PN Formulations

Electrolyte	Daily Addition to Adult Parenteral Nutrition Formulations[34]	Dietary Reference Intakes (DRI)[17,35] for adults >18 yr[a]	
Sodium	1-2 mEq/kg + replacement	500 mg/day[b]	
Potassium	1-2 mEq/kg + replacement	1000 mg/day[c]	
Calcium	10-15 mEq	1000-1200 mg/day[d]	
Phosphorus	20-40 mmol	580 mg/day[e]	700 mg/day[f]
Magnesium	8-20 mEq	♂ 330-350 mg/day[e]	400-420 mg/day[f]
		♀ 265 mg/day[e]	310-320 mg/day[f]

[a] Not pregnant or lactating.
[b] Estimated minimum requirement of healthy persons. No allowance has been made for large, prolonged losses from the skin through sweat. No evidence indicates that higher intakes confer any health benefits.[17]
[c] Estimated minimum requirement of healthy persons. Desirable intakes of potassium may considerably exceed these values.[17]
[d] AI, Adequate intake.[34]
[e] EAR, Estimated average requirement. The intake that meets the estimated nutrient needs of 50% of the individuals in a group.[34]
[f] RDA, Recommended dietary allowance. The intake that meets the estimated nutrient needs of 97% to 98% of the individuals in a group.[17]

Na^+ intake typically exceeds basal requirements. Losses occur principally through urine, sweat, and GI secretions. Maintaining Na^+ homeostasis relies on the body's ability to balance Na^+ gains with Na^+ losses. Total body Na^+ *content* is the principal determinant of ECF *volume* and Na^+ *concentration* is the principal determinant of plasma *osmolality*. Normal plasma $[Na^+]$ is 135 to 145 mmol/L. Although Na^+ and water balance are regulated independently, they are nonetheless closely intertwined. As described previously, changes in total body Na^+ content, and thus ECF volume, stimulate regulatory mechanisms to alter renal Na^+ excretion and restore ECF volume, whereas changes in $[Na^+]$, and thus plasma osmolality, stimulate a variety of regulatory mechanisms to restore water and osmolar homeostasis. Thirst perception, the ability to conserve Na^+, and the ability to dilute and concentrate urine may decline with advanced age, placing elderly patients receiving fixed amounts of fluids and electrolytes at risk for developing water and Na^+ imbalances.[14,15]

Disorders of plasma $[Na^+]$, dysnatremias, can occur concurrently with disorders of ECF volume and Na^+ balance, which have been detailed previously. However, plasma $[Na^+]$ does not, in and of itself, provide information about the fluid status of the extracellular compartment, nor does it reflect total body Na^+ stores. Hyponatremia can occur with volume excess and deficit, as can hypernatremia. Optimal treatment of dysnatremias can prove challenging. In many instances, medical nutrition therapy can be modified to support efforts directed at restoring normal plasma $[Na^+]$.

HYPONATREMIA. Hyponatremia (plasma $[Na^+]$ <135 mmol/L) represents a relative excess of water in relation to the body's total Na^+ content. Hyponatremia can be associated with low, normal, or high tonicity as well as states of low, normal, or high total body Na^+ content and ECF volume. Hyponatremia is a common clinical problem. A high prevalence of hyponatremia is found in patients hospitalized for acute illness, the risk increasing in parallel with the age of the patient.[14] Older patients in long-term care facilities are especially prone to hyponatremia. This is thought to be due in part to decreased Na^+ intake from diet or tube feedings combined with age-related impairment of renal Na^+ conservation.[14] Serious complications can arise from hyponatremia itself or from therapeutic error. Signs and symptoms relate to CNS dysfunction and may include lethargy, confusion, agitation, dysarthria, seizures, stupor, and coma.[25] During chronic hyponatremia, brain cells extrude solute, thereby reducing ICF osmolality, defending cell volume, and diminishing neurologic symptoms.[23,35] In the past, it has been assumed that the likelihood of brain damage from hyponatremia was directly related to the rapidity and degree of hyponatremia. More recently, other factors have been identified as being more important. These factors include age and gender, with children and menstruant women being the most susceptible.[27] Knowing the plasma osmolality (P_{OSM}) and urinary Na^+ (U_{NA}) is helpful in elucidating the cause of hyponatremia (Fig. 10-2).[9,36,37] Effective plasma osmolality (tonicity) determines the risk for cerebral edema.[6,30] The most common causes of severe hyponatremia in adults are thiazide diuretics,[38,39] postoperative states,[31] and other causes of syndrome of inappropriate antidiuretic hormone secretion (SIADH);[28] polydipsia in psychiatric patients, and transurethral prostatectomy (from massive absorption of Na^+-free irrigant solutions).[30]

Hypotonic hyponatremia (P_{OSM} <280 mOsm/L) represents an excess of water in relation to body Na^+ stores, which can be low, normal, or high. Dilutional hyponatremia caused by retention of water is the most common form of hyponatremia and generally reflects conditions that impair renal excretion of water.[30,35] Hyponatremia associated with impaired renal excretion of water is categorized according to status of ECF volume.

Hypovolemic hypotonic hyponatremia reflects deficits of both water and Na^+. This can occur with renal (U_{NA} >5 mmol/L) or extrarenal (U_{NA} <5 mmol/L) losses. Losses of renal origin include diuretics, salt-wasting nephropathy, bicarbonaturia, renal tubular acidosis (RTA), adrenal insufficiency, ketonuria, osmotic diuresis, and Bartter's syndrome. Extrarenal losses include vomiting, diarrhea, "third spacing" (e.g., bowel obstruction, peritonitis, pancreatitis, muscle trauma, burns), excessive sweating, and wound drainage.[8,30,35] As described previously, nursing home patients are at risk for developing depletional hyponatremia because of a combination of decreased Na^+ intake and impaired renal Na^+ conservation.

Isovolemic hypotonic hyponatremia is somewhat a misnomer and actually reflects an excess of TBW, a small proportion of which occurs in the ECF. This is associated with water intoxication (e.g., iatrogenic or psychogenic polydipsia), glucocorticoid deficiency, hypothyroidism, hypokalemia, and SIADH.[10,30,35] SIADH can be caused by CNS disorders, pulmonary disorders, tumors, postoperative state, pain, severe nausea,[30] infection with human immunodeficiency virus (HIV), and certain drugs.[26] In SIADH, antidiuretic hormone (ADH, vasopressin) is secreted inappropriately with respect to plasma osmolality. This results in inappropriately concentrated urine in the setting of decreased plasma osmolality. Continued intake of water combined with increased ADH levels causes expansion of ECF volume and dilutional hyponatremia.

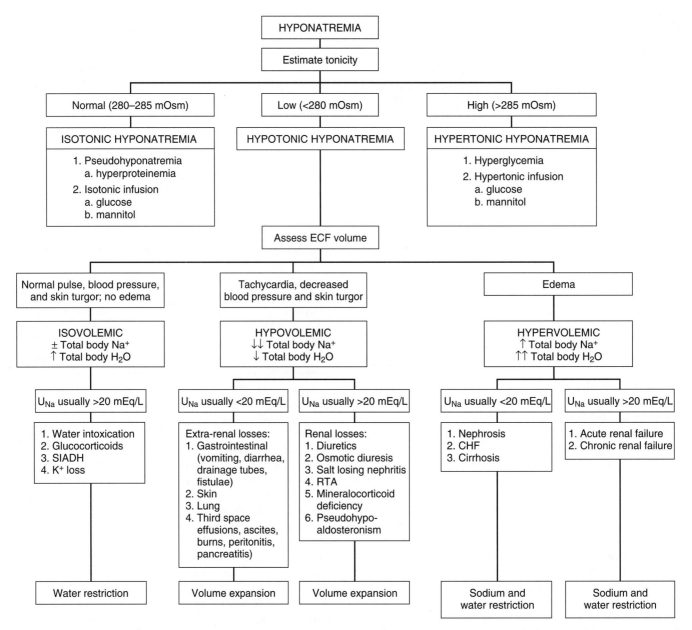

FIGURE 10-2 Evaluation of hyponatremia. *CHF,* Congestive heart failure; *ECF,* extracellular fluid; *RTA,* renal tubular acidosis; *SIADH,* syndrome of inappropriate antidiuretic hormone secretion; *TBW,* total body water. (Adapted from Avner ED: Clinical disorders of water metabolism: hyponatremia and hypernatremia, *Pediatr Ann* 24[1]:26, 1995; Narins RG, Jones ER, Stom MC, et al.: Diagnostic strategies in disorders of fluid, electrolyte and acid-base homeostasis, *Am J Med* 72:496, 1982.)

Hypervolemic hypotonic hyponatremia reflects excesses of both body water and Na^+, with a proportionately higher excess of body water. Causes include nephrotic syndrome, cirrhosis, congestive heart failure (U_{NA} <10 mmol/L), and renal failure (U_{NA} >20 mmol/L).

Isotonic hyponatremia (P_{OSM} 280 to 295 mOsm/L) usually results from hyperlipidemia or hyperproteinemia. It is often termed *pseudohyponatremia* because it results from laboratory artifact and does not represent true hyponatremia. Measurement of plasma $[Na^+]$ by flame photometry is based on total plasma volume, which includes water, protein, and lipid components. Na^+, however, is soluble only in the aqueous fraction. High levels of protein or lipid reduce the volume of the aqueous component in which the Na^+ is dissolved and, in so doing, result in an inap-

propriately low $[Na^+]$. Increasing use of ion-specific electrode measurement has all but eliminated artifactual hyponatremia.[30] Pseudohyponatremia is evident when the measured plasma osmolality is normal but the calculated osmolality is low.

Hypertonic hyponatremia (P_{OSM} >295 mOsm/L) is usually due to hyperglycemia or retention of hypertonic infusions of mannitol. The osmotic gradient that is created results in movement of water from the ICF to the ECF, thus diluting plasma $[Na^+]$.[1,6] For every 100-mg/dl increase in glucose or mannitol, plasma $[Na^+]$ decreases 1.6 mmol/L.[8]

Treatment. Optimal management of hypotonic hyponatremia dictates balancing risks of hypotonicity against those associated with treatment.[30,35] The presence and severity of symptoms determine rate of correction. Generally, symptoms of hyponatremia are not manifested until plasma concentrations reach 120 to 125 mmol/L. [35]

In cases of asymptomatic hypertonic or isotonic hyponatremia, efforts should be directed at correcting the underlying cause and replacing any Na^+, K^+, or water deficits. For example, insulin administration is appropriate treatment for hypertonic hyponatremia resulting from uncontrolled diabetes mellitus.

Asymptomatic hypovolemic hypotonic hyponatremia is appropriately managed with administration of isotonic saline solution. For the patient receiving enteral nutrition, NaCl can be added to the formula or given as NaCl tablets. [14] One teaspoon of table salt contains approximately 6 g NaCl ($\approx$ 104 mmol Na^+). Similarly, for patients receiving PN, Na^+ content can be increased using Cl^-, acetate, or phosphate salts. The Na^+ deficit can be estimated using Formula 2 in Box 10-3. Generally, no more than half this deficit should be replaced within the first 24 hours. [40] Plasma $[Na^+]$ should be monitored closely for correction rates that are more rapid than recommended. In addition to repletion of body Na^+ stores, water content of enteral or parenteral support regimens should be adjusted to help restore effective ECF volume. For hypervolemic hypotonic hyponatremia, fluid restriction is indicated. Diuresis may also be warranted. Enteral and parenteral nutrition support regimens should be adjusted to reduce water intake.

Fluid restriction is also indicated as initial treatment for isovolemic hypotonic hyponatremia, as observed in SIADH. Salt-loading results in increased urinary Na^+ wasting rather than correction of hyponatremia. Administration of isotonic saline is not suitable treatment for SIADH. It results in a transient increase in plasma $[Na^+]$, followed by an increased in Na^+ excretion, a net gain of water, and worsening of hyponatremia. The use of loop diuretics combined with a liberal NaCl intake to augment net water loss may prove beneficial in the treatment of SIADH. [30]

With severe, symptomatic hyponatremia, 3% hypertonic saline may be given judiciously until plasma $[Na^+]$ reaches 120 mmol/L or until symptoms resolve. To reduce the risk of neurologic complications resulting from rapid fluid shifts, *initial* correction should proceed at a rate no greater than 2 mmol/L per hour. This can generally be accomplished by administering 3% NaCl solution at a rate of 1 to 2 ml/kg per hour. [28,41,42] Alternatively, Formulas 2 and 3 in Box 10-3 can be used in guiding implementation of selected treatment plan as formulated by pathophysiologic and clinical considerations. [29] As symptoms subside, rate of correction should be reduced to approximately 1 mmol/L per hour. [30] Severe chronic hyponatremia, hepatic failure, alcoholism, K^+ depletion, and malnutrition increase the risk of osmotic demyelination associated with overly aggressive correction of hyponatremia. [43-45] For these patients, a slower, more conservative approach (i.e., no more than 0.5 mmol/L per hour increase in plasma $[Na^+]$) is warranted. [28] In general, targeted rate of correction should not exceed 8 to 12 mmol/L in 24 hours or 20 mmol/L in 48 hours. [26,28,30,39,46] Frequent monitoring of plasma $[Na^+]$ is imperative, especially during initial stages of treatment.

HYPERNATREMIA. Hypernatremia (plasma $[Na^+]$ >145 mmol/L) represents a deficit of water in relation to total body Na^+ content and always denotes a state of hypertonicity and cellular dehydration, at least transiently. [32] As such, signs and symptoms are primarily of CNS origin and include altered mental status, lethargy, irritability, restlessness, seizures (in children), muscle twitching, hyperreflexia, spasticity, fever, nausea, vomiting, labored breathing, and intense thirst. [25,41] Signs and symptoms are generally more pronounced when the increase in plasma $[Na^+]$ concentration is of great magnitude or occurs rapidly. [32] Hypernatremia that develops gradually allows for greater brain adaptation. Acutely, there is rapid uptake of electrolytes by brain cells, which in turn minimizes the reduction in brain cell volume. This is followed by a slower adaptive phase during which organic osmolytes accumulate and brain cell volume is restored. [18] Hypernatremia is less common than hyponatremia. Because of the effectiveness of the thirst and renal-concentrating mechanisms in defending against water depletion and hypertonicity, sustained hypernatremia is observed only in the setting of impaired thirst or inability to self-regulate water intake. [18,32] Those at risk include elderly patients, infants, patients receiving hypertonic infusions, tube feedings, osmotic diuretics, or lactulose; patients on mechanical ventilation, and those with altered mental status, uncontrolled diabetes, or underlying polyuric disorders. [14,25,33,41]

Because hypernatremia can occur with decreased, normal, or increased total body Na^+ stores, it is helpful to categorize according to total body Na^+ content (Fig. 10-3). Hypernatremia with decreased total body Na^+ results from losses of both water and Na^+, with a relatively greater proportion of water loss. Clinical presentation includes signs of hypovolemia, such as orthostatic hypotension, tachycardia, flattened neck veins, poor skin turgor, and dry mucous membranes. [41] The causes reflect renal or extrarenal loss of hypotonic fluid. Hypernatremia with normal total body Na^+ results from renal or extrarenal loss of water, the former due to a defect in vasopressin production or renal response to the hormone. Hypernatremia due to extrarenal water loss only develops in those without access to water or with neurologic deficits that preclude them from seeking water in response to thirst. [18] With no loss of total body Na^+ content, approximately two thirds of the water loss will be realized by the ICF compartment. Therefore, patients with hypernatremia and normal total body Na^+ content typically appear euvolemic. Hypernatremia with increased total body Na^+ is the least common form of hypernatremia and generally results from administration of hypertonic saline solutions, sodium bicarbonate ($NaHCO_3$), or ingestion of salt tablets. [41]

Treatment. Evaluation of hypernatremia and determination of treatment approach is depicted in Fig. 10-3. The goal of treatment is to restore normal effective ECF volume, alleviate symptoms, normalize plasma $[Na^+]$ at an acceptable rate, and restore ICF volume. Overzealous correction of hypernatremia can result in rapid fluid shifts and associated neurologic complications including cerebral edema, seizures, permanent brain injury, and death. [18,32] In general, the slower the development of hypernatremia, the greater the brain adaptation and the greater the risks associated with rapid correction. Thus, hypernatremia of gradual or unknown rate of development should be corrected more slowly than that which developed rapidly. Although there is no consensus for optimal rate of correction, suggested rates are generally on the order of 1.0 mmol/L per hour decrease in plasma $[Na^+]$ for hypernatremia of rapid (i.e., hours) development and 0.5 mmol/L per hour for hypernatremia of longer or

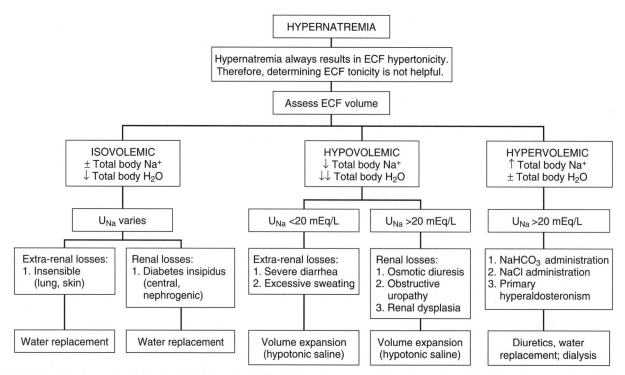

FIGURE 10-3 Evaluation of hypernatremia. *ECF,* Extracellular fluid; *TBW,* total body water. (Adapted from Avner ED: Clinical disorders of water metabolism, *Hyponatremia Hypernatremia Ann* 24[1]:28, 1995.)

unknown development.[32] Because hypernatremia is always associated with hypertonicity, measurement of plasma osmolality is not helpful in evaluation and treatment. A thorough assessment of the patient's fluid status is, however, important because hypernatremia can occur with hypovolemia, isovolemia, and hypervolemia. For the patient receiving PN, adjustments in PN formulation can be made to help restore normal plasma [Na⁺] and ECF volume.

In hypovolemic hypernatremia, total body Na⁺ content is low. The *volume* deficit should be corrected first, using isotonic saline, until hemodynamic stability is attained. Then, the *water* deficit should be corrected with water given orally or through a feeding tube, or with intravenous solutions such as hypotonic saline or 5% dextrose in water.[32,41] Estimation of water deficit is shown in Box 10-3. Formula 1 provides an adequate estimate of water deficit in hypernatremia secondary to pure water loss; however, it underestimates the deficit in patients with hypotonic fluid loss.[32] No more than half of the water deficit should be corrected within the first 24 hours.[18,41] For patients receiving PN, the Na⁺ content should be reduced so as only to replace ongoing Na⁺ losses. The volume can be increased to help correct the water deficit and replace ongoing losses.

In euvolemic hypernatremia, water losses far exceed solute losses. The water deficit should be calculated and replaced as previously described. The PN formulation should be adjusted to match water and solute losses.

In hypervolemic hypernatremia, the goal is to remove the excess Na⁺. This is achieved through the combined use of diuretics (e.g., furosemide) and 5% dextrose in water.[41] Hemodialysis may be required for renal failure. Na⁺ should be eliminated from PN formulations.

Close monitoring of plasma [Na⁺] during treatment is essential to achieve rates of correction within suggested guidelines. Treatment should be reformulated if rate of correction is too fast. Formula 3 in Box 10-3 projects the effect of 1 L retained infusate on plasma [Na⁺] and can be used to further guide implementation of selected treatment. As with correction of any deficit, care must be given to replacement of ongoing losses in addition to correction of estimated deficit.

Potassium

Potassium (K⁺) is crucial to maintaining cell volume, hydrogen ion concentration, enzyme function, protein synthesis, cell growth, and neuromuscular activity. Total body K⁺ in hospitalized patients is approximately 43 mmol/kg body weight.[47] Only a small portion of this, 2%, is located in the ECF. Normal plasma [K⁺] is 3.5 to 5.0 mmol/L. The tremendous K⁺ concentration gradient between the ICF and ECF compartments is maintained through the action of the energy-dependent Na⁺-K⁺-ATPase pump, which also maintains the ECF to ICF Na⁺ concentration gradient. The gradient of [K⁺] across the cell membrane determines the membrane potential. Changes in the ratio of intracellular to extracellular K⁺ can adversely affect neuromuscular and cardiac function by altering nerve and muscle cell resting membrane potentials. Distribution of K⁺ between the two compartments is affected by acid-base status; osmolality; and various hormones, including insulin, epinephrine, and aldosterone.[1]

The estimated minimum requirement of healthy persons and the amount typically added to PN formulations are listed in Table 10-5. K⁺ enters the body through food, medications, and K⁺-containing intravenous fluids. The body also "releases" K⁺ into the ECF whenever there is cell breakdown (e.g., tissue catabolism, rhabdomyolysis, hematoma resorption), or when ECF pH drops (i.e., acidemia). K^+ losses occur through the kidneys, GI tract, and skin. About 90% of daily K^+ intake is excreted in the urine.[47] Formed stools contain about 5 to 10 mmol/day. K^+ loss via the skin is generally negligible because sweat contains only 5 to 10 mmol/L and total daily volume is small.[1]

The kidneys are the principal regulators of K^+ balance. K^+ homeostasis is maintained by adjusting the amount excreted in the urine. The kidneys, however, do not conserve K^+ as efficiently Na^+. Even during states of K^+ depletion, appreciable amounts can still be lost in the urine. Obligatory renal K^+ loss is 5 to 10 mmol/day.[48]

HYPOKALEMIA. Hypokalemia (plasma $[K^+]$ <3.5 mmol/L) is one of the most common electrolyte abnormalities encountered in clinical practice, occurring in more than 20% of hospitalized patients.[49] Hypokalemia results from a decrease in total body K^+ or a shift of K^+ from the ECF to the ICF. K^+ depletion is rarely due to inadequate dietary K^+ intake. More often, K^+ depletion is due to increased renal or extrarenal losses. Elderly individuals, especially those living alone, and hospitalized patients receiving K^+-free intravenous fluids or PN formulas with insufficient K^+ are at greater risk.[1,49] Most GI secretions are K^+-rich (Table 10-2), so abnormally large GI losses carry the risk of hypokalemia. Such losses occur with vomiting, gastric suctioning, diarrhea, drainage, and laxative abuse. Hypokalemia due to vomiting results more from renal K^+ loss than from K^+ loss in the vomitus. Vomiting causes volume contraction and metabolic alkalosis with subsequent renal K^+ wasting.[47,50] Excessive renal K^+ loss occurs with hyperaldosteronism, excess mineralocorticoids, chronic metabolic acidosis (e.g., type I and type II renal tubular acidosis), Mg^{2+} deficiency, acute leukemia, and Liddle's syndrome.[1,47] Intracellular K^+ shifts occur with anabolism, nutritional recovery state (i.e., refeeding syndrome), alkalosis (more so with metabolic alkalosis than with respiratory alkalosis), barium poisoning, and increased levels of insulin, epinephrine, and aldosterone.[1,47,51] Plasma $[K^+]$ reflects ECF K^+ content but is not indicative of total body stores. However, at normal pH, a decrease in plasma $[K^+]$ from 4 to 3 mmol/L generally indicates a K^+ loss of 150 to 200 mmol. A 2-mmol/L decrease in plasma $[K^+]$ indicates a loss in excess of 500 mmol.[47] Clinical manifestations of K^+ depletion vary greatly among individual patients. Symptoms seldom occur unless plasma $[K^+]$ is less than 3 mmol/L[50] and include muscle weakness, leg cramps, nausea, vomiting, ileus, paresthesias, and a weak, irregular pulse.

Treatment. Treatment of hypokalemia is directed at the underlying cause. Any existing alkalosis should be corrected. In the absence of increased metabolic demand and cellular uptake of K^+ (e.g., anabolism, refeeding syndrome, insulin and glucose administration), hypokalemia is generally a result of excessive GI or renal K^+ losses. Urine K^+ levels are useful in evaluating causes of hypokalemia. Excretion of more than 40 mmol/24 hr indicates renal K^+ wasting (e.g., due to diuretics, alkalosis, increased aldosterone levels, chronic interstitial nephritis, pyelonephritis, or nephrotoxic agents). Urine K^+ excretion less than 20 mmol/24 hr signifies the kidneys are conserving K^+ appropriately and there is likely a total body

deficit.[47] The therapeutic goals are to correct the K^+ deficit and minimize ongoing losses.[50] K^+ replacement can be given orally or parenterally as any of a variety of available K^+ salts, depending on route of administration and the presence of coexisting acid-base imbalances. KCl is the preferred agent for treatment of K^+ loss associated with chloride depletion (e.g., that resulting from diuretic therapy, vomiting, or gastric drainage).[49] It is generally safer to correct hypokalemia via the oral route. Various K^+ replacement guidelines have been described in the literature. MacLaren and colleagues recently devised evidence-based guidelines for electrolyte replacement in the intensive care unit, taking into consideration degree of depletion, creatinine clearance, and route of administration.[52] Alternatively, the K^+ deficit can be estimated based on plasma $[K^+]$. Generally, only half of this amount should be replaced in the first 24 hours.[40] Intravenous K^+ is indicated when oral dosing is not feasible or when hypokalemia is severe. K^+ concentrations in solutions given by peripheral vein should not exceed 40 mmol/L.[50] Intravenous K^+ administration should not exceed 10 to 20 mmol/hr. Patients receiving this amount warrant electrocardiogram monitoring. For the patient receiving PN, the K^+ content can be increased in the form of potassium chloride, potassium acetate, or potassium phosphate (3 mmol potassium phosphate yields about 4.4 mmol K^+). The amount should be increased judiciously to replace ongoing losses and correct the deficit. For plasma concentrations less than 3.5 mmol/L, separate intravenous KCl supplementation may be indicated. A dose of 20 mmol KCl in 100 ml saline given over 1 hour usually increases plasma $[K^+]$ by 0.2 mmol/L.[40] If hypokalemia is attributed to refeeding syndrome, carbohydrate and overall caloric intake should be reduced until K^+ stores are replenished. This is accomplished by reducing the dextrose content of the PN formulation or reducing the amount of enteral formula provided. Throughout treatment, plasma $[K^+]$ should be monitored closely to avoid overcorrection. If hypokalemia is refractory to treatment, plasma $[Mg^{2+}]$ should be checked because hypomagnesemia results in increased renal secretion of K^+.[50]

HYPERKALEMIA. Hyperkalemia (plasma $[K^+]$ >5.0 mmol/L) can result from an increase in exogenous (e.g., diet, medications, blood transfusions, intravenous fluids) or endogenous K^+ load (e.g., crush injury, rhabdomyolysis, hemolysis, GI hemorrhage, catabolism, administration of cytotoxic agents), an extracellular K^+ shift (acidosis, more so with metabolic acidosis than with respiratory acidosis[47]), or inadequate K^+ excretion (e.g., renal failure, adrenal insufficiency).[1,50] Sustained hyperkalemia is almost always caused by impaired renal excretion.[47,50] GI adaptation (i.e., decreased K^+ absorption) helps maintain normal K^+ levels as renal failure progresses. Hyperkalemia is generally not seen until the glomerular filtration rate (GFR) is less than 10 ml/min.[26] Fasting can worsen hyperkalemia in patients with chronic renal failure because of the reduction in cellular K^+ uptake associated with decreased insulin levels.[26] Pseudohyperkalemia can occur with hemolyzed blood samples, leukocytosis, and thrombocytosis. Hyperosmolar states can also cause hyperkalemia. For each 10-mOsm/L increase in effective plasma osmolality, plasma $[K^+]$ can increase 0.4 to 0.8 mmol/L. As with hypokalemia, alterations in plasma $[K^+]$ represent changes in ECF K^+ content but are not indicative of total body stores. Because such a small proportion of total body K^+ resides in the ECF, even slight changes in plasma $[K^+]$ affect the concentration gradient dramatically. This in turn causes neuromuscular dysfunction and accounts for the cardiovascular and GI symptoms associated with hyperkalemia. Cardiovascular symptoms include electrocardiographic abnormalities, bradycardia, hypotension, ventricular fibrillation, and diastolic cardiac arrest. GI symptoms include nausea, vomiting, diarrhea, and intestinal colic. Additionally, symptoms such as confusion, irritability, weakness, paresthesias, and areflexia can occur.[1]

Treatment. Treatment of hyperkalemia begins with assessment of cause. Therapeutic options include reducing total body K^+ content, shifting K^+ intracellularly, and antagonizing the membrane effect of hyperkalemia. Reduction of total body K^+ can by accomplished by reduction of K^+ intake, enhancement of fecal excretion (e.g., K^+-exchange resin, sorbitol), enhancement of renal excretion (e.g., mineralocorticoids, increased salt intake/cautious volume expansion, diuretics), and dialysis. Administration of glucose and insulin, alkali, or β-agonists promotes intracellular shift of K^+. The membrane effect of hyperkalemia is antagonized by administration of calcium salts and hypertonic saline.[47] Patients with electrocardiogram signs of hyperkalemia are at risk for life-threatening arrhythmias and should receive intravenous calcium gluconate.[26]

Calcium

Calcium (Ca^{2+}) is the fifth most abundant mineral element[53] and third most abundant cation in the human body. In addition to its obvious importance in skeletal physiology, Ca^{2+} plays a vital role in many neuromuscular and enzymatic processes. Of the 1000 to 1200 g of Ca^{2+} in the average adult, approximately 98% is contained in the skeleton.[53] Only 1% of the total skeletal reservoir of Ca^{2+} is exchangeable with ECF. Normal daily intake of Ca^{2+} is 1 to 3 g.[1] The majority of this is excreted via the GI tract, 200 mg or less is excreted in the urine, and small amounts (15 to 100 mg) are lost in sweat.[1,53] In the adult, there is no persistent net gain or loss of Ca^{2+} in health.[53] The dietary reference intake (DRI) and amount typically added to PN formulations are listed in Table 10-5. Normal plasma total $[Ca^{2+}]$ is 8.0 to 11.0 mg/dl. Ca^{2+} homeostasis is regulated by various hormones that influence GI Ca^{2+} absorption, renal Ca^{2+} excretion, and skeletal Ca^{2+} resorption. Low plasma Ca^{2+} levels stimulate release of parathyroid hormone (PTH). This increases bone resorption, stimulates renal conservation of Ca^{2+}, and activates vitamin D, which in turn increases GI Ca^{2+} absorption.[1,53,54] Calcitonin is released by the thyroid gland in response to hypercalcemia and acts by inhibiting bone resorption.

Plasma Ca^{2+} exists in three forms: ionized, bound, and complexed. Ionized Ca^{2+} is the most physiologically important and accounts for approximately 45% of plasma Ca^{2+}. Approximately 40% of plasma Ca^{2+} is bound to proteins, principally albumin, and the remaining 15% is in the form of phosphate, citrate, sulfate, lactate, and bicarbonate complexes. The ratio of ionized to total Ca^{2+} is affected by plasma pH and protein levels. Acidosis increases and alkalosis decreases the ionized fraction. A pH change of 0.1 to 0.2 units can elicit a 10% change in ionized $[Ca^{2+}]$.[3] Hypoalbuminemia decreases total $[Ca^{2+}]$, but does not affect ionized $[Ca^{2+}]$. Total plasma

Ca^{2+} is the Ca^{2+} measure performed most frequently in the laboratory. Because ionized Ca^{2+} is the physiologically active form, interpretation of total Ca^{2+} values must accommodate any intercurrent hypoalbuminemia or acid-base disturbances. The total $[Ca^{2+}]$ corrected for hypoalbuminemia can be estimated as follows:

$$\text{Total } Ca^{2+}_{CORRECTED} \text{ (mg/dl)} = \text{Total } Ca^{2+}_{MEASURED} \text{ (mg/dl)} + ([4-\text{albumin (g/dl)}] \times 0.8).$$

Because this is only an approximation, measurement of ionized Ca^{2+} is often preferred, especially in cases of acid-base imbalance, hemodialysis, myeloma, renal failure, cirrhosis, treatment with thiazide diuretics, sepsis, cardiovascular instability, massive transfusions and citrated blood products, plasmapheresis, cardiopulmonary bypass, and liver transplantation.[53]

HYPOCALCEMIA. Symptomatic hypocalcemia can occur with a decrease in total body Ca^{2+} or a decrease in the fraction of ionized Ca^{2+}. Hypocalcemia (total $Ca^{2+}_{CORRECTED}$ < 8.0 mg/dL; ionized Ca^{2+} < 4.5 mg/dl) can result from many disorders that decrease Ca^{2+} absorption, increase its loss, or alter its regulation. Decreased GI Ca^{2+} absorption occurs with decreased vitamin D_3 activity (e.g., vitamin D deficiency, hyperphosphatemia, pseudohypoparathyroidism, acute or chronic renal failure), decreased mucosal mass (e.g., massive small bowel resection), menopause, advanced age, rapid intestinal transit time, and steatorrhea.[54] Other causes of hypocalcemia include decreased PTH activity (e.g., acute pancreatitis, hypomagnesemia, hypoparathyroidism), hungry-bone syndrome (e.g., parathyroidectomy, thyroidectomy), massive soft tissue damage or infection (e.g., crush injuries, rhabdomyolysis, necrotizing fasciitis), and massive blood transfusions. Symptoms of hypocalcemia are neuromuscular and include tetany, paresthesias, muscle weakness, muscle and abdominal cramps, hyperactive deep tendon reflexes, and electrocardiographic changes (prolonged QT interval). Expression of symptoms reflects both the absolute $[Ca^+]$ and its rate of fall.

Treatment. In the absence of symptoms, treatment is not emergent. The cause of hypocalcemia should be identified and treated concurrently with Ca^{2+} repletion. Oral Ca^{2+} supplementation to provide 1000 to 1500 mg elemental Ca^{2+} per day is generally adequate for patients who are asymptomatic or require long-term supplementation. Absorption of Ca^{2+} supplements improves if they are taken with food, perhaps as a result of slower gastric emptying and increased time in which the Ca^{2+}-containing chyme is in contact with the absorptive surface.[54] For patients receiving PN, the Ca^{2+} content can be increased within institution-specific compatibility guidelines for Ca^{2+}/PO_4^{3-} and Ca^{2+}/Mg^{2+} concentrations. Exceeding recommended guidelines can result in solution instability and the formation of insoluble precipitates.[33] If the Ca^{2+} cannot be increased sufficiently in the PN formulation, or if the patient is symptomatic, separate intravenous Ca^{2+} supplementation, typically in the form of calcium gluconate, is warranted.

HYPERCALCEMIA. Symptomatic hypercalcemia (total $Ca^{2+}_{CORRECTED}$ >11.0 mg/dl; ionized Ca^{2+} >5.5 mg/dl) can occur with either a rise in total $[Ca^{2+}]$ or an increase in the fraction of ionized Ca^{2+}. The critical level for emergency treatment of hypercalcemia is greater than 15 mg/dl.[1] Hypercalcemia essentially never occurs from ingestion of natural food sources, but has been reported with excessive ingestion of Ca^{2+} supplements, usually taken with absorbable alkali (i.e., Ca^{2+}-based antacids).[54] The principal causes of hypercalcemia are hyperparathyroidism and cancer with bone metastases, typically metastatic breast cancer with concomitant estrogen replacement therapy.[1] Additional causes include vitamin D toxicity, hyperthyroidism, sarcoidosis, and prolonged immobilization. Early symptoms of hypercalcemia include fatigue, muscle weakness, anorexia, nausea, vomiting, constipation, and depression. Symptoms can progress to psychosis, obtundation, coma, and death. Chronic hypercalcemia can affect renal concentrating capability and result in polyuria, polydipsia, and metastatic Ca^{2+} deposits. Metastatic soft tissue calcification is most likely to occur when the plasma calcium-phosphorous product (Ca × P) exceeds 55 mg^2/dl^2.[55]

Treatment. Symptomatic hypercalcemia is life threatening and requires immediate treatment, which typically involves expansion of the ECF so that urine output and subsequent Ca^{2+} excretion increases. Saline is the fluid of choice because Na^+ competes with Ca^{2+} for tubular reabsorption.[1] Concurrent administration of furosemide is used to induce diuresis. Patients with renal failure or life-threatening hypercalcemia may need dialysis. Ca^{2+} should be omitted from PN formulations until symptoms abate. Additional treatment after volume expansion and diuresis may include calcitonin (most effective for hypercalcemia secondary to increased parathyroid hormone) or gallium nitrate (for hypercalcemia associated with metastatic disease) to reduce bone resorption. Corticosteroids decrease intestinal Ca^{2+} absorption, renal tubular absorption, and bone resorption and may be useful in treating hypercalcemia of multiple myeloma, lymphomas, Addison's disease, or vitamin D toxicity.[1] Use of inorganic phosphates reduces plasma Ca^{2+} levels by decreasing bone resorption and forming calcium-phosphate complexes. However, this therapy can result in serious complications and is used only when other treatment proves ineffective.[1]

Phosphorus

Phosphorus (P), the most abundant intracellular anion, is critically important in every cell of the body.[56] Phosphorus is a structural component of bones and teeth, facilitates normal nerve and muscle function, and acts as an acid-base buffer in the urine. Phosphorus is a key component of virtually every enzyme system and plays a vital role in cellular bioenergetics. About 80% to 85% of the 500 to 800 g of phosphorus contained in the adult body is present in bones as hydroxyapatite crystals and is slowly exchangeable with the small fraction in the ECF (only 1%).[51,53] The remaining 14% is found in soft tissues. The DRI and amount typically added to PN formulations are listed in Table 10-5.

Phosphorus homeostasis is maintained by the small intestine, kidneys, and skeleton under the hormonal influence of PTH, vitamin D, and calcitonin. Typical intake is 800 to 1400 mg, about two thirds of which is absorbed, primarily in the jejunum.[53,57] Absorption is enhanced with decreased dietary Ca^{2+}, increased acidity of intestinal contents, and the actions of vitamin D and growth hormone. Under conditions of phosphorus balance, most of the phosphorus absorbed from the intestine is excreted in the urine. Urinary phosphorus losses increase under the influence of PTH and calcitonin. Urinary losses generally decrease with anabolism and phosphorus deficiency.

Most of the phosphorus in the ECF exists as inorganic phosphate ions, predominately HPO_4^{2-} and $H_2PO_4^-$. The relative amounts of these two ions are pH dependent. In clinical practice, the terms *phosphorus* and *phosphate* are used interchangeably, although this is not technically correct. The laboratory measures inorganic phosphorus (P_i), expressed in milligrams per deciliter or millimoles per liter.[53] Normal serum P_i concentration is 2.5 to 4.5 mg/dl. Phosphate levels are affected by intake, intestinal absorption, renal excretion, hormonal regulation associated with bone metabolism, and factors that induce transcellular shifts. Serum $[P_i]$ is not a reliable indicator of total body stores.

HYPOPHOSPHATEMIA. Hypophosphatemia (serum $[P_i]$ <2.5 mg/dl) can occur with or without depletion of body phosphate stores. Similarly, a normal serum $[P_i]$ does not exclude the possibility of phosphate depletion because the body strives to maintain normal serum concentrations despite declining stores. Hypophosphatemia with phosphate depletion occurs gradually as a result of inadequate dietary phosphorus intake or impaired absorption. This occurs with alcoholism or other diseases associated with poor nutrient intake, prolonged use of phosphorus-binding antacids, or GI disorders that result in malabsorption, maldigestion, or steatorrhea.[51,57] Hypophosphatemia that develops suddenly is far more common and can result from internal redistribution (e.g., refeeding syndrome, recovery from diabetic ketoacidosis (DKA), respiratory alkalosis, glucose and insulin administration) or increased urinary losses (e.g., hyperaldosteronism, corticosteroids, osmotic diuresis, hypomagnesemia, hypokalemia, hyperparathyroidism, thiazide diuretics, inhibition of carbonic anhydrase, alcohol abuse, renal tubule defects, acute volume expansion, vitamin D deficiency, hungry bone syndrome).[57,58] In DKA, hypophosphatemia results from glucose-induced osmotic diuresis and the intracellular shift that follows glucose and insulin administration. Hypophosphatemia associated with refeeding syndrome can be severe and results from enhanced intracellular ion transport associated with carbohydrate-stimulated insulin release and cellular anabolism.[59] Although hypophosphatemia is generally not associated with chronic renal failure, it is observed with the initiation of PN in those patients with renal failure who also have underlying malnutrition.[60] Development of hypophosphatemia is common in patients with acute renal failure treated by continuous renal replacement therapy (CCRT).[61]

Clinical manifestations of hypophosphatemia include altered bone and mineral metabolism, and disorders of muscle, cardiac, respiratory, hematologic, and central nervous systems. Proximal myopathy, dysphagia, and ileus are common alterations of skeletal and smooth muscle.[57] Weakness of the respiratory muscles can lead to respiratory fatigue and acute respiratory failure.[51] Rhabdomyolysis may complicate severe cases, particularly in alcoholic patients with phosphate depletion.[56,57] Neuromuscular manifestations include acute areflexic paralysis, paresthesias, weakness, numbness, confusion, and coma.[51]

Treatment. Recognizing patients at risk for developing hypophosphatemia is a key component of management. Any form of nutrition support, be it oral, enteral, or parenteral, should be instituted cautiously when there is a high index of suspicion for refeeding syndrome. In this setting, it has been recommended that dextrose infusions be started at a rate of 2 mg/kg per minute.[62] A similar approach is warranted for enteral feedings, for example, starting at 50% estimated caloric needs.[51] Nutrition support regimens should not be advanced until hypophosphatemia and any other attendant electrolyte imbalances have been corrected. Increased recognition of the prevalence and significance of hypophosphatemia in patients receiving nutrition support has led to more aggressive repletion regimens.[51,63] Intravenous dosing schemes have been proposed as both graduated and fixed doses. In patients receiving specialized nutrition, Clark and associates recommend a graduated dosing scheme of 0.16 mmol/kg (over 4 to 6 hours), 0.32 mmol/kg (over 4 to 6 hours), and 0.64 mmol/kg (over 8 to 12 hours) for mild, moderate, and severe hypophosphatemia, respectively. [64] For critically ill patients with moderate hypophosphatemia, Rosen and associates recommend a fixed dose of 15 mmol (over 2 hours), with repeated dosing to a maximum of 45 mmol in 24 hours.[65]

MacLaren and colleagues recently devised evidence-based guidelines for P_i and other electrolyte replacement in the intensive care unit, taking into consideration degree of depletion, creatinine clearance, and route of administration.[52] In patients receiving PN, additional phosphate can be added to the PN formulation as sodium or potassium phosphate. However, because of concentration limits imposed by calcium-phosphate compatibility guidelines, separate intravenous phosphate infusion is usually required for moderate to severe hypophosphatemia. Assignment of severity of hypophosphatemia varies among investigators, institutions, and laboratory assays; however, in general, mild hypophosphatemia is characterized by values greater than 2.0 mg/dl, moderate by values 1.0 to 2.0 mg/dl, and severe by values less than 1.0 mg/dl. Mild hypophosphatemia can be treated with oral phosphate supplements such as Phospho-Soda (sodium phosphate) or Neutra Phos (sodium and potassium phosphate). During repletion, serum $[P_i]$ concentration should be monitored closely to evaluate response to treatment. Levels should be measured several hours after supplementation to allow time for intracellular redistribution. The therapeutic end point of phosphate repletion is a sustained concentration within normal limits.[51]

HYPERPHOSPHATEMIA. Hyperphosphatemia (serum $[P_i]$ >4.5 mg/dl) can result from increased exogenous or endogenous phosphorus load, enhanced GI absorption, or decreased urinary excretion. Exogenous sources include diet (rarely), PN formulations, phosphate supplements, and phosphate-containing enemas.[56] Endogenous release of phosphate into the ECF occurs with significant cellular destruction (e.g., administration of cytotoxic agents, hypercatabolic states, hemolysis, rhabdomyolysis, and malignant hyperthermia) or extracellular redistribution (e.g., lactic acidosis, respiratory acidosis, and the early stages of DKA).[56,57] The most common cause of hyperphosphatemia is decreased urinary excretion due to acute or chronic renal failure. Decreased urinary phosphorus excretion can also occur with hypoparathyroidism, acromegaly, and thy-

rotoxicosis.[57] Hyperphosphatemia is usually asymptomatic; however, hypocalemia and tetany can occur with rapid increases in serum phosphorus. Metastatic soft tissue calcification becomes a concern as the calcium-phosphorus product exceeds 55 mg^2/dl^2.[55] Chronic hyperphosphatemia may lead to renal osteodystrophy in patients with renal failure.

Treatment. In the absence of renal insufficiency, volume expansion with isotonic saline solution will increase the fractional excretion of P_i by the kidneys.[56] Exogenous sources of phosphorus should be eliminated or minimized and phosphate binders (e.g., calcium carbonate, aluminum hydroxide) employed to reduce GI absorption. Patients with renal failure are discouraged from long-term use of aluminum hydroxide antacids because aluminum is toxic for bones, bone marrow, and the brain.[57] Dialysis may be required for patients who have kidney disease or serum P_i levels in excess of 10 to 12 mg/dl.[56]

Magnesium

Mg^{2+} is the body's fourth most prevalent cation and is second to K^+ in terms of intracellular concentration. Mg^{2+} is crucial to many cell functions. It is a critical cofactor in more than 300 enzymatic reactions involving cellular bioenergetics, as well as protein and nucleic acid synthesis.[66] Mg^{2+} is also vital in bone mineralization, transmission of neuromuscular activity, CNS activity, and myocardial function and may be cardioprotective against sudden death.[66,67] The normal total body Mg^{2+} content is about 24 g, approximately 50% to 60% of which is incorporated into bone.[53,57] Only 1% is located in the ECF. The remainder is found in soft tissues. Both intracellular and extracellular Mg^{2+} exists in three states: free or ionized (the physiologically active form); complexed (to citrate, phosphate, bicarbonate); and protein-bound. In ECF, 61% of total Mg^{2+} is ionized, 6% is complexed, and 33% is protein bound.[66] Hypoalbuminemia results in decreased total $[Mg^{2+}]$, but does not affect ionized levels. In clinical practice, serum rather than plasma $[Mg^{2+}]$ is measured because the anticoagulants used for plasma affect the assay.[53,68] The normal range for serum Mg^{2+} is 1.7 to 2.5 mg/dl (0.7 to 1.1 mmol/L). As with other ions that are found primarily intracellularly, ECF concentration is a poor indicator of total body stores.

Mg^{2+} homeostasis is regulated by GI absorption and renal excretion. Normally, only one third of dietary Mg^{2+} is absorbed. Renal excretion of Mg^{2+} varies and is affected by Na^+ and Ca^{2+} excretion, PTH, ECF volume, and plasma $[Mg^{2+}]$.[57] Mg^{2+} excretion decreases with decreased Na^+ and Ca^{2+} excretion, decreased ECF volume, decreased plasma $[Mg^{2+}]$, and increased levels of PTH.[57] The kidneys have an amazing ability to conserve Mg^{2+}. In the absence of exogenous sources, renal excretion may be as low as 0.5 mmol per day. The average daily Mg^{2+} intake in the United States ranges from 240 to 365 mg.[67] The DRI and the amount typically added to PN formulations are listed in Table 10-5.

HYPOMAGNESEMIA. Mg^{2+} deficiency is one of the most overlooked electrolyte alterations among hospitalized patients,[69] perhaps because its existence may be masked by normal serum $[Mg^{2+}]$. As of yet, there is no straightforward alternative Mg^{2+} measure other than total serum $[Mg^{2+}]$.[70] Hypomagnesemia (serum $[Mg^{2+}]$ <1.7 mg/dl; 0.7 mmol/L) can result from (1) diminished intake (e.g., protein-calorie malnutrition, alcoholism), (2) impaired GI absorption or excessive GI loss (e.g., malabsorption with steatorrhea [Mg^{2+} and Ca^{2+} combine with fatty acids to form poorly absorbable soap complexes in the intestinal lumen],[71] severe diarrhea, fistulas, nasogastric suctioning, laxative abuse), and (3) increased urinary loss (e.g., diuretic phase of acute tubular necrosis, postrenal transplant, diabetes, diuretics, alcohol, cyclosporine, digoxin, amphotericin, aminoglycoside and cisplatin nephrotoxicity, hypercalcemia, hypophosphatemia).[57,66] Hypomagnesemia can also be precipitated by various metabolic stressors that cause Mg^{2+} redistribution (e.g. high catecholamine levels [promote increased Mg^{2+} uptake by adipose tissue], major burns, sepsis, trauma, alcohol withdrawal, hypothermia, acute myocardial infarction, cardiopulmonary bypass and massive blood transfusion).[66] Hypomagnesemia is a common component of refeeding syndrome caused by decreased total body stores combined with increased cellular uptake as nutritional substrates are provided. The elderly are at risk for Mg^{2+} deficit because of a combination of marginal intake and various pathologies and treatments common to elderly persons (e.g., diabetes mellitus, use of hypermagnesuric diuretics).[72]

Most symptoms of moderate to severe hypomagnesemia are nonspecific and often associated with other ion abnormalities such as hypokalemia, hypocalcemia, and metabolic alkalosis.[57] Chronic Mg^{2+} deficiency and acute hypomagnesemia are associated with increased cardiovascular morbidity and mortality.[66] Clinical manifestations include muscle weakness, hyperactive tendon reflexes, tremors, tetany, cardiac arrhythmias, vertigo and ataxia, depression, psychosis, seizures, carbohydrate intolerance, hyperinsulinism, atherosclerosis, osteoporosis, osteomalacia, and hypokalemia that is refractory to treatment until Mg^{2+} is replaced.[57]

Treatment. Treatment of mild asymptomatic hypomagnesemia includes oral administration of Mg^{2+} salts to provide 10 to 30 mEq (5 to 15 mmol) elemental Mg^{2+} in divided doses.[57] Oral supplementation may also be warranted in patients at risk for Mg^{2+} deficiency even if serum [Mg^{2+}] is normal.[73] Parenteral magnesium sulfate (1 g $MgSO_4 \cong 8$ mEq or 4 mmol Mg^{2+}) is warranted for moderate to severe hypomagnesemia, symptomatic hypomagnesemia, and hypomagnesemia associated with refeeding syndrome.[51] Parenteral replacement is also indicated when the GI tract is nonfunctional. In patients who have severe Mg^{2+} deficiency (<1.0 mg/dl), total body deficits can be on the order of 1 to 2 mEq/kg.[74] Because patients with normal renal function retain less than half of the administered dose, a total of 2 to 4 mEq/kg may be required to replenish body stores.[1,74,75] This can be given as repeated doses of 25 mEq (3 g $MgSO_4$) over 2 to 6 hours.[40,76] For patients receiving PN, the Mg^{2+} content of the PN formulation can also be increased in accordance with manufacturer or institution-specific guidelines for maximum divalent cation concentrations. Mg^{2+} replacement should be given cautiously and in much smaller doses in the setting of oliguric renal failure. MacLaren and colleagues recently devised evidence-based guidelines for electrolyte (including Mg^{2+}) replacement in the intensive care unit, taking into consideration degree of depletion, creatinine clearance, and route of administration.[52]

HYPERMAGNESEMIA. Hypermagnesemia (serum [Mg^{2+}] >2.5 mg/dl) occurs infrequently and is usually iatrogenic (e.g., intravenous Mg^{2+} administration, Mg^{2+}-containing cathartics and antacids).[57] Those most at risk are the elderly and individuals with renal insufficiency. Other conditions that can result in hypermagnesemia include adrenocortical insufficiency, early burn injury, severe trauma or surgical stress, rhabdomyolysis, severe dehydration, and severe acidosis.[1]

Early symptoms of Mg^{2+} toxicity may occur with serum concentrations of 4.9 to 7.3 mg/dl (4 to 6 mEq/L) and include hypotension, bradycardia, respiratory depression, depressed mental status, and ECG abnormalities.[57] As serum levels approach 12 mg/dl (10 mEq/L, 5 mmol/L), symptoms progress to respiratory paralysis, narcosis, and cardiac arrhythmias.

Treatment. Treatment of hypermagnesemia consists of elimination of exogenous Mg^{2+} and correction of any coexisting acidosis or volume deficit. Slow intravenous administration of calcium chloride or calcium gluconate (5 to 10 mEq) controls symptoms temporarily as Ca^{2+} antagonizes the neuromuscular effects of Mg^{2+}.[1,76] If symptoms persist, dialysis may be necessary.

Acid-Base Balance
Normal Physiology

An acid is any substance that tends to release hydrogen ions (H^+) in solution, whereas a base is any substance that tends to accept H^+. Daily metabolism of carbohydrate, protein, and fat generates approximately 1 mmol of H^+ per kilogram body weight.[77] A variety of organic acids account for half of this amount. Sulfuric acid produced by the metabolism of sulfur-containing amino acids, such as methionine and cystine, and phosphoric acid accounts for the remainder.[47,78] Additionally, large quantities of carbon dioxide (CO_2), approximately 20,000 mmol/day, are liberated with normal tissue metabolism.[79] CO_2 in turn combines with water to form carbonic acid (H_2CO_3). Despite this large acid load, the magnitude of [H^+] is quite small compared with other electrolytes—nanomole (10^{-9} mol) versus millimole (10^{-3} mol) per liter. Acidity is more readily expressed in terms of pH units, representing $\log 1/[H^+]$. A decrease in pH signifies an increase in [H^+], and vice versa. It is essential that pH be maintained within very narrow limits for optimal functioning of the human body. Severe deviations in systemic acidity can be life-threatening. Normal arterial pH ranges from 7.35 to 7.45. Acid-base equilibrium is maintained through the action of buffer systems, the regulation of H^+ and bicarbonate (HCO_3^-) excretion and reabsorption by the kidneys, and the regulation of CO_2 elimination by the lungs. When impairments in the body's regulatory mechanisms occur or when acid-base losses or gains exceed normal regulatory capabilities, acid-base disequilibrium ensues. The term *metabolic* used in the context of acid-base balance refers to disturbances in [HCO_3^-], whereas *respiratory* refers to disturbances in P_{CO_2}, the partial pressure of CO_2 in blood. A state in which the pH is lower than 7.35 is termed *acidemia*. A state in which the pH is greater than 7.45 is termed *alkalemia*. The terms *acidosis* and *alkalosis* refer to physiologic *processes* or disease states that, if not corrected, lead to acidemia and alkalemia.[2,78] Thus, in the setting of simultaneous perturbations having opposite effects on [H$^+$], patients can be *acidotic* or *alkalotic* without being *acidemic* or *alkalemic*.

Regulation

BUFFER SYSTEMS. Buffers are present in all body fluids and respond instantaneously to changes in pH. A buffer is a weak acid or base and its corresponding salt. When a strong acid (or base) is added to the system, it reacts with the components of the buffer system to form a new acid (or base) that is weaker than the original acid (or base). The resulting change in pH is less dramatic than if the strong acid (or base) had been added to water alone.

Proteins and phosphates are important in maintaining intracellular pH. The hemoglobin-oxyhemoglobin system is the main intracellular buffer of red blood cells. The HCO_3^-/H_2CO_3 system is the principal buffer of the ECF compartment and accounts for 50% of the blood's buffering capacity. Inorganic or organic acids added to the system combine with HCO_3^-, producing H_2CO_3 and the Na$^+$ salt of the inorganic or organic acid. For example,

$$HCl_{(STRONG\ ACID)} + NaHCO_{3\ (BUFFER\ BASE)} \rightarrow$$
$$NaCl_{(INORGANIC\ SALT)} + H_2CO_{3\ (WEAK\ ACID)}$$

and

$$H_2SO_{4\ (STRONG\ ACID)} + 2\ NaHCO_{3\ (BUFFER\ BASE)} \rightarrow$$
$$Na_2SO_{4\ (INORGANIC\ SALT)} + 2\ H_2CO_{3\ (WEAK\ ACID)}$$

The H_2CO_3 dissociates into CO_2 and water. The CO_2 is subsequently eliminated through the lungs. The inorganic acid anions are excreted by the kidneys with H$^+$ or as ammonium salts. The organic acid anions are metabolized as the underlying disorder is corrected, although there may be some renal excretion.

RESPIRATORY SYSTEM. The respiratory center of the brain responds directly to changes in [H$^+$]. Alveolar ventilation (respiratory rate × tidal volume) can increase 400% to 500% of normal with increases in arterial [H$^+$]. The reduction in acid load is realized through increased elimination of CO_2. Conversely, a decrease in arterial [H$^+$] decreases respiratory drive as much as 50% to 75%, resulting in significant CO_2 retention. The ventilatory response to changes in arterial pH occurs rapidly, usually within 1 to 2 minutes.

RENAL SYSTEM. The kidneys regulate acid-base balance by adjusting HCO_3^- levels. This regulation depends on an array of mechanisms that alter Na$^+$, H$^+$, and HCO_3^- excretion and reabsorption as well as the rate of ammonia synthesis. The normal ratio of HCO_3^- to H_2CO_3 is 20:1, corresponding to a pH of 7.4. An increase in CO_2 ultimately results in renal H$^+$ excretion and HCO_3^- generation. The excess CO_2 combines with water to form H_2CO_3, which then dissociates into H$^+$ and HCO_3^-. H$^+$ ions are exchanged for Na$^+$ ions and excreted, producing acidic urine. HCO_3^-, in combination with Na$^+$, gains access to the peritubular plasma and is returned to the ECF. Thus, the proper ratio of acids to bases, and hence normal pH, is restored. This mechanism is inhibited by dehydration and Na$^+$ deficiency. When the ECF becomes alkalemic, the kidneys conserve H$^+$ and increase HCO_3^- excretion, thus producing alkaline urine. This mechanism is inhibited by a deficiency of Na$^+$ or K$^+$

because the body would not be able to maintain electroneutrality under these conditions. The renal response to changes in pH is much slower than the respiratory response and may take hours to days.

Assessing Acid-Base Status

Proper assessment of acid-base status relies on careful interpretation and integration of appropriate laboratory data with the patient's clinical picture. Determining acid-base status based on insufficient data can produce erroneous conclusions and lead to misguided treatment.

ARTERIAL BLOOD GAS ANALYSIS. An arterial blood gas (ABG) determination provides valuable information needed to assess acid-base status. The pH indirectly measures the [H$^+$] and expresses overall, or net, acid-base status. Arterial pH decreases with an increase in [H$^+$] and increases with a decrease in [H$^+$] such that a pH less than 7.35 denotes acidemia and a pH greater than 7.45 denotes alkalemia. Severe acidemia is defined as a pH less than 7.20. Severe alkalemia is defined as a pH greater than 7.60. P_{CO_2} reflects the respiratory component of acid-base balance. The partial pressure rises with decreased alveolar ventilation and resultant CO_2 retention. It decreases with increased alveolar ventilation and elimination of CO_2. The partial pressure of oxygen in arterial blood (Pa_{O_2}) is not paramount in determining acid-base status. It may, however, provide information regarding possible etiology. For instance, hypoxemia can cause hyperventilation and respiratory alkalosis. It can also result in increased anaerobic metabolism, with subsequent lactic acid production and metabolic acidosis. Oxygen saturation (Sa_{O_2}) measures the degree to which hemoglobin is saturated with oxygen. It has no direct bearing on assessment of acid-base status. The base excess or deficit reflects the amount of buffer in the blood. The [HCO_3^-] reflects the metabolic component of acid-base balance.

PLASMA ELECTROLYTES. Determination of the metabolic component of acid-base disorders requires analysis of plasma electrolytes, principally Cl$^-$ and HCO_3^- concentrations. Cl$^-$, an acid anion, may increase with metabolic acidosis and decrease with metabolic alkalosis, depending on cause. HCO_3^- decreases in metabolic acidosis and increases in metabolic alkalosis. Note that the laboratory measures and reports total CO_2 content. This can be somewhat confusing and misleading. Total CO_2 includes H_2CO_3, dissolved CO_2, and HCO_3^-. However, all but 1 to 3 mmol/L is in the form of HCO_3^-. For ease of understanding, total CO_2 content should be regarded as [HCO_3^-]. Plasma K$^+$ levels can rise and fall with changes in acid-base status secondary to transcellular shifts resulting from hydrogen ion exchange. Na$^+$, BUN, creatinine, and glucose concentrations may be beneficial in investigating possible causes of acid-base disorders.

Acid-Base Disorders

METABOLIC ACIDOSIS. Metabolic acidosis is a physiologic process or condition that results in an absolute or relative increase in acid concentration (Table 10-6). This can occur via the addition of acid from exogenous sources (e.g., diet, medications, intravenous fluid, toxic ingestion), from endogenous acid generation (e.g., lactic acidosis, DKA), or from failure to excrete the acid load (e.g., renal failure). Direct loss of HCO_3^- (e.g., diarrhea, renal tubular acidosis, pancreatic fistula) also

Causes of Acid-Base Disorders

Acid-Base Disorder	Defect	Possible Causes
Metabolic acidosis	Increased acid generation/addition of acid	Ketoacidosis (diabetic, alcoholic, pancreatic, and starvation ketoacidosis)
		Lactic acidosis (shock, cardiopulmonary arrest)
		Rhabdomyolysis
		Toxic ingestion (salicylates, methanol, ethylene glycol, paraldehyde)
		Addition of acidifying salts (ammonium chloride, lysine hydrochloride, arginine hydrochloride, hydrochloric acid)
	Retention of fixed acids	Renal insufficiency (acute or chronic renal failure, renal tubular acidosis, type I, hypoaldosteronism)
	Loss of base bicarbonate	Gastrointestinal losses (severe diarrhea, small bowel fistulas, biliary drainage, pancreatic drainage, ureterosigmoidostomy)
		Renal losses (early renal failure, renal tubular acidosis, type II, diuretic treatment with carbonic anhydrase inhibitors: acetazolamide, triameterene, spironalactone)
Metabolic alkalosis	Loss of fixed acids	Gastrointestinal losses (vomiting, gastric suctioning, villous adenoma, congenital chloridorrhea)
		Renal losses (diuretics, mineralocorticoid excess, chronic hypercapnia, hypercalcemia, hypoparathyroidism)
	Gain of base bicarbonate	Administration of bicarbonate or its precursors, massive blood transfusion, milk alkali syndrome, diuretics, volume contraction or depletion
	Intracellular H^+ shift	Severe potassium depletion, carbohydrate refeeding after starvation
Respiratory acidosis, acute	Pulmonary/thoracic	Severe pneumonia, adult respiratory distress syndrome, flail chest, pneumothorax, hemothorax, smoke inhalation
	Airway obstruction	Aspiration, asphyxiation, laryngospasm (severe hypocalcemia, anaphylaxis), prolonged acute asthma attack
	Neuromuscular abnormalities	Guillain-Barré syndrome, hypokalemia, high cervical cordotomy, drugs/toxins
	Central nervous system depression	Sedative overdose, anesthesia, cerebral trauma, cerebral infarct
	Systemic	Cardiac arrest, massive pulmonary embolus, severe pulmonary edema
	Metabolic	Extremely high-carbohydrate diet; overfeeding
Respiratory acidosis, chronic	Obstructive lung disease	Emphysema, chronic bronchitis, cystic fibrosis, obstructive sleep apnea
	Restrictive lung disease	Obesity-hypoventilation syndrome, kyphoscoliosis, hydrothorax, fibrothorax, severe chronic pneumonitis
	Neuromuscular disease	Poliomyelitis, muscular dystrophy, multiple sclerosis, amyotrophic lateral sclerosis, diaphragmatic paralysis
	Depression of respiratory center	Brain tumor, bulbar poliomyelitis, chronic sedative overdose
Respiratory alkalosis	Hypoxemia	Pneumonia, high-altitude (>6500 ft), hypotension, severe anemia, congestive heart failure
	Pulmonary disorders	Pulmonary embolus, inhalation of irritants, interstitial fibrosis, pneumonia, pulmonary edema, asthma
	Central stimulation of respiratory center	Anxiety, fever, pain drugs (salicylates), hyperventilation (voluntary or mechanical), intracerebral trauma, gram-negative septicemia, acute cerebrovascular accident
	Miscellaneous	Liver disease, hepatic encephalopathy

causes metabolic acidosis. Simple uncompensated metabolic acidosis is characterized by an arterial pH less than 7.35 (acidemia). Plasma $[HCO_3^-]$ is generally less than 25 mmol/L either because of direct loss of HCO_3^-–rich fluids or consumption of HCO_3^- in the buffering process. Strong acids react with $NaHCO_3$, forming the Na^+ salt of the acid and H_2CO_3. In this process, HCO_3^- is "consumed," resulting in decreased plasma $[HCO_3^-]$. Normal plasma $[HCO_3^-]$ may be observed with metabolic acidosis caused by administration of large amounts of saline solution (dilutional acidosis) and with acidosis resulting from an extracellular H^+ shift.[47] Hyperkalemia may also be associated with acidosis, depending on etiology. As H^+ moves from the ECF to the ICF, K^+ is exchanged to maintain electroneutrality and plasma $[K^+]$ increases. This H^+-K^+ exchange is generally not observed with organic acidoses, specifically lactic acidosis.

Anion Gap. In metabolic acidosis, the anion gap (AG) is calculated to help determine the cause of acidosis and thus direct treatment. Its use, however, is not without limitations. For instance, it may not be helpful in cases in which there is a mixture of organic and inorganic acidoses (e.g. lactic acidosis in combination with renal tubular acidosis).[80] Also, hypoalbuminemia decreases the AG, necessitating application of a correction factor. Nonetheless, it remains a clinically useful tool and merits explanation. The numbers of cations and anions in the body are equal; otherwise, electroneutrality would not be maintained. The laboratory does not routinely measure all of these ions. The AG is simply the difference in concentration between measured cations and anions. It is calculated thus:

$$AG = [Na^+] - ([Cl^-] + [HCO_3^-])$$

The normal AG of 12 ($\pm$2) mmol/L signifies that there is a difference between measured cations and anions of 12 mmol/L. Unmeasured anions include sulfate, phosphate, lactate, and other organic anions. Note that plasma proteins, especially albumin, are included in this gap. It has been suggested to adjust the AG for hypoalbuminemia as follows: calculated AG + 2.5(normal–measured albumin [g/dl]).[81]

Non-AG metabolic acidosis (AG $\approx$ 12 mmol/L) occurs when the decrease in HCO_3^- is offset by an equal, or nearly equal, increase in Cl^-. In this situation, the sum of the anions ($[Cl^-] + [HCO_3^-]$), which is then subtracted from $[Na^+]$, has not changed. Thus, the resulting AG is normal. This is also termed *hyperchloremic metabolic acidosis*. Loss of HCO_3^- may occur from the GI tract, renal excretion of HCO_3^-, or renal generation of HCO_3^- insufficient to match acid load. By metabolism to HCl, administration of NH_4Cl or chloride salts of amino acids can also result in hyperchloremic acidosis.[77] Dilutional acidosis results from a net retention of Cl^-, as observed in ECF volume depletion, CHF, or rapid intravenous saline administration. Common causes of non-AG acidosis are listed in Table 10-7.

Positive-gap metabolic acidosis occurs when the decrease in HCO_3^- is not offset by an increase in Cl^-, but rather by some other circulating acid anion. Because $[Cl^-]$ is normal and $[HCO_3^-]$ is decreased, their sum is also decreased. Thus, when this sum is subtracted from $[Na^+]$, the resulting AG is increased: AG is greater than 12 mmol/L. This is also termed *normochloremic metabolic acidosis*. An AG greater than 30 mmol/L invariably reflects accumulation of organic acids. Lactic acidosis is perhaps the most common cause of AG metabolic acidosis in critically ill patients. Historically, lactic acidosis is classified as type A—acidosis caused by hypoxia, and type B—acidosis not caused by hypoxia. Type A lactic acidosis can result from tissue hypoperfusion (e.g., circulatory failure) or reduced arterial oxygen content (e.g., carbon monoxide poisoning, pulmonary disease, severe anemia). Type B lactic acidosis results from hepatic failure, renal failure, strenuous exercise, excessive alcohol consumption in malnourished patients, biguanide toxicity, and thiamine deficiency.[83] The latter is of particular concern from a nutritional standpoint. Thiamine is essential for normal glucose metabolism. Without thiamine, pyruvate cannot undergo conversion to acetyl co-enzyme A (CoA). The excess pyruvate is converted to lactate. In this process, equimolar amounts of protons (H^+) are generated and lactic acidosis ensues. Because thiamine is water soluble, deficiency states develop fairly quickly—in less than 4 weeks.[83] Deaths caused by refractory lactic acidosis from thiamine deficiency have been reported in patients receiving PN devoid of thiamine.[84] The aforementioned lactic acidoses result from accumulation of L-lactate. Lactic acidosis of a different isomer results from colonic overproduction of d-lactic acid by d-LDH-forming bacteria.[47] This is most likely to occur in malabsorption syndromes in which a large amount of substrate is delivered to the colon and a proliferation of d-LDH-forming bacteria is present. Other possible causes of AG metabolic acidosis are listed in Table 10-7.

A decreased AG is most commonly due to hypoalbuminemia.[47] Other causes include laboratory error, dilution of ECF, multiple myeloma, hypermagnesemia, and hypercalcemia.[78,80]

Treatment. As for all types of acid-base disturbances, treatment is directed toward the underlying disorder. For instance, treatment of lactic acidosis from circulatory shock centers on volume resuscitation along with other measures to restore adequate tissue perfusion and oxygenation. The overall benefit of HCO_3^- therapy in treatment of lactic acidosis with severe acidemia remains controversial.[78,85] Possible adverse effects include increased net lactate production, hypernatremia, hyperosmolality, "overshoot" alkalemia and increased release of CO_2 ($HCO_3^- + H^+ \rightarrow H_2CO_3 \rightarrow CO_2 + H_2O$).[78] If lactic acidosis due to thiamine deficiency is suspected, replacement with 50 to 100 mg thiamine per day given intravenously or intramuscularly for 1 to 2 weeks is recommended. All patients receiving PN must be provided with adequate vitamin supplementation.[83] Management of d-lactic acidosis resulting from colonic overproduction of d-lactic acid by bacteria includes use of oral antibiotics in combination with a low carbohydrate diet to decrease substrate delivery to the colon.[47,85] DKA is treated with insulin and fluid administration. Alcohol-related ketoacidosis is treated with dextrose and fluid administration. Hyperchloremic metabolic acidosis caused by overzealous isotonic saline administration corrects with a change in intravenous fluid selection and reduction in Cl^- load. For patients receiving PN, the Cl^- content should be reduced. Na^+ and K^+ can be added as acetate salts rather than Cl^- salts. The therapeutic use of HCO_3^- (or a precursor such as acetate) is generally reserved for severe cases of acidosis or states of ongoing HCO_3^- loss. Under these circumstances, the HCO_3^- deficit can be approximated by the following formula:

$$HCO_3^- \text{ deficit (mmol)} = 0.5 \times ([HCO_3^-]_{NORMAL} - [HCO_3^-]_{MEASURED})$$

Note: This equation assumes an apparent space of distribution of 50%. The actual space of distribution of infused HCO_3^- is variable. The more severe the metabolic acidosis, the greater the HCO_3^- space.[85]

Only half of the calculated deficit should be replaced within the first 24 hours and the remainder over the next 24 to 48 hours. Serious complications can result from correcting pH too rapidly. Careful monitoring is imperative to avoid overcorrection. Addition of $NaHCO_3$ to PN admixtures is contraindicated because of formation of insoluble precipitates. Instead, acetate, a precursor to HCO_3^-, is added in the form of sodium

---

TABLE 10-7

Common Causes of Anion Gap and Non-Anion Gap Metabolic Acidosis[82]

Anion Gap Metabolic Acidosis	Non-Anion Gap Metabolic Acidosis
Methanol ingestion	**U**reterosigmoidostomy
Uremia	**S**mall bowel fistula
Diabetic ketoacidosis	**E**xtra chloride
Paraldehyde	**D**iarrhea
Iatrogenic	**C**arbonic anhydrase inhibitors
Lactic acidosis	**A**drenal insufficiency
Ethanol, ethylene glycol ingestion	**R**enal tubular acidosis
Salicylates	**P**ancreatic fistula

or potassium acetate. Acetate is subsequently converted to HCO_3^- in the liver.

METABOLIC ALKALOSIS. Metabolic alkalosis is a physiologic process or condition that results in an absolute or relative increase in base concentration (see Table 10-6). Simple uncompensated metabolic alkalosis is characterized by an arterial pH greater than 7.45 (alkalemia) and an elevated plasma $[HCO_3^-]$ level (hyperbicarbonatemia). It is usually accompanied by a decrease in plasma $[K^+]$ secondary to an intracellular shift. H^+ leaves the cell and enters the ECF, causing K^+ to move intracellularly.[1] Severe alkalemia (pH >7.60) is also associated with a reduction in plasma ionized $[Ca^{2+}]$.[85] The capacity of the kidney to excrete large amounts of HCO_3^- and the metabolic production of nonvolatile acids normally defend against metabolic alkalosis. Thus, generation of metabolic alkalosis requires both an increase in base (or loss of acid) and impairment of renal HCO_3^- excretion.[77] Extrarenal sources of base include oral or intravenous HCO_3^- administration, excessive use of antacids, administration of HCO_3^- precursors (e.g., citrate, lactate or acetate), and massive blood transfusions (citrate added as a buffer). HCO_3^- can also be generated endogenously in response to hypercapnia, increased mineralocorticoid activity, and K^+ deficiency.[77] In cases of severe hypokalemia, K^+ moves from the ICF to the ECF. Hydrogen ions are exchanged, resulting in intracellular acidosis and increased renal H^+ excretion. Absolute or relative loss of acid can occur through renal and nonrenal means. Loss of acid occurs through gastric suctioning or vomiting, particularly in patients with pyloric obstruction.[1] A relative loss of acid (i.e., more Cl^- than HCO_3^-), occurs with thiazide diuretics, chronic diarrhea, and hyperadrenocorticism. Factors that impair HCO_3^- excretion include diminished glomerular filtration, Cl^- deficiency, and stimulation of proximal tubule HCO_3^- reabsorption by hypercapnia, angiotensin II, norepinephrine, or K^+ deficiency.[77] Metabolic alkalosis can also result from hypovolemia and is thus termed "contraction alkalosis." Hypovolemia causes decreased renal perfusion, which stimulates aldosterone-mediated Na^+ reabsorption and K^+ excretion. The resultant hypokalemia leads to excretion of H^+ in place of K^+. The aciduria in turn causes metabolic alkalosis.[1]

Treatment. Treatment of metabolic alkalosis is directed toward the underlying disorder. If the causative processes are ongoing, every effort should be made to moderate or stop them. Vomiting should be countered with antiemetics and loss of acid through gastric suctioning should be reduced with H_2-blockers or proton pump inhibitors.[86] Administration of HCO_3^- or its precursors should be discontinued. Diuretic therapy should be reassessed. Any intercurrent K^+ or extracellular volume deficits should be corrected. Cl^- replacement is indicated when alkalosis results from loss of acid anions. Measurement of urinary $[Cl^-]$ performed on a spot urine sample is useful in formulating treatment. The presence of a low urinary Cl^- (<20 mmol/L) generally indicates volume and Cl^- depletion.[78] Appropriate treatment is volume and Cl^- repletion with isotonic saline solution and KCl. The deficit can be calculated as follows:

Chloride deficit (mmol) = 0.5 × body weight (kg) ×

$$(Cl^-_{NORMAL} - Cl^-_{MEASURED}).^{87}$$

In severe, refractory cases of metabolic alkalosis, or when volume or electrolyte constraints preclude adequate NaCl or KCl replacement, 0.1 N to 0.2 N hydrochloric acid (HCl) can be used effectively.[1,86] The infusion should be given over a period of 6 to 24 hours, with measurement of pH, Pco_2, and plasma electrolytes every 4 hours.[1] Addition of HCl to total nutrient admixtures containing amino acids, dextrose, and fat is contraindicated because of the effect of lowered pH on emulsion stability. Peripheral administration of HCl mixed with amino acids and coinfused with fat emulsion is similarly ill advised.[88]

RESPIRATORY ACIDOSIS. Respiratory acidosis is caused by acute or chronic retention of CO_2 (see Table 10-6). It is characterized by hypercapnia (Pco_2 >40 mm Hg) and, in the absence of adequate renal compensation, by a pH less than 7.35 (acidemia). Acute respiratory acidosis develops as a consequence of airway obstruction, status asthmaticus, pneumonia, pulmonary edema, respiratory center depression (e.g., drugs, brainstem injury), neuromuscular impairment (e.g., myasthenia, Guillain-Barré), ventilatory restriction (e.g., as occurs with rib fractures and flail chest), pneumothorax, and laryngeal spasm.[77,78,85] Hyperphosphatemia usually accompanies acute hypercapnia.[77] Chronic respiratory acidosis occurs principally in obstructive and restrictive pulmonary disease, but can also occur with chronic neuromuscular disease, thoracic deformities, obesity hypoventilation syndrome, and depression of the respiratory center.[78] In patients with chronic hypercapnia, infection and use of narcotics can result in respiratory decompensation with a superimposed element of acute CO_2 retention and acidemia.[85]

Treatment. Treatment of respiratory acidosis involves correction of the respiratory defect and restoration of adequate ventilation. In patients with underlying pulmonary disease, overfeeding must be avoided, because it could result in increased CO_2 production and ultimately exacerbate the respiratory acidosis. The effect of overfeeding on CO_2 production is far more pronounced than is the effect of a proportionately high carbohydrate intake in the absence of overfeeding.

RESPIRATORY ALKALOSIS. Respiratory alkalosis results from increased alveolar ventilation and elimination of CO_2 (Table 10-6). It is characterized by hypocapnia (Pco_2 <40 mm Hg) and, in the absence of adequate renal compensation, by a pH greater than 7.45 (alkalemia). Acute respiratory alkalosis can occur with various hypoxemic conditions, pulmonary disorders, central stimulation of the respiratory center (e.g., pain, anxiety), sepsis, and salicylate intoxication.[77,86] Chronic respiratory alkalosis occurs in pulmonary and hepatic disease. The dangers of severe respiratory alkalosis are those related to K^+ depletion, which results from entry of K^+ into cells in exchange for H^+ and excessive urinary K^+ loss in exchange for Na^+.[1]

Treatment. Treatment of respiratory alkalosis is directed at the underlying disorder and may involve reduction of anxiety, use of tranquilizers, oxygen therapy, and adjustment of ventilator settings. Any concurrent K^+ deficits should be corrected.

COMPENSATED AND MIXED ACID-BASE DISORDERS. Acute acid-base disorders are simple or uncompensated; however, the body attempts to restore pH to normal through both renal and respiratory compensatory mechanisms. Altered pH resulting from respiratory acid-base imbalance is countered by renal compensation whereby plasma [HCO_3^-] changes in the same direction as P_{CO_2}. The end result is a pH that is closer to normal. Similarly, altered pH resulting from metabolic acid-base imbalance is countered by respiratory compensation whereby P_{CO_2} changes in the same direction as plasma [HCO_3^-]. Again, the end result is a pH that is closer to normal. For example, appropriate respiratory response to metabolic acidosis is increased ventilation and elimination of CO_2, resulting in decreased P_{CO_2}. This compensatory response increases pH toward normal. Complete compensation generally does not occur. The pH remains skewed in the direction of the primary acid-base disorder. Respiratory compensation for metabolic acid-base imbalances occurs quickly, within minutes. Renal compensation occurs more slowly and may take 3 to 5 days for maximal effect. Predicted compensatory responses are listed in Table 10-8. Mixed acid-base disorders are those in which more than one primary acid-base disorder exists. For example, a patient with chronic respiratory acidosis due to chronic obstructive pulmonary disease would normally have an elevated plasma [HCO_3^-] as a result of renal compensation. Should this patient undergo abdominal surgery and sustain significant unreplaced loss of gastric acid because of suctioning, he or she would develop a primary metabolic alkalosis with a plasma [HCO_3^-] greater than what would be predicted as a compensatory response. Predicted values for compensatory responses can be used to differentiate between primary acid-base disorders and compensatory responses. Alternatively, acid-base nomograms and maps such as those devised by DuBose[89] and Goldberg[90] have been advocated.

Treatment. When treating mixed acid-base disorders it is imperative to differentiate between primary disorders and appropriate compensatory responses. *Only the primary disorders should be treated.* The primary disorder is identified by first assessing individual metabolic and respiratory acid-base status. The pH is then evaluated, remembering that it will tend to be in the direction of the primary acid-base disorder. Finally, these findings are compared with the patient's clinical picture. Is everything consistent? It is also advisable to determine predicted compensatory changes (Table 10-8). When predicted values do not agree with measured values, this may indicate the existence of a second primary acid-base disorder. Because this disorder is also a primary disorder, it too should be treated appropriately. As the primary acid-base disorder(s) is (are) treated the compensatory response diminishes accordingly.

Conclusion

Maintenance of fluid, electrolyte, and acid-base balance depends on a vast array of complex, interrelated homeostatic mechanisms that work in concert to stabilize the cellular environment and facilitate normal physiology and function. A host of factors, including illness and injury, can disrupt this delicate balance, altering cell environment and ultimately cell function. Recognition and treatment of fluid, electrolyte, and acid-base disorders is an integral part of sound nutrition support practice. Detailed knowledge in this area allows the practitioner to assess when and how medical nutrition therapy can be manipulated to help restore homeostasis.

TABLE 10-8

Acute Acid-Base Disorders and Compensatory Responses*

Acute (Primary) Disorder	HCO_3^-	P_{CO_2}	PH	Appropriate Compensatory Response	Predicted Change in Laboratory Values	Resultant pH
Metabolic acidosis	↓↓	N	↓↓	*Respiratory:* Increased ventilation and elimination of CO_2, ↓ P_{CO_2} (hypocapnea), ⇒ increase in pH	For each 1 mmol/L ↓ in HCO_3^- P_{CO_2} ↓ 1.2-1.5 mm Hg	↓
Metabolic alkalosis	↑↑	N	↑↑	*Respiratory:* Decreased ventilation and retention of CO_2, ↑ P_{CO_2} (hypercapnea), ⇒ decrease in pH	For each 1 mmol/L ↑ in HCO_3^- P_{CO_2} ↑ 0.3–0.5 mm Hg	↑
Respiratory acidosis	N	↑↑	↓↓	*Renal:* Increased reabsorption and generation of HCO_3^- increased H^+ excretion, ⇒ increase in pH	For each 10 mm Hg ↑ P_{CO_2} HCO_3^- ↑ 1-2 mmol/L *acutely* HCO_3^- ↑ 3-4 mmol/L *chronically*	↓
Respiratory alkalosis	N	↓↓	↑↑	*Renal:* Decreased reabsorption and generation of HCO_3^-, decreased H^+ excretion ⇒ decrease in pH	For each 10 mm Hg ↓ P_{CO_2} HCO_3^- ↓ 1-2 mmol/L *acutely* HCO_3^- ↓ 4-6 mmol/L *chronically*	↑

* Double arrows (↓↓/↑↑) denote changes observed with the acute, or primary, acid-base disorder. Single arrows (↓/↑) indicate change observed with the compensatory response.

REFERENCES

1. Shires III TG, Barber A, Shires TG: Fluid, electrolyte, and nutritional management of the surgical patient. In Schwartz SI (ed): *Principles of surgery,* ed 7, New York, 1999, McGraw-Hill, pp 53-75.

2. Halperin ML, Goldstein MB: *Fluid, electrolyte, and acid-base physiology: a problem-based approach,* ed 3, Philadelphia, 1999, WB Saunders.

3. Heird WC, Driscoll JM Jr, Schullinger JN, et al: Intravenous alimentation in pediatric patients, *J Pediatr* 80(3):351-372, 1972.

4. Gallagher-Allred C: Fluid and electrolyte requirements. In Krey SH, Murrar RL (eds): *Dynamics of nutrition support,* Norwalk, CT, 1986, Appleton-Century-Crofts, pp 249-275.

5. Lustig JV: Fluid and electrolyte therapy. In Hay WW, Groothius JR, Hayward AR, Levin MJ (eds): *Current pediatric diagnosis and treatment,* ed 12, East Norwalk, CT, 1995, Appleton & Lange, pp 1178-1189.

6. Oster JR, Singer I: Hyponatremia, hyposmolality, and hypotonicity: tables and fables, *Arch Intern Med* 159(3):333-336, 1999.

7. Dorwart WV, Chalmers L: Comparison of methods for calculating serum osmolality from chemical concentrations, and the prognostic value of such calculations, *Clin Chem* 21(2):190-194, 1975.

8. Bhagat CI, Garcia-Webb P, Fletcher E, et al: Calculated vs measured plasma osmolalities revisited, *Clin Chem* 30(10):1703-1705, 1984.

9. Penney MD, Walters G: Are osmolality measurements clinically useful? *Ann Clin Biochem* (Pt 6) 24:566-571, 1987.

10. Smithline N, Gardner KD Jr: Gaps in the anionic and osmolal gaps, *JAMA* 236(14):1594-1597, 1976.

11. Gennari FJ: Serum osmolality: uses and limitations, *N Engl J Med* 310(2):102-105, 1984.

12. Ambrose ML, Goldberg KE, Johnson PH et al (eds): *Fluid and electrolytes made incredibly easy,* Springhouse, PA, 1997, Springhouse Corp., p 4.

13. Horne MM, Swearingen PL: *Pocket guide to fluids, electrolytes, and acid-base balance,* ed 2, St Louis, 1993, Mosby.

14. Miller M: Hyponatremia: Age-related risk factors and therapy decisions, *Geriatrics* 53(7):32-46, 1998.

15. Beck LH: Changes in renal function with aging, *Clin Geriatr Med* 14(2):199-209, 1998

16. Kleiner SM: Water: an essential but overlooked nutrient, *J Am Diet Assoc* 99(2):200-206, 1999.

17. Food and Nutrition Board: *Recommended dietary allowances,* ed 10, Washington, DC, 1989, National Academy Press.

18. Palevsky PM: Hypernatremia, *Semin Nephrol* 18(1):20-30, 1998, pp 249-250.

19. Vogelzang JL: Overview of fluid maintenance/prevention of dehydration, *J Am Diet Assoc* 99(5):605-611, 1999.

20. Mange K, Matsuura D, Borut C, et al: Language guiding therapy: the case of dehydration versus volume depletion, *Ann Int Med* 127(9):848-853, 1997.

21. Maesaka JK, Gupta S, Fishbane S: Cerebral salt-wasting syndrome: does it exist? *Nephron* 82(2):100-109, 1999.

22. Oh MS, Carroll HJ: Cerebral salt-wasting syndrome: we need better proof of its existence, *Nephron* 82(2):110-114, 1999.

23. Singer GG, Brenner BM: Fluid and electrolyte disturbances. In Fauci SA, Braunwald E, Isselbacher KJ, et al. (eds): *Harrison's principles of internal medicine,* vol 1, ed 14, New York, 1998, McGraw-Hill, pp 265-271.

24. McGee S, Abernathy III B, Simel DL: Is this patient hypovolemic? [The rational clinical evaluation], *JAMA* 281(11):1022-1029, 1999.

25. Fried LF, Palevsky PM: Hyponatremia and hypernatremia, *Med Clin North Am* 81(3):585-609, 1997.

26. Yee J, Parasuraman R, Narins R: Selective review of key perioperative renal-electrolyte disturbances in chronic renal failure patients, *Chest* 115(5):149S-157S, 1999.

27. Fraser CL, Arieff AI: Epidemiology, pathophysiology, and management of hyponatremic encephalopathy, *Am J Med* 102(1):67-77, 1997.

28. Gross P, Reimann D, Neidel J, et al: The treatment of severe hyponatremia, *Kidney Int* 53(suppl 64):6S-11S, 1998.

29. Adrogué HJ, Madias NE: Aiding fluid prescription for the dysnatremias, *Intensive Care Med* 23:309-316, 1997.

30. Adrogué HJ, Madias NE: Hyponatremia, *N Engl J Med* 342(21):1581-1589, 2000.

31. Gowrishankar M, Lin S-H, Mallie JP: Acute hyponatremia in the perioperative period: insights into its pathophysiology and recommendations for management, *Clin Nephrol* 50(6):352-360, 1998.

32. Adrogué HJ, Madias NE: Hypernatremia, *N Engl J Med* 342(20):1493-1499, 2000.

33. National Advisory Group on Standards and Practice Guidelines for Parenteral Nutrition: Safe practices for parenteral nutrition formulations, *J Parenter Enteral Nutr* 22(2):49-66, 1998.

34. Standing Committee on the Scientific Evaluation of Dietary Reference Intakes, Food and Nutrition Board, Institute of Medicine: *Dietary reference intakes for calcium, phosphorus, magnesium, vitamin D, and fluoride,* Washington, DC, 1997, National Academy Press, pp 106-117, 141-142, 173-176, 187, 219-234, 246.

35. Verbalis J: Adaptation to acute and chronic hyponatremia: implications for symptomology, diagnosis, and therapy, *Semin Nephrol* 18(1):3-19, 1998.

36. Avner ED: Clinical disorders of water metabolism: hyponatremia and hypernatremia, *Pediatr Ann* 24(1):23-30, 1995.

37. Narins RG, Jones ER, Stom MC, et al: Diagnostic strategies in disorders of fluid, electrolyte and acid-base homeostasis, *Am J Med* 72(3):496-520, 1982.

38. Spital A: Diuretic-induced hyponatremia, *Am J Nephrol* 19(4):447-452, 1999.

39. Wilcox CS: Metabolic and adverse effects of diuretics, *Semin Nephrol* 19(6):557-568, 1999.

40. Piazza-Barnett R, Matarese LE: Electrolyte management in total parenteral nutrition, *Support Line* 21(2):8-15, 1999.

41. Kumar S, Berl T: Sodium, *Lancet* 352(9123):220-228, 1998.

42. Sterns RH, Spital A, Clark EC: Disorders of water balance. In Kokko JP, Tannen RI (eds): *Fluid and electrolytes,* Philadelphia, 1996, WB Saunders, pp 63-109.

43. Gennari FJ: Hypo-natremia: disorders of water balance. In Davison AM, Cameron JS, Grünfeld JP, Kerr DNS, Ritz E, Winearls CG (eds): *Oxford textbook of clinical nephrology,* ed 2, vol 1, Oxford, England, 1998, Oxford University Press, pp 175-200.

44. Kumar S, Berl T: Approach to the hyponatremia patient. In Berl T (ed): *Disorders of water, electrolytes, and acid-base. Part 1 of Atlas of diseases of the kidney,* vol 1, Philadelphia, 1999, Blackwell Science, pp 9-15.

45. Laureno R, Karp BI: Myelinosis after correction of hyponatremia, *Ann Int Med* 126(1):57-62, 1997.

46. Halterman RK, Berl T: Therapy of dysnatremic disorders. In Brady HR, Wilcox CS (eds): *Therapy in nephrology and hypertension,* Philadelphia, 1998, WB Saunders, pp 257-269.

47. Oh MS, Uribarri J: Electrolytes, water, and acid-base balance: In Shils ME, Olson JA, Shike M, Ross AC (eds): *Modern nutrition in health and disease,* ed 9, Baltimore, 1999, Williams & Wilkins, pp 105-137.

48. Van Zee KJ, Barie PS, Lowry SF: Electrolyte disorders. In Cameron JL (ed): *Current surgical therapy,* ed 4, St Louis, 1992, Mosby-Year Book, pp 1005-1029.

49. Cohn JN, Kowey PR, Whelton PK, Prisant LM: New guidelines for potassium replacement in clinical practice: a contemporary review by the National Council on Potassium in Clinical Practice, *Arch Intern Med* 160(16):2429-2436, 2000.

50. Singer GG, Brenner BM: Fluid and electrolyte disturbances. In Fauci SA, Braunwald E, Isselbacher KJ, et al. (eds): *Harrison's principles of internal medicine,* vol 1, ed 14, New York, 1998, McGraw-Hill, pp 271-276.

51. Brooks MJ, Melnik G: The refeeding syndrome: an approach to understanding its complications and preventing its occurrence, *Pharmacotherapy* 15(6):713-726, 1995.

52. MacLaren R, Ramsay KB, Liiva MT, et al: The development and implementation of evidence-based electrolyte replacement guidelines in the intensive care unit, *Can J Hosp Prac* 52(6):393-396, 1999.

53. Woo J, Henry JB: Metabolic intermediates and inorganic ions. In Henry JB (ed): *Clinical diagnosis and management by laboratory methods,* ed 19, Philadelphia, 1996, WB Saunders, pp 162-191.

54. Weaver CM, Heanley RP: Calcium. In Shils ME, Olson JA, Shike M, Ross AC (eds): *Modern nutrition in health and disease,* ed 9, Baltimore, 1999, Williams & Wilkins, pp 141-154.

55. Block GA, Port FK: Re-evaluation of risks associated with hyperphosphatemia and hyperparathyroidism in dialysis patients: recommendation for change in management, *Am J Kid Dis* 35(6):1226-1237, 2000.

56. Weisinger JR, Bellorin-Font E: Magnesium and phosphorus, *Lancet* 352(9125):391-396, 1998.

57. Knochel JP: Phosphorus. In Shils ME, Olson JA, Shike M, Ross AC (eds): *Modern nutrition in health and disease,* ed 9, Baltimore, 1999, Williams & Wilkins, pp 158-167.

58. Subramanian R, Khardori R: Severe hypophosphatemia: pathophysiologic implications, clinical presentations, and treatment, *Medicine* 79(1):1-8, 2000.

59. Solomon SM, Kirby DF: The refeeding syndrome: a review, *J Parenter Enteral Nutr* 14:90-97, 1990.

60. Duerksen DR, Papineau N: Electrolyte abnormalities in patients with chronic renal failure receiving parenteral nutrition, *J Parenter Enteral Nutr* 22(2):102-104, 1998.

61. Davenport A: Magnesium and phosphorus, *Lancet* 352(9138):1475, 1998 (correspondence).

62. Apovian CM, McMahon MM, Bistrian BR: Guidelines for refeeding the marasmic patient, *Crit Care Med* 18(9):130-133, 1990.

63. Maier-Dobersberger T, Lochs H: Enteral supplementation of phosphate does not prevent hypophosphatemia during refeeding of cachectic patients, *J Parenter Enteral Nutr* 18(2):182-184, 1994.

64. Clark CL, Sacks GS, Dickerson RN, et al: Treatment of hypophosphatemia in patients receiving specialized nutrition support using a graduated dosing scheme: results from a prospective clinical trial, *Crit Care Med* 23(9):1504-1511, 1995.

65. Rosen GH, Boullata JI, O'Rangers EA, et al: Intravenous phosphate repletion regimen for critically ill patients with moderate hypophosphatemia, *Crit Care Med* 23(7):1204-1210, 1995.

66. Gomez MN: Magnesium and cardiovascular disease, *Anesthesiology* 89(1):222-240, 1998.

67. Garzon P, Eisenberg MJ: Variation in the mineral content of commercially available bottled waters: implications for health and disease, *Am J Med* 105(2):125-130, 1998.

68. Elin RJ: Laboratory tests for assessment of magnesium status in humans, *Magnes Trace Elem* 10(2-4):172-181, 1991-1992.

69. Whang R, Hampton EM, Whang DD: Magnesium homeostasis and clinical disorders of magnesium deficiency, *Ann Pharmacother* 28(2):220-226, 1994.

70. Schuck P, Gammelin G, Resch KL: Magnesium and phosphorus, *Lancet* 352(9138):1474-1475, 1998 (correspondence).

71. Haderslev KV, Jeppesen PB, Mortensen PB, Staun M: Absorption of calcium and magnesium in patients with intestinal resection treated with medium chain fatty acids, *Gut* 46(6):819-823, 2000.

72. Durlach J, Bac P, Durlach V, et al: Magnesium status and the aging: an update, *Magnes Res* 11(1):25-42, 1998.

73. Durlach J, Bac P, Durlach V, et al: Neurotic, neuromuscular and autonomous form of magnesium imbalance, *Magnes Res* 10(2):169-195, 1997.

74. Flink EB: Therapy of magnesium deficiency, *Ann NY Acad Sci* 162(2):901-905, 1969.

75. Reinhart RA: Magnesium metabolism, *Arch Intern Med* 148(11):2415-2420, 1988.

76. Shils ME: Magnesium. In Shils ME, Olson JA, Shike M, Ross AC (eds): *Modern nutrition in health and disease,* ed 9, Baltimore, 1999, Williams &Wilkins, pp 169-192.

77. Gluck SL. Acid-base [electrolyte quintet], *Lancet* 352(9126):474-479, 1998.

78. Preuss HG: Fundamentals of clinical acid-base evaluation, *Clin Lab Med* 13(1):103-116, 1993.

79. Hood VL, Tannen RL: Mechanisms of disease: protection of acid-base balance and pH regulation of acid production, *N Engl J Med* 339(12): 819-826, 1998.

80. Badrick T, Hickman PE: The anion gap: a reappraisal, *Am J Clin Pathol* 98(2):249-252, 1992.

81. Gottschlich MM, Matarese LE, Shronts EP: *Nutrition support dietetics— core curriculum,* ed 2, Silver Spring, MD, 1993, American Society for Parenteral and Enteral Nutrition.

82. Wilson RF: Acid-base problems. In Tintinalli JE, Krome RL, Ruiz E (eds): *Emergency medicine: a comprehensive study guide,* ed 3, New York, 1992, McGraw-Hill, pp 35-61.

83. Romanski SA, McMahon MM: Metabolic acidosis and thiamine deficiency, *Mayo Clinic Proc* 74(3):259-263, 1999 (case report).

84. Centers for Disease Control and Prevention. Lactic acidosis traced to thiamine deficiency related to nationwide shortage of multivitamins for total parenteral nutrition-United States, 1997, *MMWR Morbid Mortal Wkly Rep* 46:523-528, 1997.

85. Adrogué HJ, Madias NE: Medical progress: Management of life-threatening acid-base disorders: first of two parts, *N Engl J Med* 338(1):26-34, 1998 (review article).

86. Adrogué HJ, Madias NE: Medical progress: management of life-threatening acid-base disorders: second of two parts, *N Engl J Med* 338(2): 107-111, 1998 (review article).

87. Inadomi DW, Kopple JD: Fluid and electrolyte disorders in total parenteral nutrition. In Narins RJ, Maxwell MH, Kleeman CR (eds): *Clinical disorders of fluid and electrolyte metabolism,* New York, 1987, McGraw-Hill, pp 1437-1462.

88. Bistrian BR, Driscoll D, McCowen KC: Acid-base disorders, *N Engl J Med* 338(22):1626-1629, 1998 (correspondence).

89. DuBose TD, et al: Acid-base disorders. In Brenner BM, Rector FC (eds): *The kidney,* ed 5, Philadelphia, 1996, WB Saunders, pp 929-998.

90. Goldberg M, et al: Computer-based instruction and diagnosis of acid-base disorders, *JAMA* 223(3):269-275, 1973.

Maria G. Boosalis, PhD, MPH, RD, LD

E VER since Dr. Casimir Funk coined the word *vitamine* to describe vital amines—substances necessary for life[1]— volumes have been written on vitamins. Of particular clinical interest is the relationship of vitamins to disease and the recent focus on the potential role of vitamins in preventing chronic diseases.[2]

This chapter reviews and summarizes the role and specific requirements for vitamins in adults receiving enteral and/or parenteral nutrition. The specific needs of neonates and the pediatric population are covered elsewhere in the text. The last of the dietary reference intakes (DRIs) for the vitamins and minerals have been completed and are included in this chapter. The DRIs are composed of four categories of reference intakes designed to reflect the latest understanding of nutrient requirements for healthy persons, based on optimizing health in individuals and groups instead of just preventing nutritional deficiencies.[3] The four DRIs categories are (1) *estimated average requirement (EAR)*, the intake that meets the estimated nutrient need of 50% of the individuals in that group and serves as the basis for developing the recommended dietary allowance; (2) *recommended dietary allowance (RDA),* the intake that meets the nutrient need of almost all (97% to 98%) individuals in that group; (3) *adequate intakes (AIs),* the average observed or experimentally derived intake by a defined population or subgroup that appears to sustain a defined nutritional state, such as normal circulating nutrient values, growth, or other functional indicators of health (If no EAR can be determined, no RDA can be set; therefore the AIs serve as a goal for intake); and (4) *tolerable upper intake level (UL),* the maximum intake by an individual that is unlikely to pose risks of adverse health effects in almost all (97% to 98%) individuals. It is important to note that this UL is not intended to be a recommended level of intake. For most nutrients, this figure refers to total intakes from food, fortified food, and nutrient supplements.

Because these revisions are recent, oral vitamin-mineral formulations may not yet have been altered to reflect these new recommendations. In addition, further research may be needed to determine if the parenteral (intravenous) recommendations will need to be adjusted as a result. Some progress toward that end has already been made, as a result of a 1985 public workshop on "Multivitamin Preparations for Parenteral Use" sponsored by the Food and Drug Administration (FDA) and the American Medical Association (AMA). As a result of the data presented at that workshop, the AMA-FDA workshop committee recommended that the dosage of certain vitamins be increased and that vitamin K be added to the intravenous for-

mulation for adults and children 11 years of age and older. This final rule was published in the April 20, 2000 *Federal Register*[4] and the proposed changes are shown in Table 11-1. The manufacturers of the adult parenteral vitamin preparations are now in the process of reformulating their products to meet these new recommendations.

Vitamin A

General Overview

Vitamin A is a fat-soluble vitamin required by humans and other vertebrates. Vitamin A consists of a family of molecules with 20 carbons, a characteristic structure, and a tetraene side chain on carbon-15. This tetraene side chain contains a hydroxyl group (retinol), an aldehyde group (retinal), a carboxylic acid group (retinoic acid), or an ester group (retinyl ester). This term also includes the provitamin A carotenoids of which three, α-carotene, β-carotene, and β-cryptoxanthin, have food composition data available. The term retinoids refers to retinol, its metabolites, and any synthetic analogues that have a similar

---

TABLE 11-1

Vitamin Intake Recommendations

Vitamin	Adult AMA[5] (Parenteral)	Dietary Reference Intakes (Female/Male)	Adult Parenteral Recommendations Per Unit Dose[4] (AMA-FDA Workshop)
A	3300 IU	700/900 μg	1 mg
D	200 IU	5 μg (19-50 yr) 10 μg (51-70 yr) 15 μg (>70 yr)	5 μg
E	10 IU	15 mg	10 mg
K	*	90/120 μg	150 μg
C	100 mg	75/90 mg	200 mg
Thiamine	3 mg	1.1/1.2 mg	6 mg
Niacin	40 mg	14/16 mg NE	40 mg
Riboflavin	3.6 mg	1.1/1.3 mg	3.6 mg
B$_6$	4 mg	1.3 mg (19-50 yr) 1.5/1.7 mg (>50 yr)	6 mg
B$_{12}$	5 μg	2.4 μg	5 μg
Folate	400 μg	400 μg DFE	600 μg
Biotin	60 μg	30 μg	60 μg
Pantothenic acid	15 mg	5 mg	15 mg

AMA, American Medical Association, parenteral guidelines; *FDA*, Food and Drug Administration; *DFE*, dietary folate equivalents; *NE*, niacin equivalents. (See text for explanation of DFE and NE.)
*Recognized as essential but guidelines not established.

structure.[6] Preformed vitamin A is only found in animal-derived products, while dietary carotenoids are found primarily in fruits, vegetables, and oils.

Vitamin A is required for epithelial cell integrity throughout the body,[7] gene expression, reproduction, normal embryonic development, growth, and immune function.[6] Vitamin A is also required for vision. For example, the transduction of light into neural signals is performed by the retinal form of vitamin A;[8] the maintenance of (1) normal differentiation of the cornea and conjunctival membranes (to prevent xerophthalmia) and (2) the photoreceptor rod and cone cells in the retina is performed by the retinoic acid form.

Signs and Symptoms of Deficiency

Xerophthalmia is the most specific clinical effect of a deficiency of vitamin A. The World Health Organization (WHO)[9] classified the stages of xerophthalmia to include night blindness (an impaired adaptation due to a slowed regeneration of rhodopsin), conjunctival xerosis, Bitot's spots, corneal xerosis, corneal ulceration, and scarring, with night blindness being the first ocular symptom observed.[6]

In animals, there is a well-documented association between impaired embryonic development and a deficiency of vitamin A.[10,11] Given the role of this vitamin in epithelial cell integrity, a deficiency of vitamin A also results in follicular hyperkeratosis, a condition that is correctable by vitamin A (retinal) or β-carotene supplementation.[12,13] Immune function is also adversely affected by a deficiency of vitamin A with reductions in lymphocyte numbers, natural killer cells, and antigen-specific immunoglobulin responses.[14,15] In addition, a decrease in leukocytes and lymphoid organ weights, a decreased resistance to immunogenic tumors, and impaired T-cell function have been observed.[16,17] Lastly, a deficiency of vitamin A has also been associated with an increased risk of infectious morbidity and mortality in both experimental animals and humans, particularly in developing countries.[6] Persons at increased risk for developing vitamin A deficiency include those with gastrointestinal dysfunction, diarrhea,[18,19] or fat malabsorption syndromes;[20] those with a long-term history of alcohol consumption;[21] those with impaired transport of vitamin A from either a protein[22,23] or zinc deficiency;[24,25] and those with increased needs or losses secondary to burn injury, major surgery,[26,27] fever, or infection.[28,29] Visual disturbances were reported in an individual on long-term home parenteral nutrition who was not receiving vitamin A supplementation.[30]

Signs and Symptoms of Toxicity

The UL, as defined in the latest DRIs, is the highest level of daily vitamin A intake that is likely to pose no risk of adverse health effects in almost all individuals.[6] As recommended, individuals in the general population should not routinely exceed the consumption of this amount. The UL for vitamin A varies with age and is 3000 μg per day of preformed vitamin A for both men and women 19 years of age and older. An acute toxicity of vitamin A (resulting from single or short-term doses) of 15,000 IU in adults[31] generally presents as nausea, vomiting, headache, blurred vision, increased cerebrospinal fluid pressure, and muscular incoordination.[32] A bulging fontanelle in infants has also been observed as a result of acute vitamin A toxicity.[33] On the

other hand, chronic toxicity of vitamin A is usually due to the ingestion of larger doses of vitamin A (30,000 IU or higher) for months or years, the effects of which are generally more varied and nonspecific. These effects include (but are not limited to) central nervous system effects, liver abnormalities, and changes in bone and skin. When the UL for vitamin A was determined, three primary adverse effects of excessive intake were considered: (1) reduced bone mineral density; (2) teratogenicity such as craniofacial malformations and abnormalities of the heart, thymus, and central nervous system except neural tube defects; and (3) liver abnormalities (i.e., elevated liver enzymes, fibrosis, cirrhosis, and sometimes death).[6]

Assessment of Status

Numerous issues are involved in determining the status of vitamin A, as discussed in the newest edition of the DRIs for this vitamin.[6] Briefly, the concentration of retinol in the plasma is not linear and, thus, over a wide range of adequate hepatic vitamin A stores, there is little change in the concentration of either retinol or retinol-binding protein (RBP).[34] Despite this, circulating levels of plasma retinol are often used clinically as an indicator of vitamin A status: levels less than 20 μg/dl (0.70 μmol/L) indicate a deficiency state, whereas levels greater than 30 μg/dl (1.05 μmol/L) are associated with satisfactory vitamin A status.[19,35,36] In addition, depleted liver stores of vitamin A would indicate a deficiency state, but liver biopsy is required for diagnosis. Marginal vitamin A status can also be determined by one of three different response assays.[6,37] For example, the relative-dose-response assay measures the percentage change in serum retinol levels 5 hours after a known dose of a retinoid. If the percentage change is greater than 20%, vitamin A status is suspected to be marginal.

Requirements

As shown in Table 11-1, the new RDA for vitamin A is 700 μg per day for women and 900 μg per day for men 19 years of age and older.[6] These values are the best guidelines for enteral replacement, as long as special conditions (i.e., increased needs or losses) are accounted for. Parenteral vitamin A requirements are also listed in Table 11-1 as established by the AMA.[5] The AMA recommends 3300 IU of vitamin A (as retinol) per day intravenously, which is in keeping with findings from other groups who recommend between 1500 and 4200 IU per day.[38,39] The nomenclature and conversion values for vitamin A activity have changed since the last revision of the RDA.[40] According to the recent Institute of Medicine (IOM) report[6] one retinol activity equivalent (RAE) = 1 μg of all-trans-retinol = 12 μg of all-trans-β-carotene = 24 μg of other provitamin A carotenoids. In addition, 1 international unit (IU) vitamin A activity = 0.3 μg of all-trans-retinol = 3.6 μg all-trans-β-carotene = 7.2 μg other provitamin A carotenoids. With this new nomenclature in mind and as also shown in Table 11-1, the new recommendations from the AMA-FDA workshop committee are for 1.0 mg of vitamin A (as retinol) per unit dose of adult parenteral vitamin preparations.[4]

Special Concerns

Loss of vitamin A through nonspecific adsorption onto the surface of the polymer tubing has been reported,[41,42] as has loss of vitamin A in parenteral solutions exposed to daylight.[43-45] Vitamin A levels seem stable in admixtures of parenteral nutrition (PN).[44]

Vitamin D

General Overview

Vitamin D (calciferol) is a group of fat-soluble seco-sterols that are either consumed in the diet or are photosynthesized in the skin of vertebrates during exposure to solar ultraviolet B radiation.[46] The two major physiologically relevant forms of vitamin D are vitamin D_2 (ergocalciferol) and vitamin D_3 (cholecalciferol).[47] Vitamin D_2 comes from ergosterol, a yeast and plant sterol, while vitamin D_3 originates from 7-dehydrocholesterol, a precursor of cholesterol, when synthesized in the skin. To become a biologically active hormone, vitamin D undergoes two hydroxylations. The first hydroxylation, on carbon 25, occurs in the endoplasmic reticulum of the liver; the second, on carbon 1, occurs in the proximal convoluted tubules of the kidney to form $1\alpha,25$-dihydroxyvitamin D $[1,25(OH)_2D]$.[48,49] As its biologically active form, vitamin D functions to maintain circulating levels of calcium and phosphorus within the normal range. It accomplishes this by increasing the small intestine's ability to absorb calcium and phosphorus and by stimulating osteoclastic stem cells to mature and increase calcium and phosphorus resorption from bone.[48,50,51] Recent work indicates that $1,25(OH)_2D$ is also involved in the growth and differentiation of other cells, including immune and hematopoietic cells.[52] Receptors for vitamin D have been found in brain, breast, gonads, mononuclear cells, pancreas, stomach, skin and certain tumor cells.[48,49,53,54]

Signs and Symptoms of Deficiency

A deficiency of vitamin D is characterized, biochemically, by a normal or low-normal level of calcium, a low-normal or low-fasting level of phosphorus, and an elevated level of parathyroid hormone (PTH) in the serum. In addition, the circulating level of alkaline phosphatase is usually elevated,[55] as is the urinary excretion of the bone collagen by-products, hydroxyproline, pyridinoline, deoxypyridinoline, and N-telopeptide.[56] Because of the inadequate mineralization or demineralization of the skeleton that accompanies a deficiency of vitamin D, osteomalacia results. In addition, the secondary hyperparathyroidism that occurs in vitamin D deficiency enhances calcium mobilization from the skeleton, resulting in porotic bone.[57] This increased susceptibility to osteoporosis is quite evident in elders who consume inadequate amounts of vitamin D. In addition to elders,[58] very young children[59] and adolescents[60] are most likely to develop a vitamin D deficiency. As reviewed by Gottschlich[61] persons with regional enteritis, tropical sprue, pancreatic insufficiency, gastric resection, or jejunoileal bypass surgery (conditions that interfere with vitamin D absorption) can also develop osteomalacia. Liver dysfunction can interfere with absorption, transport, or utilization of vitamin D,[62] and chronic renal failure can prevent the final hydroxylation to 1,25-dihydroxyvitamin D.

Signs and Symptoms of Toxicity

Hypervitaminosis D is accompanied by large increases in plasma 25(OH)D concentrations to levels of 160 to 500 ng/ml (400 to 1250 nmol/L).[63] The adverse effects of such high levels of vitamin D are primarily mediated by the resultant hypercalcemia, although some existing evidence suggests that these high levels of vitamin D may have direct toxic effects on various organ systems (i.e., kidney, bone, central nervous system, cardiovascular system).[64] Pharmacologic doses of vitamin D, in the range of 250 to 1250 µg/day (10,000 to 50,000 IU/day) over many years, have resulted in toxic effects.[65] Hypercalcemia associated with hypervitaminosis D results in many debilitating effects.[63,64] These effects include, but are not limited to, a loss in the urinary concentrating mechanism of the renal tubules[66] and the metastatic calcification of soft tissues, predominantly the kidney, blood vessels, heart, and lungs.[65,67,68] Young children are most susceptible to the toxic effects of vitamin D; as little as 1800 IU of cholecalciferol can result in hypervitaminosis D.[69]

Assessment of Status

The circulating level of 25(OH)D is the best indicator of vitamin D status because it represents a summation of both the total cutaneous production and the oral ingestion of either vitamin D_2 or vitamin D_3.[70,71] Normal values range between 20 nmol/L (8 ng/ml) and 150 nmol/L (60 ng/ml). Generally, serum values less than 25 nmol (10 ng/ml) indicate impending or frank vitamin D deficiency.[72]

Requirements

The requirements and recommendations for vitamin D have changed with the recent publication of revised DRIs.[63] As shown in Table 11-1, for men and women, 19 through 50 years of age, it is 5 µg (200 IU) per day; for those 51 through 70 years of age, it increases to 10 µg (400 IU) per day; and for those men and women older than 70 years of age, it further increases to 15 µg (600 IU) per day. The AMA adult parenteral recommendation is 200 IU per day,[5] which generally[73] but not always[39,74] maintains circulating levels within the normal range. As shown in Table 11-1, the new recommendation from the AMA-FDA workshop committee for vitamin D (as ergocalciferol or cholecalciferol) in adult parenteral vitamin preparations remains the same at 5.0 µg (200 IU).[4]

Special Concerns

Certain drugs (anticonvulsants, cimetidine, isoniazid) compromise vitamin D status and lead to a deficiency as does hypoparathyroidism, given the role of parathyroid hormone in promoting the synthesis of 1,25-dihydroxyvitamin D in the kidney.[63,75]

Metabolic bone disease has been a problem for both adults and children receiving long-term PN.[76,77] The cause of this problem is likely multifactorial, and potential mechanisms are reviewed elsewhere.[78] One known causal factor is the presence of aluminum in parenteral solutions, which results in reduced bone formation and mineralization.[78] The contribution of administered vitamin D is still uncertain; some studies reported resolution of some of the observed abnormalities,[76,79] but others did not.[80,81] Whatever the cause, the presence of preexisting bone disease, drugs, toxins, deficiencies in the solutions, and coexisting medical conditions that could predispose to bone disease must be considered.

Vitamin E

General Overview

The primary function of vitamin E is to serve as a nonspecific chain-breaking antioxidant to prevent the propagation of free-radical reactions.[82] Specifically, vitamin E is a peroxyl radical scavenger and, as such, particularly protects polyunsaturated fatty acids (PUFAs) within membrane phospholipids and in plasma lipoproteins.[83] In addition to the antioxidant effects,[82] vitamin E also inhibits protein kinase C activity (which is involved in cell proliferation and differentiation in many types of cells) and downregulates the expression of intercellular cell adhesion molecule and vascular cell adhesion molecule-1, (thereby decreasing the adhesion of blood cell components to the endothelium). Vitamin E also functions to upregulate the expression of cytosolic phospholipase A_2 and cyclooxygenase-1 (likely explaining the dose-dependent enhanced release of prostacyclin, a potent vasodilator and inhibitor of platelet aggregation in humans).

Signs and Symptoms of Deficiency

Vitamin E deficiency occurs rarely in humans. It has been observed in rare genetic abnormalities of the α-tocopherol transfer protein (α-TTP), the main transport protein for the vitamin in the circulation.[84] In addition, because vitamin E is fat soluble, its status is compromised by any condition that interferes with fat absorption. Such conditions include but are not limited to prolonged steatorrhea, pancreatitis,[85,86] cystic fibrosis,[87,88] short-bowel syndrome,[85,89] and cholestasis.[90] Premature infants[91,92] and those with severe protein-calorie malnutrition,[93] liver dysfunction,[94,95] or a β-lipoproteinemia[96] are also at risk for developing a vitamin E deficiency.

Peripheral neuropathy is the primary symptom of a vitamin E deficiency.[82] This neuropathy is characterized by the degeneration of the large-caliber axons in the sensory neurons. Other symptoms that have been observed in humans include, but are not limited to, spinocerebellar ataxia, skeletal myopathy, and pigmented retinopathy. In addition, earlier studies have reported increased platelet aggregation,[97] decreased red blood cell survival and hemolytic anemia,[85,98,99] neuronal degeneration,[87,89,100] and decreased serum creatinine with creatinuria[101] in humans with vitamin E deficiency.

Signs and Symptoms of Toxicity

There is no evidence of adverse effects from the consumption of vitamin E content that is naturally occurring in foods.[82] As reviewed,[82] three of four large-scale intervention trials reported no adverse effects with daily supplementation with vitamin E of 400 to 800 IU (equivalent to 268 mg to 567 mg) (study lengths varied between 1.4 to 4.5 years). Yet in one of these four large-scale intervention trials, the Alpha-Tocopherol Beta Carotene (ATBC) Cancer Prevention Study, when 50 mg/day of *all rac*-α-tocopherol was given to Finnish male smokers for 6 years, a significant 50% increase in mortality from hemorrhagic stroke was observed. Although findings from this study need to be confirmed, the observed increase in hemorrhagic stroke is supported by data in animals given high-dose α-tocopherol supplementation.[82] Other adverse effects of excessive vitamin E may include inhibition of platelet aggregation and adhesion in vitro.[82] This is in contrast to an earlier report of no

adverse blood coagulation effects when up to 600 mg per day of α-tocopherol was given, for up to 3 years, in apparently healthy volunteers. Nonetheless, the UL for vitamin E in individuals 19 years of age and older has been established at 1000 mg (2326 μmol) of any form of supplemental α-tocopherol per day.

Assessment of Status

The circulating level of vitamin E in the plasma is primarily used to assess vitamin E status. Plasma values less than 11.6 μmol/L (5 μg/ml) indicate poor vitamin E status and are generally accompanied by increased red blood cell fragility (as evidenced by hemolysis of erythrocytes incubated in 2% hydrogen peroxide).[82,102,103]

Requirements

As shown in Table 11-1, the RDA for both women and men 19 years of age and older is 15 mg (35 μmol) of α-tocopherol per day.[82] The vitamin E activity of α-tocopherol is defined as that available from the naturally occurring form (*RRR*-α-tocopherol) and the other three synthetic 2R-stereoisomer forms (RSR, RRS, RSS) of α-tocopherol. The synthetic forms are present in fortified foods and in vitamin supplements. The other naturally occurring forms of vitamin E (β-, γ-, δ-tocopherols and the tocotrenols) do not contribute to meeting the requirement for vitamin E because they are neither converted to α-tocopherol in humans nor are they recognized by its transport protein (α-TPP) in the liver. To help distinguish between correct and current versus incorrect and past nomenclature, the synthetic *all rac*-α-tocopherol was historically and incorrectly labeled as *dl*-α-tocopherol, while the naturally occurring stereoisomer *RRR*-α-tocopherol (i.e., "natural source" vitamin E) was historically and incorrectly labeled *d*-α-tocopherol. To interconvert milligrams from international units do the following: Milligrams of α-tocopherol in food, fortified food, or multivitamin = international units of the *RRR*-α-tocopherol × 0.67 or IU of the *all rac*-α-tocopherol compound × 0.45. The new adult parenteral recommendation from the AMA-FDA workshop committee[4] is for 10 mg of vitamin E (as α-tocopherol), which is similar to the previous AMA recommendation of 10 IU per day[5] that seemed to provide adequate replacement, barring the special circumstances discussed previously.

Special Concerns

Some reports in animals,[104] and later in humans, indicate that pretreatment with vitamin E before elective cardiopulmonary bypass reduces the amount of peroxidative damage.[105,106] This requires further validation before pretreatment with vitamin E becomes routine.

If vitamin E depletion is suspected, care should be taken to avoid iron supplementation because, as a potent free radical generator, it increases red cell hemolysis.[107] The issue of vitamin E supplementation during critical illness is covered in a separate section later in this chapter.

Vitamin K

General Overview

Vitamin K is found principally in two forms. That found in green plants is known as phylloquinone, or vitamin K_1, and that synthesized by gut microflora is known as menaquinone, or vitamin K_2. As such, vitamin K functions as a coenzyme during the synthesis of the biologically active forms of several proteins involved in blood coagulation and bone metabolism.[6] With respect to blood coagulation, vitamin K functions in the posttranslational conversion of specific glutamyl residues to γ-carboxyglutamyl (GLA) residues[108] in plasma prothrombin (coagulation factor II) and the plasma procoagulants, factors VII, IX, and X. With respect to bone metabolism, osteocalcin and matrix GLA protein are structurally related vitamin K–dependent proteins. As reviewed by Shearer,[109] vitamin K promotes conversion of protein-bound glutamate to GLA, the latter of which occurs in various tissues.

Numerous studies have looked at the relationship between vitamin K and bone disease.[6] Although many of these studies suggest vitamin K plays a role in preventing bone disease, results from studies in patients who are undergoing anticoagulant therapy with warfarin have not supported this possible relationship. A recent meta-analysis of nine studies of individuals on long-term oral anticoagulant therapy found no significant effect on bone density in the distal radius, lumbar spine, femoral neck, or femoral trochanter, even though a decrease was observed in the bone density of the distal radius.[110]

Signs and Symptoms of Deficiency

Primary deficiency of vitamin K is rare in healthy adults and has usually been associated with various lipid malabsorption syndromes.[111] Usually a clinically significant deficiency of vitamin K is defined as a vitamin K–responsive hypoprothrombinemia associated with an increase in prothrombin time (PT) and/or bleeding in severe cases. Breast-fed newborns, on the other hand, are particularly susceptible to vitamin K deficiency.[112] In addition, certain disease conditions and drugs adversely affect vitamin K status. These include malabsorption syndromes and gastrointestinal disorders such as cystic fibrosis, sprue, celiac disease, ulcerative colitis, regional enteritis, short-bowel syndrome,[111] biliary obstruction,[113] and liver disease.[114] The drugs that antagonize vitamin K include coumarin and large doses of salicylates,[113,115,116] the broad-spectrum antibiotics,[113] and megadoses of vitamins A[117,118] and E.[119,120] Cholestyramine therapy can also compromise vitamin K status.[121] Vitamin K deficiency has been reported in persons fed over the long term with parenteral nutrition,[122,123] elders,[124] and those in renal failure.[125,126]

Signs and Symptoms of Toxicity

No known adverse effects have been reported regarding the consumption of vitamin K (as menaquinone or phylloquinone) from either food or supplements in humans or animals.[6] Because a quantitative risk assessment could not be performed, a UL could not be derived for vitamin K. Administration of a synthetic form of vitamin K (menadione) has been associated with liver damage[127,128] and also caused hemolytic anemia, hyperbilirubinemia, and kernicterus in a newborn.[129]

Assessment of Status

Of all the various indicators used to assess vitamin K status in humans, only PT has been associated with any adverse clinical effects,[6] yet the concentration of circulating prothrombin must be decreased by approximately 50% before the value of a one-stage PT is outside "normal" range.[130] Because the other potential indicators of vitamin K status have only been associated with changes in dietary vitamin K intake, the physiologic significance of their diet-induced changes is lacking. Circulating levels of phylloquinone in the plasma or serum have also been used to assess vitamin K status because they reflect dietary intake and respond to dietary changes within 24 hours.[131] Normal ranges for plasma phylloquinone concentration in healthy adults aged 20 to 49 years are 0.25 to 2.55 nmol/L and 0.32 to 2.67 nmol/L for those adults 65 to 92 years of age.[132] With further investigations, several other sensitive measures of vitamin K status may be found. These include, but are not limited to, the concentration of PIVKA-II (des-γ-carboxyglutamic acid prothrombin), urinary excretion of γ-carboxyglutamic acid and undercarboxylated osteocalcin.[103]

Requirements

The AI for vitamin K is based on the median intake data from National Health and Nutrition Examination Survey (NHANES) III data.[6] As shown in Table 11-1, for women 19 years of age and older, it is 90 μg of vitamin K per day, while it is 120 μg of vitamin K per day for men in the same age range. The currently used parenteral vitamin products generally do not contain vitamin K because it may interfere with anticoagulant therapy. Yet the new recommendations from the AMA-FDA workshop committee[4] (see Table 11-1), state that 150 μg of vitamin K (as phylloquinone) should be added to any new adult parenteral formulations. This new recommendation is within the range of the previous AMA recommendation of 0.2 to 1.5 mg of vitamin K per week.[5] Other groups have recommended between 5 and 10 mg vitamin K per week be given as an intramuscular or subcutaneous dose.[69,133,134]

Special Concerns

Given the antagonistic relationship between anticoagulant therapy and vitamin K intake, whoever determines the dose of anticoagulant therapy must make sure that the patient is consuming his or her usual "diet," including any recommended commercial enteral supplement, so as to maintain a relatively consistent intake of vitamin K.

Vitamin C
General Overview

Vitamin C is the general term that refers to both ascorbic acid and dehydroascorbic acid. Ascorbic acid is the functional and primary in vivo form, which is acidic in nature and provides electrons for its function as both a reductant and antioxidant. The dehydroascorbic acid form is one of the two-electron oxidation products, the other being ascorbate. Both of these products are readily reduced back to ascorbic acid chemically and enzymatically by glutathione, nicotinamide adenine dinucleotide (NADH)–, and nicotinanide adenine dinucleotide phosphate (NADPH)–dependent reductases.[82,135,136] One known function of vitamin C is its role as an electron donor for eight human enzymes, three of which participate in collagen hydroxylation (and subsequent connective tissue synthesis), two in carnitine biosynthesis, and three in hormone and amino acid biosynthesis. The latter three enzymes are necessary for the biosynthesis of the catecholamines norepinephrine and epinephrine, the amidation of peptide hormones, and in tyrosine metabolism. Vitamin C also serves as a cofactor for hydroxylase and oxygenase metalloenzymes most likely by reducing the active metal site (generally for iron and/or copper). In addition, ascorbic acid is an effective antioxidant because of its ability to donate electrons. As such, it scavenges reactive oxygen species (ROS), reactive nitrogen species (RNS), singlet oxygen, and hypochlorite.[82] Ascorbic acid also works as a reducing agent for mixed-function oxidases in the microsomal drug-metabolizing system.

Signs and Symptoms of Deficiency

Scurvy is the classic vitamin C deficiency disease that is characterized by connective tissue defects. It generally occurs at plasma concentrations of vitamin C less than 11 μmol/L (0.2 mg/dl). The clinical features of scurvy include follicular hyperkeratosis, petechiae, ecchymosis, coiled hairs, inflamed and bleeding gums, perifollicular hemorrhages, joint effusions, arthralgia, and impaired wound healing.[82] Additional symptoms include dyspnea, edema, Sjögren's syndrome (dry eyes and mouth), weakness, fatigue, and depression.

Signs and Symptoms of Toxicity

The UL for adults is 2 g of vitamin C per day. The adverse effects of osmotic diarrhea and gastrointestinal disturbances were used as the criteria for establishing the UL.[82] This UL includes vitamin C from both food and supplements. Additional adverse effects of very high intakes are increased oxalate excretion and kidney stone formation, increased uric acid excretion, pro-oxidant effects, increased iron absorption leading to iron overload, reduced vitamin B_{12} and copper status, increased oxygen demand, and erosion of dental enamel.[82,137,138] Whether rebound vitamin C deficiency follows cessation of large doses of vitamin C (systemic conditioning) still remains controversial.[139,140] Large amounts of ascorbic acid in urine or feces can also interfere with several diagnostic tests, such as fecal occult blood and glycosuria. Vitamin C overdose may also hinder heparin or coumarin anticoagulant therapy.[141]

Assessment of Status

Currently, the most practical and reliable tests for assessing vitamin C status are plasma and leukocyte concentrations of vitamin C.[103,142] Both measurements correlate with intake of vitamin C and with each other.[143,144] Plasma and serum levels of ascorbic acid less than 11 μmol/L (20 mg/dl) represent frank vitamin C deficiency, and values of 11 to 23 μmol (0.2 to 0.4 mg/dl) are marginal;[145] others have used 28 μmol/L (0.5 mg/dl) as the lower limit of normal.[145,146]

Requirements

As shown in Table 11-1, the new RDA for vitamin C in women, 19 years of age and older is 75 mg per day and for men of the same age, it is 90 mg per day. This requirement is increased by 35 mg per day for individuals who smoke. Surgical,[147] trauma,[148] cancer,[149] and burn patients[150] may also demonstrate compromised vitamin C status. The initial AMA recommenda-

tion was for a dose of 100 mg per day[5] for adults receiving parenteral nutrition, yet reports from various groups (as discussed in Boosalis and others[148]) suggest that larger doses may be required to maintain adequate vitamin C status. In fact, the new adult parenteral vitamin recommendations from the AMA-FDA workshop committee,[4] as shown in Table 11-1, are that 200 mg vitamin C (as ascorbic acid) be provided per unit dose.

Special Concerns

Ascorbic acid is sensitive to light, oxygen, reducing agents such as copper, and elevations in temperature.[151]

Thiamin

General Overview

Thiamin is a water-soluble vitamin that, as thiamin pyrophosphate, functions as a magnesium (Mg^{++})-coordinated coenzyme for oxidative decarboxylation of α-ketoacids (e.g., pyruvate → acetyl coenzyme A (CoA); α-ketoglutarate → succinyl CoA and branched-chain keto acids) and for the activity of transketolase in the hexose and pentose phosphate reactions.[152] Thiamin might also play a role in nerve conduction as a structural component of nerve membranes.[153]

Signs and Symptoms of Deficiency

Beriberi is the classic thiamin deficiency disease. In underdeveloped countries it is generally due to a thiamin-poor diet (e.g., a diet high in polished rice), whereas in developed countries it is usually secondary to alcoholism, to omission from parenteral solutions, or to long-term parenteral nutrition.[154,155] Conditions of increased thiamin need include fever, infection, trauma, burns, hyperparathyroidism, pregnancy, lactation, strenuous physical exertion, or adolescent growth. Conditions of increased thiamin loss such as dialysis, diuresis, malabsorption, and/or prolonged antacid therapy can also precipitate thiamin deficiency, especially in persons whose thiamin status may initially have been marginal.[5,61,150,156]

Dry beriberi is a neurologic disease of peripheral neuropathy manifested by impaired sensory and motor functions, principally in the lower extremities. Specifically, paresthesias, anesthesia, and weakness (difficulty arising from a squatting position) are observed. Wet beriberi also presents as cardiac failure with dyspnea, hepatomegaly, tachycardia, and oliguria, with or without severe metabolic acidosis. Specifically, there are several reports of severe lactic acidosis in both adults and children fed by parenteral nutrition.[157-160] There has also been a recent report of thiamin correcting the nucleoside analogue–induced lactic acidosis in a female with acquired immunodeficiency syndrome (AIDS).[161]

Wernicke's encephalopathy is also due to thiamin deficiency, generally precipitated by alcohol abuse, which is associated with decreased intake and intestinal absorption of thiamin. This condition is characterized by global confusion, ophthalmoplegia, and ataxia. Other manifestations include polyneuritis, stupor, coma, hypothermia, hypotension, and other symptoms of wet or dry beriberi.[162] Wernicke's encephalopathy has also been reported in adults and children who have a large tumor burden, extensive injuries or surgery, or a life-threatening infection, and as a complication of parenteral nutrition.[163-167]

Signs and Symptoms of Toxicity

Although generally recognized safe, toxic effects of thiamin have been reported with an excess of 3 g of thiamin per day (i.e., at 50 mg/kg body weight).[103] Yet, because of a lack of suitable data, a UL could not be set.[152] Serious and often fatal responses to the parenteral administration of thiamin have been reported as reviewed by Stephen and associates.[168] The characteristics of these responses suggest an anaphylactic reaction and include anxiety, pruritus, respirator distress, nausea, abdominal pain, and shock, sometimes progressing to death.[152] There have also been two reports of an allergic sensitivity and pruritus when 500 mg thiamin was given intramuscularly[169] or 100 mg of thiamin hydrochoride was given intravenously.[170]

Assessment of Status

According to Sauberlich,[103] the preferred method for assessing thiamin status is the measurement of erythrocyte transketolase activity, with and without the in vivo addition of thiamin pyrophsophate. This test provides a sensitive, specific, biochemical functional measurement of thiamin status. Normal (i.e., acceptable thiamin status) is 0% to15%; low (or marginally deficient) is 16% to 24%, and deficient (or high risk of deficiency) status is greater than 25%. Other indicators of thiamin status are reviewed in the IOM's publications of various DRIs.[152] These include thiamin pyrophosphate effect (deficiency ≥25%), erythrocyte thiamin levels (deficiency <70 nmol/L), and the urinary excretion of thiamin (deficiency <27 µg/g creatinine or <5 µg /24 hr).

Requirements

As shown in Table 11-1, the new RDA for thiamin is 1.1 mg per day for women and 1.2 mg per day for men aged 19 and older.[152] The currently used parenteral recommendation is 3 mg,[5] but several other groups recommend between 10 and 50 mg per day.[133,171-173] As also shown in Table 11-1, the latest recommendation from the AMA-FDA workshop committee[4] is for thiamin content in any new adult parenteral vitamin formulations to be increased to 6.0 mg. Ricour and colleagues[174] recommend that children receive 100 µg of thiamin per 100 kcal infused, whereas others have suggested 0.5 mg/kg body weight.[175] In the clinical situations mentioned earlier in which increased needs and losses are both possible, careful monitoring of thiamin status is recommended.

Special Concerns

In solution, thiamin is unstable in alkaline solutions and degrades in direct sunlight.

Riboflavin

General Overview

Riboflavin functions as a component of two flavin coenzymes, flavin mononucleotide (FMN) and flavin adenine dinucleotide (FAD), that act as intermediaries in electron transport in oxidation-reduction reactions. Examples of such reactions include conversion of pyridoxine to its functional coenzyme, conversion of tryptophan to niacin, and functions in the xanthine oxidase, succinic dehydrogenase, and glutathione reductase oxidative enzyme systems.

Riboflavin is heat stable but is readily destroyed by light or exposure to strong alkaline solutions.[176] The stability and content of riboflavin in parenteral nutrition solutions are increased when lipid is added (e.g., 3:1 admixtures)[177] or when the vitamin is added to the intravenous fat emulsion and so administered.[178,179] Tissue stores of riboflavin are small.

Signs and Symptoms of Deficiency

Pure, uncomplicated dietary deficiency of riboflavin is rare and is generally accompanied by multiple nutrient deficiencies.[180] Groups at increased risk for developing riboflavin deficiency include those with malabsorption syndromes;[180] thyroid dysfunction;[181] diabetes;[182] or alcoholism;[183] cancer;[184] cardiac disease;[185] and those who are physiologically stressed, as by pregnancy, lactation, rapid growth, surgery, trauma, burns, or fractures.[61] In addition, certain drugs can affect riboflavin metabolism (e.g., psychotropic drugs and tricyclic antidepressants).[186] Some investigators,[187] but not others,[188,189] make the same claim about contraceptives.

Clinical symptoms of riboflavin deficiency include sore throat; hyperemia and edema of the pharyngeal and oral mucous membranes; oral-buccal lesions (e.g., cheilosis, angular stomatitis, glossitis or magenta tongue); generalized seborrheic dermatitis; vulvar and scrotal skin abnormalities; and normochromic, normocytic anemia associated with pure red cell cytoplasia of the bone marrow.[190] There can also be ocular disturbances such as itching, burning, dryness of the eyes, corneal inflammation or vascularization,[191] and photophobia.[61,107,190] Metabolism of glucose, amino acid, and lipid is affected during riboflavin deficiency.[192,193]

Signs and Symptoms of Toxicity

Because of insuffucient suitable data, a UL could not be set for riboflavin.[152] To date, no cases of toxicity from excessive intake of riboflavin have been reported.[40,180]

Assessment of Status

The erythrocyte glutathione reductase activity coefficient (EGR-AC) assay is the currently recommended method for assessing riboflavin nutriture.[194] EGR-AC values less than 1.2 indicate acceptable riboflavin status; 1.2 to 1.4, low; and more than 1.4, deficient. This assay cannot be used for persons who have a deficiency of glucose-6-phosphate because of increased avidity of the reductase for FAD.

Requirements

As shown in Table 11-1, the RDA for riboflavin is 1.1 mg per day for women and 1.3 mg per day for men, 19 years of age and older.[152] The currently used AMA recommendation for daily parenteral infusion is 3.6 mg, which is the same as the recommendations from the AMA-FDA workshop committee for riboflavin content[4] of the new adult parenteral vitamin formulations (see Table 11-1). Reports of normal EGR-AC levels have been made with riboflavin intakes between 1.8 and 4.2 mg per day in adults receiving parenteral nutrition.[171,195,196] Boosalis and associates[148] reported that the intravenous administration of 3.6 mg per day of riboflavin maintained circulating levels of riboflavin within normal range in a group of adult polytrauma or postsurgical patients. In addition, this infusion of riboflavin was approximately twice the amount of riboflavin that was excreted in the urine of these same individuals in a 24-hour period.

Special Concerns

Negative nitrogen balance is associated with flavoprotein breakdown and riboflavin excretion,[197] and retention of riboflavin is closely associated with nitrogen intake and nitrogen balance.[198,199]

Niacin
General Overview

Niacin is a water-soluble vitamin that includes nicotinic acid, nicotinamide, and derivatives that exhibit the biologic activity of nicotinamide. Nicotinamide serves as a component of two coenzymes, nicotinamide adenine dinucleotide (NAD) and nicotinamide adenine dinucleotide phosphate (NADP). More than 200 enzymes are dependent on NAD and NADP, the nicotinamide component functioning as either a hydrogen donor or an electron acceptor. In general, the NAD-dependent enzymes function in catabolic reactions (such as oxidation of all fuels) and NADP-dependent enzymes in reductive biosynthesis reactions (e.g., of fatty acids and steroids). In other words, as part of hydrogen transfer reactions, NAD and NADP function in the synthesis and degradation of all macronutrients. In addition, hepatic NAD stores can be hydrolyzed to nicotinamide and adenosine diphosphate ribose (ADPR); the ADPR moieties can then be transferred to acceptor proteins (poly-ADP-ribosylated proteins) and as such appear to function in DNA replication and repair, cell differentiation, and calcium mobilization.[152,200]

Niacin is unique among vitamins in that it can also be synthesized from a precursor, dietary tryptophan; 60 mg (290 μmol) of tryptophan provides an average of 1 mg (8.2 μmol) niacin or 1 mg niacin equivalent (NE).

Signs and Symptoms of Deficiency

Pellagra is the classic disease of niacin deficiency. Clinically, the three D's: dermatitis, diarrhea, and dementia, characterize it. A pigmented rash is the most characteristic sign, which presents symmetrically in areas exposed to the sun and resembles sunburn. Vomiting or diarrhea accompanies gastrointestinal tract inflammation, and the tongue becomes red. Neurologically, initial symptoms may include headaches, dizziness, insomnia, irritability, depression, and eventually disorientation, delusions, and catatonia.

A primary niacin deficiency is rare in the United States (because of enrichment of grains), yet some persons are at risk of developing a secondary niacin deficiency. These include those who have a history of alcohol abuse, thyroid disorders, cancer,[201] malabsorption, burn injury, and isoniazid therapy for tuberculosis (by depleting pyridoxine required, along with riboflavin, for conversion of tryptophan to niacin).[150,151,202]

Signs and Symptoms of Toxicity

Pharmacologic doses of niacin (as nicotinic acid) are given to reduce total cholesterol and low-density lipoprotein and

triglycerides and to increase high-density lipoprotein.[203,204] Depending on the dosage and formulation, side effects include vasodilation (manifested in flushing), itching, the sensation of heat, headaches, and gastrointestinal irritation (nausea, vomiting to fulminant hepatic failure), severe hepatitis, thrombocytopenia, and niacin-induced myopathy.[205,206]

The UL for all forms of niacin (immediate-release, slow, or sustained-release and niacinamide or nicotinamide) is set at 35 mg per day, based on flushing as the adverse effect.[152]

Assessment of Status

To date, the most reliable and sensitive method for assessing niacin status is to measure the 24-hour urinary excretion of two of its methylated metabolites (NMNs), N-methyl-nicotinamide and its 2-pyridone (N-methyl-2-pyridone-5-carboxamide). The Interdepartmental Committee on Nutrition for National Defense suggests that urine levels of NMN less than 5.8 μmol (0.8 mg) per day indicate niacin deficiency.[198] Another suggested indicator is decreased concentration of NAD in red blood cells, especially in association with a low plasma concentration of tryptophan.[207,208]

Requirements

As shown in Table 11-1, the RDA for niacin is 14 mg of niacin equivalents (NE) per day for women and 16 mg of NE per day for men, 19 years of age and older.[152] As also shown in Table 11-1, the currently followed AMA recommendation[5] is 40 mg per day for adults receiving parenteral nutrition and this amount is the same as the new adult parenteral recommendation made by the AMA-FDA workshop committee.[4] At this level of intravenous supplementation, circulating levels of niacin (in whole blood) were maintained within normal range in a group of adults (during a 7-day period of study) after polytrauma and/or postsurgery.[148] This level of intravenous supplementation also exceeded the 24-hour urinary losses of niacin in the same individuals by twentyfold.[148]

Special Concerns

Because of nutrient-nutrient interactions, inadequate levels of iron, riboflavin, and/or vitamin B_6 will decrease the conversion of tryptophan to niacin.[152] Kreisberg[209] discusses the benefits and safety of the modified-release forms (i.e., intermediate-release, slow or sustained-release) of niacin over the unmodified formulations. This discussion is of importance given the increased use of niacin for its lipid-lowering effects, ready availability, and potential for serious toxicity.[209]

Vitamin B_6
General Overview

Vitamin B_6 consists of three metabolically, chemically, and functionally related forms: pyridoxine (PN), pyridoxal (PL), and pyridoxamine (PM). In the liver, erythrocytes, and other tissues, these forms are converted to the active coenzymes pyridoxal phosphate (PLP) and pyridoxamine phosphate (PMP), which are involved in more than 100 enzymatic reactions. In its coenzyme forms, vitamin B_6 participates in protein metabolism (including transaminations, deaminations, decarboxylations, desulfhydration of amino acids, and niacin formation), gluconeogenesis, lipid metabolism, steroid receptor binding,[210] central nervous system development, synthesis of neurotransmitters,[211,212] and normal immune function.[213,214]

Signs and Symptoms of Deficiency

Seborrhatic dermatitis, microcytic anemia, epileptiform convulsions along with depression, and confusion are the classical clinical symptoms of a deficiency in vitamin B_6.[152,215,216] In controlled studies of vitamin B_6 depletion, abnormalities in electroencephalograms have also been observed. [152,217]

Signs and Symptoms of Toxicity

Adverse effects of prolonged administration of large doses of pyridoxine include sensory neuropathy and dermatologic lesions.[152,218,219] The UL is 100 mg of vitamin B_6 per day, using the development of sensory neuropathy as the critical end point.

Assessment of Status

Both direct (i.e, vitamin concentrations in plasma, blood cells, and/or urine) and indirect or functional (i.e., erythrocyte aminotransferase saturation by plasma pyridoxal phosphate [PLP] or tryptophan metabolites) measurements have been used to determine pyridoxine status.[220] Because each potential measurement has its drawbacks,[152,220] a combination of three tests was often suggested. Yet because the direct measure of PLP concentration reflects tissue stores and responds to changes in dietary B_6 intake (taking 7 to 10 days to plateau), it is probably the best single indicator of vitamin B_6 status if only one test could be performed.[221] The value of 20 nmol/L of PLP, while not accompanied by observable health risks, allows a moderate safety margin to protect against the development of sign/symptoms of a clinical deficiency and is therefore suggested as the cutoff point, as discussed.[152] Note that vitamin B_6 and protein intake, respectively, increase and decrease circulating levels of vitamin B_6. A short-term indicator of vitamin B_6 status is urinary excretion of 4-pyridoxic acid, a metabolite of B_6 made in the liver, which responds rapidly to changes in dietary intake.[217,222] In general, a 24-hour urinary excretion of 4-pyridoxic acid in excess of 3.0 μmol per day suggests adequate vitamin B_6 status. The other indirect measures of vitamin B_6 status (such as tryptophan loading or erythrocyte transaminase activity) were once the generally accepted method for vitamin B_6 assessment until the method for direct measurement of plasma PLP (or pyridoxal) was developed.

Requirements

The new RDA for vitamin B_6 is 1.3 mg per day for both women and men between 19 and 50 years of age (see Table 11-1). The RDA increases, in women, to 1.5 mg per day and, in men, to 1.7 mg per day when either are 51 years of age or older. The currently followed AMA recommendation[5] for parenteral administration of vitamin B_6 is 4.0 mg per day and is increased to 6.0 mg (of pyridoxine) per unit dose in the new adult parenteral vitamin recommendations from the AMA-FDA workshop committee[4] (see Table 11-1). Jeejeebhoy and associates[133] observed two of six patients on long-term parenteral nutrition to have reduced levels of plasma pyridoxine. Boosalis and coworkers[148] observed circulating levels of vitamin B_6 at the lower range of normal in adult polytrauma or major surgery

patients given 7 days of infusion with 4 mg vitamin B_6. Urinary excretion of this vitamin was also within normal limits even though intake exceeded urinary excretion by 50 to 60 times. Pyridoxine deficiency has also been reported in association with advanced age,[223] cancer,[224] asthma,[225] burn injury,[226] uremia,[227] malabsorption, alcoholism, and liver disease.[228]

Special Concerns

Among the drugs that interact adversely with vitamin B_6 are isoniazid, hydralazine, cycloserine, penicillamine, theophylline, ethanol, and caffeine.[229,230]

Vitamin B_{12}

General Overview

To be metabolically active, vitamin B_{12} must be converted to one of its coenzyme forms, methylcobalamin or 5'-deoxyadenosylcobalamin. As methylcobalamin, vitamin B_{12} is required for conversion of homocysteine to methionine via removal of a methyl group from methyl folate and subsequent regeneration of tetrahydrofolic acid (THFA). Without regeneration of THFA, folate would be "trapped" in its methyl (circulating) form and be unavailable to perform its numerous functions, including, for example, synthesis of thymidylate and ultimately of DNA. It is this latter defect that damages the bone marrow hematopoiesis in vitamin B_{12} and folate deficiency. In addition, the methionine generated from this reaction is needed for synthesis of S-adenosylmethionine, which in turn is needed for methylation of myelin lipid, and synthesis of myelin basic protein and the subsequent synthesis of phosphatidylcholine (lecithin) and choline. As deoxyadenosylcobalamin, vitamin B_{12} is required for conversion of methylmalonyl coenzyme A to succinyl coenzyme A, a component of the degradation pathway for certain amino acids and odd-chain fatty acids.[152]

Signs and Symptoms of Deficiency

Clinically, a deficiency of vitamin B_{12} presents with hematologic, neurologic, and/or gastrointestinal effects.[152] The hematologic effects (mechanism discussed earlier) result in a characteristic megaloblastic anemia, with macrocytosis, hypersegmentation of neutrophil nuclei, bone marrow changes, and, frequently, leukopenia and thrombocytopenia. The neurologic effects are a result of inadequate myelin synthesis, which presents as peripheral nerve, spinal cord, or cerebral damage. The various signs and symptoms include paresthesias (especially of hands and feet), diminution of vibration or position sense, unsteadiness, confusion, depression, mental slowness, poor memory, and sometimes delusions and overt psychosis. Other rapidly dividing cells, such as those of the gastrointestinal tract, exhibit megaloblastic changes, often resulting in glossitis, anorexia, flatulence, constipation and/or diarrhea.

There are six different ways to develop a deficiency of vitamin B_{12}; three involve "inadequacies" (of ingestion, absorption, utilization) and three, "increases" (of requirements, excretion, destruction).[231] Persons particularly at risk for developing vitamin B_{12} deficiency because of inadequate intake include total vegetarians;[232,233] persons who have pernicious anemia,[233] total gastrectomy, sprue, resection of terminal ileum, gastric bypass surgery, or intestinal parasitic infections;[234,235] and those who take drugs such as ethanol, neomycin, metformin colchicine, potassium chloride, and *p*-aminosalicylic acid.[236] A deficiency of vitamin B_{12} due to increased requirement can be associated with pregnancy, lactation, infancy, hyperthyroidism, alcoholism, or megadosing with vitamin C.[231,237,238]

Signs and Symptoms of Toxicity

In its naturally occurring forms, vitamin B_{12} is relatively nontoxic. Because no adverse effects were associated with either high intakes of this vitamin from food or supplements, no UL was set.[152] In contrast, a rare allergic reaction to crystalline cyanocobalamin (the form of vitamin B_{12} in pharmaceuticals) has been reported.[239] Also, in rare instances infants have a congenital defect (i.e., they lack the enzyme required to remove cyanide from cyanocobalamin) and are thus harmed by the cyanocobalamin form of vitamin B_{12}.[240]

Assessment of Status

According to Sauberlich[103] and as discussed in the DRIs,[152] there are several methods of assessing vitamin B_{12} status. The earliest serum indicator of compromised vitamin B_{12} status is a low serum concentration of holotranscobalamin II (holoTCII), the primary delivery protein for vitamin B_{12}. Yet, further studies are needed to establish this assay as the sole or commonly used procedure. Because more than 90% of vitamin B_{12} deficiencies are associated with elevated serum levels of methylmalonic acid and total homocysteine,[241,242] the serum levels of these metabolites seem to be more sensitive indicators of a vitamin B_{12} deficiency than is the serum B_{12} value. However, a deficiency of folic acid or vitamin B_6 can also raise the level of homocysteine in the serum; so of the two metabolites, serum methylmalonic acid (MMA) would be the assay of choice. Yet, again, the techniques developed to measure serum MMA are costly and may not be available at routine laboratories. Therefore measuring the concentration of vitamin B_{12} in the serum is still, for practical reasons, the method of choice to determine vitamin B_{12} status. See Sauberlich[103] for a summary of normal ranges and tentative recommendations for each assay. WHO states serum vitamin B_{12} values greater than 150 pmol/L (200 pg/ml) are considered acceptable, while others suggest that acceptable levels be 258 pmol/L (350 pg/ml) or greater.[243] Acceptable values for serum MMA are tentatively set at less than 376 nmol/L.

Requirements

As shown in Table 11-1, the RDA is 2.4 μg of vitamin B_{12} per day for both women and men, 19 years of age and older.[152] There are very few reports on the intravenous requirement for vitamin B_{12}. Daily doses of 2 to 12.5 μg of vitamin B_{12} were found to sustain normal vitamin B_{12} status.[38,133,148,171,195] The currently used AMA adult parenteral recommendation of 5 μg per day[5] is the same as the new AMA-FDA workshop committee adult parenteral recommendation[4] as shown in Table 11-1.

Special Concerns

Because of the interrelationship of vitamin B_{12} and folic acid in the development of megaloblastic anemia, care must be taken to determine the status of both vitamins before supplementing either one. If, for example, only folic acid is given when vitamin B_{12} deficiency is also present, the observed megaloblastic

changes will be corrected, but the defect in myelin synthesis will persist and eventually result in neurologic damage.

Folic Acid

General Overview

"Folate" is the generic term for this vitamin that exists in many forms,[244] with folic acid (pteroylmonoglutamic acid) being the most oxidized and stable form of folate. Although the folic acid form rarely occurs in food, it is the primary form used in vitamin supplements and in fortified food products. Most of the naturally occurring folates are pteroylpolyglutamates that have reduced (tetrahydro) pteridine rings with (as many as 11) glutamic acids (polyglutamates) attached.[40,152] Metabolically, these coenzyme forms transfer single carbon fragments from one compound to another in amino acid metabolism and nucleic acid synthesis.[40,152] Specifically, folate coenzymes are involved in the following reactions: (1) deoxyribonucleic acid (DNA) synthesis and thus cell division, (2) purine synthesis, (3) generation of formate into the formate pool, and (4) amino acid interconversions. As an example (see vitamin B_{12} discussion) folic acid is needed for the synthesis of thymidylate, and ultimately of DNA. It is this latter defect that causes the megaloblastic changes in red blood cells and other rapidly dividing cells observed in both folate and vitamin B_{12} deficiencies.

Signs and Symptoms of Deficiency

An inadequate intake of folate leads initially to a decline in folate levels in the serum. This initial decrease is then followed by a decrease in the concentration of folate in red blood cells and an increase in homocysteine concentration. Ultimately, this compromise in folate status leads to megaloblastic changes in bone marrow and other rapidly dividing cells,[152] resulting in megaloblastic or macrocytic anemia. Other features (signs) include gastrointestinal disturbances (such as diarrhea) and a smooth, sore tongue. In addition, weight loss, depression of cell-mediated immunity,[245] nervous instability, and dementia can also be present.

Increased susceptibility to folic acid deficiency occurs in alcoholics[246,247] and during periods of increased or enhanced cell division, turnover, or metabolism (as with trauma, burns, infections, cancer, chronic hemolytic anemias, hyperthyroidism, pregnancy, lactation, and early infancy).[248,249] Anticonvulsant therapy (e.g., phenytoin) and folic acid compete with each other for absorption at the gut cell membrane and perhaps even at the brain cell wall.[250,251] Therapy with folic acid antagonists such as the chemotherapeutic agents methotrexate and aminopterin[252,253] and the potassium-sparing diuretic, triamterene,[254] can also lead to folic-acid deficiency. In addition, large therapeutic doses (e.g., 3900 mg/day) of nonsteroidal antiinflammatory drugs (aspirin, ibuprofen, acetaminophen) may exert antifolate activity.[152] Routine use of these drugs, on the other hand, has not been shown to impair folate status.[152]

Signs and Symptoms of Toxicity

The consumption of excess amounts of folate via food sources has not resulted in reports of any adverse effects.[255] Therefore, any reports of adverse effects involve the synthetic folic acid. Because of the antagonistic relationship between folic acid and phenytoin therapy, excessive amounts of folic acid (100 times the RDA) can precipitate a convulsion in persons "under tight control" with continuous phenytoin therapy.[251,253] Although no sign of toxicity was observed in women given 10 mg of folate per day for 4 months,[254] precipitation in the kidney of larger doses of folate has led to renal toxicity in rats.[239] Allergic reactions to oral and parenteral folic acid have been observed.[152] Whereas an oral dose of 350 µg of folic acid per day has been reported to decrease the absorption of zinc,[256] other research studies have found no or only subtle effects on zinc absorption.[152] Because of the limited but suggestive evidence that excessive intakes of synthetic folic acid may precipitate or exacerbate a neuropathy in vitamin B_{12}–deficient individuals, a UL of 1000 µg per day of folic acid, exclusive of food folate, was established.

Assessment of Status

The concentration of folate in red blood cells is the primary indicator of folate adequacy because it reflects tissue folate stores. A value of 140 ng of folate per ml (320 nmol/L) is the cutoff point for adequate folate status.[152] A circulating level of folate in the serum of less than 7 nmol/L (3 ng/ml) indicates a negative balance of folate at the time the blood sample was drawn.[251] This decline generally occurs early in folate deprivation and is a sensitive indicator of dietary folate intake.[251] Numerous studies are currently exploring the relationship between plasma homocysteine concentrations as an ancillary indicator of folate status,[251] with an increase in circulating homocysteine levels reflecting a negative folate status. However, because the circulating level of homocysteine in the plasma is also influenced by the status of both vitamins B_{12} and B_6 as well as age, gender, race, presence of certain genetic abnormalities and renal insufficiency,[152] it cannot be used as the sole or specific indicator for folate status in an individual.

Requirements

The RDA for folic acid is 400 µg of dietary folate equivalents per day for both women and men 19 years of age and older.[152] Dietary folate equivalents are established to adjust for the nearly 50% lower bioavailability of folate from food sources versus that coming from synthetic sources: 1 µg of dietary folate equivalent (DFE) = 1 µg of food folate = 0.5 µg of folic acid taken on an empty stomach = 0.6 µg of folic acid taken with meals.[152] Several studies have reported folic acid deficiency during parenteral nutrition therapy,[234,249,257] so supplementation with this nutrient is recommended for anyone who is receiving parenteral nutrition. Following the current AMA recommendation of 400 µg per day,[5] some studies have suggested that this level of supplementation may not be adequate maintenance or replacement for a person in physiologic stress.[148,171,258] These and other studies may be in part why the recommendation for folic acid has been increased to 600 µg in the new adult parenteral recommendations from the AMA-FDA workshop committee[4] (see Table 11-1).

Special Concerns

FOLATE AND NEURAL TUBE DEFECTS. The current recommendation is that women who are capable of becoming pregnant should be taking 400 µg of synthetic folic acid daily, from fortified foods or supplements or a combination of the two, in addition to consuming food folate from a varied diet.[152] Note: Women who have a history of a conceptus with a neural tube defect should consult their physician because larger amounts of folate are recommended in this situation.

FOLATE, VASCULAR DISEASE, AND HOMOCYSTEINE LEVELS. Historically, high levels of circulating homocysteine have been connected with vascular disease.[152] As early as 1976, a study showed a significant difference in plasma concentrations of homocysteine between patients with vascular disease and normal controls.[259] Since this observation, many studies have reported an association between an elevated plasma concentration of homocysteine and an increased risk for premature occlusive vascular disease and/or coronary heart disease.[152] The mechanism by which this elevation in circulating homocysteine levels might increase the risk of developing vascular disease remains unknown. What is known is that folate (as methyltetrahydrofolate) serves as a substrate for methionine synthase, and as such, is required for the remethylation of homocysteine. Further studies are warranted to determine if folate has a direct role in reducing the risk of developing vascular disease. To date, the available evidence is not sufficiently conclusive to use risk reduction as a basis for establishing the current RDA.[152]

Biotin

General Overview

Biotin is a sulfur-containing, water-soluble vitamin. Even though intestinal microorganisms can synthesize biotin, it remains questionable if any is available for absorption.[152] In mammalian systems, biotin functions as a component of four enzymes that transport carbon dioxide (carboxyl units) to various substrates. These four biotin enzymes are acetyl CoA carboxylase (for fatty acid synthesis), pyruvate carboxylase (for gluconeogenesis), propionyl CoA carboxylase (for propionate metabolism), and 3-methylcrotonyl CoA carboxylase (for catabolism of branched-chain amino acids).

Signs and Symptoms of Deficiency

Two lines of evidence document the human requirement for biotin. The first results from the prolonged consumption of raw egg whites,[260] which contain avidin, a biotin-binding glycoprotein. This is one of the reasons why the consumption of raw eggs is not recommended. The second line of evidence comes from patients who have been on long-term parenteral nutrition without biotin supplementation.[261] Biotin deficiency may present as dermatitis, conjunctivitis, alopecia, and abnormalities of the central nervous system.[262] The observed dermatitis is dry, scaly (seborrheic) and erythematous in nature and appears quite similar to the rash seen in zinc deficiency.[152] Others at increased risk for developing biotin deficiency include pregnant and lactating women,[263] alcoholics, and persons who have undergone partial gastrectomy[264] or have a burn injury.[265] Persons who are undergoing either hemodialysis or peritoneal dialysis may also have an increased requirement for biotin.[152]

Signs and Symptoms of Toxicity

Even with intakes as high as 200 mg orally or up to 20 mg intravenously, no adverse effects of biotin were noted in humans.[152] A UL for biotin could not be set because of insufficient data.[152]

Assessment of Status

The two best indicators of biotin status include (1) an abnormally decreased excretion of biotin in the urine and (2) an abnormally increased excretion of 3-hydroxyisovalerate acid in the urine.[266] Normal values for the 24-hour excretion of biotin vary with the assay and need to be established. Normal values for the 24-hour excretion of 3-hydroxyisovalerate acid in the urine generally range between 77 to 195 µmol per 24 hours (mean +/- standard deviation = 112 +/- 38).[152]

Requirements

An AI of 30 µg of biotin per day in adults was set by extrapolating data from infants and limited estimates of biotin intake in the general population.[152] The initial AMA recommendation of 60 µg per day [5] is the same as the new adult parenteral recommendation from the AMA-FDA workshop committee[4] as shown in Table 11-1. Most[148,267,268] but not all[74] investigators have found this to be adequate replacement for biotin.

Special Concerns

Various manifestations of biotin deficiency are also associated with zinc deficiency:[269] Both present with scaly erythematous dermatitis around the eyes, nose, and mouth; anorexia; and hair loss. Therefore, it is important to determine zinc status if biotin deficiency is suspected. Deficiency of essential fatty acids (EFA) also manifests itself in a very similar erythematous dermatitis, yet the distribution differs. The dermatitis of EFA deficiency is generalized over the body; the lesions of the other two have the characteristic periorofacial distribution.

Pantothenic Acid

General Overview

Pantothenic acid is a water-soluble B vitamin that is widely distributed in foods and is relatively stable in moist heat and in the presence of both oxidizing and reducing agents. Pantothenic acid is vital to the synthesis and maintenance of CoA, a cofactor and acyl group carrier for many enzymatic processes and of acyl carrier protein, a component of the fatty acid synthase complex.[270] Structurally, pantothenic acid is composed of pantoic acid linked to β-alanine. As a component of CoA, pantothenic acid is involved in release of energy from carbohydrate, fat, and ketogenic amino acids; in gluconeogenesis; in the synthesis of heme and sterols; and in most acetylation reactions. As a component of acyl carrier protein (ACP), a component of fatty acid synthase complex, pantothenic acid is necessary for fat synthesis.[271,272]

Signs and Symptoms of Deficiency

Given the wide distribution of this vitamin in foods, a deficiency of pantothenic acid has only been observed in individuals who were either fed diets virtually devoid of the vitamin[273] or were given a metabolic antagonist to the vitamin (ω-methyl pantothenic acid).[274] The subsequent signs and symptoms of the resultant deficiency include varying degrees of irritability and restlessness, fatigue, apathy, malaise, sleep disturbances, gastrointestinal complaints (nausea, vomiting, and abdominal cramps), neurobiologic symptoms (numbness, paresthesias, muscle cramps, staggering gait), hypoglycemia,

and an increased insulin sensitivity.[152] Historically, a deficiency of pantothenic acid was implicated in the "burning feet" syndrome that affected prisoners of war in Asia during World War II because this syndrome corrected when only pantothenic acid (and not the other B vitamins) were given.[275] Chronic malnutrition or prolonged overindulgence in alcohol can lead to pantothenic acid deficiency (along with deficiencies of many other nutrients, especially the B vitamins).

Signs and Symptoms of Toxicity

Pantothenic acid is relatively safe. According to the DRIs report for this vitamin, there have been no adverse effects of oral pantothenic acid in humans or animals.[152] This is consistent with an earlier report that men given as much as 10 g per day for 6 weeks showed no untoward effects;[276] however, this is in contrast to another report of diarrhea and water retention when doses of 10 to 20 g per day were given.[277] Because a quantitative risk assessment cannot be performed, a UL could not be established for pantothenic acid.

Assessment of Status

The urinary excretion of pantothenic acid is closely related to dietary intake and likely the easiest test to conduct and interpret. A urinary excretion of pantothenic acid less than 1 mg/day (in adults) indicates poor status or nutrition of the vitamin.[103,152]

Requirements

As shown in Table 11-1, the AI for pantothenic acid is 5 mg per day in adults 19 years of age and older.[152] The currently followed AMA recommendation of 15 mg per day for persons receiving parenteral nutrition[5] is the same as the new adult parenteral recommendations from the AMA-FDA workshop committee[4] (see Table 11-1). In most studies to date, this level of supplementation has been adequate to keep both circulating levels and 24-hour urine excretion of pantothenic acid within normal limits.[73,74,148,171,195,278,279]

Antioxidants in Critical Illness

A free radical is a chemical compound that has an unpaired electron in its outer orbit, which renders it quite unstable and, thus, very reactive.[280] To pair this "unpaired" electron, the compound "reacts with" or "attacks" other molecules in its vicinity to generate a more stable compound. Derivatives of oxygen are the most important free radicals and arise as by-products of normal metabolism and by exposure to environmental pollutants (such as alcohol, tobacco smoke, ozone, radiation, and sunlight). Examples of free radicals are (1) the superoxide radical ($O_2^\bullet$) generated from either the addition of an electron (e^-) to oxygen (O_2) or oxidation of ferrous iron (Fe^{++}) to ferric iron (Fe^{+++}) in the presence of oxygen and (2) the hydroxyl radical ($OH^\bullet$), which is formed when hydrogen peroxide is in the presence of an electron and a hydrogen ion or Fe^{++}. Other reactive oxygen metabolites (ROM) include hydrogen peroxide (H_2O_2, formed nonenzymatically when superoxide is in the presence of an electron and two hydrogen ions [H^+], or enzymatically, via superoxide dismutase, when two superoxide radicals react with two hydrogen ions) and singlet oxygen (an excited state of oxygen formed by energy capture).[281]

When the body is unable to dispose of, or "neutralize," free radicals or ROM in a timely manner, they accumulate and become harmful. This condition is called *oxidative stress.* For example, lipid peroxidation occurs when free radicals "attack" polyunsaturated fatty acids and thus damage cell membranes. Normally, harmful free radicals or ROM are neutralized by the body's antioxidant mechanisms. These mechanisms include the antioxidant enzyme systems glutathione peroxidase, superoxide dismutase, and catalase (which prevent generation of toxic substances) and the antioxidant molecules, generally vitamins E, C, carotenes, glutathione, cysteine, uric acid, taurine, and flavinoids (which can intercept free radicals or ROM as they are generated). It is noteworthy that the key antioxidant enzyme systems also rely on the trace elements selenium, zinc, copper, and manganese to function. Oxidative stress also results when the balance between "prooxidants" and "antioxidants" is in favor of the "prooxidants."[282]

Besides being generated by environmental pollutants and oxygen per se, free radicals or ROM are also generated in large amounts during critical illness (e.g., trauma, surgery, ischemia/reperfusion injury, acute respiratory distress syndrome [ARDS], infection, burns). This phenomenon is likely mediated by the release of cytokines and the initiation of an acute-phase response.[283] An acute phase response, now better known as the systemic inflammatory response, can also occur in individuals who are free from acute stress (e.g., trauma, surgery) but are experiencing more chronic low-grade inflammatory processes (as reviewed in Boosalis and associates[284]). In addition to altering the circulating levels of certain visceral proteins and various minerals,[285-290] new evidence suggests that the presence of an acute phase (i.e., systemic inflammatory) response is also associated with alterations in the circulating levels of certain antioxidants.[284] Briefly, Boosalis and colleagues[284] in their study identified the presence of an acute phase response (defined by an elevation in serum C-reactive protein levels) in a subgroup of elderly women who were free of acute trauma and who had not had surgery. Along with the elevation in circulating levels of C-reactive protein were the predictable increases in the circulating levels of copper and fibrinogen and decreases in the circulating albumin and thyroxine-binding prealbumin (transthyretin) levels. Moreover and more importantly, in this study the systemic acute phase inflammatory response was also significantly and negatively correlated with plasma lycopene ($p < .05$), β-carotene ($p < .05$), α-carotene ($p < .05$), and total carotenoids ($p < .01$) concentrations. These findings suggest that antioxidant status can also be influenced by an inflammatory response that is more chronic in nature, which is consistent with the findings in the critical illness population.

For example, neutrophil granules destroy bacteria and other foreign matter by generating and mobilizing (oxygen) free radicals.[291] Several studies have implicated free radicals in the pathogenesis of ARDS,[292-294] and depressed circulating levels of both ascorbate and vitamin E have been reported in patients with ARDS.[295,296] Along with ARDS, decreased circulating levels of vitamin C or vitamin E have been reported after surgery,[297,298] polytrauma,[148] burns,[299] and sepsis,[300,301] and critical illness.[302] Reduced circulating levels of vitamins E and C have also been reported in persons on long-term parenteral nutrition.[196,303]

Given the increased generation of free radicals and the decreased circulating levels of antioxidants observed during critical illness, is there a role for additional amounts of antioxidants in these clinical settings? To date, relatively few human studies have addressed this question specifically. On the other hand, many animal studies have shown a beneficial effect of antioxidant therapy in reducing either morbidity[304,305] or mortality[306,307] associated with critical illness. In humans, more specifically those with ARDS, treatment with intravenous selenium, vitamin E, ascorbic acid, and N-acetyl cysteine reduced mortality.[308] Supplemental N-acetyl cysteine provides cysteine for glutathione synthesis and a scavenger for hydrogen peroxide and hydroxyl radicals. Yet the provision of another antioxidant, superoxide dismutase, has not been as successful,[309,310] except when given before the onset of sepsis.[283] Even though superoxide dismutase efficiently scavenges superoxide anion, if the hydrogen peroxide produced is not effectively removed, levels of hydroxyl radicals increase and further damage results. Another study reported that vitamins C and E plus allopurinol (an antioxidant), when given before coronary-artery bypass surgery, resulted in fewer perioperative infarcts and ischemic electrocardiographic events.[311]

Conclusion

In conclusion, along with studies addressing whether supplemental antioxidants should be provided during periods of critical illness, future studies should also address which combination of antioxidants and how much of each should be provided. Of particular importance in these future studies is to determine the numerous interrelationships, both synergistic as well as antagonistic, among the "antioxidant nutrients." For example, both vitamin C and β-carotene may become prooxidants in certain circumstances, and vitamin C, when supplemented to enhance the recycling of oxidized vitamin E, can promote the availability of free iron and potentially contribute to an increased risk of infection.[312] For now, it seems that circulating levels of certain antioxidants are decreased during periods of critical illness, which suggests that a compromise in their status is possible.

REFERENCES

1. Briggs GM, Calloway DH (eds): *Bogert's nutrition and physical fitness,* Philadelphia, 1979, WB Saunders, p 116.
2. How should the recommended dietary allowances be revised? A concept paper from the food and nutrition board, *Nutr Rev* 52(6):216-219, 1994.
3. National Academy of Sciences: Chapter 1, Dietary reference intakes. Reprinted with permission in *Nutr Rev* 55(9):319-351, 1997.
4. U.S. Department of Health and Human Services: Parenteral multivitamin products, *Fed Regist* 65:21200-21201, 2000.
5. American Medical Association: Multivitamin preparations for parenteral use: a statement by the Nutrition Advisory Group, *J Parenter Enteral Nutr* 3:258-262, 1979.
6. Institute of Medicine Food and Nutrition Board: Dietary reference intakes for vitamin A, vitamin K, arsenic, boron, chromium, copper, iodine, iron, manganese, molybdenum, nickel, silicon, vanadium, and zinc, Washington, DC, 2001, National Academy Press, pp 65-126, 127-154.
7. Gudas LJ, Sporn MB, Roberts AB: Cellular biology and biochemistry of the retinoids. In Sporn MB, Roberts AB, Goodman DS (eds): *The retinoids: biology, chemistry, and medicine,* ed 2, New York, 1994, Raven Press, pp 443-520.

8. Saari JC: Retinoids in photosensitive systems. In Sporn MB, Roberts AB, Goodman DS (eds): *The retinoids: Biology, chemistry, and medicine,* ed 2, New York, 1994, Raven Press, pp 351-385.

9. World Health Organization (WHO): *Control of vitamin A deficiency and xerophthalmia,* Technical Report Series No 672, Geneva, Switzerland, 1982, World Health Organization.

10. Morriss-Kay GM, Sokolova N: Embryonic development and pattern formation, *FASEB J* 10:961-968, 1996.

11. Wilson JG, Roth CB, Warkany J: An analysis of the syndrome of malformations induced by maternal vitamin A deficiency. Effects of restoration of vitamin A at various times during gestation, *Am J Anat* 92:189-217, 1953.

12. Chase HP, Kumar V, Dodds JM, Sauberlich HE, Hunter RM, Burton RS, Spalding V: Nutritional status of preschool Mexican-American migrant farm children, *Am J Dis Child* 122:316-324, 1971.

13. Sauberlich HE, Hodges HE, Wallace DL, Kolder H, Canham JE, Hood J, Raica N, Lowry LK: Vitamin A metabolism and requirements in the human studied with the use of labeled retinal, *Vitam Horm* 32:251-275, 1974.

14. Cantorna MT, Nashold FE, Hayes CE: Vitamin A deficiency results in a priming environment conducive for TH1 cell development, *Eur J Immunol* 25:1673-1679, 1995.

15. Nauss KM, Newberne PM: Local and regional immune function of vitamin A-deficient rats with ocular herpes simplex virus (HSV) infections, *J Nutr* 115:1316-1324, 1985.

16. Dawson HD, Ross AC: Chronic marginal vitamin A status effects the distribution and function of T cells and natural T cells in aging Lewis rats, *J Nutr* 129:1782-1790, 1999.

17. Wiedermann U, Hanson LA, Kahu H, Dahlgren UI: Aberrant T-cell function in vitro and impaired T-cell dependent antibody response in vivo in vitamin A-deficient rats, *Immunology* 80:581-586, 1993.

18. Sommer A, Katz J, Tarwotje I: Increased risk of respiratory disease and diarrhea in children with preexisting mild vitamin A deficiency, *Am J Clin Nutr* 40:1090-1095, 1984.

19. Feachem RG: Vitamin A deficiency and diarrhea, *Trop Dis Bull* 84: R2-R16, 1987.

20. Olson JA: Vitamin A, retinoids, and carotenoids. In Shils ME, Olson JA, Shike M (eds): *Modern nutrition in health and disease,* Malvern, PA, 1994, Lea & Febiger, pp 287-307.

21. Lieber CS: Hepatic, metabolic and toxic effects of ethanol. 1991 update, *Alcohol Clin Exp Res* 15:573-592, 1991.

22. Arroyave G, Wilson D, Mendez J, et al: Serum and liver vitamin A and lipids in children with severe protein malnutrition, *Am J Clin Nutr* 9: 180-185, 1961.

23. Smith FR, Suskind R, Thanangkul O, et al: Plasma vitamin A, retinol-binding protein and prealbumin concentrations in protein calorie malnutrition, III: response to varying dietary treatments, *Am J Clin Nutr* 28:732-738, 1975.

24. Jacob RA, Sandstead HH, Solomons NW, et al: Zinc status and vitamin A transport in cystic fibrosis, *Am J Clin Nutr* 31:638-644, 1978.

25. Smith JC, McDaniel EG, Fan FF, Halsted JA: Zinc: a trace element essential in vitamin A metabolism, *Science* 181:954-955, 1973.

26. Szebeni A, Negyesi G, Feuer L: Vitamin A levels in the serum of burned patients, *Burns* 7:313B-318B, 1980.

27. Rai K, Courtemanch AD: Vitamin A assay in burned patients, *J Trauma* 15:419B-424B, 1975.

28. Stephensen CB, Alvarez JO, Kohatsu J, et al: Vitamin A is excreted in the urine during acute infection, *Am J Clin Nutr* 60:388-392, 1994.

29. Bhaskaram P, Reddy V, Raj S, Bhatnagar RC: Effect of measles on the nutritional status of preschool children, *J Trop Med Hyg* 87:21-25, 1984.

30. Forbes GM, Forbes A: Micronutrient status in patients receiving home parenteral nutrition, *Nutrition* 13(11-12):941-944, 1997.

31. Bendich A, Langseth L: Safety of vitamin A, *Am J Clin Nutr* 49:358-371, 1989.

32. Olson JA: Adverse effects of large doses of vitamin A and retinoids, *Semin Oncol* 10:290-293, 1983.

33. Persson B, Tunell R, Ekengren K: Chronic vitamin A intoxication during the first half year of life, *Acta Paediatr Scand* 54:49-60, 1965.

34. Underwood BA: Vitamin A in animal and human nutrition. In Sporn MB, Roberts AB, Goodman DS (eds): *The retinoids,* vol 1, New York, 1984, Raven Press, pp 281-392.

35. Flores H. Frequency distributions of serum vitamin A levels in cross-sectional surveys and in surveys before and after vitamin A supplementation. In *A brief guide to current methods of assessing vitamin A status.* A report of the International Vitamin A Consultative Group (IVACG), Washington, DC, 1993, The Nutrition Foundation, pp 9-11.

36. Underwood BA: Hypovitaminosis A: international programmatic issues, *J Nutr* 124:1476S-1472S, 1994.

37. Olson JA: Needs and sources of carotenoids and vitamin A, *Nutr Rev* 52(2):S67B-S73B, 1994.

38. Lowry SF, Goodgame JT, Maher MM, Brennan MF: Parenteral vitamin requirements during intravenous feeding, *Am J Clin Nutr* 31:2149-2158, 1978.

39. Kirkemo AK, Burt ME, Brennan MF: Serum vitamin level maintenance in cancer patients on total parenteral nutrition, *Am J Clin Nutr* 35: 1003-1009, 1982.

40. Food and Nutrition Board, National Research Council: *Recommended dietary allowances,* ed 10, Washington, DC, 1989, National Academy of Sciences, p 80.

41. Shenai JP, Stahlman MT, Chytil F: Vitamin A delivery from parenteral alimentation solution, *J Pediatr* 99:661-663, 1981.

42. Henton DH, Merritt RJ: Vitamin A sorption to polyvinyl and polyolefin intravenous tubing, *J Parenter Enteral Nutr* 14:79-81, 1990.

43. Allwood MC, Plane JH: The degradation of vitamin A exposed to ultra-violet radiation, *Int J Pharmacol* 19:207-213, 1984.

44. Billion-Rey F, Guillaumont M, Frederich A, Aulagner G: Stability of fat-soluble vitamins A (retinol palmitate), E (tocopherol acetate), and K1 (phylloquinone) in total parenteral nutrition at home, *J Parenter Enteral Nutr* 17:56-60, 1993.

45. Allwood MC, Martin HJ: The photodegradation of vitamins A and E in parenteral nutrition mixtures during infusion, *Clin Nutr* 19(5):39-42, 2000.

46. Holick MF: McCollum Award Lecture, 1994: vitamin D: new horizons for the 21st century, *Am J Clin Nutr* 60:619-630, 1994.

47. Fieser LF, Fieser M: Vitamin D. In *Steroids,* New York, 1959, Reinhold, pp 90-168.

48. DeLuca HF: The vitamin D story: a collaborative effort of basic science and clinical medicine, *Fed Proc* 2:224-236, 1988.

49. Reichel H, Koeffler HP, Norman AW: The role of the vitamin D endocrine system in health and disease, *N Engl J Med* 320:981-991, 1989.

50. Holick MF: Vitamin D: biosynthesis, metabolism, and mode of action. In DeGroot LJ, Besser G, Cahill GF, et al. (eds): *Endocrinology,* vol 2, New York, 1989, Grune & Stratton, pp 902B-926B.

51. Holick MF: Vitamin D and the skin: photobiology, physiology and therapeutic efficacy for psoriasis. In Heersche NM, Kanis JA (eds): *Bone and mineral research,* vol 7, Amsterdam, 1990, Elsevier, pp 313-366.

52. Lemire JM: Immunomodulatory role of 1,25-dihydroxyvitamin D_3, *J Cell Biochem* 49:26-31, 1992.

53. Stumpf WE, Sar M, Reid FA, et al: Target cells for 1,25-dihydroxyvitamin D_3 in intestinal tract, stomach, kidney, skin, pituitary, and parathyroid, *Science* 206:1188B-1190B, 1979.

54. Bhalla AK, Amento EP, Clemens TL, et al: Specific high-affinity receptors for 1,25-dihydroxyvitamin D_3 in human peripheral blood mononuclear cells: presence in monocytes and induction in T lymphocytes following activation, *J Clin Endocrinol Metab* 57:1308B-1310B, 1983.

55. Goldring SR, Krane SM, Avioli LV: Disorders of calcification: osteomalacia and rickets. In DeGroot IJ (ed): *Endocrinology,* vol 2, ed 3, Philadelphia, 1995, WB Saunders, pp 1204-1227.

56. Kamel A, Brazier M, Picard C, Voitte F, Samson L, Desnet G, Sebert JI: Urinary excretion of pyridinolines crosslinks measured by immunoassay and HPLC techniques in normal subjects and in elderly patients with vitamin D deficiency, *Bone Miner* 26:197-208, 1994.

57. Favus MJ, Christakos S: *Primer on the metabolic bone diseases and bone mineral metabolism,* ed 3, Philadelphia, 1996, Lippincott-Raven.

58. Freaney R, McBrinn Y, McKenna MJ: Secondary hyperparathyroidism in elderly people: combined effect of renal insufficiency and vitamin D deficiency, *Am J Clin Nutr* 58:187-191, 1993.

59. Belton NR: Rickets—not only the "English Disease," *Acta Paediatr Scand* 323(suppl):68-75, 1986.

60. Stephens WP, Klimiuk PS, Warrington S, et al: Observations on the natural history of vitamin D deficiency amongst Asian immigrants, *Q J Med* 51:171-188, 1982.

61. Gottschlich MM: Micronutrients. In Skipper A (ed): *Dietitian's handbook of enteral and parenteral nutrition,* Bethesda, 1989, Aspen Publications, pp 163-203.

62. Avioli LV, Lee SW, McDonald JE, et al: Metabolism of vitamin D_3-3H in human subjects: distribution in blood, bile, feces, and urine, *J Clin Invest* 46:983-992, 1967.

63. Institute of Medicine Food and Nutrition Board: Dietary reference intakes for calcium, phosphorus, magnesium, vitamin D, and fluoride, Washington, DC, 1999, National Academy Press, pp 250-287.

64. Holmes RP, Kummerow FA: The relationship of adequate and excessive intake of vitamin D to health and disease, *J Am Coll Nutr* 2:173-199, 1983.
65. Allen SH, Shah JH: Calcinosis and metastatic calcification due to vitamin D intoxication. A case report and review, *Horm Res* 37:68-77, 1992.
66. Galla JH, Booker BB, Luke RG: Role of the loop segment in the urinary concentrating defect of hypercalcemia, *Kidney Int* 29:977-982, 1986.
67. Moncrief MW, Chance GW: Nephrotoxic effect of vitamin D therapy in vitamin D refractory rickets, *Arch Dis Child* 44:571-579, 1969.
68. Taylor CB, Hass GM, Ho KJ, Liu LB: Risk factors in the pathogenesis of arteriosclerotic heart disease and generalized atherosclerosis, *Ann Clin Lab Sci* 2:239-243, 1972.
69. American Academy of Pediatrics: The prophylactic requirement and the toxicity of vitamin D, *Pediatrics* 31:512-525, 1963.
70. Haddad JG, Hahn TJ: Natural and synthetic sources of circulating 25-hydroxyvitamin D in man, *Nature* 244:515-517, 1973.
71. Holick MF: Vitamin D: photobiology, metabolism, mechanism of action, and clinical application. In DeGroot LJ, Besser M, Burger HG, Jameson JI, Loriaux DI, Marshall JC, O'Dell WD, Potts JI, Rubenstein AH (eds): *Endocrinology*, ed 3, Philadelphia, 1995, WB Saunders.
72. Holick MF: The use and interpretation of assays for vitamin D and its metabolites, *J Nutr* 120:1464-1469, 1990.
73. Shils ME, Baker H, Frank O: Blood vitamin levels of long-term adult home total parenteral nutrition patients: the efficacy of the AMA-FDA parenteral multivitamin formulation, *J Parenter Enteral Nutr* 9:179-188, 1985.
74. Dempsey DT, Mullen JL, Rombeau JL, et al: Treatment effects of parenteral vitamins in total parenteral nutrition patients, *J Parenter Enteral Nutr* 11:229-237, 1987.
75. Bengoa JM, Bolt MJ, Rosenberg IH: Hepatic vitamin D 25-hydroxylase inhibition by cimetidine and isoniazid, *J Lab Clin Med* 104:546-552, 1984.
76. Shike M, Harrison JE, Sturtridge WC, et al: Metabolic bone disease in patients receiving long-term parenteral nutrition, *Ann Intern Med* 92:343-350, 1980.
77. Klein GL, Cannon RA, Diament M, et al: Infantile vitamin D resistant rickets associated with total parenteral nutrition, *Am J Dis Child* 136:74-76, 1982.
78. Klein GL, Coburn JW: Parenteral nutrition: effect on bone and mineral metabolism, *Annu Rev Nutr* 11:93-119, 1991.
79. Shike M, Sturtridge WC, Tam CS, et al: A possible role of vitamin D in the genesis of parenteral nutrition-induced metabolic bone disease, *Ann Intern Med* 95:560-568, 1981.
80. Lipkin EW, Ott SM, Klein GL: Heterogeneity of bone histology in parenteral nutrition patients, *Am J Clin Nutr* 46:673-680, 1987.
81. Vargas JH, Klein GL, Ament ME, et al: Metabolic bone disease of total parenteral nutrition: course after changing from casein to amino acids in parenteral solutions with reduced aluminum content, *Am J Clin Nutr* 48:1070-1078, 1988.
82. Institute of Medicine Food and Nutrition Board: Dietary reference intakes for vitamin C, vitamin E, selenium, carotenoids, Panel on Dietary Antioxidants and Related Compounds, Subcommittees on Upper Reference Levels of Nutrients and Interpretation and Uses of DRIs, Standing Committee on the Scientific Evaluation of Dietary Reference Intakes, Washington, DC, 2000, National Academy Press, pp 186-283, 95-185.
83. Burton GW, Joyce A, Ingold KU: Is vitamin E the only lipid-soluble, chain-breaking antioxidant in human blood plasma and erythrocyte membranes? *Arch Biochem Biophys* 221:281-290, 1983.
84. Cavalier I, Ouahchi K, Kayden HJ, DiDonato S, Reutenauer I, Mandel JI, Koenig M: Ataxia with isolated vitamin E deficiency: heterogeneity of mutations and phenotypic variability in a large number of families, *Am J Hum Genet* 62:301-310, 1998.
85. Binder HJ, Herting DC, Hurst V, et al: Tocopherol deficiency in man, *N Engl J Med* 273:1289-1297, 1965.
86. Braunstein H: Tocopherol deficiency in adults with chronic pancreatitis, *Gastroenterology* 40:224-231, 1961.
87. Sitrin MD, Lieberman F, Jensen WE, et al: Vitamin E deficiency and neurologic disease in adults with cystic fibrosis, *Ann Intern Med* 107:51-54, 1987.
88. Gordon HH, Nitowsky HM, Cornblath M: Studies in tocopherol deficiency in infants and children, *Am J Dis Child* 90:669-681, 1955.
89. Howard L, Ovesen L, Satya-Murti S, Chu R: Reversible neurological symptoms caused by vitamin E deficiency in patients with short bowel syndrome, *Am J Clin Nutr* 36:1243-1249, 1982.
90. Bjorneboe A, Bjorneboe GE, Drevon CA: Serum half-life, distribution, hepatic uptake and biliary excretion of alpha-tocopherol in rats, *Biochim Biophys Acta* 921:175-181, 1987.
91. Gross S, Melhorn DK: Vitamin E, red cell lipids and red cell stability in prematurity, *Ann NY Acad Sci* 203:141-162, 1972.
92. Bieri JG, Farrell PM: Vitamin E, *Vitam Horm* 34:31-75, 1976.
93. Majaj AS, Dinning JS, Azzam SA, Darby WJ: Vitamin E responsive megaloblastic anemia in infants with protein calorie malnutrition, *Am J Clin Nutr* 12:374-379, 1963.
94. Traber MG, Kayden HJ: Preferential incorporation of alpha-tocopherol vs gamma-tocopherol in human lipoproteins, *Am J Clin Nutr* 49:517-526, 1989.
95. Traber MG, Burton GW, Ingold JU, Kayden HJ: RRR- and SRR-alpha-tocopherols are secreted without discrimination in human chylomicrons, but RRR-alpha-tocopherol is preferentially secreted in very low-density lipoproteins, *J Lipid Res* 31:675-685, 1990.
96. Farrell PM, Machlin LJ: Human health and disease. In Machlin LJ (ed): *Vitamin E, A comprehensive treatise,* New York, 1980, Marcel Dekker, pp 520-620.
97. Lake AM, Stuart MJ, Oski FA: Vitamin E deficiency and enhanced platelet function. Reversal following E supplementation, *J Pediatr* 90:722-725, 1977.
98. Gordon HH, Nitowsky HM, Cornblath M: Studies in tocopherol deficiency in infants and children, *Am J Dis Child* 90:669-681, 1955.
99. Horwitt MK, Century B, Zeman AA: Erythrocyte survival time and reticulocyte levels after tocopherol depletion in man, *Am J Clin Nutr* 12:99-106, 1963.
100. Bye AM, Muller DP, Wilson J, et al: Symptomatic vitamin E deficiency in cystic fibrosis, *Arch Dis Child* 60:162-164, 1985.
101. Nitowsky HM, Tildon JT, Levin S, Gordon HH: Studies of tocopherol deficiency in infants and children. VII. The effect of tocopherol on urinary, plasma and muscle creatine, *Am J Clin Nutr* 10:368-378, 1962.
102. Farrell PM, Roberts RJ: Vitamin E. In Shils ME, Olson JA, Shike M (eds): *Modern nutrition in health and disease,* ed 8, Malvern, PA, 1994, Lea & Febiger, pp 326-341.
103. Sauberlich HE: *Laboratory tests for the assessment of nutritional status,* ed 2, Baton Rouge, 1999, CRC Press.
104. Axford-Gately RA, Wilson GJ: Myocardial infarct size reduction by single high dose or repeated low dose vitamin E supplementation in rabbits, *Can J Cardiol* 9:94-98, 1993.
105. Barsacchi R, Pelosi G, Maffei S, et al: Myocardial vitamin E is consumed during cardiopulmonary bypass: indirect evidence of free radical generation in human ischemic heart, *Int J Cardiol* 37:339-343, 1992.
106. Coghlan JG, Flitter WD, Clutton SM, et al: Lipid peroxidation and changes in vitamin E levels during coronary artery bypass grafting, *J Thorac Cardiovasc Surg* 106:268-274, 1993.
107. Grant JP: Vitamin requirements. In *Handbook of total parenteral nutrition,* ed 2, Philadelphia, 1992, WB Saunders, p 297.
108. Suttie JW: Synthesis of vitamin K-dependent proteins, *FASEB J* 7:445-452, 1993.
109. Shearer MJ: Vitamin K, *Lancet* 345:229-234, 1995.
110. Caraballo PJ, Gabriel SE, Castro MR, Atkinson EJ, Melton LJ III: Changes in bone density after exposure to oral anticoagulants: a meta-analysis, *Osteoporos Int* 9:441-448, 1999.
111. Savage D, Lindenbaum J: Clinical and experimental human vitamin K deficiency. In Lindenbaum J (ed): *Nutrition in hematology,* New York, 1983, Churchill Livingstone, pp 271-319.
112. Brinkhous KM, Smith HP, Warner ED: Plasma prothrombin level in normal infancy and in hemorrhagic disease of the newborn, *Am J Med Sci* 193:475-480, 1937.
113. Olson RE: Vitamin K. In Shils ME, Olson JA, Shike M (eds): *Modern nutrition in health and disease,* ed 8, Malvern, PA, 1994, Lea & Febiger, pp 342-357.
114. Blanchard RA, Furie BC, Jorgensen M, et al: Acquired vitamin KB-dependent carboxylation deficiency in liver disease, *N Engl J Med* 305:242-248, 1981.
115. McGehee WG, Klotz TA, Epstein DJ, Rapaport ST: Coumarin necrosis associated with hereditary protein C deficiency, *Ann Intern Med* 101:59-60, 1984.
116. Hooper CA, Harvey BB, Stone HH: Gastrointestinal bleeding due to vitamin K deficiency in patients on parenteral cefamondole, *Lancet* 1:39-40, 1980.
117. Light RF, Alsher RP, Frey CN: Vitamin A toxicity and hyperthrombinemia, *Science* 100:225-226, 1944.

118. Matshiner JT, Amelotti JM, Doisy EA: Mechanism of the effect of retinoic acid and squalene on vitamin K deficiency in the rat, *J Nutr* 91:303-306, 1967.
119. March BE, Wong E, Seier L, et al: Hypervitaminosis E in the chick, *J Nutr* 103:371-377, 1973.
120. Corrigan JJ, Marcus FI: Coagulopathy associated with vitamin E ingestion, *JAMA* 230:1300-1301, 1974.
121. Gross L, Brotman M: Hypoprothrombinemia and hemorrhage associated with cholestyramine therapy, *Ann Intern Med* 72:95-96, 1970.
122. Dudrick SJ, Wilmore DW, Vars HM, Rhoads JE: Long-term total parenteral nutrition with growth, development and positive nitrogen balance, *Surgery* 64:134-142, 1968.
123. Ryan JA: Complications of total parenteral nutrition. In Fischer E (ed): *Total parenteral nutrition,* Boston, 1976, Little, Brown, pp 55-100.
124. Hazell K, Baloch KH: Vitamin K deficiency in the elderly, *Gerontol Clin* 12:10-17, 1970.
125. Pineo GF, Gallus AS, Hirsh J: Unexpected vitamin K deficiency in hospitalized patients, *Can Med Assoc J* 109:880-883, 1973.
126. Ansell JE, Kumar R, Deykin D: The spectrum of vitamin K deficiency, *JAMA* 238:40-42, 1977.
127. Chiou TJ, Chou YT, Tzeng WF: Menadione-induced cell degeneration is related to lipid peroxidation in human cancer cells, *Proc Natl Sci Counc Repub China B* 22:13-21, 1998.
128. Badr M, Yoshihara H, Kauffman F, Thurman R: Menadione causes selective toxicity to periportal regions of the liver lobule, *Toxicol Lett* 35:241-246, 1987.
129. Owen CA: Pharmacology and toxicology of the vitamin K group. In Sebrell WH, Harris RS (eds): *The vitamins,* vol III, New York, 1971, Academic Press, pp 492-509.
130. Suttie JW: Vitamin K and human nutrition, *J Am Diet Assoc* 92:585-590, 1992.
131. Sokoll LJ, Booth SL, O'Brien ME, Davidson KW, Tsaioun KI, Sadowski JA: Changes in serum osteocalcin, plasma phylloquinone, and urinary gamma-carboxyglutamic acid in response to altered intakes of dietary phylloquinone in human subjects, *Am J Clin Nutr* 65:779-784, 1997.
132. Sadowski JA, Hood SJ, Dallal GE, Garry PJ: Phylloquinone in plasma from elderly and young adults: factors influencing its concentration, *Am J Clin Nutr* 50:100-108, 1989.
133. Jeejeebhoy KN, Langer B, Tsallas G, et al: Total parenteral nutrition at home: studies in patients surviving 4 months to 5 years, *Gastroenterology* 71:943-953, 1976.
134. Jeppson B, Gimmon Z: Vitamins. In Fischer JE (ed): *Surgical nutrition,* Boston, 1983, Little, Brown, pp 241-281.
135. May JM, Cobb CE, Mendiratta S, Hill KF, Burk RF: Reduction of the ascorbyl free radical to ascorbate by thioredoxin reductase, *J Biol Chem* 273:23039-23045, 1998.
136. Park JB, Levine M: Purification, cloning and expression of dehydroascorbic acid-reducing activity from human neutrophils: identification as glutaredoxin, *Biochem J* 315:931-938, 1996.
137. Horning DH, Moser U: The safety of high vitamin C intakes in man. In Counsell JN, Hornig DH (eds): *Vitamin C (ascorbic acid),* London, 1981, Applied Science, pp 225-248.
138. Rivers JM: Safety of high-level vitamin C ingestion, *Ann NY Acad Sci* 498:445-454, 1987.
139. Gerster H, Moser U: Is high dose vitamin C associated with systemic conditioning? *Nutr Res* 8:1327-1332, 1988.
140. Omaye ST, Skala JH, Jacob RA: Rebound effect with ascorbic acid in adult males, *Am J Clin Nutr* 48:379-380, 1988.
141. Jacob RA: Vitamin C. In Shils ME, Olson JA, Shike M (eds): *Modern nutrition in health and disease,* ed 8, Malvern, PA, 1994, Lea & Febiger, pp 432B-448B.
142. Jacob RA: Assessment of human vitamin C status, *J Nutr* 120:1480B-1485B, 1990.
143. Bates CJ, Rutishauser IH, Black AE, et al: Long term vitamin status and dietary intake of healthy elderly subjects. 2. Vitamin C, *Br J Nutr* 42:43-56, 1977.
144. Omaye ST, Schaus EE, Kutnink MA, Hawkes WC: Measurement of vitamin C in blood components by high-performance liquid chromatography. Implication in assessing vitamin C status, *Ann NY Acad Sci* 498:389-401, 1987.
145. Jacob RA, Skala JH, Omaye ST: Biochemical indices of human vitamin C status, *Am J Clin Nutr* 46:818-826, 1987.
146. Blanchard J, Conrad KA, Watson RR, et al: Comparison of plasma, mononuclear, and polymorphonuclear leucocyte vitamin C levels in young and elderly women during depletion and supplementation, *Eur J Clin Nutr* 43:97-106, 1989.
147. Crandon JH, Lennihan R, Mikal S, Reif AE: Ascorbic acid economy in surgical patients, *Ann NY Acad Sci* 92:246-267, 1961.
148. Boosalis MG, Edlund D, Moudry B, et al: Circulating blood and twenty-four hour urinary levels of water-soluble vitamins: are current intravenous multivitamin preparations adequate? *Nutrition* 4:431-438, 1988.
149. Cameron E, Pauling L, Leibovitz B: Ascorbic acid and cancer: a review, *Cancer Res* 39:663-681, 1979.
150. Lund CC, Levenson SM, Green RW, et al: Ascorbic acid, thiamine, riboflavin and nicotinic acid in relation to acute burns in man, *Arch Surg* 55:557-583, 1947.
151. Burge JC, Flancbaum L, Holcombe B: Copper decreases ascorbic acid stability in total parenteral nutrition solutions, *J Am Diet Assoc* 94:777-779, 1994.
152. Institute of Medicine Food and Nutrition Board: *Dietary reference intakes for thiamin, riboflavin, niacin, vitamin B_6, folate, vitamin B_{12}, pantothenic acid, biotin, and choline,* Standing Committee on the Scientific Evaluation of Dietary Reference Intakes, Washington, DC, 1998, National Academy Press, pp 58-389.
153. Itokawa Y, Schulz RA, Cooper JR: Thiamine in nerve membranes, *Biochem Biophys Acta* 266:293-299, 1972.
154. Kramer J, Goodwin JA: Wernicke's encephalopathy: complication of intravenous hyperalimentation, *JAMA* 238:2176-2177, 1977.
155. Harper CG: Sudden, unexpected death and Wernicke's encephalopathy: a complication of prolonged intravenous feeding, *Aust NZ J Med* 10:230-235, 1980.
156. Christakis G, Miridjianian A: Diets, drugs and their interrelationships, *J Am Diet Assoc* 52:21-24, 1968.
157. Oriot D, Wood C, Gottesman R, Huault G: Severe lactic acidosis related to acute thiamine deficiency, *J Parenter Enteral Nutr* 15:105-109, 1991.
158. Velez RJ, Myers B, Guber MS: Severe acute metabolic acidosis (acute beriberi): an avoidable complication of total parenteral nutrition, *J Parenter Enteral Nutr* 9:216-219, 1985.
159. Nakasaki H, Ohta H, Soeda J, Hakuuchi H, Tsuda H, Tajima T, Hitomi T, Fjii K: Clinical and biochemical aspects of thiamine treatment for metabolic acidosis during total parenteral nutrition, *Nutrition* 13(2):110-117, 1997.
160. Centers for Disease Control and Prevention (CDC): Lactic acidosis traced to thiamine deficiency related to nationwide shortage of multivitamins for total parenteral nutrition—United States, 1997, *MMWR Morbid Mortal Wkly Rep* 46(23):523-528, 1997.
161. Schramm C, Wanitschke R, Galle PR: Thiamine for the treatment of nucleoside analogue-induced severe lactic acidosis, *Eur J Anaesthesiol* 16(10):733-735, 1999.
162. Tanphaichitr V: Thiamin. In Shils ME, Olson JA, Shike M (eds): *Modern nutrition in health and disease,* ed 8, Malvern, PA, 1994, Lea & Febiger, pp 359B-365B.
163. Victor M, Adams RD, Collins GH: *The Wernicke-Korsakoff syndrome, and related neurologic disorders due to alcoholism and malnutrition,* ed 2, Philadelphia, 1989, FA Davis, pp 1-231.
164. Seear M, Lockitch G, Jacobson B, et al: Thiamine, riboflavin, and pyridoxine deficiencies in a population of critically ill children, *J Pediatr* 121:533-538, 1992.
165. Hahn JS, Berquist W, Alcorn DM, Chamberlain L, Bass D: Wernicke encephalopathy and beriberi during total parenteral nutrition attributable to multivitamin infusion shortage, *Pediatrics* 101(1):E10, 1998.
166. Vasconcelos MM, Silva KP, Vidal G, Silva AF, Domingues RC, Berditchevsky CR: Early diagnosis of pediatric Wernicke's encephalopathy, *Pediatr Neurol* 20(4):289-294, 1999.
167. Decker MJ, Isaacman DJ: A common cause of altered mental status occurring at an uncommon age, *Pediatr Emerg Care* 16(2):94-96, 2000.
168. Stephen JM, Grant R, Yeh CS: Anaphylaxis from administration of intravenous thiamine, *Am J Emerg Med* 10:61-63, 1992.
169. Royer-Morrot MJ, Zhiri A, Paille F, Royer RJ: Plasma thiamine concentrations after intramuscular and oral multiple dosage regimens in healthy men, *Eur J Clin Pharmacol* 42:219-222, 1992.
170. Wrenn KD, Murphy F, Slovis CM: A toxicity study of parenteral thiamine hydrochloride, *Ann Emerg Med* 18:867-870, 1989.
171. Nichoalds GE, Meng HC, Caldwell MD: Vitamin requirements in patients receiving total parenteral nutrition, *Arch Surg* 112:1061-1064, 1977.
172. Broviac JW, Scriber BH: Prolonged parenteral nutrition in the home, *Surg Gynecol Obstet* 139:24-28, 1974.
173. Dudrick SJ, MacFayden BV, Souchon EA, et al: Parenteral nutrition techniques in cancer patients, *Cancer Res* 37:2440-2450, 1977.

174. Ricour C: Techniques et indications de la nutrition parenterale exclusive chez l'enfant, *Rev Prat* 35:1105-1113, 1985.

175. Seear M, Lockitch G, Jacobson B, et al: Thiamine, riboflavin, and pyridoxine deficiencies in a population of crucially ill children, *J Pediatr* 121:533-538, 1992.

176. Chen MF, Boyce HW, Triplett L: Stability of the B vitamins in mixed parenteral nutrition solution, *J Parenter Enteral Nutr* 7:462-464, 1983.

177. Smith JL, Canham JE, Wells PA: Effect of phototherapy light, sodium bisulfite and pH on vitamin stability in total parenteral nutrition admixtures, *J Parenter Enteral Nutr* 4:394-402, 1988.

178. Baeckert PA, Green HL, Fritz I, et al: Vitamin concentrations in very low birth weight infants given vitamins intravenously in a lipid emulsion: measurement of vitamins A, D, and E and riboflavin, *J Pediatr* 113: 1057-1065, 1988.

179. Dahl GB, Svensson L, Kinnander NJG, et al: Stability of vitamins in soybean oil fat emulsion under conditions simulating intravenous feeding of neonates and children, *J Parenter Enteral Nutr* 18:234-239, 1994.

180. McCormick DB: Riboflavin. In Shils ME, Olson JA, Shike M (eds): *Modern nutrition in health and disease,* ed 8, Malvern, PA, 1994, Lea & Febiger, pp 366-375.

181. Rivlin RS: Riboflavin metabolism, *N Engl J Med* 283:463-472, 1970.

182. Cole HS, Lopez R, Cooperman JM: Riboflavin deficiency in children with diabetes mellitus, *Acta Diabetol Lat* 13:25-29, 1976.

183. Rosenthal WS, Adham NF, Lopez R, Cooperman JM: Riboflavin deficiency in complicated chronic alcoholism, *Am J Clin Nutr* 26: 858-860, 1973.

184. Rivlin RS: Riboflavin and cancer. In Rivlin RS (ed): *Riboflavin,* New York, 1975, Plenum Press, pp 369-391.

185. Steier M, Lopez R, Cooperman JM: Riboflavin deficiency in infants and children with heart disease, *Am Heart J* 92:139-143, 1976.

186. Pinto J, Huang YP, Rivlin RS: Inhibition of riboflavin metabolism in rat tissues by chlorpromazine, imipramine and amitriptyline, *J Clin Invest* 67:1500-1506, 1981.

187. Newman LJ, Lopez R, Cole HS, et al: Riboflavin deficiency in women taking oral contraceptive agents, *Am J Clin Nutr* 31:247-249, 1978.

188. Roe DA, Bogusz S, Sheu J, McCormick DB: Factors affecting riboflavin requirements of oral contraceptive users and nonusers, *Am J Clin Nutr* 35:495-501, 1982.

189. Lewis CM, King JC: Effect of oral contraceptive agents on thiamin, riboflavin, and pantothenic acid status in young women, *Am J Clin Nutr* 33:832-838, 1980.

190. Wilson JA: Disorders of vitamins: Deficiency, excess and errors of metabolism. In Petersdorf RG, Harrison TR (eds): *Harrison's principles of internal medicine,* ed 10, New York, 1983, McGraw-Hill, pp 461-470.

191. Sydenstricker VP, Sebrell WH, Cleckley HM, Kruse HD: The ocular manifestations of ariboflavinosis, *JAMA* 114:2437-2445, 1940.

192. Olpin SE, Bates CJ: Lipid metabolism in riboflavin deficient rats: effect of dietary lipids on riboflavin status and fatty acid profiles, *Br J Nutr* 47:577-596, 1982.

193. Pinto J, Dutta P, Rivlin R: Alteration in age-related decline of beta-adrenergic receptor binding in adipocytes during riboflavin deficiency, *Clin Res* 33:526A, 1985.

194. Sauberlich HE, Judd JH, Nicholalds GE, et al: Application of the erythrocyte glutathione reductase assay in evaluating riboflavin nutritional status in a high school student population, *Am J Clin Nutr* 25:756-762, 1972.

195. Stromberg P, Shenkin A, Campbell RA, et al: Vitamin status during total parenteral nutrition, *J Parenter Enteral Nutr* 5:295-299, 1981.

196. Labadarios D, O'Keefe SJ, Dicker J, et al: Plasma vitamin levels in patients on prolonged total parenteral nutrition, *J Parenter Enteral Nutr* 12:205-211, 1988.

197. Coon WW: Riboflavin metabolism in surgical patients, *Surg Gynecol Obstet* 120:1289-1295, 1965.

198. Sauberlich HD, Skala JH, Dowdy RP: *Laboratory tests for the assessment of nutritional status,* Boca Raton, 1974, CRC Press, pp 70-74.

199. Turkki PR, Degruccio GD: Riboflavin status of rats fed two levels of protein during energy deprivation and subsequent repletion, *J Nutr* 113:282-292, 1983.

200. Swendweid ME, Jacob RA: Niacin. In Shils ME, Olson JA, Shike M (eds): *Modern nutrition in health and disease,* ed 8, Malvern, PA, 1994, Lea & Febiger, pp 376-382.

201. Basu TK, Raven RW, Bates C, Williams DC: Excretion of 5-hydroxyindole acetic acid and N^1-methylnicotinamide in advanced cancer patients, *Eur J Cancer* 9:527-528, 1973.

202. Hilton JG, Wells CH: Nicotinic acid reduction of plasma volume after thermal trauma, *Science* 191:861-862, 1976.

203. Sheperd J, Packard CJ, Patsch JR, et al: Effects of nicotinic acid therapy on plasma high density lipoprotein subfraction distribution and composition and on apolipoprotein A metabolism, *J Clin Invest* 63:858-867, 1979.

204. Cashin-Hemphill L, Mack WJ, Pogoda JM, et al: Beneficial effects of colestipol-niacin on coronary atherosclerosis: a 4-year follow-up, *JAMA* 264(23):3013-3017, 1990.

205. Etchason JA, Miller TD, Squires RW, et al: Niacin-induced hepatitis: a potential side effect with low-dose time-release niacin, *Mayo Clin Proc* 66:23-28, 1991.

206. Gharavi AG, Diamond JA, Smith DA, Phillips RA: Niacin-induced myopathy, *Am J Cardiol* 74:841-842, 1994.

207. Jacob RA, Swendseid ME, McKee RW, et al: Biochemical markers for assessment of niacin status in young men: urinary and blood levels of niacin metabolites, *J Nutr* 119:591-598, 1989.

208. Fu CS, Swendseid ME, Jacob RA, McKee RW: Biochemical markers for assessment of niacin status in young men: levels of erythrocyte niacin coenzymes and plasma tryptophan, *J Nutr* 119:1949-1955, 1989.

209. Kreisberg RA: Niacin: a therapeutic dilemma "one man's drink is another's poison," *Am J Med* 97:313-316, 1994.

210. Compton MM, Cidlowski JA: Vitamin B_6 and glucocorticoid action, *Endocrin Rev* 7:140-148, 1986.

211. Dakshinamurti K, Paulose CS, Siow YL: Neurobiology of pyridoxine. In Reynolds RD, Leklem JE (eds): *Vitamin B_6: its role in health and disease,* New York, 1985, Alan R Liss, pp 99-121.

212. Kirksey A, Morre DM, Wasynczuk AZ: Neuronal development in vitamin B_6 deficiency, *Ann NY Acad Sci* 585:202-218, 1990.

213. Chandra RK, Au B, Heresi G: Single nutrient deficiency and cell-mediated immune responses, II: Pyridoxine, *Nutr Res* 1:101-106, 1981.

214. Axelrod AE, Trakatellis AC: Relationship of pyridoxine to immunological phenomena, *Vitam Horm* 22:591-607, 1964.

215. Weintraub LR, Conrad ME, Crosby WH: Iron-loading anemia. Treatment with repeated phlebotomies and pyridoxine, *N Engl J Med* 275:169-176, 1966.

216. Hines JD, Harris JW: Pyridoxine-responsive anemia: description of three patients with megaloblastic erythropoiesis, *Am J Clin Nutr* 14:137-146, 1964.

217. Leklem JE: Vitamin B_6 metabolism and function in humans. In Leklem JE, Reynolds RD (eds): *Clinical and physiological applications of vitamin B_6,* New York, 1987, Alan R Liss, pp 3-28.

218. Schaumburg H, Kaplan J, Windebank A, et al: Sensory neuropathy from pyridoxine abuse. A new megavitamin syndrome, *N Engl J Med* 309: 445-448, 1983.

219. Dalton K, Dalton MJ: Characteristics of pyridoxine overdose neuropathy syndrome, *Acta Neurol Scand* 76:8-11, 1987.

220. Leklem LE: Vitamin B_6: a status report, *J Nutr* 120:1503-1507, 1990.

221. Lui A, Lumeng L, Aronoff GR, Li T-K: Relationship between body store of vitamin B6 and plasma pyridoxal-P clearance: metabolic balance studies in humans, *J Lab Clin Med* 106:491-497, 1985.

222. Brown RR, Rose DP, Leklem JE, et al: Urinary 4-pyridoxic acid, plasma pyridoxal phosphate, and erythrocyte aminotransferase levels in oral contraceptive users receiving controlled intakes of vitamin B_6, *Am J Clin Nutr* 28:10-19, 1975.

223. Rose CS, Gyorgy P, Butler M, et al: Age differences in vitamin B_6 status of 617 men, *Am J Clin Nutr* 29:847-853, 1976.

224. Potera C, Rose DP, Brown RR: Vitamin B_6 deficiency in cancer patients, *Am J Clin Nutr* 30:1677-1679, 1977.

225. Reynolds RD, Natta CL: Depressed plasma pyridoxal phosphate concentrations in adult asthmatics, *Am J Clin Nutr* 41:684-688, 1985.

226. Barlow GB, Wilkinson AW: Plasma pyridoxal phosphate levels and tryptophan metabolism in children with burns and scalds, *Clin Chim Acta* 64:79-82, 1975.

227. Kopple JD, Swenseid ME: Vitamin nutrition in patients undergoing maintenance hemodialysis, *Kidney Int* 7(suppl):79-84, 1975.

228. Baker H, Frank O, Zetterman RK, et al: Inability of chronic alcoholics with liver disease to use food as a source of folates, thiamin and vitamin B_6, *Am J Clin Nutr* 28:1377-1380, 1975.

229. Bhagavan HN: Interaction between vitamin B_6 and drugs. In Reynolds RD, Leklem JE (eds): *Vitamin B_6: its role in health and disease,* New York, 1985, Alan R Liss, pp 401-415.

230. Ubbink JB, Bissbort S, Vermaak WJH, Delport R: Inhibition of pyridoxal kinase by methylxanthines, *Enzyme* 43:72-79, 1990.

231. Herbert V: Staging vitamin B_{12} (cobalamin) status in vegetarians, *Am J Clin Nutr* 59(suppl):1213S-1222S, 1994.

232. Winawer SJ, Streiff R, Zamcheck N: Gastric and hematological abnormalities in a vegan with nutritional vitamin B_{12} deficiency. Effect of oral vitamin B_{12}, *Gastroenterology* 53:130-135, 1967.

233. Baker SJ: Human vitamin B$_{12}$ deficiency, *World Rev Nutr Diet* 8:52-69, 1967.

234. Kahn SB: Recent advances in the nutritional anemias, *Med Clin North Am* 54:631-645, 1970.

235. Boylan LM, Sugerman HJ, Driskell JA: Vitamin E, vitamin B$_6$, vitamin B$_{12}$, and folate status of gastric bypass surgery patients, *J Am Diet Assoc* 88:579-585, 1988.

236. Shaw S, Jayatilleke E, Bauman W, Herbert V: Mechanism of B$_{12}$ malabsorption and depletion due to metformin discovered by using serial serum holo-transcobalamin II (holo TCII) (B112 on TCII) as a surrogate for serial Schilling tests, *Blood* 82(10 suppl 1):432A, 1993.

237. Herbert V, Drivas G, Foscaldi R, et al: Multivitamin/mineral food supplements containing vitamin B$_{12}$ may also contain analogues of vitamin B$_{12}$, *N Engl J Med* 307:255-256, 1982.

238. Shaw S, Herbert V, Colman N, Jayatilleke E: Effect of ethanol-generated free radicals on gastric intrinsic factor and glutathione, *Alcohol* 7:153-157, 1990.

239. Herbert V, Das KC: Folic acid and vitamin B$_{12}$. In Shils ME, Olson JA, Shike M (eds): *Modern nutrition in health and disease,* ed 8, Malvern, PA, 1994, Lea & Febiger, pp 402-425.

240. Fenton WA, Rosenberg L: Inherited disorders of cobalamin transport and metabolism. In Stanbury JB, Wyngaarden JB, Frederickson DS, et al. (eds): *Metabolic basis of inherited disease,* ed 6, New York, 1989, McGraw-Hill, pp 2065-2082.

241. Allen RH, Stabler SP, Savage DG, Lindenbaum J: Diagnosis of cobalamine deficiency I: usefulness of serum methylmalonic acid and total homocysteine concentrations, *Am J Hematol* 34:90-98, 1990.

242. Lindenbaum J, Savage DG, Stabler SP, Allen RH: Diagnosis of cobalamine deficiency II: relative sensitivities of serum cobalamin, methylmalonic acid, and total homocysteine concentrations, *Am J Hematol* 34:99-107, 1990.

243. Lindenbaum J, Savage DG, Stabler SP, Allen RH: Prevalence of cobalamin deficiency in the Framingham elderly population, *Am J Clin Nutr* 60:2-11, 1994.

244. Wagner C: Symposium on the subcellular compartmentation of folate metabolism, *J Nutr* 126:1228S-1234S, 1996.

245. Gross RL, Reid JV, Newberne PM, et al: Depressed cell-mediated immunity in megaloblastic anemia due to folic acid deficiency, *Am J Clin Nutr* 28:225-232, 1975.

246. Hartshorn EA: Food and drug interactions, *J Am Diet Assoc* 70:15-19, 1977.

247. Halsted CH, Robles EA, Mezey E: Intestinal malabsorption in folate-deficient alcoholics, *Gastroenterology* 64:526-532, 1973.

248. Barlow GB, Wilkinson AW: 4-amino-imidazole-5-carboxamide excretion and folate status in children with burns and scalds, *Clin Chim Acta* 29:355-358, 1970.

249. Steinberg D: Folic acid deficiency: early onset of megaloblastosis, *JAMA* 222:490, 1972.

250. Druskin MS, Wallen MH, Bonagura L: Anticonvulsant associated megaloblastic anemia, *N Engl J Med* 267:483-485, 1962.

251. Colman N, Herbert V: Dietary assessments with special emphasis on prevention of folate deficiency. In Botez MI, Reynolds EH (eds): *Folic acid in neurology, psychiatry, and internal medicine,* New York, 1979, Raven Press, pp 23-33.

252. Hellman S, Iannotti AT, Bertino JR: Determinations of the levels of serum folate in patients with carcinoma of the head and neck treated with methotrexate, *Cancer Res* 24:105-113, 1964.

253. Werkheiser WC: The biochemical, cellular and pharmacological action of folic acid antagonists, *Cancer Res* 23:1277-1285, 1963.

254. Lieberman FL, Bateman JR: Megaloblastic anemia possibly induced by triamterene in patients with alcoholic cirrhosis, *Ann Intern Med* 68:168-173, 1968.

255. Butterworth CE, Tamura T. Folic acid safety and toxicity: a brief review, *Am J Clin Nutr* 50:353-358, 1989.

256. Herbert V: Recommended dietary intakes (RDI) of vitamin B$_{12}$ in humans, *Am J Clin Nutr* 45:671-678, 1987.

257. Shah PC, Zafar M, Patel AR: Folate deficiency during intravenous hyperalimentation, *J Med* 8:383-392, 1977.

258. Boles JM, Garo B, Morin JF, Garre M: Comparison between two regimens of folic acid supplementation in intensive care patients, *Clin Nutr* 5:88, 1986.

259. Wilcken DE, Wilcken B: The pathogenesis of coronary artery disease. A possible role for methionine metabolism, *J Clin Invest* 57:1079-1082, 1976.

260. Baugh CM, Malone JW, Butterworth CE Jr: Human biotin deficiency. A case history of biotin deficiency induced by raw egg consumption in a cirrhotic patient, *Am J Clin Nutr* 21:173-182, 1968.

261. Mock DM, deLorimer AA, Liebman WM, et al: Biotin deficiency: an unusual complication of parenteral alimentation, *N Engl J Med* 304:820-823, 1981.

262. Mock DM: Biotin. In Ziegler EE, Filer LJ, Jr (eds): *Present knowledge in nutrition,* ed 7, Washington, DC, 1996, International Life Sciences Institutes Nutrition Foundation, pp 220-235.

263. Bhagavan HN, Coursin DB: Biotin content of blood in normal infants and adults, *Am J Clin Nutr* 20:903-906, 1967.

264. Markkanen T: Studies on the urinary excretion of thiamine, riboflavin, nicotinic acid, pantothenic acid and biotin in achlorhydria and after partial gastrectomy, *Acta Med Scand (Suppl)* 360:1-56, 1960.

265. Barlow GB, Dickerson JA, Wilkinson AW: Plasma biotin levels in children with burns and scalds, *J Clin Pathol* 29:58-59, 1976.

266. Mock NI, Malik MI, Stumbo PJ, Bishop WP, Mock DM: Increased urinary excretion of 3-hydroxyisovaleric acid and decreased urinary excretion of biotin are sensitive early indicators of decreased status in experimental biotin deficiency, *Am J Clin Nutr* 65:951-958, 1997.

267. McClain CJ, Baker H, Onstad GR: Biotin deficiency in an adult during home parenteral nutrition, *JAMA* 247:3116-3117, 1982.

268. Nichoalds GE, Luther RW, Sykes TR, et al: Biotin status of adult TPN patients, *J Parenter Enteral Nutr* 6:577, 1982.

269. Moynahan EJ: Acrodermatitis enteropathica: a lethal inherited human zinc-deficiency disorder, *Lancet* 2:399-400, 1974.

270. Tahiliani AG, Beinlich CJ: Pantothenic acid in health and disease, *Vitam Horm* 46:165-228, 1991.

271. Abiko Y: Metabolism of coenzyme A. In Greenburg DM (ed): *Metabolism of sulfur compounds,* vol 7, *Metabolic pathways,* New York, 1975, Academic Press, pp 1-25.

272. Goldman P, Vagelos PR: Acyl-transfer reactions (CoA-structure, function). In Florkin M, Stotz EH (eds): *Comprehensive biochemistry,* vol 15, *Group-transfer reactions,* Amsterdam,1964, Elsevier, pp 71-92.

273. Fry PC, Fox HM, Tao HG: Metabolic response to a pantothenic acid deficient diet in humans, *J Nutr Sci Vitaminol* 22:339B-346B, 1976.

274. Hodges RE, Bean WB, Ohlson MA, Bleiler R: Human pantothenic acid deficiency produced by omega-methylpantothenic acid, *J Clin Invest* 38:1421-1425, 1959.

275. Glusman M: The syndrome of "burning feet" (nutritional melagia) as a manifestation of nutritional deficiency, *Am J Med* 3:211-223, 1947.

276. Ralli EP, Dumm ME: Relation of pantothenic acid to adrenal cortical function, *Vitam Horm* 11:133-158, 1953.

277. Harris RS: Pantothenic acid. In Sebrell WH Jr, Harris RS (eds): *The vitamins: chemistry, physiology, pathology,* vol 2, New York, 1954, Academic Press, pp 591-694.

278. Bradley JA, King RF, Schorah CJ, Hill GL: Vitamins in intravenous feeding: a study of water-soluble vitamins and folate in critically ill patients receiving intravenous nutrition, *Br J Surg* 65:492-494, 1978.

279. Inculet RI, Norton JA, Nichoalds GE, et al: Water soluble vitamins in cancer patients on parenteral nutrition: a prospective study, *J Parenter Enteral Nutr* 11:243-249, 1987.

280. Rose RC, Bode AM: Biology of free radical scavengers: an evaluation of ascorbate, *FASEB J* 7:1135-1142, 1993.

281. Sardesai VM: Role of antioxidants in health maintenance, *Nutr Clin Pract* 10:19-25, 1995.

282. Sies H: Oxidative stress: introduction. In Sies H (ed): *Oxidative stress: oxidants and antioxidants,* San Diego, 1991, Academic Press, pp. xv-xvi.

283. Goode HF, Webster NR: Antioxidants in intensive care medicine, *Clin Intensive Care* 4:265-269, 1993.

284. Boosalis MG, Snowdon DA, Tully CL, Gross MD: Acute phase response and plasma carotenoid concentrations in older women: findings from the nun study, *Nutrition* 12:475-478, 1996.

285. Stahl WM: Acute phase protein response to tissue injury, *Crit Care Med* 15:545-550, 1987.

286. Wilmore DW: Nutrition and metabolism following thermal injury, *Clin Plast Surg* 1:603-619, 1974.

287. Boosalis MG, Solem L, McCall JT, et al: Serum zinc response in thermal injury, *J Am Coll Nutr* 7:69-76, 1988.

288. Boosalis MG, McCall JT, Solem LD, et al: Serum copper and ceruloplasmin levels and urinary copper excretion in thermal injury patients, *Am J Clin Nutr* 44:899-906, 1986.

289. Boosalis MG, McCall JT, Ahrenholz DH, et al: Serum and urinary silver levels in thermal injury patients, *Surgery* 101:40-43, 1987.

290. Boosalis MG, Ott L, Levine AS, et al: Relationship of visceral proteins to nutritional status in chronic and acute stress, *Crit Care Med* 17:741-747, 1989.

291. Pesanti EL, Nugent KM: Modulation of pulmonary clearance of bacteria by antioxidants, *Infect Immun* 48:57-61, 1985.

292. Weiland JE, Davis WB, Holter JF, et al: Lung neutrophils in the adult respiratory distress syndrome. Clinical and pathophysiologic significance, *Am Rev Respir Dis* 133:218-225, 1986.

293. Cochrane CG, Spragg RG, Revak SD: Pathogenesis of the adult respiratory distress syndrome: Evidence of oxidant activity in bronchoalveolar lavage fluid, *J Clin Invest* 71:754-761, 1983.

294. Leff JA, Parsons PE, Day CE, Taniguchi N, Jochum M, Fritz H, Moore PA, Moore EE, McCord JM, Repine JE: Serum antioxidants as predictors of adult respiratory distress syndrome in patients with sepsis, *Lancet* 341:777-780, 1993.

295. Takeda K, Shimada Y, Amano M: Plasma lipid peroxides and alpha-tocopherol in critically ill patients, *Crit Care Med* 12:957-959, 1984.

296. Cross CE, Forte T, Stocker R, et al: Oxidative stress and abnormal cholesterol metabolism in patients with adult respiratory distress syndrome, *J Lab Clin Med* 115:396-404, 1990.

297. Louw JA, Werbeck A, Louw ME, et al: Blood vitamin concentrations during the acute phase response, *Crit Care Med* 20:934-941, 1992.

298. Agarwal N, Norkus E, Garcia C, et al. Effect of surgery on serum antioxidant vitamins, *J Parenter Enteral Nutr* 20(suppl):32S, 1996.

299. Nguyen TT, Cox CS, Traver DL, et al: Free radical activity and loss of plasma antioxidants, vitamin E, and sulfhydryl groups in patients with burns: the 1993 Moyer award, *J Burn Care Rehabil* 14:602-609, 1993.

300. Goode HF, Cowley HC, Walker BE, et al: Decreased antioxidant status and increased lipid peroxidation in patients with septic shock and secondary organ dysfunction, *Crit Care Med* 23:646-651, 1995.

301. Downing C, Piripitsi A, Bodenham A, Schorah CJ: Plasma vitamin C in critically ill patients, *Proc Nutr Soc* 52:314A, 1993.

302. Schorah CJ, Downing C, Piripitsi A, et al: Total vitamin C, ascorbic acid, and dehydroascorbic acid concentrations in plasma of critically ill patients, *Am J Clin Nutr* 63:760, 1996.

303. Lemoyne M, Van Gossum A, Kurian R, Jeejeebhoy KN: Plasma vitamin E and selenium and breath pentane in home parenteral nutrition patients, *Am J Clin Nutr* 48:1310-1315, 1988.

304. Kunimoto F, Morita T, Ogawa R, Fujita T: Inhibition of lipid peroxidation improves survival rate of endotoxemic rats, *Circ Shock* 21:15-22, 1987.

305. McKechnie K, Furman BL, Parratt JR: Modification by oxygen free radical scavengers of the metabolic and cardiovascular effects of endotoxin infusion in conscious rats, *Circ Shock* 19:429-439, 1986.

306. Fuller RN, Henson EC, Shannon EL, et al: Vitamin C deficiency and susceptibility to endotoxin shock in guinea pigs, *Arch Pathol* 92:239-243, 1971.

307. Nonaka A, Manabe T, Tobe T: Effect of a new synthetic free radical scavenger, 2-octadecyl ascorbic acid, on the mortality in mouse endotoxemia, *Life Sci* 47:1933-1939, 1990.

308. Sawyer MAJ, Mike JJ, Chavin K, Marino PL: Antioxidant therapy and survival in ARDS, *Crit Care Med* 17:S153, 1989.

309. Hoffman H, Siebeck M, Welter HF, Schweiberer L: High dose superoxide dismutase potentiates respiratory failure in septicemia, *Am Rev Respir Dis* 135:A78, 1987.

310. Traber DL, Adams T, Sziebert L, et al: Potentiation of lung vascular response to endotoxin by superoxide dismutase, *J Appl Physiol* 58:1005-1009, 1985.

311. Sisto T, Paajanen H, Metsa-Ketela T, et al: Pretreatment with antioxidants and allopurinol diminishes cardiac onset events in coronary artery bypass grafting, *Ann Thorac Surg* 59:1519-1523, 1995.

312. Fuhrman MP: Antioxidant supplementation in critical illness: what do we know? *Nutrition* 16:470-471, 2000.

Minerals and Trace Elements

12

Michele A. DeBiasse-Fortin, MS, RD, LDN, CNSD

SIXTEEN mineral elements are considered essential nutrients for humans: calcium, phosphorus, potassium, sulfur, sodium, chlorine, magnesium, iron, zinc, selenium, manganese, copper, iodine, molybdenum, cobalt, and chromium. The first seven of these are classified as macronutrient minerals because they contribute more than 0.005% of body weight. They are discussed in Chapter 10 in detail. The remaining nine mineral elements are classified as micronutrients, or trace elements, because they are present in the body only in "trace" amounts (less than 0.005% of body weight).[1] The minerals discussed in this chapter include iron, zinc, copper, selenium, chromium, manganese, molybdenum, and aluminum. Each mineral's function, metabolism, characteristics of deficiency and toxicity, and requirements are reviewed, with an emphasis on the effect of critical illness. In addition, methods for assessment of status and guidelines for supplementation are presented.

Recommendations for supplementation of trace minerals fall under the guidelines of the recommended dietary allowances (RDAs) or the estimated safe and adequate daily dietary intakes (ESADDIs) both set by the Food and Nutrition Board. RDAs are "the levels of intake of essential nutrients considered to be adequate to meet the known nutritional needs of practically all healthy individuals."[2] When the data are sufficient to establish a range of nutritional requirements, but inadequate to set an RDA, the ESSADI may be recommended.[3] In both cases, these standards have been set for healthy persons. They are not requirements set for an individual, but for a population. In addition, they are established to prevent deficiency, not to affect potential therapy or disease prevention. Given the foundations of both the RDA and ESSADI, the clinician is often left with little guidance for prescribing vitamins and minerals to critically ill individuals, especially those receiving enteral and parenteral nutrition (PN) support. The savvy practitioner has a keen understanding of the functions, metabolism, deficiency and toxicity levels, and the safety and efficacy of the nutrients he or she "prescribes" and uses this information to guide the decisions for patients under his or her care.

Iron

Function

The most important function of iron is as a carrier of oxygen. Iron can be characterized as either functional or nonfunctional. Functional iron is present in hemoglobin, myoglobin, and in various iron-containing enzymes. Nonfunctional iron is found stored in the liver, spleen, and bone marrow.[1] Apotransferrin, a globulin produced by the liver, complexes with ferric iron to form transferrin, which is the main transport protein for iron.[4] In the cell, iron is stored on ferritin. Free iron, especially in the ferrous state, is toxic because it can significantly increase free oxygen radical production.

Metabolism

Iron stores have a strong regulatory influence on the amount of iron absorbed.[4] Absorption of iron rises slowly as stores decline and demonstrates a steep rise when stores reach depletion. Absorption also increases in iron deficiency anemia as iron requirements for erythropoiesis are unmet. Body iron content is regulated mainly through changes in the amount of iron absorbed by the intestinal mucosa.[5] The absorption of iron is regulated by the mucosal cells in the upper small intestine[6] and occurs mainly in the duodenum and proximal jejunum. Heme and nonheme iron are absorbed via different mechanisms.[5] Heme iron is highly bioavailable and readily absorbed (40% of that ingested).[1] Nonheme iron absorption is quite variable (10% to 50% of that ingested) and can be enhanced by several factors, including acid environment (from vitamin C, citric acid, lactic acid, hydrochloric acid, and acid amino acids) and the presence of animal tissue proteins.[1] Inhibitors of nonheme iron absorption include phytates, oxalic acid, polyphenols, calcium, reduced gastric acidity, and magnesium-based antacids.[1,5,7] Most investigators suggest that the absorption of iron is reduced after injury or during inflammation.[1] Apotransferrin, a globulin produced by the liver, complexes with ferric iron to form transferrin, which is the main transport protein for iron.[4] Transferrin binds to transferrin receptors on the surface of cells, and with the reduction of iron to its ferrous form, iron then readily crosses the cell membrane. In the cell, iron is stored on ferritin, or it can be used for the synthesis of iron-containing enzymes.

After injury or infection, iron transport is dramatically altered.[1] Within hours, serum iron is depressed and the storage form of iron is elevated. Transferrin concentrations and total iron-binding capacity (TIBC) demonstrate a more gradual decline. This shift in iron that occurs during the acute-phase response that follows injury or infection has been postulated to benefit the host by moving the exchangeable iron to a sequestered storage form, thereby reducing its availability to microorganisms; however, this theory has also been questioned.[8] In the absence of blood loss, iron is excreted in small amounts.[5] Basal obligatory losses of iron are primarily from

Acknowledgment: A special thank you is extended to Carol Braunschweig, PhD, RD, who contributed to the first edition chapter.

superficial gastrointestinal (GI) blood loss and desquamation of surface cells from the skin and GI and urinary tracts. This total daily loss is increased in menstruating women.

Assessment of Status

The status of iron stores can be assessed by measuring the levels of serum ferritin, TIBC, and iron.[1,5] Reduced serum ferritin and iron concentrations, combined with elevated serum TIBC concentrations, indicate iron depletion. During the acute-phase response, serum iron, transferrin, and TIBC concentrations become depressed, and ferritin levels become elevated.[1] By obtaining each of these measurements, it is possible to differentiate iron deficiency resulting from need versus that resulting from stress or infection.

Deficiency and Toxicity

Iron deficiency is one of the most common nutritional problems in both developing and developed areas of the world.[6] Typically, iron deficiency results in microcytic, hypochromic anemia.[1] Signs and symptoms include tachycardia, fatigue, pallor, reduced work capacity, and alterations in mental and motor development. Impaired temperature regulation and decreased resistance to infection have also been reported.[9] Chronic iron overdosage can result in hemachromatosis,[4] a disorder characterized by cirrhosis, diabetes, and hyperpigmentation of the skin. Iron overload can also lead to increased oxidant activity as excess iron is released from its storage form. The result is the production of free radicals that can then lead to cell damage. Other features of iron overload include fatigue, sterility, changes in skin color, arthropathy, cardiac arrhythmias, hypothyroidism and testicular atrophy.[1] Of note, patients with infection tend to sequester exogenously administered iron in their lungs.[4]

Requirements and Supplementation

The RDAs for iron for adult men and women are 10 mg and 15 mg, respectively. In pregnancy, iron requirements are increased to 30 mg to allow for expansion of red cell mass, to provide iron to the fetus and placenta, and to replace blood loss during delivery.[5] Iron supplementation is used for the prevention and treatment of iron deficiency. It is important to recognize that iron supplementation will not correct erythropoietic abnormalities caused by conditions other than iron deficiency and is not indicated for the treatment of anemia resulting from causes other than iron deficiency; therefore, correct diagnosis of the cause of anemia is imperative.[5] The optimal method to replete iron stores is oral supplementation because it is safer, more convenient, and less expensive than other methods, and some evidence indicates that it is used more efficiently. Unfortunately, the use of large doses of iron orally may be complicated by nausea and therefore lead to noncompliance. Taking the supplement with food can reduce nausea. Ferrous sulfate (20% elemental iron), 320 mg twice daily is the standard supplemental oral dose.[1] Given the slow replenishment of iron stores, supplementation is generally required for 6 to 12 months to treat a deficiency.

Indications for the parenteral administration of iron (intramuscularly or intravenously) are limited. The parenteral use of iron dextran has resulted in fatal anaphylactic-type reactions and other significant side effects, and its use therefore should be restricted to situations in which the indication is clearly established, and the patient is not responsive to oral iron therapy.[5] Parenteral nutrition formulations have been used as a vehicle for the administration of iron dextran in both maintenance and therapeutic replacement doses.[10-12] In patients who are not iron deficient and require parenteral nutrition (PN) for a limited time, the supplementation of iron is clearly not indicated. In patients requiring long-term PN, because iron is not a component of the standard trace element preparation, the need for iron supplementation is less clear.[5] The use of maintenance doses of parenteral iron in patients receiving long-term PN is common practice among some clinicians, but it is not fully supported. Confusion involves the decision of whether or not to supplement with low, maintenance doses of iron in an effort to prevent deficiency or to wait and treat a deficiency when it occurs. Another recognized issue is the physical compatibility of iron dextran in parenteral nutrition formulations. In a study by Wan,[13] minimal changes were observed in a nonlipid-containing PN solution observed over an 18-hour period at room temperature after iron dextran was added at a concentration of 100mg/L. Unfortunately, PN solutions generally are infused over a 24-hour period, leaving further study necessary before this can be recommended. Studies of iron dextran added to 3-in-1 PN solutions (dextrose, amino acid, and lipid) demonstrate eye-apparent destabilization of the lipid fraction after 24 hours at room temperature, making this vehicle inappropriate for iron dextran administration.

Zinc

Function

Zinc is widely distributed in the body and is second to iron in total body content.[14] It is involved in many biochemical processes including cellular respiration, immune function, wound healing, membrane stability, antioxidant function, membrane transport of calcium, synthesis of proteins, deoxyribonucleic acid (DNA) and ribonucleic acid (RNA), carbohydrate metabolism, utilization of nitrogen and sulfur, cell division and growth, pituitary and adrenal gland function, enzyme detoxification of free radicals, and bone metabolism.[14-16] Zinc functions as a cofactor of more than 200 enzyme systems.[14,16] Zinc plays an important role in appetite regulation.[17] Zinc deficiency decreases appetite, while zinc supplementation increases appetite. It is postulated that this effect is the result of zinc-induced alterations in neurotransmitter metabolism. In a recent study by Mantzoros and others, serum zinc status was shown to affect serum leptin levels with the magnitude of change proportional to the changes in cellular zinc.[17] Zinc status has also been shown to have an effect on lipid metabolism, in that high levels of zinc supplementation have been shown to increase concentrations of total serum cholesterol, low-density lipoprotein cholesterol, and triacylglycerol.[18] In a recent study by Jern and colleagues, a positive correlation was observed between serum zinc concentrations and protein catabolic rate, such that supplementing the diet of hemodialysis patients with zinc led to an improvement in protein catabolic rate.[19] Parenteral zinc supplementation has also been shown to precipitate an exaggerated acute-phase response as evidenced by a significantly higher febrile response in patients experiencing a mild acute-phase reaction.[20] Zinc can exist in several different valence states, but usually is divalent.[4]

Metabolism

Absorption of zinc occurs in the small intestine, especially the jejunum, via simple diffusion and specific ligands that transport zinc with them into the mucosal cells.[1,14] Zinc absorption from a supplement administered 3 or more hours after ingestion of a meal has been shown to range between 40% and 90%, while a supplement administered with a meal results in an absorption rate of 8% to 38%.[19] Animal proteins, amino acids, and unsaturated fatty acids enhance zinc absorption, whereas phytates; folates; high levels of copper, cadmium, and iron; and consumption of a high-calcium diet decrease zinc absorption.[14,21,22] With increasing amounts of zinc in a meal, the amount of zinc absorbed increases. Long-term zinc intake (i.e., zinc status) can also affect absorption of dietary zinc, in that prolonged low-zinc diets increase zinc absorption and retention.[21] In addition, protein-energy malnutrition results in an alteration in small intestine mucosal absorptive capacity for zinc, promoting zinc malabsorption. This can lead to a self-perpetuating cycle of poor zinc absorption, and further compromise of zinc stores.[23,24] Zinc is absorbed into the intestinal epithelial cells and transported via the plasma carrier proteins macroglobulin, albumin, transferrin, glycoprotein, and transthyretine.[1,14] Once in the blood, 80% to 90% of zinc can be found within the erythrocytes, 10% to 17% in the plasma, and 3% or less in white blood cells. From the circulation, zinc is taken up by the liver and other tissues[4] where zinc ions form complexes with metalloenzymes, membrane proteins, and metallothionein. Excretion of zinc is mainly via the bile, although a small amount is excreted in urine, sweat, desquamation of skin, and hair losses. Urinary zinc excretion is enhanced with the use of diuretics and in diabetic patients.[18,25] It is also increased after injury during the acute-phase response.[26,27]

Assessment of Status

Plasma zinc concentration, the most commonly measured index of zinc status, is insensitive and therefore unreliable.[4,16] Other methods for determining zinc status have been explored and include measurement of zinc concentrations in white blood cells, measurement of 5'NT activity, measurement of zinc kinetics, and determination of relationships between physiologic functions and zinc nutrition. Of these, measurement of zinc or 5'NT in white blood cells (or plasma) appears to be the most applicable to clinical situations.[16]

Deficiency and Toxicity

Because of zinc's role in cellular growth and differentiation, the effects of zinc deficiency are especially pronounced in tissues and organs with rapid turnover and during periods of rapid growth.[24] Organ systems known to be affected by severe zinc deficiency include the skin, GI tract, central nervous, immune, skeletal, and reproductive.[28] Symptoms of severe zinc deficiency include delayed wound healing, hair loss, diarrhea, growth failure, poor appetite, and impaired vision.[24,29] Secondary zinc deficiency can occur in many conditions including human immunodeficiency virus (HIV), chronic liver disease, diabetes, cancer, and chronic inflammatory diseases such as rheumatoid arthritis. Neurologic diseases such as Alzheimer's disease and Down syndrome are associated with redistribution or sequestration of zinc.[24] Zinc deficiency is common in the critically ill because of decreased intake, increased losses from the GI tract, and increased urinary losses resulting from hypoalbuminemia.[4] Zinc toxicity is uncommon and usually occurs in accidental intake or occupational exposure.[14,19] Symptoms include metallic taste, nausea, vomiting, stomach cramps, fever, diarrhea, and renal failure. Excess zinc can retard wound healing,[30,31] and it reduces both phagocyte and lymphocyte functions, thereby reducing immune responses.[1,32] Chronic zinc intake can lead to copper deficiency and anemia.[1,4] Recently, an association between high intakes of serum zinc and a faster disease progression and death in HIV-1-infected men has been shown.[33,34]

Requirements and Supplementation

The current RDA for zinc is 12 mg/day in adult women and 15 mg/day in adult men.[22,31] The RDA is lower for females because of their lower body weight. Current guidelines for parenteral trace elements recommend supplementing with the standard daily dose of 5 mg elemental zinc.[20] The American Medical Association (AMA) guidelines for parenteral zinc supplementation for catabolic patients include an additional 2 to 4 mg of zinc per day.[1]

Copper
Function

Copper is an essential trace element, third in total body content after iron and zinc. It is widely distributed throughout human tissues and organs, with the highest concentrations present in the liver.[35] Copper plays a role in many physiologically important pathways. It is required for proper erythropoiesis and leucopoiesis, skeletal mineralization, myelin formation, immune function, connective tissue synthesis, cardiac function, and glucose regulation.[35,36] All metaloenzymes of copper possess oxidative reductase activity. A number of the key enzymes include cytochrome-C-oxidase, required for energy production; superoxide dismutase, a key cytosolic antioxidant; and lysyloxidase, which catalyzes the oxidation of lysyl residues on collagen.[4,35] Copper is also an essential component of the oxidation enzyme ceruloplasmin, which oxidizes ferrous to ferric ion so it can be transported on ceruloplasmin to other tissues.[4]

Metabolism

Copper is thought to be absorbed readily throughout the upper GI tract, including the stomach, duodenum, and jejunum by both an active and passive transport system.[35,36] The biologic availability of copper is enhanced significantly by dietary protein and decreased by high doses of zinc and vitamin C.[1,36] Copper transport from the intestinal mucosa to the liver and other tissues is poorly understood.[35] It is thought that once in the blood, copper is carried on transcuprein and albumin to the liver and secondarily to the kidneys.[37] In the liver, most plasma copper is bound to ceruloplasmin and is secreted into the blood for transport to other tissues or is excreted.[1] The primary route of copper excretion is via the biliary tract; therefore, conditions that lead to chronic biliary obstruction impair copper excretion and may promote hepatic accumulation. The amount of copper excreted in the bile increases or decreases proportionately with the amount of copper intake.[1]

Assessment of Status

Traditionally, plasma or serum copper concentration has been used to measure copper status. This is most likely the least reliable indicator of copper status, except in cases of severe copper deficiency.[38] Most changes observed in plasma copper concentrations are associated with changes in ceruloplasmin. As with plasma or serum copper concentration, ceruloplasmin concentrations are depressed during severe copper deficiency; however, in instances of marginal deficiency or in short-term studies of copper deprivation, ceruloplasmin responses are variable, rendering its measurement insensitive.[38] Currently, it appears that study of the copper-containing enzymes erythrocyte Cu/Zn superoxide dismutase and platelet cytochrome-C-oxidase may be better indicators of metabolically active copper and copper stores than plasma concentrations of copper or ceruloplasmin because the enzyme activities are sensitive to changes in copper stores and are not as sensitive to factors unrelated to copper status.[37,38]

Deficiency and Toxicity

Acquired copper deficiency is an extremely rare occurrence because of the ubiquitous nature of copper in various foods, but it has been described in patients receiving PN since 1972.[35,36] Low serum copper levels have also been described in patients recovering from major burn injury.[39,40] Copper deficiency is characterized by anemia; neutropenia; and rarely, thrombocytopenia.[36] Coronary artery disease has been observed in patients with the inherited form of copper deficiency (Menkes' syndrome), but it has not been observed in acquired copper deficiency. Toxicity from excess copper intake has not been well documented.[4] A recent study by Ford cites several studies, including his own, that have found elevated serum copper concentrations to be associated with cardiovascular disease, but it is unclear whether copper directly affects atherogenesis or is a marker of the inflammation associated with cardiovascular disease.[37]

Requirements and Supplementation

The ESSADI for copper is set between 1.5 and 3.0 mg/day.[38] This recommendation is based on copper requirements that have been estimated between 1.2 and 2.0 mg/day. The AMA recommendation for parenteral nutrition supplementation of copper is 0.5 to 1.5 mg/day.[41] Fleming[42] recommends reducing copper supplementation in PN to 0.155 mg/day when a patient develops chronic hyperbilirubinemia. Unfortunately, reduction of a single trace element in a PN solution is problematic because trace elements are usually added as a preparation that contains several trace elements. Fuhrman suggests that it may be more clinically feasible to reduce copper supplementation by providing a trace element preparation no more than three times per week when a patient develops chronic hyperbilirubinemia.[35]

Selenium

Function

Selenium functions within mammalian systems primarily in the form of selenoproteins. Selenoproteins contain selenium and selenocysteine and perform various physiologic roles.[43] Eleven selenoproteins have been identified and include both classical (cellular) glutathione peroxidase and plasma (extracellular) glutathione peroxidase. Selenium plays a vital role in the cellular antioxidant defense system. This system protects the integrity of the cell membrane and the immune system.[14] It is interesting to note that selenium can spare vitamin E and vice versa. As a result, the need for selenium declines as vitamin E intake increases.[1]

Metabolism

Selenium is well absorbed throughout the small bowel.[1,14] The organic forms of selenium are better absorbed than the inorganic forms. Absorption of selenium is probably by active transport, but the exact mechanism for absorption and transport is not well understood. Selenium is widely distributed in the body, with high concentrations in the liver, kidney, and testes. The primary route for excretion of selenium is via the kidneys,[14,43] although ingested selenium is also exhaled by the lungs.[14] Lower doses of selenium should be given when renal function is impaired.[43]

Assessment of Status

Estimates of selenium status can be accomplished through a variety of means, including the measurement of specific selenoproteins; estimation of selenium intake; measurement of selenium concentrations in blood, tissues, or excreta; and determination of glutathione peroxidase activity in various blood components.[1,43]

Deficiency and Toxicity

Human selenium deficiencies are rare. The primary group who has developed selenium deficiency includes those who received PN for prolonged periods without selenium supplementation. Low selenium levels have often been reported in the critically ill.[44] Symptoms seen in this population include muscle weakness and pain.[1,43] Selenium toxicity has occurred in areas where soil concentrations of selenium are great or, in one case in the United States, when a manufacturing error of a selenium supplement resulted in a product that contained 182 times the amount of selenium declared on the label.[45] Signs of toxicity include nausea, vomiting, hair loss, peripheral neuropathy, fatigue, and changes in nails and teeth.[1,45]

Requirements and Supplementation

The recently published dietary reference intakes[46] fixed the new RDA for selenium at 55 μg/day for both men and women. This level was chosen because it was associated with the highest level of glutathione peroxidase activity.[47,48] Given the documented increased requirements for the critically ill, it is recommended that selenium supplementation be increased for this population.[4,44]

Chromium

Function

The metabolic functions for chromium are not well defined.[49] The biologic functions of chromium include its involvement in both carbohydrate and lipid metabolism. Specifically, chromium functions in the regulation of insulin by increasing insulin binding to cells through increased insulin receptor numbers.[50] Chromium is thought to be the active component in glucose tolerance factor (GTF).[1] Chromium exists in several forms, of which hexavalent and trivalent are the most prevalent. The hexavalent form is recognized as toxic, whereas trivalent chromium is not.[51]

Metabolism

Chromium absorption and metabolism depend on its oxidation state, whether the chromium is complexed, and the intestinal contents. Very little of trivalent chromium is absorbed (less than 2% of the dose), although when complexed with picolinate or nicotinate, absorption is improved.[51] The exact mechanism of absorption is unclear, but factors such as oxalate intake, iron and zinc deficiency, and diabetes increase absorption, whereas phytate and aging decrease absorption. Following absorption, chromium is bound to transferrin; albumin; and, possibly, globulin proteins for transport throughout the system. Chromium is excreted mainly in the urine, and excretion increases as the result of a glucose load, stress conditions, strenuous exercise, physical trauma, pregnancy, and lactation.[1] Chromium excretion is also elevated in diabetics after insulin administration.[51] Hexavalent chromium is better absorbed, and blood levels are three to five times greater than those following administration of trivalent chromium. After absorption, hexavalent chromium enters the erythrocytes and binds to the globulin fraction of hemoglobin where it then becomes reduced to the trivalent form. Because trivalent chromium cannot cross the erythrocyte membrane, it remains irreversibly trapped in the cell.[51]

Assessment of Status

Currently no good method is available to determine chromium status. Plasma levels do not reflect tissue levels because tissue levels are ten times higher than plasma. In addition, balance studies show that there can be a negative chromium balance in the presence of raised plasma levels.[51] The best way to diagnose chromium deficiency currently is to observe whether the hyperglycemia and neuropathy that develop unexpectedly in patients on PN responds to chromium infusion.[1]

Deficiency and Toxicity

Signs of chromium deficiency include impaired glucose tolerance, increased levels of circulating insulin, elevated cholesterol and triglyceride levels, and decreased high density lipoprotein levels. No credible data or reports have shown adverse effects of trivalent chromium in humans. It is extraordinarily safe and has a wide margin of safety.[45] As previously mentioned, hexavalent chromium is recognized as toxic.

Requirements and Supplementation

The ESSADI for trivalent chromium is between 50 to 200 µg/day.[51] The reference dose set by the U.S. Environmental Protection Agency (EPA) for trivalent chromium is 1.47 mg/kg. This conservative estimate is 350 times the upper limit of the ESSADI, which is a much larger safety factor than almost any other nutrient.[50] Recommendations from the American Medical Association Panel suggest the daily administration of 10 to 15 µg of chromium per day in PN solutions. More recently, Fleming recommended 10 to 20 µg/day be added to PN.[42]

Anderson, in his review article on chromium, suggests that both amounts may not be adequate for severely stressed patients, an assertion also made by Demling and DeBiasse in their review of micronutrients in critical illness.[4,50] It also should be noted that the basal chromium content of PN solutions varies widely and should be monitored.[50]

Manganese
Function

Manganese is known to be involved in enzyme activation as a component of several metalloenzymes including arginase, pyruvate carboxylase, and manganese superoxide dismutase. Enzymes activated by manganese frequently can also be activated by magnesium.[1] As a component of various enzymes, manganese assists in energy release, fatty acid and cholesterol synthesis, release of lipid from the liver, and production of procollagen fibers and ground substance for wound healing.[1,4]

Metabolism

Relatively little is known about manganese absorption. The total percentage of dietary manganese absorbed from a meal is small, with most studies suggesting that humans absorb less than 5%.[52] High dietary iron has been shown to decrease manganese absorption and status in rats, and there is a strong negative association between ferritin status and the absorption and retention of manganese.[52] Once absorbed, manganese is bound to α2-macroglobulin and transported to the liver where a portion of it is oxidized to Mn 3+, bound to transferrin and transported throughout the body.[1] Virtually 100% of manganese is excreted mainly in bile, although nonbiliary routes of manganese excretion are known to exist.[53]

Assessment of Status

There is still no clearly defined method for assessing manganese status.[54] Many authors suggest that the concentration of manganese in red cells is a better indicator of manganese tissue accumulation than plasma manganese concentrations.[53,54]

Deficiency and Toxicity

Descriptions of manganese deficiency in humans are not conclusive. Some of the symptoms reported include neuromuscular dysfunction, dermatitis, and hypocholesterolemia.[1,4] No toxicity from dietary manganese has been reported,[1] but a number of studies have demonstrated significant neurotoxicity and elevated blood manganese concentrations when manganese is provided in conjunction with parenteral nutrition to patients with chronic liver and/or cholestatic disease.[1,53-56] The earliest toxic phase is characterized by general symptoms of weakness, anorexia, apathy, and somnolence. This is followed by signs of basal ganglia dysfunction that resemble Parkinson's disease. The final phase is characterized by muscular rigidity, staggered gait, and fine tremor.[53,56] There is apparently a greater susceptibility to manganese toxicity in elderly patients.

Requirements and Supplementation

The ESADDI for manganese has been established at 2 to 5 mg/day.[52,54] Manganese is routinely administered to patients receiving PN at 100 to 800 µg daily. It is also contained in PN components in trace amounts.[56] Recently, there has been some suggestion that 100 μg/day should be the maximum amount provided in PN, and careful monitoring of manganese levels should be a part of the routine practice for those patients receiving PN for more than 30 days. In addition, manganese should be eliminated from the PN of patients with cholestasis[54,56] because trace amounts of manganese are associated with the components of the PN solution in amounts that will likely prevent deficiency.[56]

Molybdenum

Function

Molybdenum may exist in several oxidation states (+3, +4, +5, and +6), and as a result, it functions as a facilitator of electron transfer reactions.[14] Molybdenum serves as a cofactor for various enzymes, including xanthene oxidase, aldehyde oxidase, and sulfite oxidase. Xanthene oxidase catalyzes the oxidative hydroxylation of purines and pyrimidines. Aldehyde oxidase oxidizes purines, pyrimidines, and pteridines and may be involved in nicotinic acid metabolism. Sulfite oxidase, an enzyme essential to humans, catalyzes the oxidation of sulfite to sulfate. This reaction is necessary for the metabolism of sulfur amino acids.[57]

Metabolism

Molybdenum is absorbed well in the GI tract by both passive and active transport.[14] Absorption of molybdenum is inhibited by copper, and increased molybdenum and sulfur levels decrease serum copper levels.[4] Molybdenum is transported in the blood bound to α_1-macroglobulin and is loosely associated with erythrocytes during transport. It is present in the highest concentrations in the liver, kidney, skin, and bones. Molybdenum is excreted primarily in the urine (90%) and to a lesser extent in the bile (10%).[14] A recent study by Turnlund and colleagues demonstrated that very little molybdenum is excreted into the GI tract (<1% per day), and urinary molybdenum appears to be the only point of regulation of molybdenum retention.[57]

Assessment of Status

No current method offers a good assessment of molybdenum status.[4] Neutron activation analysis would achieve the sensitivity needed to assess molybdenum status, but this technique is limited to facilities with nuclear reactors and is not widely available.

Deficiency and Toxicity

Molybdenum deficiency is difficult to diagnose because the low end of the reference range is not well defined.[14] Deficiency states are characterized by mouth and gum disorders, hypouricemia, hyperoxypurinemia, mental disturbance, and coma. Chronic exposure to molybdenum results in loss of appetite, listlessness, diarrhea, anemia, and slow growth.

Requirements and Supplementation

An ESADDI of 0.15 to 0.5 mg/day for adults was introduced in the ninth edition of the recommended dietary allowances. This level was revised downward to 0.075 to 0.250 mg/day in the tenth edition on the basis of newer reports of usual dietary intake.[14]

Aluminum

Function

Aluminum is the third most abundant naturally occurring element and the most common metallic element, composing approximately 8.8% of the earth's crust.[58] Aluminum has no known physiologic function in either humans or animals, and it is regarded as a potential toxin, particularly in patients with compromised renal function.[58,59] Although ubiquitous in nature, aluminum is largely insoluble, and the lungs, skin, and GI tract act as barriers to prevent it from entering the body. As a result, the estimated total body content of aluminum is less than 50 mg.[60]

Metabolism

The metabolism of aluminum in normal subjects has been studied by only a few investigators. Aluminum appears to be very poorly absorbed from the GI tract, such that only a small amount of aluminum has been found in the urine of subjects consuming a normal diet.[61] Aluminum absorption from the intestinal lumen is initially into the intestinal mucosal cells, and only a small proportion of this uptake continues into the blood.[62] Several factors have been shown to enhance aluminum absorption including citrate, pH, parathyroid hormone, 1,12-dihydroxyvitamin D_3, and uremia. Inhibitors of absorption include fluoride and calcium.[62]

The primary route of aluminum excretion is the kidneys, with only trivial amounts excreted in bile.[60,63] Several studies have shown that with the ingestion of large quantities of aluminum-containing antacids, urinary aluminum can be increased in normal subjects fivefold to fifteenfold.[60]

Assessment of Status

Blood levels of aluminum are not always predictive of tissue pathology and depend, among other factors, on length of time exposed and dose.[64] One source suggests that a plasma aluminum level greater than 10 μg/dl put individuals at risk for aluminum toxicity.[58] In a special report published jointly by the American Society for Clinical Nutrition (ASCN) and the American Society for Parenteral and Enteral Nutrition (ASPEN), it was suggested that determinations of aluminum content in fluid or tissues be performed by flameless or electrothermal atomic absorption spectroscopy or inductively coupled plasma emission spectroscopy.[63]

Deficiency and Toxicity

As stated previously, there is no known requirement for aluminum, and no deficiency has been reported. In contrast, toxicity states that result from the accumulation of aluminum have been noted in the literature since the mid-1970s. These first cases were observed in patients with end-stage renal disease who were receiving hemodialysis therapy when aluminum was found as a contaminant of the water used in the dialysis process. These patients exhibited a low-turnover vitamin D–resistant osteomalacic bone disease, and an encephalopathy with dementia that existed in conjunction with elevated tissue levels of aluminum and accumulation of aluminum at the mineralization front of bone.[63] Since that time, numerous studies have been published investigating the role of aluminum in bone disease and dementia states.[58-60,64-66] Many of these studies have focused on the role of long-term PN in inducing these toxicity effects because metabolic bone disease was observed with significant frequency in this population. As a result, the aluminum content of parenteral nutrition solutions was evaluated, and it was discovered that casein hydrolysate amino acid solutions contained a significantly greater amount of aluminum than crystalline amino acid solutions. In one such study, the concentration difference was 100-fold.[60] These investigations lead to the use of deionized water for both hemodialysis and peritoneal dialysis for those patients with end-stage renal disease, and the substitution of crystalline amino acids for casein hydrolysate amino acids in parenteral nutrition solutions. Both interventions have resulted in decreased incidence of aluminum toxicity in the populations using these therapies.[63]

In addition to the previously listed disorders, microcytic hypochromic anemia has also been found to be a manifestation of

aluminum toxicity.[64] Aluminum may also accumulate in the parathyroid gland, although its functional effects are unknown.[60]

Requirements and Supplementation
There is no known requirement for aluminum. The average adult dietary intake of aluminum is about 3 to 5 mg/day, of which only 15 μg (0.3% to 0.5%) is absorbed. There are no recommendations for aluminum supplementation.

Conclusion
Table 12-1 contains a summary of each of the minerals presented in this chapter. When recommending supplementation of minerals and trace elements, it is important for the clinician to remember how closely regulated they are. While it is impor-

TABLE 12-1
Summary of Minerals and Trace Elements

Mineral	RDA/ESADDIs[†]	Deficiency Symptoms	Toxicity Symptoms	Laboratory Assessment	Oral Supplement	Parenteral Supplement
Iron	10-15 mg	Microcytic hypochromic anemia, pallor, fatigue, low serum iron and ferritin, high TIBC	Hyperpigmentation of the skin, cirrhosis, diabetes, sterility, arthropathy, cardiac arrhythmias	Serum iron, TIBC, and ferritin	Ferrous sulfate, 320 mg twice/day for 6 mo to 1 yr	Not supported
Zinc	12-15 mg	Diarrhea, hair loss, delayed growth and wound healing, impaired taste	Copper deficiency, microcytic anemia, reduced immune response, renal failure	WBC zinc concentration, 5'NT activity	Zinc sulfate, 20-40 mg/day	2-4 mg/day*
Copper	1.5-3.0 mg[†]	Microcytic hypochromic anemia, neutropenia	Vomiting, hepatic necrosis, ataxia, cirrhosis	Erythrocyte Cu/Zn superoxide dismutase and platelet cytochrome-C-oxidase activity	Cupric sulfate, 2 mg/day	0.5-1.5 mg/day
Selenium	55 μg/day	Cardiomyopathy, muscle pain, weakness	Hair loss, peripheral neuropathy, fatigue, nail and teeth changes	Selenoprotein measurement, serum selenium, glutathione peroxidase activity	Selenium sulfate, 50-200 μg/day	≤100 μg/day
Chromium	50-200 μg/day[†]	Glucose intolerance, elevated cholesterol and triglyceride levels, reduced HDL cholesterol	None reported from dietary intake	Glucose tolerance test	Chromium chloride, 200 μg/day	10-20 μg/day
Manganese	2-5 mg/day[†]	Dermatitis, hypocholesterolemia, neuromuscular dysfunction	Weakness, anorexia, somnolence, basal ganglia dysfunction, muscular rigidity, staggered gait, fine tremor	RBC manganese concentration	2-5 mg/day	≤100 μg/day
Molybdenum	0.075-0.250 mg/day[†]	Mouth and gum disorders, hypouricemia, hyperoxypurinemia, mental disturbance, coma	Anorexia, listlessness, diarrhea, anemia, slow growth	No good method	None specified	None specified
Aluminum	None	None	Vitamin D–resistant osteomalacic bone disease, dementia, microcytic hypochromic anemia	Flameless or electrothermal atomic absorption spectroscopy	None recommended	None recommended

HDL, High-density lipoprotein; *RBC,* red blood cell; *TIBC,* total iron-binding capacity; *WBC,* white blood cell.
*Amount to supplement in addition to the standard maintenance trace element preparation.
[†]Estimated safe and adequate daily dietary intake.

tant to provide appropriate individual mineral supplements, the interrelationship between the various trace minerals should not be forgotten. Caution should especially be used with the parenteral administration of minerals because the natural regulatory mechanism of the GI tract is bypassed. In addition, because many of these minerals are not readily excreted, there is a potential for toxicity. Supplementation regimens that fail to consider these facts can induce nutrient imbalances that could harm rather than benefit the patient.[1]

REFERENCES

1. Braunschweig C: Minerals and trace elements. In *Contemporary nutrition support practice: a clinical guide,* St Louis, 1998, WB Saunders, pp 163-173.
2. DeBiasse MA, Wilmore DW: What is optimal nutrition support? *New Horizons* 2(2):122-130, 1994.
3. Olin SS: Between a rock and a hard place: methods for setting dietary allowances and exposure limits for essential minerals, *J Nutr* 128 (suppl 2):364S-367S, 1998.
4. Demling RH, DeBiasse MA: Micronutrients in critical illness, *Crit Care Clin* 11(3):651-673, 1995.
5. Kumpf VJ: Parenteral iron supplementation, *Nutr Clin Pract* 11(4):139-146, 1996.
6. Monson ER: The ironies of iron, *Am J Clin Nutr* 69(5):831-832, 1999.
7. Minihane AM, Fairweather-Tait SJ: Effect of calcium supplementation on daily nonheme-iron absorption and long-term iron status, *Am J Clin Nutr* 68(1):96-102, 1998.
8. Weinberg ED: Iron withholding: a defense against infection and neoplasia, *Physiol Rev* 64(1):65-102, 1984.
9. Beard JL, Borel MJ, Derr J: Impaired thermoregulation and thyroid function in iron-deficiency anemia, *Am J Clin Nutr* 52(5):813-819, 1990.
10. Norton JA, Peters ML, Wesley R, et al. Iron supplementation of total parenteral nutrition: a prospective study, *J Parent Enteral Nutr* 7(5):457-461, 1983.
11. Porter KA, Blackburn GL, Bistrian BR: Safety of iron dextran in total parenteral nutrition: a case report, *J Am Coll Nutr* 7(2):107-110, 1988.
12. Dudrick SJ, O'Donnell JJ, Raleigh DP, et al: Rapid restoration of red blood cell mass in severely anemic surgical patients who refuse transfusion, *Arch Surg* 120(6):721-727, 1985.
13. Kwong KW, Tsallas G: Dilute iron dextran formulation for addition to parenteral nutrient solutions, *Am J Hosp Pharm* 37(2):206-210, 1980.
14. Chan S, Gerson B, Subramaniam S: The role of copper, molybdenum, selenium and zinc in nutrition and health, *Clin Lab Med* 18(4):673-685, 1998.
15. Wilson RF, Tyburski JG: Metabolic responses and nutritional therapy in patients with severe head injuries, *J Head Trauma Rehabil* 13(1):11-27, 1998.
16. Sandstead HH, Alcock NW: Zinc: an essential and unheralded nutrient, *J Lab Clin Med* 130(2):116-118, 1997.
17. Mantzoros CS, Prasad AS, Beck FWJ, et al: Zinc may regulate serum leptin concentrations in humans, *J Am Coll Nutr* 17(3):270-275, 1998.
18. Sandstead HH, Egger NG: Is zinc nutriture a problem in persons with diabetes mellitus? *Am J Clin Nutr* 66(3):681-682, 1997.
19. Jern NA, VanBeber AD, Gorman MA, et al: The effects of zinc supplementation on serum zinc concentration and protein catabolic rate in hemodialysis patients, *J Ren Nutr* 10(3):148-153, 2000.
20. Braunschweig CL, Sowers M, Kovacevich DS, et al: Parenteral zinc supplementation in adult humans during the acute phase response increases the febrile response, *J Nutr* 127(1):70-74, 1997.
21. Lonnerdal B: Dietary factors influencing zinc absorption, *J Nutr* 130(suppl 5S):1378S-1383S, 2000.
22. Wood RD, Zheng JJ: High dietary calcium intakes reduce zinc absorption and balance in humans, *Am J Clin Nutr* 65(6):1803-1809, 1997.
23. Wapnir RA: Zinc deficiency, malnutrition and the gastrointestinal tract, *J Nutr* 130(suppl 5S):1388S-1392S, 2000.
24. Costello RB, Grumstrup-Scott J: Zinc: what role might supplements play? *J Am Diet Assoc* 100(3):371-375, 2000.
25. Saltzman JR, Russell RM: The aging gut, *Gastro Clin North Am* 27(2):309-324, 1998.
26. Askari A, Long CL, Blakemore WS: Urinary zinc, copper, nitrogen, and potassium losses in response to trauma, *J Parenter Enteral Nutr* 3(3):151-156, 1979.
27. Fell GS, Fleck A, Cuthbertson DP, et al: Urinary zinc levels as an indication of muscle catabolism, *Lancet* 1(7798):280-282, 1973.
28. Hambridge M: Human zinc deficiency, *J Nutr* 130(suppl 5S):1344S-1349S, 2000.
29. Prasad AS: Zinc deficiency in humans: a neglected problem, *J Am Coll Nutr* 17(6):542-543, 1998.
30. Klein CJ: Zinc supplementation (letter to the editor), *J Am Diet Assoc* 100(10):1137-1138, 2000.
31. Andrews J, Gallagher-Allred C: The role of zinc in wound healing, *Adv Wound Care* 12(3):137-138, 1999.
32. Chandra RK: Nutrition in the immune system: an introduction, *Am J Clin Nutr* 66:460S-463S, 1997.
33. Tang AM, Graham NM, Kirby A, et al: Dietary micronutrient intake and risk of progression to acquired immunodeficiency syndrome (AIDS) in human deficiency virus type 1 (HIV-1)-infected homosexual men, *Am J Epidemiol* 138(11):937-951, 1993.
34. Tang AM, Graham NMH, Saah AJ: Effects of micronutrient intake on survival in human immunodeficiency virus type 1 infection, *Am J Epidemiol* 143(12):1244-1256, 1996.
35. Fuhrman MP, Herrmann V, Masidonski P, et al: Pancytopenia after removing copper from total parenteral nutrition, *J Parenter Enteral Nutr* 24(6):361-366, 2000.
36. Spiegel JE, Willenbucher RF: Rapid development of severe copper deficiency in a patient with Crohn's disease receiving parenteral nutrition, *J Parent Enteral Nutr* 23(3):169-172, 1999.
37. Ford ES: Serum copper concentration and coronary heart disease among US adults, *Am J Epidemiol* 151(12):1182-1188, 2000.
38. Milne DB: Copper intake and assessment of copper status, *Am J Clin Nutr* 67(suppl):1041S-1045S, 1998.
39. Gosling P, Rothe HM, Sheehan TMT, et al: Serum copper and zinc concentrations in patients with burns in relation to burn surface area, *J Burn Care Rehabil* 16(5):481-486, 1995.
40. Cunningham JJ, Lydon MK, Emerson R, et al: Low ceruloplasmin levels during recovery from major burn injury: influence of open wound size and copper supplementation, *Nutrition* 12(2):83-88, 1996.
41. Cordano A, Placko RP, Graham GG: Hypocupremia and neutropenia in copper deficiency, *Blood* 28(2):280-283, 1966.
42. Fleming R: Trace elements metabolism in adult patients requiring TPN, *Am J Clin Nutr* 49(3):573-579, 1989.
43. Holben DH, Smith AM: The diverse role of selenium within selenoproteins: a review, *J Am Diet Assoc* 99(7):836-843, 1999.
44. Metnitz PGH, Bartens C, Fischer M, et al: Antioxidant status in patients with acute respiratory distress syndrome, *Intensive Care Med* 25(2):180-185, 1999.
45. Hathcock JN: Vitamins and minerals: efficacy and safety, *Am J Clin Nutr* 66(2):427-437, 1997.
46. Food and Nutrition Board, Institute of Medicine. *DRI: Dietary reference intakes for vitamin C, vitamin E, selenium and carotenoids,* Washington, DC, 2000, National Academy Press, pp 284-324.
47. Neve J: New approaches to assess selenium status and requirement, *Nutr Rev* 58(12):363-369, 2000.
48. Monson ER: Dietary reference intakes for the antioxidant nutrients: vitamin C, vitamin E, selenium, and carotenoids, *J Am Diet Assoc* 100(6):637-640, 2000.
49. Lukaski HC: Magnesium, zinc, and chromium nutriture and physical activity, *Am J Clin Nutr* 72(suppl):585S-593S, 2000.
50. Anderson RA: Chromium, glucose intolerance and diabetes, *J Am Coll Nutr* 17(6):548-555, 1998.
51. Jeejeebhoy KN: The role of chromium in nutrition and therapeutics and as a potential toxin, *Nutr Rev* 57(11):329-335, 1999.
52. Finley JW: Manganese absorption and retention by young women is associated with serum ferritin concentration, *Am J Clin Nutr* 70(1):37-43, 1999.
53. Wardle CA, Forbes A, Roberts NB, et al: Hypermaganesemia in long-term intravenous nutrition and chronic liver disease, *J Parenter Enteral Nutr* 23(6):350-355, 1999.
54. Bertinet DB, Tinivella M, Balzola FA, et al: Brain manganese deposition and blood levels in patients undergoing home parenteral nutrition, *J Parenter Enteral Nutr* 24(4):223-227, 2000.
55. Ono J, Harada K, Kodaka R, et al: Manganese deposition in the brain during long-term total parenteral nutrition, *J Parenter Enteral Nutr* 19(4):310-312, 1995.
56. Fitzgerald K, Mikalunas V, Rubin H, et al: Hypermagnesemia in patients receiving total parenteral nutrition, *J Parenter Enteral Nutr* 23(6):333-336, 1999.
57. Turnland JR, Keyes WR, Peiffer GL, et al: Molybdenum absorption, excretion, and retention studied with stable isotopes in young men during depletion and repletion, *Am J Clin Nutr* 61(5):1102-1109, 1995.

58. Davis A, Spillane R, Zublena L: Aluminum: a problem trace metal in nutrition support, *Nutr Clin Pract* 14(5):227-231, 1999.

59. Koo WWK: Parenteral nutrition-related bone disease, *J Parenter Enteral Nutr* 16(4):386-394, 1992.

60. Klein GL, Alfrey AC, Miller NL, et al: Aluminum loading during total parenteral nutrition, *Am J Clin Nutr* 35(6):1425-1429, 1982.

61. Greger JL, Baier MJ: Excretion and retention of low or moderate levels of aluminium by human subjects, *Fd Chem Toxic* 21(4):473-477, 1983.

62. Lote CJ, Saunders H: Aluminum: gastrointestinal absorption and renal excretion, *Clin Sci* 81(3):289-295, 1991.

63. ASCN/ASPEN Working Group on Standards for Aluminum Content of Parenteral Nutrition Solutions: Parenteral drug products containing aluminum as an ingredient or a contaminant: response to Food and Drug Administration notice of intent and request for information, *J Parenter Enteral Nutr* 15(2):194-198, 1991.

64. Novak M, Freundlich M, Gaston Z: Aluminum exposure and toxicity, *J Pediatr Gastroent Nutr* 9(3):267-268, 1989.

65. Gray G: Nutrition and dementia, *J Am Diet Assoc* 89(12):1795-1801, 1989.

66. Klein GL, Ott SM, Alfrey AC, et al: Aluminum as a factor in the bone disease of long-term parenteral nutrition, *Trans Assoc Am Physicians* 95:155-164, 1982.

Joanne Slavin, PhD, RD

Historical Background

The term *dietary fiber* was not coined until 1953, but the anticonstipating effects of high-fiber foods have been long appreciated. In 430 BC, Hippocrates compared the superior laxative effects of coarse wheat and refined wheat.[1] Graham (of graham cracker fame) denounced the harmful effects of refined carbohydrate foods during the nineteenth century, and the first Kellogg's and Post cereals were formulated in response to increasing interest in dietary fiber. In the 1920s, J. H. Kellogg published extensively on the attributes of bran, claiming it increased stool weight, promoted laxation, and prevented disease.[2] Dietary fiber was studied throughout the 1930s and then forgotten.

Denis Burkitt is usually credited with popularizing the contemporary idea that dietary fiber may protect against the development of Western diseases, including diabetes, hypercholesterolemia, heart disease, diverticular disease, and colon cancer.[3] Whether isolated dietary fiber has the same physiologic properties as the dietary fiber found naturally in grains, fruits, and vegetables with associated substances is not known and is difficult to study.

Research in the role of dietary fiber in human nutrition has progressed slowly because of disagreement about what fiber is and how it can be measured. In this chapter I define dietary fiber, explain how it is measured, compare food sources and isolated dietary fiber sources, summarize studies of physiologic effects of dietary fiber, and finally review literature relevant to dietary fiber and enteral nutrition.

What Is Dietary Fiber?

Dietary fiber has been defined in many ways. The most abundant compounds identified as fiber are in plant cell walls; other fibers are part of the intracellular cement; and still others are secreted by plants in response to injury.[4] Thus, dietary fiber cannot be *equated* to the plant cell wall. A physiologic definition for dietary fiber is generally accepted. Dietary fiber is plant cell material that resists digestion by the endogenous enzymes of humans. Starch that resists pancreatic enzyme action and passes into the colon is considered dietary fiber. Dietary fiber has been defined as the sum of polysaccharides and lignin not digested by the endogenous secretions of the human gastrointestinal tract.[5] Lignin is not a carbohydrate, but a polyphenolic compound that is associated with dietary fiber.

Dietary fiber is not an accurate term because many of its components are not fibrous. Gums and mucilages, for example,

are classified as dietary fiber because mammalian enzymes or secretions do not digest them. Only one component of dietary fiber, cellulose, is truly fibrous; yet *dietary fiber* is the accepted term for describing the roughage or residue in the human diet.

Research shows that not all dietary fiber is created equal, and attempts have been made to describe components of dietary fiber that might explain its physiologic effectiveness. Dietary fiber can be divided into three major fractions:

- Structural polysaccharides are associated with the cell wall and include noncellulose polysaccharides (hemicellulose and some pectins) and cellulose.
- Structural nonpolysaccharides are predominantly lignin.
- Nonstructural polysaccharides include gums and mucilages secreted by cells and polysaccharides from algae and seaweed.

For simplicity, dietary fiber can be divided into noncellulose polysaccharides, cellulose, and lignin. Human foodstuffs contain mainly noncellulose polysaccharides, some cellulose, and little lignin. The average proportions of noncellulose polysaccharides, cellulose, and lignin for common foodstuffs are about 70%, 20%, and 10%, respectively.

Overall, fruits and vegetables tend to contain more cellulose than cereals. Lignin is most abundant in fruits with edible seeds (e.g., strawberries) and in mature vegetables such as carrots and other root vegetables. The dietary fiber composition of a plant food depends on its species, maturity, and structure (i.e., leaf, root, or stem).

The human diet contains, in addition to polysaccharides and lignin, plant-derived materials similar to fiber that resist digestion in the small bowel. These include cutin, waxes, small amounts of protein and lipids, and phenolic compounds. Nonenzymatic browning products are often indigestible and are considered dietary fiber. Dietary fibers have also been classified by water solubility because water-soluble and water-insoluble fibers have distinctive physiologic effects.

Solubility of polysaccharides is defined analytically as solubility in 80% ethanol. Branching of monosaccharides does affect solubility in ethanol. Indigestible oligosaccharides such as the raffinose family or fructans are neither included in the dietary fiber concept nor counted as dietary fiber in any of the current analytic methods. This omission is currently being discussed because these oligosaccharides have dietary fiberlike physiologic effects.

Fermentability of dietary fiber is another property that has been linked to physiologic effects. It is difficult to measure the fermentation of fibers because it is determined by breakdown of fiber in the gut, and no accepted methods exist to measure fermentability in vivo. Generally, very soluble fibers such as oat bran, guar gum, and pectin are extensively fermented, whereas insoluble fibers such as cellulose are not. The fermentability of most fiber products is not known. Processing can enhance or limit fermentability of dietary fiber. For example, "oat fiber" may be mostly insoluble dietary fiber if that fiber is extracted from oat hulls rather than oat bran.

Methods for determining fermentability of fibers in vitro have been developed. Eleven fiber-rich substrates were subjected to incubation in vitro with fecal bacteria, and fermentation and short-chain fatty acid (SCFA) production were measured.[6] Citrus pectin was 83% fermentable, oat fiber, about 6% fermentable. SCFA production was correlated to fermentability in the in vitro system.

The Food and Nutrition Board, under the oversight of the Standing Committee on the Scientific Evaluation of Dietary Reference Intakes, assembled a panel on the definition of dietary fiber to develop a proposed definitions(s) of dietary fiber. Based on the panel's deliberations, the following definitions are proposed:[7]

- *Dietary fiber* consists of nondigestible carbohydrates and lignin that are intrinsic and intact in plants.
- *Added fiber* consists of isolated, nondigestible carbohydrates that have beneficial physiologic effects in humans.
- *Total fiber* is the sum of *dietary fiber* and *added fiber.*

Two categories of fiber are described: (1) *dietary fiber*, fiber that is in its natural state, and (2) *added fiber*, fiber that is isolated, manufactured, synthetic, or enzyme-produced. *Added fiber* does not have to be plant-based. Other important recommendations of the committee are that *added fiber* must show a beneficial physiologic effect in order to be classified as *added fiber.* In addition, the committee recommended phasing out the terms *soluble* and *insoluble dietary fiber.* Two properties, viscosity and fermentability, were recommended as meaningful alternative characteristics for the terms *soluble* and *insoluble fiber.*

Methods for Measuring Dietary Fiber

When we accept a physiologic definition of dietary fiber, measuring dietary fiber becomes problematic. Originally, values were given as *crude fiber,* a method that seriously underestimates the total dietary fiber content of food, recovering only 50% to 80% of the cellulose, 10% to 50% of the lignin, and 20% of the hemicellulose.[4] Dietary fiber values are usually three to five times the crude fiber values, but no correction factors can be used because the relationship between crude fiber and dietary fiber varies, depending on the various chemical components. Bran flakes, for example, contain 6 times more dietary fiber than crude fiber; strawberries, only 1.6 times more dietary than crude fiber.

Despite enormous scientific interest in dietary fiber, few reliable values are available for the dietary fiber content of human foods and enteral nutrition products.[8] Unfortunately, the values that are available are generated with different methods and, so, are not comparable. Nutrient databases contain some dietary fiber values, but many are missing.

The difficulty in devising a method for assessing total dietary fiber can be appreciated if one considers the diverse nature of dietary fiber. A simple, reproducible method for removing protein, fat and soluble sugars and starch from food while retaining both water-soluble and water-insoluble components of dietary fiber is difficult from an analytic standpoint.

Nutrition labels list total dietary fiber values that are generated with the dietary fiber method developed by the Association of Official Analytical Chemists (AOAC). Methods are available for measuring soluble and insoluble dietary fiber. Measurement values for dietary fiber vary greatly, depending on the laboratory doing the analysis, sample issues, and other variables. The largest compilation of published dietary fiber values was generated with a modified Theander method, so these values cannot be compared directly with values generated with the AOAC method.[9] Further, when the dietary fiber content and composition of different forms of fruits were measured by a modified Theander method and the AOAC method, the two sets of fiber data were significantly different.[10]

Fiber Sources and Intake

Dietary fiber is found only in plant products such as fruits, vegetables, nuts, beans, legumes, and grains. The most concentrated sources of dietary fiber are the bran layers of grains, like wheat bran. Because of their higher water content, fruits and vegetables provide less dietary fiber per gram of ingested material than drier grains and cereals. The effect of cooking on the fiber content of foods is not clear. Cooking foods can cause browning reactions that increase their apparent fiber content because the browning products are analyzed as lignin. Cooking also drives out water that would increase the percentage of dietary fiber in the product. Heat processing of enteral formulas with fiber does not appear to alter physiologic response.[11]

In the United States average dietary fiber intakes continue to be less than recommended amounts. Recommendations for adult dietary fiber intake generally fall in the range of 20 to 35 g per day.[12] Others have recommended dietary fiber intakes based on kilocalorie intake, 10 to 13 g of dietary fiber per 1000 kcal.[13] Attempts have been made to define recommended dietary fiber intakes for children and adolescents. Although based on limited clinical data, the recommendation for children older than 2 years is to increase dietary fiber intake to an amount equal to or greater than their age plus 5 g/day[14] to achieve intakes of 25 to 35 g/day after age 20 years. Specific recommendations for the elderly have not been published, although a safe recommendation would be encourage intake of 10 to 13 g dietary fiber per 1000 kcal.

Usual intakes of dietary fiber in the United States average only 11 g per day, so few people get the recommended amount. One obvious reason is that most of the popular foods we consume contain little dietary fiber. For example, most servings of grains, fruits, and vegetables contain 1 to 3 g of dietary fiber.[4] Thus, to get the recommended amounts of dietary fiber one would need to consume at least 10 servings of the fiber-containing foods per day. If consumers were eating according to the United States Department of Agriculture Food Guide Pyramid and were choosing cereals, whole grains, and intact fruits and vegetables, it would be possible for them to obtain the recommended levels of dietary fiber, but despite the efforts of nutrition educators, dietary fiber intake averages only half the recommended amount and does not appear to be increasing.

Physiologic Effects

Dietary fiber affects the digestive tract from mouth to anus and has other important physiologic functions. The effect of dietary fiber on the intestinal tract is affected by the type of fiber ingested, the health status of the subject, previous diet, and other components of the diet. Thus, the confusion in the field of dietary fiber is the result of the many variables that are not controlled in research studies. For this chapter, only research that was conducted in humans is described because it is believed that the fate of dietary fiber is much different in humans than in experimental animals that have large cecums.

Digestible carbohydrates, including starches, are hydrolyzed by enzymes and broken down to component sugars ready for absorption. Although it was generally believed that this process was complete, new research suggests that some 3% to 20% of starch is not completely digested and absorbed in the small intestine. That which escapes into the large intestine is termed *resistant starch* and probably functions much as dietary fiber does in the gut, although it is a highly fermentable dietary fiber.[15] Some oligosaccharides also escape digestion, as does lactulose (an indigestible disaccharide) and lactose in lactose-intolerant persons.

When carbohydrates reach the cecum, they are fermented. The products of this fermentation are SCFA and gas, including carbon dioxide, hydrogen, and methane. These gases escape through the lungs or the rectum (as flatus). This active fermentation process in the gut is difficult to study in vivo. Dietary fiber fermentation has been estimated by measuring the dietary fiber in food and in feces and comparing the amounts. Researchers have also estimated breath hydrogen and methane production as means of determining fiber fermentation. SCFA production has been measured by having subjects swallow dialysis bags and collecting these bags in freshly passed feces or measuring SCFAs in stool samples. None of these methods is ideal, and little information is available on the fate of dietary fiber in the body.

Gastrointestinal Tract Effects

MOUTH AND STOMACH. In the mouth, fiber stimulates the flow of saliva, principally by increasing the volume of the food bolus. When dietary fiber reaches the stomach, it dilutes the contents and (perhaps) prolongs storage. Pectin and guar gum generally increase gastric emptying time, whereas other fibers have no effect. Viscosity of the fiber source may be the important variable in gastric emptying, although the data are confusing.

SMALL INTESTINE. Dietary fiber is thought to dilute the contents of the small intestine, and the most viscous dietary fibers may delay absorption of carbohydrates and fats in the small intestine. This is one possible explanation of why viscous fibers (soluble) are usually more effective than insoluble fibers in lowering serum cholesterol and moderating glucose response. Changes in absorption of macronutrients seen with fiber feeding are of little practical significance in the United States, but they may be significant in countries where food is scarce.

Fiber can affect pancreatic enzyme activity, although data are confusing. In vitro, insoluble fiber reduced the activity of amylase, lipase, and trypsin, whereas pectin had no effect. It is generally accepted that dietary fiber in typically consumed doses has little effect on mineral absorption in the small intestine. Persons whose diet is low in minerals may be at risk for deficiencies, and additional fiber should not be recommended unless adequate minerals are consumed.

Fibers also can lower serum cholesterol by binding bile acids. Bile acids bound to fiber may not be reabsorbed in the small intestine, instead being lost in feces. Because the body can resynthesize bile acids, it is unlikely that binding of bile acids by certain fibers is a principal mechanism of the effect of fiber on serum cholesterol. In the colon, bacteria convert primary bile acids into smaller secondary bile acids, which may increase the risk of colon cancer. Insoluble fibers, which may dilute the concentration of secondary bile acids in the colon, might therefore protect against colon cancer.

Dietary fiber also affects small intestine morphology and epithelial cell regeneration. The intestinal villi of vegetarians are broad and leaf-shaped, whereas jejunal villi of humans who consume a "typical American diet" are fingerlike and regular. Animal studies have also shown that the level and type of dietary fiber consumed can alter the structure of the small intestine.

LARGE INTESTINE. More than 75% of dietary fiber in an average American diet disappears during transit, resulting in production of carbon dioxide, hydrogen, methane, and SCFAs. SCFAs include butyrate, propionate, and acetate. Propionate and acetate are thought to be metabolized in colonic epithelial cells or peripheral tissue. Butyrate may regulate colon cell proliferation and serve as an energy source for colon cells. Propionic acid is transported to the liver, and some research suggests that propionic acid may suppress cholesterol synthesis. This could be another potential explanation of how soluble dietary fiber lowers serum cholesterol. Fecal excretion of SCFAs may not reflect colon levels, and other methods for measuring SCFAs in the large intestine have not been studied well. Production of SCFAs lowers the pH of the colon, which may be important in the role of fiber in the prevention of gastrointestinal diseases, including colon cancer.

If approximately 20 g of fiber are fermented in the colon each day, approximately 200 mmole of SCFA is produced, of which 62% is acetate, 25% propionate, and 16% butyrate. Colonic absorption of SCFAs is concentration dependent and shows no evidence of a saturable process. The mechanism by which SCFAs cross the colonic mucosa is thought to be passive diffusion of the un-ionized acid into the mucosa cells. SCFAs are respiratory fuel for the colonic mucosa. In isolated human colonocytes, butyrate is actively metabolized to both carbon dioxide and ketone bodies, which process accounts for about 80% of the oxygen consumption of colonocytes. Butyrate is consumed almost completely by the colonic mucosa, whereas acetate and propionate enter the portal circulation, extending the effects of dietary fiber beyond the intestinal tract.

Butyrate may provide important protection against colon carcinoma.[16] Trophic effects on normal colonocytes in vitro and in vivo are induced by butyrate. In contrast, butyrate arrests the growth of neoplastic colonocytes and inhibits the preneoplastic hyperproliferation induced by some tumor promoters in vitro. Butyrate induces differentiation of colon cancer cell lines and regulates expression of molecules involved in colonocyte growth and adhesion. Resistant starch may be a better substrate than nonstarch polysaccharide in increasing production of butyrate,[17] although the lack of a generally accepted analytic procedure to measure SCFA limits research in this area.

Epidemiologic Evidence for Relationship Between Dietary Fiber and Disease

LARGE BOWEL CANCER. Extensive epidemiologic evidence supports the theory that dietary fiber may protect against large bowel cancer. Correlation studies that compare colorectal cancer incidence or mortality rates among countries with estimates of national dietary fiber consumption suggest that fiber in the diet may protect against colon cancer.[18] Case-control studies are considered stronger than population-based correlation studies because individual exposure to dietary variables can be related to individual outcome.

Data collected from 20 populations in 12 countries showed that average stool weight varied from 72 to 470 g per day and was inversely related to colon cancer risk.[19] When results of 13 case-control studies of colorectal cancer rates and dietary practices were pooled, the authors concluded that the results provided substantive evidence that consumption of fiber-rich foods is inversely related to risks of both colon and rectal cancer.[20] The authors estimate that the risk of colorectal cancer in the U.S. population could be reduced by about 31% with an average increase in fiber intake from food sources of about 13 g per day.

Two recently published intervention studies do not support the protective properties of dietary fiber against colon cancer.[21,22] The studies found no significant effect of high fiber intakes on the recurrence of colorectal adenomas. Both papers described well-planned dietary interventions to determine whether high-fiber food consumption could lower colorectal cancer risk, as measured by a change in colorectal adenomas, a precursor of most large-bowel cancers. Perhaps the fiber interventions were not long enough, the fiber dose was not high enough, and recurrence of adenoma is not an appropriate measure of fiber's effectiveness in preventing colon cancer. Yet the results from the studies are clear. Increasing dietary fiber consumption over 3 years did not alter recurrence of adenomas.

Despite the inconsistency in the results of fiber and colon cancer studies, the scientific consensus is that there is enough evidence on the protectiveness of dietary fiber against colon cancer that health professionals should be promoting increased consumption of dietary fiber.[23]

BREAST CANCER. Limited epidemiologic evidence has been published on fiber intake and human breast cancer risk because the fat and fiber content of the diet are generally inversely related, it is difficult to separate the independent effects of these nutrients, and most research has focused on the fat and breast cancer hypothesis. International comparisons show an inverse correlation between breast cancer death rates and consumption of fiber-rich foods. An interesting exception to the high-fat diet hypothesis in breast cancer was observed in Finland, where intake of both fat and fiber is high and the breast cancer mortality rate is considerably lower than in the United States and other Western countries where the typical diet is high in fat. The large amount of fiber in the rural Finnish diet may modify the breast cancer risk associated with a high-fat diet.[24]

A meta-analysis of 12 case-control studies of dietary factors and risk of breast cancer found that high dietary fiber intake was associated with reduced risk of breast cancer.[25] Dietary fiber intake has also been linked to lower risk of benign proliferative epithelial disorders of the breast.[26] Not all studies find a relationship between dietary fiber intake and breast cancer incidence, including a prospective cohort study reported by Willett and colleagues.[27]

Considerable evidence suggests that both breast and colon cancers are hormone-mediated diseases.[28] Few studies have examined the effects of dietary fiber on hormone metabolism while fat content of the diet was held constant. Rose and colleagues[29] reported that when wheat bran was added to the usual diet of premenopausal women, it significantly reduced serum estrogen concentrations, whereas neither corn bran nor oat bran had an effect. Dietary fiber intake was increased from about 15 g per day to 30 g per day in this study, an increase similar to that recommended by the National Cancer Institute. Goldin and associates[30] reported that a high-fiber, low-fat diet significantly decreased serum concentrations of estrone, estrone sulfate, testosterone, and sex hormone–binding globulin in premenopausal women. Dietary fiber also caused prolongation of the menstrual cycle by 0.72 day and of the follicular phase by 0.85 day, changes thought to reduce overall risk of developing breast cancer.

Dietary Fiber and Other Diseases

Dietary fiber has also been shown to be effective in reducing serum cholesterol, and it may decrease risk of coronary heart disease by decreasing serum lipids, lowering blood pressure, improving glucose metabolism, and aiding in weight control. Soluble fibers appear to be most effective in lowering serum cholesterol. Meta-analysis of 10 trials that evaluated the lipid-lowering effects of oats supports the notion that oats have hypocholesterolemic effects, independent of other dietary changes.[31] Both oats and psyllium have FDA-accepted health claims for their ability to lower blood cholesterol and reduce risk of heart disease. Less dramatic cholesterol-lowering effects are observed for vegetables, fruits, barley, and rice bran. Large epidemiologic studies document protection against cardiovascular disease from vegetable, fruit, and cereal fiber.[32]

Soluble fibers have greater potential to alter serum lipid levels than do insoluble fibers. Soluble fibers also decrease low-density lipoproteins (LDL) while maintaining high-density lipoproteins (HDL) Further, soluble fibers lower serum cholesterol even when the main dietary modifiers of blood lipids, saturated fats and cholesterol, are greatly reduced in the diet.[33] Multiple mechanisms appear to be involved in the hypocholesterolemic response, and mechanisms for lowering cholesterol may vary considerably among the various sources of dietary fiber.

Some clinical research suggests that dietary fiber may play a role in improving blood sugar control in diabetes. Dietary fiber, especially soluble fiber, can delay glucose absorption and reduce insulin requirements in both insulin-dependent and non–insulin-dependent diabetes mellitus. Obese persons with diabetes often respond to a high-fiber diet with weight loss and decreased insulin requirements. Guevin and colleagues[34] compared postprandial glucose, insulin, and lipid response when non–insulin-dependent diabetes patients consumed one of four fiber diets. The fiber diets contained two levels of total dietary fiber (10 or 20 g) and soluble and insoluble fiber in two ratios (1:4 and 2:3). The incremental area under the curve for glucose and insulin was lower for those who consumed 20 g of dietary fiber as compared with 10 g but was not affected by the soluble-insoluble fiber ratio. The authors conclude that the proportions of soluble and insoluble fiber in cereal and fruit do not necessarily predict the effects of fiber on glycemic response, whereas the overall quantity of fiber does appear to affect postprandial glucose metabolism in non–insulin-dependent diabetes.

Jenkins and colleagues[35] discuss the factors in foods that are important in insulin-resistant diseases. Fiber-rich foods contain many types of dietary fiber in addition to other potentially beneficial compounds. Glycemic index may be an important variable, as is the food form. For instance, is the food intact or has it been processed or milled? The protective effect of high fiber foods may be associated with an increased protein-to-carbohydrate ratio. Increased vegetable protein intake may act directly to reduce clotting factors and oxidized LDL-cholesterol levels. It is clear that not all dietary fibers are useful in treatment of insulin resistance because isolated fibers often do not alter glucose or insulin levels.

Intake of dietary fiber above recommended levels may be needed to improve glycemic control in patients with type 2 diabetes. In a randomized, crossover study, 13 patients with type 2 diabetes were fed diets containing 24 and 50 g per day of dietary fiber.[36] The high-fiber diet reduced plasma total cholesterol concentration by 6.7%, triglyceride concentrations by 10.2%, and VLDL-cholesterol concentrations by 12.5%. In addition, the high-fiber diet improved glycemic control and decreased hyperinsulinemia.

High-fiber diets tend to be lower in fat, and thus lower in calories, and should be appropriate for weight control. In one study, subjects who ate a high-fiber cereal at breakfast chose a lower-calorie buffet lunch than the subjects who did not eat a high-fiber breakfast.[37] Thus, a high-fiber diet may affect satiety, but whether that translates into weight loss is not known. Despite theoretic reasons why high-fiber diets should promote weight loss, results from clinical trials are inconsistent, and long-term clinical trials have not been conducted.

Enteral Formulas with Fiber

Two types of formulas that contain dietary fiber are currently marketed: (1) blenderized formulas made from whole foods and (2) formulas supplemented with purified fiber sources. The amount of dietary fiber in these products varies: published values range from 1.9 to 3.3 g of total dietary fiber (TDF) per 250 ml of "blenderized" formula and from 2.5 to 5.9 g of TDF per 250 ml of formulas containing soy polysaccharides.[8] The quantity of soluble and insoluble fiber in enteral products has been determined, and the blenderized formulas generally contain a higher ratio of soluble fiber to insoluble fiber, as determined by the AOAC procedure.[8]

Purified fiber sources used in enteral products include oat, pea, hydrolyzed guar gum, and sugar beet fibers, as well as others. Some formulas use a mixture of fiber sources. No recommendations exist for fiber intake in various disease states or for patients in long-term care facilities.

A recent addition to enteral formulas is fructooligosaccharides (FOSs). FOSs are short-chain oligosaccharides (usually 2 to 10 monosaccharide units) that are not digested in the upper digestive tract and therefore have physiologic effects similar to those of soluble fiber.[38] FOSs are fermented to SCFAs, which should stimulate water and electrolyte absorption and aid in the treatment of diarrhea. FOS also helps maintain and restore the balance of healthy gut flora.[38] FOS is a preferred energy source for bifidobacteria but are not used by potentially pathogenic bacteria. FOS is not isolated by the currently accepted method for dietary fiber, so it cannot technically be called dietary fiber. The newly proposed definitions of dietary fiber, if implemented, should allow FOS to make a label claim as added fiber.

Bowel Function with Fiber-Containing Enteral Formulas

The original rationale for adding dietary fiber to enteral formulas was to normalize bowel function. Dietary fiber is usually promoted as a preventive against constipation for the normal healthy population. Enteral formulas containing fiber are also used in the acute-care setting to prevent diarrhea associated with tube feeding. Bowel function is affected by more than fiber level, and there is much individual variation in the amount of fiber needed for optimal bowel function.

Studies on the biologic effects of enteral formulas containing fiber are few, and even less information is available on patients. Soy polysaccharide (about 22 and 44 g of TDF) added to an enteral formula significantly increased stool weights of healthy male adults.[11] Sixty grams of soy polysaccharide was not tolerated well by the subjects. Heymsfield and colleagues compared enteral formulas containing soy polysaccharide and found no difference in stool weight between Sustacal (with 1.4 g of TDF per 250 kcal) and Enrich (3.4 g of TDF per 250 kcal).[39] Fisher and coworkers reported no difference in stool weight or stool frequency when soy polysaccharide was added to the enteral formula of patients in a long-term care facility.[40] Thus, existing clinical studies do not definitively support the assertion that the addition of dietary fiber to an enteral formula improves bowel function.

Dietary fiber is thought to normalize bowel function in healthy subjects, and there is anecdotal evidence of reduction of diarrhea in patients receiving fiber-containing formulas. No convincing data have been published to document that fiber-containing enteral formulas prevent diarrhea in tube-fed patients.[41] Unfortunately, there are no standard, accepted ways of defining diarrhea.[41] The reported incidence of diarrhea in tube-fed patients ranges from 2% to 63%. Stool frequency, stool consistency, and stool quantity are the three features of bowel elimination usually used to define diarrhea. In addition to fiber, oral agents such as sorbitol and magnesium have been suggested as important intake variables affecting stool consistency.

Dietary fiber may improve fecal incontinence. Bliss and colleagues[42] found that patients with fecal incontinence who consumed dietary fiber as psyllium or gum arabic had significantly fewer incontinent stools than with placebo treatment. Improvements in fecal incontinence or stool consistency did not appear to be related to unfermented dietary fiber.

Fiber-enriched formula was used as a treatment for infant colic.[43] Because infants with colic appear to have abdominal pain similar to that of adults with irritable bowel syndrome, additional fiber may relieve colic symptoms. Infants were fed either Isomil or Isomil plus soy polysaccharide in a blinded design. The authors concluded that fiber did not affect colicky behavior in the majority of infants, who continued to cry and fuss excessively.

Brown and colleagues[44] measured the effect of soy polysaccharide on the severity, duration, and nutritional outcome of acute, watery diarrhea in children. The subjects were hospitalized. Peruvian male infants between 2 and 24 months of age were randomly assigned to receive a soy protein isolate, lactose-free formula with added soy polysaccharide, or the same diet without added fiber. Soy polysaccharide, although it did not affect stool output, macronutrient absorption, or nutritional status during acute, watery childhood diarrhea, significantly and markedly reduced the duration of liquid stool excretion.

Kapadia and colleagues[45] compared bowel function and SCFA production in healthy subjects whose diets contained either no fiber or 15 g of soy oligosaccharide fiber, oat fiber, or soy polysaccharide. The soy oligosaccharide fiber was associated with production of more butyrate than were the other fibers. Compared with a fiber-free polymeric enteral diet, daily consumption of an enteral diet supplemented with 30 g of total dietary fiber derived from a poorly fermentable oat fiber, a highly fermentable soy oligosaccharide fiber, or a moderately fermentable soy polysaccharide fiber had little, if any, impact on bowel function measures, according to the authors. The study suffers from short feeding periods (4 to 7 days), but the results support the assertion that enteral formulas should not include just any dietary fiber source but rather a fiber source that best meets the needs of the patient (e.g., bowel function, SCFA production, cholesterol lowering, glucose control).

Scheppach and Bartram[46] conclude that the results of clinical studies with dietary fiber have been disappointing, although the model proposed—that fiber is fermented, generating SCFAs, which serve as nutrition for colonic mucosal cells—is correct. To study the physiologic effects of dietary fiber, especially in a sick population, is extremely difficult. Studies have been too short, measurements are semiquantitative, and methods such as measuring dietary fiber and SCFAs are not well developed. In vivo, researchers must depend on feces as a source of SCFAs or must have subjects swallow dialysis bags and retrieve the bags in feces and measure SCFAs in the dialysate. It is not clear that results from in vitro fermentation studies have direct application in vivo. Despite the lack of compelling clinical data, dietary fiber is the treatment of choice for many bowel disorders.

Potential Negative Effects of Dietary Fiber

Potential negative effects of dietary fiber include reduced absorption of vitamins, minerals, proteins, and calories. It is unlikely that healthy adults who consume fiber in amounts within the recommended ranges will have problems with nutrient absorption; however, dietary fiber recommendations of 25 g per day may not be appropriate for children and elderly persons because so little research has been conducted in these populations.

Generally, dietary fiber in recommended amounts is thought to normalize transit time and should help when either constipa-

tion or diarrhea is present; however, case histories have reported diarrhea when excessive amounts of dietary fiber are consumed,[47] so it is difficult to individualize fiber intake based on bowel function measures. Thus, stool consistency cannot be used as a benchmark of appropriate dietary fiber intake. Fiber-containing tube feedings caused intestinal obstruction from cecal bezoar in a seriously ill male who was also receiving intestinal motility suppressing medications.[48] A large fiber bezoar developed and resulted in mesenteric hemorrhage.

Dietary fiber fermented in the gut produces gas, including hydrogen, methane, and carbon dioxide, which may be related to complaints of distention or flatulence. In a trial in our laboratory,[11] subjects who were consuming enteral diets reported no significant differences in subjective measures of bowel function among diets containing 0, 30, and 60 g of soy polysaccharide per day. Patil and associates[49] found that both fiber-free and fiber-containing diets were tolerated equally well. Generally, the gas and bloating sometimes associated with fiber consumption subside as the body adapts to increased fiber. When dietary fiber is increased, fluid intake should be also, and fiber should be increased gradually to allow the gastrointestinal tract time to adapt. Further, normal laxation may be achieved with smaller amounts of dietary fiber, and the smallest dose that results in normal laxation should be accepted.

Another potential concern is the effect of dietary fiber on micronutrient absorption, especially of minerals. Heymsfield and colleagues found reduced rates of apparent absorption for phosphorus, magnesium, and zinc when 12.4 g of soy polysaccharide was added to a fiber-free elemental diet.[39] Taper and coworkers[50] found that 40 g of soy fiber caused a negative balance for copper and iron, whereas zinc, calcium, and magnesium remained in positive balance. When mineral intake exceeds the recommended dietary allowances (RDAs), the effects of fiber on mineral absorption appear to be insignificant.

Even less information is available on the effect on vitamin absorption of dietary fiber in enteral products. Shinnick and coworkers[51] found that 15 g per day of soy fiber added to a fiber-free formula reduced apparent folate absorption. In this study the folate content of the diet was twice the RDA. No data are available on the effects of long-term feeding with fiber-enriched enteral formula and vitamin absorption.

Another concern for acutely ill persons is the potential interaction of dietary fiber in enteral formulas with drug absorption. Few data are available, but Kasper and associates[52] gave β-acetyldigoxin together with an enteral diet containing either no fiber or cellulose, pectin, carrageenan, and carob seed flour. Fiber did not reduce the digoxin concentration in serum. Carboxymethyl cellulose may reduce absorption of tranquilizers and hypotensive agents.

Another concern with fiber-enriched enteral formulas is the potential difficulty with small-bore feeding tubes. This is most problematic with gums and other viscous fibers. Soy polysaccharide and other fibers used in enteral formulas can be used in normal feeding tubes. Patil's group[49] fed a formula diet supplemented with soy fiber through a No. 8 French nasogastric tube and reported no problems with tube blockage.

Formulas containing fiber tend to be more expensive than standard formulas, making them a difficult choice in the absence of compelling clinical data. Few data have been published on the effectiveness of fiber-containing formulas in the long-term setting, and less expensive and more effective laxation aids are available.

Candidates for Fiber-Supplemented Enteral Formulas

Research-based recommendations about which patients are good candidates for fiber-containing enteral formulas cannot be made. Tube-fed patients with constipation or diarrhea who are known to have otherwise healthy gastrointestinal tracts should be considered candidates for fiber-containing enteral formulas. Because of the potential protective role of fiber against diverticulosis, colon cancer, diabetes, and heart disease, a fiber-enriched enteral formula may be indicated for patients in long-term enteral feeding. Dietary recommendations consistently support the need to increase the fiber content of the American diet.

Conclusion

Dietary fiber is not a panacea, and the popularity of fiber in nutrition often gets ahead of the scientific base. Fiber-containing enteral formulas may work better for certain patients, and they should be used if they produce positive results. Clinicians should be cautious in prescribing fiber-containing enteral products. Because of the wide individual variability of responses to dietary fiber and the potential problems with large doses, the smallest dose of dietary fiber that gives the desired result should always be used.

REFERENCES

1. McCance RA, Widdowson EM: Old thought and new work on breads white and brown, *Lancet* 2(6882):205-210, 1955.
2. Kellogg J: *The new dietetics,* Battle Creek, MI, 1921, Modern Medicine Publishing, pp 1-933.
3. Burkitt DP, Walker ARP, Painter NS: Dietary fiber and disease, *J Am Med Assoc* 229:1068-1074, 1974.
4. Slavin JL: Dietary fiber: classification, chemical analyses, and food sources, *J Am Diet Assoc* 87(9):1164-1171, 1987.
5. Trowell H: Definitions of fibre, *Lancet* 1(856):503, 1974.
6. McBurney MI, Thompson LU: In vitro fermentabilities of purified fiber supplements, *J Food Sci* 54(2):347-350, 1989.
7. Institute of Medicine, Dietary Reference Intakes: *Proposed definition of dietary fiber, food and nutrition board,* Washington, DC, 2001, National Academy Press.
8. Fredstrom SB, Baglien KS, Lampe JW, Slavin JL: Determination of the fiber content of enteral feedings, *J Parenter Enteral Nutr* 15(4):450-453, 1991.
9. Marlett JA: Content and composition of dietary fiber in 117 frequently consumed foods, *J Am Diet Assoc* 92(2):175-186, 1992.
10. Marlett JA, Vollendorf NW: Dietary fiber content and composition of different forms of fruits, *Food Chem* 51(1):39-44, 1994.
11. Slavin JL, Nelson NL, McNamara EA, Cashmere K: Bowel function of healthy men consuming liquid diets with and without dietary fiber, *J Parenter Enteral Nutr* 9(3):317-321, 1985.
12. Marlett JA, Slavin JL: Position of the American Dietetic Association: Health implications of dietary fiber, *J Am Diet Assoc* 97(10):1157-1159, 1997.
13. Pilch S: Physiological Effects and Health Consequences of Dietary Fiber, Bethesda, MD, 1987, Life Sciences Research Office, Federation of American Societies for Experimental Biology, pp 1-236.
14. Williams CL, Bollella M, Wynder EL: A new recommendation for dietary fiber intake in childhood, *Pediatrics* 96(suppl 5S):985S-988S, 1995.
15. Stephen AM, Haddad AC, Phillips SF: Passage of carbohydrate into the colon: direct measurement in humans, *Gastroenterology* 85(3):589-595, 1983.
16. Valazquez OC, Lederer HM, Rombeau JL: Butyrate and the colonocyte: implications for neoplasia, *Dig Dis Sci* 14(4):727-739, 1996.
17. Topping DL, Clifton PM: Short-chain fatty acids and human colonic function: roles of resistant starch and nonstarch polysaccharides, *Physiol Rev* 81(3):1031-1064, 2001.
18. Bingham SA: Mechanisms and experimental and epidemiological evidence relating dietary fibre (non-starch polysaccharides) and starch to protection against large bowel cancer, *Proc Nutr Soc* 49(2):153-171, 1990.
19. Cummings JH, Bingham SA, Heaton KW, Eastwood MA: Fecal weight, colon cancer risk and dietary intake of nonstarch polysaccharides (dietary fiber), *Gastroenterology* 103(6):1783-1789, 1992.
20. Howe GR, Benito E, Castelleto R, et al: Dietary intake of fiber and decreased risk of cancers of the colon and rectum: evidence from the combined analysis of 13 case-control studies, *J Natl Cancer Inst* 84(24):1887-1896, 1992.
21. Schatzkin A, Lanza E, Corle D, Lance P, Iber F, Cann B, Shike M, Weissfeld J, Burt R, Cooper MR, Kikendall JW, Cahill J, and the Polyp Prevention Trial Study Group. Lack of effect of a low-fat, high-fiber diet on the recurrence of colorectal adenomas, *N Engl J Med* 342(16): 1149-1155, 2000.
22. Alberts DS, Marinez ME, Kor DL, Guillen-Rodriguez, Marshall JR, Van Leeuwen JB, Reid ME, Ritenbaugh C, Vargas PA, Bhattacharyya AB, Earnest DL, Sampliner RE, and the Phoenix Colon Cancer Prevention Physicians' Network: Lack of effect of a high-fiber cereal supplement on the recurrence of colorectal adenomas, *N Engl J Med* 324(16):1156-1162, 2000.
23. Kim YI: AGA technical review: Impact of dietary fiber on colon cancer occurrence, *Gastroenterology* 118(6):1235-1257, 2000.
24. Rose DP: Dietary fiber, phytoestrogens, and breast cancer, *Nutrition* 8(1):47-51, 1992.
25. Howe GR, Hirohata T, Hislop TG, et al: Dietary factors and risk of breast cancer: Combined analysis of 12 case-control studies, *J Natl Cancer Inst* 82(7):561-569, 1990.
26. Baghurst PA, Rohan TE: Dietary fiber and risk of benign proliferative epithelial disorders of the breast, *Int J Cancer* 63(4):481-485, 1995.
27. Willett WC, Hunter DJ, Stampfer MJ, et al: Dietary fat and fiber in relation to risk of breast cancer. An 8-year follow-up, *JAMA* 268(15):2037-2044, 1992.
28. Rose DP: Diet, hormones, and cancer, *Annu Rev Publ Health* 14:1-17, 1993.
29. Rose DP, Goldman M, Connolly JM, Strong LE: High-fiber diet reduces serum estrogen concentrations in premenopausal women, *Am J Clin Nutr* 54(3):520-525, 1991.
30. Goldin BR, Woods MNL, Spiegelman D, et al: The effect of dietary fat and fiber on serum estrogen concentrations in premenopausal women under controlled dietary conditions, *Cancer* 74(suppl 3):1125-1131, 1994.
31. Ripsin CM, Keenan JJ, Jacobs DR, et al: Oat products and lipid lowering: a meta-analysis, *JAMA* 267(24):3317-3325, 1992.
32. Rimm EB, Ascherio A, Giovannucci E, et al: Vegetable, fruit, and cereal fiber intake and risk of coronary heart disease among men, *JAMA* 275(6):447-451, 1996.
33. Jenkins DJA, Wolever TMS, Rao AV, et al: Effect on blood lipids of very high intakes of fiber in diets low in saturated fat and cholesterol, *N Engl J Med* 329(1):21-26, 1993.
34. Guevin N, Jacques H, Nadeau A, Galibois I: Postprandial glucose, insulin, and lipid responses to four meals containing unpurified dietary fiber in noninsulin-dependent diabetes mellitus (NIDDM), hypertriglyceridemic subjects, *J Am Coll Nutr* 15(4):389-396, 1996.
35. Jenkins DJ, Axelsen M, Kendall CW, Augustin LS, Vuksan V, Smith U: Dietary fibre, lente carbohydrates and the insulin-resistant diseases, *Br J Nutr* 83 (suppl 1):S157-S163, 2000.
36. Chandalia M, Garg A, Lutjohann D, von Bergmann K, Grundy SM, Brinkley LJ: Beneficial effects of high dietary fiber intake in patients with type 2 diabetes mellitus, *N Engl J Med* 342(19):1392-1398, 2000.
37. Levine AS, Tallman JR, Grace MK, et al: Effect of breakfast cereals on short-term food intake, *Am J Clin Nutr* 50(6):1303-1307, 1989.
38. Roberfroid M, Slavin JL: Nondigestible oligosaccharides, *Crit Rev Food Science Nutr* 40(6):461-480, 2000.
39. Heymsfield SB, Roongspisuthipong C, Evert M, et al: Fiber supplementation of enteral formulas: effects on the bioavailability of major nutrients and gastrointestinal tolerance, *J Parenter Enteral Nutr* 12(3):265-273, 1988.
40. Fischer M, Adkins W, Hall L, et al: The effects of dietary fibre in a liquid diet on bowel function of mentally retarded individuals, *J Ment Defic Res* 29(Pt 4):373-381, 1985.

41. Bliss DZ, Guenter PA, Settle RG: Defining and reporting diarrhea in tube-fed patients: what a mess! *Am J Clin Nutr* 55(3):753-759, 1992.

42. Bliss DZ, Jung HJ, Savik K, Lowry A, LeMoine M, Jensen L, Werner C, Schaffer K: Supplementation with dietary fiber improves fecal incontinence, *Nurs Res* 50(4):203-213, 2001.

43. Treem WR, Hyarms JS, Blankschen E, et al: Evaluation of the effect of a fiber-enriched formula on infant colic, *J Pediatr* 119(5):695-701, 1991.

44. Brown KH, Perez F, Peerson JM, et al: Effect of dietary fiber (soy polysaccharide) on severity, duration, and nutritional outcome of acute, watery diarrhea in children. *Pediatrics* 92(2):241-247, 1993.

45. Kapadia SA, Raimundo AH, Grimble GK, et al: Influence of three different fiber-supplemented enteral diets on bowel function and short-chain fatty acid production, *J Parenter Enteral Nutr* 19(1):63-68, 1995.

46. Scheppach WM, Bartram HP: Experimental evidence for and clinical implications of fiber and artificial enteral nutrition, *Nutrition* 9(5):399-405, 1993.

47. Saibil F: Diarrhea due to fiber overload, *N Engl J Med* 320(9):599, 1989.

48. Cooper SG, Tracey EJ: Small bowel obstruction caused by oat bran bezoar, *N Engl J Med* 320(7):1148-1149, 1989.

49. Patil DH, Grimble GK, Keohane P, et al: Do fibre-containing enteral diets have advantages over existing low residue diets? *Clin Nutr* 4:67, 1985.

50. Taper LJ, Milam RS, McCallister MS, et al: Mineral retention in young men consuming soy-fiber augmented liquid-formula diets, *Am J Clin Nutr* 48(2):305-311, 1988.

51. Shinnick FL, Hess RL, Fischer MH, Marlett J: Apparent nutrient absorption and upper gastrointestinal transit with fiber-containing enteral feedings, *Am J Clin Nutr* 49(3):471-475, 1989.

52. Kasper H, Zilly W, Fassl H, Fehle F: The effect of dietary fiber on postprandial serum digoxin concentration in man, *Am J Clin Nutr* 32(12):2436-2438, 1979.

Determining the Nutrition Support Regimen

14

Robert S. DeChicco, MS, RD, LD, CNSD

Laura E. Matarese, MS, RD, LD, FADA, CNSD

DETERMINING the nutrition support regimen involves deciding whether a patient requires nonvolitional feeding and, if so, selecting the most efficacious method. Benefits of nutrition support (NS) include improved clinical outcome and shorter hospitalizations; however, as with any therapy, it has the potential for adverse effects that must be considered.

Once the decision has been made to initiate NS, the route of feeding must be chosen along with the formula and method of administration. This is influenced by the type of intravenous (IV) or enteral access and the patient's clinical status, nutritional status, and underlying disease.

Determining the Need for Nutrition Support

The first step in determining the need for NS is to assess whether the patient can consume adequate nutrients orally. This requires evaluation of the integrity and functional capability of the gastrointestinal (GI) tract and the patient's ability and willingness to eat.

Oral consumption of a standard diet is always the first option when the GI tract is functional, accessible, and "safe to use." The patient who has an appetite should receive an individualized diet with oral supplements or snacks between meals if needed. The composition and consistency of the diet should be altered if the patient has trouble chewing or swallowing. Food preferences, allergies and intolerances, and religious and cultural food habits should be taken into consideration. Psychologic obstacles to eating, such as dementia and depression, should be evaluated and treated.

Assessing oral intake is necessary to determine what percentage of nutritional requirements can be consumed by mouth. At times, this process relies heavily on clinical judgment rather than on objective evidence because methods used to assess oral intake are inexact. Retrospective methods such as a diet history, 24-hour recall, and food frequency questionnaire can be used to estimate past oral intake, but these techniques are only as good as the interviewer's skill and the subject's memory and may more accurately reflect past, rather than current, intake. Prospective methods, such as calorie counts, are inherently inaccurate because of failure to record food consumed and variations in intake on recording days.[1] The usefulness of this method is further decreased because of the delay between the time calorie counts are ordered and the availability of the results. Oral intake can be estimated from nursing documentation of fluid intake, but this can be misleading because it is based strictly on volume, not calories.

If the patient's diet order is *nil per os* (NPO), it is necessary to estimate when oral feedings will begin and when return to normal intake might be expected. Signs of a functioning GI tract include the presence of bowel sounds; a soft, nontender abdomen; passage of flatus or stool; and an intact appetite. In patients who require nasogastric tubes for decompression, secretions should diminish. When the integrity of the GI tract has been compromised by trauma or surgery, an upper GI and a small bowel x-ray study may be required before initiating feedings.

The presence and degree of malnutrition should be evaluated because malnourished patients tend to have higher rates of morbidity and mortality[2-4] and longer hospitalizations[5] than adequately nourished patients. This is compounded by the fact that a large percentage of hospitalized patients are malnourished at the time of admission;[2,4,6] oral intake is often suboptimal, especially among the elderly;[7] and nutritional status tends to decline with length of hospital stay.[5] Therefore, timely intervention is necessary for patients with preexisting malnutrition to prevent nutritional depletion from becoming worse.

In spite of its benefits, the provision of NS can cause adverse effects and therefore should not be routinely administered to all patients who cannot eat. A meta-analysis by Heyland and colleagues[8] of 26 randomized clinical trials involving over 2000 surgical and critically ill patients since 1980 concluded that providing parenteral nutrition (PN) does not significantly influence mortality compared with standard care. The authors noted a trend toward lower major complications with PN, but the treatment effect was not as great in studies published since 1989 and in studies with a higher quality score. PN has been associated with poorer outcomes compared with patients receiving standard therapy in several studies.[9,10] The Veterans Affairs Total Parenteral Nutrition Cooperative Study[9] reported that mildly malnourished patients receiving preoperative PN for 1 to 2 weeks had a significantly greater number of infectious complications during the first 30 postoperative days after major abdominal or thoracic surgery than did a control group who consumed an oral diet *ad libitum*. In a study by Brennan and colleagues[10] involving postoperative NS, malnourished patients who were to undergo major pancreatic resection for malignancy were randomized to receive either PN or IV fluids. The PN group suffered significantly more major complications without any clinical benefit in minor complications or length of stay as compared with the IV-fluid group.

NS appears to be the most beneficial in patients who are severely malnourished. Patients in the Veterans Affairs Total Parenteral Nutrition Cooperative Study[9] were categorized according to nutritional status as borderline malnourished, mildly malnourished, or severely malnourished. Only the severely malnourished patients who received PN had significantly fewer noninfectious complications than patients who received standard therapy. When the meta-analysis by Heyland[8] analyzed studies including only malnourished patients, the complication rate was significantly lower with PN compared with standard therapy. No such difference existed in studies with adequately nourished patients.

The length of time a hospitalized patient should endure without adequate nutritional intake before NS becomes necessary is unclear. It depends on a number of factors including the patient's clinical and nutritional status and when resumption of an oral diet is anticipated. Most unstressed or mildly stressed hospitalized patients with intact nutritional stores can forego adequate intake for at least several days without adversely affecting their outcome. This time frame may be shortened in patients with preexisting malnutrition or elevated metabolic requirements due to disease, surgery, or trauma. Guidelines from the American Society for Parenteral and Enteral Nutrition (ASPEN) suggest that NS should be initiated in patients with inadequate oral intake for 7 to 14 days, or in whom inadequate intake is anticipated for that time period.[11]

The practice of administrating NS to malnourished patients before surgery to promote nutritional repletion is controversial (see Chapter 21). While some studies demonstrate no clear benefit,[12] several well-designed randomized clinical trials suggest that preoperative NS, when administered in adequate amounts for a sufficient length of time to malnourished patients, can reduce postoperative morbidity and mortality.[9,13,14] It has been suggested that NS is effective in this manner when provided in adequate amounts for 7 to 14 days.[11]

Determining the Route of Nutrition Support

Enteral nutrition (EN) delivered via a feeding tube is the method of choice for patients with a functional GI tract who require NS. EN promotes comparable or better outcomes[15-17] and is less costly[18] compared with PN. The superiority of tube feedings over PN is primarily due to a reduction in septic complications.[15-19] Although the mechanism is not totally understood, it is believed that nutrients administered enterally help maintain the gut mucosal barrier, which prevents bacterial translocation. The benefits of EN may be realized even if it does not meet the patient's full nutritional requirements. Kudsk and coworkers[19] reported that trauma patients randomized to receive enteral feedings received approximately 50% of goal calories, which was significantly less than a matched group who received PN. In spite of this, the enteral group suffered significantly fewer septic complications than the PN group. Although tube feedings are generally recognized as safer than PN, they are not totally innocuous and carry their own unique set of complications (see Chapter 17). Many of these complications can be minimized by proper tube placement and administration along with regularly scheduled maintenance and monitoring.

EN is indicated in patients with adequate digestive and absorptive capacity of the GI tract but who cannot or will not eat enough. Specific indications for EN include psychiatric disorders, severe dysphagia or esophageal obstruction, neurologic impairment, major burns or trauma, organ system failure, radi-

ation or chemotherapy for cancer, acquired immunodeficiency syndrome (AIDS), and low-output enterocutaneous fistulas.[11]

PN remains effective therapy in cases of a nonfunctional GI tract or the need for bowel rest. Specific indications for PN include massive small bowel resection, radiation enteritis, intractable vomiting or diarrhea, severe acute pancreatitis, intestinal obstruction, GI ischemia, diffuse peritonitis, ileus, high-output enterocutaneous fistula, and hyperemesis gravidarum.[11] PN may also be warranted in spite of a functional GI tract when it is impossible to obtain or maintain enteral access, as when patients repeatedly pull out feeding tubes or when it is not possible to place a feeding tube into the small bowel of a patient at risk for aspiration. PN is contraindicated when the GI tract is functional, dependence on therapy is expected to last less than 5 days, and a poor prognosis does not warrant aggressive nutritional intervention (see Chapter 18).

Enteral Nutrition Support

Once the decision to provide EN via a feeding tube has been made, the type and route of access, type of formula, and method of administration must be determined. Tube feedings should be delivered by the least invasive and most physiologic method available. Timing is also important because EN delivered immediately after injury may improve wound healing[20] and limit the degree of hypermetabolism[21] and infectious complications.[15,17,22]

FEEDING ACCESS AND ROUTE OF ADMINISTRATION. The type of access and route of administration for tube feedings are usually determined by the expected length of therapy and risk of aspiration. Nasogastric or nasoenteric feeding tubes are generally used when therapy is expected to be short lived (i.e., less than 4 to 6 weeks) or for interim access before the placement of a long-term feeding tube. Long-term access requires a percutaneous or surgically placed feeding tube.

Nasogastric or nasoenteric feeding tubes are the most common devices for short-term enteral access because they are relatively inexpensive and easy to place and are safer than venous access devices. Feeding into the stomach, rather than the small bowel, is usually preferred in patients with an intact gag reflex and normal gastric function because it is more physiologic. Transpyloric feeding tubes should be reserved for patients at risk for aspiration or who have gastroparesis. This practice is based on the belief that patients are more likely to aspirate when fed into the stomach as compared with the small bowel, although most studies report no difference.[23-25] Simultaneously decompressing the stomach while feeding into the small bowel may also decrease the risk of aspiration.

The most common complication associated with placement of nasogastric and nasoenteric feeding tubes is tube malposition. Ghahremani and coworkers[26] reported a complication rate of 7.6% in 340 hospitalized patients who required bedside nasogastric tube placement without fluoroscopic guidance. Tube malposition comprised 58% of total complications. Nasoenteric feeding tubes can be placed intraoperatively, with endoscopic or fluoroscopic guidance, or blindly at bedside. Intraoperative placement requires the feeding tube to be placed manually during surgery, but this is not common practice in most institutions. Using an endoscope or fluoroscope requires special equipment and may necessitate transporting the patient off the floor, which may be impractical for patients in intensive care units. Several techniques for the blind placement of nasoenteric feeding tubes at bedside have been described,[27,28] but all have shortcomings. Zaloga[27] describes a technique for placing transpyloric tubes at bedside, but it requires removing, bending, and reinserting the stylet after the tube is placed into the stomach. Reinserting a stylet with the tube in place is not recommended because it could perforate the tube or extend through the infusion hole. Placing a feeding tube into the stomach and allowing it to migrate spontaneously into the small bowel, with or without prokinetic agents, has met with varying degrees of success. In one study,[29] feeding tubes passed spontaneously beyond the pylorus in only one third of patients within 24 hours. Others have reported higher rates of spontaneous passage after premedication with metoclopramide[30,31] or erythromycin.[32-34]

Nasogastric and nasoenteric feeding tubes differ in material and the location and size of exit ports (see Chapter 16). Some feeding tubes have weighted tips to aid in transpyloric placement and prevent retrograde migration into the stomach, but data to support this is equivocal. Evidence suggests that unweighted tubes have equal or better placement rates[31,32,35] and stay in position longer than weighted tubes.[29]

Percutaneous or surgically placed feeding tubes are usually reserved for when EN is expected to continue longer than 4 to 6 weeks. Percutaneous endoscopic gastrostomy (PEG) tubes are more popular compared with surgically placed tubes because they are less costly, have decreased procedure-related morbidity and mortality, usually do not require general anesthesia, and allow enteral feeding to be initiated more quickly.[36,37] Others argue that there is no cost advantage to PEG tubes over surgical gastrostomies placed under local anesthesia because many of the percutaneous tubes require replacement.[38] Also, upper GI strictures or obstruction may prohibit use of an endoscope to place percutaneous tubes. The advantage of percutaneously placed over surgically placed tubes is even less apparent when feeding into the small bowel is required because of high failure rates of percutaneous endoscopic jejunostomy (PEJ) tubes or percutaneous endoscopic gastrostomies with a jejunal extension tube (PEG/JETs).[39,40] In a follow-up study of PEJ tubes,[39] 84% of the tubes failed and were functional for an average of only 39.5 days (range 1 to 480 days). Separation of the inner PEJ tube from the outer gastrostomy tube and clogging because of the PEJ tube's smaller lumen were the major reasons for failure. More recent studies report lower rates of tube dysfunction and better tube durability with PEG/JETs,[41] probably as a result of improved tube design.

A direct percutaneous endoscopic jejunostomy (DPEJ) or needle catheter jejunostomy (NCJ) can also be used to access the small bowel for EN. A DPEJ is placed endoscopically, as a PEG, except that the endoscope is passed through the duodenum, past the ligament of Treitz, into a loop of jejunum adjacent to the abdominal wall. A regular pull-through PEG tube is used for access. The procedure is technically more difficult than a PEG because of the peristaltic action and narrow lumen of the jejunum, but most studies report a high percentage of successful placements with low complication rates.[42,43] Rumalla and Baron[43] reported successful DPEJ placement in 26 of 32 patients (72%) with no reintervention for tube mal-

function or displacement during a mean follow-up period of 107 days. A DPEJ has several potential advantages over a standard PEJ. A wide-diameter tube can be used for the DPEJ to decrease the incidence of clogging, and it will not migrate or kink as a standard PEJ tube might. An NCJ is placed intraoperatively and involves inserting a small catheter into the lumen of the jejunum proximal to the ligament of Treitz. The advantage of an NCJ is that it has a low complication rate,[44] nutrients can be administered almost immediately, and the catheter can easily be removed when it is no longer needed. Sarr[44] reported only three major complications with the insertion and use of 500 consecutive NCJs placed over a 10-year period. Unfortunately, the small lumen of the catheter may occlude more readily than larger-bore feeding tubes.

In many cases, feeding into the small bowel can be initiated almost immediately after location is confirmed, even in the absence of bowel sounds. Although many critically ill patients cannot be fed into the stomach because of gastric atony, the small bowel usually continues to function and can tolerate enteral nutrients. This was demonstrated in a study by Moore and associates[15] examining the effects of early enteral feedings. NCJs were placed at the time of operation in critically injured trauma patients randomized to receive enteral nutrition. The enteral feedings, started 12 to 18 hours postoperatively and advanced to the goal rate within 72 hours, were tolerated well by 86% of the subjects.

FORMULA SELECTION. The selection of an enteral formula is based on matching the patient's clinical status and nutritional requirements with the nutritional composition of a formula (Fig. 14-1). This can be difficult because of the proliferation of commercially available products. The choices can be narrowed down by answering a few basic questions:
1. Are the patient's digestive and absorptive capabilities intact?
2. Does the patient have significant organ dysfunction?
3. Does the patient have high metabolic requirements?
4. Does the patient require a fluid restriction?

Evaluating the patient's digestive and absorptive capacity helps determine whether to use a polymeric or a predigested formula. Polymeric formulas contain intact nutrients and are appropriate for most patients with normal gut function. Predigested formulas contain hydrolyzed protein in the form of peptides and free amino acids, carbohydrates as glucose oligosaccharides, and fat in varying combinations of long- and medium-chain triglycerides. Predigested formulas are indicated for patients with compromised GI tracts because hydrolyzed nutrients require less active digestion than intact components. The optimal composition of peptides and free amino acids is not known. Predigested formulas are also sometimes used as starter regimens for patients who have not received enteral feedings for long periods, but evidence is not sufficient to support their widespread use. As a general rule, polymeric formulas should be the first line of treatment for most patients who require tube feeding. Predigested formulas should be reserved until the patient has demonstrated intolerance to a standard formula.

Disease-specific enteral formulas have to be designed for patients with severe liver or kidney dysfunction (see Chapter 20). Formulas for liver failure are enriched in branched-chain amino acids and contain smaller amounts of aromatic amino

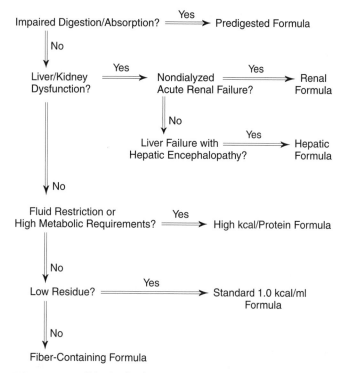

Impaired Digestion/Absorption? →(Yes)→ Predigested Formula

↓No

Liver/Kidney Dysfunction? →(Yes)→ Nondialyzed Acute Renal Failure? →(Yes)→ Renal Formula

↓No

Liver Failure with Hepatic Encephalopathy? →(Yes)→ Hepatic Formula

↓No

Fluid Restriction or High Metabolic Requirements? →(Yes)→ High kcal/Protein Formula

↓No

Low Residue? →(Yes)→ Standard 1.0 kcal/ml Formula

↓No

Fiber-Containing Formula

FIGURE 14-1 Tube feeding formula selection. (Adapted from DeChicco RS, Matarese LM: Selection of nutrition support regimens, *Nutr Clin Prac* 7:239-245, 1992.)

acids. They are intended to improve hepatic encephalopathy in patients who cannot tolerate standard solutions, but evidence to support their use is equivocal.[45] The use of branched-chain amino acid enriched diets is recommended only in chronic encephalopathy unresponsive to pharmacotherapy.[11] Formulas for renal failure are low in protein but contain a large percentage of essential amino acids (EAA). They are intended for short-term use in patients with acute renal failure who are not undergoing dialysis. However, the efficacy of formulas with predominantly EAA is unclear.[46,47] It is recommended that patients with acute renal failure who require NS should receive a balance of essential and nonessential amino acids.[11] Other products are available that are designed for use in various disease states such as diabetes mellitus and pulmonary insufficiency (see Chapters 15 and 20).

Fluid restriction or high metabolic requirements may require the use of a calorically dense formula to provide adequate nutrients without exceeding the patient's fluid limits. These products tend to contain moderate levels of electrolytes, which may also make them useful for patients with renal insufficiency.

Formulas supplemented with fiber have been advocated to improve bowel function and glucose control (see Chapter 13). While short-term studies have failed to demonstrate a consistent effect on constipation, diarrhea,[48] or blood sugar,[49] evidence of improved bowel function with long-term enteral feeding is more compelling.[50,51] The efficacy of fiber-supplemented formulas in hospitalized patients may be improved by efforts to incorporate a combination of soluble and insoluble fiber to take advantage of the unique characteristics of each. Although evidence to support the routine use of fiber supplemented formulas is lacking, it should be considered in patients

with diarrhea or constipation with an otherwise normal GI tract, and in patients requiring long-term tube feedings.

Osmolality should not be a factor in formula selection. The osmolality of enteral formulas has little discernible effect on GI tolerance for gastric[52] or duodenal feedings.[53] The practice of diluting hyperosmolar formulas when instituting tube feedings simply delays provision of adequate nutrients to the patient.

Location of the enteral feeding tube within the GI tract should not affect formula selection. Although the use of predigested formulas for feeding into the small bowel was common practice in the past, polymeric formulas, including products supplemented with fiber, can be infused into the jejunum via percutaneously or surgically placed tubes with good results. Some clinicians prefer to use predigested formulas with an NCJ because these formulas generally have lower viscosity than polymeric formulas and are therefore less likely to occlude the small tube lumen. A polymeric formula can, however, be infused through an NCJ with an infusion pump.

ADMINISTRATION TECHNIQUES. Administration techniques for EN are limited by the type and site of access. Tube feedings can be administered via bolus, intermittent, or continuous methods. Bolus feedings are administered by gravity over a short time, usually 5 minutes or less. Intermittent feedings are administered over a longer period of time, usually 20 to 30 minutes, using a feeding container and gravity drip. Although bolus feedings can be administered faster than intermittent feedings, they are more likely to cause adverse GI effects because of the shorter time interval. The bolus and intermittent methods are usually reserved for gastric feeding because the stomach can act as a reservoir to handle relatively large volumes of formula over a short time. The feedings are usually administered via a percutaneous or operative gastrostomy because of the large lumen, but they can also be given through small-bore nasogastric tubes. Bolus and intermittent feedings are the most physiologic methods of administration because the gut can rest between feedings, and they are the easiest to administer because an infusion pump is not required. For these reasons, bolus and intermittent feedings are desirable for patients who are going home or to an extended care facility on enteral feedings.

Continuous feedings are delivered slowly over 12 to 24 hours, usually with an infusion pump. The use of an infusion pump is more desirable than gravity drip because a constant infusion rate can be sustained and accidental bolus delivery is less likely to occur. Continuous administration is usually the feeding technique tolerated best[54] and may be necessary when patients cannot tolerate bolus or intermittent methods. Transpyloric feedings require continuous infusion because the small bowel cannot act as a reservoir for large volumes of fluid delivered within a short time.

Tube feedings can be cycled for patients who are making the transition from tube to oral feedings, in an attempt to stimulate appetite, or for those receiving home enteral nutrition, to allow bowel rest and time away from the pump. The feedings may be administered at night and discontinued during the day to afford the patient greater mobility and an opportunity to eat.

Parenteral Nutrition

Although tube feedings are the preferred method of NS, PN remains a necessary and effective option for patients who require gut rest. The route of administration and formula selection are determined by the expected duration of therapy and nutritional requirements. PN can also be used in combination with tube feedings for patients who cannot tolerate full enteral feedings (see Chapters 18 and 22).

FEEDING ACCESS AND ROUTE OF ADMINISTRATION. The type of access and route of administration for PN are usually determined by the anticipated duration of therapy and the patient's nutritional status and venous presentation (Table 14-1). PN via a peripheral vein is generally reserved for patients who require short-term therapy (i.e., less than 5-7 days), do not suffer from severe malnutrition or metabolic stress, are not fluid restricted, and have good peripheral venous access. The advantages of peripheral PN are that (1) venous access can be obtained at bedside by standard venipuncture methods and (2) there are fewer complications with peripheral compared with central venous catheters.[55] The drawback of peripheral PN is that venous access must be changed frequently and that it is difficult to provide the full nutritional requirement for many patients because of limits on the osmolarity of the solution to prevent thrombophlebitis. PN via a central vein is indicated for patients who need long-term therapy or fluid restriction or have high metabolic requirements. The advantage of central PN is that the catheter, once placed, can remain in place for an extended period and there is no limit on osmolarity of the solution because it is infused into a large vein. Central PN is also preferable to peripheral PN if there is intolerance to intravenous lipids, poor peripheral access, or if central access is already in place.

The preferred access sites for a central venous catheter are the subclavian or internal jugular veins. Accessing the subclavian vein is associated with a higher rate of pneumothorax but lower rates of infection than the jugular approach.[56] If the subclavian and jugular veins are not available, the femoral vein can be used. Femoral access is usually the least desirable option because it is associated with a higher incidence of thrombophlebitis and infection than are the subclavian and jugular veins.[57]

The access device is usually determined by the duration and type of therapy. A percutaneous central venous catheter is considered temporary, and its use is usually confined to hospitalized patients. A permanent (tunneled) catheter such as a Broviac, Hickman, or Groshong is placed surgically or under fluoroscopy and is designed for long-term therapy. An implanted port is also considered permanent and offers the theoretic advantage of improved body image and less risk of infec-

tion because it is completely subcutaneous. The discomfort of "accessing" a port may render this approach impractical if daily access is required, as for PN.

A peripherally inserted central catheter (PICC) is another alternative for long-term central access for PN. A PICC is a long, flexible silicone catheter designed to be inserted into the median basilic or cephalic vein via the antecubital space and advanced until the tip rests in the subclavian vein or in the superior vena cava.[58] Although used principally for long-term antibiotic therapy, PN has been infused through PICC lines with good results.[58-60] The advantage of a PICC line over other permanent catheters is that it can be inserted in a patient's room by a specially trained registered nurse or under fluoroscopy, making it more cost effective than catheters placed in an operating room. More importantly, while PICCs tend to have more minor complications than other permanent catheters, there is less risk of serious complications, such as pneumothorax.[61] Duerksen and colleagues[60] reported that PICCs had more local complications such as malpositioned or leaking catheters and phlebitis, but they had no difference in thrombosis or line sepsis compared with both tunneled and nontunneled central venous catheters used for PN over a 10-year period.

PARENTERAL NUTRITION PRESCRIPTION. The type of solution is determined by the patient's IV access and clinical status. PN can be delivered as a dextrose and amino acid solution, called a *two-in-one*, or an admixture of dextrose, amino acids, and lipids, referred to as a *total nutrient admixture (TNA)*, *all-in-one*, or *three-in-one* (see Chapter 18).

A *two-in-one* solution has advantages over a TNA because it is more stable and because dextrose-based solutions are generally tolerated well by most patients. *Two-in-one* solutions are usually more cost effective compared with TNAs because dextrose is a less expensive calorie source than lipids. Most patients receiving a standard dextrose and amino acid solution have IV lipids administered 1 to 3 times per week to supply essential fatty acids. This practice delivers approximately 10% to 15% of total calories from fat.

The use of a TNA is desirable in patients who require a reduced carbohydrate load because of glucose intolerance or hypercapnia. Lipids are also an important calorie source for peripheral PN because fat has a minimal contribution to the osmolarity of the solution. Most TNAs administered via a central venous catheter contain 20% to 40% of nonprotein calories as fat, while peripheral solutions can contain up to 70% or more. Excessive administration of IV lipids is not desirable because of concerns about solution stability and possible immunosuppressive effects; in addition, IV lipids should not be administered to patients with severe hypertriglyceridemia or allergy to eggs.

Amino acid solutions used in PN can be categorized as standard or disease-specific. Standard amino acids contain physiologic amounts of essential and nonessential amino acids and are designed for patients with normal organ function. Disease-specific amino acid solutions are designed for patients with severe liver and kidney disease, but evidence to support their efficacy is lacking (see Chapter 20). The decision to use a disease-specific amino acid solution depends largely on tolerance to standard solutions. Patients with hepatic encephalopathy caused by liver disease may not tolerate the levels of

---

TABLE 14-1

Indications for Peripheral and Central Parenteral Nutrition

Peripheral	Central
Length of therapy <5-7 days	Length of therapy >5-7 days
Not hypermetabolic	Hypermetabolic
No fluid restriction	Fluid restriction
	Intolerance/allergy to IV lipids
	Poor peripheral access
	Central access already in place

methionine and aromatic amino acids in standard solutions, making it impossible to achieve positive nitrogen balance without inducing hepatic encephalopathy or coma. An amino acid solution designed for liver failure should be used if the patient needs intravenous feeding *and* the encephalopathy does not respond to standard or usual treatment. Once the encephalopathy improves, a trial of standard amino acids is in order. Provision of NS to patients with acute renal failure is best accomplished with standard amino acid solutions and dialysis; however, renal failure solutions enriched with EAAs can be used for short periods (generally less than a week) to inhibit the rise in blood urea nitrogen (BUN) with acute renal failure until dialysis can be instituted.

ADMINISTRATION TECHNIQUES. PN is usually administered continuously to hospitalized patients because this makes it easier to tolerate the fluid and carbohydrate load and to monitor and correct metabolic alterations. It also requires less nursing time and manipulation of the catheters and IV tubing. Although continuous PN is recognized as safe and is tolerated well, continuous infusion of nutrients is contrary to the normal circadian cycle of eating and fasting. Patients who are stable with continuous PN and who will require long-term therapy may benefit from shortening the infusion time to 12 to 18 hours. Cyclic PN appears to be as effective as continuous PN in maintaining nutritional status.[62,63] Potential advantages of cyclic infusion include reversal of hepatic steatosis and liver enzyme changes associated with continuous infusion[63] and better quality of life and psychic well-being (because the patient can spend time away from the infusion pump). On the other hand, cyclic PN may be more difficult to tolerate because it requires the patient to tolerate greater fluid and dextrose loads because of the shorter infusion period.

Conclusion

The goal in determining the nutrition support regimen is to evaluate whether a patient needs NS, and, if so, choose the best route and method of administration. This process involves assessing the accessibility and functional capacity of the GI tract and the clinical and nutritional status of the patient. NS should not be provided routinely to patients who cannot eat unless the potential benefits exceed the potential risks of the therapy.

REFERENCES

1. Dwyer JT: Assessment of dietary intake. In Shils ME, Young VR (eds): *Modern nutrition in health and disease,* Philadelphia, 1988, Lea & Febiger, pp 887-905.
2. Mullen JL, Gertner MH, Buzby GP, et al: Implications of malnutrition in the surgical patient, *Arch Surg* 114:121B-125B, 1979.
3. Seltzer MH, Slocum BA, Cataldi-Betcher ML, et al: Instant nutritional assessment: absolute weight loss and surgical mortality, *J Parenter Enteral Nutr* 6:218B-221B, 1982.
4. Naber TH, Schermer T, de Bree A, et al. Prevalence of malnutrition in non-surgical hospitalized patients and its association with disease complication, *Am J Clin Nutr* 66:1232-1239, 1997.
5. Weinsier RL, Hunker EM, Krumdieck CL, et al: Hospital malnutrition. A prospective evaluation of general medical patients during the course of hospitalization, *Am J Clin Nutr* 32:418B-426B, 1979.
6. Bistrian BR, Blackburn GL, Vitale J, et al: Prevalence of malnutrition in general medical patients, *JAMA* 235:1567B-1570B, 1976.

7. Sullivan DH, Sun S, Walls R: Protein-energy undernutrition among elderly hospitalized patients: a prospective study, *JAMA* 281:2013-2019, 1999.
8. Heyland DK, MacDonald S, Keefe L, et al: Total parenteral nutrition in the critically ill patient. A meta-analysis, *JAMA* 280:2013-2019, 1998.
9. The Veterans Affairs Total Parenteral Nutrition Cooperative Study Group: Perioperative total parenteral nutrition in surgical patients, *N Engl J Med* 325:525-532, 1991.
10. Brennan MF, Pisters PW, Posner M, et al: A prospective randomized trial of total parenteral nutrition after major pancreatic resection for malignancy, *Ann Surg* 220:436-444, 1994.
11. Guidelines for the use of parenteral and enteral nutrition in adult and pediatric patients, *J Parenter Enteral Nutr* 26:1SA-138SA, 2002.
12. Thompson BR, Julian TB, Stremple JF. Perioperative total parenteral nutrition in patients with gastrointestinal cancer, *J Surg Res* 30:497-500, 1981.
13. Bellantone R, Doglietto GB, Bossola M, et al. Preoperative parenteral nutrition in the high risk surgical patient, *J Parenter Enteral Nutr* 12:195-197, 1988.
14. Fan S, Lo C, Lai E, et al: Perioperative nutritional support in patients undergoing hepatectomy for hepatocellular carcinoma, *N Engl J Med* 331:1547-1552, 1994.
15. Moore FA, Moore EE, Jones TN, et al: TEN versus TPN following major abdominal trauma-reduced septic morbidity, *J Trauma* 29:916-922, 1989.
16. Kudsk KA, Croce MA, Fabian TC, et al: Enteral versus parenteral feeding: effects on septic morbidity after blunt and penetrating abdominal trauma, *Ann Surg* 215:503-513, 1992.
17. Moore EE, Jones TN: Benefits of immediate jejunostomy feeding after major abdominal trauma: a prospective randomized study, *J Trauma* 26:874-881, 1986.
18. Bower RH, Talamini MA, Sax HC, et al: Postoperative enteral vs. parenteral nutrition. A randomized, controlled trial, *Arch Surg* 121:1040-1045, 1986.
19. Kudsk KA, Carpenter G, Petersen S, et al: Effect of enteral and parenteral feeding in malnourished rats with *E. coli*-hemoglobin adjuvant peritonitis, *J Surg Res* 31:105-110, 1981.
20. Schroeder D, Gillanders L, Mahr K, et al: Effect of immediate postoperative enteral nutrition on body composition, muscle function, and wound healing, *J Parenter Enteral Nutr* 15:376-383, 1991.
21. Mochizuki H, Trocki O, Dominioni L, et al: Mechanism of prevention of postburn hypermetabolism and catabolism by early enteral feeding, *Ann Surg* 200:297-310, 1984.
22. Grahm TW, Zadrozny DB, Harrington T: The benefits of early jejunal hyperalimentation in the head-injured patient, *Neurosurgery* 25:729-735, 1989.
23. Strong RM, Condon SC, Solinger MR, et al: Equal aspiration rates from postpylorus and intragastric-placed small bore nasoenteric feeding tubes: a randomized, prospective study, *J Parenter Enteral Nutr* 16:59-63, 1992.
24. Montecalvo MA, Steger KA, Farber HW, et al: Nutritional outcome and pneumonia in critical care patients randomized to gastric versus jejunal tube feedings, *Crit Care Med* 20:1377-1387, 1992.
25. Kearns PJ, Chin D, Mueller L, et al: The incidence of ventilator-associated pneumonia and success in nutrient delivery with gastric versus small intestinal feeding: a randomized clinical trial, *Crit Care Med* 8:1742-1746, 2000.
26. Ghahremani GG, Gould RJ: Nasoenteric feeding tubes: radiographic detection of complications, *Dig Dis Sci* 31:574-585, 1986.
27. Zaloga GP: Bedside method for placing small bowel feeding tubes in critically ill patients. A prospective study, *Chest* 100:1643-1646, 1991.
28. Thurlow PM: Bedside enteral feeding tube placement into duodenum and jejunum, *J Parenter Enteral Nutr* 10:104-105, 1986.
29. Rees RG, Payne-James JJ, King C, et al: Spontaneous transpyloric passage and performance of "fine bore" polyurethane feeding tubes: a controlled clinical trial, *J Parenter Enteral Nutr* 12:469-472, 1988.
30. Whatley K, Turner WW, Dey M, et al: When does metoclopramide facilitate transpyloric intubation? *J Parenter Enteral Nutr* 8:679-681, 1984.
31. Lord LM, Weiser-Maimone A, Pulhamus M, et al: Comparison of weighted vs. unweighted enteral feeding tubes for efficacy of transpyloric intubation, *J Parenter Enteral Nutr* 17:271-273, 1993.
32. Komenaka IK, Giffard K, Miller J, et al: Erythromycin and position facilitated placement of postpyloric feeding tubes in burned patients, *Digest Surg* 17:578-580, 2000.
33. Kalliafas S, Choban PS, Ziegler D, et al: Erythromycin facilitates postpyloric placement of nasoduodenal feeding tubes in intensive care unit patients: randomized double-blinded, placebo-controlled trial, *J Parenter Enteral Nutr* 20:385-388, 1996.

34. Stern MA, Wolf DC: Erythromycin as a prokinetic agent: a prospective, randomized, controlled study of efficacy in nasoenteric tube placement, *Am J Gastroenterol* 89:2011-2013, 1994.

35. Levenson R, Turner WW, Dyson A, et al: Do weighted nasoenteric feeding tubes facilitate duodenal intubations? *J Parenter Enteral Nutr* 12:135-137, 1988.

36. Kirby DF, Craig RM, Tsang T, et al: Percutaneous endoscopic gastrostomies: a prospective evaluation and review of the literature, *J Parenter Enteral Nutr* 10:155-159, 1986.

37. Jarnagin WR, Duh QY, Mulvihill SJ, et al: The efficacy and limitations of percutaneous endoscopic gastrostomy, *Arch Surg* 127:261-264, 1992.

38. Steigmann GV, Goff JS, Silas D, et al: Endoscopic versus operative gastrostomy: final results of a prospective randomized trial, *Gastrointest Endosc* 36:1-5, 1990.

39. Kaplan DS, Murthy UK, Linscheer, WG: Percutaneous endoscopic jejunostomy: long-term follow-up of 23 patients, *Gastrointest Endosc* 35:403-406, 1989.

40. Simon T, Fink AS: Recent experience with percutaneous endoscopic gastrostomy/jejunostomy (PEG/J) for enteral nutrition, *Surg Endosc* 14:436-438, 2000.

41. Mathus-Vliegen LM, Koning H. Percutaneous endoscopic gastrostomy and gastrojejunostomy: a critical reappraisal of patient selection, tube function and the feasibility of nutritional support during extended follow-up, *Gastrointest Endosc* 50:746-754, 1999.

42. Shike M, Latkany L, Gerdes H, et al: Direct percutaneous endoscopic jejunostomies for enteral feeding, *Gastrointest Endosc* 44:536-540, 1996.

43. Rumalla A, Baron TH. Results of direct percutaneous endoscopic jejunostomy, an alternative method for providing jejunal feeding, *Mayo Clin Proc* 75:807-810, 2000.

44. Sarr MG. Appropriate use, complications and advantages demonstrated in 500 consecutive needle catheter jejunostomies, *Br J Surg* 86:557-561, 1999.

45. Fabbri A, Magrini N, Bianchi G, et al. Overview of randomized clinical trials of oral branched-chain amino acid treatment in chronic hepatic encephalopathy, *J Parenter Enteral Nutr* 159-164, 1996.

46. Mirtallo JM, Schneider PJ, Mavko K, et al. A comparison of essential and general amino acid infusions in the nutrition support of patients with compromised renal function, *J Parenter Enteral Nutr* 6:109-113, 1982.

47. Kopple JD, Swendseid ME: Nitrogen balance and plasma amino acid levels in uremic patients fed on essential amino acid diet, *Am J Clin Nutr* 27:806-812, 1974.

48. Frankenfield DC, Beyer PL: Soy-polysaccharide fiber: effect on diarrhea in tube-fed, head-injured patients, *Am J Clin Nutr* 50:533-538, 1989.

49. Peters AL, Davidson MB: Effects of various enteral feeding products on postprandial blood glucose response in patients with type I diabetes, *J Parenter Enteral Nutr* 16:69-74, 1992.

50. Liebl BH, Fischer MH, Van Calcar SC, et al: Dietary fiber and long-term large bowel response in enterally nourished nonambulatory profoundly retarded youth, *J Parenter Enteral Nutr* 14:371-375, 1990.

51. Shankardass K, Churchmach S, Chelswick K, et al: Bowel function of long-term tube-fed patients consuming formulae with and without dietary fiber, *J Parenter Enteral Nutr* 14:508-512, 1990.

52. Keohane PP, Attrill H, Love M, et al: Relation between osmolality of diet and gastrointestinal side effects in enteral nutrition, *Br Med J* 288:678-680, 1984.

53. Zarling EJ, Parmar JR, Mobarhan S, et al: Effect of enteral formula infusion rate, osmolality, and chemical composition upon clinical tolerance and carbohydrate absorption in normal subjects, *J Parenter Enteral Nutr* 10:588-590, 1986.

54. Hiebert JM, Brown A, Anderson RG, et al: Comparison of continuous vs. intermittent tube feedings in adult burn patients, *J Parenter Enteral Nutr* 5:73-75, 1981.

55. Collignon PJ. Intravascular associated sepsis. A common problem, *Med J Aust* 161:374-378, 1994.

56. Sznajder JI, Zveibil FR, Bitterman H, et al: Central vein catheterization, failure and complication rates by three percutaneous approaches, *Arch Intern Med* 146:259-261, 1986.

57. Goetz AM, Wagener MM, Miller JM, et al: Risk of infection due to central venous catheters: effect of site of placement and catheter type, *Inf Control Hospital Epidemiol* 19:842-845, 1998.

58. Lam S, Scannell R, Roessler D, et al: Peripherally inserted central catheters in an acute-care hospital, *Arch Intern Med* 154:1833-1877, 1994.

59. Hoshal VL: Total intravenous nutrition with peripherally inserted silicone elastomer central venous catheters, *Arch Surg* 110:644-646, 1975.

60. Duerksen DR, Papineau N, Siemens J, et al: Peripherally inserted central catheters for parenteral nutrition: a comparison with centrally inserted catheters, *J Parenter Enteral Nutr* 23:85-89, 1999.

61. Alhimyary A, Fernandez C, Picard M, et al: Safety and efficacy of total parenteral nutrition delivered via a peripherally inserted central venous catheter, *Nutr Clin Prac* 11:199-203, 1996.

62. Lerebours E, Rimbert A, Hecketsweiler B, et al: Comparison of the effects of continuous and cyclic nocturnal parenteral nutrition on energy expenditure and protein metabolism, *J Parenter Enteral Nutr* 12:360-364, 1988.

63. Maini B, Blackburn GL, Bistrian BR, et al: Cyclic hyperalimentation: an optimal technique for preservation of visceral protein, *J Surg Res* 20:515-525, 1976.

Enteral Formulations 15

Susan T. Fussell, PhD, RD, CNSD

SINCE the first commercially produced enteral formulas were introduced in the 1940s, the number of products has increased dramatically to include a spectrum of formulas from oral supplements to tube-feeding formulations so specialized they may be suitable for only a few patients. The earliest enteral feedings were made on-site from whole foods, but nearly all tube feeding is now done with products purchased in liquid form in cans, bottles, brick-packs, or ready-to-hang containers. (A few adult and pediatric formulas are available in powdered form.) Most of these formulas are an emulsion of macronutrients and micronutrients known as a defined formula. Feedings still made from whole foods are called blenderized formulas. Any of the enteral products can be used for tube feeding, but only a few are acceptable for use as an oral supplement. Generally, the more hydrolyzed the macronutrients and the more calorically dense the product, the less palatable it is.

Blenderized formulas may be prepared by the institution or caregiver or purchased in cans. Their major advantage is that the whole foods from which they are prepared contain flavonoids, dietary fibers, and other phytochemicals whose role in human nutrition has not been studied sufficiently to warrant their addition to defined formulas. Blenderized formulas are generally high in fiber and residue and may contain cow's milk and lactose. Making blenderized formulas on-site is rarely done because of labor costs, the increased risk of bacterial contamination, and the uncertain nutrient content. Homemade blenderized mixtures are also more likely to occlude feeding tubes because of incomplete homogenization.

Defined formulas are nutritionally complete mixtures of carbohydrate, protein, fat, micronutrients, and water (Table 15-1). Standard formulas are made with polymeric macronutrients: intact proteins, large carbohydrate polymers, and triglycerides. More specialized formulas with partially or completely hydrolyzed macronutrients are also available. Whether these hydrolyzed macronutrients are beneficial remains controversial. Pediatric enteral formulas (intended for ages 1 to 10 years) (see Chapter 27) are similar to adult defined and blenderized formulas, but there are fewer variations in caloric density and macronutrient proportions. While adult formulas vary in caloric density and protein content, pediatric formulas all provide 1.0 kcal/ml and 12% of total calories from protein, with the exception of Vivonex Pediatric (0.8 kcal/ml) and

Compleat Pediatric (15% protein). Pediatric formulas also have similar levels of micronutrients and are all lactose and gluten free. Several specialized pediatric formulas are available with fiber, partially hydrolyzed proteins or free amino acids, or a high proportion of medium-chain triglycerides (Table 15-2).

Finally, there are adult formulas with compounds added that are not traditionally considered essential nutrients or with nutrients added in unusual amounts or ratios. These include certain amino acids and fatty acids, antioxidants, dietary fibers, and nucleotides. Unfortunately, data are lacking in many areas including optimal levels of nutrients in disease states, optimal forms of nutrients, nutrient-nutrient interactions, and potentially beneficial but nonessential components. When new components have been considered for addition to enteral feeding, many of the clinical trials have compared one product against another, often with multiple variations in nutrient content of the products being studied. Although these studies may show efficacy of a product, they do not provide information about the effects of individual nutrients.

Standard enteral formulas (Table 15-3) are the least expensive products and even in tertiary-care hospitals meet the needs of most patients. Products with hydrolyzed macronutrients or special additives can cost up to 20 times as much as standard formulas. The cost of enteral formulas is a significant portion of the total expenditure for enteral feeding. In a study of 11 teaching hospitals, formula cost was 43% of total costs even when labor, waste, and other miscellaneous costs were considered.[1] Chapter 20 provides a detailed discussion of the uses of specialized enteral formulas. The choice of formula for a patient should be based on a complete assessment of the individual's needs, considering nutrient requirements, metabolic abnormalities, gastrointestinal function, and medical condition. Choosing a formula by matching the patient's diagnosis with the name or marketing of a formula may lead to inappropriate feeding or increased cost.

Water and Caloric Density

Enteral formulas can be divided into three categories of caloric density: 1 kcal/ml (about 85% water), 1.2 to 1.5 kcal/ml (78% to 82% water), and 2 kcal/ml (71% water).[2] The 1 kcal/ml formulas are appropriate for patients with no fluid restrictions. The most concentrated formulas may be necessary for patients with renal failure, pulmonary edema, liver failure, congestive heart failure, or other conditions where fluid intake must be restricted. Formulas with intermediate caloric density may be

Acknowledgment: A special thank you is extended to Elaine Trujillo, MS, RD, who contributed to the first edition chapter.

TABLE 15-1

Macronutrient Sources in Enteral Formulas and Modular Components

Macronutrient	Polymeric Formulas	Partially Hydrolyzed Formulas	Blenderized Formulas	Modular Components
Protein	Casein Ca, Mg, or Na caseinate Lactalbumin Milk protein concentrate Soy protein isolate Whey protein concentrate	Casein hydrolysate Crystalline L-amino acids Hydrolyzed lactalbumin Hydrolyzed meat Hydrolyzed whey or whey protein Soy protein hydrolysate	Beef Casein Nonfat milk	Calcium caseinate Whey protein concentrate
Carbohydrate	Corn syrup Corn syrup solids Fructose Maltodextrin Modified cornstarch Sucrose	Cornstarch Fructose Maltodextrin Modified cornstarch	Fruit Nonfat milk Vegetables	Hydrolyzed cornstarch Maltodextrin
Fat	Borage oil Canola oil Corn oil High oleic sunflower oil MCTs Monoglycerides and diglycerides Safflower oil Soybean oil Soy lecithin	Acetylated monoglycerides Fatty acid esters Fish oil MCTs Safflower oil Sardine oil Soybean oil Soy lecithin Structured lipids	Beef Corn oil	Fish oil MCTs Safflower oil Soy lecithin

MCTs, Medium-chain triglycerides.

TABLE 15-2

Pediatric Enteral Formulas*

Formula	Protein Source	Fat/CHO (% kcal)	MCT (% of fat)	Fiber (g/L) (Insoluble:Soluble)	Fiber Source
Compleat Pediatric	Caseinates	35/50	18	4.4 (73:27)	Fruits and vegetables
Kindercal	Caseinates, milk protein	37/51	20	5.9 (97:3)	Gum arabic, soy fiber
Nutren Junior	Milk protein, whey protein	37/51	25	0	—
Nutren Junior with Fiber	Milk protein, whey protein	37/51	25	6 (100:0)	Soy polysaccharides
Pediasure	Caseinate, whey protein	44/44	19.5	0	—
Pediasure with Fiber	Caseinate, whey protein	44/44	19.5	5 (94:6)	Soy fiber
Peptamen Junior	Hydrolyzed whey protein	33/55	60	0	—
PRO-Peptide for Kids	Hydrolyzed whey protein	33/55	18.5	0	—
Resource Just for Kids	Caseinates, whey protein	44/44	20	0	—
Resource Just for Kids with Fiber	Caseinates, whey protein	44/44	20	6 (50:50)	Soy fiber, partially hydrolyzed guar gum
Vivonex Pediatric	Free amino acids	25/63	68	0	—

CHO, Carbohydrate.
*See text for caloric density, protein content, and other information of pediatric formulas.

useful for partial fluid restriction or as concentrated oral supplements for patients with impaired oral intake or when there is gastrointestinal volume intolerance. When comparing the nutrient content of formulas of different caloric densities, nutrients should be expressed per 1000 kcal rather than per liter. If nutrients are expressed per liter, the higher caloric density formulas appear to offer greater amounts of nutrients when the actual daily intake may be the same or even less than from the lower density formula.

Even enteral formulas with the highest water content (1 kcal/ml) do not provide enough water to meet usual fluid needs. Additional water must be given intravenously, orally, or administered through the feeding tube. When using concentrated formulas in patients with normal fluid needs, the risk of dehydration is increased because of miscalculation of fluid

needs, caregiver misunderstanding of the importance of additional water, or patient intolerance to water boluses. When calculating fluid intake from enteral products, the solute volume of the formula should be subtracted from the total volume of formula consumed.[2] For example, 2000 ml of a 1.0 kcal/ml product contains 1700 ml of fluid and 300 ml of solutes. A patient with normal fluid needs (1 ml/kcal) would need an additional 300 ml of water or other fluids.

The more concentrated formulas may contribute to constipation because they deliver less water to the gastrointestinal tract. The higher caloric density of these formulas may also delay gastric emptying, and they may be more likely to occlude small-bore feeding tubes. Finally, it is usually more difficult to keep added modular macronutrients in suspension in more concentrated formulas.

TABLE 15-3

Representative Standard Adult Enteral Formulas

Formula	Caloric Density (kcal/ml)	Protein (% kcal)	CHO (% kcal)	Fat (% kcal)
Boost	1.01	17	67	16
Boost High Protein	1.01	24	55	21
Boost Plus	1.52	16	50	34
Comply	1.5	16	48	36
Deliver 2.0	2.0	15	40	45
Ensure	1.06	14.1	63.9	22
Ensure High Protein	0.095	21.3	54.7	24
Ensure Plus	1.5	14.7	56.4	29
Ensure Plus HN	1.5	16.7	53.3	30
Isocal	1.06	13	50	37
Isocal HN	1.06	18	46	37
Isocal HN Plus	1.2	17	48	35
Isosource	1.2	14	57	29
Isosource HN	1.2	18	53	29
NovaSource 2.0	2.0	18	43	39
NuBasics	1.0	14	60	20
NuBasics Plus	1.5	14	47	39
NuBasics VHP	1.0	25	45	30
NuBasics 2.0	2.0	16	39	45
Nutren 1.0	1.0	16	51	33
Nutren 1.5	1.5	16	39	45
Nutren 2.0	2.0	16	39	45
Osmolite	1.06	14	57	29
Osmolite HN	1.06	16.7	54.3	29
Osmolite HN Plus	1.2	18.5	52.5	29
Promote	1.0	25	52	23
Replete	1.0	25	45	30
Traumacal	1.5	22	38	40

CHO, Carbohydrate.

Physical Properties

Osmolality

Osmolality and osmolarity are measures of the concentration of molecules in an aqueous solution. *Osmolality* is defined as milliosmoles per kilogram of solvent. *Osmolarity* is the milliosmoles per liter of solution. Osmolality is the appropriate term for describing solutes in enteral formulas and is used by manufacturers of these products. The major contributors to osmolality in enteral formulas are electrolytes, minerals, and small organic compounds.

Enteral product osmolality ranges from 270 mOsm/kg to about 700 mOsm/kg, depending on the concentration of water-soluble components. The higher the caloric density, the less water in the formula and the higher the osmolality. Smaller molecules contribute more to osmolality, so products with hydrolyzed macronutrients tend to have the highest osmolality. Sucrose, commonly added to products used as oral supplements, also increases osmolality.

Osmolality was once considered a major factor in gastrointestinal intolerance to enteral feeding. High osmolality formulas were diluted to improve tolerance, but this can lead to bacterial contamination of the formula and inadequate nutrient intake. Studies have shown that in patients with normal gastrointestinal function, side effects of enteral feeding, including nausea, bloating, cramps, and diarrhea, are not related to

osmolality,[3,4] even with duodenal feeding.[5] Other causes of diarrhea during tube feeding are discussed in Chapter 17.

Viscosity

The viscosity of a formula depends on the concentration and characteristics of the macronutrients and fiber. Higher viscosity products may affect the rate of delivery of feeding pumps and are more likely to occlude small-bore feeding tubes. The relative viscosity of isolated fibers has so far limited the caloric density of fiber-containing formulas to 1.5 kcal/ml. At least one manufacturer now offers oral nutritional supplements that have been prethickened to nectar- or honey-consistency for patients with dysphagia.

Protein

Dietary protein provides amino acids for synthesis of structural proteins, enzymes, antibodies, and signaling proteins. Amino acids are also precursors for neurotransmitters and nucleic acids, and they act as important metabolic intermediates. Amino acids are oxidized for energy and contribute to the caloric value of the diet. Chapter 7 describes in detail the roles of amino acids and protein in nutrition support. Protein in enteral formulas may be in the form of intact proteins, peptides, or free amino acids. The amount of protein in enteral formulas varies from about 6% of calories in very protein-restricted formulas intended for patients with renal failure to 25% of calories. It is important to provide adequate water for excretion of nitrogenous waste to patients receiving high-protein formulas (Tables 15-4 and 15-5).

Determination of protein quality is a complex process involving assessment of the amino acid profile, protein and amino acid digestibility, and the effects of other diet components (see Chapter 7). In 1991, the FAO/WHO Expert Consultation proposed a protein-digestibility amino acid score (PDCAAS). The protein scores calculated by this method predict the ability of a protein to provide indispensable amino acids at a low level of intake (0.7 g/kg per day).[6] Further research is necessary to compare this method with more traditional approaches, but it is likely that this newer method will be applied to enteral formulas in the future. Sources of protein in enteral formulas are generally from foods with high-quality protein—milk, beef, and soy beans. Most enteral formulas are gluten free. Individual amino acids may be added to formulas to improve protein quality or provide increased amounts of conditionally essential amino acids. When amino acids such as L-glutamine or L-arginine are added at therapeutic levels, they should not be considered in assessment of the formula's protein content or quality.[7]

Amino Acids

Enteral formulas called *elemental formulas* have individual amino acids as their sole source of protein. Elemental formulas are among the most expensive products and have the highest osmolality. Their use is usually restricted to tube feeding because of the unpleasant odor and taste.

At the time elemental formulas were developed, it was thought that amino acids would provide better absorption and utilization for some patients. Subsequent research identifying carrier-mediated absorption of dipeptides and tripeptides lead

TABLE 15-4

Protein and Amino Acid Content of Specialized Enteral Formulas

Formula	Protein (% kcal)	Arginine (g/1000 kcal)	Carnitine (mg/1000 kcal)	Glutamine (g/1000 kcal)	Taurine (mg/1000 kcal)
STANDARD FORMULAS					
	13-25	1.2-2.4	0-150	3-8	0-211
INTACT PROTEIN FORMULAS (+ AMINO ACIDS)					
Immun-Aid	32	15.4	100	12.5	200
Impact	22	12.5	0	5.9	0
Impact 1.5	22	12.5	93	6	187
Impact with Fiber	22	12.5	0	6	0
PEPTIDE-BASED FORMULAS					
Advera	18.7	3.2	99	5.4-6.4	166
Alitraq	21.1	4.5	112	14.2-15.5	200
Criticare HN	14	1.4	0	1.6-2.4	0
Crucial	25	10.0	100	4.8	100
Glutasorb	21	5.26	0	10.52	0
Impact Glutamine	24	12.5	108	11.5	108
Optimental	20.5	5.5	110	4.4	110
Peptamen 1.5	16	1.1	100	3.0	100
Peptamen	16	1.2	100	3.0	100
Peptamen VHP	25	1.9	100	4.6	100
Perative	20.5	11.3	108	5.4	108
ProBalance	18	1.7	83	3.9-5.7	83
PRO-Peptide	16	1.12	130	3	130
PRO-Peptide VHN	25	1.76	130	4.7	130
Reabilan	12.5	1.0	80	5.0	140
Reabilan HN	17.5	1.4	80	9.3	140
SandoSource Peptide	20	5.0	100	4.7	200
Subdue	20	1.5	79	3.7	100
Vital HN	16.7	2.1	0	1.8-2.2	0
AMINO ACID FORMULAS					
Amin-Aid	4	0	0	0	0
f.a.a.	20	12	100	0	100
L-Emental	15	2.9	0	4.9	0
Tolerex	8	1.8	0	3.5	0
Vivonex T.E.N.	15	2.9	60	19	60
Vivonex Plus	18	5.0	67	10.0	67

TABLE 15-5

Formulas Intended for Use in Renal Disease*

Formula	Protein (% kcal)	Protein Source	Micronutrients	Potassium (mg/L)
Magnacal Renal	15	Intact protein	Vitamin D restricted	1270
Nepro	14	Intact protein	Vitamin D restricted	1060
Novasource Renal	15	Intact protein, L-arginine	Vitamins A and D restricted	810
NutriRenal	14	Intact protein	Vitamins D and K restricted	1256
Renalcal	6.9	L-amino acids (67% EAAs), intact protein	No fat-soluble vitamins, electrolytes, or minerals except zinc and selenium	0
Suplena	6.0	Intact protein	Vitamins A and D restricted	1120

EAAs, Essential amino acids.
*All formulas are 2.0 kcal/ml, 35%-46% fat, 790-900 mg Na/L, and Ca:P ratio approximately 2:1.

to the development of peptide-based formulas. Recent studies have shown that even patients with gastrointestinal disease can benefit from enteral feeding with intact protein or peptides. Intact proteins may help maintain intestinal integrity when compared with diets of crystalline amino acids.[8] In a randomized, double-blind study of patients with Crohn's disease, comparing formulas with intact protein versus amino acids, both were equally effective at promoting remission.[9]

Peptides

Peptide-based enteral formulas contain protein that has been partially hydrolyzed to mixtures of peptides of varying chain lengths. Absorption may be improved with peptides compared with amino acids and intact protein, which may be useful in patients with inadequate digestive enzymes, short bowel syndrome, or other forms of malabsorption, although more research is needed to define the optimal use of these products. Improved absorption as defined by a lower incidence of diarrhea has been difficult to document in other patients. In a small study of critically ill patients, a peptide-based formula resulted in about the same incidence of diarrhea as a whole-protein formula.[10] Other studies have confirmed that the incidence of diarrhea between peptide or whole-protein formulas differs little.[11-13]

The availability of the amino acids from peptide-based formulas appears to be the same as for intact proteins. In one study, there was no difference between a standard formula and a peptide-based formula in their effect on serum albumin concentration.[10] The same peptide-based formula also did not increase serum proteins or nitrogen balance in a group of critically ill patients.[12] In another study, Heimburger found only a small but significant increase in serum fibronectin concentration in patients fed peptide-based formula.[11]

Branched-Chain Amino Acids

Formulas specifically designed for patients with hepatic encephalopathy (HE) contain increased amounts of the branched-chain amino acids (BCAA), valine, leucine, and isoleucine and decreased amounts of the aromatic amino acids (AAA), phenylalanine, tyrosine, and tryptophan (Table 15-6). In these formulas, BCAAs make up 45% to 50% of total protein compared with 20% in standard formulas. Patients with HE often have an altered plasma amino pattern with higher than normal AAA concentrations and lower than normal BCAA concentrations. Exogenous sources of BCAAs can help normalize the plasma amino pattern. However, the effectiveness of BCAAs in actually reversing HE is still under debate.[14] (See Chapter 20 for a detailed discussion of the proposed mechanism of BCAAs role in HE.) A review of clinical studies concluded that treatment with BCAAs was most appropriate for patients in whom HE developed or continued while consuming adequate amounts of standard protein and for critically ill patients with chronic HE.[15] Continuing investigation into the basic mechanisms of BCAA metabolism may result in improved ability to predict which patients with HE would benefit from BCAA-supplemented, low-AAA enteral formulas.[16]

Plasma amino acid patterns are altered in critically ill patients, resulting in a similar change in the ratio of AAAs to BCAAs. However, studies of high-BCAA enteral formulas have not been able to show an improvement in the morbidity or mortality of these patients. This is also discussed in detail in Chapter 20. Currently, the only high-BCAA enteral formulas available are intended for patients with HE and contain only 11% to 15% protein. This may not provide adequate protein for other critically ill patients.

Glutamine

Glutamine has been found to be a primary fuel for the gastrointestinal tract. An exogenous source of glutamine may be beneficial during the stress response in reducing skeletal muscle breakdown to provide glutamine to the liver. Numerous studies have shown benefits of adding glutamine to parenteral nutrition; however, it has been more difficult to show benefit of enteral glutamine supplementation. In one study of enteral feeding in the 3 days following trauma, a formula with additional glutamine failed to alter nitrogen balance or protein turnover. Preliminary studies indicate that enteral glutamine may improve acid-base balance by increasing plasma bicarbonate and renal acid secretion.[17] In 19 critically ill patients, a peptide-based enteral formula supplemented with glutamine did not improve nitrogen balance, serum albumin or transthyretin concentration, or immune function, although differences in plasma amino acids were noted.[18] Authors of a recent study of oral glutamine supplementation in patients undergoing bone marrow transplantation failed to find improvements in outcome in spite of the positive studies in similar patients who received glutamine-enhanced parenteral nutrition.[19] Oral glutamine also failed to improve intestinal permeability when fed to patients with Crohn's disease for 4 weeks.[20] Although glutamine appears to be safe in doses up to at least 30 g/day, the best route, dose, and duration of oral glutamine supplementation are not clear (see Chapters 7 and 20.)

Because all intact proteins contain glutamine, enteral formulas with intact proteins or hydrolyzed proteins contain glutamine. Amounts of glutamine in enteral formulas have been calculated from the glutamine content of their protein sources. Values are 2.8 to 7.3 g/1000 kcal for standard enteral formulas[21] (see Table 15-4). Until recently, therapeutic amounts of glutamine were only available in powdered products because glutamine is not completely soluble or stable in aqueous solu-

---

TABLE 15-6

Enteral Formulas With Increased Branched-Chain Amino Acids

Formula	Caloric Density (kcal/ml)	Protein (% kcal)	Arginine (g/1000 kcal)	BCAAs (% of Total Protein)	Carnitine (mg/1000 kcal)	Taurine (mg/1000 kcal)
STANDARD FORMULAS						
	1.0-2.0	13-25	1.2-2.4	19-23	0-150	0-211
HIGH BRANCHED-CHAIN AMINO ACID FORMULAS						
Hepatic-Aid II	1.2	15	3.3	46	0	0
L-Emental Hepatic	1.2	15	5.2	46	0	0
NutriHep	1.5	11	3.2	50	80	80

tions. Currently, one manufacturer has added glutamine in the form of peptides to a liquid enteral formula. Glutamine is also available as a powdered single-nutrient supplement that can be mixed with water, food, or enteral formula and used within 24 hours.[22]

Glutamine and arginine both have two amine groups that must be excreted as urea when the amino acids are oxidized. This can add significantly to the renal solute load of high-protein formulas containing therapeutic levels of these amino acids. Because they cannot be incorporated into body proteins, it is not appropriate to include them in calculations of protein intake.

Arginine

Arginine can be synthesized by humans and was not originally considered an essential amino acid, but is now thought to be required for growth and in certain disease states. In addition to its role as a component of proteins, arginine is a precursor of urea; creatinine; and ornithine, itself a precursor of polyamines. Arginine stimulates release of several hormones, including glucagon, prolactin, insulin, and growth hormone. In cell culture, arginine is required for maximal cell growth and optimal lymphocyte function. Interest in arginine metabolism in critical illness is based on its role as the precursor of nitric oxide.[23] Nitric oxide appears to regulate blood pressure, blood flow, and platelet aggregation and adhesion. Chapters 7 and 20 give further detail on arginine. Unfortunately, many of the clinical trials of arginine supplementation were conducted with formulas containing several additives, so that arginine's role in improving immune function could not be determined.[24] When arginine was fed alone as a supplement to oral or enteral feeding, there was no improvement in immune function of elderly patients with decubitus ulcers.[25] Arginine is present in all enteral formulas made from intact proteins. Additional arginine is added to several formulas intended to enhance immune function (see Table 15-4). It is also available as a powdered supplement.

Taurine

Taurine is a β-amino acid found in nearly all human tissue, but not incorporated into proteins. Although the biochemical mechanisms have not all been elucidated, taurine acts as an antioxidant, neuromodulator, and regulator of calcium homeostasis, and is probably important for immune function and the inflammatory response. Although taurine can be synthesized in the liver and brain, dietary sources provide a significant portion of the body's taurine. Plasma taurine levels may become elevated in renal failure or decreased in trauma, sepsis, or cancer.[26] Currently, most adult formulas are supplemented with taurine (see Table 15-4).

Carbohydrate

Carbohydrate, in the form of glucose, is the primary source of fuel for mammalian metabolism. Polysaccharides, oligosaccharides, disaccharides, and monosaccharides are all carbohydrate forms used to provide energy and glucose in enteral formulas (see Table 15-1). (See Chapter 8 for a discussion of carbohydrate metabolism and requirements.) Polysaccharides are carbohydrate polymers containing more than 10 monosaccharide

units. An inability to digest or absorb polysaccharide is extremely rare, so polysaccharides provide the majority of energy in nearly all enteral formulas. Polysaccharides may be hydrolyzed to increase solubility resulting in maltodextrin, maltose, modified starches, and disaccharides and monosaccharides. Oligosaccharides contain 3 to 10 monosaccharides and are more soluble than larger polysaccharides. Disaccharides, while generally rapidly digested and absorbed, are not usually the primary carbohydrate source because of their high osmolality. Sucrose is the most commonly used disaccharide, mostly to sweeten formulas used as oral supplements. As the carbohydrate molecules become smaller, the sweetness and osmolality of the formula increase. Only a few enteral formulas contain lactose, although both patients and medical staff may believe they do because of a formula's milky appearance. Some lactose-free formulas still contain galactose and cannot be used for patients with galactosemia.

The amount of carbohydrate in enteral formulas ranges from about 40% to 80% of total calories. Formulas with fiber and a reduced carbohydrate content have been developed to improve blood glucose control in patients with diabetes mellitus or stress-induced hyperglycemia. While the carbohydrate content of formulas appears to be the major factor in glycemic response, there is a large individual variability in response to enteral products,[27,28] and many patients with diabetes mellitus can achieve good glucose control on standard products. Products with low carbohydrate content are necessarily higher in fat (Table 15-7). Because patients with diabetes mellitus have an increased risk of cardiovascular disease, formulas with reduced carbohydrate and increased fat may not be appropriate for long-term use.

Studies of patients with respiratory failure noted carbon dioxide retention and increased work of breathing with high-carbohydrate enteral formulas, leading to development of so-called pulmonary formulas that have reduced carbohydrate calories and increased fat calories. Subsequent research has shown that these observations were probably a result of overfeeding rather than an effect of the proportion of carbohydrate in the formula. If overfeeding is avoided, standard formulas are unlikely to affect respiratory function. Some of the pulmonary formulas also contain ω-3 fatty acids and/or higher levels of antioxidants. See Chapter 20 for further discussion of specialized nutrition support in diabetes mellitus and pulmonary disease.

Fat

It is well established that fat provides energy and essential fatty acids in both oral diets and enteral formulas. However, in the last several decades, several more specialized functions of lipids have been identified. (See Chapter 9 for discussion of fat metabolism and requirements.) The fat content of enteral formulas varies from 5% (the minimum amount to meet essential fatty acid requirements) to 55% in formulas intended to reduce carbohydrate intake in patients with carbon dioxide retention, diabetes mellitus, or glucose intolerance. Standard formulas contain 15% to 35% of total calories as fat. The optimal amount for various conditions is not clear. Formulas with high fat content may delay stomach emptying.[29]

TABLE 15-7

Formulas With Altered Carbohydrate-To-Fat Ratio or Sources

Formula	Caloric Density (kcal/ml)	Protein (% kcal)	Carbohydrate (% kcal)	Carbohydrate (Sources)	Fat (% kcal)
Choice dm	0.93	17	40	Maltodextrin, sugar	43
Choice dm TF	1.06	17	40	Maltodextrin	43
Diabetasource	1.0	20	36	Maltodextrin, fructose, vegetables, fruits	44
Glucerna	1.0	16.7	34.3	Maltodextrin, fructose	49.0
Glytrol	1.0	18	40	Maltodextrin, fructose, modified corn starch	42
Lipisorb Liquid	1.35	17	48	Maltodextrin, sugar	35
NovaSource Pulmonary	1.5	20	40	Corn syrup, sucrose	40
NutriVent	1.5	18	27	Maltodextrin	55
Oxepa	1.5	16.7	28.1	Sugar, maltodextrin	55.2
Pulmocare	1.5	16.7	28.2	Sugar, maltodextrin	55.1
Resource Diabetic	1.06	24	36	Hydrolyzed corn starch	40
Respalor	1.5	20	40	Maltodextrin	40

The fat in enteral formulas is added in the form of triglycerides, either naturally occurring or structured (see below), in an emulsion within the aqueous phase. Because of the large molecular weight of triglycerides, fat does not contribute to formula osmolality. Their constituent fatty acids are a varying mixture of polyunsaturated (both ω-6 and ω-3), monounsaturated, and medium-chain fatty acids. The sources of fat in enteral formulas are shown in Table 15-8. The size of the fat droplets in the emulsion is known to affect fat digestion in healthy subjects, although no manufacturer has capitalized on this yet.[30]

ω-3 Fatty Acids

The ω-3 fatty acids currently being studied for their potential to alter disease include linolenic (18:3n-3) acid, eicosapentaenoic acid (20:5n-3), and docosapentaenoic (22:6n-3) acid. Linolenic acid is an essential fatty acid found in significant amounts in soybean oil and rapeseed oil. The other two fatty acids, found mainly in fish oils, are not considered essential because humans can synthesize them from linolenic acid. However, increased exogenous intake can alter the fatty acid composition of cell membranes and affect prostaglandin and cytokine production and cell-mediated immunity.[31-33] Patients with various acute or chronic diseases may have abnormal plasma fatty acid profiles that could be corrected by providing ω-3 fatty acids.[34] While it is possible to alter animal or human phospholipids and prostaglandins by feeding oral ω-3 fatty acids, whether this improves clinical outcome still needs to be investigated.[35-38] Omega-3 fatty acids also have a range of effects on cardiovascular disease[39] and hemodynamics, which could influence their use in enteral formulas.[40]

Medium-Chain Triglycerides

Medium-chain triglycerides (MCTs) are glycerol esterified with medium-chain fatty acids (6 to 12 carbons), which are responsible for the special characteristics of MCTs. The MCTs used in enteral formulas and modules are prepared from palm or coconut oil. Their major advantage is an absorption mechanism that does not require pancreatic enzymes, bile, transport in the lymphatic system, or carnitine-dependent transport into mitochondria. Thus, they can be used to provide a concentrated source of energy to patients with fat malabsorption or damage to lymphatic vessels. Medium-chain fatty acids are metabolized in the liver and form ketones if fed in excess. This can be a disadvantage in patients who already produce excess ketones or can be exploited in a ketogenic diet. Many adult formulas and all pediatric formulas contain some MCTs. Modular MCTs can be added to formulas and have been prescribed for increasing the caloric density of oral diets, but many patients find them unpalatable. MCTs can cause gastrointestinal discomfort and diarrhea, possibly by accelerating small bowel transit.[41]

Structured Lipids

Structured lipids are triglycerides made by hydrolyzing a mixture of MCTs and long-chain triglycerides (LCTs) together and allowing random reesterification, resulting in a triglyceride with the desired combination of fatty acids. This can have varying effects on absorption depending on the chain length of fatty acids in the three positions on the glycerol moiety. Numerous animal studies and some human studies have shown improved fat absorption with certain structured lipids, but further research is needed to prove other benefits in humans of this rather costly process[42] (see Chapter 9). At least one enteral formula contains structured lipid.

Fiber

Dietary fiber has always been present in blenderized formulas because it is a component of fruits and vegetables, but the addition of isolated fibers to defined formulas began in the 1980s with the addition of soy polysaccharide. As knowledge increases about the variety of fibers and their physiolgic effects, other fibers have been included in enteral formulas (see Chapter 13). Some confusion remains over the terminology used to describe nondigested material in diets and formulas. The term *residue* refers to the increase in fecal weight caused by undigested food material. Residue is assumed to include not only some of the dietary fibers but also other compounds not digested by human or bacterial enzymes and then absorbed, such as tough meat fibers. The term has become less meaningful as knowledge increases about the specific structures and characteristics of dietary fiber. Dietary fiber is defined as a heterogeneous group of compounds that are not digested by human enzymes; they may be digested by bacterial enzymes and absorbed in the colon. Enteral formulas without added fiber are considered very low in residue because their macronutrients are highly digestible.[43]

TABLE 15-8

Fat Content of Selected Enteral Products*

Formula	Fat (g/L)	Fat (source)	Fat (% kcal)	Linoleic Acid (g/L)	MCTs (g/L)	ω-3 Fatty Acids (g/L)
TUBE FEEDING						
Advera	22.8	Canola oil, MCTs, sardine oils	15.8	3.4	4.0	1.16
Alitraq	15.5	MCTs, safflower oils	13.0	6.6	6.5	1.55
Amin-Aid	46.2	Soybean oil, lecithin, monoglycerides and diglycerides	21.2	10.2	0.0	0.92
Boost	17.8	Canola, high-oleic sunflower, corn oils	16.0	4.0	0.0	0.80
Boost High Protein	23.0	Canola, high-oleic sunflower, corn oils	21.0	5.1	0.0	1.10
Boost Plus	58.0	Canola, high-oleic sunflower, corn oils	34.0	12.8	0.0	2.70
Boost with Fiber	17.8	Canola, high-oleic sunflower, corn oils	16.0	3.9	0.0	0.80
Choice dm TF	51.0	Canola, high-oleic sunflower, corn, MCTs oils	43.0	10.2	4.9	2.10
Compleat	37.0	Beef fat, canola oil	31.0	6.4	0.0	1.84
Comply	61.0	Corn, canola, high-oleic sunflower, MCTs oils	36.0	10.8	11.8	2.30
Criticare HN	5.3	Safflower oil, emulsifiers	4.5	3.4	0.0	0.10
Crucial	67.6	MCTs, fish, soybean oils, lecithin	39.0	7.7	33.8	3.80
Deliver 2.0	101.0	Soybean, MCTs oils	45.0	37.0	29.0	5.50
DiabetiSource	49.0	Sunflower, canola oils, beef fat	44.0	5.0	0.0	2.10
Ensure	25.0	High-oleic safflower, canola, corn oils	21.6	20.0	0.1	0.46
Ensure Plus	53.3	Canola, high-oleic safflower, corn oils	32.0	28.6	0.1	0.66
Ensure Plus HN	49.0	High-oleic safflower, canola, corn oils	30.0	6.7	9.8	0.62
Ensure with Fiber	25.0	High-oleic safflower, canola, corn oils	21.6	20.0	Trace	0.46
Fibersource Std.	39.0	MCTs, canola oils	29.0	7.2	8.4	2.70
Fibersource HN	39.0	MCTs, canola oils	29.0	7.2	8.4	2.70
Glucerna	54.4	High-oleic safflower, canola oils	49.0	7.7	0.1	0.69
Glytrol	47.5	MCTs, canola, high-oleic safflower, soybean oils, lecithin	42.0	5.4	9.5	1.80
Hepatic-Aid II	36.2	Soybean oil, lecithin, monoglyceride and diglycerides	27.7	8.0	0.0	0.72
Immun-Aid	22.0	Canola, MCTs oils	20.0	2.1	11.0	1.20
Impact	28.0	Refined menhaden, palm kernel, sunflower oils	25.0	2.5	7.6	1.70
IntensiCal	42.0	Canola, MCTs, high-oleic sunflower, corn, menhaden oils	29.0	6.6	10.3	1.90
Introlite	18.4	MCTs, corn, soybean oils	30.0	5.8	7.2	0.16
Isocal	44.0	Soybean, MCTs oils	37.0	19.4	8.9	2.70
Isocal HN	45.0	Soybean, MCTs oils	37.0	14.6	17.3	2.30
Isocal HN Plus	40.0	Canola, MCTs, high-oleic sunflower, corn oils	29.0	6.1	11.5	1.30
Isosource Std.	39.0	MCTs, canola oils	29.0	7.2	8.4	2.70
Isosource HN	39.0	MCTs, canola oils	29.0	7.2	8.4	2.70
Isosource VHN	29.0	MCTs, canola oils	25.0	2.9	15.1	1.20
Jevity	34.7	High-oleic safflower, canola, MCTs oils	29.0	4.7	6.4	1.20
Jevity Plus	39.3	High-oleic safflower, MCTs oils, lecithin	29.0	5.4	7.3	1.30
Kindercal	44.0	Canola, high-oleic sunflower, MCTs, corn oils	37.0	7.8	8.7	1.60
Lipisorb Liquid	57.0	MCTs, soybean oils	35.0	4.5	48.0	0.70
Magnacal Renal	101.0	Canola, high-oleic sunflower, MCTs, corn oils	45.0	17.9	20.0	3.70
Modulen IBD	47.6	Milkfat, MCTs, corn, soy oils, lecithin	42.0	4.4	11.6	Not available
Nepro	95.6	High-oleic safflower, canola oils	43.0	15.5	Trace	2.80
NovaSource Pulmonary	68.0	MCTs, canola oils	40.0	11.5	14.5	4.70
NovaSource Renal	100	High-oleic sunflower, corn, MCTs oils	45.0	16.6	14.0	0.00
NuBasics	36.7	Canola, corn oils, soy lecithin	33.0	10.6	0.0	2.3
NuBasics Plus	64.8	Canola, corn oils, lecithin	39.0	18.6	0.0	4.08
NuBasics 2.0	106.0	MCTs, canola, corn oils, soy lecithin,	45.0	7.2	79.5	1.60
NuBasics VHP	34.0	Canola, corn oils, lecithin	30.0	9.6	0	2.08
Nutren 1.0	38.0	MCTs, canola, corn oils, lecithin	33.0	8.2	9.6	1.74
Nutren 1.0 with Fiber	38.0	Canola, MCTs, corn oils, lecithin	33.0	8.2	9.6	1.74

Continued.

TABLE 15-8

Fat Content of Selected Enteral Products*—cont'd

Formula	Fat (g/L)	Fat (source)	Fat (% kcal)	Linoleic Acid (g/L)	MCTs (g/L)	ω-3 Fatty Acids (g/L)
Nutren 1.5	67.5	MCTs, canola, com oils, lecithin	39.0	9.8	33.2	2.51
Nutren 2.0	106	MCTs, canola, corn oils, lecithin	45.0	7.8	78.0	1.51
Nutren Junior	42.0	Soybean, MCTs, canola oils, soy lecithin	37.0	11.7	10.5	2.40
NutriFocus	48.7	Canola, corn, high-oleic safflower oils	29.6	Not available	Not available	Not available
NutriHep	21.0	MCTs, canola, corn oils, lecithin	12.0	1.6	14.0	0.40
NutriVent	94.8	Canola, MCTs, corn oils, lecithin	55.0	15.4	39.4	3.50
Optimental	28.4	Sardine, structured MCTs oils	25.0	3.9	4.9	4.30
Osmolite	34.7	High-oleic safflower , canola oils, MCTs	29.0	4.8	6.4	1.10
Osmolite HN	34.7	High-oleic safflower, canola, MCTs oils	29.0	4.8	6.4	1.10
Osmolite HN Plus	39.3	High-oleic safflower, canola, MCTs oils, lecitin	2.9	5.4	7.2	1.20
Oxepa	93.7	Canola, MCTs, borage, sardine oils	55.2	15.0	23.8	17.50
Pediasure	50.0	Safflower, MCTs, soybean oils	44.1	10.7	9.5	9.90
Pediasure with Fiber	50.0	Safflower, MCTs, soybean oils	44.1	10.7	9.5	1.00
Peptamen	39.0	MCTs, soybean oils, soy lecithin, residual milkfat	33.0	3.9	27.3	0.56
Peptamen Junior	38.5	MCTs, soybean, canola oils, lecithin, residual milkfat	33.0	4.7	23.1	0.94
Peptamen VHP	39.0	MCTs, soybean oils, lecithin, residual milkfat	33.0	3.2	27.3	0.40
Peptamen 1.5	58.5	MCTs, soybean oils, lecithin, residual milkfat	33.0	6.1	41.2	0.90
Perative	37.4	Canola, MCTs, corn oils	25.0	6.8	14.8	1.20
ProBalance	40.6	Canola, MCTs, corn oils, lecithin	30.0	8.3	8.1	2.40
Promote	26.0	High-oleic safflower, canola, MCTs oils	23.0	3.9	4.5	0.76
Promote with Fiber	28.2	High-oleic safflower, canola, MCTs oils	25.0	4.2	5.2	0.78
Protain XL	30.0	Canola, MCTs, high-oleic sunflower, corn oils	26.0	5.3	5.7	1.10
Pulmocare	93.3	Canola, MCTs, corn, high-oleic safflower oils	55.1	18.4	18.5	4.80
Reabilan	40.5	MCT, soybean, canola oils, lecithin	35.0	6.7	20.0	1.20
Reabilan HN	51.9	MCT, soybean, canola oils, lecithin	35.0	9.1	26.5	1.60
Renalcal	34.4	MCTs, canola oils	35.0	6.3	24.1	1.80
Replete	34.0	Canola, MCTs oils, lecithin	30.0	5.1	8.5	2.10
Replete with Fiber	34.0	Canola, MCTs oils, lecithin	30.0	5.1	8.5	2.10
Resource Std.	25.0	Corn, high-oleic sunflower, soybean oils	22.0	7.0	0.0	0.50
Resource Plus	46.0	Corn, high-oleic sunflower, soybean oils	28.0	13.0	0.0	0.90
Respalor	68.0	Canola, MCTs, high-oleic sunflower, corn oils	40.0	10.3	20.0	2.20
Subdue	34.0	MCTs, canola, high-oleic sunflower, corn oils	30.0	3.1	18.0	0.70
Subdue Plus	51.0	MCTs, canola, high-oleic sunflower, corn oils	30.0	5.5	24.0	1.20
Suplena	95.6	High-oleic safflower, soy oils	43.0	18.9	Trace	0.80
Tolerex	1.5	Safflower oil	1.0	1.2	0.0	0.00
TraumaCal	68.0	Soybean, MCTs oils	40.0	25.0	20.0	3.70
TwoCal HN	90.9	High-oleic safflower, MCTs, canola oils	40.1	10.8	17.3	1.21
Ultracal	39.0	Canola, MCTs, high-oleic sunflower, corn oils	37.0	5.9	11.5	1.30
Ultracal HN Plus	40.0	Canola, MCTs, high-oleic sunflower, corn oils	29.0	6.1	11.5	1.30
Vital High Nitrogen	10.8	Safflower, MCTs oils	9.4	4.0	3.5	0.08
Vivonex Pediatric	24.0	MCTs, soybean oils	25.0	3.9	16.3	0.50
Vivonex Plus	6.7	Soybean oil	6.0	3.4	0.0	0.50
Vivonex TEN	2.8	Safflower oil	3.0	2.2	0.0	0.00
MODULES						
MCTs Oil	930.0	MCTs oil	100.0	0.0	933.0	0.00
Microlipid	510.0	Safflower oil	100.0	400.0	0.0	2.00
Super MaxEPA	333.3	Fish oil	71.4	0.0	0.0	111.33

*Product information verified by manufacturers 10/01 by Michele Gottschlich and Theresa Mayes.
Adapted with permission from Gottschlich MM: Selection of optimal lipid sources in enteral and parenteral nutrition, *Nutr Clin Prac* 1992;7(4):152-165.

Fibers used in enteral formulas include soy polysaccharide, gums, pectin, and fructooligosaccharides. There is a large body of research on the effects of many isolated fibers, but most of the studies of fiber added to enteral formulas have been done with soy polysaccharide or hydrolyzed guar gum. Fiber sources listed on ingredient labels are not 100% dietary fiber (e.g., soy polysaccharide is 75% dietary fiber). Most manufacturers now also give the grams per liter of dietary fiber on product labels. Fiber content of enteral formulas is limited by the difficulty of keeping it in suspension. So far fiber has not been added to formulas with a caloric density greater that 1.5 kcal/ml. Table 15-9 shows the fiber content of representative products.

Plant fibers have been classified by solubility in water and fermentability by intestinal bacteria. The ability of soluble fibers to form gels and hold water in the gastrointestinal tract has important effects on gastrointestinal motility and stool properties. Most soluble fibers are fermented by intestinal bacteria, producing hydrogen gas, carbon dioxide, and short-chain fatty acids, but concordance between the two classifications is not 100%. Some insoluble hemicelluloses are fermented. The total fiber and soluble and insoluble fractions have been independently analyzed in some enteral formulas, or they may be available from the manufacturer.[44]

Chapter 13 includes a more complete discussion of dietary fiber and its effects on gastrointestinal physiology and stool consistency. Fiber-free enteral formulas tend to slow gastrointestinal transit, decrease total stool output, and decrease water content of the stool compared with a typical oral diet. Healthy subjects changed from their self-selected diets to fiber-free enteral formulas experienced a significant increase in transit time and a decrease in wet stool weight. The addition of oat fiber, soy polysaccharide, or soy oligosaccharide to the enteral formula had little influence on transit time and stool weight.[45] Another study showed shortened transit time with a soy polysaccharide fiber compared with fiber-free formula.[46] Addition of soy polysaccharide to enteral feeding resulted in increased stool water content, dry weight, and frequency in a year-long study of profoundly disabled youth.[47] The effects of fiber on bowel function in hospitalized patients have been more difficult to quantify because the research is complicated by the different definitions of diarrhea used in various studies and the difficulty of collecting data. Most studies do not show improvements in bowel function in patients who are receiving antibiotics.[48-52]

Short-chain fatty acids (SCFAs) from the fermentation of dietary fiber by colonic bacteria provide energy to colonocytes and other cells. This may be especially important to people with short bowel syndrome but a preserved colon.[53] The potential energy value of fermentable fiber varies by the degree of fermentation, but it is estimated that the average available energy is about 2 kcal/g dietary fiber. In typical Western diets this may contribute up to 12% of total energy intake.[54] SCFAs also stimulate mucosal blood flow and cell proliferation and enhance water and electrolyte absorption.[55]

Fructooligosaccharides (FOS) are forms of dietary fiber that occur naturally or can be produced enzymatically from sucrose. Natural FOS occur in plants including onions, chicory, and Jerusalem artichokes. They are fermented to SCFAs, mainly acetate, by intestinal bifidobacteria.[56-58] This has lead to interest in adding FOS to enteral formulas as a "prebiotic" or growth stimulant of desirable bacterial species.

TABLE 15-9
Fiber Source and Amount in Adult Enteral Formulas

Formula	kcal/ml	Fiber Source*	Total Dietary Fiber (TDF) (g/1000 kcal)	Insoluble Fiber (% of TDF)	Soluble Fiber (% of TDF)
Boost with Fiber	1.01	Soy fiber	11.0	79	21
Choice dm Oral	1.01	Soy fiber, acacia, microcrystalline cellulose, carrageenan	11.8	73	27
Choice dm Tube Feeding	1.06	Microcrystalline cellulose, soy fiber, acacia, carrageenan	13.6	77	23
Compleat	1.07	Fruits and vegetables	4.0	74	26
Diabetisource	1.0	Fruits and vegetables	4.3	74	26
Ensure Fiber with FOS	1.06	Oat fiber, fructooligosaccharides, soy fiber	11.2	67	33
Ensure Glucerna OS	0.93	Soy polysaccharide	8.3	NA	NA
Fibersource	1.2	Partially hydrolyzed guar gum	8	75	25
Glucerna	1.0	Soy fiber	14.1	94	6
Glytrol	1.0	Gum arabic, soy polysaccharides, pectin	15	33	67
Impact w/ Fiber	1.0	Soy fiber, partially hydrolyzed guar gum	10	50	50
Isosource 1.5	1.5	Soy fiber, partially hydrolyzed guar gum	5	48	52
Isosource VHN	1.0	Soy fiber, partially hydrolyzed guar gum	10	48	52
Jevity	1.06	Soy fiber	13.6	94	6
Jevity Plus	1.2	Fructooligosaccharides, oat fiber, soy fiber, gum arabic	10	75	25
Novasource Pulmonary	1.5	Soy fiber, partially hydrolyzed guar gum	5	48	52
Nutren 1.0 Fiber	1.0	Soy polysaccharides	14	95	5
ProBalance	1.2	Soy polysaccharides, gum arabic	8	75	25
Promote w/ Fiber	1.0	Oat fiber, soy fiber	14.4	94	6
Protain XL	1.0	Soy fiber	9.1	94	6
Replete with Fiber	1.0	Soy polysaccharides	14	95	5
Resource Diabetic	1.06	Partially hydrolyzed guar gum, soy fiber	12.1	25	75
TwoCal HN	2.0	Fructooligosaccharides	5	0	100
Ultracal	1.06	Microcrystalline cellulose, soy fiber, acacia, carrageenan	13.6	72	28
Ultracal HN Plus	1.2	Microcrystalline cellulose, soy fiber, acacia, carrageenan	8	73	27

*Listed in order of appearance on product labels.

Are there disadvantages to fiber in enteral formulas? Adding fiber to enteral formulas does increase viscosity, which could make them more likely to occlude feeding tubes. There has been some concern that fiber might decrease macronutrient and micronutrient absorption. While soy polysaccharide appears to have no effect on macronutrient absorption,[59] it does increase fecal mineral and nitrogen excretion, although this may not be clinically significant at the current levels of fiber.[60,61] A study of three different nondigestible oligosaccharides showed no effect on calcium and iron absorption.[62]

A few cases of bowel obstruction that may have been associated with the use of fiber-containing enteral formulas have been reported. One group described four patients with burn injuries or toxic epidermal necrolysis who required surgery for bowel obstruction or perforation after early enteral feeding with fiber-supplemented formulas.[63] In patients at risk for bowel obstruction or ischemia, it may be safest to initiate feeding with fiber-free formula.

Micronutrients
Vitamins

Enteral formulas are intended to provide complete nutrition, so most will meet 100% of the recommended daily intakes (RDIs) for vitamins and minerals when the patient receives 1000 to 1600 kcal/day. Notable exceptions are the formulas intended for patients with renal failure, which may contain reduced amounts of fat-soluble vitamins that are not dialyzed and increased amounts of water-soluble vitamins that are lost during dialysis.[64]

Antioxidants

Oxidative stress may be a contributing factor in chronic and degenerative diseases as well as critical illness. Nutrients considered antioxidants include ascorbic acid, vitamin A, vitamin E, carotenes, and selenium. Antioxidants maintain cell membrane integrity by preventing lipid peroxidation. They appear to be necessary for optimal immune function. Patients who have been starved or experienced catabolic illnesses may be depleted of antioxidants, and higher amounts of free radicals may be generated during certain critical illnesses.[65] See Chapter 11 for a more detailed discussion of vitamins and antioxidants.

Enteral products intended for use during critical illness or immunosuppression may be described by the manufacturer as having increased amounts of antioxidants, but the concentrations vary widely and often overlap with concentrations of these nutrients in standard formulas. For example, most standard formulas provide 140 to 250 mg/1000 kcal of ascorbic acid, while products with increased antioxidants have 200 to 700 mg/1000 kcal. Selenium content in standard formulas is 40 to 60 µg/1000 kcal and 45 to 70 µg in specialized formulas. Betacarotene has been added to some standard formulas, but not all high antioxidant formulas. There are few clinical studies of the effectiveness of individual antioxidants or varied combinations in enteral formulas, so it is impossible to determine optimal supplementation.

Minerals

Most formulas will meet major mineral requirements in 1000 to 1500 ml/day; however, the amount of calcium currently in enteral formulas varies from 500 to 1300 mg/1000 kcal. Formulas at the low end of this range may not meet current recommendations for calcium intake, especially in patients with low energy needs, although calcium absorption from a standard fiber-free enteral formula appears to be about 40%,[66] somewhat higher than absorption from a mixed diet (23% to 30%).[67] Most formulas provide adequate trace minerals, although not all contain the ultratrace minerals selenium, chromium, and molybdenum (see Chapter 12).

Other Components
Carnitine

Carnitine is an amine synthesized by the body from lysine and S-adenosylmethionine, but also provided in the diet in animal products. A typical Western diet usually provides 100 to 300 mg/day. Carnitine transfers long-chain fatty acids into mitochondria for β-oxidation. Carnitine also transports other acyl groups and free coenzyme A in a number of reactions.[68] Numerous hereditary and acquired disorders of carnitine metabolism have been described.[69] Acquired carnitine deficiency may be caused by inadequate intake; increased losses, usually through renal failure; or decreased synthesis, seen in hepatic and renal failure and premature infants. Patients may have increased needs during critical illness or hemodialysis.[69] Optimal carnitine intake during these states has not been determined, but many enteral formulas now contain an amount comparable to the usual intake from an oral diet (see Table 15-4).

Nucleotides

Recently, there has been interest in adding nucleosides and nucleotides to enteral formulas (see Chapter 20). A nucleotide consists of a base (adenine, guanine, cyosine, and uracil in ribonucleic acid [RNA] or thymine in deoxyribonucleic acid [DNA]) bonded to a phosphorylated monosaccharide (ribose in RNA or deoxyribose in DNA). A nucleoside contains a base and an unphosphorylated monosaccharide. Nucleotides participate in energy-transfer reactions as high-energy intermediates and coenzymes. They serve as second messengers, enzyme regulators, and precursors of RNA and DNA. In animals, dietary nucleotides appear to be important in maintaining cellular and humoral immunity and supporting intestinal development.[70,71] Nucleotide-containing diets may also alter intestinal flora in favor of bifidobacteria.[72]

Under normal conditions, humans synthesize adequate amounts of nucleotides, mostly in the liver, in a series of reactions requiring folic acid, glutamine, and other amino acids. Exogenous nucleotides may be an important source of nucleosides and bases in rapidly dividing tissues such as the intestinal mucosa and lymphoid tissues. Enterally ingested nucleotides are digested by intestinal enzymes, then absorbed as nucleosides or free bases and monosaccharides.[73] Data on effects of enteral nucleotides in humans are very limited. Although there are positive studies of "immune-enhancing" enteral formulas containing fish oil, antioxidants, arginine, and nucleotides, to my knowledge there are no clinical trials of enteral feeding in which the only variable was addition of nucleotides to the formula.[74,75] Further research is needed to identify the specific benefits of nucleotides. Only a few adult enteral formulas contain nucleotides.

Modular Products

Modular products, or modules, are single nutrients or combinations of several nutrients that can be used to customize commercial formulas or supplement an oral diet. Products are available that provide intact fat, carbohydrate, protein, some amino acids, and micronutrients. Over-the-counter foods such as vegetable oil, corn syrup, and nonfat milk powder may also be used to provide additional energy and protein. Generally, modules are used to alter the macronutrient proportions of existing formulas or add an amino acid or micronutrient for a patient with unusual needs. Although it is possible to design and mix entire formulas customized to meet a patient's specific needs, few institutions find this cost-effective. There may also be an increased risk of bacterial contamination of formulas that are mixed de novo or altered with modules. Care must be taken in measuring modules and calculating nutrients because products vary in energy density and nutrient composition. Detailed information on the composition and use of these products has been published.[76]

Conclusion

The majority of enteral formulations are nutritionally complete mixtures of isolated macronutrients, micronutrients, and water. The caloric density varies from about 1 to 2 kcal/ml, corresponding to water content of about 85% to 70%. Formulas with higher caloric density are generally used for patients who require fluid restriction. Although patients with normal fluid requirements are usually fed formulas with lower caloric density (and high water content), they may require additional fluid to meet their fluid needs. Osmolality of enteral products ranges from 270 mOsm/kg to 700 mOsm/kg, but studies have shown that osmolality has little effect on gastrointestinal tolerance to feeding. Protein in enteral formulas can be in the form of intact protein, small peptides, or amino acids. Specialized products are available for patients with altered amino acid metabolism. These include formulas high in branched-chain amino acids; formulas with added glutamine, arginine, or taurine; and products without nonessential amino acids. Carbohydrate sources include glucose and other monosaccharides, disaccharides, oligosaccharides, and large, naturally occurring polymers such as cornstarch. Fat sources are generally vegetable oils that provide energy and essential fatty acids. Many enteral formulas also contain medium-chain triglycerides that bypass the normal mechanisms for fat absorption and transport. Products with a high proportion of medium-chain triglycerides may be useful for patients with deficiencies of exocrine pancreatic or bile secretion or chylothorax. Finally, most manufacturers offer products supplemented with fiber, which can alter gastrointestinal function and provide precursors for short-chain fatty acids. Choosing the appropriate enteral formulation for a patient should begin with a complete assessment of the patient's nutritional status and requirements, medical condition, and gastrointestinal function. A comparison of this information with the properties of the various formulas available will help identify the product that most closely meets the patient's nutritional needs.

REFERENCES

1. Silkroski M, Allen F, Storm H: Tube feeding audit reveals hidden costs and risks of current practice, *Nutr Clin Prac* 13(6):283-290, 1998.
2. Lipp J, Lord LM, Scholer LH: Fluid management in enteral nutrition, *Nutr Clin Prac* 14(5):232-237, 1999.
3. Gottschlich MM, Warden GD, Michel M, Havens P, Kopcha R, Jenkins M, Alexander JW: Diarrhea in tube-fed burn patients: incidence, etiology, nutritional impact, and prevention, *J Parenter Enteral Nutr* 12(4):338-345, 1988.
4. Keohane PP, Attrill H, Love M, Frost P, Silk DBA: Relation between osmolality of diet and gastrointestinal side effects in enteral nutrition, *Br Med J* 288(6418):678-680, 1984.
5. Zarling EJ, Parmar JR, Mobarhan S, Clapper M: Effect of enteral formula infusion rate, osmolality, and chemical composition upon clinical tolerance and carbohydrate absorption in normal subjects, *J Parenter Enteral Nutr* 10(6):588-590, 1986.
6. Reeds P, Schaafsma, G, Tome D, Young V: Criteria and significance of dietary protein sources in humans: summary of the workshop with recommendations, *J Nutr* 130(7):1874S-1876S, 2000.
7. Harper AE, Yoshimura NN: Protein quality, amino acid balance, utilization, and evaluation of diets containing amino acids as therapeutic agents, *Nutrition* 9(5):460-469, 1993.
8. Zeigler TR, Estivariz CF, Jonas CR, Gu LH, Jones DP, Leader LM: Interactions between nutrients and peptide growth factors in intestinal growth, repair, and function, *J Parenter Enteral Nutr* 23(suppl 6): S174-S183, 1999.
9. Verma S, Brown S, Kirkwood B, Giaffer MH: Polymeric versus elemental diet as primary treatment in active Crohn's disease: a randomized, double-blind trial, *Am J Gastroenterol* 95(3):735-739, 2000.
10. Heimburger DC, Geels WJ, Thiesse KT, Bartolucci AA: Randomized trial of tolerance and efficacy of a small-peptide enteral feeding formula versus a whole-protein formula, *Nutrition* 11(4):360-364, 1995.
11. Heimburger DC, Geels WJ, Bilbrey J, Redden DT, Keeney C: Effects of small-peptide and whole-protein enteral feedings on serum proteins and diarrhea in critically ill patients: a randomized trial, *J Parenter Enteral Nutr* 21(3):162-167, 1997.
12. Mowatt-Larssen CA, Brown RO, Wojtysiak SL, Kudsk K: Comparison of tolerance and nutritional outcome between a peptide and a standard enteral formula in critically ill, hypoalbuminemic patients, *J Parenter Enteral Nutr* 16(1):20-24, 1997.
13. Viall C, Porcelli K, Teran JC, Varma RN, Steffe WP: A double-blind clinical trial comparing the gastrointestinal side effects of two enteral feeding formulas, *J Parenter Enteral Nutr* 14(3):265-269, 1990.
14. Skeie B, Kvetan V, Gil KM, Rothkopf MM, Newsholme EA, Askanazi J: Branch-chain amino acids: their metabolism and clinical utility, *Crit Care Med* 18(5):549-571, 1990.
15. Fabbri A, Magrini N, Bianchi G, Zoli M, Marchesini G: Overview of randomized clinical trials of oral branched-chain amino acid treatment in chronic hepatic encephalopathy, *J Parenter Enteral Nutr* 20(2):159-164, 1996.
16. Suryawan A, Hawes JW, Harris RA, Shimomura Y, Jenkins AE, Hutson SM: A molecular model of human branched-chain amino acid metabolism, *Am J Clin Nutr* 68(1):72-81, 1998.
17. Welbourne T, Claville W, Langford M: An oral glutamine load enhances renal acid secretion and function, *Am J Clin Nutr* 67(4):660-663, 1998.
18. Jensen GL, Miller RH, Talabiska DG, Fish J, Gianferante L: A double-blind, prospective, randomized study of glutamine-enriched compared with standard peptide-based feeding in critically ill patients, *Am J Clin Nutr* 64(4):615-621, 1996.
19. Dickson TMC, Wong RM, Negrin RS, Shizuru JA, Johnston LJ, Hu WW, Blume KG, Stockerl-Goldstein KE: Effect of oral glutamine supplementation during bone marrow transplantation, *J Parenter Enteral Nutr* 24(2):61-66, 2000.
20. Den Hond E, Hiele M, Peeters M, Ghoos Y, Rutgeerts P: Effect of long-term oral glutamine supplements on small intestinal permeability in patients with Crohn's disease, *J Parenter Enteral Nutr* 23(1):7-11, 1999.
21. Swails WS, Bell SJ, Borlase BC, Forse RA, Blackburn GL: Glutamine content of whole proteins: implications for enteral formulas, *Nutr Clin Prac* 7(2):77-80, 1992.
22. Savy GK: Enteral glutamine supplementation: clinical review and practical guidelines, *Nutr Clin Prac* 12(6):259-262, 1997.
23. Kelly E, Morris SM, Billiar TR: Nitric oxide, sepsis, and arginine metabolism, *J Parenter Enteral Nutr* 19(3):234-238, 1995.
24. Clark RH, Feleke G, Din M, Yasmin T, Singh G, Khan FA, Rathmacher JA: Nutritional treatment for acquired immunodeficiency virus-associated wasting using β-hydroxy β methylbutyrate, glutamine, and arginine: a

randomized, double-blind, placebo-controlled study, *J Parenter Enteral Nutr* 24(3):133-139, 2000.

25. Langkamp-Henken B, Herrlinger-Garcia KA, Stechmiller JK, Nickerson-Troy JA, Lewis B, Moffatt L: Arginine supplementation is well tolerated but does not enhance mitogen-induced lymphocyte proliferation in elderly nursing home residents with pressure ulcers, *J Parenter Enteral Nutr* 24(5):280-287, 2000.

26. Stapleton PP, O'Flaherty L, Redmond P, Boucher-Hayes DJ: Host defense—a role for the amino acid taurine? *J Parenter Enteral Nutr* 22(1):42-48, 1998.

27. Milla C, Doherty L, Raatz S, Schwarzenberg SJ, Regelmann W, Moran A: Glycemic response to dietary supplements in cystic fibrosis is dependent on the carbohydrate content of the formula, *J Parenter Enteral Nutr* 20(3):182-186, 1996.

28. Peters AL, Davidson MB: Effects of various enteral feeding products on postprandial blood glucose response in patients with type I diabetes, *J Parenter Enteral Nutr* 16(1):69-74, 1992.

29. Akrabawi SS, Mobarhan S, Stoltz RR, Ferguson PW: Gastric emptying, pulmonary function, gas exchange, and respiratory quotient after feeding a moderate versus high fat enteral formula meal in chronic obstructive pulmonary disease patients, *Nutrition* 12(4):260-265, 1996.

30. Armand M, Pasquier B, Andre M, Borel P, Senft M, Peyrot J, Salducci J, Portugal H, Jaussan V, Lairon D: Digestion and absorption of 2 fat emulsions with different droplet sizes in the human digestive tract, *Am J Clin Nutr* 70(6):1096-1106, 1999.

31. Caughey GE, Mantzioris E, Gibson RA, Cleland LG, James MJ: The effect on human tumor necrosis factor α and interleukin 1β production of diets enriched in n-3 fatty acids from vegetable oil or fish oil, *Am J Clin Nutr* 63(1):116-122, 1996.

32. Hughes DA, Pinder AC, Piper Z, Johnson IT, Lund EK: Fish oil supplementation inhibits the expression of major histocompatibility complex class II molecules and adhesion molecules on human monocytes, *Am J Clin Nutr* 63(2):267-272, 1996.

33. Wu D, Meydani SN, Meydani M, Hayek MG, Huth P, Nicolosi RJ: Immunologic effects of marine- and plant-derived n-3 polyunsaturated fatty acids in nonhuman primates, *Am J Clin Nutr* 63(2):273-280, 1996.

34. Peck LW, Monsen ER, Ahmad S: Effect of three sources of long-chain fatty acids on the plasma fatty acid profile, plasma prostaglandin E_2 concentrations, and pruritus symptoms in hemodialysis patients, *Am J Clin Nutr* 64(2):210-214, 1996.

35. Adams S, Yeh Y, Jensen GL: Changes in plasma and erythrocyte fatty acids in patients fed enteral formulas containing different fats, *J Parenter Enteral Nutr* 17(1):30-34, 1993.

36. Palombo JD, DeMichele SJ, Lydon EE, Gregory TJ, Banks PL, Forse RA, Bistrian BR: Rapid modulation of lung and liver macrophage phospholipid fatty acids in endotoxemic rats by continuous enteral feeding with n-3 and gamma-linolenic fatty acids, *Am J Clin Nutr* 63(2):208-219, 1996.

37. Prisco D, Filippini M, Francalanci I, Paniccia R, Gensini GF, Abbate R, Serneri GGN: Effect on n-3 polyunsaturated fatty acid intake on phospholipid fatty acid composition in plasma and erythrocytes, *Am J Clin Nutr* 63(6):925-932, 1996.

38. Swails WS, Kenler AS, Driscoll DF, DeMichele SJ, Babineau TJ, Utsunamiya T, Chavali S, Forse RA, Bistrian BR: Effect of a fish oil structured lipid-based diet on prostaglandin release from mononuclear cells in cancer patients after surgery, *J Parenter Enteral Nutr* 21(5):266-274, 1997.

39. Schaefer EJ: Effects of dietary fatty acids on lipoproteins and cardiovascular disease risk: summary, *Am J Clin Nutr* 65(5 suppl):1655S-1666S, 1997.

40. Grimsgaard S, Bonaa KH, Hansen J, Myhre ESP: Effects of highly purified eicosapentaenoic acid and docosahexaenoic acid on hemodynamics in humans, *Am J Clin Nutr* 68(1):52-59, 1998.

41. Ledeboer M, Masclee AAM, Biemond I, Lamers CBHW: Effect of intragastric or intraduodenal administration of a polymeric diet on gallbladder motility, small-bowel transit time, and hormone release, *Am J Gastroenterol* 93(11):2089-2096, 1998.

42. Hyltander A, Sandstrom R, Lundholm K: Metabolic effects of structured triglycerides in humans, *Nutr Clin Prac* 10(3):91-97, 1995.

43. Palacio JC, Rombeau JL: Dietary fiber: a brief review and potential application to enteral nutrition, *Nutr Clin Prac* 5(3):99-106, 1990.

44. Fredstrom SB, Baglien KS, Lampe JW, Slavin JL: Determination of the fiber content of enteral feedings, *J Parenter Enteral Nutr* 15(4):450-453, 1991.

45. Kapadia SA, Raimundo AH, Grimble GK, Aimer P, Silk DBA: Influence of three different fiber-supplemented enteral diets on bowel function and short-chain fatty acid production, *J Parenter Enteral Nutr* 19(1):63-68, 1995.

46. Slavin JL, Nelson NL, McNamara EA, Cashmere K: Bowel function of healthy men consuming liquid diets with and without dietary fiber, *J Parenter Enteral Nutr* 9(3):317-321, 1985.

47. Liebl BH, Fischer MH, Van Calcar SC, Marlett JA: Dietary fiber and long-term large bowel response in enterally nourished nonambulatory profoundly retarded youth, *J Parenter Enteral Nutr* 14(4):371-375, 1990.

48. de Kruif JTCM, Vos A: The influence of soyfibre supplemented tube feeding on the occurrence of diarrhoea in postoperative patients, *Clin Nutr* 12(6):360-364, 1993.

49. Dobb GJ, Towler SC: Diarrhoea during enteral feeding in the critically ill: a comparison of feeds with and without fibre, *Intensive Care Med* 16(4):252-255, 1990.

50. Frankenfield DC, Beyer PL: Soy-polysaccharide fiber: effect on diarrhea in tube-fed head-injured patients, *Am J Clin Nutr* 50(3):533-538, 1989.

51. Guenter PA, Settle RG, Perlmutter S, Marino PL, DeSimone GA, Rolandelli RH: Tube feeding-related diarrhea in acutely ill patients, *J Parenter Enteral Nutr* 15(3):277-280, 1991.

52. Homann HH, Kemen M, Fuessenich C, Senkal M, Zumtobel V: Reduction in diarrhea incidence by soluble fiber in patients receiving total or supplemental enteral nutrition, *J Parenter Enteral Nutr* 18(6):486-490, 1994.

53. Nordgaard I, Hansen BS, Mortensen PB: Importance of colonic support for energy absorption as small-bowel failure proceeds, *Am J Clin Nutr* 64(2):222-231, 1996.

54. Behall KM, Howe JC: Contribution of fiber and resistant starch to metabolizable energy, *Am J Clin Nutr* 62(5 suppl):1158S-1160S, 1995.

55. Scheppach W: Effects of short chain fatty acids on gut morphology and function, *Gut 35* (1 suppl):S35-S38, 1994.

56. Bouhnik Y, Vahedi K, Achour L, Attar A, Salfati J, Pochart P, Marteau P, Flourie B, Bornet F, Rambaud J: Short-chain fructo-oligosaccharide administration dose-dependently increases fecal bifidobacteria in healthy humans, *J Nutr* 129(1):113-116, 1999.

57. Menne E, Guggenbuhl N, Roberfroid M: Fn-type chicory inulin hydrolysate has a prebiotic effect in humans, *J Nutr* 130(5):1197-1199, 2000.

58. Molis C, Flourie B, Ouarne F, Gailing MF, Lartigue S, Guibert A, Bornet F, Galmiche JP: Digestion, excretion, and energy value of fructooligosaccharides in healthy humans, *Am J Clin Nutr* 64(3):324-328, 1996.

59. Ehrlein, H, Stockmann A: Intestinal absorption of nutrients is not influenced by soy fiber and does not differ between oligomeric and polymeric enteral diets, *Dig Dis Sci* 43(9):2099-2110, 1998.

60. Heymsfield SB, Roongspisuthipong C, Evert M, Casper K, Heller P, Akrabawi SS: Fiber supplementation of enteral formulas: effects on the bioavailability of major nutrients and gastrointestinal tolerance, *J Parenter Enteral Nutr* 12(3):265-273, 1988.

61. Taper LJ, Milam RS, McCallister MS, Bowen PE, Thye FW: Mineral retention in young men consuming soy-fiber-augmented liquid-formula diets, *Am J Clin Nutr* 48(2):305-311, 1988.

62. van den Heuvel EGHM, Schaafsma G, Muys T, van Dokkum W: Nondigestible oligosaccharides do not interfere with calcium and nonheme-iron absorption in young, healthy men, *Am J Clin Nutr* 67(3):445-451, 1998.

63. Scaife CL, Saffle JR, Morris SE: Intestinal obstruction secondary to enteral feedings in burn trauma patients, *J Trauma* 47(5):859-863, 1999.

64. Makoff R, Gonick H: Renal failure and the concomitant derangement of micronutrient metabolism, *Nutr Clin Prac* 14(5):238-246, 1999.

65. Sardesai VM: Role of antioxidants in health maintenance, *Nutr Clin Prac* 10(1):19-25, 1995.

66. van Dokkum W, De La Gueronniere V, Schaafsma G, Bouley C, Luten J, Latge C: Bioavailability of calcium of fresh cheeses, enteral food and mineral water. A study with stable calcium isotopes in young adult women, *Br J Nutr* 75(6):893-903, 1996.

67. Mahan LK, Escott-Stump S (eds): *Food, nutrition, & diet therapy,* Philadelphia, 1996, WB Saunders, pp 125-126.

68. Boehm KA, Helms RA, Christensen ML, Storm MC: Carnitine: a review for the pharmacy clinician, *Hospital Pharmacy* 28(9):843-850, 1993.

69. Pons R, De Vivo DC: Primary and secondary carnitine deficiency syndromes, *J Child Neurol* 10(S):2S8-2S24, 1995.

70. Bustamante SA, Sanches N, Crosier J, Miranda D, Colombo G, Miller MJS: Dietary nucleotides: effects on the gastrointestinal system in swine, *J Nutr* 124(1 suppl):149S-156S, 1994.

71. Carver JD: Dietary nucleotides: cellular immunity, intestinal and hepatic system effects, *J Nutr* 124(1 suppl):144S-148S, 1994.

72. Uauy R: Nonimmune system responses to dietary nucleotides, *J Nutr* 124 (1 suppl):157S-159S, 1994.

73. Rudolph FB: The biochemistry and physiology of nucleotides, *J Nutr* 124 (1 suppl):124S-127S, 1994.

74. Beale RJ, Bryg DJ, Bihari DJ: Immunonutrition in the critically ill: a systematic review of clinical outcome, *Crit Care Med* 27(12):2799-2805, 1999.

75. Zaloga GP: Immune-enhancing enteral diets: Where's the beef? *Crit Care Med* 26(7):1143-1146, 1998.

76. Davis A, Baker S: The use of modular nutrients in pediatrics, *J Parenter Enteral Nutr* 20(3):228-236, 1996.

Enteral Equipment 16

Lucinda K. Lysen, RD, LD, RN, BSN

Historical Perspective

Tube feeding is often perceived as a development of modern nutritional medicine, but nutrients have been delivered by tubes or catheters for many centuries. The ancient Egyptians used nutrient enemas to coat inflamed intestines and provide nutrients.[1] One of the earliest known records of tube feeding dates back to 1617, when Aquapendente, a monk, used a tube made of silver for nasogastric feeding.[2] Tubes of silver, leather, or rubber were used in the seventeenth, eighteenth, and nineteenth centuries, and it is documented that in 1882 it took four strong men to insert a feeding tube into an uncooperative patient.[3]

Nasogastric feeding tubes did not appear in the American literature until 1879.[4] Use of soft rubber tubes for gavage feeding of pediatric patients was first described in the late 1800s.[5] The Levin tube of 1921, which is still in use (although it is thick and uncomfortable), led in the 1950s to development of polyethylene tubes.[6-8] Many changes have occurred since then in developing feeding tubes that are more easily inserted, more comfortable, and have various other feature and equipment improvements.

Equipment Selection

Many factors must be considered when selecting an enteral feeding delivery system (Box 16-1). Enteral feeding equipment—tubes, containers, administration systems, and pumps—must be selected on an individual basis. Many manufacturers of feeding tubes provide these enteral access and delivery devices for a total enteral delivery system.[9]

Tube feedings can be delivered into almost any access site in the proximal gastrointestinal (GI) tract. Selecting the access site is determined by the status of the GI tract, the risk of aspiration (e.g., in a patient with diminished mental status or lower esophageal reflux), the expected duration of tube feeding, and whether surgical feeding tube placement is an option.

Feeding Routes

The commonly used routes for enteral feeding of pediatric and adult patients include nasogastric, nasoduodenal, nasojejunal, gastrostomy, gastrojejunostomy, and jejunostomy tubes.

Acknowledgment: A special thank you is extended to Patricia Queen Samour, MMSc, RD, who contributed to the first edition chapter.

BOX 16-1
Factors in Enteral Feeding

Enteral access route
Rate of feeding
Volume of feeding
Stability of patient (critical or noncritical illness)
Gastric emptying rate
GI tolerance of tube feeding
Age of patient
Type of formula
Calorie and protein needs
Ease of administration
Patient cooperation and mobility

Cervical pharyngostomy tube feedings are not often used today, owing to the vascularity of this area and the risk of hemorrhage. The indications for enteral feeding and advantages and disadvantages of various feeding routes are shown in Table 16-1.

Nasogastric feeding is often indicated when tube feeding is expected to be used on a short-term basis—generally for less than 4 weeks—or for the patient who requires only supplemental nocturnal feedings. Orogastric intubation is used in premature infants because a nasogastric tube would occlude the airway of these obligate nose breathers.[10] Both are also used in adults in the intensive care unit for gastric decompression or when nasal intubation is not desirable, as in patients with maxillofacial trauma. Generally the nasogastric or orogastric routes can be used for bolus or continuous feeding. They do require a functional GI tract and an unobstructed passage from the oral or nasal cavity to the stomach. The use of nasogastric and orogastric tubes is discouraged in the presence of vomiting or gastroesophageal reflux.

Gastrostomy tubes are usually indicated for long-term use. They can be used in the presence of impaired swallowing or esophageal obstruction if the stomach and small bowel are functional. Nasojejunal tubes should be considered for patients with slow gastric emptying (e.g., premature infants) or short-term feeding in those persons or patients with an obstruction above the jejunum. For long-term use, a jejunostomy may be warranted and is associated with reduced risk of aspiration and of aspiration pneumonia. Continuous infusion feedings are usually recommended; bolus feedings often result in diarrhea and feeding intolerance because the jejunum has no reservoir capacity.

201

TABLE 16-1

Enteral Feeding Routes: Indications, Advantages, Disadvantages

Feeding Route	Indications	Advantages	Disadvantages
Nasogastric (NG) Nasoduodenal (ND)	Requires functioning gut and gag reflex Useful when aspiration, reflux, gastroparesis present	Reservoir capacity permits bolus feeding Reduces aspiration risk	Risk of pulmonary aspiration May require fluoroscopic tube placement (spontaneous with weighted tubes) May require continuous infusion technique Not appropriate for long-term feedings
Nasojejunal (NJ)	Useful when aspiration, reflux, gastroparesis present	Allow earlier postoperative or posttrauma feeding Reduces aspiration risk	May require fluoroscopic tube placement (spontaneous with weighted tubes) May require continuous infusion technique Not appropriate for long-term feedings
Gastrostomy (GT)	Recommended for long-term feeding Requires functioning stomach and gag reflex	Percutaneous endoscopic gastrostomy (PEG) requires no surgery Reservoir capacity permits bolus feeding	Risk of pulmonary aspiration Stoma care necessary
Jejunostomy (JT)	Recommended for long-term feeding Useful when access to or functioning of stomach is impaired, if patient is high risk for aspiration, or if patient has had intestinal surgery above the jejunum	Percutaneous endoscopic jejunostomy (PEJ) requires no surgery Allows earlier postoperative or posttrauma feeding	Stoma care necessary May require continuous infusion

Adapted from Ideno KT: Enteral nutrition. In Gottschlich MM, Matarese LE, Shronts EP (eds): *Nutrition support dietetics core curriculum*, ed 2, Silver Spring, MD, 1995, ASPEN, p 84.

Feeding Tube Characteristics

The past 20 years have seen major improvements in enteral feeding tubes, particularly in the size and materials of which they are made.[11] The newer feeding tubes are smaller, softer, and more pliable, and so pose less risk of oropharyngeal and esophageal irritation.[12] In the elderly population, small-bore (No. 10 French or smaller), pliable (e.g., silicone or polyurethane) feeding tubes are desirable because of the increased fragility of the GI mucosa. [13-16]

Considerations in selecting a feeding tube include tube material and length, diameter (lumen), ports, weights, feeding guides or stylets, and tips (Box 16-2). In selecting a feeding tube for a pediatric patient, consideration should be given to the patient's age and size, the viscosity of the formula, and whether an infusion pump will be used (Box 16-3). Many feeding tubes are available in today's marketplace (Table 16-2).

Length

Tubes are available in various lengths for pediatric patients (Table 16-3) and adults and to allow passage into the duodenum or jejunum. Transnasal tubes for adults are available for gastric (36 inches) or intestinal (up to 60 inches or 132 cm) feeding.

BOX 16-2

Important Considerations in Tube Selection

MATERIAL
Largest flow lumen per outer diameter
Ease of insertion (mechanical and comfort)
Resistance to kinking
Ability to aspirate residuals
Comfort and lack of irritation to tissues
Durability

WEIGHTS
Weighted versus nonweighted
Tungsten versus silicone weights

TIP SIZE AND SHAPE
Bolus versus smooth
Water-activated lubricant coating

EYELETS
Location in tip

Size, shape, and number

TUBE LENGTH
Pediatric versus adult
Gastric versus small bowel

STYLETS
Steel wire versus plastic
Ease of removal
Potential for replacement
Internal versus external
No stylet

TUBE PATENCY

ADMINISTRATION SET CONNECTORS
Side port for medication and flush

COST

BOX 16-3

Desirable Features of a Pediatric Nasogastric Tube

1. Made of silastic or polyurethane
2. Available in small diameters (No. 10 F or smaller)
3. Available in variety of lengths with markings to facilitate measuring depth of tube insertion
4. Weighted tip to prevent dislodgment
5. Smooth bolus to facilitate easy insertion and removal
6. Stylet that remains in place during insertion, is prelubricated for easy removal, and is flow-through to determine proper tube placement with stylet still in place
7. Radiopaque for placement verification
8. Compatible with administration sets and with feeding containers in a variety of sizes to accommodate use in neonates and older children

From Cooning SW: Unique aspects in pediatric care. In Lang CE (ed): *Nutrition support in critical care*, Gaithersburg, MD, Aspen Publishers, Inc., copyright 1987, p 399.

TABLE 16-2

Nasoenteral Feeding Tubes

Manufacturer	Product	Material	Weight (g)	Eyelet Placement	Length (in)	French Size	Features
Cook Company	Frederick Miller Tube (nasoduodenal)	Polyvinyl chloride	0.1	Side	45	8	Uses guideware for fluoroscopic placement
Corpak MedSystems	Corflo-Ultra (nasogastric)	Polyurethane	Tungsten 1, 1.5 3 7	Tip	22 36 36 43	6* 6*, 8* 6†, 8†, 10†, 12† 8†, 10†, 12†	Hydrophilic lubricant on internal and external lumen
							1-g and 1.5-g weights available for pediatric patients (Ultra)
							Available in traditional pill shape or a smooth bolus designed to prevent clogs
	Corflo-Ultra Lite (nasogastric)		Unweighted	Tip	22 36 43	5†, 6†, 8† 5*, 6‡, 8‡, 10†,12* 8‡, 10†, 12‡	Color-coded flow-thru stylet
							Braided design reduces stylet removal friction
							Outflow through exit port has anti-clog bolus (Ultra)
	Corflo Controller (nasogastric)	Polyurethane	Tungsten 3 7	Tip	43 43 55	8†, 10† 8†, 10†, 12† 10†	Stiff stylet for ease of manipulation under fluoroscopy (Controller)
							Y-access port
Radius International, LP	Radius Tube (nasoduodenal)	Polyurethane	Unweighted	Side	45	5*, 6*, 8*, 10*, 12*	Exit port larger than comparable tubes to prevent clogging
							Lubricant
							One piece Y set connector
Ross Products Division, Abbott Laboratories	Ross Nasoenteric Tubes (nasogastric, nasoduodenal, nasojejunal)	Polyurethane	Tungsten 3	Side, end	36 45 60	8†, 12*, 14*, 16* 8*, 8†, 10†, 12† 10*	Patented interlock between tube and adapter to minimize separation and leakage
							Patented weighted, open-end bolus with 1-2 side ports
							Flow-thru stylet with water-activated lubricant designed to ease placement
							Uses guidewire for fluoroscopic placement
							Y-access port
							Radiopaque
Novartis	Compat (nasogastric)	Polyurethane	Tungsten 4 Unweighted	Side, tip	42 42	8†, 10†, 12†, 14* 12*, 14*	Stretch-Lok Strap on the Y-adapter locks feeding set in place
							Prelubricated stylet (Stayput)
							Patented suture string attached to bolus tip facilitates endoscopic manipulation (Stayput)
	Stayput (nasojejunal)	Polyurethane	Unweighted	Side, tip	55	9†	Long length decreases risk of nasal irritation (Stayput)
							Y-access port
							Radiopaque
Kendall	Dobhoff (nasogastric)	Polyurethane	Tungsten 3,5 5 3, 5	Side, tip	43 55 43 43	8‡ 8‡ 12‡ 10	Hydrophilic lubricant on inside and tip of lumen
							With and without Y-access port (Pedi-Tube)
	Entriflex (nasogastric)	Polyurethane	7 7 7 5	Side, tip	55 43 43 43	8‡ 8‡ 10‡, 12‡ 8‡	For endoscopic placement (Endo-Tube)
							Radiopaque
	Kangaroo (nasoduodenal)	Polyurethane	Unweighted	Side, end	36	8‡, 10‡, 12‡, 14‡	
	Endo-tube (nasojejunal)	Polyurethane	Tungsten 7	Side, end	60	12‡	
	Pedi-Tube (nasogastric)	Polyurethane	1.5	Side	20, 36	6‡	

TABLE 16-2
Nasoenteral Feeding Tubes—cont'd

Manufacturer	Product	Material	Weight (g)	Eyelet Placement	Length (in)	French Size	Features
ZEVEX Incorporated	EnteraFlo (Dual Port: nasogastric, duodenal, jejunal)	Polyurethane	Unweighted	Side	22 36 36 45 36 45 36 45	6† 6† 8† 8† 10† 10† 12* 12†	Exit port larger than comparable tubes to prevent clogging Available in wide range of sizes for pediatric and adult patients Tubes may be used for NG, ND, or NJ feedings One piece Y set connector Flow-thru stylet Lubricant Radiopaque

Product information verified by manufacturers in October, 1996. Data compiled by Michele Gottschlich, PhD, RD; Cindy Lysen, RD, RN; and Theresa Mayes, RD.
* Stylet free.
† Stylet.
‡ Available with or without stylet.

Diameter

The diameter of the outer lumen, known as "outer diameter" or OD, is designated by French (F) units; No. 1 F is 0.33 mm. The selection of tube lumen depends on the type of formula and tube-feeding delivery system. The smaller diameters No. 5 to 8 F usually can be used for commercially prepared formulas. Different tubes of a given French size can have different internal diameters (ID) (Table 16-4). The larger the ID is, the less chance of tube clogging because the ID of the tubing directly affects formula flow. Silicone tubes have a thicker wall than polyurethane tubes for any given French size and thus have a smaller ID.

A tube lumen size of No. 8 F or larger is usually suggested for formulas containing fiber and for other very viscous formulas administered by infusion pump. A tube lumen of 10 F or larger may be needed for fiber formulas or very viscous ones administered by gravity or bolus methods.

For patient comfort, the smallest tube diameter through which a formula will flow should be used. A small-bore, nasoenteric tube (No. 8 to 12 F) is usually tolerated well by adults. Typical enterostomy tube lumens are larger than 12 F for gastrostomy tubes, are 6 F for jejunostomy tubes, and smaller than 8 F for needle catheter jejunostomy tubes.

Material

Selection of nasoenteric tube material is based on patient comfort and tube performance (Table 16-5).[11-14] Historically, feeding tubes were made from rubber, latex, or polyvinyl chloride. These tubes were very stiff and uncomfortable. Exposure to gastric acid causes polyvinyl chloride to become stiffer and brittle and thus is not recommended for tube feedings. Tubes today are likely to be made from polyurethane or silicone. Although silicone is softer and more comfortable, it is difficult to aspirate gastric contents because the walls of the tube can collapse. Polyurethane is much stronger and such tubes have larger lumens, so polyurethane is the preferred material in most cases.

TABLE 16-3
Nasoenteric Pediatric Tube Selection Guide

	Tube Length (in)	
Age (yr)	Nasogastric	Transpyloric
<1	22	22-36
1-18	36	36-43
	Tube Diameter (French No.)	
Formula Categories	Gravity	Pump
Infant formula	5-8	5-6
Blenderized	12-18	8-10
Milk-based	8-10	6-8
Lactose-free	8	6-8
Fiber-enriched	10	6-8
Elemental	6	6
High-density	8-10	6-10

Adapted from Del Rio D, Williams K, Esvelt B: *Handbook of enteral nutrition: A practical guide to tube feeding*, Medical Specifics Publishing, copyright 1982, p 71.

TABLE 16-4
Inner and Outer Feeding Tube Diameters

Material	PVC	PU	PVC	PU	PVC	PU	S	PU	PVC	PU	S	PVC
French size	5	5	6	6	8	8	9.6	10	12	12	14	14
ID (mm)	0.96	1.10	1.10	1.37	1.55	2.03	1.98	2.61	2.51	2.71	2.64	3.12
OD (mm)	1.65	1.65	2.10	2.10	2.67	2.79	3.18	3.30	4.01	4.06	4.88	4.62
Internal area (mm²)	0.72	0.95	0.95	1.47	1.89	2.98	3.08	5.30	4.95	5.77	5.46	7.64

PVC, Polyvinylchloride; *PU*, polyurethane; *S*, silicone; *ID*, inner diameter; *OD*, outer diameter.

TABLE 16-5

Comparison of Nasoenteric Feeding Tube Materials

Characteristic	Rubber and Polyvinyl Chloride Tubes	Silicone and Polyurethane Tubes
MATERIAL AND EFFECT ON:		
Pliability	(−) Limited	(+) Enhanced
Flexibility	(−) Limited	(+) Enhanced
Comfort	(−) Decreased	(+) Increased
Oropharynx	(−) Increased irritation	(+) Decreased irritation
Esophagus	(−) Increased irritation	(+) Decreased irritation
Life span or integrity of tube	(−) Decreased after exposure to digestive secretions	(+) Not affected by exposure to digestive secretions
Ease of insertion	(+) Stiff for easy insertion	(−) May require stylet for easier insertion
TUBE BORE SIZE AND EFFECT ON:	(−) Larger bore size	(+) Smaller bore size
Pulmonary aspiration	(−) Increased risk	(+) Decreased risk
Lower esophageal sphincter	(−) Increased risk of compromise	(+) Decreased risk of compromise
Tube occlusion	(+) Decreased risk	(−) Increased risk
Ability to swallow	(−) Hindered	(+) Unhindered
Ability to check gastric residuals	(+) Tube does not collapse with external suction	(−) Tube may collapse with external suction

(−), Disadvantage; (+), advantage.
Ideno KT: Enteral nutrition. *In* Gottschlich MM, Matarese LE, Shronts EP (eds): *Nutrition support dietetics core curriculum,* Silver Spring, MD, ASPEN, 1993, p 87.

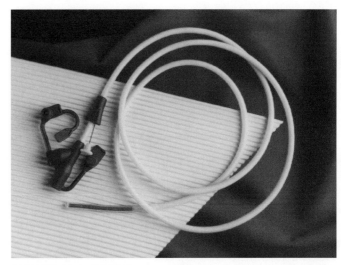

FIGURE 16-1 Kendall Kangaroo polyurethane feeding tube with tungsten segments. (Courtesy of Tyco Healthcare/Kendall.)

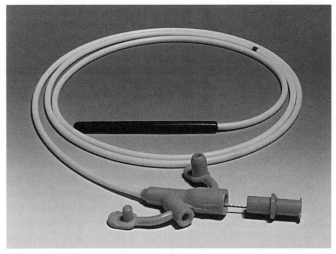

FIGURE 16-2 Ross nasoenteric feeding tube. Tungsten-weighted bolus. Open-end feeding port and at least one side port for good fluid flow, Y-connector site. Graduated length reference markings aid in intubation. (Photo used with permission of Ross Products Division, Abbott Laboratories, Columbus, OH.)

Gastrostomy tube material may consist of silicone, polyurethane, rubber, or latex; and a Foley catheter may be used for a Stamm, Witzel, or Janeway gastrostomy. Jejunostomy tube (J-tube) catheter material may be rubber, latex, silicone, polyvinyl, silicone rubber, or polyethylene.[13-17]

Weights

In theory, a weighted feeding tube facilitates transpyloric passage and holds the tube in position. Studies indicate, however, that unweighted feeding tubes are as effective as weighted ones at maintaining feeding tube placement.[18] Consequently, a large selection of both weighted and nonweighted tubes is available. Weights at the distal end of tubes consist predominantly of inert tungsten, usually in 3-, 5-, or 7-g amounts (Figs. 16-1 and 16-2). Weights are available as pellets or cylinders, in slices or segments, or as powder. Less frequently used materials include stainless steel and silicone.

Other reported methods of promoting transpyloric feeding tube passage include the use of a magnet-tipped feeding tube that is dragged into proper position using an external magnet.[19] In a recent study, a small balloon located at the tip of a nasojejunal tube improved transpyloric migration and spontaneous small bowel positioning.[20]

Stylets

Stylets can be used to facilitate placement of soft, flexible feeding tubes. Wire stylets or guidewires are stiff and straight and provide good insertion and duodenal placement under fluoroscopic guidance. Most stylets are of uncoated stainless steel and are preinserted into the feeding tube to prevent inadvertent puncture or weakening of the tube wall. Guidewires should not be reinserted into the feeding tube in situ owing to the risk of esophageal perforation. Blunt loop and spring tips have been designed to further decrease the risk of tube puncture. Some stylets also come color-coded to match tube connectors. Most feeding tubes are designed so that the stylet cannot accidentally exit a feeding port and perforate surrounding tissue during tube placement. Most stylets are characterized as *flow-through,* meaning that a hole in the adapter at the proximal end allows for attachment of a syringe or for aspiration of stomach contents or checking placement by injecting air for abdominal auscultation. Some of the new stylets have a Teflon or water-activated lubricant coating to ease removal.

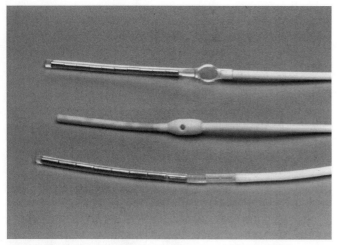

FIGURE 16-3 Three nasoenteral feeding tubes with three different types of exit ports. (Courtesy of Rusch, Inc.)

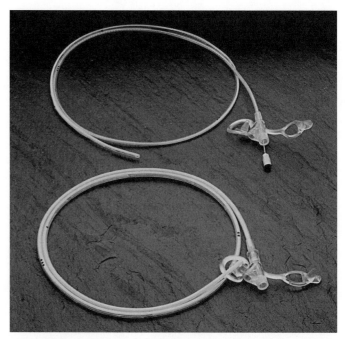

FIGURE 16-4 Nasogastric feeding tubes. Note incremental markings for placement guidance and special Y-port features. (Courtesy of Novartis Nutrition.)

Tips

With increasing use of small-bore feeding tubes, tube clogging has become a significant problem. Several ways to alleviate this problem are regular flushing of the feeding tube and avoiding administering crushed medications through the tube. Tube manufacturers have attempted to redesign certain aspects of feeding tubes to minimize clogging. As a result, tube tips have been modified. Many tubes now have multiple feeding ports or eyelets to help prevent kinking and clogging. Some have "staggered eyelets" a few centimeters from the end of the tube to prevent backflow and clogging. Other tubes have one large "anticlog" exit port, which helps to prevent tube occlusion from formula sediment and medications. Some feeding tubes have an exit port on either side of the tube that allows for uniform flow of formula out of both sides of the tube (Fig. 16-3). Regardless of what tube is used, the practitioner should always evaluate the tube to ensure that the feeding exit port allows unimpeded outflow of formula. Since a case report of tip detachment in recent literature, potential for this problem also has become a consideration in feeding tube selection.[21]

Ports

Some nasoenteral feeding tubes contain an additional port for irrigation and medication administration without disconnecting the feeding administration set tubing. These Y ports can accommodate a feeding set or Luer syringe. Other feeding tube Y ports are "port specific"; that is, the main port accommodates only the feeding set and the side port the syringe (Figs. 16-4 and 16-5). Some gastrostomy tubes have 3 ports: balloon, feeding, and medication ports (Fig. 16-6).

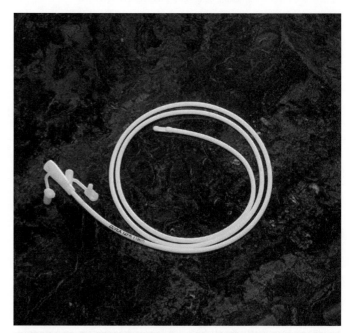

FIGURE 16-5 ZEVEX EnteraFlo nasoenteric feeding tube. Y port facilitates irrigation and medication delivery. (Courtesy of ZEVEX International.)

Nasoenteral Feeding Tube Insertion

The nasoenteral feeding tube is inserted through the nares and via the esophagus, enters the stomach or small intestine, depending on the desired position.[22] Nasoenteral feeding tubes are used most for patients who will require tube feedings for less than a few weeks. Nasogastric feeding tubes are appropriate for alert patients who have an intact gag reflex. Nasoduodenal and nasojejunal feeding tubes are appropriate when the potential for aspiration is great or when functioning of the proximal GI tract is impaired.

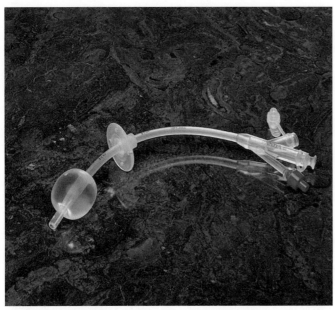

FIGURE 16-6 ZEVEX PANDA tri-funnel gastrostomy tube with three ports—balloon, feeding set, and hydration/medication. Comes in color-coded No. 14 to 24 F sizes. (Courtesy of ZEVEX International.)

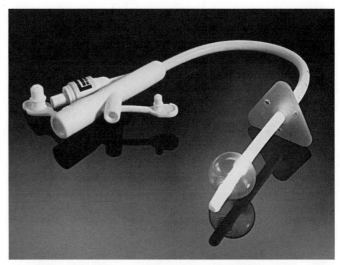

FIGURE 16-7 Ross gastrostomy tube used for replacement or primary gastrostomy. Triangular skin disk maintains correct tube placement after insertion. Open tip minimizes clogging. Y port for flushing. (Photo used with permission of Ross Products Division, Abbott Laboratories, Columbus, OH.)

Most nasoenteral feeding tubes have incremental markers for placement guidance (see Fig. 16-4). They are also radiopaque, for x-ray confirmation of proper placement. Often tubes are made of medical-grade radiopaque polyurethane, which is flesh tinted and can be identified on x-ray images. Markings on the tubes at set intervals facilitate accurate placement and monitoring of tube position.

It is essential that proper feeding tube placement be checked before initiating a feeding. Unfortunately it is relatively easy to inadvertently insert a small-bore feeding tube into a lung, which can result in pneumothorax, aspiration, and death, so every precaution must be taken. Feeding tube position can be verified by auscultation, aspiration, and pH testing, and by x-ray imaging. X-ray confirmation, the one definitive method, should be used when the feeding tube's location is in question.

Surgically and Endoscopically Inserted Feeding Tubes

Surgically inserted feeding tubes include (1) the cervical esophagostomy, (2) gastrostomy, (3) jejunostomy, (4) percutaneous endoscopic gastrostomy (PEG), and (5) percutaneous endoscopic jejunostomy (PEJ).

The cervical pharyngostomy or esophagostomy is made with a stab wound into the esophagus or larynx through which a feeding tube is passed into the esophagus or stomach. This procedure has been used in in postoperative head and neck surgery patients. However, owing largely to the high risk of aspiration, the potential for hemorrhage in this densely vascular area and the possibility of nerve damage associated with this type of tube insertion and maintenance, the use of this technique has decreased.

The gastrostomy is created by a surgical incision into the stomach for long-term feeding; the jejunostomy is created by

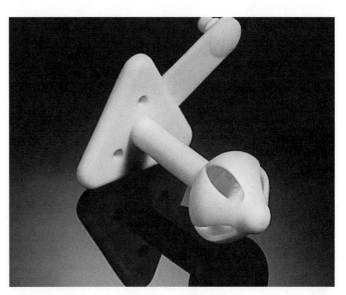

FIGURE 16-8 Ross Stomate low-profile gastrostomy tube for use in patients with an established gastrocutaneous fistula tract from a previously placed gastrostomy tube. (Photo used with permission of Ross Products Division, Abbott Laboratories, Columbus, OH.)

surgical incision into the jejunum. These procedures are usually performed under general anesthesia. Several gastrostomy tubes are commercially available (Figs. 16-7, 16-8).

The gastrostomy and PEG tubes are used principally for long-term feeding of patients who have adequate gut function and are not at risk for aspiration. PEG tubes can also be placed for gastric decompression.

The PEG tube is placed after introducing an endoscope into the stomach. A local anesthetic is administered through the abdominal wall, and a stab wound is created. A catheter is then introduced into the stomach lumen and secured. Low-profile G-tubes (named for their size and configuration; [see Fig. 16-8])

TABLE 16-6

Comparison of Types of Gastrostomies

Type	Description	Features
Janeway	Gastric tube is made and transferred through the abdominal wall to create a permanent stoma	Simple surgical procedure; decreased risk of gastric content leakage
Percutaneous endoscopic (PEG)	Tube inserted percutaneously after endoscopic guidance	Often done with local anesthesia; easy closure after removal of tube (usually within a few hr)
Stamm	Insertion and suturing of a catheter into opening established between the sutured stomach and abdominal wall surface	Simple to perform; easy closure after removal of tube (usually within a few hr)
Witzel	In addition to the Stamm gastrostomy, the tube is sutured in a seromuscular tunnel	Seromuscular tunnel reduces risk of reflux around gastrostomy tube

From Ideno KT: Enteral nutrition. *In* Gottschlich MM, Matarese LE, Shronts EP (eds): *Nutrition support dietetics core curriculum*, ed 2, Silver Spring, MD, 1995, ASPEN, p 86.

and "button" PEG tubes (named for their shape) are now available that are more aesthetically pleasing.

Features of PEG tubes vary, and selection of the appropriate tube takes careful consideration. In a pediatric oncology population studied recently, the level of pain associated with accessing the stoma and ease of tube care were more important issues in the outcome of tube selection than the mechanical complications associated with tube use.[23] Some button PEG tubes now include a rigid tube introducer and stoma-length measuring device, touted to provide easier access/placement, although other PEGS are noted for long-term comfort and aesthetic appeal.[24]

The PEJ tube may be used in postoperative patients with a dysfunctional GI tract or in those who are at high risk for aspiration. With the PEJ, the tubing is advanced through the stomach and into the proximal small intestine. The PEJ is used for patients who have gastroesophageal reflux and are at risk for aspiration. Both procedures are cost-effective because they are performed under local anesthesia. They are commonly used for long-term and home care patients because they can remain in place for extended periods. A gastrostomy with a jejunal extension can also be used for jejunal feeding.[25-26] Comparisons of types of gastrostomies and jejunostomies are shown in Table 16-6.

The needle catheter jejunostomy, smaller in F size, is used postoperatively when a predigested formula is fed. It is often placed during upper abdominal surgery when it is anticipated that the patient will require enteral feedings postoperatively. The needle catheter jejunostomy has been associated with mechanical complications, including kinking and clogging, that require operative replacement.

Securing Nasal Feeding Tubes

A number of nasal tube fasteners for enteral feeding tubes are available to maintain enteral tube position. Instead of using white adhesive tape, many of the nasal tube fasteners have a

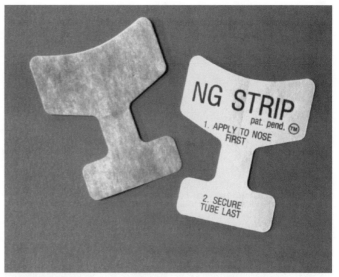

FIGURE 16-9   NG strips to affix feeding tube to bridge of nose.

BOX 16-4

Important Characteristics of Enteral Feeding Containers

Easy to fill, close, and hang
Easy-to-read calibrations and directions
Appropriate size
Adaptable tubing port
Compatible with pump
Easy to clean
Leakproof
Requires minimal storage space
Recyclable

flexible material coated with a hypoallergenic adhesive that minimizes irritation, blistering, and skin shear. This type of material remains securely in place even in the presence of perspiration or phlegm and helps prevent tissue necrosis by avoiding tube pressure on the nose. Fasteners with macropores are advantageous because they increase vapor transmission, resulting in less trapped moisture (Fig. 16-9). Other holding devices are available, such as nasotube clips, modified oxygen nasal cannulas, and rubber tourniquets.[13,27]

Enteral Feeding Containers

A variety of enteral feeding containers that vary in ease of use and cost are on the market today. Some containers are specifically designed as part of a tube feeding "kit;" many are universally compatible. Factors to evaluate in feeding container selection include type of material, volume capacity, entry port location, packaging, and the option of prefilled or ready-to-fill. The characteristics of the ideal enteral feeding container are listed in Box 16-4. Because containers currently available vary considerably, they should be carefully evaluated before they are used. For example, some are difficult and cumbersome to fill. Rigid containers are easier to fill than soft collapsible ones but require more storage space.

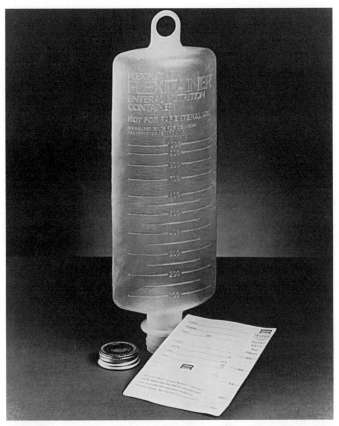

FIGURE 16-10 Flexitainer enteral nutrition container (1000 ml or less) for convenient administration of large-volume enteral feedings. (Photo used with permission of Ross Products Division, Abbott Laboratories, Columbus, OH.)

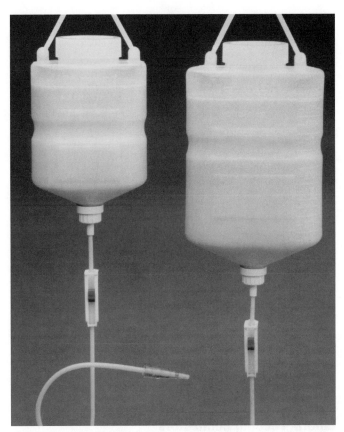

FIGURE 16-11 COMPAT Baggle semirigid container. Comes with a choice of preattached pump sets or gravity sets in two convenient sizes and features an oversized top-fill system with dual hanger rings to allow refilling while hanging. (Courtesy of Novartis Nutrition.)

Feeding containers are usually made from vinyl or polyvinyl chloride and range in capacity from 500 to 2000 ml (Fig. 16-10). Some feeding bags are made of ethyl vinyl acetate, which is stronger than vinyl and does not stretch. The gradations are usually marked in 50- or 500-ml increments. The filling entry is either on top or in front, and mouth size varies. A wide mouth opening is preferred for filling, with less spilling. Large-volume prefilled or "closed-system" containers decrease nursing time required for tube feeding management and may reduce the risk of microbial contamination; however, studies have demonstrated that system hang time and cleanliness of hands while handling the system are potentially influential factors.[28,29] For small-volume feeding, 8-ounce prefilled bottles are useful. Closed-system feeding containers often contain a spike buretral and hanger that slips over an IV pole. This feature eliminates dosing error, may reduce formula contamination, and cuts nursing time. Closed systems do have some clear disadvantages: The formula selection is limited, formula dilutions are impossible, and medication and other additives cannot be added directly to the formula. Regardless of which container is used, strict adherence to a clean technique is essential to reduce the risk of bacterial contamination. Figures 16-10 through 16-13 show some enteral feeding containers on the market.

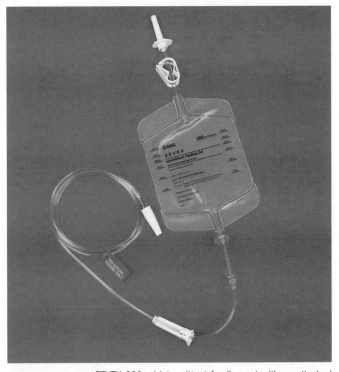

FIGURE 16-12 ZEVEX 300-ml intermittent feeding set with preattached gravity administration set. (Courtesy of ZEVEX International.)

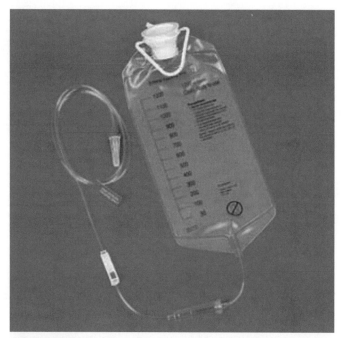

FIGURE 16-13 ZEVEX 1200-ml top-fill container with preattached gravity administration set. (Courtesy of ZEVEX International.)

BOX 16-5

Considerations for Pump Selection

Simple to use
Alarm system
Lightweight
Long battery life
Portable
Quiet
Intravenous pole attachment
Clear instructions on pump use
Easy to read
Volume-infused indicator
Inexpensive
Compact
Easy to clean
Flow rate accurate to within ±10%

Enteral Feeding Connectors

Enteral feeding set connectors are designed for gavage or gravity feeding and for enteral pump use. Often they are not interchangeable or detachable from their feeding bags. Most sets are compatible with a specific pump or several pumps, which increases cost but also improves safety and accuracy of the delivery system and may be essential with J-tube feedings and in other circumstances. Additionally, most distal ends of connectors do not attach to IV needles or Luer connectors, making it impossible to administer enteral formulas intravenously. The "screw cap administration set" is often used with closed-system feedings. Spike sets contain a pin at the proximal end of the set that spikes into the container. A roller clamp regulates formula flow when used for gravity feeding. Some spike sets can be used with pump delivery systems as well.

The Y-extension set is used in addition to Y-port tubes to deliver fluids or medications to the patient without disconnecting the administration set from the feeding tube. The Y port can be used for enteral irrigation or medication administration when indicated.

Gravity Feeding

Gravity feeding is acceptable and should be considered for a medically stable patient when a large volume of enteral feeding formula is necessary, when its viscosity is low, when the internal feeding tube diameter is wide, and when the patient has adequate absorptive capacity to tolerate inconsistent formula flow. Gravity feeding is usually administered over a 20- to 30-minute period intermittently throughout the day. Some feeding delivery sets have roller clamps to control gravity feeding flow rate (see Figs. 16-11 through 16-13).

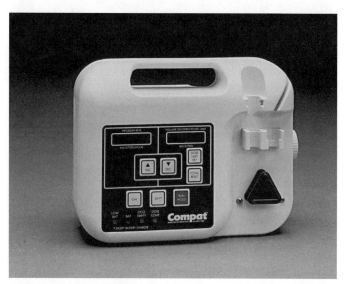

FIGURE 16-14 COMPAT enteral delivery pump. Reliability, ease of use, and special features engineered from the input of nurses make the COMPAT pump an effective device to deliver formula. (Courtesy of Novartis Nutrition.)

Bolus Feeding

Bolus feedings are administered with a syringe or bulb. For an adult patient, 250 to 500 ml per feeding is generally administered at several feedings per day. The ability to absorb nutrients using this type of feeding depends on the access site and functional capability of the gut.

Enteral Feeding Pumps

An infusion pump allows safe, accurate delivery of formulas of varying viscosities. An enteral feeding pump should be considered when a controlled rate of infusion is required for maintenance of formula flow through a small-bore feeding tube, to prevent GI intolerance, to minimize the risk of aspiration by reflux from high residuals or a weakened lower esophageal sphincter, or when feeding into the jejunum.

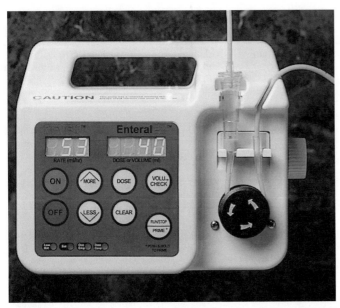

FIGURE 16-15   ZEVEX EnteralEZ enteral feeding pump. (Courtesy of ZEVEX International.)

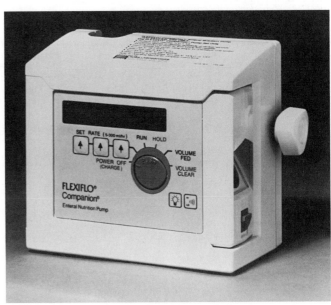

FIGURE 16-16   Ross Companion enteral nutrition pump. For controlled, accurate delivery of enteral feedings. Small, easy-to-use volumetric pump. Also suitable for ambulatory use. (Photo used with permission of Ross Products Division, Abbott Laboratories, Columbus, OH.)

Enteral feeding pumps come with an array of sophisticated features (Box 16-5). The pump should allow for a variety of infusion rates and the ability to advance in small increments, particularly for infants and young children. Most pumps are designed with rate settings from 1- to 500-ml increments and have microprocessors that ensure accuracy rates of ± 5%. Many can be programmed for total intended dose and total volume set. Most pumps have audible alarms and visual displays that indicate occlusion, malfunction, low battery, empty container, or inadvertent rate change (Figs. 16-14 through 16-16). If a patient is ambulatory or home bound, pump weight, size, and portability are important. The pump should be lightweight, compact, and easy to carry (preferably with a handle). It should have long battery life up to 24 hours and a backup current that recharges batteries. It should be easy to read, particularly in a dimly lit room; quiet; and easy to clean.

Some ambulatory pumps have carrying cases that can be worn over the shoulder, holding the pump and formula while it is infused (Table 16-7). Others have special features, including automatic flushing, that prevent tube clogging and decrease nursing time.

Conclusion

Enteral equipment has become increasingly sophisticated over the past 15 years.[30] Ease of administration and improvement in accuracy are among the features that have made enteral feeding delivery systems more user friendly than ever. With the contributions of specialists working together in nutrition support, in and out of the hospital setting, equipment will continue to be modified to improve patient comfort while attempting to achieve precise delivery.

TABLE 16-7
Enteral Infusion Pumps

Manufacturer	Product	Size	Weight (lb)	Accuracy (%)	Flow Rate (ml/hr)	Volume Limits (ml)	Occlusion Pressure (Psi)	Power Source
Ross Laboratories	Flexiflo III	9.7" x 7.0" x 5.5"	7.5	+10	1-300	1-9999	23 (nominal)	Rechargeable battery or AC
	Companion	4.3" x 6.0" x 1.7"	1.5	+10	5-300	N/A	24 (mean)	Rechargeable battery or AC
	Companion Clearstar	4.3" x 6.0" x 1.7"	1.5	+10	1-300	1-9999 in 1-ml increments	25 (nominal)	Rechargeable battery or AC
	Patrol	8.5" x 6.5" x 4.8"	6.6	+10	1-300	1-9999 in 1-ml increments	18 (nominal)	Rechargeable battery or AC
	Quantum	8.25" x 7.5" x 6.0"	7.2	+10	1-300	1-9999	15 (mean)	Rechargeable battery or AC
Novartis	COMPAT Enteral Pump 235 and 240 models	7.4" x 9.5" x 5.3"	5.7	+10	1-295	0-9995 in 5-ml increments	15	Rechargeable battery or AC
Kendall	Kangaroo 224	7.25" x 5.5" x 4.25"	3.5	Not stated	5-300 in 5-ml increments	N/A	12	Rechargeable battery or AC
	Kangaroo 324	7.25" x 5.5" x 4.25"	3.5	Not stated	1-300, or 1-50 in 1-ml increments and 50-300 in 5 ml increments	5-2000	12	Rechargeable battery or AC
	Kangaroo Pet	5.75" x 3.75" x 2.0"	1.4	+10	1-75 in 1-ml increments; 75-400 in 5-ml increments	1-2000	15 (nominal)	Rechargeable battery or AC
	Kangaroo EntriFlush Pump	10.03" x 6.1" x 4.2"	5.2	+10	1-150 in 1-ml increments; 150-2000 in 5-ml increments	1-150 in 1-ml increments; 150-2000 in 5-ml increments	12 (nominal) 15 (maximum)	Rechargeable battery or AC
	Kangaroo Control	6.9" x 4.3" x 5.0"	3.3	+10	1-400 in 1-ml increments	1-3000 in 1-ml increments	12 (nominal) 15 (maximum)	Rechargeable battery or AC
ZEVEX	EnteraLite	5" x 4.5" x 2"	1.3	+5	1-600	1-3000 in 10-ml increments	8 (low), 12 (high)	Rechargeable battery or AC
	EnteralEZ	7.3" x 9" x 5"	5.6	+10	1-295	1-2000 in 1-ml increments; 2005-9999 in 5-ml increments	15	Rechargeable battery or AC
	2200	7.3" x 9" x 5"	5.6	+10	1-295	1-2000 in 1-ml increments; 2005-9999 in 5-ml increments	15	Rechargeable battery or AC

Battery Life (hr)	Recharge Time (hr)	Alarms	Disposables	Additional Comments
8 @ 300 ml/hr	12	Tube occlusion, empty container, open cover, low battery, completed dose	Proprietary set line	Computer controlled with easy-to-use touch controls and clearly visible number display. Displays both the volume fed and selected dose to be fed.
8 @ 150 ml/hr	1.5 for every hr of battery use	Occlusion, empty, select run, reset rate, low battery	Proprietary set line	Cassette is designed to prevent accidental product free flow due to improper set loading. The cassette design helps minimize alarm conditions. Can be worn by an ambulatory patient in a carrying case.
16 @ 125 ml/hr	8	Occlusion, empty, select run, reset rate, low battery, dose complete	Proprietary set line	Cassette is designed to prevent accidental product free flow due to improper set loading. The cassette design helps minimize alarm conditions. Can be worn by an ambulatory patient in a carrying case.
8 @ 125 ml/hr	4.5 while off; 12 if operating	Free flow, no flow, dose fed, low battery, select rate, select run	Proprietary set line	Incorporates a Safe-T-Valve designed to protect against runaway feeding if set is improperly loaded or becomes dislodged. Has a programmable hold for up to 90 minutes. Has a lock-out feature to temporarily disable set rate, set dose, and clear volume dial settings.
8 @ 125 ml/hr	8 while off; 12 if operating	Occlusion, empty, dose complete, turn to run, low battery, door/cassette (not closed), set rate	Proprietary set line	Has automatic set-priming feature, cassette is designed to prevent accidental free flow due to improper loading. Does not utilize a drop sensor to monitor flow. The pump can program a preset dose and has memory retention when turned off, automatic flush feature.
8 @ 100 ml/hr	12	Battery, low battery, occlusion/empty/freeflow, rate change, hold (model 235 only), dose complete, self test	Proprietary set line	Has memory retention of infusion rate, dose limit, volume and accumulated volume; also has a dose limit for intermittent feedings with 3 selectable alarm models.
24 @ 125 ml/hr	15	No set, flow error, low battery, hold error, system error	Proprietary set line	Has a safety feature to safeguard against overinfusion, has touch panel for ease of setup and operation and large easy-to-read LED displays.
24 @ 125 ml/hr	15	No set, flow error, low battery, hold error, system error, dose delivered	Proprietary set line	Has a safety feature to safeguard against overinfusion, has touch panel for ease of setup and operation and large easy-to-read LED displays. Also has the ability to preset the dose to be delivered.
14	8	No set, flow error, low battery, hold error, dose delivered, system error, internal problem	Proprietary set line	Small and lightweight, does not require the use of a special set, memory capable of retaining rate, dose, volume delivered, and interval setting for up to 16 hr after pump has been turned off.
8 @ 125 ml/hr	12	Feed error, flush error, low battery, hold error, no set, system error, dose delivered, internal circuit problem, bad set	Proprietary set line	Has the ability to set the flush interval and has a flush now capability, has an autopriming of the pump set feature and integral valves on the sets to provide anti-free flow protection. Has easy-to-read LED display and a 16 hr memory for all settings once the pump is turned off.
16 @ 125 ml/hr	16	Flow error, low battery, system error, hold error, load set, volume to be delivered	Proprietary set line	Has safety loading arm. Self-priming. Pump has message center for volume delivered, volume remaining, and time remaining.
24 @ 125 ml/hr	5	Dose complete, set improperly, loaded upstream/downstream occlusion, empty set, check, jam, low battery, error, 2 min. timeout	Proprietary set line	Patented disposable set allows for operation in any orientation, set prime button, automatic anti-free flow, interval feed allows automatic repetition of dose delivery, 24-hour service and pump replacement program, machine washable carrying packs.
6 @ 125 ml/hr	12	Battery on, low battery, dose complete, free flow, occlusion, empty set, 2.5 min. timeout	Proprietary set line	Convenient push-button set priming, pump retains memory and settings when turned off, VoluCheck accumulated dose feature, built in carry hand and pole clamp, built in administration cap holder, adjustable alarm control, except free flow alarm.
6 @ 125 ml/hr	12	Battery on, low battery, dose complete, free flow, occlusion, empty set, 2.5 min. timeout	Proprietary set line	Pump has nonvolatile memory, VoluCheck accumulated dose feature, built-in carry hand and pole clamp, built-in administration cap holder, adjustable alarm control.

REFERENCES

1. Bliss DW: Feeding per rectum, *Med Rec* 22:64-67, 1882.
2. Pareira MD, Conrad EJ, Hicks W, Elman R: Therapeutic nutrition with tube feeding, *JAMA* 156:810-816, 1954.
3. Rankin DN: Three cases of nasal alimentation, *Arch Laryngol* 3:355-358, 1882.
4. Gallagher TJ: On the different methods of artificial alimentation, *NY Med J* 30:141-149, 1879.
5. Holt LE: Gavage (forced feeding) in the treatment of acute diseases of infancy, and childhood, *Med Red* 45:542-551, 1894.
6. Levin AL: A new gastroduodenal catheter, *JAMA* 76:1007, 1921.
7. Royce S, Tepper C, Watson W, Day R: Indwelling polyethylene nasogastric tube for feeding premature infants, *Pediatrics* 8:79-81, 1951.
8. Wagner EA, Jones DV, Koch CA, Smith GD: Polyethylene tube feeding in premature infants, *J Pediatr* 41:79-83, 1952.
9. *Clinical and economic evaluation of enteral delivery systems in nutrition support.* Proceedings of the Third Annual Ross Enteral Device Conference, *NCP* 13(3)SI-S60, 1998.
10. Hohenbeink K, Nicol JJ: Pediatrics. In Gottschlich MM, Matarese LE, Shronts EP (eds): *Nutrition support dietetics core curriculum,* ed 2, Silver Spring, MD, 1993, ASPEN, pp 182-183.
11. *Enteral nutrition and device use in alternate care settings.* Proceedings of the Second Annual Ross Medical Nutrition and Device Roundtable, *NCP* 15(6):S1-S80, 2000.
12. Paine JS: Practical aspects of nasogastric feeding in pediatric patients from a ward nursing perspective, *Nutr Supp Serv* 6-11-14, 1986.
13. Forlaw L, Chernoff R, Guenter P: Enteral delivery systems. In Rombeau JL, Caldwell MD (eds): *Enteral and tube feeding,* Philadelphia, 1990, WB Saunders, pp 174-191.
14. Bernard M, Forlaw L: Complications and their prevention. In Rombeau JL, Caldwell MD (eds): *Enteral and tube feeding,* Philadelphia, 1984, WB Saunders, pp 542-569.
15. Silk DBA, Payne-James JJ: Complications of enteral nutrition. In Rombeau JL, Caldwell MD (eds): *Enteral and tube feeding,* Philadelphia, 1990, WB Saunders, pp 510-531.
16. Campbell SM, Geraghty M, Behr S: In Silverman E (ed): *Enteral nutrition handbook,* Columbus, OH, 1991, Ross Laboratories.
17. Rombeau JL, Palacio JC: Feeding by tube enterostomy. In Rombeau JL, Caldwell MD (eds): *Enteral and tube feeding,* Philadelphia, 1990, WB Saunders, pp 230-249.
18. Levenson R, Turner WW, Dyson A, et al: Do weighted feeding tubes facilitate duodenal intubations? *J Parenter Enteral Nutr* 12(2):135-137, 1988.
19. Soivin M, Levy CMH, Hayes J: A multicenter, prospective study of the placement of transpyloric feeding tubes with assistance of a magnetic device, *J Parenter Enteral Nutr* 24(5):304-307, 2000.
20. Cohen LD, Alexander DJ, Catto J, Mannion R: Spontaneous transpyloric migration of a ballooned nasojejunal tube: a randomized controlled trial, *J Parenter Enteral Nutr* 24(4):240-243, 2000.
21. Sood AK, Pardubsky PD, Gacuson M, et al: Nasoenteric tube complication: a case report of tip detachment, *NCP* 13(1):40-42, 1998.
22. Hanson RL: Predictive criteria for length of nasogastric tube insertion for tube feeding, *J Parenter Enteral Nutr* 3(3):160-163, 1979.
23. Ringwald-Smith K, Hale G, Williams R, et al: Comparison of two different low profile gastrostomy enteral feeding devices in pediatric oncology patients, *NCP* 15(4):189-192, 2000.
24. Dormann AR, Wejda B, Huchzemeyer H, Malfertheiner P: Skin-level gastrostomy using a novel balloon-type device: long-term results in oncological patients, *NCP* 16(6):355-358, 2001.
25. Strife JL, Dunbar JS, Rice S: Jejunal intubation via gastrostomy catheters in pediatric patients, *Radiology* 154:249, 1985.
26. Mukkerjee D, Emmens RW, Putham TC: Nonoperative conversion of gastrostomy to feeding jejunostomy in children and adults, *Surg Gynecol Obstet* 154:881, 1982.
27. Meer JA: A new nasal bridle for securing nasoenteral feeding tubes, *J Parenter Enteral Nutr* 13:331-334, 1989.
28. Vanek VW: Closed versus open enteral delivery systems: a quality improvement study, *NCP* 15 (5):234-243, 2000.
29. Storm HM, Skipper A: Closed-system enteral feedings: point-counterpoint, *NCP* 15(4):193-202, 2000.
30. Minard G, Lysen LK: Enteral access devices. In Gottschlich M, Gurman P, et al (eds): *The science and practice of nutrition support: a case-based core curriculum,* ed 1, Silver Spring, MD, 2001, ASPEN, pp 167-188.

Complications of Enteral Nutrition 17

Peter L. Beyer, MS, RD

ENTERAL nutrition is the preferred route for providing nutrition support when the gastrointestinal (GI) tract is functional. Compared with conventional central venous feeding, enteral feeding is associated with fewer serious complications, is more nutritionally complete, is more effective in maintaining or restoring host immune response, and takes advantage of normal physiologic and metabolic processes. In addition, delivery of nutrients by way of the GI tract allows maintenance of physical and immune-mediated barriers; decreases risk of sepsis; reduces the risk of cholestasis; and stimulates dozens of gut peptides, which affect far more than the GI tract.[1-5] The cost of feeding tube placement, administration, equipment, and formula is also considerably less than parenteral nutrition.

Most of the complications associated with enteral feeding are minor, but some can be quite serious. The incidence and severity of complications, however, can be reduced by assessment of the patient's clinical status and nutritional needs, careful placement of the feeding tube, monitoring the feeding process, and proper selection and advancement of the formula. In this chapter, the more common complications of enteral nutrition are discussed along with guidelines for their prevention and treatment. Complications can be categorized in several ways, but we have grouped them under three main headings: (1) problems encountered during the placement of feeding tubes and delivery of enteral formulas (2) clinical and metabolic problems, and (3) nutritional problems.

Complications with Initial Placement of Feeding Tubes

Nasogastric and Nasoenteric Tubes

Complications that can occur during the placement of nasogastric or nasoenteric tubes include nasopharyngeal irritation and pain; misplacement of the tube; and in patients who are confused or upset, further agitation and combativeness. The smaller, softer, and more flexible types of feeding tubes used today can easily coil or kink during placement. Patients who are alert can swallow small amounts of water to facilitate tube passage.[6-8] Lidocaine or other topical anesthetic is sometimes used to reduce patient discomfort.[9] When the patient cannot participate in tube placement, a stylet can be used to stiffen the tube or the small tube can be attached to or passed inside a larger one to be withdrawn after placement. Perforation of the lung, esophagus, stomach, or small intestine can result from using stylets, rigid tubes, or endoscopes to place, clear, or advance the feeding tubes.[7,8] Intracranial entry has been

reported in cranial trauma and nontrauma patients.[7,10] Fortunately, perforation rarely occurs and can be prevented by enlisting the patient's cooperation, using a lubricated tube to facilitate passage, and stopping advancement of the tube if resistance is encountered. Newer tubes are now available that prevent the stylet from exiting the distal end of the feeding tube.

When tubes are inadvertently placed into the lung, patients usually demonstrate some form of respiratory distress (coughing, shortness of breath, inability to speak), but some patients never exhibit symptoms. In some cases patients may not be able to communicate or may not exhibit a normal reaction to respiratory insults. Initial position of nasogastric/nasoenteric tubes is verified automatically when placed by endoscope, fluoroscopy, sonography, or electromyograms. These methods are also considered the best ways to verify feeding tube position after traditional placement, but they may not be available or practical for frequent use at the bedside or home setting. Several "bedside" methods are used to verify tube placement, but because no single method is foolproof, at least two techniques are usually recommended: (1) asking the patient to speak, (2) auscultation (listening at the abdomen for "gurgling" while air is introduced into the tube) or (3) withdrawing fluid to check for volume, appearance, acid pH, or the presence of bilirubin or digestive enzymes[11,12] Another technique being evaluated is the use of a colorimetric sensor for the presence of carbon dioxide, which would indicate that the tube is in the lung.[13]

Recommendations for frequency of checking the position of enteral tubes vary, depending on institutional protocol. Because feeding tubes may become displaced, coiled, or kinked, some institutions recommend daily verification of placement when continuous feedings are used and before starting bolus or intermittent feeding. Common nursing practice is to color tube feedings with blue food coloring to differentiate the presence of the feeding from other fluids and secretions. Another technique used to determine aspiration of tube feeding includes use of glucose-oxidase strips to detect presence of sugars in the tube feeding.[14] The sensitivity and specificity of both techniques in proving presence of tube feeding in lung aspirates appears to be marginal, and the blue dye used may not always be safe. Clinical features, such as presence of fever, purulent aspirates, or radiographic evidence of pulmonary infiltrates, can be used to determine aspiration.[15]

Placement of feeding tubes into the duodenum or jejunum has been recommended in persons at increased risk of reflux and aspiration and in patients who may have impaired gastric emptying or upper GI obstruction. Although not all investigators agree that transpyloric placement is superior in preventing aspiration,[6,15] the consensus appears to be that jejunal placement may decrease the frequency of aspiration in at least high-risk patients. Patients considered at increased risk for reflux, aspiration, or aspiration pneumonia include those with delayed gastric emptying, dysphagia, altered mental status, inadequate cough and swallowing reflexes, and lower esophageal sphincter dysfunction.[6,8,16] Use of large diameter tubes may also allow more reflux of feeding.[17]

Feeding tubes can be passed beyond the stomach and into duodenum or jejunum by allowing the tube to migrate through the pylorus by natural peristalsis. However, the process may take several days even with the aid of prokinetic medications, and success is marginal. Nasoenteric placement may also be performed intraoperatively, laparoscopically, endoscopically, or aided by use of magnets.[11] When feeding into the jejunum, more attention should be paid to feeding rate, caloric density, and osmolarity because several digestive, absorptive, and coordinating functions of the stomach and proximal small bowel are bypassed (Box 17-1).

Complications with Placement of Gastrostomy and Jejunostomy Tubes

Nasogastric tubes are not usually considered acceptable for prolonged use (> 4 weeks), not only because of esthetic concerns, but also because of potential problems with rhinitis, tissue erosions, tube deterioration, and increased risk of reflux and aspiration. Alternatives include surgically placed or endoscopically placed gastrostomy and jejunostomy tubes. Each has its indications and limitations.

Surgically Placed Gastrostomy and Jejunostomy (Open and Laparoscopic Gastrostomy and Jejunostomy)

Surgically placed gastrostomy or jejunostomy tubes are usually now reserved for persons with pharyngeal, esophageal, or gastric obstructions; upper GI tumors or when abdominal surgery is already being performed for other purposes. Surgical placement of gastrostomy tubes is relatively expensive; requires the use of a sterile setting; and may include

---

BOX 17-1

Preventing Problems During Nasogastric and Nasojejunal Tube Placement

- Explain the procedure to the patient.
- Check for clear nasal passages; position patient correctly.
- Have the patient participate to the degree possible, swallow to aid passage, and so on.
- Use lubricated feeding tube.
- Use silicone-based polyurethane or other tubes that are soft and do not harden.
- Use caution with stiff tubes, stylets, and guidewires.
- Use a tube that will not allow stylet to pass through distal end.
- Stop when resistance is met.
- Use connectors for feeding bags/sets that are incompatible with IV tubing or are labeled *"not for IV use."*
- Verify placement initially and at least daily thereafter.
- Use restraints, mitts, or bridles only when necessary and only to limit access to the feeding tube.

---

several complications related to the surgical procedure, anesthesia, the type of tubes employed, or establishing and maintaining the insertion site. Published complication rates vary widely, from 2% to greater than 50%, with an overall complication rate of approximately 15%.[7,18,19] The most common complications associated with open gastrostomy feeding tube placement include local wound infection, catheter leakage, and tube dislodgment. Wound dehiscence, peritonitis, aspiration, bleeding, and GI obstruction are more serious but less frequent complications.[7,18]

Laparoscopic placement of gastrostomy and jejunostomy may result in many of the same complications as surgical gastrostomy tube placement. Laparoscopic gastrostomies and jejunostomies are usually less invasive and result in less tissue trauma and scarring. Jejunal placement of a large intraluminal balloon, "bumper," or T-tube in some cases can result in a higher incidence of obstruction because the lumen of the jejunum is considerably smaller than the stomach. If the loop of jejunum is not immobilized during the procedure, risk of volvulus may also be increased. Feeding into the jejunum also requires more caution in the rate and concentration of enteral formulas, and tube placement too far into the jejunum may also increase risk of GI distress.

Needle Catheter Jejunostomy

Needle catheter jejunostomy is a placement technique used during abdominal surgery.[19,20] A small catheter is placed into the jejunum over a wire placed via needle puncture through the abdominal wall. Because the catheter is small, placement results in less trauma, and consequently is less likely to cause fistula, bowel obstruction, or volvulus than other jejunostomy techniques. It may also be removed more easily than most feeding devices. Because of the small tube size (5 to 6 Fr), clogging is more common, unless lower viscosity feedings are used and tubes are irrigated appropriately. Replacement of dislodged tubes may also be more difficult.

Complications Associated with Percutaneous Endoscopic Gastrostomy, Gastrojejunostomy, and Direct Endoscopic Jejunostomy

Percutaneous endoscopic gastrostomy (PEG) is a type of tube placement performed with the aid of an endoscope. The tube is placed by one of several "push" techniques (abdominal wall punctured from outside the stomach) or "pull" techniques (wall of the stomach and abdomen punctured from inside the stomach). The tube is normally secured on the inside of the stomach/jejunum by a balloon, collar, or T-tube and on the outside by a flange, button, or collar to prevent movement and leakage of the tube. Newer techniques and equipment have allowed endoscopic placement of tubes orally or nasoenterically into the stomach or the jejunum (PEG/J), or direct placement into the jejunum.[18,19,21-25] Placement and use of PEG/J tubes are associated with complication rates ranging from less than 10% to greater than 30%, depending on the type of apparatus, the patient's clinical status, and the experience of the clinicians who place the tube and care for the patient. Endoscopically placed gastrostomies, and PEG/J tubes in general, appear to be superior to surgically placed gastrostomies and jejunostomies in terms of overall morbidity and mortality and cost. PEG tubes are now considered the route of choice for long-term enteral feeding.[18,19,23]

Complications associated with PEG/PEJ feedings include leakage, irritation or infection around the feeding site; peritonitis; fistulas; dislodgment of the tube, collars, or buttons; GI obstruction from dislodged components of the tube; abdominal pain; and aspiration pneumonia.[18,21-25] Medical conditions that increase the apparent risk of complications for placement of feeding gastrostomies include severe malnutrition, malignancies, significant obesity, ascites, coagulopathies, abdominal trauma, and active inflammatory disease. Newer tubes and placement strategies are being developed to reduce the risk of obstruction, dislodgment, and complications related to anesthesia with surgical and endoscopically placed gastrostomies and jejunostomies.

Mechanical Problems During Tube Feeding

Nasogastric and Enteric Tubes

After the feeding tube has been placed, the tube may be displaced by coughing, retching, or vomiting or as a result of the patient or other health care personnel pulling the feeding tube, purposely or inadvertently. Removal is quite common in confused or demented patients or those who are not convinced of the necessity of enteral feedings. Feeding tubes, especially the small silicone or urethane type, can kink or knot, even after placement. When rubber or polyvinyl chloride (PVC) feeding tubes are used for prolonged periods, they may become stiff and brittle, and subsequently crack. Large tubes of any type are more likely to cause mucosal irritation and erosions. PVC or rubber tubes of any size are more likely to stiffen and cause mucosal irritation or erosion. Sometimes a feeding tube or the distal segment of tube that contains the weight becomes enlarged with time. Rarely, portions of the feeding tube break and may result in obstruction of the GI tract. By far, however, clogging, displacement, and removal of nasogastric and nasoenteric tubes are the most common of the mechanical complications.[8,21,26]

OBSTRUCTION OF FEEDING TUBES. Obstructed or clogged feeding tubes are one of the most common mechanical problems associated with nasogastric and nasoenteric feeding tubes. Tubes are more likely to become occluded when (1) small diameter tubes are used, (2) powdered or crushed medications are passed through the tubes, (3) acidic or alkaline medications are passed through the tube, (4) tubes are not routinely flushed after feedings are stopped, or (5) blenderized food formulas containing particulate matter are used.[21,27-31] Congealing or clumping of formula in the tube can also result from interaction of the formula with acid and proteolytic enzymes in the stomach. Withdrawal of gastric residuum often results in clumping and obstruction when acid gastric secretions are mixed with formula in the feeding tube. When tube feedings are introduced into the small intestine, the tube is exposed to digestive enzymes and alkaline secretions, but because the overall pH is closer to neutral and the enzymes are more active digestants, clogging is not as likely as with intragastric feeding.[27,28] Microbial growth and colonization of the feeding tube can result in clogging if formula is not rinsed from the tube after the feeding is stopped. The risk of clogging can be minimized by relatively simple procedures that are sometimes difficult to achieve in practice without monitoring. One of the primary preventive measures is to flush with enough water to keep the tube clear. During continuous feeding, tubes should be routinely flushed with water every 4 hours, whenever the feeding is stopped, and whenever (liquid or powdered) medications must be given through the feeding tube.[29-31] Using liquid forms of medication does not insure that clogging will not occur. Acidic or alkaline medications or viscous elixirs can cause the formula to clump or thicken.[30,31]

In clinical practice, a great deal of credence has been placed in using a variety of fluids to rinse or open feeding tubes. Cola beverages, cranberry juice, and warmed tea have been purported to be useful for unclogging feeding tubes. In truth, the ingredients in these fluids that are commonly believed to be "digestants" are weak and ineffective when compared with more potent pancreatic enzymes, such as pancrelipase (Viokase) and pancreatin, to unclog tubes.[21,27-29] Furthermore, when soft drinks and juices are used as rinsing agents, their dried residues can further narrow the lumen of the tube and contribute to clogging. Warm water is far superior as a solvent and rinsing agent and leaves little or no residue.[21,29]

Once the tube is clogged, the options are to remove the tube or attempt to clear the obstruction. Several methods have been recommended, and the success rates probably depend on the cause of the obstruction, the amount of tube occluded, and how long the tube has been clogged. Irrigating the tube with a syringe filled with warm water can be attempted, but with only gentle pressure. Excessive pressure can rupture or break the feeding tube. Small, hollow tubes can be passed inside the feeding tubes to deliver warm water to more distal sites. A mixture of pancreatic enzyme and sodium bicarbonate can be used to dissolve clots, using a smaller tube to deliver the mixture to the obstruction.[21,27] Generally, use of water or digestive enzyme solutions have been superior to commonly used cranberry juice and cola beverages in clearing feeding tubes.[21,27-29] In an earlier study, routine irrigation with 30 ml of water proved far superior in maintaining patency to irrigation compared with cranberry juice. Eleven of 15 tubes became occluded when routinely flushed with cranberry juice, while none of 15 irrigated with water became clogged.[29] Stylets used with tube placement, newer corkscrew stylets, endoscopy brushes, and endoscopic retrograde cholangio pancreatography (ERCP) tubes have been used to physically break up the obstructions.[21,26,32] In the past, stiff wires were sometimes used to open feeding tubes, but perforation of the tube and mucosal surfaces have been reported.[26] Caution must be used to prevent perforation of the GI mucosa using any stylet, and wires should not be used. When kinked or knotted tubing is the cause of obstruction, the tube must either be repositioned or removed (Box 17-2).

Feeding Sets and Pumps

In most cases, when continuous feeding is desired the formula is poured into a feeding bag or rigid bottle or the formula may be prepackaged in feeding containers. The feeding bag is hung on a pole or stand similar to those used for intravenous solutions. The feeding bag is typically connected to a pump to control flow rate. In the past, gravity drip was the primary

Preventing Obstruction of Feeding Tubes

- With continuous feeding, routinely flush feeding tubes every 4 hours.
- Flush feeding tubes with water whenever feedings are stopped.
- Flush feeding tubes before and after gastrointestinal contents are withdrawn.
- Avoid giving powdered, crushed, highly acidic, or alkaline medications through the feeding tube whenever possible.
- If medications must be given through the tube, flush it with water before and after.
- Prevent contamination of enteral feeding.
- Avoid passing viscous foods and fiber supplements through small tubes.
- If blended foods are used, be sure foods are finely divided, and use larger tubes.

mode of delivery for continuous feeding and clips or screws attached to the tubing from the reservoir were used to regulate flow rates. Establishing and maintaining a consistent flow rate was difficult, and the tubing often became permanently crimped at the site of the regulator. Most of the tubing used currently with feeding bags and pumps is too narrow to allow gravity drip at acceptable rates with most standard enteral formulas. Gravity drip is now primarily used when bolus or intermittent feedings are used without a pump. Larger tubes or using a disposable syringe barrel is used as the reservoir. Rapid administration becomes more of a concern when bolus feedings are given.

Commercial feeding bags and tubing "sets" currently used in combination with enteral pumps rarely cause problems, but a few complications can still occur. The outlet ports from feeding bags and connecting tubes can become occluded if the tubing lines become kinked; if medications, viscous foods, or fibrous materials are added to the bags; or if bacterial growth is significant (at least 10^7 organisms per milliliter).[33]

Other problems with feeding sets include difficulty opening and closing the reservoirs, bursting open if dropped, leaking from the fill site or connectors, and incompatibility with feeding pumps. "Generic" feeding sets are available, but sometimes only the sets sold with the pump fit properly. In some facilities with a large volume of enteral feeding, feedings are poured into the containers and frozen for later use. Some types of containers, however, may crack or leak after being frozen. Fewer complications appear to occur with prefilled, ready-to-hang feeding bags or bottles. The prefilled, ready-to-feed formulas are economical, can be stored for long periods of time at room temperature, reduce the chance for delivery of excessively concentrated or dilute formula, discourage the addition of other fluids and medications to the reservoir, and reduce (but not eliminate) the chance of contamination and longer "hang time."[34-36] Disadvantages include the inability to modify the feeding solutions and limited variety of the products available in ready-to-feed form.

Institutions or purchasing groups can establish criteria for selecting desired tube feeding reservoirs and sets, such as (1) a rigid neck that allows filling without requiring manipulation with the operator's fingers to open the reservoir, (2) filled reservoirs that do not leak after freezing or during storage and transport, (3) filled reservoirs that are sturdy enough to be dropped from a reasonable height without breaking or opening, and (4) filled reservoirs that are compatible with feeding pumps and feeding method.

Connection of distal ends of feeding sets to intravenous lines is a rare but obviously serious complication. It could potentially occur in a critical care setting when a number of intravenous lines are being used.[37,38] The problem can be prevented by requiring that tubing connectors be incompatible with intravenous sets or that the manufacturer attach a tag to the distal end of the feeding set labeled *"not for IV use."*

Mechanical problems that may occur with feeding pumps include electrical failures (motor, switches, alarms, sensors, battery), breakage after being dropped, or becoming inoperable after becoming wet. Feeding tubes can break or kink, and the flexible section of the tubing that is stretched around cam-driven models can be pulled apart. Excessively high or low pressures can be generated within the tubing, especially with distal feeding tube obstructions. Flow rates can be inaccurate when changes occur in the viscosity of the feeding or when the tubing becomes bent or twisted as the patient moves about. Most pumps are fairly reliable, and accuracy is generally within 10% of stated rates, but flow rates should be evaluated at different settings, with different formulas, and under various conditions.[39,40]

Clinical Problems Related to Tube Feeding

Diarrhea—Incidence and Definition

In the acute care setting, the reported incidence of diarrhea in tube-fed patients ranges from less than 5% to greater than 60%.[41-43] The higher figures are more likely to be reported in the intensive care unit (ICU) setting. In these settings, diarrhea occurs with such frequency that it is assumed to be a natural consequence of enteral feeding. On the other hand, in the long-term or home care settings, constipation or impaction may be problematic with use of the same enteral feeding formulas—even when similar or less stringent protocols for advancement, rate, and concentration of feedings are used. Coexisting physiologic stressors, medications, and treatments in acute care settings likely contribute to the higher incidence of diarrhea. The incidence of diarrhea can also vary depending on the definition of diarrhea and conditions under which enteral feedings are used. Diarrhea can simply be a descriptor of stool volume and texture or a life-threatening medical problem. Significant diarrhea is more likely related to factors other than the use or composition of the enteral feeding.[42-45]

Diarrhea is usually defined by at least two of three descriptors. Typically it is characterized by stool weight greater than 250 to 300 g, watery consistency, and/or more than three stools per day.[41-45] Sometimes the term *diarrhea* is used by patients or caretakers to describe watery or frequent stools but the 24-hour stool weight may actually be less than 200 g. Frequent small stools may still be a clinical problem, but their occurrence and resolution may not be related to tube feeding. Diarrhea may result from osmotic, secretory and or infectious etiologies.[42-45]

The stools resulting from patients receiving enteral formulas, specifically from defined formula diets, tend to be "mushy" and may be mistaken for diarrhea. Diarrhea definitely occurs more frequently in tube-fed, acute care patients than in a normal population, but, in evaluating reports of diarrhea, descriptors such as *consistency, frequency,* and *volume* of stools should be included.[43]

DIARRHEA—ASSOCIATED CAUSES AND RISK FACTORS. The long list of causes and contributors to diarrhea includes medications, rate of delivery of the tube feeding, composition of the feeding formula, malnutrition (involving both micronutrients and macronutrients), aggressive refeeding, patient's concomitant clinical problems, and opportunistic infection. In hospitalized patients, most cases of diarrhea can probably be attributed, directly or indirectly, to medications and the severity of the patient's illness (Box 17-3).[41-46]

Medications, specifically antibiotics, may contribute to diarrhea in several ways. Antibiotics can reduce the usual "salvage" by colon bacteria of small amounts of malabsorbed foodstuffs. Antibiotics such as penicillins, cephalosporins, and gentamycin can alter colonic flora or drastically reduce the numbers of colonic bacteria that normally convert osmotically active molecules (e.g., carbohydrate and amino acids) to gases and short-chain fatty acids (SCFAs). The SCFAs are normally absorbed rapidly and efficiently from the lumen of the colon as long as the amount produced is close to normal.[43-46] Absorption of the SCFAs also aids absorption of electrolytes and water from the colon. Eradication of the bacteria from the colon results in accumulation of osmotically active molecules and reduced absorption of electrolytes and water. If more substrates than usual are malabsorbed, as often occurs in hospitalized patients, the resulting accumulation of osmols can result in considerable fluid loss.[47]

Antibiotics can also have direct effects on GI function. Erythromycin, for example, increases the migrating motor complex activity of the proximal gut, resulting in more rapid gastric emptying and movement of proximal small bowel contents. Erythromycin is also poorly absorbed and like clarithromycin and others, is considered an enteric irritant.[46] Clindamycin increases biliary secretion and is considered a GI mucosal irritant.[48] Finally, some antibiotics may effect opportunistic proliferation of pathogenic organisms normally suppressed by competitive organisms in the GI tract. The organisms or the toxins produced can result in large fluid losses by decreasing absorption and increasing secretion of fluid and electrolytes.[46,49] *Clostridium difficile* is most commonly associated with antibiotic-related diarrhea and accounts for 10% to 25% of cases, but *Clostridium perfringens, Salmonella, Shigella, Campylobacter, Yersinia enterocolitica,* and *Escherichia coli* organisms have also been implicated.[46,49,50] The specific cause of *Clostridium difficile* infection cannot always be isolated, but it is associated with the number of antibiotics used, the duration of exposure to antibiotics, the number of days in the hospital, and specific types of antibiotics. Clindamycin, penicillins, and cephalosporins are implicated most often, but tetracycline, erythromycin, chloramphenicol, sulfonamides, quinolones, and trimethoprim have also been associated with the occurrence of *C. difficile*.[46-50] Increased risk of *C. difficile* infection is also associated with use of antineoplastic agents, especially methotrexate, doxorubicin, and cyclophosphamide.[51,52] Patients with human immunodeficiency virus (HIV) and immune deficiencies may have several contributors to the etiology of the diarrhea, including toxic effects of medications, proliferation of opportunistic organisms, and GI manifestations of the disease itself.[53,54]

Antacids, (especially magnesium salts), histamine H_2-receptor blockers,[42,43,45,55] and proton pump inhibitors[56-57] have been implicated in cases of diarrhea. At least in theory, reducing gastric acid can allow proliferation and colonization of microbes in the stomach and small intestine normally held in check by acid. Although use of acid-suppressing medications may not always be a direct cause, their use has been associated with diarrhea individually or in combination with other medications.[42,56,57]

Hyperosmolar medications and sorbitol elixirs can also contribute to diarrhea.[31,42] Liquid forms of medications such as acetaminophen, cimetidine, dextromethorphan, ferrous sulfate, multivitamins, potassium chloride, and theophylline may be hypertonic, with osmolarities in the range of 800 to more than 6000 mOsm/L. The liquid medications may also contain significant amounts of sorbitol, a sugar with a "cool," sweet taste that is poorly absorbed.[31,42] Only 5 to 20 g of sorbitol is sufficient to cause diarrhea in children and adults.[58] Antacids and other medications that contain significant amounts of magnesium can also contribute to diarrhea. "Standing" orders for laxatives, stool softeners, and acid-suppressing medications sometimes are not discontinued, and occasionally a patient may take laxatives covertly.

Impaction, which most often occurs in immobilized, chronic-care patients, can be manifested by symptoms of diarrhea. Passage or secretion of fluid around the impaction may be responsible for the loose stool. The volume of stool usually is not great, and the patient may intermittently pass small volumes of liquid stool and experience abdominal distention and cramping.

Malnutrition can contribute to diarrhea in several ways.[59-61] It can result in reduced gastric acid secretion; decreased secretion of enzymes from the stomach, pancreas, and brush border; and decreased proliferation, height, and maturity of intestinal villi. The net effect is reduced efficiency and effectiveness of digestion and absorption. Malnutrition can compromise overall host immunity, decrease levels of secretory immunoglobulin A (IgA) in the GI tract, and may increase the potential for microbial proliferation and entry of microbes across the mucosal

---

BOX 17-3
Potential Causes of Diarrhea

- Medications: Antibiotics; H_2-receptor antagonists, antacids; medications containing significant amounts of sorbitol, magnesium; hypertonic medications; antineoplastic agents
- GI disorders or dysfunction, including gastric or small bowel resection, inflammatory bowel disease, pancreatic insufficiency, radiation enteritis, sprue, protein-losing gastroenteropathies
- Malnutrition, including hypoproteinemia and micronutrient deficiencies.
- Excessive rate of feeding, concentration, volume, or osmolality, especially in malnourished patients and patients whose GI tract has not been used for several days
- Opportunistic GI infection: Immunosuppression from disease or medications, hypochlorhydria; infusion of significant amounts of contaminated feeding formula; altered GI flora
- Physiologic stress
- Bowel impaction
- Intolerance or allergy to feeding formula
- Diabetes
- Hyperthyroidism

barrier. In a severely compromised host, transfer of microbes from the GI tract is considered a significant source for septic complications. Significant hypoalbuminemia is associated with decreased tolerance to enteral feedings, which theoretically is due to gut edema or decreased oncotic gradient across the bowel wall. Hypoalbuminemia may also reflect significant malnutrition or physiologic stress, either of which could decrease tolerance to enteral feeding. Low serum albumin does not contraindicate tube feeding but may require that rate, osmolality, and volume of feedings must be increased cautiously.

MANAGEMENT OF DIARRHEA. The first steps in resolving diarrhea are to evaluate the severity, duration, and pattern of occurrence and then to investigate possible causes including secretory, osmotic, or infectious sources. Where possible and as appropriate, the physician should withdraw or substitute the offending medications (e.g., magnesium-based antacids can sometimes be replaced with calcium or aluminum salts). Hypertonic elixirs or sorbitol-containing medications can often be diluted or replaced. With malnourished patients or patients with jejunal feedings or compromised GI function, feeding rate or concentration can be reduced or continuous feedings can be used instead of bolus. If specific offending ingredients are causal (e.g., lactose or allergens), the enteral formula may be changed. After preventable causes of diarrhea have been addressed, medications such as opiates, loperamide, or paregoric may reduce or resolve many cases of mild to moderate diarrhea. In cases of diarrhea caused by stasis and bacterial overgrowth, however, drugs that slow motility may worsen the situation.[45,46]

Diarrhea has also been associated with proliferation of microbes in enteral feeding solutions. Safe, clean handling of feeding formula, tubes, and reservoirs; addition of stabilizers; and acidification of the formula all may help prevent contamination and growth of microbes in the formula.[62]

Severe diarrhea (generally considered more than 1 L of stool per day) usually indicates significant malabsorption, maldigestion, or secretory or infectious causes. Maldigestion or malabsorption, for example, might respond to decreasing the concentration, osmolarity, or rate of the formula, or changing the composition of the formula, (e.g., using medium-chain triglycerides or pancreatic enzymes) or changing to a chemically defined diet to enhance absorption. Secretory diarrhea may result from infectious agents such as C. *difficile* or other agents, viral gastroenteritis, inflammatory states, and/or as a result of malabsorbed bile acids. Osmotic diarrheas are typically more rectified by dietary modification than secretory and other forms of diarrhea, although diet may help attenuate other forms.

Infectious diarrhea, as in C. *difficile* infection or the patient with acquired immunodeficiency syndrome (AIDS) who may be suffering from several opportunistic infections such as giardiasis, cryptosporidiosis, amebiasis, salmonellosis, or shigellosis, may require specific antimicrobial therapy.[53,54] In HIV, the disease, medications used to treat the GI infection, and malnutrition may contribute to the diarrhea.

Various forms of foodstuffs or prebiotic and probiotic supplements have been used to prevent or treat diarrhea with varying degrees of success. Prebiotic supplements or foods that contain oligosaccharides, fibers, or resistant starches have a role in "stabilizing or normalizing" GI flora and function.[41,62-66] The prebiotic materials tend to soften stools in cases of constipation and firm stools during diarrhea. Continuous supplies of some prebiotics alter fecal flora, increase water absorption, help maintain the unstirred water layer along the mucosa, and are fermented by colonic microbes to SCFAs. SCFAs serve as a primary fuel for colonocytes, are trophic to enterocytes, and enhance colonic absorption of water and sodium. The more acid milieu favors the proliferation of "beneficial" bifidobacteria and lactobacilli that prevent adherence or colonization of organisms such as C. *difficile* and, in underdeveloped countries, cholera. Pectin, fructose oligosaccharides, inulin, psyllium, soy fibers, and banana flakes all have been claimed to be helpful in firming stools and preventing or treating diarrhea, but additional study in humans and specifically enteral applications are warranted.[41,63-66] Addition of prebiotics may be relatively ineffective in treating more severe cases of infectious, secretory, or osmotic diarrheas. Whenever possible, enteral products should probably contain dietary fiber or prebiotic materials for normal health maintenance.

Supplementation of formulas with probiotics (nonpathogenic organisms that exert positive effects on health) also holds promise for prevention and treatment of diarrhea and other GI and systemic problems. Applications in enteral nutrition are limited, but ingestion of several strains of probiotic organisms has been at least partially effective in the prevention of antibiotic- and rotavirus-associated diarrhea and gastroenteritis. Lactobacillus rhamnosus GG, lactobacillus acidophilus, and Saccharomyces boulardii are examples of probiotics that have been used in controlled human trials with some success.[68,69]

Aspiration

Aspiration is one of the most serious and potentially life-threatening complications of tube feeding.[2] This is especially true in the patient compromised by disease, trauma, neurologic disorders, immune deficits, or malnutrition.[21,43,70] The term *aspiration*, in this context, refers to entry of tube feeding or GI secretions into the lungs. The incidence of aspiration ranges greatly from less than 4% to greater than 70%, depending on the criteria used to define aspiration, the population studied, and the method(s) employed to verify the complication. Consequences range from coughing and wheezing to infection, tissue necrosis, and respiratory failure. The consequences of aspiration depend on the volume, pH, particle size, composition, and microbial content of the aspirated material and the prior health of the patient. Some minor degree of pharyngeal aspiration of gastric secretions occurs in normal, healthy individuals with little consequence. With tube feedings, however, the likelihood for significant aspiration and adverse sequelae is greater.

Factors that increase the risk of clinically significant aspiration include the supine position of the patient, delayed gastric emptying, reflux, use of large diameter feeding tubes, tracheal intubation, age of the patient, neuromuscular disorders, decreased consciousness, increased concentration of microbes in the aspirate, aspiration of gastric contents (acid and digestive enzymes), and decreased intensity of nursing care.[15-17,21,70] Ileus, GI obstruction, and a host of other medical and surgical problems can also cause vomiting, which, especially in a compromised patient, further increases the risk of aspiration. Use of bolus feedings or rapid infusion of enteral feedings, especially those of higher osmolality or caloric concentration, can increase the risk of reflux, vomiting, and aspiration, even when infused transpylorically or by gastrostomy tube.

As mentioned earlier, aspiration can also occur as a result of misplacement or dislocation of the feeding tube. Typically, if the feeding tube enters the airway while it is being placed, the patient coughs and expresses discomfort; however, patients who are sedated or obtunded may not be able to respond normally.

Several measures have been advocated to prevent aspiration, but each has limitations. To further prevent aspiration in tube-fed patients, elevating the head of the bed to at least 30 degrees, checking residual gastric volume, and use of prokinetic agents such as metoclopramide and erythromycin to enhance gastric emptying have been recommended, especially in patients at high risk.[6,7,15,70] In general, aspiration is less of a risk with continuous than with bolus or intermittent feedings.[6,15,70] Placing tubes transpylorically, especially at or beyond the ligament of Treitz, may reduce (but not eliminate) the risk of aspiration. Whether and the degree to which enteric placement of feeding tubes prevents aspiration have been controversial but may depend on the placement and feeding protocols and the risk of the population studied.[15,21,23,70]

The volume of fluid remaining in the stomach or small intestine depends on the rate at which the tube feeding is administered, amount of fluids secreted from the GI tract, rate of GI transit, and GI absorptive rate. Each factor must be considered when deciding to start and advance enteral feedings. In most settings, protocols for routine checks of gastric residuum are used, especially for high-risk patients or when increasing rate and concentration of bolus feedings. Use of a cutpoint for volume of gastric or intestinal residuum as a decision tool to limit subsequent feedings is a common and logical clinical practice. However, the association between gastric or enteric volume and aspiration has not been well documented and the cutpoints are not well correlated with gastric emptying. Recommendations range from 150 to 250 ml for intragastric feedings and approximately 100 ml for gastrostomies placed on the anterior wall,[15,38,43,71] but even these recommendations might vary depending on the degrees of patient risk. The higher the flow rate, volume, caloric concentration, osmolality, and viscosity of the feeding, the greater the potential for increased gastric residuals.

Contamination of Feeding Solutions

Ready-to-feed commercial enteral products, unlike modular or tube feedings prepared from regular foods, are essentially sterile until opened (Box 17-4). Contamination of enteral formulas decanted into feeding bags, however, is common in the hospital setting. Contamination and proliferation of microbes in the formula may simply result in altered color, consistency, or clumping of the feeding, but in some cases, contamination may be manifested in colonization of the GI tract and diarrhea.[33,71-73] The typical hospitalized, tube-fed patient is at greater risk than a free-living, healthy person for adverse consequences of contaminated foods. The patient may be immunologically compromised as a result of malnutrition, disease, or

---

BOX 17-4

Reducing Risk of Microbial Contamination

- Use prefilled, ready-to-feed enteral feeding when possible.
- Wash hands before handling enteral feeding products.
- Check for out-of-date, swollen, or leaking enteral formula containers,
- When filling enteral formulas into feeding bags, avoid touching fluid path, openings, and spikes.
- Discard unused portions of feedings or refrigerate unused portions immediately after decanting; label unused portion with time, date, and patient's identification.
- Watch for change in color and consistency in enteral formulas during delivery.
- Avoid unnecessary opening/additions to tube feeding.
- If not using prefilled enteral feeding, discard remainder of formula after 8 to 12 hours hang time; rinse feeding bag and all tubing with water; refill with fresh product.
- In hospital, discard feeding bag or set every 24 hours.
- If reuse of feeding bag cannot be avoided, use bag that does not have crevices or corners that cannot be cleaned. Insufficient data are available regarding safety of reusing enteral feeding bags.
- If blended food formula is used, employ safe handling practices from start to finish; avoid using for immunosuppressed patients.

---

medications. In a patient fed directly into the small bowel, the bacteriostatic effects of gastric acid and digestive enzymes are bypassed, further increasing the risks associated with contaminated formula. If the patient is receiving medications to block or neutralize gastric acid secretions, the chances for gastric and intestinal colonization may also be increased.

When commercially prepared enteral products are found to contain significant concentrations of microbes during administration to the patient, the primary source is typically the hands of persons who open, fill, and connect the feeding reservoirs.[62,71-75] Microbes are typically transferred from nursing staff who perform routine patient care activities and then fill the feeding bags. The types of microbes found in enteral feedings in the clinical setting are not those typically associated with food-borne illness, but rather are nosocomial organisms normally found in hospital units.

Most enteral feedings provide excellent media for microbial growth but hyperosmolar tube feedings, those that have a more acidic pH and those that contain microbial inhibitors, are less likely to support microbial growth than typical isotonic formulas.[33,72-76] Potassium sorbate, methylparaben, and sodium benzoate, all common food additives, have been used by one enteral formula company to inhibit growth of at least some organisms, but effectiveness data are not available.

Because normal enteral feedings bags may be relatively expensive, they are sometimes reused in clinical and home settings. The safety and cost effectiveness of reusing enteral feeding bags, however, has probably not been adequately evaluated. Few studies have been published regarding rinsing and cleaning procedures, degree of contamination, and patient outcomes. Published reports are limited, conflicting, and far from complete.[76-77] Some enteral feeding reservoirs are difficult to clean completely, and the same concerns that face food service managers regarding clean equipment, safe food preparation, and storage apply to reuse of enteral feeding products.[33,35,62,78-80] Additional study is required regarding which types of enteral formulas and bags can be rinsed and reused and with what procedures and for what duration. Guidelines for one institution may not apply for all formulas, feeding apparatus, patients, or situations.

Contamination is less likely to occur with commercial enteral feeding formulas, which are prefilled into feeding bags.[34,35,80-83] Because the prefilled products come in a limited number of concentrations and nutrient mixtures, they may not be used in acute care as often as they might in extended care facilities or the home setting after the patient is more stable. The bags are normally 1 to 2 L in volume and, if handled with reasonable care, can be hung by the bedside for 24 to 36 hours. Contamination can still occur in prefilled containers when (1) spikes are inserted to connect the tubing; (2) when medications or other additives are introduced; or (3) theoretically, from retrograde seeding of microbes in bags that do not have drip chambers that separate tubing and fresh enteral product in the feeding bag.[80-84]

A primary reason that enteral formulas are rarely made from regular foods is the significant risk of contamination during preparation. Although commercial products are now used almost exclusively, patients or their caretakers sometimes insist on using tube feedings made from regular foods. In addition to organisms found naturally on or in foods, employees or patient caregivers in the home must practice sanitation and safety measures at each step from purchase of the individual ingredients to preparation and storage.[62,75,76,78-80,82] Each piece of equipment used for measuring, mixing, and storing the products must be clean. Ensuring a safe, blenderized tube feeding delivered to the patient's bedside is an institutional food service nightmare. Because commercial products are less likely to become contaminated if rather simple guidelines are followed, they are the preferred choice when safety and sanitation are concerns.

Underfeeding

ENERGY AND PROTEIN INTAKE. Tube-fed patients often receive less than the prescribed or desired amount of feeding.[8,15,43] Errors can be made in the original estimate of nutrient needs, the product can be diluted or improperly mixed, or the initial feeding rate and volume may not have been increased. The most common reason for underfeeding, however, is interruptions in the feeding schedule. Feedings are stopped for various reasons—diagnostic and therapeutic procedures, ambulation, infusion of medications, clogged or misplaced tubes, occurrence of diarrhea, excess residual volume or other complications, personal care and hygiene, or when visitors come. The patient or caretakers may purposely or accidentally change the rate, time, or volume or replace the formula with liquids of lower nutrient density. Patients or caretakers may be concerned about the cost of the product or excessive weight gain or may simply be confused about the intent or composition of feeding. If patients are underfed for long periods or have high nutritional needs, the resulting undernutrition, including macronutrients and micronutrients, may be significant.

MICRONUTRIENT DEFICIENCIES. Deficiencies of vitamins, minerals, and electrolytes as a result of enteral feedings are now relatively rare, as a result of the widespread use of commercial products, which usually provide adequate levels of most nutrients. Some patients, however, may be at increased risk because of poor intake before starting enteral feedings, malabsorption,

increased requirements, or drug-nutrient interactions. Some patients may need therapeutic levels of micronutrients in addition to standard feedings.

Blenderized, modular, and standard tube feedings that are diluted or modified can also be deficient in vitamins or minerals. A patient who has unusually low energy requirements (e.g., <1500 kcal) or receives fewer calories than are needed might also receive too few micronutrients. Some of the more serious deficiencies are discussed next.

HYPONATREMIA. Hyponatremia typically is not a result of too little sodium in the diet; usually it reflects a hypervolemic state such as congestive heart failure, cirrhosis, or nephrotic syndrome; it may also reflect a euvolemic state as seen with excess antidiuretic hormone, thiazide diuretics, cortisol deficiency, or hypothyroidism. Because our diet is typically excessive in sodium, hyponatremia related to excess loss of sodium in relation to water is relatively uncommon, but may occur with GI suctioning, vomiting, malabsorption syndromes (including short-bowel syndrome), excessive renal losses, or long-term use of dilute or very low-sodium tube feedings or thiazide diuretics. Caretakers using infant formulas or making home-prepared formulas from unsalted foods for enteral feeding may unknowingly create very low-sodium formulas. Diet and medical history, urinary sodium, and serum osmolality help determine the etiology. Prevention and treatment of hyponatremia typically involves identification of the potential causes and, when appropriate, fluid restriction for dilutional hyponatremia or provision of supplemental sodium for true sodium depletion.[85-87]

HYPOKALEMIA AND HYPOPHOSPHATEMIA. Hypokalemia and hypophosphatemia often go hand-in-hand because they typically occur with combinations of prolonged nutrition depletion, catabolic stress, alcoholism, rapid refeeding, or and/or insulin therapy.[43,85,87-92] A potassium-wasting diuretic or long-term diarrhea increases the risk of hypokalemia. Treatment of mild hypokalemia includes increased dietary potassium (e.g., 20 to 40 mEq of potassium chloride) and correction of factors that might have contributed to the hypokalemia. More severe cases of hypokalemia require careful intravenous replacement.

Medications associated with increased phosphorus losses include aluminum hydroxide, theophylline, sucralfate, and foscarnet.[85,87-90] Treatment of hypophosphatemia includes therapeutic replacement of phosphorus and withdrawal or substitution of agents that contribute to hypophosphatemia. With milder hypophosphatemia, 20 to 40 mmol of phosphorus can be provided in the form of 5 to 10 ml of Fleets phosphosoda in 500 to 1000 ml of formula.[88] If hypophosphatemia is significant (e.g., serum phosphorus < 1.6 mg/dl), intravenous phosphorus should be provided.

Overfeeding

Unlike overfeeding with parenteral nutrition, providing excessive calories or carbohydrate by way of enteral feeding is somewhat limited by decreasing GI tolerance. Significant overfeeding with standard enteral formulas typically results in increased gastric residuals, abdominal bloating, cramping, diarrhea, or reflux, especially in a malnourished patient or one whose GI function is compromised.[41-43,91,92] Overfeeding may lead to gradual weight gain and hyperglycemia; hyperlipidemia;

and increased fat deposition in long-term, tube-fed patients, especially those who are bedridden. Patients with neuromuscular disease may appear normal weight but may have replaced lost muscle mass with gains in fat mass. Accurate initial assessment of calorie requirements followed by periodic reassessment prevents overfeeding.[90] Use of indirect calorimetry, measures of body composition, and weight histories can be used when height-weight relationships may not be helpful.

Overfeeding results in increased metabolic rate, cardiac demand, respirations, and carbon dioxide production. Increased carbon dioxide production can result from either excessive calorie intake or high-carbohydrate intake. Overfeeding and the potential for increased respiratory demand can be monitored by the respiratory quotient (RQ), the ratio of carbon dioxide produced to oxygen consumed by metabolic processing of energy substrates. This value is measured with a metabolic cart while performing indirect calorimetry.[93] RQ resulting from the oxidation of carbohydrate is approximately 1, whereas the RQ from processing fat is only 0.7. The act of converting excess carbohydrate calories to fat has an RQ of 8, and significant overfeeding can result in net RQs greater than 1.0.[93]

Concern for overfeeding carbohydrate or calories is usually directed toward patients with chronic obstructive pulmonary disease (COPD) or those on ventilators who are retaining carbon dioxide and struggling to breathe with, or be weaned from, respirators. Reducing excessive calorie intake is far more therapeutic than reducing the carbohydrate content of the feeding, but if the calorie level is acceptable, reducing carbohydrate content and increasing lipid calories may be beneficial in reducing carbon dioxide load.

Hyperglycemia

Compared with its relative frequency in association with central venous feeding, hyperglycemia is relatively rare in patients fed by enteral feedings, especially by continuous drip. The relatively slow rate of formula infusion, combined with the normal GI and endocrine mechanisms for processing the energy substrates, make hyperglycemia less likely. Overfeeding of energy and glucose is also somewhat self-limited by GI tolerance. Most hyperglycemia secondary to enteral feeding is likely the result of combinations of other factors commonly seen in the acute care setting, including diabetes, medications (notably steroids), and physiologic stressors. Treatment of hyperglycemia includes making certain that calories and rate of administration are appropriate, using insulin or oral hypoglycemic agents when necessary, reducing or eliminating (when possible) medications associated with hyperglycemia, and adjusting the timing of enteral "meals" with the onset, peak, and duration of hypoglycemic agents. Specialty products that contain fiber and greater proportions of monounsaturated fatty acids may help control glycemia and lipemia for persons fed long term by tube.[94]

For patients with diabetes who require insulin, use of enteral pumps and intermittent feedings can be used quite effectively to regulate blood sugar and control lipids. The patient or caregiver can adjust insulin doses and enteral feeding rates and schedules to produce acceptable levels of glycemia over a 24-hour period. The frequency and composition of the feedings can be tailored to fit the profile to the hypoglycemic agent.

Initial monitoring typically includes blood glucose measures every 6 to 8 hours (continuous feeding); daily blood urea nitrogen, electrolytes, creatinine, and a record of energy intake; and weekly serum triglyceride and cholesterol levels.[94,95] When the patient's condition stabilizes, the frequency can be decreased.

Refeeding Syndrome

Patients who have a long history of poor caloric intake as a result of anorexia, maldigestion, or malabsorption and are then aggressively refed are at risk for *refeeding syndrome*.[43,91,92] Long-term undernutrition causes gradual loss of skeletal muscle mass and of functional tissues from organ systems—heart, lungs, liver, and GI tract. In addition, patients lose total body stores of biologic catalysts and electrolytes, including several vitamins, phosphorus, potassium, magnesium, zinc, and trace elements. Overfeeding a malnourished patient adds to the physiologic burden by increasing cardiac output, respirations, substrate interconversions, and synthesis of adenosine triphosphate and protein. When refeeding, levels of anabolic hormones increase and levels of circulating nutrients move to serve intracellular functions. Overfeeding and the hypermetabolic state it produces can severely burden the cardiovascular and respiratory systems of previously depleted patients. Overfeeding substrate without sufficient micronutrients can precipitate serious hypokalemia, hypophosphatemia, hypomagnesemia, and other micronutrient deficiencies. Depleted patients have reduced body cell mass and may have very low calorie requirements. Prevention of refeeding syndrome involves ensuring that feeding begins slowly at calorie levels below maintenance needs and that they are gradually advanced to maintenance needs. Micronutrient requirements (particularly for phosphorus, potassium, and magnesium) should be anticipated, closely monitored, and corrected as needed. Restoration of body cell mass can then be targeted with physical therapy and additional calories as the patient improves.

Azotemia, Hypernatremia, and Dehydration (Tube Feeding Syndrome)

Tube feeding syndrome includes azotemia, hypernatremia, and dehydration that result from use of high-protein tube feedings with a high renal solute load, typically with inadequate amounts of water. Classic cases involved elderly patients given concentrated, high-protein feedings, but the problem has also occurred with misuse of modular products and powdered formulas.[96,97] In some cases, the concentration and osmolality of the tube feeding may have resulted in diarrhea, which increased water losses. Because many of the patients were obtunded or unable to speak, they could not express thirst. The combination of high solute load and negative fluid balance resulted in dehydration and subsequent increases in blood urea nitrogen and hypernatremia. Hypernatremia occurred, not because of excessive sodium intake, but rather as a result of hemoconcentration. Most commercial products have safe renal solute loads, but use of modular protein sources, concentrated powdered enteral feedings, and "homemade" high protein tube feedings can create opportunities for excess solute load. Prevention simply requires the provision of adequate fluid (at least 1 ml/kcal plus any unusual respiratory, renal, or GI losses) and avoiding protein loads greater than 1.5 g/kg of desirable body weight. In particular, infants, the elderly, and those who cannot communicate or control feedings should be carefully monitored.

Constipation

The occurrence of constipation is less common in the acute care setting than in long-term care settings, but in one series of 400 tube-fed patients, 15% required intervention for constipation.[41] The more common risk factors for constipation include inadequate hydration, inactivity, immobilization, neuromuscular disorders, hypothyroidism, inadequate fiber intake, hypokalemia, previous misuse of laxatives, and GI motility disorders. Use of medications such as anticholinergics, nonsteroidal antiinflammatory agents, narcotics, bile acid sequestrants, furosemide, nitroglycerine, and antidepressants has been associated with constipation.[98-100] Satisfactory resolution may not always be possible, but encouraging the patient to ambulate as much as possible and providing adequate water and fiber in feedings may help. Pharmacologic interventions—stool softeners, appropriate laxatives, or prokinetic agents—may be required.

Risk-Benefit Decisions in Enteral Feeding

Generally speaking, when typical indications for tube feeding are met, the benefits of enteral nutrition support outweigh the potential complications (Box 17-5). Frequency and severity of complications related to the placement and use of enteral feedings can be reduced considerably by interdisciplinary quality improvement protocols and guidelines. In some cases, risks of complications are inherently greater than the benefits associated with tube feeding, regardless of the quality of care provided, and these must be anticipated. Patients at increased risk for complications include those with significant malnutrition, GI dysfunction or malignancies, metabolic disease, advanced age, dementia and obtundation, unprotected airway, tracheal intubation, reflux, compromised immune function, persons receiving multiple medications, and patients under the care of persons not trained in placement and delivery of tube feeding.[6,7,15,43] The number of potential problems underscores the need for caution in the placement, delivery, and monitoring of the patients feeding apparatus and formula.

In some cases, complications associated with enteral feedings can be significant. Potential morbidity and mortality associated with enteral feeding complications must be weighed against the realistic expectations for improvements in nutrition,

functional status, and quality of life. Caretakers and patients need to be informed about risks, benefits, and costs.[101-103]

Quality Assurance and Improvement in Enteral Nutrition

The objectives of total quality management programs in health care are to evaluate and improve important aspects of patient care. Emphasis is on outcomes, rather than evaluating processes in patient care. Certainly, enteral nutrition qualifies as an important aspect of patient care. Systematic evaluation of enteral feeding practices can improve documentation of care, decrease morbidity and mortality, improve patient satisfaction and confidence in the health care team, and decrease health care costs. Protocols, standards of care, clinical indicators, and clinical pathways can be used as guides measuring practice.[104-107]

Quality improvement in enteral nutrition is best tailored to the specific setting or patient mix. Examples of aspects to be evaluated in quality improvement programs include significant mechanical, metabolic, and GI complications. Examples of indicators used in evaluating enteral nutrition programs include the adequacy of support, prevalence of aspiration, diarrhea, hyperglycemia, or hypophosphatemia; use of rectal tubes; tube replacements; and documentation of patient instruction regarding placement and use of feedings. The results of quality improvement programs can (1) point out the need for changes in policies, procedures, equipment, communication tools or training; (2) recognize good care; (3) document justified expenditures of resources; and (4) create solutions and innovations in patient care.

BOX 17-5

Increased Risk of Complications with Enteral Feeding

- Gastrointestinal dysfunction
- Prior abdominal surgeries
- Dementia, decreased level of consciousness
- Advanced age
- Tracheal intubation, unprotected airway
- Dysphagia, lower esophageal sphincter dysfunction, reflux
- Compromised immune function
- Significant malnutrition
- Caretakers unfamiliar with enteral placement and delivery

REFERENCES

1. Romand JA, Suter PM: Enteral nutrition: the right stuff at the right time in the right place, *Crit Care Med* 28(7):2671, 2000.
2. Kudsk KA: Importance of enteral feeding in maintaining gut integrity, *Tech Gastroent Endosc* 3(2):22, 2001.
3. Mercadante S: Parenteral versus enteral nutrition in cancer patients: indications and practice, *Support Care Cancer* 6(2):85, 1998.
4. Minard G, Kudsk KA: Nutritional support and infections: does the route matter? *World J Surg* 22(2):213, 1998.
5. Rehfeld JF: The new biology of gastrointestinal hormones, *Phys Rev* 78(4):1087, 1998.
6. Jolliet P, et al: Enteral nutrition in intensive care patients: a practical approach, *Clin Nutr* 18(1):47, 1999.
7. Minard G: Enteral access, *Nutr Clin Pract* 9(5):172, 1994.
8. Mobarhan S, Trumbore LS: Enteral tube feeding: a clinical perspective on recent advances, *Nutr Rev* 49(5):129, 1991.
9. Wolfe RT, Fosnocht DE, Linscott MS: Atomized lidocaine as topical anesthesia for nasogastric tube placement: a randomized double blind, placebo-controlled trial, *Ann Emerg Med* 35(5):421, 2000.
10. Freij RM, Mullett ST: Gastrointestinal insertion of a nasogastric tube in a non-trauma patient, *J Accid Emerg Med* 14(1):45, 1997.
11. Levy H: Nasogastric and nasoenteric feeding tubes, *Gastroentest Endosc Clin North Am* 8(3):529, 1998.
12. Gharpure V, et al: Indicators of postpyloric feeding tube placement in children, *Crit Care Med* 28(8):2962, 2000.
13. Thomas BW, Falcone RE: Confirmation of nasogastric tube placement by colormetric indicator detection of carbon dioxide: a preliminary report, *J Am Coll Nutr* 17(2):195, 1998.
14. Metheny NA, Aud MA, Wunderlich RJ: A survey of methods used to detect pulmonary aspiration of enteral formula in intubated tube-fed patients, *Am J Crit Care* 8(3):160, 1999.
15. Echevarria CG, Winkler MF: Enteral feeding challenges in critically ill patients, *Top Clin Nutr* 16(1):37, 2000.

16. Lucas CE, Yu P, Vlakos A, Ledgerwood AM, et al: Lower esophageal sphincter dysfunction often precludes safe gastric feeding in stroke patients, *Arch Surg* 134(1):55, 1999.

17. Noviski N, Yehuda YB, Serour F, Gorenstein A, Mandelberg A, et al: Does the size of nasogastric tubes affect gastroesophageal reflux in children? *J Pediatr Gastroenterol Nutr* 29(4):448, 1999.

18. Faries MB, Rombeau JL: Use of gastrostomy and combined gastrojejunostomy tubes for enteral feeding, *World J Surg* 23(6):603, 1999.

19. Allen JW, Spain DA: Open and laparoscopic surgical techniques for obtaining enteral access, *Tech Gastroent Endosc* 3(1):50, 2001.

20. Sarr MG: Appropriate use, complications and advantages demonstrated in 500 consecutive needle catheter jejunostomies, *Br J Surg* 86(4):557, 1999.

21. McClave SA: Managing complications of percutaneous and nasoenteric feeding tubes, *Tech Gastroent Endosc* 3(1):62, 2001.

22. De Baere T, Chapot R, Kuoch V, Chevallier P, et al: Percutaneous gastrostomy with fluoroscopic guidance: single-center experience in 500 consecutive cancer patients, *Radiology* 210(3):651, 1999.

23. Mathus-Vliegen LMH, Koning H: Percutaneous endoscopic gastrostomy and gastrojejunostomy: a critical reappraisal of patient selection, tube function and the feasibility of patient support during extended follow-up, *Gastroentest Endosc* 50(6):746, 1999.

24. De Legge M: Enteral access—the foundation of feeding: endoscopic nasoenteric tube placement, *Tech Gastroent Endosc* 3(1):22, 2001.

25. Ginsberg GG: Direct percutaneous endoscopic jejunostomy, *Tech Gastroent Endosc* 3(1):42, 2001.

26. Monturo CA: Enteral access device selection, *Nutr Clin Prac* 5(5):207, 1990.

27. Marcuard SP, Stegall KS: Unclogging feeding tubes with pancreatic enzymes, *J Parenter Enteral Nutr* 14(2):198, 1990.

28. Nicholson LJ: Declogging small-bore feeding tubes, *J Parenter Enteral Nutr* 11(6):594, 1987.

29. Wilson MF, Haynes-Johnson V: Cranberry juice or water? A comparison of feeding-tube irrigants, *Nutr Supp Serv* 7(7):23, 1987.

30. Cutie AJ, Altman E, Lenkel L: Compatibility of enteral products with commonly employed drug additives, *J Parenter Enteral Nutr* 7(2):186, 1983

31. Estoup M: Approaches and limitations of medication delivery in patients with enteral feeding tubes, *Crit Care Nurs* 14(1):68, 1994.

32. Golioto M, Lytle J, Jowell P: Re-establishing patency of a small bore feeding tube with complete occlusion—a novel use for an ERCP catheter, *Nutr Clin Prac* 16(5):284, 2001.

33. Byrum B: *Characteristics of bacterial growth in ready-to-feed liquid nutritional products. Report of the Ross Workshop on Contamination of Enteral Feeding Products During Clinical Usage,* Columbus, OH, 1983, Ross Laboratories.

34. Beattie TK, Anderton A: Microbial evaluation of four enteral feeding systems which have been deliberately subjected to faulty handling procedures, *J Hosp Infect* 42(1):11, 1999.

35. Storm HM: Closed-system enteral feedings: point-counterpoint, *Nutr Clin Prac* 15(4):193, 2000.

36. Orvieto A, Kirsch J, Goldberger J: Evaluation of enteral delivery systems, *Nutr Supp Serv* 3(4):44, 1983.

37. Malone M, Aftahi S, Howard L: Inadvertent intravenous administration of an elemental enteral nutritional formula, *Ann Pharmacother* 27(10):1187, 1993.

38. Ulicny KS, Korelitz JL: Multiorgan failure from the inadvertent intravenous administration of enteral feeding, *J Parenter Enteral Nutr* 13(6):658, 1989.

39. Goff KL: The nuts and bolts of enteral infusion pumps, *Medsurg Nurs* 6(1):9, 1997.

40. Dietscher JE, Foulks CJ, Watts M: Accuracy of enteral pumps: in vitro performance, *J Parenter Enteral Nutr* 18(4):359, 1994.

41. Montejo JC: Enteral nutrition-related gastrointestinal complications in critically ill patients: a multicenter study, *Crit Care Med* 27(8):1447, 1999.

42. Smith CE, Marien L, Brogdon C, et al: Diarrhea associated with tube feeding in mechanically ventilated critically ill patients, *Nurs Res* 39(3):148, 1990.

43. Mallampalli A, McClave SA: Monitoring patients on enteral tube feeds, *Tech Gastroent Surg* 3(1):55, 2001.

44. Frankenfield DC, Beyer PL: Dietary fiber and bowel function in tube-fed patients, *J Am Diet Assoc* 91(5):590, 1991.

45. Eisenberg PG: Causes of diarrhea in tube-fed patients: a comprehensive approach to diagnosis and management, *Nutr Clin Prac* 8(3):119, 1993.

46. Cunha BA: Nosocomial diarrhea, *Crit Care Clin* 14(2):329, 1998.

47. Clausen MR, Bonnan H, Tvede M, Mortensen PB: Colonic fermentation to short-chain fatty acid is decreased in antibiotic-associated diarrhea, *Gastroenterology* 101(6):1497, 1991.

48. Grossman RF: The relationship of absorption characteristics and gastrointestinal side effects of oral antimicrobial agents, *Clin Ther* 13(1):189, 1991.

49. Vogel LC: Antibiotic-induced diarrhea, *Orthop Nurs* 14(2):38, 1995.

50. Kelly CP, Lamont JT: *Clostridium difficile* infection, *Annu Rev Med* 49:375, 1998.

51. Job ML, Jacobs NF: Drug induced *Clostridium difficile*-associated disease, *Drug Saf* 17(1):37, 1997.

52. Kkornblau S, et al: Management of cancer treatment-related diarrhea. Issues and therapeutic strategies, *J Pain Symptom Manage* 19(2):118, 2000.

53. Ramakrisna BS: Prevalence of intestinal pathogens in HIV patients with diarrhea: implications for treatment, *Indian J Pediatr* 66(1):85-91, 1999.

54. Moe G: Enteral feeding and infection in the immunocompromised patient, *Nutr Clin Pract* 6(2):55-64, 1991.

55. Edes TE, Walk BE, Austin JL: Diarrhea in tube-fed patients: feeding formula not necessarily the cause, *Am J Med* 88(2):91, 1990.

56. Reilly JP: Safety profile of the proton-pump inhibitors, *Am J Health Sys Pharm* 56(54):S11.

57. Shah S, et al: Gastric acid suppression does not promote clostridial diarrhea in the elderly, *Q J Med* 93(3):175-181, 2000.

58. Hyams JS: Sorbitol intolerance: an unappreciated cause of functional gastrointestinal complaints, *Gastroenterology* 84(1):30, 1983.

59. Mora RJL Malnutrition: organic and functional consequences, *World J Surg* 23(6):530, 1999.

60. Cunningham-Rundles S, Lin DH: Nutrition and the immune system of the gut, *Nutrition* 14(7-8):573, 1998.

61. Welsh FK, et al: Gut barrier function in malnourished patients, *Gut* 42(3):396, 1998.

62. Patchell CJ, et al: Reducing contamination of enteral feeds, *Arch Dis Child* 78(2):166, 1998.

63. Van-Loo J, et al: Functional food properties of non-digestible oligosaccharides: a consensus report from the ENDO project, *Br J Nutr* 81(2):121, 1999.

64. Gibson GR: Dietary modulation of the human gut microflora using prebiotics, *Br J Nutr* 80(2):S209, 1998.

65. Ward PB, Young GP: Dynamics of *Clostridium difficile* infection. Control using diet, *Adv Exp Med Biol* 412:63, 1997.

66. Emery EA et al: Banana flakes control diarrhea in enterally fed patients, *Nutr Clin Prac* 12(2):72, 1997.

67. Cummings JH, Macfarlane GT, Englyst HN: Prebiotic digestion and fermentation, *Am J Clin Nutr* 73:S415, 2001.

68. Marteau PR, et al: Protection from gastrointestinal diseases with the use of probiotics, *Am J Clin Nutr* 73:S430.

69. Cresci GA: The use of probiotics with the treatment of diarrhea, *Nutr Clin Prac* 16(1):30, 2001.

70. Elpern EH: Pulmonary aspiration in hospitalized adults, *Nutr Clin Prac* 12(1):5, 1997.

71. Zaloga GP: Blind placement of enteric feeding tubes, *Tech Gastroent Endosc* 3(1):9, 2001.

72. Belnap, DC, Davidson LJ, Flournoy DJ: Microorganism and diarrhea in enterally fed intensive care unit patients, *J Parenter Enteral Nutr* 14(6):622, 1990.

73. Bussy V, Marechal F, Masca S: Microbial contamination of enteral feeding tubes occurring during nutritional treatment, *J Parenter Enteral Nutr* 16(6):552-557, 1992.

74. Heyland DK, Wood G: Effect of acid feeds on feeding system contamination, *Nutr Clin Prac* 13(3):S33, 1998.

75. Fagerman KE: Limiting bacterial contamination of enteral nutrient solutions: 6-year history with reduction of contamination at two institutions, *Nutr Clin Prac* 7(1):31, 1992.

76. Oie S, Kamiya A, Hironaga K, Koshiro A, et al: Microbial contamination of enteral feeding solution and its prevention, *Am J Infect Control* 21(1):34, 1993.

77. Kohn-Keeth C, Shott S, Olree K: The effects of rinsing enteral delivery sets on formula contamination, *Nutr Clin Prac* 11(6):269, 1996.

78. Lucia-Rocha-Carvalho M, et al: Hazard analysis and critical control point system approach in the evaluation of environmental and procedural sources of contamination of enteral feedings in three hospitals, *J Parenter Enteral Nutr* 24(5):296, 2000.

79. Oliviera MH, et al: Microbial quality of reconstituted enteral formulations used in hospitals, *Nutrition* 16(9):729, 2000.
80. Beattie TK, Anderton A: Decanting versus sterile pre-filled nutrient containers—the microbial risks in enteral feeding, *Int J Environ Health Res* 11(1):81, 2001.
81. Dentinger B, Faucher KJ, Ostrom SM, Schmidl MK, et al: Controlling bacteral contamination of an enteral formula through the use of a unique closed system: contamination, enteral formulas, closed system, *Nutrition* 11(6):747, 1995.
82. Mathus-Vliegen LM, Binnekade JM, deHaan RJ: Bacterial contamination of ready-to-use 1-L feeding bottles and administration sets in severely compromised intensive care patients, *Crit Care Med* 28(1):67, 2000.
83. Moffitt et al: Clinical and laboratory evaluation of a closed enteral feeding system under cyclic feeding conditions, *Nutrition* 13(7-8):622, 1997.
84. Bott L, et al: Contamination of gastrostomy feeding systems in children in a home-based enteral nutrition program, *J Pediatr Gastroenterol Nutr* 33(3):266, 2001.
85. Breach C, Saldanha LG: Tube feeding complications, Part III: Metabolic, *Nutr Supp Serv* 8(8):16, 1988.
86. Fall PJ: Hyponatremia and hypernatremia. A systematic approach to causes and their correction, *Postgrad Med* 107(5):75, 2000.
87. Mathews JJ, Aleem RF, Gamelli RL: Cost reductions strategies in burn nutrition services: adjustments in dietary treatment of patients with hyponatremia and hypophosphatemia, *J Burn Care Rehabil* 20(1):80-4.
88. Sacks GS, Walker J, Dickerson RN, et al: Observations of hypophosphatemia and its management in nutrition support, *Nutr Clin Pract* 9(3):105, 1994.
89. Ogawa T, Kamikubo K: Hypokalemic periodic paralysis associated with hypophosphatemia in a patient with hyperinsulinemia, *Am J Med Sci* 318(1):69, 1999.
90. Gearhart MO, Sorg TB: Foscarnet-induced severe hypomagnesemia and other electrolyte disorders, *Ann Pharmacother* 27(3):285, 1993.
91. Klein KJ, Stanek GS, Wiles CE: Overfeeding macronutrients to critically ill adults: metabolic complications, *J Am Diet Assoc* 98(7):795, 1998.
92. Fisher M, Simpser E, Schneider M: Hypophosphatemia secondary to oral refeeding in anorexia nervosa, *Int J Eat Disord* 28(2):181, 2000.
93. Talpers SS, Romberger DJ, Bunce SB, Pingleton SK: Nutritionally associated increased carbon dioxide production. Excess total calories vs high proportion of carbohydrate calories, *Chest* 102(2):551, 1992.
94. Coulston AM: Clinical experience with modified enteral formulas for patients with diabetes, *Clin Nutr* 17(S2):S46, 1997.
95. Campbell SM, Schiller MR: Considerations for enteral nutrition support of patients with diabetes, *Topics Clin Nutr* 7(1):23, 1991.
96. Gault HM, Dixon ME, Doyle M, Cohen WM: Hypernatremia, azotemia, and dehydration due to high-protein tube feeding, *Ann Intern Med* 68(4):778, 1968.
97. Masterton JP, Dudley HAF: Design of tube feeds for surgical patients, *Br Med J* 5362:909, 1963.
98. Rao SC: Functional colonic and anorectal disorders, *Postgrad Med* 98(5):115, 1995.
99. Stewart RB, Moore MT, Marks RG, Hale WE, et al: Correlates of constipation in an ambulatory elderly population, *Am J Gastroent* 87(7):859, 1992.
100. Wilson JA: Constipation in the elderly, *Clin Geriatr Med* 15(3):499, 1999.
101. Callahan CM, Haag KM, Weinberger M, Buchanan NN, et al: Outcomes of percutaneous endoscopic gastrostomy among older adults in a community setting, *J Am Geriatr Soc* 48(9):1048, 2000.
102. Mitchell SL, Berkowitz RE, Lawson FM, Lipsitz LA, et al: A cross-national survey of tube-feeding decisions in cognitively impaired older persons, *J Am Geriatr Soc* 48(4):391, 2000.
103. Rabeneck L, McCullough LB, Wray NP: Ethically justified, clinically comprehensive guidelines for percutaneous endoscopic gastrostomy tube placement, *Lancet* 349(9050):496, 1997.
104. Kushner RF, Ayello EA, Beyer PL, et al: National Coordinating Committee clinical indicators of nutrition care, *J Am Diet Assoc* 94(10):1168, 1994.
105. Gallagher AL, Onda RM: Using quality assurance procedures to improve compliance with standards of nutrition care for patients receiving isotonic tube feedings, *J Am Diet Assoc* 93(6):678, 1993.
106. Clemmer TP, et al: Results of a collaborative quality improvement program on outcomes and costs in a tertiary critical care unit, *Crit Care Med* 27(9):1768, 1999.
107. Wilmore DW: Nutrition and metabolic support in the 21st century, *J Parenter Enteral Nutr* 24(1):1, 2000.

Parenteral Nutrition 18

Annalynn Skipper, MS, RD, FADA, CNSD

PARENTERAL nutrition (PN) has been designated a major medical advance of the twentieth century, both because it enabled feeding of many patients who formerly would have died of malnutrition and because it focused attention on nutrition in medicine. PN was developed to provide intravenous nutrition to patients who were unable to tolerate gastrointestinal feedings. Formulas are composed of protein, carbohydrate, lipids, vitamins, minerals, and electrolytes in amounts specific to the patient's needs. PN can be provided through a central vein that can accommodate more concentrated solutions in smaller volumes or through a peripheral vein that accommodates larger volumes of dilute solution.

Historical Overview

Provision of PN that contained adequate amounts of protein, carbohydrate, fat, and micronutrients has been technically feasible only since the late 1960s; however, PN has been a subject of experimentation since the 1600s, when sharpened quills were used to administer a mixture of milk and wine into the veins of dogs.[1] A significant advance came in the 1800s, when intravenous saline was administered to humans as a treatment for cholera. By the 1930s a 5% glucose solution was also available for maintenance of fluid balance. Protein hydrolysates for intravenous administration were developed in Sweden during the 1940s.[2] These two macronutrient sources could be administered via peripheral veins, but the calories were inadequate to spare protein. Dextrose solutions in concentrations greater than 10% were not tolerated well, because of their high osmolarity. Therefore, administration of adequate dextrose to meet calorie needs also resulted in large volumes of fluid being given to patients who were least able to tolerate them.[3]

A search for a concentrated calorie source ensued. Two potential energy sources were alcohol, which contains 7 kcal/g, and fat, which contains 9 kcal/g. Early experiments with alcohol demonstrated undesirable side effects, including hepatotoxicity when alcohol was administered in amounts large enough to provide adequate calories, so investigations of alcohol were discontinued.

Initial experience with lipid emulsions was also discouraging. Emulsions prepared from cottonseed oil became commercially available in 1957 but were removed from the U.S. market following reports of jaundice, fever, and bleeding.[4] In Europe, however, experimentation with lipids continued, and emulsions made from soybean oil were administered successfully through peripheral veins.[2]

Another significant advance occurred in 1967, when Mogil and others demonstrated that the subclavian vein could be cannulated.[5] This enabled administration of concentrated nutrient solutions and set the stage for the development of parenteral formulas made from concentrated dextrose and protein hydrolysates. A 1968 report by Dudrick and others[6] documented growth in beagle puppies receiving nutrition by vein and was the genesis of PN. The first report of PN in a human came the next year when it was administered to an infant girl with intestinal atresia.[7]

Subsequent developments quickly advanced toward the solutions in use today. During the mid 1970s crystalline amino acids synthesized from soybeans replaced protein hydrolysates.[2] Recommendations for standard amounts of vitamins and minerals were published in 1975 and 1979, respectively.[8,9] Lipids were reintroduced in the United States in 1976. In 1983, total nutrient admixture of amino acids, dextrose, and lipids was approved by the U.S. Food and Drug Administration (FDA).[10] Throughout the 1970s and 1980s specialized amino acid formulations were developed for renal[11-13] and hepatic failure[14] and for sepsis and stress.[15] Development of new access devices and delivery systems continued throughout the 1980s as well.[16] Proliferation of nutrition support teams, dissemination of nutrition knowledge, and experience with PN dramatically reduced the complications described in early reports, making PN safe when administered by appropriately trained clinicians.

Rationale for Parenteral Feeding

PN was originally developed to nourish individuals whose gastrointestinal tract was not capable of digesting and absorbing nutrients. The ultimate indication for PN continues to be a nonfunctioning gastrointestinal tract and documented inability to tolerate enteral feeding. In addition, the patient should be at nutritional risk. This can be defined as a loss of at least 10% of preillness weight in a patient who has taken nothing by mouth for 5 to 7 days.[17] PN is not thought to be beneficial unless used for at least 7 to 14 days.[17] Therefore, it is selected when a particular indication is expected to continue for more than 7 to 14 days.

Guidelines for Patient Selection

The potential for serious complications, and the expense of PN, have led several organizations to develop guidelines to help clinicians select patients who will benefit from PN. The first of these guidelines was published by the American Society for Parenteral and Enteral Nutrition (ASPEN) in 1986[18] and revised and expanded in 1993.[19] The third edition of these guidelines was released in 2002.[17] The American College of Physicians (ACP) published a meta-analysis of perioperative PN studies in 1987[20] and a subsequent meta-analysis of PN studies with cancer chemotherapy in 1989.[21] Also in 1989, the American Gastroenterology Association (AGA) published guidelines for PN.[22] These initiatives resulted in practice guidelines for PN that have helped identify inappropriate PN and may have improved practice.[23,24] A significant meta-analysis was published in 1997,[25] and more recently, the Institute of Medicine prepared a report entitled "The Role of Nutrition in Maintaining Health in the Nation's Elderly,"[26] which reviews the efficacy of PN. The AGA guidelines were updated in 2001.[27] A summary of these guidelines follows.

Malignant Disease

Cancer patients comprise the largest percentage of patients receiving long-term PN.[28] PN may be useful for cancer patients if nutritional compromise is suspected[22] or if treatment is expected to cause gastrointestinal disturbances that will last longer than 1 week.[17, 27] As compared with those who did not receive PN, cancer patients who did had four times greater risks of infection, a lower survival rate (81%), and no difference in toxicity from chemotherapy.[21,27] PN is unlikely to benefit patients whose malignancy is documented to be unresponsive to chemotherapy or radiation therapy. It is agreed that PN is not a treatment for cancer but for the associated malnutrition.[17,27]

Perioperative Parenteral Nutrition

Preoperative PN is recommended for severely malnourished patients who are having surgery that is expected to render them *nil per os* (NPO) for more than 7 to 10 days and for previously well-nourished patients who develop postoperative complications that are usually associated with NPO for more than 7 to 10 days. It is agreed that routine use of preoperative PN is not indicated unless patients are severely malnourished and that PN should be initiated at the time of surgery or within 3 days afterward.[17,25]

Inflammatory Bowel Disease

PN facilitates remission in 60% to 80% of patients with acute exacerbations of Crohn's disease, but nutrition support does not affect disease activity with acute exacerbations of ulcerative colitis.[17,25] Enteral nutrition is generally preferred with acute Crohn's disease unless high-output fistulas are present.[17] If enteral feeding is not possible, PN can be used to preserve lean body mass while surgery is being considered.[25]

Short-Bowel Syndrome

PN should be administered to patients with short-bowel syndrome who cannot absorb adequate nutrients by mouth. For those with less than 60 cm of small bowel,[17] PN may be necessary for an indefinite period and is lifesaving therapy for these individuals.[25]

Hepatic Disease

PN has been recommended for nutritionally compromised patients with advanced chronic liver failure. Branched-chain amino acid (BCAA) formulas may enable greater protein intake in patients with chronic encephalopathy who are intolerant to standard amino acid formulas, but they have not been shown to be superior to standard amino acid formulas.[17, 25]

Pancreatitis

PN has been recommended if abdominal pain, ascites, or increases in the serum amylase value preclude enteral nutrition. An additional indication is increased fistula output caused by enteral feedings.[17] Lipid emulsions are considered safe in pancreatitis if serum triglycerides remain below 400 mg/dl during the infusion.[17,25]

Critical Care

Nutrition support should be initiated in patients who are not expected to resume oral feeding for 7 days.[17,22]

Renal Failure

For patients with renal failure, PN can be used as indicated to maintain optimal calorie intake. Amino acid formulations that contain essential amino acids alone are no longer recommended.[17]

Acquired Immunodeficiency Syndrome

Data are insufficient to support the routine use of PN for patients who have acquired immunodeficiency syndrome (AIDS). [17,26,27] It is suggested that the risks and benefits of PN should be explained to patients before therapy is instituted.[22] Care should be taken to minimize the risk of infection for this patient population.[17]

Respiratory Failure

Manipulation of carbohydrate-lipid ratios can reduce carbon dioxide production but are unlikely to modify the respiratory quotient or to benefit patients who are not overfed.[17] Thus routine use of modified carbohydrate and fat formulations is not warrented. [1]

Eating Disorders

PN may be useful for patients with eating disorders who have severe malnutrition (as demonstrated by less than 70% of ideal body weight or greater than 30% recent weight loss) and who cannot tolerate enteral feeding for physical or emotional reasons. Because these patients are at risk for complications associated with refeeding syndrome, gradual initiation of PN is recommended.[17, 1]

Other Clinical Indications

PN is safe in pregnancy and is recommended for patients with intestinal pseudoobstruction.[19] It is also recommended for neurologic problems in patients without a functioning gastrointestinal tract.[19] PN is used in many situations that fall outside existing guidelines. Current guidelines will continue to be updated as knowledge and practice advance.

Contraindications to Parenteral Nutrition

The most important contraindication to PN is a functioning gastrointestinal tract.[17] Additionally, PN should not be used when the patient's prognosis does not warrant aggressive nutrition support or when the risks outweigh the benefits.

Ethical Considerations

Because, when compared to starvation, PN has the potential to prolong life, withholding or withdrawing it is often the subject of debate. In recent years, increased attention has been focused on decisions to withhold or withdraw nutrition from critically ill or comatose patients. Failure of the judicial system to provide a consistent approach in these cases has led to confusion about withholding and withdrawing parenteral feeding.

Ethical issues are less likely to surface when the patient's wishes are known. In many states, patients can provide advanced directives about their care. Prepared in advance of illness, such documents usually refer to ventilator support, surgical intervention, medications, and feeding; however, the wording in these documents rarely distinguishes among oral feeding, tube feeding, and PN, and few patients are aware of the advantages, disadvantages, and costs of the various options.

When ethical questions about feeding arise, it is appropriate to avoid investing PN with social or symbolic meaning. It is recommended that PN be regarded as treatment for malnutrition rather than as a food source.[18] It is also agreed that responsible decisions (made together by the patient, family members, physician, nurse, and nutrition support team members) to withhold or withdraw PN cannot be construed as causing death. In addition, there is no legal or ethical requirement that, once started, a treatment must continue. The point could be made that to withdraw support is no different from the decision not to initiate it[19] (see Chapter 44).

Economic Considerations

Studies documenting the benefits of PN are limited by the ethical impropriety of withholding feeding from those who are malnourished, but PN costs can be evaluated by two methods.[28] Cost-benefit analysis determines the cost of a particular therapy and then quantifies the results of its use in dollars. Cost-effectiveness analysis also determines the cost of a therapy and then determines the cost or savings by measuring a related effect. For example, the costs of PN would be determined in both cost-benefit analysis and cost-effectiveness analysis. In cost-benefit analysis the benefits of using PN would be measured by determining reduced wound infection, length of stay, or another predetermined benefit. In cost-effectiveness analysis, the cost of a wound infection or hospital stay would be determined and the costs of PN compared to them.

To perform cost-benefit or cost-effectiveness analysis, it is essential to determine accurate costs of PN. Less expensive than many other common therapies, long-term PN can nevertheless generate significant charges to third-party payers.[29] Charges for PN are based on raw materials, labor, and overhead. These charges for PN may also be inflated to cover fees for professional and technical staff, fees for laboratory or other tests, and fees for pumps, tubing, and other accessories of nutrient delivery.[30]

Costs of raw materials used to compound PN have declined steadily as production costs have decreased and hospitals have negotiated favorable prices. Labor costs for compounding have declined with increased use of pharmacy technicians and automated compounders. Overhead costs vary greatly from one institution to another and throughout the country. Costs also vary by product and equipment selection, type of professional service performed, level of clinicians' training, and customary professional fees. It is appropriate to consider these factors to ensure that cost comparisons are fair and accurate.

Selecting and Establishing Parenteral Access

Before initiating PN, venous access is established. Venous access is selected according to how long it is expected to be used, the limitations presented by the patient's condition, and the availability of equipment and facilities. Central or peripheral veins may be used to provide PN. *Peripheral access* uses the small veins of the extremities, usually hands or forearms. The term *central access* refers to the large veins in the trunk. Central veins that can be used for PN include the subclavian, internal jugular, and femoral veins. Because central venous access is most often used for PN, it is discussed first.

Central Access

Orr and Ryder[31] describe four types of central venous access devices: tunneled catheters, implanted ports, short-term catheters, and peripherally inserted central catheters (PICCs). Tunneled catheters are placed in the operating room by a surgeon. They most often enter the vein on the upper chest wall and are tunneled away from the vein to an exit site near the xiphoid process or the axilla or on the abdominal wall. They are considered permanent and with proper care can be left in place for several years. Tunneled catheters are available in single-, double-, or triple-lumen models. Multiple-lumen models accommodate infusions of medications, fluids, or blood products in addition to PN. They are useful for patients who require continuous pain medications or who receive frequent doses of intravenous medications.

Implantable ports are similar to tunneled catheters in that they must be placed in the operating room by a surgeon. They are available with single or double ports and are suitable for long-term access. Unlike tunneled catheters, they lie completely under the skin, and they may be accepted well by patients with body image concerns. Because they are usually placed just below the clavicle on the chest wall, they may be difficult for the patient to cannulate. Nursing intervention may be required to change needles used to gain access to these ports.

Short-term access is provided via a central catheter inserted percutaneously at the bedside under local anesthesia. These catheters are available in single- or multiple-lumen configurations.

The risk of catheter infection in patients receiving PN was greater with triple-lumen catheters than with single-lumen catheters.[32] Another study[33] found no difference between the two in a critically ill patient population, but not all were used for PN. Management of catheters by a team of trained personnel has been shown to reduce the rate of catheter infection.[19]

Percutaneously inserted central catheters enter the antecubital vein and are threaded into the subclavian vein. In many states, nurses may place these catheters at the bedside, thus avoiding the expense of an operative fee generated with tunneled catheters. Because they ultimately reside in a vein of suitable size to accommodate concentrated solutions, they may be used for PN.[34] At least one study demonstrated that infections are not increased with PICC catheters, but that mechanical complications such as leaking are common.[35]

Peripheral Access

Peripheral access with conventional intravenous needles may also be used for nutrition support; however, peripheral veins are easily sclerosed by hypertonic parenteral solutions.[36] To minimize irritation to the vein, it is recommended that the osmolarity of peripheral parenteral nutrition (PPN) solutions be limited to 900 mOsm/L.[37] Addition of heparin and hydrocortisone has been shown to improve tolerance to PPN.[38] Even with appropriate PPN, intravenous sites may have to be changed frequently to maintain venous patency.[39]

The volume of fluid required for nutrient delivery limits the clinical utility of PPN. For example, 3 L of the PPN solution shown in Table 18-1 provides 1634 calories with the addition of 250 ml of 20% lipids (3.25 L total). PPN may be useful when the outcome of the situation necessitating nutrition support is unclear, and it is desirable to provide some nutrition without the risk and expense of inserting a central line. One example is a malnourished patient who has a bowel obstruction that might either resolve or progress to surgery within a few days. Another example is the first or second admission for hyperemesis gravidarum during the first trimester of pregnancy because resolution of symptoms may be reasonably expected.

TABLE 18-1

Examples of Typical Parenteral Nutrition Solutions

FOR PERIPHERAL ADMINISTRATION:*

Amino acids	35 g
Dextrose	70 g
Sodium chloride	15 mEq
Potassium acetate	30 mEq
Sodium phosphate	20 mEq
Magnesium sulfate	8 mEq
Calcium gluconate	9.4 mEq
Multiple vitamins	10 ml
Trace elements	3 ml
Heparin	200 units

Administer 250 ml of 20% lipids daily to provide 878 kcal and 35 g of protein in 1250 ml of fluid.

FOR CENTRAL ADMINISTRATION:*

Amino acids	60 g
Dextrose	250 g
Sodium chloride	35 mEq
Potassium acetate	30 mEq
Sodium phosphate	20 mEq
Magnesium sulfate	8 mEq
Calcium gluconate	9.4 mEq
Multiple vitamins	10 ml
Trace elements	3 ml
Heparin	1000 units

Administer 250 ml of 20% lipids daily to provide 1590 kcal and 60 g of protein in 1250 ml of fluid.

*Nutrient content expressed per liter.

Parenteral Macronutrients

PN formulas are usually composed of protein in the form of amino acids, carbohydrate as dextrose, and fat as lipid emulsion in ratios tailored to the needs of the individual patient.

Protein

The primary function of protein in PN is to maintain nitrogen balance, thus preventing skeletal muscle from being degraded for gluconeogenesis. Normal, healthy adults' protein requirement is well-defined: 0.8 g/kg per day.[40] Recommendations for protein intake in critical illness vary. Cerra found that 2.0 g of protein per kilogram body weight per day was optimal in severe stress.[41] Shaw observed maximum protein synthesis when severely septic patients were given 1.5 g of protein per kilogram of body weight.[42] Larsson found no improvement in nitrogen balance when nitrogen was administered in amounts greater than 1.25 g/kg.[43] For most patients, a range of 1.2 to 2.0 g/kg per day of protein is appropriate.

Recommended protein intake in renal disease varies according to the stage of renal failure and the type of treatment. With peritoneal dialysis, 1.2 to 1.5 g of protein per kilogram of ideal body weight per day is recommended for maintenance or repletion. For hemodialysis, 1.1 to 1.4 g/kg of ideal body weight per day is recommended for maintenance or repletion.[44]

Protein restrictions have been recommended for patients with hepatic failure but may be contraindicated in association with catabolism or critical illness.[45,46] The appropriate protein intake depends on the stage of encephalopathy and the proposed medical treatment. Formulations that contain 35% of amino acids as branched chains have been used to supplement protein intake for hepatic failure patients receiving PN; however, because of their dilute amino acid concentration, these formulas may not provide adequate protein given the fluid restrictions usually imposed on hepatic failure patients. For patients who do not respond as expected when given the recommended protein intake, nitrogen balance studies or urea kinetic modeling can help identify protein requirements.

Commercial amino acids are available in concentrations of 3.5%, 5.5%, 7%, 7.5%, 8.5%, 10%, 11%, 15%, and 20%. The dilute solutions (3.5% and 5.5%) are most often used for peripheral administration. The more concentrated amino acid solutions (8.5%, 10%, 11%, 15%, and 20%) are most often used for central administration. Amino acid profiles for parenteral solutions are based on recommendations by the Food and Agricultural Organization/World Health Organization (FAO/WHO) for optimal proportions of essential amino acids. Arginine and histidine are included because they are essential during stress. Representative profiles for commercial amino acid solutions are shown in Table 18-2. Modified products have been developed for renal failure, hepatic failure, and stress (Tables 18-3 and 18-4).

Future directions in parenteral protein nutrition will probably involve improved amino acid profiles. One intriguing suggestion is that amino acid solutions be modeled on the profile of amino acids released from muscle in persons who were fasted, *then* stressed.[47] In addition, technologic advances are necessary to ensure compatibility and stability of parenteral

TABLE 18-2

Examples of Crystalline Amino Acid Infusions

	Travasol	FreAmine III	Aminosyn II
Manufacturer	Clintec	B. Braun	Abbott
Concentration	10%	10%	10%
Nitrogen (g/100 ml)	1.65	1.53	1.53
Essential amino acids (mg/100 ml)			
Isoleucine	600	690	660
Leucine	730	910	1000
Lysine	580	730	1050
Methionine	400	530	172
Phenylalanine	560	560	298
Threonine	420	400	400
Tryptophan	180	150	200
Valine	580	660	500
Nonessential amino acids (mg/100 ml)			
Alanine	2070	710	993
Arginine	1150	950	1018
Histidine	480	280	300
Proline	680	1120	722
Serine	500	590	530
Taurine	0	0	0
Tyrosine	40	0	270
Aminoacetic acid (glycine)	1030	1400	500
Glutamic acid	0	0	738
Aspartic acid	0	0	700
Cysteine	0	<24	0
Electrolytes (mEq/L)			
Sodium	0	10	45.3
Potassium	0	0	0
Chloride	40	<3	0
Acetate	87	~89	71.8
Phosphate (mmol/L)	0	10	0
Osmolarity (mOsm/L)	1000	~950	873

Drug facts and comparisons, ed 56, St. Louis, 2001, Facts and Comparisons.

TABLE 18-3

Examples of Renal Failure Formulas

	Aminosyn-RF	Aminess	NephrAmine	RenAmin
Manufacturer	Abbott	Clintec	B. Braun	Clintec
Concentration (%)	5.2	5.2	5.4	6.5
Nitrogen (g/100 ml)	0.79	0.66	0.65	1
Essential amino acids (mg/100 ml)				
Isoleucine	462	525	560	500
Leucine	726	825	880	600
Lysine	535	600	640	450
Methionine	726	825	880	500
Phenylalanine	726	825	880	490
Threonine	330	375	400	380
Tryptophan	165	188	200	160
Valine	528	600	640	820
Histidine	429	412	250	420
Nonessential amino acids (mg/100 ml)				
Cysteine			<20	
Arginine	600			630
Alanine				560
Proline				350
Glycine				300
Serine				300
Tyrosine				40
Electrolytes (mEq/L)				
Sodium			5	
Acetate	~105	50	~44	60
Potassium	5.4			
Chloride			<3	31
Osmolarity (mOsm/L)	475	416	435	600

Drug facts and comparisons, ed 56, St. Louis, 2001, Facts and Comparisons.

amino acids. For example, exact compliance with the optimal amino acid profile is currently hindered by the fact that some amino acids are insoluble in water (cystine and tyrosine). Until recently, glutamine was thought to be unstable in amino acid solutions; however, studies showing its stability have been conducted,[48] and amino acid solutions containing glutamine dipeptide are available.

Carbohydrate

The primary function of parenteral carbohydrate is to serve as an energy source. Requirements for carbohydrate have not been clearly delineated, but a minimum figure of 100 g per day is often used. This figure was derived from the finding that administration of 2 L of fluid with 50 g of carbohydrate per liter suppresses gluconeogenesis and, therefore, protein catabolism. The maximum oxidation rate for glucose is 5 mg/kg per minute.[49] When calculated for individuals, this figure translates to 7 g/kg body weight. For critically ill patients, it is suggested that carbohydrate intake be reduced to 4 mg/kg per minute.[19]

Optimum carbohydrate is an amount adequate to spare protein without exacerbating hyperglycemia. If questions about the appropriate carbohydrate intake arise, measurement of the respiratory quotient is recommended to afford insight into carbohydrate utilization.

Commercial carbohydrate consists of anhydrous dextrose monohydrate in sterile water. These solutions are available in concentrations ranging from 5% to 70% and contain 3.4 calories per gram of dextrose (Table 18-5).

Future directions in carbohydrate administration will probably involve commercial development of alternative energy sources that minimize the hyperglycemia sometimes associated with dextrose administration. For example, animal studies suggest that xylitol may be a useful calorie source in carbohydrate intolerance or insulin resistance.[50] Glycerol may also be used to reduce hyperglycemia and improve nitrogen retention following trauma.[51]

Fat

Parenteral lipids are provided as a source of essential fatty acids and calories. They can be substituted to some extent for dextrose calories for patients with glucose intolerance or used as a concentrated calorie source for patients who require volume restriction.

Lipid requirements can be met by providing 4% of calories as linoleic acid or approximately 10% of calories as a commercial lipid emulsion from safflower oil. As commercial lipid emulsions containing alternate lipid sources are introduced, the minimum amount given is based on the linoleic acid content of the emulsion rather than the percentage of total calories.

TABLE 18-4
Examples of Branched-Chain Amino Acid Formulas for Stress and Hepatic Failure

BranchAmine		Stress Formulations		Hepatic Formulation
	BranchAmine	FreAmine-HBC	Aminosyn	HepatAmine
Manufacturer	Clintec	B. Braun	Abbott	B. Braun
Concentration (%)	4.0	6.9	7	8
Nitrogen (g/100 ml)	0.443	0.97	1.12	1.2
Essential amino acids (mg/100 ml)				
Isoleucine	1380	760	789	900
Leucine	1380	1370	1576	1100
Lysine	0	410	265	610
Methionine	0	250	206	100
Phenylalanine	0	320	228	100
Threonine	0	200	272	450
Tryptophan	0	90	88	66
Valine	1240	880	789	840
Nonessential amino acids (mg/100 ml)				
Alanine	0	400	660	770
Arginine	0	580	507	600
Histidine	0	160	154	240
Proline	0	630	448	800
Serine	0	330	221	500
Tyrosine	0	0	33	0
Glycine	0	330	660	900
Cysteine	0	<20	0	<20
Electrolytes (mEq/L)				
Sodium	0	10	7	10
Chloride	0	<3	0	<3
Acetate	0	~57	72	~62
Phosphorus	0	0	0	10
Osmolarity	316	620	665	785

Drug facts and comparisons, ed 56, St. Louis, 2001, Facts and Comparisons.

TABLE 18-5
Osmolarity and Calorie Content of Dextrose Solutions

Dextrose Concentration %	Osmolarity (mOsm/L)	Calories* (kcal/L)	Carbohydrate (g/L)
5	250	170	50
10	500	340	100
20	1000	680	200
50	2500	1700	500
70	3500	2380	700

*Based on the calorie value of dextrose monohydrate used in commercial preparations (3.4 kcal/g).

Recommendations for optimal lipid intake have evolved over the past decade. Since the 1970s, intravenous lipid emulsions have been used to provide as much as 70% of calories in peripheral parenteral regimens without complications.[2] In 1982, Allardyce noted that lipid administration in excess of 3 g/kg per day was associated with the development of cholestasis.[52] At that time, it was often recommended to provide 30% to 50% of calories as lipid. More recently, the negative impact of a high linoleic acid intake on immune function has been appreciated.[53] Concerns that long-chain fatty acids impair neutrophil function, endotoxin clearance, and complement synthesis have resulted in the recommendation to limit lipid administration to 1 g/kg per day[54] or 25% to 30% of total calories.[55] A recent trial found no difference in infectious complications when immunocompromised bone marrow transplantation patients were randomized to receive 30% versus 6% of calories from lipid.[56]

Commercial lipid preparations are aqueous emulsions of soybean or safflower oil. They are composed principally of long-chain triglycerides. Three concentrations, 10%, 20%, and 30% are available. In addition to fatty acids, lipids contain glycerol emulsifiers, which raise the calorie concentration of the 10% emulsion to 1.1 kcal/ml, 20% emulsion to 2.0 kcal/ml, and 30% emulsion to 3.0 kcal/ml. Egg yolk phospholipid is also present in lipid preparations and may contribute to the phosphorus intake of patients who receive more than 500 ml of lipids per day. Fatty acid profiles of common commercial lipids are listed in Table 18-6.

Future considerations in lipid nutrition include physical mixtures of long- and medium-chain triglycerides that are described as *structured lipids*. These emulsions may not depress reticulothelial function as much as long-chain triglycerides do and may therefore have the potential to decrease sepsis rates.[57] Fish oils also have the potential to reduce sepsis because they profoundly decrease endotoxin. Products based on fish oil and olive oil may soon be available commercially in the United States.

Parenteral Additives

Once macronutrients are compounded, vitamins, minerals, and electrolytes are added to provide complete nutrition. In some

TABLE 18-6

Fatty Acid Content of Intravenous Lipid Preparations*

	Intralipid		Liposyn II		Liposyn III	
Manufacturer	Clintec Nutrition		Abbott		Abbott	
Concentration (%)	10	20	10	20	10	20
Oil (%)						
Safflower			5	10		
Soybean	10	20	5	10	10	20
Fatty acid content (%)						
Linolenic	50	50	65.8	65.8	54.5	54.5
Oleic	26	26	17.7	17.7	22.4	22.4
Palmitic	10	10	8.8	8.8	10.5	10.5
Linoleic	9	9	4.2	4.2	8.3	8.3
Stearic	3.5	3.5	3.4	3.4	4.2	4.2
Osmolarity (mOsm/L)	260	260	276	258	284	292

Drug facts and comparisons, ed 56, St. Louis, 2001, Facts and Comparisons.
*Each emulsion contains 1.2% egg yolk phospholipid and 2.21% to 2.5% glycerin.

TABLE 18-7

Parenteral Electrolyte Recommendations for Patients with Normal Function

	Sheldon	Schlichtig	NAG
Potassium	120-160 mmol/d	70-100 mEq	1-2 mEq/kg
Sodium	125-150 mmol/d	70-100 mEq	1-2 mEq/kg + replacement
Phosphate	12-25 mmol/1000 kcal	20-30 mmol	20-40 mmol
Magnesium	7.5-10 mmol/d	15-20 mEq	8-20 mEq
Calcium		10-20 mmol	10-15 mEq
Chloride			As needed to maintain acid-base balance

Data from Sheldon GF, Kudsk KA, Morris JA: Electrolyte requirements in total parenteral nutrition. In Deitel M (ed): *Nutrition in clinical surgery,* Baltimore, 1985, Williams & Wilkins; Schlichtig R, Ayers SM: *Nutritional support of the critically ill,* Chicago, 1988, Year Book, p 130; National Advisory Group: Safe practices for parenteral nutrition formulations, *J Parenter Enteral Nutr* 22:49-66, 1998.

institutions, PN has also been used as a vehicle for drug delivery. For patients with stable electrolyte losses or increased electrolyte needs, PN can provide supplemental electrolytes.

Electrolytes

Electrolyte requirements for patients receiving PN vary depending on body weight, the presence of malnutrition or catabolism, the degree of electrolyte depletion, changes in organ function, ongoing electrolyte losses, and the disease process. In addition, several common drugs exert a profound effect on electrolyte requirements. Electrolyte management is described in detail in Chapter 10.

Guidelines for electrolyte management of patients receiving PN should be used in conjunction with the clinical judgment of an experienced practitioner. The wide variety of electrolytes provided to patients receiving PN is illustrated by the recommendations in Table 18-7. The potential for small adjustments in electrolyte intake to affect patient morbidity and even mortality demands careful electrolyte monitoring for patients receiving PN.

During compounding, electrolytes are added to parenteral solutions as salts. Sodium and potassium are available as chloride, acetate, phosphate, or lactate. Potassium and sodium combine with chloride, acetate, or lactate in a 1:1 molar ratio. The phosphate salts have a different ratio. For sodium phosphate the ratio is 4 mEq of sodium to each 3 mMol of phosphate. For potassium phosphate the ratio is 4.4 mEq of potassium for every 3 mMol of phosphate. Magnesium is most often available as the sulfate salt. Several calcium preparations are available, but calcium gluconate is the most soluble and thus is used most frequently.[58] The amino acid solutions used in PN may include small amounts of inherent electrolytes as well as acetate added to the amino acid solutions as a buffer.

Although electrolytes increase the osmolarity of parenteral solutions, large amounts can be added to PN solutions containing amino acids and dextrose alone without negatively affecting solution stability. There are, however, limits to the amounts of electrolytes that can be added to PN solutions containing lipids.[59]

An important potential hazard of excess cations in PN is the insoluble precipitate that forms when excessive amounts of calcium and phosphorus are added to PN. Precipitate formation in PN solutions has resulted in crystal deposition in the lungs of patients who subsequently died.[60] The solubility of calcium and of phosphorus varies with the volume of the solution, its pH (which depends on the amount of amino acids added), the type of calcium preparation, the temperature at which the solutions are stored, and the order of admixture. Warming of solutions as they enter the body during administration or as they enter the incubators of neonates can also result in precipitation.[61] Solutions for neonates or infants are more likely to precipitate because they contain relatively large amounts of calcium in relation to phosphorus and are provided in small volumes with relatively low concentrations of amino acids.[62] Amino acid manufacturers publish solubility curves to help clinicians avoid precipitate formation. Alternatively, solutions can be prepared with a range of calcium and phosphorus contents as long as the product of calcium (in milliequivalents) and phosphorus (in millimoles) is less than 200.[61]

Bicarbonate has not traditionally been added to PN because of concerns that it changes the pH of the solution and forms insoluble precipitate with calcium and magnesium. One study[63] does document the acceptability of adding 50 ml or 150 ml of sodium bicarbonate to a PN solution of 8.5% FreAmine III with less than 10% loss of bicarbonate and no change in pH; however, because of the potentially lethal result of precipitate, many pharmacies continue to avoid the practice. Thus acetate, a bicarbonate precursor, is added to the PN. The amount of acetate and chloride in PN can be manipulated in response to acid-base imbalance of metabolic origin. For patients who have severe metabolic acidosis, bicarbonate can be administered using a separate line. More details on acid-base balance are provided in Chapter 10.

Vitamins

The need for vitamins and minerals was illustrated early in the history of PN, when vitamin-free PN resulted in deficiency sates rarely seen in patients who ate a normal diet. More recently, during a nationwide vitamin shortage, beriberi from thiamine-free PN resulted in several deaths.[64]

Current recommendations for parenteral vitamin administration are changing. The 1975 American Medical Association

TABLE 18-8

Recommendations for Parenteral Vitamin Intake

Vitamin	AMA	FDA
Vitamin A	3300 IU	5000 IU
Vitamin D	200 IU	400 IU
Vitamin E	10 IU	30 IU
Vitamin K		150 µg
Ascorbic acid	100 mg	200 mg
Folacin	400 µg	600 µg
Niacin	40 mg	40 mg
Riboflavin	3.6 mg	3.6 mg
Thiamine	3 mg	6 mg
B$_6$ (pyridoxine)	4 mg	6 mg
B$_{12}$ (cyanocobalamin)	5 µg	5 µg
Pantothenic acid	15 mg	15 mg
Biotin	60 µg	60 µg

Adapted from Multivitamin preparations for parenteral use. A statement by the National Advisory Group, *J Parentr Enter Nutr* 3:258-262, 1979 and *Federal Register* April 20, 2000.
AMA, American Medical Association; *FDA*, Food and Drug Administration.

(AMA) guidelines have been updated by the FDA (Table 18-8).[8,65] New formulations will include Vitamin K as well as increased amounts of Vitamin C, thiamine, pyridoxine, and folic acid. Commercial preparations are available that parallel the current recommendations for parenteral vitamins. If supplementation with individual vitamins is needed, these preparations are available.

Minerals

Initial recommendations for parenteral trace mineral supplementation were developed by the AMA in 1977 (Table 18-9).[9] A commercial preparation containing the recommended amounts of zinc, manganese, copper, and chromium was developed to facilitate PN compounding. For those with increased zinc requirements because of small bowel losses, parenteral zinc is available for supplementation. While the original AMA recommendations did not include selenium, a trace mineral preparation containing selenium in combination with the original four minerals is now available. A similar preparation containing the original four minerals plus selenium and iodide is also available, although the need for parenteral iodide supplementation is not clearly established. Molybdenum has not routinely been included in PN regimens, but based on a single case study, recommendations of 100 to 200 µg per day for adults[66] and 0.25 µg/kg per day for preterm and term infants on long-term PN[67] were published. Commercial trace mineral preparations are available in different concentrations.

Recently, reports of manganese toxicity in PN patients have appeared in the literature,[68,69] and concerns have been expressed in relation to the potentially reduced needs for trace elements that are excreted via the biliary tract for patients who have biliary stasis with long-term PN. Current recommendations for mineral intakes may be revised in the near future. Chapter 12 contains a more detailed discussion of this topic.

Owing to the potential for an anaphylactic reaction during intravenous administration, iron has not been included in commercial mineral preparations; however, difficulties with intramuscular iron injections have fostered interest in iron-

TABLE 18-9

Recommendations for Parenteral Mineral Intake

Mineral	Amount(mg)
Zinc	2.5-5.0 (additional amounts as follows: 2.0 mg/day in acute catabolism 12.2 mg/L of small bowel fluid losses 17.1 mg/L of stool or ileostomy output)
Copper	0.3-0.5 mg
Chromium	10.0-15.0 µg
Manganese	60-100 µg
Selenium	20-60 µg

Adapted from Guidelines for essential trace element preparations for parenteral use: A statement by an expert panel, *JAMA* 24:2051-2054, 1979.
ASPEN Board of Directors: Guidelines for the use of parenteral and enteral nutrition in adult and pediatric patients, *J Parenter Enteral Nutr* 26(1):1SA–138SA, 2002.

supplemented PN. Small amounts of iron dextran (0.5 to 1.5 mg per day) have been added to dextrose and amino acids without adverse effects;[70] however, conflicting compatibility reports are available for iron and PN solutions that contain lipids.[71,72] According to package inserts, newer iron preparations such as sodium ferric gluconate and iron sucrose are incompatible with PN.

Medications

As central access and continuous infusion facilitate administration of some drugs, the temptation to add medication to PN is great. Using PN as a drug delivery vehicle can also facilitate fluid management by eliminating the need for a separate diluent for each drug administered. Considerations when adding drugs to PN include compatibility of a medication with PN constituents, the effect of pH changes on PN compatibility and drug effectiveness, whether the infusion schedule of the PN is appropriate to achieve therapeutic levels of the drug, and the potential for drug-drug interactions if more than one drug is added to PN. It is also appropriate to note that visual inspection of PN formulas for compatibility is inadequate for detecting dangerous particles or evaluating drug potency. The complexity of these issues frequently mandate referral to institutional policy governing addition of medications to PN or referral to texts on the topic, consultation with a pharmacist experienced in PN compounding and compatibility, or contact with drug manufacturers. Medications that are sometimes added to PN include albumin, aminophylline, cimetidine, famotidine, ranitidine, heparin, hydrochloric acid, or regular insulin.[73]

Insulin

Despite optimal carbohydrate intake, hyperglycemia is frequently observed in patients receiving PN. To achieve blood sugar control during continuous infusions of concentrated dextrose, insulin can be added to the PN formula. Adsorbance of insulin to glass bottles, polyvinyl chloride bags, and tubing used for PN administration has been documented.[74] Insulin loss from PN solutions occurs during the first hour of PN infusion, then no further losses occur.[74] These data suggest that a limited number of insulin-binding sites exist for each container. It is assumed that a similar amount of insulin would bind to individual containers made from the same material. Wide variations in the amount of bound insulin have been reported; the results may be related to the type of container studied.

Fifty percent of insulin was lost from polyolefin bottles with polyvinyl chloride administration sets,[75] whereas as little as 5% to 15% of human insulin was lost in ethyl vinyl acetate bags containing crystalline amino acids.[76] It is appropriate to remember that insulin adsorbance can result in increased insulin requirement; however, addition of insulin to PN can result in excellent blood sugar control.

Heparin

Heparin is often added to PN in an attempt to reduce the complications of catheter occlusion related to fibrin formation around the catheter tip. According to Grant,[1] the addition of 1000 units per liter of heparin greatly reduces the incidence of catheter occlusion but has no anticoagulant effect on serum. Greater amounts of heparin may be used for PPN.

Histamine H$_2$-Receptor Blockers

Because patients receiving PN usually eat nothing by mouth, they are at increased risk for stress ulcers. Stress ulcer prophylaxis may be achieved by the addition of H$_2$-receptor blockers to PN. Famotidine (20 and 40 mg/L) has been shown to be stable in PN and in the total nutrient admixture.[77,78] Ranitidine hydrochloride has also been shown to be stable in PN solutions and three-in-one admixtures.[79,80] As much as 5 g of cimetidine has been shown to be compatible with PN solutions.[81] Smaller amounts may be appropriate in total nutrient admixture.

Physical Characteristics of Parenteral Nutrition Solutions

The method the pharmacy uses to compound PN preparations is critical to the delivery of PN. For institutions where the demand for PN is insufficient or pharmacy staffing does not allow individualized compounding of solutions, commercial formulas with standard electrolyte profiles can be purchased. This system may decrease pharmacy labor costs, but it prevents individualization of parenteral formulas and may increase costs if standard formulas necessitate peripheral electrolyte supplementation.

In some institutions, the pharmacy compounds a predetermined range of solutions (e.g., standard, high-potassium, high-protein, renal). This is a workable alternative for a homogeneous patient population, if care is taken to design solutions that truly match the needs of the patients served.

Since the advent of automated compounding equipment and bulk packaging of concentrated macronutrients, most hospitals provide individualized formulas that are adjusted daily to the needs of the patient. The prescription is checked electronically then transferred to an automated compounder, which measures nutrients into a single container adequate for a 24-hour infusion.

Automated compounders can be used to manufacture conventional nutrient solutions, which combine dextrose and amino acids (two-in-one) or total nutrient admixtures, which combine protein, carbohydrate, and lipid (three-in-one).[82] For the two-in-one system, lipids are administered peripherally by using an additional container, pump, and tubing or by "piggybacking" them into the central line. Each system has advantages and disadvantages. The two-in-one system provides greater flexibility in the amounts of dextrose and amino acids that can be given; however, lipid administration is usually based on available container sizes (100, 250, 500 ml). Because formulas containing dextrose and amino acids alone are clear, gross precipitate or other particulates can be observed. These solutions can also be filtered using a 0.22-μm bacteria-retentive filter.

The total nutrient admixture (TNA) system uses concentrated stock solutions that can be diluted to an almost indefinite variety of macronutrient contents. With TNA, the need for extra equipment is eliminated and costs are reduced;[83] however, this system requires substantial pharmacologic expertise to institute and maintain. Adding lipids increases the fragility of the emulsion; thus, restrictions on the number and types of additives make it more challenging to produce an acceptable prescription. In addition, the opacity of the emulsions prevents observation of precipitate, thus increasing the risk of particulate being infused into the patient. Because of the larger size of lipid particles, TNA is filtered through a 1.2-μm filter that is not bacteria retentive.

Osmolality and Osmolarity

Osmolality and *osmolarity* are two terms used to describe the density of particles in a solution. *Osmolality* refers to the number of water-attracting particles per weight of water in kilograms. *Osmolarity* refers to the number of millimoles of liquid or solid in a liter of solution. While osmolality is most often used in reference to enteral feedings and is the standard for blood, osmolarity is the preferred term for parenteral solutions. The body maintains serum osmolality in a narrow range (280 to 300 mOsm/kg). Changes in osmolality above or below this range can result in serious metabolic disturbances. Although PN administration might potentially change serum osmolality, the large volume of blood, rapid blood flow, and renal regulatory mechanisms mediate this process. To avoid irritation to the veins, solutions with an osmolarity greater than 900 mOsm/L are not usually administered peripherally. Solutions with greater osmolarity may be administered via a central vein. The osmolarity of parenteral solutions is commonly greater than 1800 mOsm/L. Osmolarity can be measured in the laboratory, or a rough estimate can be obtained using the calculations shown in Box 18-1.

BOX 18-1

Osmolarity Calculations for Parenteral Solutions

The osmolarity of 1 L of parenteral nutrient solution can be estimated according to the following calculations:

For amino acids, multiply the concentration (%) by 100.
For dextrose, multiply the concentration (%) by 50.
For electrolytes, multiply the number of millimoles as follows:

Sodium	× 2
Potassium	× 2
Magnesium	× 1
Calcium	× 1.4

Example:

Amino acids 6%	6 × 100	= 600 mOsmol
Dextrose 25%	25 × 50	= 1250 mOsmol
Sodium 35 mEq	35 × 2	= 70 mOsmol
Potassium 30 mEq	30 × 2	= 60 mOsmol
Magnesium 5 mEq	5 × 1	= 5 mOsmol
Calcium 5 mEq	5 × 1.4	= 7 mOsmol
Total		1992 mOsmol

Parenteral Nutrition Compounding

PN prescriptions can be calculated by the patient's nutrient requirements, the available macronutrients, and the available compounding system. Several concepts are central to this process. Nutrient concentration is expressed as the ratio of solute to diluent. This percentage is equivalent to the number of grams per deciliter of solution. As the volume of diluent changes, so does the concentration or percentage of nutrients in solution. The terms *initial concentration* and *final concentration* are used to describe the nutrients as they come from the manufacturer (initial concentration) or after admixture (final concentration). Sample calculations for developing a PN prescription are given in Box 18-2.

Methods of Administration

PN may be initiated in several ways. Two that have worked well are described here. For adult patients whose fluid tolerance is unknown, 1 L of PN may be given for the first 24 hours. Macronutrients are maximally concentrated into 1 L unless hyperglycemia indicates dextrose restriction. If fluid status and glucose control are acceptable, PN is advanced to goal on the second day. For patients who do not require volume restriction, the full volume of a dilute solution can be given on the first day. Then, if glucose control is acceptable, dextrose is increased to the goal amount. Regardless of what method is selected to increase macronutrients, proportional increases are made in carbohydrate-dependent electrolytes such as magnesium and phosphorus, in protein-dependent electrolytes such as potassium, and in volume-dependent electrolytes such as sodium. Exceptions to this protocol are based on changes in patient management, disease process, the results of laboratory or other tests, and the clinical judgment of the clinician providing the PN.

For patients who have insulin-dependent diabetes, are taking steroids, or are at risk for refeeding syndrome, dextrose may initially be restricted to 100 to 150 g per day. For patients with marasmus or edema, initial restriction of sodium has been recommended.[84] Supplemental phosphorus, magnesium, and, if appropriate, potassium are provided to patients at risk for refeeding syndrome.[85]

For all patients, capillary glucose measurements are taken three or four times daily until the values are normal for 2 consecutive days. Regular insulin may be administered according to a sliding scale (Table 18-10).[86]

When appropriate expertise is available, a continuous insulin infusion or drip can be substituted for sliding scale insulin. Regardless of what method is selected, the goal is to control blood sugar between 120 and 200 mg/dl.

For patients who needed insulin before institution of PN, approximately half of the established insulin requirement may be included as regular insulin in the initial bag of PN formula.[86] If the blood sugar value is less than 200 mg/dl, approximately two thirds of the previous day's subcutaneous insulin dose is added to the PN as regular insulin. If sugar is not well-controlled, an amount equal to the previous day's subcutaneous insulin dose is added to the PN as regular insulin.

Changes in medications that affect blood sugar control or changes in amounts of exogenous glucose may necessitate

TABLE 18-10

Suggested Doses of Regular Insulin Administered Subcutaneously

Capillary Glucose (mg/dl)	Dose (units)		
	IDDM	NIDDM	Stress Diabetes
200-250	3	5	5
251-300	6	10	10
301-350	9	15	15
351-400	12	20	20

adjustments in this protocol. Once the blood sugar value is less than 200 mg/dl, the dextrose content of the PN is gradually increased toward goal. If serum glucose levels fall below 120 mg/dl, the amount of insulin in the PN is reduced.

Lipids can be given in the first PN infusion unless serum triglyceride values are elevated. It is recommended that triglyceride levels of less than 400 mg/dl should be maintained while lipids are being infused.[17] Hypertriglyceridemia precluding lipid infusion is rare, and when it exists it usually resolves over the first several days of fat-free PN. For patients with normalizing triglycerides, lipids can be administered in amounts that prevent essential fatty acid deficiency. For persistent or severe hyperlipidemia or for patients with egg allergy, oral or topical safflower oil can be administered to alleviate the topical symptoms of essential fatty acid deficiency.[87]

Twenty-four-hour infusion of lipids does not stimulate glucose production and may reduce the effect of lipids on the reticulothelial system.[54] Because of the potential for infection, however, it is recommended that lipids be infused over 12 hours unless they are incorporated into a total nutrient admixture.[88]

Increasing Parenteral Nutrition to Goal

PN is often administered over 24 hours daily. This minimizes manipulation of the lines and facilitates blood sugar control. During PN, circulating insulin levels remain high, and this condition reduces the amount of carbohydrate that enters the cell and favors hepatic lipogenesis. Therefore, cyclic PN has been suggested as a means of decreasing hepatic complications of PN.[89]

Lerebours and coworkers[90] compared continuous and cyclic PN and found no differences in nitrogen balance or energy expenditure when nutrient intakes of the two regimens were held constant. Cyclic PN also allows some time off the pump so that patients can move about. For those with limited vascular access (e.g., single-lumen catheters), cyclic PN may be necessary to allow administration of medications or blood products.

Generally, cyclic schedules are achieved over 2 or 3 days, during which glucose is monitored carefully to avoid increased blood sugar levels that can occur with increased dextrose infusion and to avoid rebound hypoglycemia when infusions are stopped for the day. Stable patients usually tolerate cyclic PN over 12 to 14 hours.

Discontinuing Parenteral Nutrition

At some point, most patients regain adequate gastrointestinal function to tolerate enteral or oral feedings. Enteral or oral

BOX 18-2

Parenteral Nutrient Calculations†

The following illustrates calculations for parenteral nutrition solutions compounded by four different methods. All calculations are based on a patient whose estimated needs are 1700 kcal and 70 g protein. The preferred method for PN calculations, orders, and labels is in grams per liter. Conversion to percent is included for understanding only.

I. Calculating macronutrient concentrations.
A. 2-in-1 solution calculations:
Calculate 2-in-1 solution using 2000 ml fluid (this volume includes lipid emulsion)
1. Determine kcal to be provided as fat.
   Estimated kcal × desired percentage of fat = kcal as fat
   1700 kcal × 30% = *510 kcal from fat*
2. Convert fat kcal to volume of lipid emulsion.
   Fat kcal ÷ kcal/ml lipid emulsion = volume of lipid emulsion
   510 kcal ÷ 1.1 [10% emulsion] kcal/ml = *463 ml* of 10% lipid emulsion, *or*
   510 kcal ÷ 2.0 [20% emulsion] kcal/ml = *255 ml* of 20% lipid emulsion
   Some institutions prefer lipid to be ordered in volumes as packaged by the supplier (i.e., 100, 250, or 500 ml).
   In this example, *500 ml of 10% lipid* is used, leaving 1500 ml for the remaining PN solution.
3. Determine kcal to be provided from protein.
   Estimated protein need × kcal/g protein = 70 g protein × 4 kcal/g = *280 kcal protein.*
4. Determine amino acid concentration (AA).

   $$\frac{\text{Protein g}}{\text{PN volume}} \times 100 = \% \text{ AA}$$

   $$\frac{70 \text{ g}}{1500 \text{ ml}} \times 100 = 4.7\% \text{ AA}$$

5. Determine kcal to be provided from carbohydrate.
   Estimated kcal need − (kcal as fat + kcal as protein) = carbohydrate kcal
   1700 kcal − (510 kcal + 280 kcal) = *910 kcal carbohydrate*

Substrate	Usual Amount	Maximum Units of Substrate
Carbohydrate	40%-60% of total kcal	<5 mg/kg/min
Protein	1.0-2.0 g/kg/day	2.0-2.5 g/kg/day
Fat	20%-40% of total kcal	1-2 g/kg/day

6. Determine carbohydrate concentration.
   a. Carbohydrate kcal ÷ kcal/g dextrose* = g dextrose
      910 kcal ÷ 3.4 kcal/g = 268 g dextrose
      Dextrose solutions are 3.4 kcal/g rather than 4 kcal/g.
   b. $\dfrac{\text{g dextrose}}{\text{volume PN}} \times 100 = \% \text{ dextrose}$

   $$\frac{268 \text{ g}}{1500 \text{ ml}} \times 100 = 17.9\% \text{ dextrose}$$

7. Final order: 1500 ml 4.7% AA, 17.9% dextrose, 500 ml 10% lipid (lipid volume was rounded from 463 to 500 ml).

B. Calculate a 2-in-1 solution with a fluid restriction of 1250 ml.
1. Determine kcal to be provided as fat.
   Estimated kcal × desired % = fat kcal
   1700 kcal × 30% = *510 kcal fat*
2. Convert fat kcal to volume of lipid emulsion.
   A 20% lipid solution is preferred for fluid-restricted patients.
   kcal as fat ÷ kcal/ml lipid emulsion = lipid volume
   510 kcal 2 kcal/ml ÷ (20% emulsion) = *255 ml*
   This can be rounded to 250 ml, leaving 1000 ml for the remaining PN solution.
3. Determine kcal to be provided from protein.
   Estimated protein needs × kcal/g protein = kcal protein
   70 g × 4 kcal/g = *280 kcal protein*

4. Determine amino acid (AA) concentration.

   $$\frac{\text{g protein}}{\text{PN volume}} \times 100 = \% \text{ AA}$$

   $$\frac{70 \text{ g}}{100 \text{ ml}} \times 100 = 7.0\% \text{ AA}$$

5. Determine kcal to be provided from carbohydrate.
   Estimated kcal needs − (fat kcal + protein kcal = carbohydrate kcal
   1700 kcal − (510 kcal + 280 kcal) = 910 kcal carbohydrate
6. Determine carbohydrate concentration.
   a. Carbohydrate kcal ÷ kcal/g dextrose = g dextrose
      910 kcal ÷ 3.4 kcal/g = 268 g dextrose
   b. $\dfrac{\text{g dextrose}}{\text{volume PN}} \times 100 = \% \text{ dextrose}$

   $$\frac{268 \text{ g}}{1000 \text{ ml}} \times 100 = 26.8\% \text{ dextrose}$$

7. Final order:
   1 L 7% AA, 26.8% dextrose, and 250 ml 20% lipid. This solution will not compound, so the dextrose must be reduced to 17.5% until fluid restrictions are lifted. (If the pharmacy uses a 15% AA stock solution, it will compound. See Compounding Guidelines below for specific calculations.)

C. Calculate a 3-in-1 solution with 2000 ml fluid.
1. Determine kcal to be provided as fat.
   Estimated kcal × desired percentage = kcal fat
   1700 kcal × 30% = *510 kcal fat*
2. Convert fat kcal to volume of lipid emulsion.
   a. Fat kcal ÷ kcal/g = g fat
      510 kcal ÷ 9 kcal/g* = 56.7 g fat
   b. $\dfrac{\text{g fat}}{\text{PN volume}} \times 100 = \% \text{ lipid}$

   $$\frac{56.7 \text{ g}}{200 \text{ ml}} \times 100 = 2.8\% \text{ lipid}$$

3. Determine kcal to be provided from protein.
   g protein × kcal/g = protein as kcal
   70 g × 4 kcal/g = *280 kcal protein*
4. Determine amino acid concentration (AA).

   $$\frac{\text{g protein}}{\text{PN volume}} \times 100 = \% \text{ AA}$$

   $$\frac{70 \text{ g}}{2000 \text{ ml}} \times 100 = 3.5\% \text{ AA}$$

5. Determine kcal to be provided from carbohydrate.
   Estimated kcal needs − (fat as kcal + protein kcal) = carbohydrate kcal
   1700 kcal − (510 kcal + 280 kcal) = *910 kcal carbohydrate*
6. Determine carbohydrate concentration.
   a. kcal dextrose ÷ kcal/g dextrose = g dextrose
      910 kcal ÷ 3.4 kcal/g = 26.8 g dextrose
   b. $\dfrac{\text{g dextrose}}{\text{PN volume}} \times 100 = \% \text{ dextrose}$

   $$\frac{268 \text{ g}}{2000 \text{ ml}} \times 100 = 13.4\% \text{ dextrose}$$

7. Final order:
   2 L 3.5% AA, 13.4% dextrose, and 2.8% lipid.

---

*Nine kcal/g is used as an estimate; however, lipid emulsions are actually 10 kcal/g because of components other than fat in the emulsion.

Continued.

BOX 18-2

Parenteral Nutrient Calculations†—cont'd

D. Calculate a 3-in-1 solution with 1250 ml fluid restriction.
1. Determine kcal to be provided as fat.
   Estimated kcal × desired percent = fat kcal
   1700 kcal × 30 = *510 kcal fat*
2. Convert fat kcal to volume of lipid emulsion.
   a. kcal fat ÷ kcal/g = g fat
      510 kcal ÷ 9 kcal/g = 56.7 g fat

   b. $\dfrac{\text{g fat}}{\text{PN volume}} \times 100\% = \%\ \text{lipid}$

   $\dfrac{56.7\ \text{g}}{1250\ \text{ml}} \times 100 = 4.5\%\ \textit{lipid}$

3. Determine kcal to be provided from protein.
   g protein × kcal/g = kcal as protein
   70 g × 4 kcal/g = 280 kcal protein
4. Determine kcal to be provided from carbohydrate.
   Estimated kcal needs − (fat kcal + protein kcal) = carbohydrate kcal
   1700 kcal − (510 kcal + 280 kcal) = *910 kcal carbohydrate*
5. Determine carbohydrate concentration.
   a. kcal dextrose ÷ kcal/g dextrose = g dextrose
      910 kcal ÷ 3.4 kcal/g = 268 g dextrose

   b. $\dfrac{\text{g dextrose}}{\text{PN volume}} \times 100 = \%\ \text{dextrose}$

   $\dfrac{268\ \text{g}}{1250\ \text{ml}} \times 100 = 21.4\%\ \textit{dextrose}$

6. Final Order: 1.25 L 5.6% AA, 21.4% dextrose, and 4.5% lipid. This solution will not compound, the dextrose will have to be reduced to *12.3%* until fluid restrictions are listed. See compounding guidelines below for specific calculations. If the pharmacy uses a 15% amino acid stock solution, it will compound.

II. Compounding Parenteral Nutrition
Assume stock solutions of 70% dextrose, 10% amino acids, and 20% lipids.
1. Determine PN volume and grams of carbohydrate, protein, and fat.
2. Determine volume of 70% dextrose stock solution.
3. Determine volume of 10% amino acid stock solution.
4. Determine volume of 20% lipid.
5. Determine volume of sterile water and additives.
6. Adjust dextrose or other substrates if solution cannot be compounded at the desired volume.

Sample Calculations
A. A 2-in-1 solution with fluid restriction 1250 ml
1. Determine PN volume and grams of carbohydrate, protein, and fat (see I.B.).
   Volume 1250 ml
   Lipid 250 ml 20%
   Carbohydrate 268 g
   Protein 70 g
2. Determine volume of 70% dextrose solution.
   g dextrose ÷ g/100 ml stock solution = volume of stock solution
   268 g ÷ 70 g/100 ml = *383 ml 70% dextrose solution*
3. Determine volume of 10% AA solution.
   g protein ÷ g/100 ml stock solution = volume of stock solution
   70 g ÷10 g/100 ml = *700 ml 10% AA solution*
4. Determine volume of 20% lipid.
   250 ml (see I.B.2.)
   In a 2-in-1 solution, this is separate from the PN solution.
   This leaves 1000 ml for AA and dextrose

5. Determine volume of sterile water and additives.
   Volume PN solution − (volume of dextrose + volume AA) = volume for water and additives
   1000 ml − (383 ml + 700 ml) = − *83 ml*
   These volumes of stock solution do not fit into the desired PN volume.
6. Adjust solution.
   a. Determine the volume available for dextrose.
      Volume desired − (volume of AA solution + volume for additives*) = volume available for dextrose.
      1000 ml − (700 ml + 50 ml) = *250 ml*
   b. Determine new grams of dextrose.
      Volume of dextrose × solution concentration = g dextrose stock solution
      250 ml × 70 g/100 ml = *175 g dextrose*
   c. Determine dextrose concentration.

   $\dfrac{\text{g dextrose}}{\text{PN volume}} \times 100 = \%\ \text{dextrose}$

   $\dfrac{175\ \text{g}}{1000\ \text{ml}} \times 100 = 17.5\%\ \textit{dextrose}$

B. 3-in-1 solution with fluid restriction of 1250 ml.
1. Determine PN volume and grams of carbohydrate, protein, and fat (see I.D.).
   Volume 1250 ml
   Carbohydrate 268 g
   Protein 70 g
   Fat 56 g
2. Determine volume of 70% dextrose solution.
   g dextrose ÷ g/100 ml stock solution = volume of stock solution
   268 g ÷ 70 g/100 ml = *383 ml 70% dextrose solution*
3. Determine volume of 10% AA solution.
   g protein ÷ g/100 ml stock solution = volume of stock solution
   70 g ÷10 g/100 ml = 700 ml 10% AA solution
4. Determine volume of 20% lipid.
   g fat ÷ g/100 ml stock solution = volume of stock solution
   56 ÷ 20 g/100 ml = *280 ml 20% lipid.*
5. Determine volume of sterile water and additives.
   Desired PN volume − (volume dextrose solution + volume AA solution + volume lipids) = volume of water and additives
   1250 ml − (383 ml + 700 ml + 280 ml) = 113 ml
   This solution will not compound.
6. Adjust solution.
   a. Determine the volume available for dextrose.
      Desired volume − (volume of AA solution + volume lipid + volume additives) = volume available for dextrose
      1250 ml − (700 + 280 + 50) = *220 ml*
   b. Determine new grams of dextrose.
      Volume of dextrose × solution concentration = g dextrose stock solution
      220 ml × 70 g/100 ml = *154 g dextrose*
   c. Determine new dextrose concentration.

   $\dfrac{\text{g dextrose}}{\text{PN solution}} \times 100 = \%\ \text{dextrose}$

   $\dfrac{154\ \text{g}}{1250\ \text{ml}} \times 100 = 12.3\%\ \textit{dextrose}$

---

*Usually 50-100 ml.

---

†Adapted from Fish J: Worksheets for calculating total parenteral nutrition, *Support Line* 17:10-13, 1995.

feedings should begin when the gastrointestinal tract is long enough and in good enough condition for nutrient absorption. This may be assessed by evaluating the patient's history for a diagnosis or surgical procedures that could interfere with nutrient absorption. In addition, the patient should demonstrate adequate gastrointestinal motility as evidenced by normoactive bowel sounds, passage of flatus or stool, and minimal nasogastric drainage or vomiting. Incremental reductions in PN can be made as enteral or oral feedings are increased. When enteral or oral feedings are tolerated at 65% to 75% of goal calories, parenteral feedings can be discontinued.

For those who do not eat well, the effect of PN on appetite is often a concern. An early paper showed that parenteral nutrients delayed gastric emptying and increased feelings of satiety.[91] Several papers have since shown that PN impairs appetite.[92-94] This appears to be dose related because gastric emptying and oral intake were normal when serum glucose was below 120 g/dl or when PN was fed at 50% of calorie needs.[94] Increasing PN to 100% of energy needs, in combination with hyperglycemia, blunted the appetite. In addition, parenteral glucose may impair appetite more than fat.[94] Further studies are needed to confirm the impact of these findings on resumption of oral intake for PN patients.

Rebound hypoglycemia with discontinuation of PN is a potential concern; however, the only study on the topic found no detrimental effects on serum insulin or glucagon levels when PN was abruptly discontinued.[95] For patients who are eating, PN can be reduced and stopped over 24 to 48 hours. If PN is inadvertently but abruptly discontinued in patients who are not eating, all insulin should be stopped and blood sugar values monitored for 30 minutes after discontinuation of PN. Based on blood sugar levels, appropriate therapy should be implemented.

A third concern arises when PN has served as a vehicle for electrolyte supplementation or administration of medication. The need for continued electrolyte supplementation should be evaluated. Consultation with a pharmacist may help establish appropriate doses and forms of medications.

Conclusion

PN, one of the major medical advances of the last three decades, enables feeding of patients who formerly would have succumbed to starvation. The techniques for PN have been refined, and ongoing research will facilitate appropriate utilization of the therapy. In the future, PN will be used in combination with other therapies to provide even more disease-specific therapy and as a vehicle for nutritional modulation of disease.

REFERENCES

1. Grant JP: *Handbook of total parenteral nutrition,* ed 2, Philadelphia, 1992, WB Saunders, p 1.
2. Wretlind A: Parenteral nutrition, *Surg Clin North Am* 58(5):1055-1070, 1978.
3. Rhoads JE, Dudrick SJ, Vars HM: History of intravenous nutrition. In Rombeau JL, Caldwell MD (eds): *Parenteral nutrition,* Philadelphia, 1986, WB Saunders, pp 1-10.
4. Meyer CE, Fancher JA, Schurr PE, Webster HD: Composition, preparation and testing of an intravenous fat emulsion, *Metabolism* 6:591-596, 1957.
5. Mogil RA, DeLaurentis DA, Rosemond GP: The infraclavicular venipuncture, *Arch Surg* 95:320-324, 1967.
6. Dudrick SJ, Wilmore DW, Vars HM, Rhoads JE: Long-term total parenteral nutrition with growth, development, and positive nitrogen balance, *Surgery* 64(1):134-142, 1968.
7. Dudrick SJ, Wilmore DH, Vars HM, Rhoades JE: Can intravenous feeding as the sole means of nutrition support growth in the child and restore weight loss in an adult? An affirmative answer, *Ann Surg* 169(6):974-984, 1969.
8. American Medical Association Department of Foods and Nutrition: Multivitamin preparations for parenteral use; a statement by the Nutrition Advisory Group, *J Parenter Enteral Nutr* 3(4):258-262, 1979.
9. American Medical Association Department of Foods and Nutrition: Guidelines for essential trace element preparations for parenteral use, *JAMA* 241(19):2051-2054, 1979.
10. Driscoll DF, Baptista RJ, Bistrian BR, Blackburn GL: Practical considerations regarding the use of total nutrient admixtures, *Am J Hosp Pharm* 43(2):416-419, 1986.
11. Abel RM, Abbott WM, Beck CH, et al: Essential L-amino acids for hyperalimentation in patients with disordered nitrogen metabolism, *Am J Surg* 128(3):317-323, 1974.
12. Blumenkrantz MJ, Kopple JD, Koffler A, et al: Total parenteral nutrition in the management of acute renal failure, *Am J Clin Nutr* 31(10):1831-1840, 1978.
13. Mirtallo JM, Schneider PJ, Mavko K, et al: A comparison of essential and general amino acid infusions in the nutritional support of patients with compromised renal function, *J Parenter Enteral Nutr* 6(2):109-113, 1982.
14. Millikan WJ, Henderson JM, Warren WD, et al: Total parenteral nutrition with F080 in cirrhotics with subclinical encephalopathy, *Ann Surg* 197(3):294-304, 1983.
15. Bower RH, Muggia-Sullam M, Vallgren S, et al: Branched chain amino-acid enriched solutions in the septic patient, *Ann Surg* 203(1):13-20, 1986.
16. Meguid MM, Eldar S, Wahba A: The delivery of nutritional support, *Cancer* 55(1 suppl):279-289, 1985.
17. ASPEN Board of Directors:Guidelines for the use of parenteral and enteral nutrition in adult and pediatric patients, *J Parenter Enteral Nutr* 26(1):1SA-137SA, 2002.
18. ASPEN Board of Directors: Guidelines for the use of total parenteral nutrition in the hospitalized adult patient, *J Parenter Enteral Nutr* 10(5):441-445, 1986.
19. ASPEN Board of Directors: Guidelines for the use of parenteral and enteral nutrition in adult and pediatric patients, *J Parenter Enteral Nutr* 17(4): 1SA-52SA, 1992.
20. Anonymous: Perioperative parenteral nutrition, *Ann Intern Med* 107(2):252-253, 1987.
21. Anonymous. Parenteral nutrition in patients receiving cancer chemotherapy, *Ann Intern Med* 110(9):734-736, 1989.
22. Sitzman JV, Pitt HA: Statement on guidelines for total parenteral nutrition, *Dig Dis Sci* 34(4):489-496, 1989.
23. Maurer J, Weinbaum F, Turner J, et al: Reducing the inappropriate use of parenteral nutrition in an acute care teaching hospital, *J Parenter Enteral Nutr* 20(4):272-274, 1996.
24. Anderson CF, MacBurney MM: Application of ASPEN clinical guidelines: parenteral nutrition use at a university hospital and development of a practice guideline algorithm, *Nutr Clin Pract* 11(2):53-58, 1996.
25. Klein S, Kinney J, Jeejeebhoy K, et al: Nutrition support in clinical practice: review of published data and recommendations for future directions, *Am J Clin Nutr* 66(3):683-706, 1997.
26. Committee on Nutrition Services for Medicare Beneficiaries, Food and Nutrition Board: *The role of nutrition in maintaining health in the nation's elderly,* Washington DC, 2000, Institute of Medicine National Academy Press.
27. American Gastroenterological Association. American Gastroenterological Association medical position statement: parenteral nutrition, *Gastroenterology* 121(4):966-969, 2001.
28. Ofman J, Koretz RL: Clinical economics review: nutritional support, *Aliment Pharmacol Ther* 11(3):453-471, 1997.
29. Howard L, Heaphey L, Fleming CR, et al: Four years of North American registry home parenteral nutrition outcome data and their implications for patient management, *J Parenter Enteral Nutr* 15(4):384-393, 1991.
30. Twomey PL, Patching SC: Cost-effectiveness of nutritional support, *J Parenter Enteral Nutr* 9(1):3-10, 1985.
31. Orr ME, Ryder MA: Vascular access devices: perspectives on designs, complications, and management, *Nutr Clin Pract* 8(4):145-152, 1993.
32. McCarthy MC, Shives JK, Robinson RJ, Broadie TA: Prospective evaluation of single and triple lumen catheters in total parenteral nutrition, *J Parenter Enteral Nutr* 11(3):259-262, 1987.

33. Gil RT, Kruse JA, Thill-Baharozian MC, Carlson RW: Triple- vs single-lumen central venous catheters. A prospective study in a critically ill population, *Arch Intern Med* 149(5):1139-1143, 1989.

34. Duerksen DR, Papineau N, Siemens J, Yaffe C: Peripherally inserted central catheters for parenteral nutrition: a comparison with centrally inserted catheters, *J Parenter Enteral Nutr* 23(1):85-89, 1999.

35. Loughran SC, Borzatta M: Peripherally inserted central catheters: a report of 2506 catheter days, *J Parenter Enteral Nutr* 19(2):133-136, 1995.

36. Gazitua R, Wilson K, Bistrian BR, Blackburn GL: Factors determining peripheral vein tolerance to amino acid infusions, *Arch Surg* 114(8):897-900, 1979.

37. Isaacs JW, Millikan WJ, Stackhouse J, et al: Parenteral nutrition of adults with a 900 milliosmolar solution via peripheral veins, *Am J Clin Nutr* 30(4):552-559, 1977.

38. Tighe MJ, Wong C, Martin IG, McMahon MJ: Do heparin, hydrocortisone, and glyceryl trinitrate influence thrombophlebitis during full intravenous nutrition via peripheral vein? *J Parenter Enteral Nutr* 19(6):507-509, 1995.

39. Gianino MS, Brunt LM, Eisenberg PC: The impact of a nutrition support team on the cost and management of multilumen central venous catheters, *J Intravenous Nurs* 15(6):327-332, 1992.

40. Food and Nutrition Board: *Recommended dietary allowances,* ed 10, Washington, DC, 1989, National Academy Press, p 3.

41. Cerra FB, Blackburn G, Hirsh J, et al: The effect of stress level, amino acid formula, and nitrogen dose on nitrogen retention in traumatic and septic stress, *Ann Surg* 205(3):282-287, 1987.

42. Shaw JH, Wildbore M, Wolf RR: Whole body protein kinetics in severely septic patients. The response to glucose infusion and total parenteral nutrition, *Ann Surg* 205(3):288-294, 1987.

43. Larsson J, Lenmarken C, Martenson J, et al: Nitrogen requirements in severely injured patients, *Br J Surg* 77(4):413-416, 1990.

44. Stover J (ed): *A clinical guide to nutrition care in end stage renal disease,* Chicago, 1994, American Dietetic Association, pp 28, 43.

45. Nompleggi DJ, Bonkovsky HL: Nutritional supplementation in chronic liver disease: an analytical review, *Hepatology* 19(2):518-533, 1994.

46. Mullen KD, Weber FL: Role of nutrition in hepatic encephalopathy, *Semin Liver Dis* 11(4):292-304, 1991.

47. DeBiasse MA, Wilmore DW: What is optimal nutritional support, *New Horizons* 2(2):122-130, 1994.

48. Lowe DK, Benefell K, Smith RJ, et al: Safety of glutamine-enriched parenteral nutrient solutions in humans, *Am J Clin Nutr* 52(6):1101-1106, 1990.

49. Wolfe RR, O'Donnell TF, Stone MD, et al: Investigation of factors determining the optimal glucose infusion rate in total parenteral nutrition, *Metabolism* 29(9):892-900, 1980.

50. Karlstad MD, DeMichele SJ, Bistrian BR, Blackburn GL: Effect of total parenteral nutrition with xylitol on protein and energy metabolism in thermally injured rats, *J Parenter Enteral Nutr* 15(4):445-449, 1991.

51. Singer P, Burszstein S, Kirveld O, et al: Hypercaloric glycerol in injured patients, *Surgery* 112(3):509-514, 1992.

52. Allardyce DB: Cholestasis caused by lipid emulsions, *Surg Gynecol Obstet* 112(5):509-514, 1992.

53. Kinsella JE, Lokesh B: Dietary lipids, eicosanoids and the immune system, *Crit Care Med* 18(2 suppl):S94-S113, 1990.

54. Seidner DL, Mascioli EA, Istfan NW, et al: Effects of long-chain triglyceride emulsions on reticuloendothelial system function in humans, *J Parenter Enteral Nutr* 13(6):614-619, 1989.

55. Jensen GL, Mascioli EA, Seidner DL, et al: Parenteral infusion of long- and medium-chain triglycerides and reticulothelial system function in man, *J Parenter Enteral Nutr* 14(5):467-471, 1990.

56. Lenssen P, Bruemmer BA, Bowden RA, et al: Intravenous lipid dose and incidence of bacteremia and fungemia in patients undergoing bone marrow transplantation, *Am J Clin Nutr* 67(5):927-933, 1998.

57. Bell SJ, Mascioli EA, Bistrian BR, et al: Alternative lipid sources for enteral and parenteral nutrition: long- and medium-chain triglycerides, structured triglycerides, and fish oils, *J Am Diet Assoc* 91(1):74-78, 1991.

58. Henry RS, Jurgeons RW, Sturgeons R, Athanikar AN: Compatibility of calcium chloride and calcium gluconate with sodium phosphate in a mixed TPN solution, *Am J Hosp Pharm* 37(5):673-674, 1980.

59. Parry VA, Harrie KR, McIntosh NL, Lowe NL: Effect of various nutrient ratios on emulsion stability of total nutrient admixtures, *Am J Hosp Pharm* 43(12):3017-3022, 1986.

60. Lumpkin MM, Burlington DB: FDA safety alert: hazards of precipitation associated with parenteral nutrition, *Am J Hosp Pharm* 51(1): 1427-1428, 1994.

61. Driscoll DF, Newton DW, Bistrian BR: Precipitation of calcium phosphate from parenteral nutrient fluids, *Am J Hosp Pharm* 51(22):2834-2836, 1994.

62. Dunham B, Marcuard S, Khazanie PG, et al: The solubility of calcium and phosphorus in neonatal total parenteral nutrition solutions, *J Parenter Enteral Nutr* 15(6):608-611, 1991.

63. Henann NE, Jacks TT: Compatibility and availability of $NaHCO_3$ in total parenteral nutrition solutions, *Am J Hosp Pharm* 42(12):2718-2720, 1985.

64. Deaths associated with thiamine-deficient total parenteral nutrition, *MMWR Morbid Mortal Weekly Rep* 38(3):43-46, 1989.

65. Shils ME, Baker H, Frank O: Blood vitamin levels of long-term adult home total parenteral nutrition patients: the efficacy of the AMA-FDA parenteral multivitamin formation, *J Parenter Enteral Nutr* 9(2):179-188, 1985.

66. Flemming CR: Trace element metabolism in adult patients requiring total parenteral nutrition, *Am J Clin Nutr* 49(3):573-579, 1989.

67. Greene HL, Hambridge KM, Schanler R, et al: Guidelines for the use of vitamins, trace elements, calcium, magnesium and phosphorus in infants and children receiving total parenteral nutrition: report of the Subcommittee on Pediatric Parenteral Nutrient Requirements from the Committee on Clinical Practice Issues of the American Society for Clinical Nutrition, *Am J Clin Nutr* 48(5):1324-1342, 1988.

68. Reynolds AP, Kiely E, Meadows N: Manganese in long term paediatric parenteral nutrition, *Arch Dis Child* 71(6):527-528, 1994.

69. Fredstrom S, Rogosheske J, Gupta P, Burns LJ: Extrapyramidal symptoms in a BMT recipient with hyperintense basal ganglia and elevated manganese, *Bone Marrow Transplant* 15(6):989-992, 1995.

70. Kwong KW, Tsallas G: Dilute iron dextran formulation for addition to parenteral nutrient solutions, *Am J Hosp Pharm* 37(2):206-210, 1980.

71. Vaughan LM, Small C, Plunkett V: Incompatibility of iron dextran and total nutrient admixture, *Am J Hosp Pharm* 47(8):1745-1746, 1990.

72. Tu YH, Knox NL, Biringer JM, et al: Compatibility of iron dextran with total nutrient admixture, *Am J Hosp Pharm* 49(9):2233-2235, 1992.

73. Driscoll DF, Baptista RJ, Mitrano FP, et al: Parenteral nutrient admixtures as drug vehicles: theory and practice in the critical care setting, *Drug Intelligence and Clinical Pharmacy* 25(3):276-282, 1991.

74. Weber SS, Wood WA, Jackson EA: Availability of insulin from parenteral nutrient solutions, *Am J Hosp Pharm* 34(4):353-357, 1977.

75. Hirsch JT, Wood JH, Thomas RB: Insulin adsorption to polyolefin infusion bottles and polyvinyl chloride administration sets, *Am J Hosp Pharm* 38(7):995-997, 1981.

76. Marcuard SP, Dunham B, Hobbs A, Caro JF: Availability of insulin from total parenteral nutrition solutions, *J Parenter Enteral Nutr* 14(3):262-264, 1990.

77. Bullock L, Fitzgerald JF, Glick MR: Stability of famotidine 20 and 40 mg/L and amino acids in total parenteral nutrition solutions, *Am J Hosp Pharm* 46(1):2321-2325, 1989.

78. Montoro JB, Pou L, Salvador P, et al: Stability of famotidine 20 and 40 mg/L in total nutrient admixtures, *Am J Hosp Pharm* 46(11):2329-2332, 1989.

79. Williams MF, Hak LJ, Dukes G: In vitro evaluation of the stability of ranitidine hydrochloride in total parenteral nutrition mixtures, *Am J Hosp Pharm* 47(7):1547-1579, 1990.

80. Cano SM, Montoro JB, Pastor C, et al: Stability of ranitidine hydrochloride in total nutrient admixture, *Am J Hosp Pharm* 45(5):1100-1102, 1988.

81. Moore RA, Feldman S, Treuting J, et al: Cimetidine and parenteral nutrition, *J Parenter Enteral Nutr* 5(1):61-63, 1981.

82. Driscoll DF: Total nutrient admixtures: Theory and practice, *Nutr Clin Pract* 10(3):114-119, 1995.

83. Eskew JA: Fiscal impact of a total parenteral nutrient admixture program at a pediatric hospital, *Am J Hosp Pharm* 44(1):111-114, 1987.

84. Apovian CM, McMahon MM, Bistrian BR: Guidelines for refeeding the marasmic patient, *Crit Care Med* 18(9):1030-1033, 1990.

85. Brooks MJ, Melnik G: The refeeding syndrome: an approach to understanding its complications and preventing its occurrence, *Pharmacotherapy* 15(6):713-725, 1995.

86. McMahon M, Manji N, Driscoll DF, Bistrian BR: Parenteral nutrition in patients with diabetes mellitus: theoretical and practical considerations, *J Parenter Enteral Nutr* 13(5):545-553, 1989.

87. Miller DG, Williams SK, Palombo JD et al: Cutaneous application of safflower oil in preventing essential fatty acid deficiency in patients on home parenteral nutrition, *Am J Clin Nutr* 46(1):419-423, 1987.

88. Brown DH, Simkover RA: Maximum hang times for IV fat emulsions, *Am J Hosp Pharm* 44(2):282-284, 1987.

89. Maini B, Blackburn GL, Bistrian BR, et al: Cyclic hyperalimentation: an optimal technique for preservation of visceral protein, *J Surg Res* 20(6):515-525, 1976.

90. Lerebours E, Rimbert A, Hecketsweiler B, et al: Comparison of the effects of continuous and cyclic nocturnal parenteral nutrition on energy expenditure and protein metabolism, *J Parenter Enteral Nutr* 12(4):360-364, 1988.

91. MacGregor IL, Wiley ZD, Lavigne ME, Way LW: Slowed rate of gastric emptying of solid food in man by high calorie parenteral nutrition, *Am J Surg* 138(5):652-654, 1979.

92. Reifen R, Khoshoo V, Dinari G: Effect of parenteral nutrition on oral intake, *Pediatr Endocrinol Met* 12(2):203-205, 1999.

93. Gil KM, Skeie B, Kvetan V, et al: Parenteral nutrition and oral intake: effect of glucose and fat infusions, *J Parenter Enteral Nutr* 15(4):426-432, 1991.

94. Bursztein-De Myttanaere S, Gil KM, Heymsfield SB, et al: Gastric emptying in humans: Influence of different regimens of parenteral nutrition, *Am J Clin Nutr* 60(2):244-248, 1994.

95. Wagman LD, Newsome HH, Miller KB, et al: The effect of acute discontinuation of total parenteral nutrition, *Ann Surg* 204(5):524-529, 1986.

Complication Management in Parenteral Nutrition
19

M. Patricia Fuhrman, MS, RD, LD, FADA, CNSD

THIS chapter reviews the various complications associated with parenteral nutrition (PN)— technical, septic, gastrointestinal (GI), and metabolic (Tables 19-1 to 19-3). Emphasis is given to catheter-related, hepatic, and macronutrient complications. An understanding of the causes and treatment of the complications associated with PN is necessary to provide optimal nutrition support.

Catheter-Related Complications

Peripheral or central venous access is required to deliver nutrients with parenteral solutions. Placement of an intravenous (IV) catheter is the most commonly performed invasive procedure.[1] Thirty-eight potential complications are related to catheterization.[2] Table 19-1 outlines common complications associated with intravenous catheters. Catheters vary according to the number of lumens available for use, tunneled versus percutaneous venous access, material, and size (diameter and length). The number of catheter lumens is determined by anticipated need for different infusates. Tunneled catheters and implanted ports are placed when long-term need for central venous access is expected. Catheter materials (i.e., silastic, polyurethane, silicone elastomer, polyethylene, polyvinyl chloride, and hydrogel) depend on the manufacturer and the size of the catheter. Silicone elastomer is the most often used material for IV catheters.

TABLE 19-1
Catheter-Related Complications of Parenteral Nutrition

Complications	Possible Etiology	Symptoms	Treatment	Prevention
Pneumothorax	Catheter placement by inexperienced personnel	Tachycardia, dyspnea, persistent cough, diaphoresis	Small pneumothorax may spontaneously resolve; larger pneumothorax may require chest tube	Catheter placement by experienced personnel
Air embolism	Air inspired while line is interrupted or uncapped	Cyanosis, tachypnea, hypotension, churning heart murmur (classic sign)	Immediately place patient on left side and lower HOB to try to keep air in apex of right ventricle until it is reabsorbed.	Catheter placement by experienced personnel
Catheter embolization	Pulling catheter back through needle used for insertion	Cardiac arrhythmias	Surgical removal of catheter tip	Avoid withdrawing catheter through insertion needle
Venous thrombosis	Mechanical trauma to vein, hypotension, solution osmolarity, hypercoagulopathy, sepsis	Swelling or pain in one or both arms or shoulders or neck	Anticoagulation therapy with urokinase, reteplase, TPA, or streptokinase; catheter removal	Silicone catheter, addition of heparin, low-dose warfarin, urokinase
Catheter occlusion	Hypotension, failure to maintain line patency, formation of fibrin sheath on catheter exterior, solution precipitates	Inability to infuse or withdraw blood through catheter	Anticoagulation therapy with urokinase or streptokinase	Larger diameter catheter, routine flushing of catheter, monitor solution for precipitation
Improper tip location	Venous vasculature anomalies, catheter placement by inexperienced personnel	Phlebitis, severe cardio respiratory distress, possible thrombosis	Catheter removal	Proper catheter placement by experienced personnel
Phlebitis	Peripheral administration of hypertonic solution (>900 mOsm), line infiltration	Erythema, swelling, pain at peripheral site	Change peripheral line site; start central PN, if appropriate	Minimize osmolarity of peripheral solution with lipids as primary kcal source; decrease additives in PN
Catheter-related sepsis	Inappropriate technique for line placement, poor catheter site care, contaminated solution	Unexplained fever, chills, erythemic indurated catheter insertion site	Remove catheter and replace at another site (see Fig. 19-2)	Develop and implement strict protocols for line placement and catheter care

Adapted from Skipper A, Marian MJ: Parenteral nutrition. In Gottschlich MM, Matarese LE, Shronts EP (eds): *Nutrition support dietetics core curriculum*, ed 2, Silver Spring, MD, ASPEN, 1993, pp105-123.
HOB, Head of bed; *PN,* parenteral nutrition; *TPA,* tissue plasminogen activator.

Gastrointestinal Complications Associated with Parenteral Nutrition

Complication	Possible Cause	Symptoms	Treatment	Prevention
Fatty liver	Cause unclear; theories include infusion of carbohydrate in excess of hepatic oxidative capacity, overfeeding of calories or fat, excess infusion of amino acids, EFAD, choline and carnitine deficiency	Elevation of liver enzymes within 1-3 wk after PN initiation	Reduce calories or carbohydrate fraction	Cyclic PN: rule out other causes; use mixed substrate; avoid overfeeding; avoid glucose infusion >5-7 mg/kg/min
Cholestasis	Precise cause unknown; theories include impaired bile flow; absence of intraluminal nutrients to stimulate hepatic bile secretion; excess glucose, lipids, and amino acid infusion; toxic tryptophan metabolites; choline deficiency	Progressive increases in serum bilirubin; elevated serum total alkaline phosphatase; jaundice	Avoid over-feeding; rule out other causes	Early use of GI tract
Gastrointestinal atrophy	Atrophy of villi, colonic hypoplasia	Presence of enteric bacteria in mesenteric lymph nodes; development of enteric bacteremia and sepsis without clear source	Transition to enteral or oral feedings, as tolerated	Early use of GI tract
Gastric hyperacidity	Gastric acid secretion without enteral intake	Development of gastritis or stress ulcers	H_2-receptor antagonists	Early use of GI tract

Adapted from Skipper A, Marian MJ: Parenteral nutrition. In Gottschlich MM, Matarese LE, Shronts EP (eds): *Nutrition support dietetics core curriculum*, ed 2, Silver Spring, MD, 1993 ASPEN, pp 105-123.
EFAD, Essential fatty acid deficiency; *GI*, gastrointestinal; *PN*, parenteral nutrition.

Placement

PERIPHERAL ACCESS. A small vessel in the hand or forearm is cannulated for peripheral access. Peripheral vessels have a limited tolerance for hypertonic infusates. Generally infusates do not exceed 900 mOsm. This limits the composition of the parenteral solution.

CENTRAL VENOUS ACCESS. Central venous access commonly originates from the subclavian, jugular, basilic or femoral vein (Fig. 19-1). Subclavian and jugular access originates in the chest and neck, respectively. A peripherally inserted central catheter (PICC) is placed into the antecubital fossa or the mid-humeral area of the arm and the tip of the catheter threaded into the superior vena cava or right atrium of the heart. Femoral access originates in the groin area.

PLACEMENT COMPLICATIONS. Reported technical complications of placement of central venous access include pneumothorax, catheter embolism, air embolism, vessel injury, and malposition of the catheter tip.[1-6] The incidence of pneumothorax can be reduced if experienced personnel place catheters and if the number of required catheter insertions is minimized.[4,5,7] Catheter replacement over a guidewire has been reported to decrease the incidence of mechanical complications.[4] Placement of an IV catheter by interventional radiology and using a venous cutdown approach are both associated with a decrease in IV catheter placement complications.[5]

Vascular erosion associated with central venous catheters was found to be related to catheters placed on the left side of the body and the use of large-bore catheters (14-gauge or larger).[3] The problem with left-sided catheter insertion is the acute angle between the brachiocephalic vein and the superior vena cava. This angle increases the risk of placing the catheter adjacent to a vessel wall (and perhaps puncturing it) or perpetually spraying the vessel wall with the hypertonic IV solution.

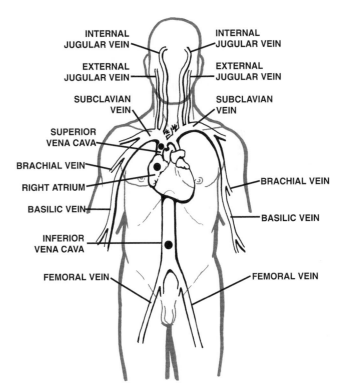

FIGURE 19-1 Sites of central venous access for parenteral nutrition.

Larger catheters are generally more rigid and may perforate the vessel and may be less responsive to respiratory and cardiac motion.[3]

Catheter malposition is identified by radiography when verifying catheter placement after insertion. Because malposition of the catheter can result in serious complications such as

TABLE 19-3

Metabolic Complications Associated with Parenteral Nutrition

Complication	Possible Cause	Symptoms	Treatment	Prevention
Hypervolemia	Excess fluid administration, renal dysfunction, congestive heart failure, hepatic failure	Dyspnea, bounding pulse, moist rales, edema, weight gain	Fluid restriction, diuretics, dialysis in extreme cases	Initiate PN once fluid balance stable; monitor input/output; monitor serum and urine osmolality
Hypovolemia	Inadequate fluid administration, overdiuresis	Dehydration, thirst, dry mucous membranes, low urine output, weight loss	Increase fluid intake	Monitor daily intake/output; monitor serum and urine osmolality
Hyperkalemia	Renal dysfunction, excessive potassium administration, metabolic acidosis, potassium-sparing medications	Diarrhea, tachycardia, cardiac arrest, oliguria, paresthesias	Decrease potassium intake, provide potassium binders	Monitor serum levels for trends; assess for drug-nutrient interactions, especially potassium-sparing diuretics
Hypokalemia	Inadequate potassium provision; increased potassium losses (diarrhea, diuretics, intestinal fistulas)	Nausea, vomiting, confusion, arrhythmias, cardiac arrest, respiratory depression	Increase PN or IV potassium.	Provide 40 mEq of potassium daily unless contraindicated; 3 mEq of potassium/g nitrogen required for anabolism
Hypernatremia	Inadequate free water administration, excessive sodium intake, excessive water losses (fever, burns, hyperventilation)	Thirst, decreased skin turgor, mild irritability in some cases, elevated serum sodium, BUN, and hematocrit	Decrease sodium intake, replenish fluids	Avoid excess sodium intake; monitor fluid status; monitor urine sodium
Hyponatremia	Excessive fluid administration, nephritis and/or adrenal insufficiency, dilutional states (congestive heart failure, SIADH, cirrhosis of the liver with ascites)	Confusion, hypotension, irritability, lethargy, seizures	Restrict fluid intake; increase sodium intake as dictated by clinical status	Avoid overhydration; provide 60-100 mEq/day of sodium unless contraindicated by cardiac, renal, or fluid status; monitor urine sodium
Hyperglycemia	Rapid infusion of concentrated dextrose solution; sepsis, pancreatitis postoperative stress; chromium deficiency; use of steroids; advanced age; multiple sources of dextrose from both oral and intravenous routes	Blood glucose >200 mg/dl, metabolic acidosis polyuria, polydipsia	Insulin; reduce dextrose concentration in PN	Slow initiation and advancement of PN; use mixed substrate solution
Hypoglycemia	Abrupt discontinuation of PN, insulin overdose	Weakness, sweating, palpitations, lethargy, shallow respirations	Dextrose	Taper PN solution; with abrupt discontinuation of PN, hang 10% dextrose at the same rate as the PN to prevent rebound hypoglycemia; monitor serum glucose when insulin is being given
Hypertriglyceridemia	Lipid provision exceeds ability to clear lipids from bloodstream (>4 mg/kg/min); sepsis, multisystem organ failure, pathologic hyperlipidemia, lipoid nephrosis; medication use alters fat metabolism (e.g., cyclosporin)	Serum level >400 mg/dl Lipemic serum	Decrease lipid volume administered, lengthen infusion time, simultaneously infuse glucose	Assess for history of hyperlipidemia before initiation of PN, avoid lipid administration >2.5 g/kg/day or >60% of total calories
Hypercalcemia	Renal failure, tumor lysis syndrome, bone cancer, excess vitamin D administration, prolonged immobilization and stress, hyperparathyroidism	Confusion, dehydration, muscle weakness, nausea, vomiting, coma	Isotonic saline, inorganic phosphate supplementation, corticosteroids, mithramycin	Encourage weight-bearing activity; evaluate vitamin D intake
Hypocalcemia	Decreased vitamin D intake, hypoparathyroidism, citrate binding of calcium because of excessive blood transfusion, hypoalbuminemia	Parasthesias, tetany, irritability, ventricular arrhythmias	Calcium supplementation	Provide calcium, 0.2 to 0.3 mEq/kg/day
Hypermagnesemia	Excessive magnesium administration, renal insufficiency	Respiratory paralysis, hypotension, premature ventricular contractions, lethargy, cardiac arrest, coma, liver dysfunction	Decrease magnesium provision	Monitor serum levels for trends
Hypomagnesemia	Refeeding syndrome, alcoholism, diuretic use, increased losses (e.g., diarrhea), medication (e.g., cyclosporin), diabetic ketoacidosis, chemotherapy	Cardiac arrhythmias, tetany, convulsions, muscle weakness	Magnesium supplementation	Monitor serum levels for trends; provide 0.25-0.45 mEq/kg/day

Continued.

TABLE 19-3

Metabolic Complications Associated with Parenteral Nutrition—cont'd

Complication	Possible Cause	Symptoms	Treatment	Prevention
Hyperphosphatemia	Excess phosphate administration, renal dysfunction.	Parasthesias, flaccid paralysis, mental confusion, hypertension, cardiac arrhythmias, soft tissue calcification with prolonged elevated levels	Decreased phosphate administration, phosphate binders	Monitor serum levels for trends
Hypophosphatemia	Refeeding syndrome, alcoholism, phosphate-binding antacids, dextrose infusion, overfeeding, secondary hyperparathyroidism, insulin therapy	Neurologic changes, respiratory muscle fatigue, diaphragmatic contractility, erythrocyte hemolysis, leukocyte dysfunction	Phosphate supplementation, stop phosphate-binding antacids, avoid overfeeding, initiate calories at BEE	Provide 7-9 mMol phosphate/1000 kcal, monitor serum phosphorus, and replete beforeand during PN as needed
Prerenal azotemia	Dehydration, excess protein provision, inadequate nonprotein calorie provision with mobilization of own protein stores	Elevated serum BUN	Increased fluid intake, decreasd protein load, increased nonprotein calories	Monitor serum BUN for trends; perform nitrogen balance study
Overfeeding	Excess carbohydrate and/or protein administration	Excess carbohydrate: CO_2 retention, cardiac tamponade, liver dysfunction. Excess protein: elevated BUN, excess nitrogen excretion, elevated BUN to creatinine ratio	Decreased carbohydrate, protein provision, as needed	Avoid excess carbohydrate/protein administration
Essential fatty acid deficiency	Inadequate fat intake	Dermatitis, alopecia, alterations in pulmonary, neurologic, and red cell membranes	Lipid administration	Provide 2%-4% of kcal as linoleic acid, or 8%-10% of kcal as fat, especially in patients with severe malnutrition, fat malabsorption, or expected not to take food by mouth for >2 wk

Adapted from Skipper A, Marian MJ: Parenteral nutrition. In Gottschlich MM, Matarese LE, Shronts EP (eds): *Nutrition support dietetics core curriculum,* ed 2, Silver Spring, MD, 1993, ASPEN, pp 105-123.
BEE, Basal energy expenditure; *BUN,* blood urea nitrogen; *IV,* intravenous; *PN,* parenteral nutrition; *SIADH,* syndrome of inappropriate antidiuretic hormone.

thrombophlebitis, perforation of the vessel or heart, and infusion of fluid into the mediastinum or pleural space, it is vital to verify proper placement with a radiograph before infusion of PN or any other intravenous fluids.[8] Malposition of central venous catheters has also been reported to result in back pain secondary to positioning of the catheter in the azygos vein[9] and acute pharyngitis secondary to phlebitis when the catheter was placed in the internal jugular vein rather than the subclavian vein, as intended.[10] Air embolism, a rare but lethal complication, can occur during catheter insertion or removal but more often is associated with damage or disconnection of the catheter at the hub.[11]

Catheter Care

To prevent catheter occlusion and maintain patency, routine flushing of the IV catheter is recommended.[12] Many institutions use a preservative-free saline solution for routine flushing of IV catheters. Other agents used prophylactically to prevent occlusion of IV catheters include heparin,[13] warfarin,[14] and urokinase.[15] A study in AIDS patients on home PN showed no difference in thrombotic complications when prophylactic low-dose warfarin (1 g/day)was given.[16] There is no consensus about the proper dose of heparin to reduce the risk of catheter occlusion without precipitating hemorrhagic complications in susceptible patients. Doses of 1000 U/L were not found to be effective, and 5000 U every 6 hours has resulted in GI bleeding.[12] A meta-

analysis by Randolph and others reported that 3 U heparin/ml PN, 5000 U every 6 or 12 hours, or a daily dose of 2500 U of low molecular weight heparin effectively reduced the incidence of major vein thrombosis.[13]

Needleless IV access devices have been introduced to decrease the risk of exposure to blood-borne infections that occur from needle-stick injuries.[17] However, with the increased use of needless access has come a concomitant increase in reports of bloodstream infections in home care,[18] surgical,[19] and pediatric patients.[20] The Intravenous Nurses Society has revised standards of practice to recommend changing needleless devices every 24 hours, disinfecting the IV access port with alcohol before puncture and injection, and securing all junctions with luer-locks, clasps or threaded devices.[21]

Catheter Occlusion

Catheter occlusion is the most common noninfectious complication of long-term IV catheters.[22,23] Occlusion is defined as the inability to infuse or aspirate blood without resistance from an IV catheter.[22] Inability to withdraw blood from the catheter was characteristic of both thrombotic and nonthrombotic occlusions.[24] Factors that contribute to loss of catheter patency include mechanical malfunction of the catheter, occlusion of the catheter lumen, and encasement of the catheter tip by fibrin formation. Compher and colleagues reported an increased risk of venous thrombosis in patients with short bowel syndrome with hyperhomocysteinemia, which in turn was associated with vitamin B_{12} deficiency.[25] The clinical impact of vitamin supplementation and reduction of total homocysteine levels on the incidence of venous thrombosis, particularly catheter-related thrombosis, is currently unknown. Treatment such as anticoagulation therapy, thrombolytic therapy, elevation of the affected limb, and removal of the catheter, depends on the etiology because lytic therapy will not eliminate a nonthrombotic occlusion.[24] It is also important to determine the causative agent of the catheter occlusion because different treatments are indicated for different occluding agents: urokinase, heparin, tissue plasminogen activator (TPA,) and reteplase for blood; ethanol and sodium hydroxide for lipids; hydrochloric acid for calcium/phosphate precipitates; and sodium bicarbonate for precipitant formed by giving basic pH medications.[26]

THROMBOTIC COMPLICATIONS. According to Hoch, 95% of catheter occlusions are thrombotic in etiology.[23] The factors contributing to the occurrence of thrombosis are known as the Triad of Virchow and were described in the nineteenth century: damage to the vessel wall, changes in blood flow, and alterations in the composition of the blood.[27,28] Symptoms associated with catheter-related venous thrombosis are neck vein distention, edema, pain in the affected area, tingling of the throat, and a prominent venous pattern on the chest.[22] Fibrin deposition on the catheter results when the body "perceives" an indwelling catheter as a foreign body and defends itself by depositing fibrin and platelets on the catheter. Within 48 hours of placement, the catheter develops fibrin deposits, which increase the risk of catheter thrombosis each day the catheter is in place. Development of a fibrin sleeve is suspected when blood cannot be aspirated from the catheter, but infusate flows through the catheter without difficulty. Eventually the catheter could become totally occluded if not treated. Thrombolytic therapy with urokinase, heparin, and TPA have been shown to be effective in treating thrombosis, resolving symptoms, and permitting continued use of the affected catheter.[26,29] Prophylatic treatment of home PN catheters with urokinase (5000 U instilled for 4 to 8 hours once a month) resulted in a reduction of catheter infections and replacements as well as reduced hospitalizations for catheter-related complications.[30] There has been a shortage of urokinase because of inadequate availability of raw materials for production. Therefore clinicians rely on heparin, TPA , and reteplase. Thrombolytic agents are contraindicated with active internal bleeding and central nervous system (CNS) or vascular injury such as aneurysm, cerebrovascular accident, or injury or surgery within the CNS.[31]

NONTHROMBOTIC COMPLICATIONS. Another possible cause of venous catheter occlusion is pinch-off syndrome, a mechanical complication that occurs when a tunneled silastic central venous catheter placed percutaneously via the subclavian vein is compressed between the first rib and the clavicle.[32] Although this is rare (1.1%), it should be considered as a cause when intermittent occlusion occurs with infusion and withdrawal from central venous catheters.[32] Treatment is removal of the catheter. Catheter fracture, catheter tip location, catheter dislodgement, and catheter migration can all contribute to loss of catheter patency and necessitate repositioning or removal of the IV catheter.[26]

Catheter Location

PERIPHERAL ACCESS. Peripheral venous access infusate osmolarity tolerance is limited to 700 to 900 mOsm/L.[33] This limitation necessitates the use of a lipid-based nutrient system because lipids are fairly isotonic and well tolerated by the peripheral veins. The lipid-based infusate may protect the vascular endothelium of the peripheral veins, which in conjunction with heparin infusion, may control the development of thrombophlebitis.[34] Phlebitis and thrombosis are concerns when nutrition is provided via a peripheral access. Phlebitis can result from bacterial, chemical, or mechanical etiologies and is characterized by erythema, edema, hardness of the vein, or pain. Factors that may result in phlebitis include cannula size, material, colonization, insertion site, infusion components, vein size, and duration of infusion.[35] Phlebitis prophylaxis includes buffering the solution to maintain the pH between 7.2 to 7.4, providing glycerol or lipids as a calorie source, adding heparin-hydrocortisone to the solution, rotating of the cannula site every 48 to 72 hours, using topical nonsteroidal antiinflammatory medications or glyceryl trinitrate patches to the cannula site, and monitoring by a nutrition support team. When peripheral nutrition solutions with osmolarities of 1200 and 1700 mMol/L were compared, the risk of thrombophlebitis was no different between the two solutions.[36] Although thrombophlebitis developed in 30% of the lines inserted, patency of the lines was maintained for an average of 6.3 days.

PERIPHERALLY INSERTED CENTRAL CATHETERS. PICC lines are becoming increasingly popular for long-term, nontunneled, central IV access because of their low cost and reduced incidence of complications as compared with traditional central access catheters. A study by Loughran and Borzatta reported a less than 1% rate of infectious and thrombotic complications.[37] Phlebitis, which occurred in 10% of the patients, was either an early complication resulting from placement mechanics or a late complication resulting from chemical or patient-specific causes. A retrospective study of 800 catheters compared PICCs to tunneled catheters and found a statistically significant increase in overall complications with the PICC.[38] Duerksen and associates reported that increased use of PICCs resulted in a decrease in septic complications and an increase in phlebitis and catheter leaking and malposition.[39] Confirmation of tip placement in the superior vena cava or right atrium is necessary before infusing PN and other hyperosmolar solutions through a PICC.

CENTRAL VENOUS ACCESS. The subclavian vein is associated with a lower risk of catheter-related infection than the jugular or femoral vein.[40] Femoral catheters have been associated with increased risk of complications, such as thrombophlebitis and infection, and they are generally not used unless cannulation of the subclavian or internal jugular veins is contraindicated. Catheter placement verification in the inferior vena cava is required to prevent thrombophlebitis secondary to infusion of hyperosmolar solutions through the small veins proximal to the inferior vena cava. Harden, Kemp, and Mirtallo retrospectively evaluated the complication rates with triple-lumen catheters and femoral or nonfemoral access.[41] They reported a higher incidence of bacteremia (16.7% versus 1.8%, respectively) in the femorally inserted catheters. Another study reported that femoral catheters had a lower incidence of complications, despite the fact that 20% of patients had complications that necessitated catheter removal.[42] A larger prospective study of 52 patients demonstrated that aggressive dressing care and monitoring were effective in controlling infectious complications: 53% of the catheters were used longer than 7 days. There were no reports of thrombophlebitis or other noninfectious complications.[43] Recommendations for the use of femoral access include aseptic insertion and catheter care, use of catheters with a small diameter and long length, verification of tip placement in the inferior vena cava, diligent monitoring for bacterial and thrombogenic complications, and avoidance of the site unless other venous sites are contraindicated.[41,42]

Sepsis

Catheter-related sepsis is the leading complication of intravenous catheters and is the most frequent cause of long-term morbidity in home PN patients.[44] *Staphylococcus epidermis* (33.5%), *Staphylococcus aureus* (13.4%), enterococcus (12.8%) and *Candida albicans* (5.8%) are the most common infectious organisms of central venous catheters.[40] Fever in a patient who has no other identifiable source of infection raises suspicion of a catheter-related infection. Catheter-related infections can be categorized as either local or systemic. Local infections are confined to the insertion site and are manifested as erythema, purulent drainage, and induration around the catheter exit site. Colonization is the identification of microorganism growth from the tip or indwelling part of the catheter. The patient may or may not exhibit signs of local infection. Catheter colonization is common and occurs in approximately 25% of patients with a central venous catheter for less than or equal to 10 days.[45] Catheter-related blood stream infection (CR-BSI) is defined as a positive blood culture and clinical or microbiologic evidence that the catheter is the most probable source of the infection.[46] Approximately one out of every 20 patients with a short-term central venous catheter will develop CR-BSI with an associated mortality rate varying between 4% and 20%.[45] Indications that the catheter is the source of the infection are obtaining the same microorganism identified from the catheter exit site or catheter tip as from the peripheral blood or resolution of symptoms (i.e., fever, leukocytosis, hypotension) with catheter removal.[46,47] It is important to distinguish between incidence of colonization and documented CR-BSI when reviewing articles on prevention and treatment of catheter-related septic complications. Table 19-4

lists the Center for Disease Control definitions for exit site, tunnel, pocket, and bloodstream infections and provides treatment options.[48,49]

Many factors are believed to contribute to catheter-related sepsis: duration of catheterization, severity of illness, type of catheter inserted, location of the catheter, number of catheter lumens, intended use of the catheter, and type of catheter dressing.[1,40] *Staphylococci* can produce a biofilm that adheres to the surface of medical devices inserted into the body. Plasma proteins, fibrin, and hematocytes combine with the slime produced by the biofilm to produce a complex that is resistant to degradation and antibiotic therapy. It is also important to consider whether sepsis might already have been established at the time of catheter insertion.

Duration of catheterization is reported to be one of the most important risk factors for catheter-related infection;[50,51] however, three studies have shown that the duration of catheterization is not related to the risk of catheter-related sepsis.[52-54] Guidewire changes have been proposed as a way of removing a possibly contaminated catheter for culturing without interrupting infusion therapy. Routine guidewire changes have been suggested to prevent catheter-related sepsis. Studies have shown that changing a catheter over a guidewire does not decrease the incidence of infection but may decrease the incidence of mechanical complications associated with insertion of a new central line.[53,55] Several studies suggest that catheters should not be changed routinely but only in the event of a complication or a problem that necessitates a change.[52-54] Tunneled catheters have been correlated with a decreased incidence of infection.[47] However, meticulous site care provided by an IV team to nontunneled catheters resulted in a catheter-related infection rate comparable to tunneled catheters.[56]

Introduction of contaminants from the skin is reduced when the catheter is inserted with aseptic technique.[45] Aseptic technique should also be used for dressing and tubing changes. The type of dressing can also contribute to infection risk. Transparent, occlusive dressings have been reported to increase the risk of catheter-related sepsis;[44,50,52] however, others have reported no difference in sepsis associated with transparent dressing.[57] A study that looked at gauze, conventional polyurethane, and highly permeable polyurethane dressings for site care of pulmonary artery catheters reported that cutaneous colonization was the least with gauze, but differences in colonization and infection did not reach significance among the

TABLE 19-4
Catheter-Related Infections

Infection Type	Exit Site	Tunnel	Pocket	Bloodstream
CDC definition	Erythema, tenderness, or purulence within 2 cm of site	Erythema, tenderness, or purulence >2 cm from site	Erythema and necrosis over port reservoir or purulent exudates in subcutaneous pocket	Same isolate on semiquantitative/quantitative catheter culture and blood; no other sign of infection, defervescence with catheter removal, paired blood samples: central fivefold to tenfold greater than peripheral
Treatment options	Warm compresses, daily site care, oral antibiotics	Catheter removal	Port removal, antibiotic therapy	Antibiotic lock, systemic antibiotics, catheter removal; yeast, *S. aureus*, polymicrobial, recurrent infection, persistent bacteremia

From Krzywda EA, Andris DA, Edminston CE, et al: Parenteral access devices. In Gottschlich MM (ed): *The science and practice of nutrition support: a case-based core curriculum,* Parenteral and Enteral Nutrition, p 236. Reprinted with permission of the American Society for Parenteral and Enteral Nutrition three types of dressings.[58] Recommendations for routine catheter dressing changes range from 48 hours to 5 days.[52,58]

The risk of catheter-related sepsis has been reported to be greater with the use of multilumen catheters than with single-lumen catheters.[50,59] It is believed that the increased catheter manipulation, more severe illness in patients who require triple-lumen catheters, and infusion of PN increase the risk of infection. Pemberton reported a sixfold greater prevalence of infections with triple-lumen catheters than with single-lumen ones;[60] however, other studies have not found an association between catheter sepsis and number of catheter lumens.[54, 61] PN was not a risk factor for development of catheter-related sepsis in single (1.4%, historic controls), double (2%), or triple lumen catheters 1.9%).[62]

Treatment of infection in IV catheters often results in removal of the catheter, which necessitates insertion of another catheter at a different site. Intravenous catheters should be removed when the infection is a tunnel infection or the pathogen is a fungus or a persistent bacterium.[50,59,63] In situ treatment with antibiotics for 2 to 4 weeks with broad gram-positive and gram-negative coverage has successfully treated catheter infections without necessitating catheter removal.[63,64] Identification of the pathogen determines the specific treatment. Figure 19-2 depicts an algorithm for treatment of catheter-related sepsis.

The best "treatment" for catheter-related sepsis is prevention. It is important to identify the origin of the pathogens and to prevent their migration into the bloodstream. Resistant strains such as methicillin-resistant *S. epidermis* (MRSE), methicillin-resistant *S. aureus* (MRSA) and vancomycin-resistant enterococci (VRE) reduce current treatment options and increase the demand for prevention and control.[65] One proposed theory is that the offending organisms migrate from the skin at the catheter insertion site along the catheter tract into the bloodstream.[50,59, 66] Preventing contamination of the catheter from the insertion site begins with aseptic catheterization and catheter care.[45,59,67] Topical antiseptic solutions[68,69] and dressings[70] and antiseptic-[71,72] and antibiotic-[73,74] impregnated catheter and catheter cuffs have been identified as being protective against infection. The antiseptic, chlorhexidine, has been used as a topical disinfectant,[68,69] incorporated into dressings,[70] combined with silver sulfadiazine and impregnated onto the catheter.[71,72] Each of these studies reported reduced incidence of CR-BSI with chlorhexidine. Chlorhexidine-impregnated medical devices have been associated with cases of hypersensitivity in Japan.[75] However, no reports have been noted in the United States. Another group has found a reduction in infection and colonization with IV catheters impregnated with antibiotics, rifampin, and minocycline.[73,74] A review of the available literature determined that insertion of central venous catheters with antibacterial/antiseptic activity is cost-effective, particularly because treatment of a local infection costs $400 to $10,000 per episode.[45] For home PN patients, adherence to catheter care protocols and aseptic technique were found to be the most important factors in preventing catheter-related infections.[44,50,63] Placement and maintenance of the intravenous catheter by an intravenous therapy team has been shown to be a cost-effective method to reduce CR-BSI.[50,57,59] The occurrence of catheter-related sepsis was reduced during a

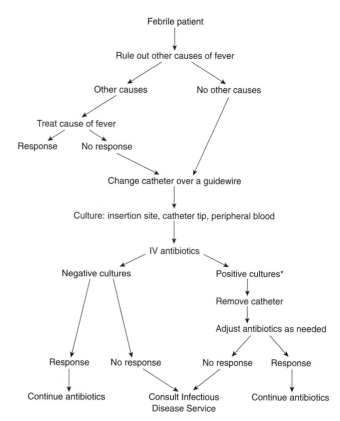

FIGURE 19-2 Algorithm for treatment of catheter-related sepsis. (Adapted from O'Keefe SJD, Burnes JU, Thompson RL: Recurrent sepsis in home parenteral nutrition patients: an analysis of risk factors, *J Parenter Enteral Nutr* 18:256-263, 1994.)

randomized controlled trial that combined self-monitoring, diary therapeutic writing, massage, and problem-solving techniques with the standard home PN regimen.[76]

Hepatic Complications Associated with Parenteral Nutrition

Incidence

It is difficult to isolate hepatic complications that result solely from PN infusion. The cause of hepatic dysfunction can be multifactorial, especially in critically ill patients who require PN support. Medications, treatments, the disease process, and the degree of malnutrition can contribute to hepatic derangements. Elevations of liver enzymes within the first 3 weeks of PN infusion are associated with hepatic steatosis.[77,78] In PN-associated hepatic dysfunction, laboratory abnormalities often develop in a particular sequence: (1) aspartate aminotransferase (AST), (2) alkaline phosphatase (AP), and (3) bilirubin.[79] Patients who are malnourished before initiation of PN are more likely to exhibit early AP elevations and associated cholestasis.[80] The interpretation of liver enzyme abnormalities and hyperbilirubinemia should include examination of hepatic histologic changes or more extensive tests of hepatic synthetic and excretory function. The prevalence of hepatic enzyme abnormalities in conjunction with PN infusion ranges from 25% to 100%. For hyperbilirubinemia, which occurs less frequently and later, it is 0% to 46%.[77] Infusion of PN for less than 1 month is associated with mild and transient elevations in liver enzymes with no evidence of permanent hepatic damage.[77,78]

Long-term PN has been associated with cholelithiasis,[81] steatohepatitis, and cholestasis.[82] Patients who after massive small bowel resection are dependent on PN may benefit from prophylactic cholecystectomy, in view of the increased incidence of gallstones in this population.[83] A 15% rate of persistent abnormal liver tests has been reported in long-term PN patients, three of whom developed chronic liver disease.[82] PN-associated hepatic dysfunction is not a benign condition for long-term home PN patients and should be treated aggressively to avoid permanent liver damage. Various nutrient deficiencies (e.g., choline,[84,85] and L-carnitine[86]) have been studied for an association with long-term PN. The development of gallbladder sludge may be a result of the severity of illness in patients fed by PN. Inflammation of the gallbladder, which results in mucous hypersecretion and cell desquamation along with cholestasis secondary to PN and absence of enteral stimulation, sets the stage for the formation of sludge, which can precede gallstone formation in these patients.[87]

Factors Reported to Affect Hepatic Function

Virtually all components of PN have been implicated as agents in the development of hepatic steatosis and cholestasis. It has been proposed that the PN solution itself may be directly toxic to the liver.[88] Other proposed causes of hepatic derangement are deficiencies of essential fatty acids,[89] nitrogen,[90] amino acids,[91] choline,[84,85] and L-carnitine[86] and excesses of calories,[90] glucose,[92] lithocholic acid,[93] tryptophan,[94] bilirubin production,[95] and fat.[96] Malnutrition,[80] elevated portal insulin-glucagon ratio,[97] and impairment of GI integrity[98] have also been implicated with hepatic dysfunction. Hepatic complications of PN have also been reported to occur more often in patients with preexisting ileal disease,[82,99] massive small bowel resection,[100,101] liver or kidney disease, or sepsis.[102] It is also hypothesized that extended duration of PN infusion increases the risk of liver-related complications.[79,96] The hepatic complications associated with PN may be related to lack of stimulation of the GI tract and absence of the first pass of nutrients through the liver.

MACRONUTRIENTS AND HEPATIC COMPLICATIONS. Introduced in 1967, PN was a glucose-based formula until 1978, when intravenous lipids were approved for use in the United States. The addition of lipids to PN has been shown to activate peripheral lipolytic enzymes, decrease hepatic triglyceride uptake, increase fatty acid oxidation, increase peripheral plasma triglyceride oxidation, and decrease the insulin-glucagon ratio.[97] However, providing more than 50% of calories as fat was associated with hepatic steatosis secondary to a decreased capacity of the liver to eliminate the excess fat.[103] Fatty liver occurs when there is an imbalance between uptake and oxidation of fatty acids and their synthesis and release as lipoproteins by the liver. Insulin resistance as seen with critical illness, type 2 diabetes mellitus, preexisting hyperlipidemia, obesity, protein-calorie malnutrition, and jejunal-ileal bypass, is a common denominator for a reduction in hepatic lipid release.[104] Initial reports of hepatic abnormalities with PN were probably

related to the large amount of calories provided and the degree of malnourished[79] and critically ill patients in the studies.

Although there was a reported case of steatosis reversed by adding lipid to the PN of a patient receiving prolonged lipid-free PN,[92] another study found no difference in steatosis between patients given a lipid-based and those fed a dextrose-based PN solution.[105] Balderman and colleagues compared the effects of lipid emulsions containing long-chain triglycerides (LCTs) versus a mixture of medium-chain triglycerides (MCTs) and LCTs in 14 patients and postulated that providing a mixture of MCTs and LCTs can prevent hepatic steatosis associated with PN.[106]

A prospective, randomized trial demonstrated that providing one third of the PN calories as lipid improved glucose tolerance and reduced hepatic complications.[96] When a glucose-lipid PN (60% dextrose, 40% lipid) was compared with a glucose PN with lipids twice a week (92.5% dextrose, 7.5% lipid), the lipid-limited group of patients had significantly higher levels of bilirubin, AST, and triglyceride.[107] This study avoided provision of excessive calories and found that AP and gamma-glutamyl transpeptidase (GGT) were elevated, regardless of the calorie source but less than in previous studies that provided higher-calorie solutions. Finding a strong correlation between liver abnormalities and excessive carbohydrate and nitrogen, Lowry and Brennan suggested the calorie-nitrogen ratio be reduced to 100:1 to prevent overfeeding.[108] Keim reported that greater caloric loads were significantly related to the development of steatosis within 5 days of initiating PN and that fatty infiltration was greater in patients who received inadequate nitrogen along with a high-fat PN solution.[90] Therefore, Keim suggested not only that excess calories be avoided in PN but also that when a larger percentage of calories is provided as lipid it may be important to give adequate nitrogen to avoid development of fatty liver.

GLUTAMINE, CHOLINE, CARNITINE. Glutamine, choline, and carnitine are not routinely added to PN and have been proposed as possible treatment options for hepatic steatosis. The addition of glutamine, a gluconeogenic amino acid, to lipid-free PN prevented hepatic steatosis in rats.[109] Glutamine may decrease hepatic uptake of fat and increase the flow of alanine through the portal vein, promoting normalization of hepatic metabolism. Although carnitine deficiency has been proposed as a possible cause of steatosis, an intravenous supplement of 1 g per day given to home PN patients failed to demonstrate a change in steatosis, despite increased serum carnitine levels.[86] Choline, a precursor of phospholipid biosynthesis, may be necessary for the liver to form lipoproteins for the transport of triglyceride in the body.[85] Patients on long-term PN have been shown to have low plasma choline levels. When lecithin was supplemented in a group of choline-deficient PN patients, there was a significant increase in serum choline levels and a decrease in fatty hepatic infiltration.[84] It was also found that hepatic steatosis improved with lecithin supplementation even though the plasma carnitine level did not change.[84]

URSODEOXYCHOLIC ACID, CHOLECYSTOKININ, METRONIDAZOLE. Ursodeoxycholic acid (UDCA) has been used to treat patients with chronic cholestatic liver disease. In a study of nine patients receiving 11 to 12 mg/kg per day of UDCA for one to two 2-month periods, decreases were seen in GGT and alanine aminotransferase but no change in AP, AST, or bilirubin.[110] It is hypothesized that UDCA replaces hepatotoxic bile salts and thus reduces cholestasis. Cholecystokinin (CCK) given intravenously every day prevented formation of biliary sludge and development of cholelithiasis in long-term PN patients.[111] Neonates receiving PN treated with prophylactic CCK had lower direct bilirubin levels than matched historic controls.[112] The effect of metronidazole on cholestasis in patients on PN suggests a role for intestinal overgrowth of anaerobic bacteria in the development of PN-related cholestasis.[93,113] It is hypothesized that the overgrowth of anaerobic bacteria is responsible for the production of hepatotoxic substances (endotoxin or lithocholic acid) that precipitate morphologic and functional changes in the liver.[93] The lithocholic acid levels have been reported to be high in patients who are beginning to show signs of liver dysfunction.[114]

Treatment of Parenteral Nutrition–Related Hepatic Dysfunction

Cyclic PN (12- to 16-hour infusions) has been shown to improve liver enzymes within the first week and has been associated with clinical resolution of hepatomegaly.[115] Cyclic PN mimics the physiologic effects of the postabsorptive state of feeding and fasting. Interrupting PN infusion allows the body to convert to the oxidation of fat, as opposed to the oxidation of carbohydrate that dominates during continuous PN. This promotes mobilization of lipid, transport of fat out of the liver, and positive nitrogen balance with decreased lipid storage.[116]

Hepatic complications associated with PN continue to be an enigma, despite ongoing research. Correction of nutrient or hormone deficiencies, excesses, or imbalances has been studied and shown to be effective and ineffective in the treatment of hepatic steatosis. Early studies may have been flawed by large calorie loads. In patients who received PN for less than a month, it has been noted that the elevations in the laboratory parameters, the fatty infiltration of the liver, and cholestasis were transient and resolved whether PN was continued, adjusted, or stopped; however, when a patient develops liver enzyme abnormalities or hyperbilirubinemia, it is imperative to assess his or her current status and to determine if calorie, protein, and micronutrient needs are being met. Special attention should be given to the calorie mix of the parenteral formula and to the total amount of calories it provides. Patients who require PN for extended periods may be at greater risk for permanent liver damage. Patients with short-bowel syndrome who meet eligibility criteria may benefit from small bowel rehabilitation and thus avoid the long-term complications of PN, including hepatic dysfunction.[117] Infusion of PN may not be the cause of hepatic dysfunction but may contribute along with many other insults that critically or chronically ill patients suffer. When liver enzymes increase, a systematic and critical evaluation of the patient's PN regimen, disease, medications, and medical treatment is necessary (Box 19-1).

Gastrointestinal Complications

The GI tract, the physiologic route by which the body obtains the nutrients to sustain life, also functions as an immune organ to prevent entry of bacteria and toxins into the body. To function as an immune barrier, the GI tract must maintain its structural, functional, and environmental integrity. GI atrophy,

---

BOX 19-1

Steps to Follow When Hepatic Dysfunction Occurs with PN Infusion[84-86, 93, 96, 108, 109, 111-120]

1. Examine kilocalorie load to avoid overfeeding.
   a. Recalculate estimated needs based on current status
   b. Perform indirect calorimetry to identify total kilocalorie requirements
2. Examine distribution of carbohydrate, fat, and protein.
   a. Provide 70:30 carbohydrate-to-fat ratio
   b. Decrease calorie to nitrogen ratio to 100:1
3. Cycle PN infusion over 12-16 hours.
   a. Monitor tolerance to infusion of total volume over shorter time period
   b. Do not cycle if glycemic control not achieved with 24-hour infusion
4. Review current medications and disease state for possible hepatotoxic impact.
5. If patient is NPO, consider providing the following:
   a. Antibiotic therapy
      1. Metronidazole
      2. Polymyxin B
   b. Glutamine for intestinal mucosal stimulation
   c. Enteral stimulation with 15%-20% of kilocalories via GI tract
6. Consider possible nutrient deficiencies. More research is needed in this area before definitive recommendations can be made. Monitor serum levels before and during supplementation.
   a. Choline
   b. L-Carnitine
   c. Glucagon
   d. Cholecystokinin

---

bacterial overgrowth, and bacterial translocation have all been attributed to the detrimental effects of PN infusion.

Gastrointestinal Atrophy

Mucosal thickness, villus height, and nitrogen content of the intestinal tract are decreased with PN-associated GI atrophy, despite adequate PN. The proposed causes of GI atrophy secondary to PN are lack of villus stimulation by enteral nutrients, inadequate secretions from the pancreas and gallbladder, and decreased stimulation by gastric hormones. GI atrophy has been shown to occur during starvation and provision of PN.

Bacterial Overgrowth and Translocation

Bacterial overgrowth, the proliferation of bacteria in the GI tract, is believed to occur as a result of GI atrophy and absence of GI stimulation by enteral nutrition. Bacterial overgrowth is thought to increase the risk of bacteria's entering the systemic circulation (bacterial translocation) through a permeable bowel. In parenterally fed rats, providing 6% to 10% of calories enterally did not affect translocation, but an increase to 20% to 25% of calories as chow decreased the incidence of bacterial translocation,[118,119] but did not affect macromolecular permeability.[119] A study of infants on PN suggested that a minimum of 18% to 21% of total kilocalories given enterally is enough to stimulate and maintain GI tract integrity, improve immune function, and prevent infection.[120] The actual presence of bacterial translocation and endotoxemia from the GI tract has not been conclusively proved in humans.[121] The association of GI atrophy with PN is detailed in Chapter 21.

Gastric Hyperacidity

To prevent gastric erosion secondary to gastric acid production without enteral intake, histamine H₂-receptor antagonists are added to PN formulas. H_2-blockers are effective in patients with massive small bowel resections, who demonstrate gastric hypersecretion and elevated serum gastrin levels.[122] The addition of H_2-receptor antagonists to the PN as opposed to being given as a separate IV can reduce costs by decreasing the number of intravenous bags, administration sets, and intravenous accesses. Continuous infusion may also help keep the gastric pH above 4.[123] Cimetidine (standard dose 1200 mg/day), ranitidine (standard dose 150 mg/day), and famotidine (standard dose 40 mg/day) have been shown to be compatible with PN and total nutrient admixture (TNA) solutions.[124-126] The dose of H_2-receptor antagonists should be decreased by 50% in patients with impaired renal clearance.

Macronutrient-Related Complications

Substrate Composition

The macronutrient components of PN can be provided as a dextrose-amino acid mixture with lipids infused separately (piggybacked) or as a TNA (dextrose-amino acid-lipid combination). Each system of nutrient delivery has advantages and disadvantages. A distinct advantage of a separate infusion of lipids is the increased stability of the infusates and the ability to visualize precipitants in the dextrose and amino acid mixture; however, even without lipids, crystalline particles are not always visible.[127] A separate infusion of lipids allows use of a smaller (0.2 to 0.4 μm) filter to remove contaminants, precipitates, and microorganisms. The TNA system provides a continuous lipid infusion, which diminishes the adverse effects of short-term lipid infusion, but TNA solutions are less stable and limit the provision of additives. A larger 1.2 μm, in-line filter is necessary to prevent occlusion of the filter with lipid particles. There is concern that this may allow entry of undesirable contaminants and infectious organisms into the bloodstream.

Calories

OVERFEEDING. Overfeeding can contribute to adverse consequences. When PN was introduced in 1968, patients' nutritional needs were overestimated because it was thought that stress and injury resulted in severe hypermetabolism and that patients needed large amounts of calories to survive. Malnourished patients were often aggressively repleted with more calories than they could effectively utilize. Although repletion and restoration of body cell mass is a long-term goal of nutrition support, there are indications that a gradual conservative approach to nutrition support causes fewer metabolic abnormalities and may decrease morbidity and mortality associated with overfeeding. Repletion of malnourished patients with PN is more likely to increase fat than lean body mass unless exercise or anabolic agents are provided as part of the regimen.[128]

Underfeeding can also be detrimental if it is prolonged. Inadequate nutrition has been associated with respiratory dysfunction, poor wound healing, increased infection risk, and poor prognosis.[127,129,130] Patients receiving PN must have a thorough nutrition assessment to determine calorie, protein, and nutrient requirements based on the extent of malnutrition, disease activity, associated organ and metabolic derangements, and prognosis. See Part II: Assessment of Nutritional Status for a thorough review of how to estimate nutritional needs.

Providing calories in excess of 25 to 35 kcal/kg body weight has been associated with hypercapnia, lipogenesis, hyperglycemia, electrolyte abnormalities, impaired phagocytosis, and increased metabolic rate.[127] A study by Talpers and colleagues examined the difference in carbon dioxide production between two groups. Ten patients received an isocaloric PN solution of incremental carbohydrate-to-lipid ratios (40:40, 60:20, 75:5) with 20% of calories as protein in all three regimens; 10 other patients received an increasing amount of total calories (1.0, 1.5, 2.0 times resting energy expenditure [REE]) with identical carbohydrate, lipid, and protein ratios (60:20:20).[131] As the total calories increased from 1.0 to 2.0 times the REE, the V_{CO_2} increased from 181 ± 23 ml/min to 244 ± 40 ml/min. When the percentage of carbohydrate calories was increased from 40% to 75% of total calories, there was no increase in the V_{CO_2}. For patients with hypercapnia and increased carbon dioxide production, a metabolic cart study can identify calorie needs and substrate utilization.

Overfeeding increases the metabolic rate, which in turn requires greater oxygenation and cardiopulmonary effort. Eventually this can progress to respiratory and cardiac failure.[129] Providing excess calories also contributes to increased fluid volume infused with the PN. Extremely malnourished patients retain fluid and sodium when fed.[129] These factors contribute to hyponatremia and edema. The effect of overfeeding on hepatic function is addressed in earlier sections of this chapter. It is also important to be aware of calorie sources that may not be as obvious as the components of PN. Peritoneal dialysis can deliver 40 to 250 kcal, depending on dextrose concentration in each 2-L exchange, and IV fluids containing 5% or 10% dextrose, 170 to 340 kcal/L, respectively. Continuous venous-venous or arterial-venous hemodialysis (CVVHD/CAVHD) uses dianeal as the osmotic gradient to remove toxins from the blood. Infusion of 1.5% dianeal at 900 ml/min has the potential to provide 474 kcal/24 hours. Propofol, a 10% lipid-based sedative, provides 1.1 kcal/ml. Although it is generally given at variable rates throughout the day and for short periods (1 to 3 days), it can significantly affect calorie intake and substrate distribution.

REFEEDING SYNDROME. Related to overfeeding is the refeeding syndrome observed when malnourished patients, particularly marasmic patients, are given overaggressive nutrition support. The body adapts to starvation by decreasing reliance on gluconeogenesis and carbohydrate for calories and increasing utilization of ketones and fatty acids, which do not require intermediates containing phosphate to produce energy. Insulin, thyroid, and adrenergic endocrine systems decrease activity with starvation.[130,131] When refeeding occurs, there is a sudden shift to glucose as a primary fuel, these endocrine systems are revitalized, and the metabolic rate accelerates. However, insulin levels may not increase enough to balance dextrose infusion. Hyperglycemia can result in further metabolic derangements of osmotic diuresis, dehydration, hypotension, hyperosmolar nonketotic coma, and metabolic acidosis.[132,133] The switch to carbohydrate-based fuel creates a sudden demand for phosphorus, which has been depleted during starvation. Hypophosphatemia is the most frequently reported consequence of refeeding syndrome.[131] The combination of hyperinsulinemia, depleted total body phosphorus stores, carbohydrate availability, and the demand for phosphorus in adenosine triphosphate synthesis contribute to the severe hypophosphatemia of the refeeding syndrome. Potassium, decreased during starvation with the loss of lean body mass, responds to refeeding and increased insulin levels by moving into the cells and, in turn, causes hypokalemia. Hypomagnesemia, along with hypokalemia and hypocalcemia, occurs with starvation and anabolic metabolism. Extracellular fluid retention with refeeding is believed to be related to hypoalbuminemia, carbohydrate metabolism, and sodium balance. Refeeding can cause abrupt development of hyperinsulinemia, which results in antinatriuresis that in turn promotes an antidiuretic effect and expansion of extracellular volume.[133] Marasmic patients with reduced cardiac mass can experience cardiac decompensation. Thiamine deficiency is also believed to be a component of refeeding syndrome. Patients who have experienced prolonged starvation or who have a history of alcohol abuse may require thiamine supplementation before receiving PN. When initiating nutrition support, it is important to correct any existing vitamin and mineral deficiencies before initiating PN with basal energy needs (20 kcal/kg or 100% to 120% basal energy expenditure [BEE]) and adequate protein (1.2 to 1.5 g/kg).[132] Calories are increased to goal over 5 to 7 days with ongoing surveillance of electrolyte, mineral, and vitamin status. The patient's weight and pulse rate can be monitored to assess fluid status. Weight gain greater than 1 kg per week probably reflects fluid retention and should be avoided.[132]

Dextrose Metabolism

The body needs a minimum of 100 to 150 g of glucose per day to provide fuel for the brain and red blood cells. Without glucose in the diet, the body catabolizes protein and obtains the required fuel via gluconeogenesis. Although it is important to provide glucose in PN to meet this metabolic demand, provision of too much glucose is associated with adverse effects. Hyperglycemia is often seen in conjunction with PN. When dextrose is the sole source of nonprotein calories, metabolic complications have been reported: insulin-stimulated lipogenesis, fatty liver, elevated liver enzymes, increased carbon dioxide production, hyperglycemia, increased metabolic rate, and increased sympathetic activity.[134,135] Levels of adrenocorticotropic hormone, cortisol, epinephrine, and norepinephrine are elevated during critical illness and increase hepatic production of glucose and glycogenolysis.[136] As more dextrose is provided as fuel, oxidation of glucose increases and can result in lipogenesis and a respiratory quotient (RQ) greater than 1.0. Wolfe and colleagues examined the effect of three glucose infusion rates, 4, 7, and 9 mg/kg per minute, and found that all three suppressed hepatic glucose release, but the 4 mg/kg per minute rate maximized glucose oxidation.[135] Addition of lipids to the parenteral formula can help provide the necessary calories without exceeding the oxidative capacity of dextrose. In critically ill patients, the maximum rate of glucose oxidation appears to be 5 to 7 mg/kg per minute.[136] Exceeding this amount can promote hyperglycemia and it is associated with adverse metabolic sequelae. Critically ill patients generally tolerate a substrate mix of 60% dextrose, 20% lipid, and 20% protein.

Glucose intolerance can be secondary to diabetes mellitus or to metabolic stress induced by trauma, infection, or steroid

therapy. Regular insulin can be provided subcutaneously (SQ) according to a sliding scale, insulin drip, and/or added directly to PN, as needed.[134,136] Patients with a normal blood glucose before initiation of PN can be started with 200 to 300 g of dextrose and increased to calorie goal, as tolerated. Blood glucose levels should be monitored every 4 to 6 hours for the first 3 days and, if well-controlled, once or twice a day thereafter.[134]

Patients with diabetes mellitus are intolerant of glucose, and hyperglycemia caused by dextrose infusion is anticipated. Severely ill patients are often intolerant to IV dextrose and require close monitoring with initiation of PN. PN should begin with 100 to 150 g of dextrose for patients with serum glucose values greater than 200 mg/dl before PN starts. The total dextrose infusion goal should not exceed 4 mg/kg per minute.[137] A general guideline for adding insulin to PN for a patient who is hyperglycemic before starting dextrose-containing PN is to add 0.1 unit of insulin for each gram of dextrose provided (e.g., add 20 units of insulin to an infusion of 200 g dextrose).[134] It had been reported that 50% of the insulin provided in the PN adhered to the infusate container and tubing and was rendered metabolically inactive;[138] however, more recent studies of currently available PN solutions and infusion materials have shown that the availability of insulin added to PN is closer to 90% to 95%.[139] Therefore, provision of insulin should be done very carefully in order to avoid hypoglycemia. Additional insulin requirements as determined by serum glucose levels can be treated with SQ sliding scale insulin or direct addition to the PN bag. If serum glucose levels exceed 200 mg/dl, additional regular insulin (0.05 units/g dextrose) can be added each day. If insulin requirements exceed 0.2 units/g dextrose in PN, a continuous insulin infusion is probably warranted.[134] Insulin in PN should be adjusted as the amount of dextrose is increased or decreased. If hyperglycemia is not successfully controlled, calorie needs must be reassessed and all potential sources of dextrose evaluated. A continuous insulin infusion may be required so that insulin can be titrated to metabolic demands; however, insulin drips are generally given only in intensive care units (ICUs). Insulin needs decrease as the patient's metabolic stress resolves and steroid dose is tapered. When estimating insulin requirements, it is also important to consider the effect of renal function, steroid doses, diffuse anasarca, medications, and the dextrose content of intravenous fluids and dialysates.

To diminish hyperinsulinemia that can occur with continuous PN infusions, it may be beneficial to cycle the PN and create a more physiologic pattern of feeding and fasting. A diabetic patient transitioning to cycled PN may require a gradual decrease from a 24-hour to a 12-hour infusion period. As more dextrose is given in a shorter time, insulin should be adjusted to keep serum glucose levels below 200 mg/dl. Tapering the PN infusion rate can be accomplished by decreasing the maximum infusion rate by half or decreasing it to 40 to 60 ml/hr for the last hour of infusion. Some patients (e.g., those with severe diabetes) may require a 2-hour taper to control rebound hypoglycemia. If PN is interrupted without opportunity for tapering and the patient's blood glucose is below 150 mg/dl, a solution of 10% dextrose in water should be provided to prevent rebound hypoglycemia.[137] If a patient experiences hypoglycemia while receiving PN with added insulin, the 10% dextrose solution can be infused concurrently to maintain blood glucose levels until the PN prescription can be modified. Studies suggest that tapering PN is not necessary.[140,141] However, tapering the infusion at the end of the cycle period or when stopping PN completely can prevent rebound hypoglycemia in susceptible patients or those receiving more than 100 g of dextrose per liter. An individualized approach based on clinical judgment is needed until more research on this subject becomes available.

Hypercapnia can occur with increased carbon dioxide production, to which healthy subjects adjust by increasing ventilation. Patients with compromised ventilatory status are unable to eliminate the excess carbon dioxide and may be difficult to wean from the ventilator. Indirect calorimetry measures the respiratory quotient (RQ), the ratio of carbon dioxide produced to oxygen consumed. The RQ is used to determine substrate utilization. Glucose has an RQ of 1.0 and therefore produces more carbon dioxide than fat (RQ, 0.7); however, studies that showed increased carbon dioxide production with higher proportions of dextrose infusion were also providing excess total calories.[131] Therefore an elevated RQ can be more indicative of excess total calories rather than the distribution of calories between dextrose and fat. When a ventilated patient has hypercapnia, it is reasonable to reassess the patient's calorie needs and decrease total calories as indicated. If the RQ remains greater than 1.0 after a decrease in total calories, the substrate mix can then be adjusted to increase the proportion of lipid and decrease dextrose while meeting estimated or measured calorie needs. Every effort should be made to avoid overfeeding a ventilated patient because this promotes lipogenesis, carbon dioxide production, and respiratory acidosis. (See Chapter 6 for a more detailed discussion of indirect calorimetry).

Alternative carbohydrate calorie sources, including xylitol, glycerol, and fructose, are being studied.[142] Utilization of alternative carbohydrate sources may alleviate adverse effects of dextrose infusion; however, with the introduction of intravenous lipids and more realistic calorie goals, it is possible to meet a patient's calorie needs without exceeding the patient's oxidative capacity of dextrose.

Amino Acid Metabolism

Currently available crystalline amino acid solutions are well tolerated by patients with adequate renal and hepatic function. Patients who develop prerenal azotemia, renal failure, hepatic encephalopathy, or hyperammonemia may benefit from a reduction in the amount of amino acids provided or a change to a specialized amino acid formula. A discussion of the appropriateness of specialized amino acid formulas is addressed in Chapters 32 and 33. When protein intolerance does develop, it may be more cost-effective to limit standard amino acids to 0.6 to 1.0 g/kg until the underlying cause of the intolerance is corrected than to use a more expensive specialty formula, that may or may not be effective.

A study by Buchman and coworkers described decreased renal function associated with long-term PN.[143] The marked decrease in creatinine clearance and tubule function could not be explained completely by factors such as age, nutritional status, nephrotoxic drugs, or the number of cases of bacteremia or fungemia. The protein load provided had no effect on renal function. The authors speculated that the acidity of the PN might

promote nephropathy. Another study reported that nine of 16 patients on long-term, cycled PN demonstrated a reduction in glomerular filtration rate.[144] Patients on long-term PN should be monitored for possible development of renal impairment.

Studies on healthy adult male volunteers have shown that plasma and skeletal amino acid levels are adversely affected by starvation and that PN could not fully correct the amino acid abnormalities within 2 weeks.[145,146] When recombinant human growth hormone was provided in conjunction with PN to trauma patients, nitrogen metabolism improved and plasma free amino acid levels were corrected.[147] Recombinant human growth hormone may exert a direct effect on amino acid metabolism or may be indirectly beneficial through its effect on increased production of insulin-like growth factor-1.

Lipid Metabolism

Until the approval of intravenous lipids for commercial use in the United States in 1978, there were reports of essential fatty acid deficiency (EFAD) in patients receiving glucose-only PN for 1 to 3 weeks.[148,149] EFAD is identified biochemically by a triene-tetraene ratio greater than 0.4 or by an increase in oleic and palmitoleic acids and a decrease in linoleic and arachidonic acids.[150,151] EFAD is prevented by providing 4% of total calories as fat.[151] Although there have been reports of correcting EFAD with topical vegetable oils,[152] other studies have not been successful.[148,149]

Hypertriglyceridemia can occur with the infusion of intravenous lipids and can contribute to pancreatitis, glucose intolerance, displacement of bilirubin from albumin by free fatty acids, interference with hemoglobin saturation determination, and suppression of humoral and cellular immunity.[153] Plasma triglycerides should be monitored before initiation of PN and routinely throughout lipid administration when hyperlipidemia is suspected. Acceptable serum triglyceride levels are less than 400 mg/dl.[154]

The effect of PN LCTs on the immune system continues to receive considerable attention. The LCTs used in lipid emulsions are high in the ω-6 fatty acids, which are the precursors for arachidonic acid. Arachidonic acid is metabolized to immunomodulating eicosanoids. An abundance of ω-6 eicosanoids causes an increase in prostaglandin E_2 (PGE_2), which inhibits the cell-mediated immune response.[155] In rats, PN infusion with lipids has been shown to interfere with normal lipid metabolism and to impair production of tumor necrosis factor (TNF) in macrophages.[156,157] Changes in macrophage phospholipid membranes may result in variations in prostaglandin and leukotriene production, which in turn can affect production of TNF secondary to increased PGE_2. Studies of cottonseed oil lipid emulsions used previously reported decreased platelet adhesiveness in adults. This same effect was reported in adults who received 100 g of intralipid;[158] however, in other studies the infusion of lipid was not found to adversely affect platelet count or aggregation.[159,160]

Impairment of the reticuloendothelial system (RES) was demonstrated after 3 days of PN with lipids piggybacked over a 10-hour period.[161] The authors suggested cautious use of LCT in patients with known or potential impairments of the RES such as burn injuries, hepatic disease, sepsis, and blunt trauma. A similar study compared the effect on RES function of continuous LCT infusion and intermittent infusion of MCTs and LCTs.[162] The authors reported that lipids provided either continuously with LCT (three-in-one admixture) or intermittently with primarily MCTs were well tolerated and were associated with increased fat removal without RES dysfunction. Critically ill patients with organ failure and sepsis received a constant infusion of a conventional lipid emulsion at 0.3 g fat/kg per hour for 0 to 120 minutes and demonstrated effective metabolism of lipids with no evidence of impaired gas exchange or glucose metabolism.[163] The triglycerides were hydrolyzed and the fatty acids were oxidized and therefore did not affect the RES. The authors postulate that infusion of lipids at low rates for extended periods of time eliminates the side effects reported when lipids were given as 500 ml over 4 to 6 hours.

The adverse effects associated with the infusion of LCTs has created interest in the use of MCTs as an alternative lipid fuel. Clinically, the benefits of MCTs are rapid clearance from the blood and carnitine-independent transport into the mitochondria. MCTs can be neurotoxic, may not spare nitrogen as well as LCTs, and do not provide essential fatty acids. Developments in lipid formulation include the physical mixture of MCTs and LCTs and the creation of structured lipids that utilize the glycerol backbone with a combination of attached MCTs and LCTs. Structured lipids were found to be safe, well-tolerated, and efficacious compared with LCT in patients following colorectal surgery.[164] Another study reported that an MCT/LCT emulsion and a pure MCT emulsion increased neutrophil expression, adhesion, and degranulation in vitro.[165] These effects were not seen with structured lipids or an LCT emulsion. Dicarboxylic acids have been investigated as possible alternative lipid fuels.[166] The advantages of this alternative fuel are its low cost and water solubility. More studies are needed to justify the replacement of lipid since it is associated with relatively few complications, provides essential fatty acids, and can be combined with dextrose and amino acids in a single container.[167]

Recommendations for providing lipid infusions while limiting adverse effects are as follows: (1) provide no more than 30% of total calories as lipid (no more than 20% during sepsis); (2) provide no more than 1 g/kg per day of fat; (3) provide a continuous lipid infusion; (4) monitor triglyceride levels; (5) provide at least 500 ml of 10% lipids twice a week to prevent EFAD when daily lipids are contraindicated.

Micronutrient-Related Complications
Fluid and Electrolytes

FLUID STATUS. Fluid volume tolerance is often an issue for patients in the ICU. Commonly used calculations for estimating fluid requirements may not be applicable for patients with renal, liver, or cardiac dysfunction. Patients may need fluid volume restriction, which can limit the total amount of calories that can be given per day via PN. Medications, blood products, and nutrition support compete for the fluid volume that the patient can tolerate. Fluid needs are increased for patients with polyuria and extrarenal volume losses, such as GI, wound, and respiratory tract excretions. It is important to assess the patient's fluid status so that realistic nutrition support goals can be determined. Inputs and outputs (I/O), weight versus dry weight, pulse rate, blood pressure, serum sodium, hematocrit,

and blood urea nitrogen (BUN) should be monitored closely. A thorough physical assessment of the patient is necessary to determine the patient's fluid status. Refer to Chapter 10 for a detailed discussion of fluid and electrolyte management.

Hypovolemic patients often present with decreased weight, elevated serum sodium and BUN values, diminished urine output with elevated specific gravity, complaints of thirst, and dry mouth and skin.[168] Patients reliant solely on PN are at risk for volume depletion and dehydration when they are receiving no other IV fluids and are unable to drink fluids by mouth. It is imperative to monitor fluid I/O closely to ensure that the fluid content of PN is adequate to compensate for urinary, GI, or insensible fluid losses. Sterile water can be added to the PN according to the patient's estimated fluid needs. Peripheral PN formulas contain a larger volume of fluid (2 to 4 L) to provide the osmolality that the peripheral veins can tolerate. Hypovolemia generally is not a consequence of providing peripheral PN.

Hypervolemia can be a problem when providing PN in the ICU, for any patient on peripheral PN and for patients with renal, liver, and cardiac failure. Patients with volume excess can have increased weight, extremity edema, polyuria with decreased specific gravity (unless oliguria or anuria is present), and decreased serum sodium.[168] Hyponatremia secondary to volume excess should not be treated with sodium supplementation because this only compounds the problem with additional fluid retention. Patients with volume excess should be restricted in fluid volume, including the provision of nutrition support. The maximum concentrations of dextrose, lipids, and amino acids should be used. It may be necessary to decrease the total calories provided in order to adhere to the total volume limitation. It may even be necessary to stop the PN temporarily for patients with severe hypervolemia. Peripheral PN is contraindicated for patients with fluid volume overload.

ELECTROLYTES

Sodium. Sodium status is closely related to fluid distribution. A detailed discussion of hyponatremia and hypernatremia is found in Chapter 10. It is imperative to determine the etiology of the abnormal sodium level before treating. In patients receiving PN, hyperosmolar hyponatremia is usually associated with hyperglycemia that, when corrected, corrects the serum sodium level. Hypoosmolar hyponatremia is the most common type of hyponatremia. The patient can be either hypovolemic and require volume expansion, euvolemic and require water restriction, or hypervolemic and require sodium and water restriction.[169] Hypernatremia can occur in patients receiving inadequate maintenance fluids or too much sodium. Volume requirements are increased for patients with inadequate free water, which can occur when patients cannot drink fluids; do not respond to thirst; or have large fluid volume losses, as with burns, fistula, fever, or hyperventilation. Sterile water or saline solutions, depending on the content of the lost fluids, can be added to the PN or given as a separate IV infusion. If the patient is receiving excessive sodium, sodium intake should be decreased if possible. The PN solution's maintenance dose of sodium, 1.0 to 1.5 mEq/kg per day, may need to be adjusted according to the patient's fluid status, sodium requirements, and organ function.[168]

Potassium. Potassium, the major intracellular cation, is involved in glucose and nitrogen metabolism. Hypokalemia is generally associated with increased losses or a shift to and from the extracellular and intracellular spaces.[169] An extensive discussion of the etiologies of hyperkalemia and hypokalemia is presented in Chapter 10. Serum potassium levels, sources of losses, and supplementation should be evaluated daily. For patients with normal renal function, the maintenance potassium content of PN can be 0.7 to 1.5 mEq/kg per day;[151,168] however, potassium needs should be assessed by examining the patient's renal function, medication profile, disease state, and lean body mass. Hyperkalemia is associated with decreased renal excretion, excessive potassium administration, hyperglycemia, potassium-sparing medications, and metabolic acidosis. Because hyperkalemia is associated with life-threatening cardiac abnormalities, treatment should not be delayed. The cause of the hyperkalemia should be identified and treated; meanwhile, the potassium content of the PN can be eliminated or decreased, depending on serum potassium level trends.

Chloride and Acetate. Chloride and acetate are often considered together because of their relationship in acid-base balance. A detailed description of acid-base balance in presented in Chapter 10. Chloride (acid) and acetate (base) are provided as salts in combination with sodium and potassium. Acetate is a precursor for bicarbonate and is rapidly converted by the liver to bicarbonate. Bicarbonate cannot be added to PN because it results in formation of insoluble carbonate salts with calcium and magnesium. Amino acid solutions contain various proportions of chloride and acetate, depending on the manufacturer. If an acid-base imbalance occurs and the primary cause of the imbalance is metabolic, the salts in PN can be adjusted to compensate for losses of chloride (e.g., metabolic alkalosis secondary to nasogastric output) or loss of bicarbonate (e.g., metabolic acidosis secondary to small intestinal fluid losses);[169] however, if the primary source of the acid-base imbalance is respiratory, an attempt to correct the compensatory metabolic imbalance will not succeed and may exacerbate the primary disorder. In the case of patients who have respiratory acidosis and are on a ventilator, it may be prudent to examine the total calories provided and the proportion of dextrose being infused in the PN, since these can contribute to excessive carbon dioxide production. No matter what causes the acid-base imbalance, it is important to treat the precipitating factor, if possible, and not just the resulting imbalance.

Minerals

CALCIUM. Calcium is added routinely to PN formulas to provide 0.2 to 0.3 mEq/kg per day, although the actual parenteral requirements and optimal dosage have not been well studied.[168] When monitoring calcium, it is better to monitor ionized calcium concentrations because 60% of serum calcium is bound to albumin, which can affect measurable serum calcium levels. If serum ionized calcium is not available, an adjusted serum calcium value can be calculated as follows:

[(4–actual serum albumin g/dl) × 0.8] + actual serum calcium mg/dl

Because calcium affects parathyroid hormone secretion, excessive calcium infusion can lead to hypophosphatemia and hyperchloridemic acidosis. Excess infusion of vitamin D or calcium can also precipitate pancreatitis and metabolic bone disease.[168] In critically ill patients, hypocalcemia occurs secondary to septic shock, blood transfusion (citrate in the blood binds calcium), renal failure, hypoalbuminemia, or hypomagnesemia.[170] When hypomagnesemia occurs with hypocalcemia, the magnesium should be supplemented along with the calcium. Hypercalcemia occurs less often in critically ill persons and is related to immobilization, vitamin D excess, and acute renal failure. Chapter 10 provides more information on calcium.

PHOSPHORUS. Phosphate is involved in transfer of energy, utilization of oxygen, and mineralization of bone. As mentioned earlier, hypophosphatemia occurs with refeeding syndrome or with overfeeding without adequate phosphate supplementation.[132,171] Preexisting hypophosphatemia should be corrected before PN is begun. The standard amount of phosphorus added to PN is 7 to 9 mMol per 1000 kcal.[168] Guidelines for supplementing hypophosphatemia are given in Chapter 10. It may be necessary to stop the PN infusion to correct a severe deficit. When starting a patient on PN, it is important to monitor for a possible intracellular flux of phosphorus with a concomitant decrease in extracellular phosphorus. Other causes of hypophosphatemia include phosphate-binding antacids, GI losses, respiratory alkalosis, and secondary hyperparathyroidism.[169] Risk factors for developing hypophosphatemia are diabetes, alcoholism, marasmus, burns, and hypothermia. When initiating nutrition support for these patients, begin at basal energy needs and increase to goal slowly, according to the patient's tolerance, while monitoring serum phosphorus and providing supplemental phosphate as indicated. Hyperphosphatemia is associated with renal insufficiency or excess phosphate administration.[172] The phosphorus in the PN can be either eliminated or decreased and the serum phosphorus level monitored in the event hypophosphatemia ensues. When treating refractory hyperphosphatemia, it is important to consider that lipid emulsions, including propofol, contain phospholipid and provide 7.5 mMol phosphate in 500 ml. Several amino acid solutions, particularly those enriched with branched chain amino acids, contain 5 mMol phosphate per 500 ml.

CALCIUM/PHOSPHORUS STABILITY IN PARENTERAL NUTRITION. The stability of calcium and phosphate in parenteral solutions is affected by a multitude of factors including the concentration of calcium, phosphate, magnesium, dextrose, and amino acids; the form of calcium salt added; the composition of amino acids; the pH of the solution; the temperature of the solution; other additives in the solution; the order of mixing components in the solution; and the interval from compounding to infusion.[173,174] When the serum calcium level is multiplied by the serum phosphorus level and the product is greater than 4.8 mMol/L (70 mg/dl), there is a risk of soft tissue calcification.[175] An unintentional excess provision of phosphate in PN resulted in hyperphosphatemia, calcification of subcutaneous arteries, and skin necrosis in a patient without renal failure.[172] Precipitation of calcium-phosphate salts is more likely when there is a high concentration of calcium and phosphate in the solution, an elevated pH, a small amount of amino acids, an elevated temperature, inclusion of calcium chloride, addition of calcium before adding phosphate, a slow infusion rate, or an extended standing or hang time.[174] In 1994 the U.S. Food and Drug Administration issued a safety alert concerning the involvement of a peripheral nutrient admixture infusion and the precipitation of calcium phosphate in two deaths and at least two cases of respiratory distress.[176] Therefore, if a patient requires IV phosphorus or calcium in addition to the standard amounts in the parenteral solution, supplementation may need to be given through a line other than the one through which PN is being infused.

MAGNESIUM. Sixty percent of the body's magnesium is found in the bones and the remaining portion as intracellular cations.[169] Although serum levels do not accurately reflect total body magnesium, serum magnesium levels are used to determine supplementation needs because deficiency syndromes are related to serum levels.[168] Magnesium is discussed in Chapter 10. Magnesium depletion contributes to hypokalemia, hypocalcemia, and hypophosphatemia. Correction of the magnesium deficiency must be concurrent with correction of the other deficiencies. The standard amount of magnesium added to PN is 0.25 to 0.45 mEq/kg per day.[151,168] Replacement therapy may take several days because rapid infusion of large doses can cause hypermagnesemia with resulting neuromuscular and respiratory depression, flushing, and hypotension.[177] It is also important to note that approximately half of infused magnesium is excreted in the urine.[168,169]

Vitamins

Patients receiving PN should receive a daily source of water and fat-soluble vitamins evenly distributed throughout the total infusion volume.[168] Patients receiving PN without multivitamins have been reported to develop thiamine deficiency and metabolic acidosis in less than 2 weeks.[178] Measurements of vitamin levels should look at functional indices rather than serum levels, which are not as accurate for total body vitamin content. Specific vitamin requirements may be enhanced or diminished because of inflammation, stress, disease, substrate utilization, increased losses or retention, or preexisting deficiencies or toxicities. Several studies indicate a reduction of vitamin levels in critically ill[179,180,181] and elderly patients.[182] For a more detailed discussion of vitamins refer to Chapter 11. A standard, complete multivitamin should be given daily to all patients. Monitor vitamin A and other fat-soluble vitamin levels in patients with renal failure who are dependent on PN for nutrient requirements.[183] For renal failure patients, an IV B and C vitamin complex, if available, may be appropriate when PN is given over a long period, particularly for patients who are malnourished and have diminished retinol-binding capacity.

The Food and Drug Administration has mandated that multivitamin infusions for adults make the following changes: increase riboflavin and thiamin to 6 mg, increase vitamin C to 200 mg, increase folic acid to 600 μg, and add 150 μg vitamin K.[184] It will be important to monitor the international normalized ration (INR) in patients who begin or stop PN during warfarin therapy. The vitamin K content of lipid solutions is variable (0 to 290 μg/L)[185] and should also be considered when determining anticoagulation therapy. The additional 100 mg vitamin C could potentially contribute to increased availability of free iron with subsequent microorganism proliferation and development of renal calculi.[186]

Trace Elements

Parenteral preparations of trace elements are available as separate nutrients or as a trace element mixture to PN formulas.

Because Chapter 12 provides an extensive discussion of trace elements and nutrition support, only a few issues are addressed here. As with multivitamins, trace element nutrition should be determined by functional assays.

IRON. Compatibility of iron dextran with PN is controversial. Compatibility with TNA has been shown with 2 mg/L[187] but not with 50 mg/L.[188] There is also concern that supplementation of parenteral iron will increase the proliferation of microorganisms. Critically ill patients should not be given parenteral iron unless a deficiency is documented and enteral iron supplementation is not feasible.[186] Iron deficiency anemia can be prevented in patients on long-term PN with the addition of iron dextran once a week to a nonlipid-containing PN solution. The recent development of less antigenic products such as iron sucrose and iron gluconate reduce the risk of providing iron to PN patients.

ZINC. The amount of parenteral zinc recommended for a stable adult patient is 2.5 to 4.0 mg per day.[189] Zinc status is affected by medications, disease state, urinary and GI excretion, and degree of physiologic stress. Zinc supplementation has been recommended for patients with excessive GI losses. For every liter of nasogastric output, an additional 10 mg zinc has been suggested. Recommended zinc replacement amounts for each liter of output from the small intestine are 12 mg zinc per liter and 10 mEq magnesium per liter, and for stool or ileostomy are 17 mg/L.[189,190] Because plasma zinc is affected by various factors and assessing zinc status can be difficult, clinicians often rely on a positive response to supplementation as an indication of zinc deficiency. However it is important to monitor patients receiving supplemental parenteral zinc to avoid adverse effects. Supplementation with 30 mg zinc resulted in an increased febrile response and is associated with an increased risk of infection.[191] Another factor to consider when adding supplemental zinc to a total nutrient admixture is the effect of the divalent cation on the stability of the TNA.

MANGANESE, COPPER, SELENIUM. Hypermanganesemia has been reported in patients on long-term PN and those with chronic liver disease.[192,193] A study that looked at manganese levels and brain deposition in home PN patients reported that supplementation with 0.1 mg manganese/day resulted in increased incidence of alterations in brain magnetic resonance images.[192] When manganese supplementation was stopped, serum levels and brain deposition significantly dropped. The authors found that intraerythrocyte manganese level was a good indicator of manganese status. Hypermanganesemia was also reported in a study that looked at short-term and long-term effects with a standard supplementation of 0.5 mg/day.[194] The authors suggested monitoring manganese levels in all patients on PN more than 30 days. Another study in home PN patients without cholestasis or neurologic symptoms found that serum manganese levels were elevated in 61% of patients with standard supplementation.[195] Omission of manganese and copper is suggested for chronic hyperbilirubinemia.[194,196] However, total elimination of copper resulted in copper deficiency and pancytopenia.[101,197] It may be more prudent to reduce the provision of the trace element affected and periodically monitor serum levels or functional indices.[101,197]

When deleting individual trace elements, it is important to provide the other trace elements that are not elevated to prevent a possible trace element deficiency, especially in patients with malabsorption syndromes, small bowel resection, or poor oral intake.[101] Selenium deficiency has been reported in critically ill patients and those on long-term PN.[198,199] Factors to consider when deliberating alteration of the multivitamin and trace element contents of PN are availability of micronutrient alternatives, anticipated duration of PN, patient's nutritional state before PN, patient's current clinical condition, and compatibility and stability of the reformulated solution.

Cycling Parenteral Nutrition Infusions

The goal of cyclic PN is to infuse the nutrients the patient requires in a shorter time period. The proposed advantages of cyclic PN are the physiologic benefit of mimicking the fasting and fed states and the psychosocial benefit of giving the patient "time off" from the infusion for normal activities of daily living. To infuse all the nutrients needed, however, the infusion rates are increased over 8 to 18 hours. Patients with cardiovascular, hepatic, or renal disorders may not tolerate rapid infusion of 1.5 to 3 L over a shorter time. Glucose intolerance may preclude cyclic PN infusion (see section on dextrose metabolism). Cycling of PN generally is not recommended for critically ill patients. This patient population is at increased risk for sepsis, which can be compounded by hyperglycemia and its association with nosocomial infections.[200] Discontinuous lipid infusion has been associated with impairment of the RES function,[167] whereas continuous infusion has not.[162,163] Cycled lipids have also been associated with worsening pulmonary function in patients with severe acute respiratory distress syndrome (ARDS) and impairment of hepatic function.[200] Although cyclic PN may be contraindicated for critically ill patients, it has been used effectively and safely for stable, chronically ill patients who require long-term PN.

Long-Term Complications of Parenteral Nutrition

Metabolic Bone Disease

Metabolic bone disease is reported as a complication of long-term PN infusion.[201-203] Abnormalities in bone remodeling seen in long-term PN patients have been related to vitamin D, increased urinary losses of calcium, aluminum toxicity, parathyroid hormone (PTH) levels, and D-lactate toxicity.[201,202] Increased urinary losses of calcium, phosphorus, and magnesium have been associated with loop diuretics; cycled PN; and excess protein, calcium, phosphorus, magnesium, sodium, vitamin D, and fluid.[201,202] Continuous PN appears to promote mineral homeostasis better than cycled PN.[202] The role of vitamin D in the development of metabolic bone disease is unclear.[202] A reduction of vitamin D, provided parenterally, from 1000 to 200 IU/day resulted in a change of the primary form, in which the vitamin D circulated in the blood from the plant form of D_2 to the cholesterol derivative in the skin, D_3.[202] The implications of this difference are not clear. When patients receive nutrients parenterally, the impact of removing vitamin D from the PN should be minimal because the primary action of vitamin D is to enhance calcium absorption in the GI tract.[201] In a prospective study of nine patients with initial decreased levels of PTH on long-term home PN, vitamin D was omitted from the

PN for a 4- to 5-year period. Removal of vitamin D resulted in an increase in lumbar spine bone mineral content, normalization of PTH and $1,25(OH)_2D$, and minimal change in calcium, phosphorus, magnesium, and 25-hydroxyvitamin D.[201] A study that provided 15 versus 45 mMol/day of inorganic phosphorus to patients on cyclic PN reported a decrease in urinary calcium excretion with the higher dose of phosphorus.[204] The decrease in calciuria was attributed to increased renal tubular resorption of calcium and not changes in PTH and vitamin D activity. A study of patients with inflammatory bowel disease (IBD) consuming an oral diet found that low bone turnover was associated with low bone formation despite normal levels of hormones involved in calcium regulation.[205] Because patients with IBD are likely to receive home PN as their disease progresses, they may experience acceleration of bone disease with dependence on long-term PN. Prevention and treatment of metabolic bone disease are confined to minimizing nutrient losses and maximizing nutrient retention with careful monitoring of nutrient and medication use.

Cost Issues

One of the issues associated with PN is the cost of infusion: financial, ethical, and social. As the health care dollar shrinks, the need to justify the high cost and high risk of nutrition support grows.[206] Efforts made to reduce inappropriate use of PN has resulted in significant cost savings and improved patient care.[207, 208] It is often difficult to differentiate the effectiveness or benefit of PN from concurrent medical care and to identify the intangible costs and benefits of nutrition support. Does the patient improve because of nutrition support or does nutritional status improve because of decreased metabolic stress and aggressive medical treatment? PN is an expensive feeding modality, and without answers to its costs versus benefits or its cost-effectiveness, fiscal and ethical issues will determine its use. There are patients for whom PN is appropriate, cost-effective, and cost-beneficial, but it is imperative to limit complications and demonstrate outcomes in these patient populations.

Conclusion

Complications of PN can be technical, septic, gastrointestinal, or metabolic. Technical complications are related to catheter placement, care, and removal. Catheter-related sepsis is the most common complication of intravenous catheters. To reduce the risk of catheter-related sepsis in patients receiving PN, protocols for aseptic placement and catheter care must be followed.

GI complications of PN include hepatic dysfunction and GI atrophy and bacterial overgrowth. Virtually every component of the parenteral solution has been implicated as a cause of hepatic steatosis and cholestasis. Careful evaluation of calories, nutrients, and medications provided may help prevent hepatic dysfunction with PN. It has been postulated that GI atrophy and bacterial overgrowth promote translocation of toxins from the GI tract into the systemic circulation. To maintain the integrity of the GI tract, 15% to 20% of total calories should be given enterally whenever feasible.

Metabolic complications encompass macronutrient and micronutrient abnormalities. Macronutrient complications include overfeeding and excesses or deficiencies of dextrose, protein, and lipids in the infusate. Micronutrient-related complications are excesses and inadequacies of fluids, electrolytes, vitamins, trace elements, and minerals. The composition of PN should be individualized to the nutrient requirements and tolerance of the patient.

A final consideration in the monitoring of the complications of parenteral support is the cost of providing PN. With health care dollars shrinking, nutrition support resources must be used efficiently and conservatively. Providing parenteral support only to those for whom it is indicated and providing the amounts of macronutrients and micronutrients necessary for optimal recovery contribute to the control of health care costs. Evidence-based standards of care, individualized patient care, and close monitoring of the infusion of PN can ensure that resources are used wisely and effectively.

REFERENCES

1. Ryder M: The future of vascular access: will the benefits be worth the risk? *Nutr Clin Prac* 14:165-169, 1999.
2. Collin GR, Ahmadinejad AS, Misse E: Spontaneous migration of subcutaneous central venous catheters, *Am J Surg* 63:322-326, 1997.
3. Mukau L, Talamini MA, Sitzman JV: Risk factors for central venous catheter-related vascular erosions, *J Parenter Enteral Nutr* 15:513-516, 1991.
4. Mueller BU, Skelton J, Callender DPE, et al: A prospective randomized trial comparing the infectious and noninfectious complications of an externalized catheter versus a subcutaneously implanted device in cancer patients, *J Clin Oncol* 10:1943-1948, 1992.
5. Denny DF: Placement and management of long-term central venous access catheters and ports, *Am J Radiol* 161:385-393, 1993.
6. Hagley MT, Martin B, Gast P, Traeger SM: Infectious and mechanical complications of central venous catheters placed by percutaneous venipuncture and over guidewires, *Crit Care Med* 20:1426-1430, 1992.
7. Wendt JR: Avoiding serious complications with central venous access, *Surg Rounds* 7:637-642, 1992.
8. Yerdel MA, Karayalcin K, Aras N, et al: Mechanical complications of subclavian vein catheterization. A prospective study, *Int Surg* 76:18-22, 1991.
9. Rosa UW, Foreman M, Willsie-Ediger S: Intermittent back pain after central venous catheter placement, *J Parenter Enteral Nutr* 17:91-93, 1993.
10. Sakaguchi M, Taguchi K, Ishiyama T: Acute pharyngitis, an unusual complication of intravenous hyperalimentation, *J Laryngol Otol* 108:159-160, 1994.
11. Waggoner SE: Venous air embolism through a Groshong catheter, *Gynecol Oncol* 48:394-396, 1993.
12. Mailloux RJ, DeLegge MH, Kirby DF: Pulmonary embolism as a complication of long-term total parenteral nutrition, *J Parenter Enteral Nutr* 17:578-582, 1993.
13. Randolph AG, Cook DJ, Gonzales CA, et al: Benefit of heparin in central venous and pulmonary artery catheters. A meta-analysis of randomized controlled trials, *Chest* 113:165-171, 1998.
14. Boraks P, Seale J, Price J, et al: Prevention of central venous catheter associated thrombosis using minidose warfarin in patients with haematological malignancies, *Br J Haematology* 101:483-486, 1998.
15. Ray CE, Shenoy SS, McCarthy PL, et al: Weekly prophylactic urokinase instillation in tunneled central venous access devices, *J Vascular Interventional Radiology* 10:1330-1334, 1999.
16. Duerksen DR, Ahmad A, Doweiko J, et al: Risk of symptomatic central venous thrombotic complications in AIDS patients receiving home parenteral nutrition, *J Parenter Enteral Nutr* 20:302-305, 1996.
17. Bliss DZ, Dysart M: Using needleless intravenous access devices for administering total parenteral nutrition (TPN): practice update, *Nutr Clin Prac* 14:299-303, 1999.
18. Do AN, Ray BJ, Banerjee SN, et al: Bloodstream infection associated with needleless device use and the importance of infection-control practices in the home health care setting, *J Infect Dis* 179:442-448, 1999.
19. Cookson ST, Ihrig M, O'Mara EM et al: Increased bloodstream infection rates in surgical patients associated with variation from recommended use and care following implementation of a needleless device, *Infect Control Hosp Epidemiol* 19:23-27, 1998.
20. McDonald LC, Banerjee SN, Jarvis WR: Line associated bloodstream infections in pediatric intensive-care-unit patients associated with a needleless device and intermittent intravenous therapy, *Infect Control Hosp Epidemiol* 19:772-777, 1998.
21. Intravenous Nurses Society: Infusion nursing standards of practice, *J Intraven Nurs* 23(suppl):S5-S81, 2000.
22. Andris DA, Krzywda EA: Central venous access: clinical practice issues, *Nurs Clin North Am* 32(4):719-740, 1997.
23. Hoch JR: Management of the complications of long-term venous access, *Semin Vasc Surg* 10:135-143, 1997.
24. Stephens LC, Haire WD, Kotulak GD: Are clinical signs accurate indicators of the cause of central venous catheter occlusion? *J Parenter Enteral Nutr* 19:75-79, 1995.
25. Compher CW, Kinosian BP, Evans-Stoner N, et al: Hyperhomocysteinemia is associated with venous thrombosis in patients with short bowel syndrome, *J Parenter Enteral Nutr* 25:1-8, 2001.
26. Hadaway LC: Major thrombotic and nonthrombotic complications, *J Intraven Nurs* 21(55):S143-S160, 1998.
27. Mammen EF: Pathogenesis of venous thrombosis, *Chest* 102(6):640S-644S, 1992.
28. Bertina RM: Introduction: hypercoagulable states, *Semin Hematol* 34(3):167-169, 1997.
29. Borg FT, Timmer J, deKam SS, Sauerwein HP: Use of sodium hydroxide solution to clear partially occluded vascular access ports, *J Parenter Enteral Nutr* 17:289-291, 1993.
30. Siepler J, Diamantidis R, Nishikawa RA, et al: Monthly urokinase in home parenteral nutrition patients reduces the incidence of hospital admissions, *J Parenter Enteral Nutr* 25:S7-S8, 2001 (abstract).
31. Stephens MB: Deep venous thrombosis of the upper extremity, *Am Fam Physician* 55(2):533-539, 1997.
32. Andris DA, Krzywda EA, Schulte W, et al: Pinch-off syndrome: a rare etiology for central venous catheter occlusion, *J Parenter Enteral Nutr* 18:531-533, 1994.
33. Mirtallo JM: Introduction to parenteral nutrition. In Gottschlich MM (ed): *The science and practice of nutrition support: a case-based core curriculum,* Dubuque, IA, 2001, Kendall-Hunt Publishing Company, pp 211-223.
34. Kohlhardt SR, Smith RC, Wright CR: Peripheral versus central intravenous nutrition: comparison of two delivery systems, *Br J Surg* 81:66-70, 1994.
35. Payne-James JJ, Khawaja HT: First choice for total parenteral nutrition: the peripheral route, *J Parenter Enteral Nutr* 17:468-478, 1993.
36. Kane KF, Cologiovanni J, McKiernan, et al: High osmolality feedings do not increase the incidence of thrombophlebitis during peripheral IV nutrition, *J Parenter Enteral Nutr* 20:194-197, 1996.
37. Loughran SC, Borzatta M: Peripherally inserted central catheters: a report of 2506 catheter days, *J Parenter Enteral Nutr* 19:133-136, 1995.
38. Smith JR, Friedell ML, Cheathan ML, et al: Peripherally inserted central catheters revisited, *Am J Surg* 176:208-211, 1998.
39. Duerksen DR, Papineau N, Siemans J, et al: Peripherally inserted central catheters for parenteral nutrition: a comparison with centrally inserted catheters, *J Parenter Enteral Nutr* 23:85-89, 1999.
40. Krzywda KA, Andris DA, Edminston: Catheter infections: diagnosis, etiology, treatment, and prevention, *Nutr Clin Prac* 14:178-190, 1999.
41. Harden JL, Kemp L, Mirtallo J: Femoral catheters increase risk of infection in total parenteral nutrition patients, *Nutr Clin Prac* 10:60-66, 1995.
42. Curtas S, Bonaventura M, Meguid MM: Cannulation of inferior vena cava for long term central venous access, *Surg Gynecol Obstet* 168:121-124, 1989.
43. Friedman B, Kanter G, Titus D: Femoral venous catheters: a safe alternative for delivering parenteral alimentation, *Nutr Clin Prac* 9:69-72, 1994.
44. O'Keefe SJ, Burnes JU, Thompson RL: Recurrent sepsis in home parenteral nutrition patients: an analysis of risk factors, *J Parenter Enteral Nutr* 18:256-263, 1994.
45. Saint S, Veenstra DL, Lipsky BA: The clinical and economic consequences of nosocomial central venous catheter-related infection: are antimicrobial catheters useful? *Infect Control Hosp Epidemiol* 21:375-380, 2000.
46. Raad I, Body GP: Infectious complications of indwelling vascular catheters, *Clin Infect Dis* 15:197-208, 1992.
47. Pearson ML: Guideline for prevention on intravascular device-related infections. Hospital Infection Control Practices Advisory Committee, *Infect Control Hosp Epidemiol* 17:438-473, 1996.

48. CDC NNIS System: National Nosocomial Infection Surveillance (NNIS) report, data summary from Oct 1989-April 1997, issued May 1997, *Am J Infect Control* 25:477-487, 1997.
49. Krzywda EA, Andris DA, Edmiston CE, et al: Parenteral access devices. In Gottschlich MM (ed): *The science and practice of nutrition support: a case-based core curriculum,* Dubuque, IA, 2001, Kendall-Hunt Publishing Company, pp 225-250.
50. Raad II, Bodey GP: Infectious complications of indwelling vascular catheters, *Clin Infect Dis* 15:197-208, 1992.
51. Bach A, Bohrer H, Motsch J, et al: Prevention of catheter-related infections by antiseptic bonding, *J Surg Res* 55:640-646, 1993.
52. Eyer S, Brummitt C, Crossley K, et al: Catheter-related sepsis: prospective, randomized study of three methods of long-term catheter maintenance, *Crit Care Med* 18:1073-1079, 1990.
53. Cobb DK, High KP, Sawyer RG, et al: A controlled trial of scheduled replacement of central venous and pulmonary-artery catheters, *N Engl J Med* 15:1062-1068, 1992.
54. Savage AP, Picard M, Hopkins CC, Malt RA: Complications and survival of multilumen central venous catheters used for total parenteral nutrition, *Br J Surg* 80:1287-1290, 1993.
55. Olson ME, Lam K, Bodey GP, et al: Evaluation of strategies for central venous catheter replacement, *Crit Care Med* 20:797-804, 1992.
56. Raad II, Davis S, Becker M, et al: Low infection rate and long durability of non-tunneled catheters: a safe and cost effective alternative for long-term use of venous access devices in patients with cancer, *Ann Intern Med* 153:1791-1796, 1993.
57. Williams N, Carlson GL, Scott NA, Irving MH: Incidence and management of catheter-related sepsis in patients receiving home parenteral nutrition, *Br J Surg* 81:392-394, 1994.
58. Maki DG, Stolz SS, Wheeler S, et al: A prospective, randomized trial of gauze and two polyurethane dressings for site care of pulmonary artery catheters: implications for catheter management, *Crit Care Med* 22:1729-1737, 1994.
59. Corona ML, Peters SG, Narr BJ, Thompson RL: Infections related to central venous catheters, *Mayo Clin Proc* 65:979-986, 1990.
60. Pemberton LB, Lyman B, Lander V, Covinsky J: Sepsis from triple- vs single-lumen catheters during total parenteral nutrition in surgical or critically ill patients, *Arch Surg* 121:591-594, 1986.
61. Farkas J, Liu N, Bleriot J, et al: Single- versus triple-lumen central catheter-related sepsis: a prospective randomized study in a critically ill population, *Am J Med* 93:277-282, 1992.
62. Ma TY, Yoshinaka R, Banaag A, et al: Total parenteral nutrition via multilumen catheters does not increase the risk of catheter-related sepsis: a randomized, prospective study, *Clin Infect Dis* 27:500-503, 1998.
63. Buchman AL, Moukarzel A, Goodson B, et al: Catheter-related infections associated with home parenteral nutrition and predictive factors for the need for catheter removal in their treatment, *J Parenter Enteral Nutr* 18:297-302, 1994.
64. Benoit JL, Carandang G, Sitrin M, et al: Intraluminal antibiotic treatment of central venous catheter infection in patients receiving nutrition at home, *Clin Infect Dis* 21:286-288, 1995.
65. Schaberg DR, Culver DH, Gaynes RP: Major trends in the microbial etiology of nosocomial infection, *Am J Med* 91(suppl 3B):72S-75S, 1991.
66. Maki DG, Cobb L, Garman JK, et al: An attachable silver-impregnated cuff for prevention of infection with central venous catheters: a prospective randomized multicenter trial, *Am J Med* 85:307-314, 1988.
67. Raad II, Hohn DC, Gilbreath J, et al: Prevention of central venous catheter-related infections using maximal sterile barrier precautions during insertion, *Infect Control Hosp Epidemiol* 15:231-238, 1994.
68. Mimoz O, Pieroni L, Lawrence C, et al: Prospective, randomized trial of two antiseptic solutions for prevention of central venous or arterial catheter colonization and infection in intensive care unit patients, *Crit Care Med* 24:1818-1823, 1996.
69. Maki DG, Ringer M, Alvarado CJ: Prospective randomized trial of povidone-iodine, alcohol, and chlorhexidine for prevention of infection associated with central venous and arterial catheters, *Lancet* 338:339-343, 1991.
70. Hanazaki K, Shingu K, Adachi W, et al: Chlorhexidine dressing for reduction in microbial colonization of the skin with central venous catheters: a prospective randomized controlled trial, *J Hosp Infect* 42(2):165-168, 1999 (letter).
71. Maki DG, Stolz SM, Wheeler S, et al: Prevention of central venous catheter-related bloodstream infection by use of an antiseptic-impregnated catheter. A randomized, controlled trial, *Ann Intern Med* 127:257-266, 1997.

72. Veenstra DL, Saint S, Sullivan SD: Cost-effectiveness of antiseptic-impregnated central venous catheters for the prevention of catheter-related bloodstream infection, *JAMA* 282:554-560, 1999.
73. Darouiche RO, Raad II, Heard SO, et al: A comparison of two anti-microbial-impregnated central venous catheters, *N Engl J Med* 340:1-8, 1999.
74. Raad I, Darouiche R, Dupuis J, et al: Central venous catheters coated with minocycline and rifampin for the prevention of catheter-related colonization and bloodstream infections. A randomized, double-blind trial, *Ann Intern Med* 127:267-274, 1997.
75. FDA Public Health Notice: Potential hypersensitivity reaction to chlorhexidine impregnated medical devices, March 11, 1998. Retrieved April 17, 2002 from http://www.fda.gov/cdrh/chlorhex.html.
76. Curtas S, Smith C, Seidner D, et al: A randomized controlled trial demonstrates decreased catheter related infection and reactive depression and increased problem solving using complimentary therapies, *J Parenter Enteral Nutr* 25:S8, 2001 (abstract).
77. Quigley EMM, Marsh MN, Shaffer JL, et al: Hepatobiliary complications of total parenteral nutrition, *Gastroenterology* 104:286-301, 1994.
78. Clarke PJ, Ball MJ, Kettlewell MGW: Liver function tests in patients receiving parenteral nutrition, *J Parenter Enteral Nutr* 15:54-59, 1991.
79. Tayek JA, Bistrian B, Sheard NF, et al: Abnormal liver function in malnourished patients receiving total parenteral nutrition: a prospective randomized study, *J Am Coll Nutr* 9(1):76-83, 1990.
80. Leaseburge LA, Winn NJ, Schloerb PR: Liver test alterations with total parenteral nutrition and nutritional status, *J Parenter Enteral Nutr* 16:348-352, 1992.
81. Pitt HA, King W, Mann LL, et al: Increased risk of cholelithiasis with prolonged total parenteral nutrition, *Am J Surg* 145:106-111, 1983.
82. Bowyer BA, Fleming CR, Ludwig J, et al: Does long-term home parenteral nutrition in adult patients cause chronic liver disease? *J Parenter Enteral Nutr* 9:11-17, 1985.
83. Manji N, Bistrian BR, Mascioli EA, et al: Gallstone disease in patients with severe short bowel syndrome dependent on parenteral nutrition, *J Parenter Enteral Nutr* 13:461-464, 1989.
84. Buchman AL, Dubin M, Jenden D, et al: Lecithin increases plasma free choline and decreases hepatic steatosis in long-term total parenteral nutrition patients, *Gastroenterology* 102:1363-1370, 1992.
85. Shronts EP: Essential nature of choline with implication for total parenteral nutrition, *J Am Diet Assoc* 97:639-649, 1997.
86. Bowyer BA, Miles JM, Haymond MW, Fleming CR: L-carnitine therapy in home parenteral nutrition patients with abnormal liver tests and low plasma carnitine concentrations, *Gastroenterology* 94:434-438, 1988.
87. Lee SP: Diseases of the liver and biliary tract. In Kinney JM, Jeejeebhoy KN, Hill GL, Owen OE (eds): *Nutrition and metabolism in patient care,* Philadelphia, 1988, WB Saunders, pp 313-341.
88. Moss RL, Das JB, Raffensperger JG: Total parenteral nutrition-associated cholestasis: clinical and histopathological correlation, *J Pediatr Surg* 28:1270-1275, 1993.
89. Nakagawa M, Hiramatsu Y, Mitsuyoshi K, et al: Effect of various lipid emulsions on total parenteral nutrition-induced hepatosteatosis in rats, *J Parenter Enteral Nutr* 15:137-143, 1991.
90. Keim NL: Nutritional effectors of hepatic steatosis induced by parenteral nutrition in the rat, *J Parenter Enteral Nutr* 11:18-22, 1987.
91. Shattuck KE, Grinnell CD, Rassin DK: Biliary amino acid and glutathione secretion in response to amino acid infusion in the isolated rat liver, *J Parenter Enteral Nutr* 18:119-127, 1994.
92. Reif S, Tano M, Oliverio R, et al: Total parenteral nutrition-induced steatosis: reversal by parenteral lipid infusion, *J Parenter Enteral Nutr* 15:102-104, 1991.
93. Freund HR, Muggia-Sullam M, LaFrance R, et al: A possible beneficial effect of metronidazole in reducing TPN-associated liver function derangements, *J Surg Res* 38:356-363, 1985.
94. Grant JP, Cox CE, Kleinman LM, et al: Serum hepatic enzyme and bilirubin elevations during parenteral nutrition, *Surg Gynecol Obstet* 145:573-580, 1977.
95. Culebras JM, Garcia-Vielba J, Garcia-Diez F, et al: The effects of total parenteral nutrition on the hepatic handling of bilirubin in the rat, *J Parenter Enteral Nutr* 17:125-129, 1993.
96. Meguid MM, Akahoshi MP, Jeffers S, et al: Amelioration of metabolic complications of conventional total parenteral nutrition, *Arch Surg* 119:1294-1298, 1984.
97. Nussbaum MS, Li S, Bower RH, et al: Addition of lipid to total parenteral nutrition prevents hepatic steatosis in rats by lowering the portal venous insulin/glucagon ratio, *J Parenter Enteral Nutr* 16:106-109, 1992.

98. Pappo I, Bercovier H, Berry E, et al: Antitumor necrosis factor antibodies reduce hepatic steatosis during total parenteral nutrition and bowel rest in the rat, *J Parenter Enteral Nutr* 19:80-82, 1995.

99. Abad-Lacruz A, Gonzalez-Huix F, Esteve M, et al: Liver function tests abnormalities in patients with inflammatory bowel disease receiving artificial nutrition: a prospective randomized study of total enteral nutrition vs total parenteral nutrition, *J Parenter Enteral Nutr* 14:618-621, 1990.

100. Stanko RT, Nathan G, Mendelow H, Adibi SA: Development of hepatic cholestasis and fibrosis in patients with massive loss of intestine supported by prolonged parenteral nutrition, *Gastroenterology* 92:197-202, 1987.

101. Fuhrman MP, Herrmann VM, Masidonski P, et al: Pancytopenia following removal of copper from TPN, *J Parenter Enteral Nutr* 24:361-366, 2000.

102. Wolfe BM, Walker BK, Shaul DB, et al: Effect of total parenteral nutrition on hepatic histology, *Arch Surg* 123:1084-1088, 1988.

103. Freund HR: Abnormalities of liver function and hepatic damage associated with total parenteral nutrition, *Nutrition* 7:1-6, 1991.

104. O'Connor BJ, Kathbamma B, Tavill AS: Non-alcoholic fatty liver (NASH syndrome), *Gastroenterologist* 5:316-329, 1997.

105. Wagner WH, Lowry AC, Silberman H: Similar liver function abnormalities occur in patients receiving glucose-based and lipid-based parenteral nutrition, *Am J Gastroenterol* 78:199-202, 1983.

106. Baldermann H, Wicklmayr M, Rett K, et al: Changes of hepatic morphology during parenteral nutrition with lipid emulsion containing LCT or MCT/LCT quantified by ultrasound, *J Parenter Enteral Nutr* 15:601-603, 1991.

107. Buchmiller CE, Kleiman-Wexler RL, Ephgrave KS, et al: Liver dysfunction and energy source: results of a randomized clinical trial, *J Parenter Enteral Nutr* 17:301-306, 1993.

108. Lowry SF, Brennan MF: Abnormal liver function during parenteral nutrition: relation to infusion excess, *J Surg Res* 26:300-307, 1979.

109. Li S, Nussbaum MS, McFadden DW, et al: Addition of L-glutamine to total parenteral nutrition and its effects on portal insulin and glucagon and the development of hepatic steatosis in rats, *J Surg Res* 48:421-426, 1990.

110. Beau P, Labat-Labourdette J, Ingrand P, et al: Is ursodeoxycholic acid an effective therapy for total parenteral nutrition-related liver disease? *J Hepatol* 20:240-244, 1994.

111. Sitzman JV, Pitt HA, Steinborn PA, et al: Cholecystokinin prevents parenteral nutrition induced biliary sludge in humans, *Surg Gynecol Obstet* 170:25-31, 1990.

112. Teitelbaum DH, Han-Markey T, Drongowski RA, et al: Use of cholecystokinin to prevent the development of parenteral nutrition-associated cholestasis, *J Parenter Enteral Nutr* 21:100-103, 1997.

113. Capron JP, Gineston JL, Herve MA, Braillon A: Metronidazole in prevention of cholestasis associated with total parenteral nutrition, *Lancet* 1:446-447, 1983.

114. Fouin-Fortunet H, Quernec LL, Erlinger S, et al: Hepatic alterations during total parenteral nutrition in patients with inflammatory bowel disease: a possible consequence of lithocholate toxicity, *Gastroenterology* 82:932-937, 1982.

115. Maini B, Blackburn GL, Bistrian BR, et al: Cyclic hyperalimentation: an optimal technique for preservation of visceral protein, *J Surg Res* 20:515-525, 1976.

116. Just B, Messing B, Darmaun D, et al: Comparison of substrate utilization by indirect calorimetry during cyclic and continuous total parenteral nutrition, *Am J Clin Nutr* 51:107-111, 1990.

117. Byrne TA, Morrissey TB, Ziegler TR, et al: Growth hormone, glutamine, and fiber enhance adaptation of remnant bowel following massive intestinal resection, *Surg Forum* 43:151-153, 1992.

118. Shou J, Lappin J, Minnard EA, Daly JM: Total parenteral nutrition, bacterial translocation, and host immune function, *Am J Surg* 167:145-150, 1994.

119. Sax H, Illig KA, Ryan CK, et al: Low-dose enteral feeding is beneficial during TPN, *Am J Surg* 171:587-590, 1996.

120. Okada Y, Klein N, van Saene HK, et al: Small volumes of enteral feedings normalize immune function in infants receiving parenteral nutrition, *J Pediatr Surg* 33(1):16-19, 1998.

121. Lipman TO: Bacterial translocation and enteral nutrition in humans: an outsider looks in, *J Parenter Enteral Nutr* 19:156-165, 1995.

122. Murphy JP, King DR, Dubois A: Treatment of gastric hypersecretion with cimetidine in the short-bowel syndrome, *N Engl J Med* 300:80-81, 1979.

123. Baptista RJ: Role of histamine (H₂)-receptor antagonists in total parenteral nutrition patients, *Am J Med* 83(6A):53-57, 1987.

124. Moore RA, Feldman S, Treuting J, et al: Cimetidine and parenteral nutrition, *J Parenter Enteral Nutr* 5:61-63, 1981.

125. Williams MF, Hak LJ, Dukes G: In vitro evaluation of the stability of ranitidine hydrochloride in total parenteral nutrient admixtures, *Am J Hosp Pharm* 47:1574-1579, 1990.

126. Bullock L, Fitzgerald JF, Glick MR: Stability of famotidine 20 and 50 mg/L in total nutrient admixtures, *Am J Hosp Pharm* 46:2326-2329, 1989.

127. Foresta K: Use of total nutrient admixtures should not be limited, *Am J Health Syst Pharm* 52:893-895, 1995 (letter).

128. Matarese LE: Body composition changes in cachetic patients receiving home parenteral nutrition, *J Parenter Enteral Nutr* 25:S6, 2001 (abstract).

129. Murciano D, Rigaud D, Pingleton S, et al: Diaphragmatic function in severely malnourished patients with anorexia nervosa. Effects of renutrition, *Am J Respir Crit Care Med* 150:1569-1574, 1994.

130. Chandra RK: Protein-energy malnutrition and immunological response, *J Nutr* 122:597-600, 1992.

131. Talpers SS, Romberger DJ, Bunce SB, et al: Nutritionally associated increased carbon dioxide production, *Chest* 102:551-555, 1992.

132. Solomon SM, Kirby DF: The refeeding syndrome: a review, *J Parenter Enteral Nutr* 14:90-97, 1990.

133. Apovian CM, McMahon MM, Bistrian BR: Guidelines for refeeding the marasmic patient, *Crit Care Med* 18:1030-1033, 1990.

134. Hurley DL, Neven A, McMahon MM: Diabetes mellitus. In Gottschlich MM (ed): *The science and practice of nutrition support: a case-based core curriculum,* Dubuque, IA, 2001, Kendall-Hunt Publishing Company, pp 663-675.

135. Wolfe RR, O'Donnell TF Jr, Stone MD, et al: Investigation of factors determining the optimal glucose infusion rate in total parenteral nutrition, *Metabolism* 29:892-900, 1980.

136. Michael SR, Sabo CE: Management of the diabetic patient receiving nutritional support, *Nutr Clin Pract* 4:179-183, 1989.

137. McMahon M, Manji N, Driscoll DF, et al: Parenteral nutrition in patients with diabetes mellitus: theoretical and practical considerations, *J Parenter Enteral Nutr* 13:545-553, 1989.

138. Weber SS, Wood WA, Jackson EA: Availability of insulin from parenteral nutrient solutions, *Am J Hosp Pharm* 34:353-357, 1977.

139. Marcuard SP, Dunham B, Hobbs A, Caro JF: Availability of insulin from total parenteral nutrition solutions, *J Parenter Enteral Nutr* 14:262-264, 1990.

140. Krzywda EA, Andris DA, Whipple JK, et al: Glucose response to abrupt initiation and discontinuation of total parenteral nutrition, *J Parent Enteral Nutr* 17(1):64-67, 1993.

141. Eisenberg PG, Gianino S, Clutter WE, et al: Abrupt discontinuation of cycled parenteral nutrition is safe, *Dis Colon Rectum* 38:933-939, 1995.

142. Karlstad MD, DeMichele SJ, Bistrian BR, et al: Effect of total parenteral nutrition with xylitol on protein and energy metabolism in thermally injured rats, *J Parenter Enteral Nutr* 15:445-449, 1991.

143. Buchman AL, Moukarzel A, Ament ME, et al: Serious renal impairment is associated with long-term parenteral nutrition, *J Parenter Enteral Nutr* 17:438-444, 1993.

144. Boncompain-Gerard M, Robert D, Fouque D, et al: Renal function and urinary excretion of electrolytes in patients receiving cyclic parenteral nutrition, *J Parenter Enteral Nutr* 24:234-239, 2000.

145. Legaspi A, Roberts JP, Albert JD, et al: The effect of starvation and total parenteral nutrition on skeletal muscle amino acid content and membrane potential difference in normal man, *Surg Gynecol Obstet* 166:233-240, 1988.

146. Tracey KJ, Legaspi A, Albert JD, et al: Protein and substrate metabolism during starvation and parenteral refeeding, *Clin Sci* 74:123-132, 1988.

147. Jeevanandam M, Ali MR, Holaday NJ, Petersen SR: Adjuvant recombinant human growth hormone normalizes plasma amino acids in parenterally fed trauma patients, *J Parenter Enteral Nutr* 19:137-144, 1995.

148. McCarthy MC, Turner WW, Whatley K, Cottam GL: Topical corn oil in the management of essential fatty acid deficiency, *Crit Care Med* 11:373-375, 1983.

149. Sacks GS, Brown RO, Collier P, Kudsk KA: Failure of topical vegetable oils to prevent essential fatty acid deficiency in a critically ill patient receiving long-term parenteral nutrition, *J Parenter Enteral Nutr* 18:274-277, 1994.

150. Holman RT: The ratio of trienoic:tetraenoic acids in tissue lipids as a measure of essential fatty acid requirement, *J Nutr* 70:405-410, 1960.

151. McCarthy MC: Nutritional support in the critically ill surgical patient, *Surg Clin North Am* 71:831-841, 1991.

152. Press M, Hartop PJ, Prottey C: Correction of essential fatty acid deficiency in man by the cutaneous application of sunflower-seed oil, *Lancet* 1:597-598, 1974.

153. Howdieshell TR, Bhalla N, DiPiro JT, et al: Effects of free glycerol contained in intravenous fat emulsion on plasma triglyceride determination, *J Parenter Enteral Nutr* 19:125-126, 1995.

154. ASPEN Board of Directors and The Clinical Guidelines Task Force: Guidelines for the use of parenteral and enteral nutrition in adult and pediatric patients, *J Parenter Enteral Nutr* (suppl):1SA-138SA, 2002.

155. Grimm H, Tibell A, Norrlind B, et al: Immunoregulation by parenteral lipids: impact on the n-3 to n-6 fatty acid ratio, *J Parenter Enteral Nutr* 18:417-421, 1994.

156. Ekelund M, Roth B, Trelde H, et al: Effects of total parenteral nutrition on lipid metabolism in rats, *J Parenter Enteral Nutr* 18:503-509, 1994.

157. Vazquez WD, Arya G, Garcia VF: Long-chain predominant lipid emulsions inhibit in vitro macrophage tumor necrosis factor production, *J Parenter Enteral Nutr* 18:35-39, 1994.

158. Kapp JP, Duckert F, Hartmann G: Platelet adhesiveness and serum lipids during and after intralipid infusion, *Nutr Metab* 13:92-99, 1971.

159. VanWay CW, Dunn EL, Hamstra RD: The effect of intravenous safflower oil emulsion on the clotting mechanism, *Am J Surg* 49:460-464, 1983.

160. Herson VC, Block C, Eisenfeld L, et al: Effects of intravenous fat infusion on neonatal neutrophil and platelet function, *J Parenter Enteral Nutr* 13:620-622, 1989.

161. Seidner DL, Mascioli EA, Istfan NW, et al: Effects of long-chain triglyceride emulsions on reticuloendothelial system function in humans, *J Parenter Enteral Nutr* 13:614-619, 1989.

162. Jensen GL, Mascioli EA, Seidner DL, et al: Parenteral infusion of long- and medium-chain triglycerides and reticuloendothelial system function in man, *J Parenter Enteral Nutr* 14:467-471, 1990.

163. Druml W, Fischer M, Ratheiser K: Use of intravenous lipids in critically ill patients with sepsis without and with hepatic failure, *J Parenter Enteral Nutr* 22:217-223, 1998.

164. Bellantone R, Bossola M, Carriero C, et al: Structured versus long-chain triglycerides: a safety, tolerance, and efficacy randomized study in colorectal surgical patients, *J Parenter Enteral Nutr* 23:123-127, 1999.

165. Wanten GJ, Geijtenbeek TB, Raymakers RA, et al: Medium-chain, triglyceride-containing lipid emulsions increase human neutophil β_2-integrin expression, adhesion, and degranulation, *J Parenter Enteral Nutr* 24:228-233, 2000.

166. Raguso CA, Mingrone G, Greco AV, et al: Dicarboxylic acids and glucose utilization in humans: effect of sebacate, *J Parenter Enteral Nutr* 18:9-13, 1994.

167. Lang CH, Abumrad NN: Dicarboxylic acids as energy substrates in parenteral nutrition, *J Parenter Enteral Nutr* 18:1-3, 1994 (editorial).

168. Grant JP: *Handbook of total parenteral nutrition,* ed 2, Philadelphia, 1992, WB Saunders 171-202.

169. Whitmire SJ: Fluid and electrolytes. In Gottschlich MM (ed): *The science and practice of nutrition support: a case-based core curriculum,* Dubuque, IA, 2001, Kendall-Hunt Publishing Company, pp 53-83.

170. Forster J, Querusio L, Burchard KW, Gann DS: Hypercalcemia in critically ill surgical patients, *Ann Surg* 202:512-518, 1985.

171. Dwyer K, Barone JE, Rogers JF: Severe hypophosphatemia in postoperative patients, *Nutr Clin Prac* 7:279-283, 1992.

172. Janigan DT, Perey B, Marrie TJ, et al: Skin necrosis: an unusual complication of hyperphosphatemia during total parenteral nutrition, *J Parenter Enteral Nutr* 21:50-52, 1997.

173. National Advisory Group on Standards and Practice Guidelines for Parenteral Nutrition: Safe practices for parenteral nutrition formulations, *J Parenter Enteral Nutr* 22:49-66, 1998.

174. Trissel LA: *Handbook on injectible drugs,* ed 11, Bethesda, MD, 2001, American Society of Health-System Pharmacists.

175. Parfitt AM: Soft-tissue calcification in uremia, *Arch Intern Med* 124:544-556, 1969.

176. Lumpkin MM, Burlington DB (Food and Drug Administration, Department of Health & Human Services): Hazards of precipitation associated with parenteral nutrition, *Safety Alert* April 18:1-3, 1994.

177. Faber MD, Kupin WL, Heilig CW, Narins RG: Common fluid-electrolyte and acid-base problems in the intensive care unit: selected issues, *Semin Nephrol* 14:8-22, 1994.

178. Velez RJ, Myers B, Guber MS: Severe acute metabolic acidosis (acute beriberi): an avoidable complication of total parenteral nutrition, *J Parenter Enteral Nutr* 9:216-219, 1985.

179. Agarwal N, Norkus E, Garcia C, et al: Effect of surgery on serum antioxidant vitamins, *J Parenter Enteral Nutr* 20:32S, 1996 (abstract).

180. Borelli E, Roux-Lombard P, Grau GE, et al: Plasma concentrations of cytokines, their soluble receptors, and antioxidant vitamins can predict the development of multiple organ failure in patients at risk, *Crit Care Med* 24:392-397, 1996.

181. Schorah CJ, Downing C, Piripitsi A, et al: Total vitamin C, ascorbic acid, and dehydroascorbic acid concentrations in plasma of critically ill patients, *Am J Clin Nutr* 63:760-765, 1996.

182. Boosalis MG, Snowdon DA, Tully CL, et al: Acute phase response and plasma carotenoid concentrations in older women: findings from the nun study, *Nutrition* 12:475-478, 1996.

183. Wolk R: Nutrition in renal failure. In Gottschlich MM (ed): *The science and practice of nutrition support: a case-based core curriculum,* Dubuque, IA, 2001, Kendall-Hunt Publishing Company; pp 575-599.

184. Parenteral multivitamin products; drugs for human use; drug efficacy study implementation; amendment (21 CFR 5.70), *Federal Register* 65:21200-21201, April 20, 2000.

185. Chambrier C, Leclercq M, Saudin F, et al: Is vitamin K supplementation necessary in long-term parenteral nutrition? *J Parenter Enteral Nutr* 22:87-90, 1998.

186. Fuhrman MP: Antioxidant supplementation in critical illness: what do we know? *Nutrition* 16:470-471, 2000.

187. Tu YH, Knox NL, Biringer JM et al: Compatibility of iron dextran with total parenteral nutrient admixtures, *Am J Hosp Pharm* 49:2233-2235, 1992.

188. Vaughan LM, Small C, Plunkett V: Incompatibility of iron dextran and a total nutrient admixture, *Am J Hosp Pharm* 47:1745-1746, 1990.

189. Expert Panel for Nutrition Advisory Group, AMA Department of Foods and Nutrition: Guidelines for essential trace element preparations for parenteral use, *JAMA* 241:2051-2054, 1979.

190. Arenas-Marquez H, Anaya-Prado R, Gonzalez-Ojeda A, et al: Gastrointestinal fistulas: clinical and nutritional management. In Rombeau JL, Rolandelli RH (eds): *Clinical nutrition: parenteral nutrition,* ed 3, Philadelphia, 2001, WB Saunders, pp 258-281.

191. Braunschweig CL, Sowers M, Kovacevich DS, et al: Parenteral zinc supplementation in adult humans during the acute phase response increases the febrile response, *J Nutr* 127:70-74, 1997.

192. Bertinet DB, Tinivella M, Balzola FA, et al: Brain manganese deposition and blood levels in patients undergoing home parenteral nutrition, *J Parenter Enteral Nutr* 24:223-227, 2000.

193. Wardle CA, Forbes A, Roberts NB, et al: Hypermanganesemia in long-term intravenous nutrition and chronic liver disease, *J Parenter Enteral Nutr* 23:350-355, 1999.

194. Fitzgerald K, Mikalunas V, Rubin H, et al: Hypermanganesemia in patients receiving total parenteral nutrition, *J Parenter Enteral Nutr* 23:333-336, 1999.

195. Siepler J, Nishikawa RA, Diamantidis T, et al: Elevated manganese levels in long-term home parenteral nutrition patients are not predicted by dose, *J Parenter Enteral Nutr* 25:S7, 2001 (abstract).

196. Matarese LE: Metabolic complications of parenteral nutrition therapy. In Gottschlich MM (ed): *The science and practice of nutrition support: a case-based core curriculum,* Dubuque, IA, 2001, Kendall-Hunt Publishing Company, pp 269-286.

197. Spiegel JE, Willenbucher RF: Rapid development of severe copper deficiency in a patient with Crohn's disease receiving parenteral nutrition, *J Parenter Enteral Nutr* 23:169-172, 1999.

198. Forceville F, Vitoux D, Gauzit R, et al: Selenium, systemic immune response syndrome, sepsis, and outcome in critically ill patients, *Crit Care Med* 26:1536-1544, 1998.

199. Angstwurm MA, Schottdorf J, Schopohl J, et al: Selenium replacement in patients with severe systemic inflammatory response syndrome improves clinical outcome, *Crit Care Med* 27:1807-1813, 1999.

200. Gramlich LM, Bistrian BR: Cyclic parenteral nutrition: considerations of carbohydrate and lipid metabolism, *Nutr Clin Prac* 9:49-50, 1994 (editorial).

201. Verhage AH, Cheong WK, Allard JP, et al: Increase in lumbar spine bone mineral content in patients on long-term parenteral nutrition without vitamin D supplementation, *J Parenter Enteral Nutr* 19:431-436, 1995.

202. Klein G: Metabolic bone disease of total parenteral nutrition, *Nutrition* 14:149-152, 1998.

203. Koo WWK: Parenteral nutrition-related bone disease, *J Parenter Enteral Nutr* 16:386-394, 1992.

204. Berkelhammer C, Wood RJ, Sitrin MD: Inorganic phosphorus reduces hypercalciuria during total parenteral nutrition by enhancing renal tubular calcium absorption, *J Parenter Enteral Nutr* 22:142-146, 1998.

205. Abitbol V, Roux C, Chaussade S, et al: Metabolic bone assessment in patients with inflammatory bowel disease, *Gastroenterology* 108: 417-422, 1995.
206. Perry S, Pillar B, Radany MH: The appropriate use of high-cost, high-risk technologies: the case of total parenteral nutrition, *Qual Rev Bulletin* 16(6):214-217, 1990.
207. Speerhas RA, Seidner DL, Steiger E: Five year follow-up of a program to minimize inappropriate use of parenteral nutrition, *J Parenter Enteral Nutr* 25:S4-S5, 2001 (abstract).
208. Trujillo EB, Young LS, Chertow GM, et al: Metabolic and monetary costs of avoidable parenteral nutrition use, *J Parenter Enteral Nutr* 23:109-113, 1999.

Rationale and Efficacy of Specialized Enteral and Parenteral Formulas

20

Laura E. Matarese, MS, RD, LD, FADA, CNSD

THE technologic advances of the late 1960s have afforded us an unprecedented capability for improving and sustaining the nutritional status of patients. Over the years they included advances in the methods of delivery and in the formulas themselves. We are now entering an era when enteral nutrition and parenteral nutrition are administered not only as a source of substrates for the body but also for their pharmacologic value. The rationale for the design of these formulas is based on physiologic and medical principles. There are data to show that these formulas are safe and suitable for use in various disease states. The challenge remains to document the efficacy of these formulas in specific patient populations.[1]

Medical Foods

Many of the specialty enteral products are classified as medical foods. According to the U.S. Food and Drug Administration (FDA), a medical food is prescribed by a physician when a patient has special nutrient needs and the patient is under the physician's ongoing care. The label must clearly state that the product is intended to be used to manage a special medical disorder or condition.[2] The FDA has divided these products into four separate categories: (1) nutritionally complete formulas that can be used as sole-source nutrition; (2) nutritionally incomplete formulas, i.e., modular products composed of protein, fat, or carbohydrates; (3) oral rehydration products that are used as fluid and electrolyte replacements for dehydration; and (4) disease-specific nutritional formulas that are specifically developed to help manage conditions such as kidney disease.

The purpose of this chapter is to describe the rationale for the use of disease-specific formulas and to evaluate the research that has been used to document the efficacy of therapy.

Renal Disease

Most of the early research on disease-specific formulas was related to renal disease. It began with an investigation of the benefits of essential amino acids (EAAs) for persons in renal failure. The goal was to improve nitrogen balance, reduce catabolism, decrease or eliminate the need for dialysis, and improve outcome. Acute renal failure (ARF) occurs in approximately 5% of hospitalized patients and is often associated with a mortality rate of 60% or greater (see Chapter 33).[3] The incidence of malnutrition in patients with renal failure is high.[4-6] Many are unable to eat because of anorexia, early satiety, nausea, or vomiting. There may also be nutrient losses from

dialysis therapy. The situation is further complicated by hypercatabolism and increased metabolic demands.

Provision of formulas composed of EAAs to patients with oliguria or anuria was based on the work of Rose, who established the requirements for amino acids (AAs) in healthy men.[7] The rationale for their use in renal disease was that if only EAAs were provided, urea could be recycled as a nitrogen source in the gastrointestinal lumen by bacterial urease, which degrades the urea to its carbon and ammonia fragments (Fig. 20-1). These fragments are then reabsorbed and converted to nonessential amino acids (NEAA) in the liver.[8] Giordano demonstrated lowered blood urea nitrogen (BUN) levels and reduction of uremia symptoms in affected patients fed 2 g of EAA nitrogen as the sole source of nitrogen along with adequate calories, vitamins, and minerals.[9] Similar results were reported by Giovannetti and Maggiore.[10]

Parenteral EAAs, hypertonic glucose, and vitamins were first administered to a single patient with renal failure by Wilmore and Dudrick in 1969, in an attempt to ameliorate the patient's symptoms and clinical condition.[11] They reported weight gain, improved wound healing, positive nitrogen balance, and reduced serum concentrations of urea nitrogen, potassium, and phosphorus. The requirement for dialysis was also decreased. Positive results of the use of EAA therapy for ARF were demonstrated in other case reports.[12-14]

The research up to this point had largely been limited to case reports of nonrandomized trials. In 1973, Abel and associates, in a prospective randomized trial, demonstrated reduced morbidity and increased survival rate for patients receiving EAAs

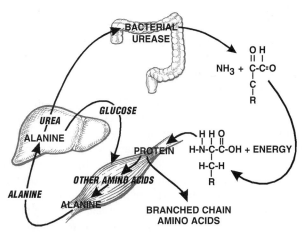

FIGURE 20-1 Urea recycling.

(Nephramine) plus 70% dextrose as compared with those receiving only 70% dextrose.[15] They also showed decreases in serum potassium, phosphorus, and magnesium concentrations without dialysis in the EAA group. Additionally, the duration of the ARF was decreased in the group of patients who received EAAs; however, it is important to note that the control group received only hypertonic dextrose and no AAs.

The theory that provision of EAAs results in urea recycling has been challenged. Patients who receive only EAAs do not have significantly decreased urea concentrations as compared with patients receiving a combination of EAAs and NEAAs. Varcoe and coworkers reported that only 3.2% of N-labeled urea nitrogen is incorporated into albumin of uremic patients.[16] Others have shown that the urea-recycling pathway of protein synthesis is not sufficient to maintain levels of all AAs.[17-19] Freund and colleagues, in a retrospective study, compared patients given a combination of EAAs and NEAAs in a dextrose solution, with those of Abel's study receiving only EAAs and dextrose.[20] Patients who received the combined AAs showed stabilization of BUN but still had a significantly higher mortality rate than the patients receiving just the EAAs; however, those who received the combined AA solutions were sicker and had a greater rate of renal failure.

Feinstein and colleagues, in a controlled double-blind study, compared three groups of patients receiving either hypertonic dextrose and no AAs, EAAs and dextrose, or a combination of EAAs and NEAAs plus dextrose.[21] Protein intake in the EAA group was 21 g per day and in the combined group was 42 g per day, 50% from EAAs and 50% from NEAAs. They reported a high degree of catabolism with no improvement in serum proteins in all groups. Nitrogen balance remained negative throughout the study. They found greater urinary nitrogen values in the combined AA group than in the EAA group. There was no difference in recovery of renal function or overall survival between the treatment groups. These data suggest that larger quantities of AAs and possibly calories are required to meet the metabolic demands of hypercatabolism. In a later study, giving 84 g per day of AAs also effected no improvement in nitrogen balance or survival.[22]

Similar findings were reported by Mirtallo and associates.[23] In a prospective trial, 44 patients were randomized to receive either EAAs or an isonitrogenous standard AA solution. Nitrogen intake was similar for both groups. There was no difference in BUN concentrations, urea appearance rate, net protein use, or nitrogen balance. They concluded that no clinical advantage was associated with the use of EAAs over standard AA solutions.

Other studies evaluated use of EAAs as part of a diet or enteral formula. Kopple and Swendseid conducted a trial to evaluate the effects of oral EAAs.[24] They fed three patients 22 g of high biologic value protein for 28 to 48 days, followed by 13 to 33 days of a diet of 21 g of EAAs. Nitrogen balance improved in the patients on the 22 g per day high-biologic protein diet, but only one patient actually exhibited positive nitrogen balance. The EAA diet contained less nitrogen and resulted in decreased BUN concentrations, but the nitrogen balances were more negative. The authors concluded that EAAs are used more efficiently than high-biologic value egg protein.

Commercial enteral formulas were also available for patients with renal failure. The early products released con-

tained EAAs and glucose. Sofio and associates gave Amin-Aid as the sole source of nitrogen or as part of a low-protein diet to 24 patients with ARF and 31 with chronic renal failure (CRF).[25] Measurements included nitrogen balance, daily rate of BUN increase, and serum potassium, phosphorus, and magnesium. The EAA formula decreased the rate of rise of BUN, stabilized serum potassium and phosphorus concentrations, and improved nitrogen balance in ARF and positive nitrogen balance in CRF.

In another study, patients with advanced renal failure were given a diet containing 20 g protein per day supplemented with EAAs plus histidine (Aminess).[26] The supplements were given as 1.3 and 2.6 g nitrogen per day intravenously and 1.3 g orally. Nitrogen balance improved with all levels of supplementation but was best when 1.3 g nitrogen was given orally.

Many studies have confirmed the benefits of dietary protein restriction and the use of high–biologic value protein for patients with CRF;[27-32] however, there are very few data to support prolonged protein restriction and EAAs, particularly for critically ill patients. It appears that both EAAs and NEAAs are needed for adequate protein synthesis. The use of special formulas that contain only EAAs or are supplemented with higher concentrations of EAAs may be indicated for patients for whom dialysis is temporarily contraindicated. Once dialysis is initiated, standard formulas should be used to provide a full complement of AAs. Because many of the renal failure formulas contain small amounts of electrolytes (if any) and fat-soluble vitamins, they may be useful in situations in which electrolytes or fat-soluble vitamins need to be restricted.[33]

Liver Disease

Patients with liver disease are often malnourished, especially those who have alcoholic liver disease (see Chapter 32).[34] When injured, these patients are likely to have complications such as gastrointestinal bleeding, sepsis, and multisystem organ failure. They require increased amounts of protein during such periods of stress, yet nutrient metabolism, particularly of protein, is impaired by liver damage, and the result is often hepatic encephalopathy (HE).[35] The exact cause of HE is not known. Affected patients usually have an abnormal plasma AA pattern characterized by elevated levels of methionine and aromatic AAs (AAAs), phenylalanine, tyrosine, free tryptophan, and decreased levels of branched-chain AAs (BCAAs), leucine, isoleucine, and valine. The molar ratio between the BCAAs and the AAAs is decreased from the normal value of 3.0 to 3.5 to less than 1.0. A molar ratio of 1.0 or less has been correlated with HE.[36] AAAs are substrates for amine synthesis in the brain, and BCAAs, substrates for muscle protein. These two groups of AAs compete for transport across the blood-brain barrier. The altered molar ratio may increase uptake of AAAs by the brain. These AAAs then act as false neurotransmitters, and HE results (Fig. 20-2).[37,38]

The rationale for developing special enteral and parenteral formulas for patients with hepatic disease was to normalize the AA pattern, which would improve or reverse HE. Thus these solutions were formulated to contain larger amounts of BCAAs and smaller quantities of AAAs and methionine. The efficacy of these formulas remains controversial.[33,35,39,40]

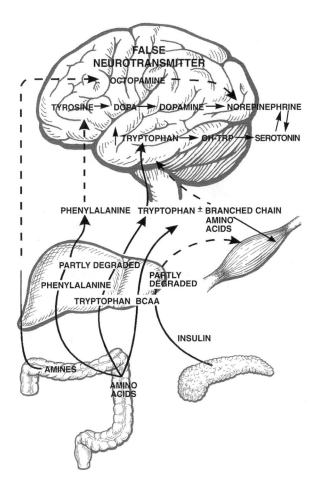

FIGURE 20-2 Branched-chain amino acids in hepatic coma.

BCAAs have been given orally to patients with chronic HE. In three studies patients were randomized to receive diets enriched with BCAAs or a control diet and were then "crossed over."[41-43] The BCAA-supplemented diet was not found to be clinically superior to the control diet. In another randomized crossover study, BCAA supplements promoted nitrogen balance that was equal to that with the control diet but did not precipitate HE.[44]

There have been very few prospective randomized multi-center controlled trials of BCAA-enriched enteral formulas in the treatment of HE. In one prospective randomized multicenter controlled trial, cirrhotic patients who had chronic portal-systemic encephalopathy were studied to compare the clinical and nutritional effects of dietary supplements of BCAAs or isonitrogenous casein.[45] Both groups received a moderately protein-restricted diet and lactulose. The patients who received the supplemental BCAAs showed improvement in encephalopathy and nitrogen balance as well as slight improvement in nutritional parameters and liver function tests. The patients who received the casein supplements and who did not improve were eventually crossed over and given BCAAs, in response to which they showed rapid improvement.

In another prospective randomized controlled trial, Cabre and colleagues gave severely malnourished cirrhosis patients continuous enteral infusion of a polymeric diet containing whole protein enriched with BCAAs or a standard low-sodium hospital diet.[46] Serum albumin concentration and Child's score

improved in the enteral-feeding group, as compared with the control group. Mortality in hospital was 12% for the enteral group and 47% for the control group.

There have been a number of studies in which patients were given BCAA supplements by various routes in a single study. Smith and associates gave high-calorie, low calcium, and low- to moderate-protein formulas enterally to three malnourished cirrhosis patients with ascites and parenterally to seven for 10 to 60 days.[47] Nine patients showed improved serum albumin, creatinine-height index, and midarm muscle and fat.

Calvey and associates randomized 64 patients with acute alcoholic hepatitis to receive a controlled diet, either alone or supplemented with 2000 kcal and 10 g nitrogen.[48] The nitrogen given orally, by nasogastric tube, or parenterally was supplied as 20 g BCAAs plus 45 g of standard AAs or 65 g of mixed protein. There were no differences in nutritional and biochemical parameters between the two groups and no consistent effect on encephalopathy.

There have been other reviews of these data. Eriksson and Conn reviewed 18 randomized controlled trials of the use of BCAAs for treatment or prevention of HE in cirrhosis patients.[49] Thirteen of these studies involved acute, chronic, or subclinical HE; three evaluated the effects of BCAAs on nitrogen metabolism; and two investigated the treatment of HE with branched-chain ketoacids. Seven of the studies in which BCAAs were given parenterally suggested that BCAA therapy was as effective as, but not better than, conventional therapy with lactulose or neomycin. They concluded that although AA profiles were corrected, no improvement was observed in acute, chronic, or subclinical HE. It was noted, however, that dietary protein was tolerated better by cirrhosis patients as BCAAs.

In a parenteral feeding study, Rossi-Fanelli and colleagues randomized 37 patients with acute HE to receive either 57 g of BCAA in hypertonic dextrose or an isocaloric amount of dextrose and lactulose.[50] Within 2 days of administration of the solutions, arousal was observed in 70% of the patients treated with BCAAs and 49% of the controls; however, this difference was not statistically significant.

In a multicenter trial, 50 patients with hepatic cirrhosis and encephalopathy, previously treated with conventional therapy, were given parenteral BCAAs in a 5% dextrose solution or 5% dextrose alone for 5 days or until HE was reversed.[51] There was no statistically significant difference in rate of arousal or mortality at 5 days; however, the BCAA solution contained 70% leucine, which may have caused a toxic imbalance of AAs.

In a larger multicenter trial, 80 patients with HE received a parenteral formula enriched with BCAAs (FO80) or an isocaloric amount of dextrose and neomycin.[52] Rate of arousal was more rapid and nitrogen balance improved in the BCAA-treated group. Additionally, survival improved in the BCAA group.

Naylor and associates evaluated nine randomized control trials of parenterally administered BCAAs to patients with chronic liver dysfunction and HE using meta-analysis.[53] When five studies' findings were pooled, a statistically significant improvement in the degree of HE was observed; however, it is not clear whether this is due to the nutrient content of the solutions or to a pharmacologic effect of the BCAA. There were also differences in the types of calorie sources used in the studies and in the various protocols. Additionally, the mortality data differed so widely among the studies that pooling of these data was impossible. Follow-up was short and the side effects and complications of treatment were not evaluated. The authors concluded that although the aggregate results suggest that BCAAs have a beneficial effect on HE, their effect on mortality is not conclusive and does not support routine use of BCAAs for nutrition support in patients with HE.

In 1994, Fan and colleagues published data showing improved outcome with the use of BCAAs.[54] They performed a prospective study to investigate whether periopertive nutrition support could improve outcome in 124 patients undergoing hepatectomy for hepatocellular carcinoma. Patients were randomly assigned to receive perioperative intravenous nutrition support in addition to their oral diet or to the control group (regular diet). The perioperative nutrition therapy consisted of a solution enriched with 35% BCAA, dextrose, and lipid emulsion given intravenously for 14 days. There was a reduction in the overall postoperative morbidity rate in the preoperative nutrition group as compared with the control group, primarily because of a reduction in septic complications. The need for diuretic therapy to control ascites was significantly lower in the perioperative nutrition group than in the control. Hospital mortality was 8% in the perioperative nutrition group and 15% in the control group.

Standard enteral or parenteral formulas can be used for most patients with liver disease.[33] Use of BCAA formulas in protein-intolerant patients with severe liver disease to improve nitrogen balance and reverse HE remains controversial. BCAA formulas may provide more protein to patients who are intolerant of conventional therapy. They have been shown to decrease mortality in patients undergoing hepatectomy for hepatocelluar carcinoma.

Pulmonary Disease

Malnutrition is common in patients with pulmonary disease (see Chapter 30).[55-58] This can adversely affect respiratory function by reducing muscle mass and causing generalized weakness.[59-62] Ventilatory drive may be reduced as a consequence of muscle atrophy.[63] Additionally, hypoalbuminemia can contribute to pulmonary edema by reducing oncotic pressure and the resulting shifts of fluid into the interstitial space.[64] Poor nutrition can also compromise immune function, which can increase susceptibility to infection.[65] These factors may contribute to prolonged intubation and failure to wean from mechanical ventilation. Consequently, it is important to provide adequate calories and protein to improve respiratory muscle function and endurance and decrease the incidence of infections.[66,67]

As glucose is oxidized, production of carbon dioxide increases. There are reports of respiratory failure precipitated by high-carbohydrate feedings,[68,69] and high-carbohydrate feedings have also been associated with respiratory quotients greater than 1.0 and impairment of ability to wean from mechanical ventilation.[70-73] As a result, nutrition therapy has been aimed at decreasing the carbohydrate load and substituting fat calories because oxidation of fat produces less carbon

dioxide and a lower respiratory quotient.[74-76] Many of the enteral formulas designed specifically for the patient with pulmonary failure contain 40% to 55.2% of the calories in the form of fat compare to standard formulas, which generally have 30% to 38% fat.

In a randomized, double-blind crossover trial, Angelillo and coworkers evaluated the effects of varying carbohydrate loads on patients with chronic obstructive pulmonary disease and hypercapnia for 15 days.[77] Patients received as the sole source of nutrition one of three enteral formulas: high fat (55.2% of calories; Pulmocare); moderate fat (30% of calories) formula; and low fat (9.4% of calories). Patients who received Pulmocare showed lower carbon dioxide production, lower respiratory quotient, and arterial carbon dioxide pressure ($Paco_2$).

Goldstein and associates compared the effects of refeeding malnourished patients with chronic obstructive pulmonary disease with a high-fat formula (Pulmocare) or a high-carbohydrate formula.[78] The patients were fed for approximately 20 days at 1.7 times the resting energy expenditure (REE). Pulmocare resulted in lower oxygen consumption and carbon dioxide production than the high-carbohydrate formula. Skeletal muscle function and endurance were improved, but these changes appeared to be related to feeding duration and not to the composition of the diet. This same group performed a prospective randomized trial to evaluate the effects of varying nonprotein calories during hypercaloric feeding and exercise.[79] Eight ambulatory malnourished patients who had chronic obstructive pulmonary disease and emphysema and eight ambulatory malnourished patients without lung disease were given a diet containing 53% carbohydrate or 55% fat for 1 week. The protein portion was kept constant. The diets were crossed over after 1 week. Ventilation and gas exchange were measured using supine cycle ergometry. Patients with emphysema exhibited 12% to 15% greater oxygen consumption, lower respiratory quotients, and larger oxygen debts than the malnourished patients without lung disease. Resting ventilation was higher with the carbohydrate-based diet than with the fat-based diet for both groups. Ventilatory response was exaggerated while the emphysema patients were fed the carbohydrate-based formula.

Al-Saady and colleagues compared the effects of a high-fat, low-carbohydrate formula with a standard high-calorie formula in a prospective double-blind trial.[80] Twenty ventilator-dependent patients were randomized to receive either Pulmocare or Ensure Plus. Calorie and protein requirements were calculated using the Fleisch standard and were modified for disease and stress. The regimens were isocaloric and isonitrogenous. Initial ventilator settings were adjusted according to the patient's clinical condition. The patients were considered eligible to remain in the study after they had been fed continually at their optimal rate for a minimum of 48 hours during ventilation. Enteral feeding was continued for 24 to 48 hours after weaning. Those patients receiving Pulmocare showed a 16% decrease in $Paco_2$, whereas the control group showed a 4% increase. Average time spent on the ventilator was 62 hours less for the Pulmocare group.

It is important to note that other factors could have affected the results of this study. The amount of sedative and muscle relaxants used may have influenced the rate of weaning from mechanical ventilation. Also the clinical diagnosis and underlying lung pathology could have affected the duration of ventilation.

Many of these studies have associated the adverse effects of providing excessive carbohydrate to patients with compromised pulmonary function; however, others maintain that overfeeding is more detrimental to these patients than is carbohydrate load. Carbon dioxide production is the index that best reflects ventilatory demand.[81] Talpers and associates looked at carbon dioxide production in mechanically ventilated patients whose isocaloric regimens contained carbohydrate as 40%, 60%, or 75% of total calories.[82] There was no significant difference in carbon dioxide production among the three groups; however, when the carbohydrate content was 60% but total number of calories varied from fasting to 1.0 time REE, 1.5 times REE, and 2.0 times REE, a significant increase in carbon dioxide production was observed. Although a high-fat formula may reduce the respiratory quotient (RQ), ventilatory demand is reduced only if carbon dioxide production is decreased. Thus to minimize carbon dioxide production it is probably more important to avoid hypercaloric regimens. The clinical benefit to gas exchange and ventilatory weaning by manipulation of carbohydrate:fat ratios when total calorie intake approximates energy requirements has not been unequivocally demonstrated to benefit patients with respiratory failure.[33]

Metabolic Stress

The phrase *metabolic stress* has been used to characterize patients who are catabolic, hypermetabolic, and critically ill (see Chapters 39 and 42). The metabolic response to stress increases the metabolic rate and produces insulin resistance and proteolysis, resulting in autocanabolism of lean muscle mass. Serum concentrations of glucocorticoids, catecholamines, glucagon, and growth hormone also increase. This response is mediated partially by cytokines, including interleukin-1, tumor necrosis factor, and interleukin-6.[83] Various nutrients have been administered individually or supplemented in parenteral and enteral formulas in an attempt to blunt the hypermetabolic response, prevent progressive deterioration of lean muscle mass, and enhance immune function.

Branched-Chain Amino Acids

Special solutions enriched with BCAAs for parenteral or enteral use have been formulated for use in critical illness.[84] Use of BCAAs is based on two clinical observations. The first is due to the stress response that, with critical illness, causes AAs to be released from skeletal muscle, gut, and connective tissue and transported to the liver for gluconeogenesis. BCAAs, especially leucine, have been shown to stimulate protein synthesis and minimize protein degradation because they are used preferentially by the skeletal muscle.[85] Second, critically ill patients have been shown to have elevated concentrations of AAAs and decreased levels of BCAAs. This may be due partly to the incidence of hepatic failure in this group of patients. Thus the rationale for the use of BCAAs in metabolic stress was to provide the body with what appeared to be a preferential fuel and to normalize the AA patterns of these patients.

Several investigators have examined the use of BCAAs during periods of metabolic stress. Cerra and colleagues, in a prospective randomized double-blind study, compared BCAA-enriched enteral formulas with formulas containing standard crystalline AAs. The patients receiving the BCAAs showed improvements in nitrogen retention, visceral protein status, and serum transferrin concentrations.[86] In another randomized prospective trial, Cerra and coworkers compared BCAA-enriched parenteral solutions with standard AA solutions in a group of 23 critically ill patients.[87] Parenteral nutrition was started within 24 hours of admission and continued for 7 days. The solutions contained 1.5 g/kg per day of amino acids, 30 kcal/kg per day of dextrose, and 7 kcal/kg per day as fat. The patients who received the BCAAs had exhibited improved nitrogen retention, total lymphocyte count, and transferrin levels. Additionally, 60% of the patients who received BCAAs showed reversal of skin test anergy; however, no differences in morbidity or mortality were reported. Bower and colleagues evaluated the effects of two different BCAA solutions during surgical stress in a nonblinded prospective randomized trial.[88] Thirty-seven patients received either a standard AA solution or a BCAA solution enriched with valine. Total parenteral nutrition (PN) was administered to provide 1.5 g/kg per day as protein, 25% of nonprotein calories as fat, and the other 75% as dextrose. When no differences were noted after the first 9 patients had been enrolled in each group, the BCAA solution was changed to a leucine-enriched formula and the study completed. The results indicated marginal improvements in nitrogen retention but no statistically significant cumulative effect. There was, however, a statistically significant increase in retinol-binding protein, but not the other visceral proteins, and there was no difference in clinical outcome. Chiarla and associates randomized 16 septic trauma patients to receive either a BCAA-enriched or a standard AA solution. They observed decreased proteolysis and AA catabolism and increased production of acute-phase proteins;[89] however, there was no difference in morbidity or mortality between the two groups. Kuhl and coworkers studied the effects of BCAA-enriched solutions on visceral protein synthesis and nitrogen balance in a prospective randomized study.[90] Twenty intensive care patients were followed for 7 days. There was no significant difference in nitrogen balance, fibronectin, thyroxine-binding prealbumin, or somatomedin-C concentrations between the patients who received the standard AAs and those who received the BCAAs.

Other investigators have not been able to demonstrate significant advantages for BCAAs over standard AAs in metabolic stress. Yu and colleagues studied the effects of BCAA-enriched enteral formulas on severely burned patients. They were unable to demonstrate any advantages of the BCAA-enriched formula over a standard egg protein formulation.[91] Freund and associates questioned whether the benefits of BCAAs were dose related. They varied the BCAA content of solutions from 22% up to 100% and found no difference in nitrogen retention.[92] Lenssen and colleagues compared a leucine-enriched solution of 45% BCAAs with a 23% BCAA solution in patients who had undergone bone marrow transplantation for leukemia.[93] The patients were observed for 1 month, but there were no differences in nitrogen retention between the two groups. The effects of BCAA-enriched total parenteral nutrition solutions on nitrogen balance, 3-methylhistidine excretion, morbidity, and mortality were evaluated in 131 septic, traumatized patients.[94] Fifty-two patients received a standard solution, and 49 patients a BCAA-enriched solution. Both formulas were isocaloric and isonitrogenous. No significant differences were found between the two groups in nitrogen balance, 3-methylhistidine excretion, morbidity, or mortality.

When evaluating the studies on the use of BCAAs in patients experiencing metabolic stress, it is important to realize that the protocols and patient populations varied significantly. The studies often included small samples. The number of calories provided in each of these studies differed, as did the percentage of calories derived from carbohydrate and fat. Even the ratios of BCAAs administered were different. There were also differences in the degrees and types of metabolic stress. Many of the investigations did not control for the presence of sepsis. All of these factors can affect outcome. Thus it is difficult to determine if the BCAAs have any beneficial effect. To date, BCAAs have not been shown to reduce morbidity or mortality in humans.[95]

Glutamine

Although glutamine is classified as an NEAA, recent studies indicate that it may be conditionally essential during periods of stress, injury, sepsis, or starvation (see Chapter 7).[96,97] It is the most abundant AA in plasma and skeletal muscle and thus constitutes approximately half of the total free AA pool in the body.[98] The small intestine is the principal site of glutamine uptake.[99] Glutamine metabolism is regulated by two enzymes: glutaminase, which catalyzes the hydrolysis of glutamine to glutamate and ammonia, and glutamine synthetase, which catalyzes the synthesis of glutamine from glutamate. Glutamine is a major carrier of circulating AA nitrogen from skeletal muscle to visceral organs because of its two nitrogen moieties.[97] In addition, it aids in the regulation of acid-base balance through the reduction of ammonia; is a precursor for the synthesis of nucleic acids and nucleotides; exerts a trophic effect on the intestinal mucosa; supplies precursors and nitrogenous end products for gluconeogenesis and urea synthesis; is a substrate for renal ammoniagenesis; acts as a regulator of glycogen synthesis and protein turnover; and is the preferred fuel for rapidly proliferating cells such as enterocytes, colonocytes, macrophages, and lymphocytes.[98] Glutamine concentrations in the blood and skeletal muscle are decreased after injury, stress, starvation, and other catabolic states.

It is glutamine's effect on the small bowel that has been of greatest interest. Glutamine exerts trophic effects on the bowel[100] and stimulates nutrient absorption.[101,102] It has been shown, principally in animal studies, to promote intestinal mucosal integrity.[97,103] It promoted healing of radiation-induced lesions of the small bowel[104] and reduced bacterial translocation from the gastrointestinal tract.[105,106] Glutamine has also been shown to maintain intestinal mucosa during chemotherapy and high-dose radiation when administered parenterally to rats.[107] Similar results have been reported in the enteral nutrition literature.[108,109] Glutamine has also been administered in combination with growth hormone and a diet

modified with fiber to enhance nutrient absorption for patients with severe short-bowel syndrome.[110] Many of these patients have been able to discontinue home total parenteral nutrition or intravenous fluids. Two prospective randomized clinical trials compared parenteral nutrition with and without glutamine in 45 and 29 bone marrow transplant patients, respectively.[111,112] There was no difference in survival rate in either trial; however, Ziegler and colleagues were able to demonstrate fewer infections and decreased length of stay for the patients who received the glutamine.[111] Because glutamine is not stable for long periods in parenteral solutions, it has not been added to commercially available parenteral AA solutions. It is also important to note that glutamine supplementation may be contraindicated in patients with liver failure or HE because intestinal glutamine metabolism results in the production of ammonia, which is subsequently released into the portal vein.[113]

Free glutamine is available in some predigested enteral formulas. Although all protein sources in enteral formulas contain glutamine, the glutamine is protein bound and it is difficult to determine the exact glutamine content because whole proteins are hydrolyzed with heat and acid to determine their AA composition. This results in hydrolysis of glutamine to glutamate. Recently, newer methods for the determination of protein- and peptide-bound glutamine have been developed.[114] There are no data to suggest that protein-bound glutamine supports gut mucosal integrity as well as free glutamine does. Most commercially available enteral formulas contain less than 14% of the total protein as glutamine.[115] This may be less than the dose required to produce the pharmacologic effect.

Arginine

Arginine is another NEAA that has been investigated for its possible pharmacologic value in enhancing immune function, accelerating wound healing, and increasing nitrogen retention (see Chapter 7). Many of these effects have been demonstrated in the rat model.[116-119] Arginine has been shown to decrease the incidence of infection and improve survival in burned guinea pigs.[120] Increased blood mononuclear response to concanavalin A and phytohemagglutinin has been demonstrated in animals receiving arginine supplementation.[121]

Some literature has also demonstrated beneficial effects of arginine supplementation in humans. Arginine has been shown to increase mitogenic blastogenesis in healthy humans.[122] In a randomized prospective trial Daly and colleagues evaluated the effects of supplemental arginine in enteral feedings on 30 cancer patients undergoing major surgical procedures.[123] Patients receiving the arginine showed increased thymic weight and lymphocyte content, improved thymic lymphocyte response to mitogen stimulation, and slowed thymic involution following injury. Arginine supplementation also resulted in enhanced lymphocyte blastogenesis and increased CD4 lymphocyte (helper T cell) concentrations. Alexander and Gottschlich randomized burn patients to receive either a standard enteral formula or a special modular feeding enriched with 2% arginine and other immune-enhancing components.[124] Patients receiving the arginine-enriched formula had fewer wound infections, shorter hospital stays (per percentage of burn area), and lower mortality rates. Arginine supplementation also has been shown to stimulate wound healing and immune function in the elderly.[125]

Nucleotides

Recently some attention has been given to the relationship between dietary nucleotides and infection.[126,127] Nucleotides are degraded to purines and pyrimidines. Purines and pyrimidines are nitrogen-containing bases that can occur as free bases, as a sugar derivative (riboses or deoxyribose) nucleoside, or with one or more phosphate groups attached to the sugar-terminal nucleotide. These nucleotides are the building blocks of RNA and deoxyribonucleic acid (DNA). The formation of new cells requires synthesis of DNA to carry genetic information. Rapidly growing tissues, especially lymphoid cells and intestinal epithelium, require purines and pyrimidines for synthesis of DNA and RNA. These must either be supplied from dietary sources or synthesized de novo in the liver.[128] It had been previously assumed that humans and animals were able to synthesize nucleotides for normal growth, development, and maintenance. The requirement for nucleotides during physiologic stress remains unknown. Thus a variety of experiments have been conducted in attempts to elucidate the nucleotide requirement that maintains normal host defenses and to determine whether supplementation would enhance the response to an infectious challenge.

Most of the research in this area has been conducted on animals. Van Buren and associates documented decreased or suppressed T cell–mediated immune response in mice, including cardiac and tumor allograft rejection,[129] delayed hypersensitivity skin test response,[130] and decreased interleukin 2 lymphokine production.[131] Kulkarni and colleagues studied the influence of dietary nucleotide restriction on resistance to bacterial challenge in mice.[132,133] Mice were given a nucleotide-free diet or a nucleotide-free diet supplemented with adenine, uracil, or RNA. Mice fed RNA- or uracil-supplemented diets had the highest survival rates after a bacterial challenge with *Staphylococcus aureus*. Adenine-supplemented diets provided some protection, but not as much as the RNA- and uracil-supplemented diets. Macrophages from the mice fed the nucleotide-free diet showed decreased bacterial phagocytosis as compared with mice fed the adenine-, uracil-, or RNA-supplemented diet.[132] Decreased survival was also observed in mice fed a nucleotide-free diet following an injection of *Candida albicans*.[127] Nucleotides have also been administered to mice in an attempt to reverse depressed immune function.[134]

Lipids

Some data suggest that altering the type and amount of lipids in both enteral and parenteral solutions affect immune function (see Chapters 9 and 35). Previously, enteral lipids and intravenous lipid emulsions were composed of long-chain triglycerides (LCTs), which were sources of both calories and essential fatty acids; however, when macrophages become overloaded with fat, their ability to remove microorganisms from circulation is impaired.[135] As a result, there may be increased translocation of bacteria, more infectious episodes, and possibly organ failure.[136,137] Parenterally administered LCTs have been shown to impair the reticuloendothelial system when they are infused too rapidly.[138] Medium-chain triglycerides (MCTs) have been included in many enteral formulas and some European intravenous lipid emulsions because they

result in more positive nitrogen balance, do not require carnitine, are a source of calories, and do not negatively affect the reticuloendothelial system less.[139-141]

Research efforts began to focus on structured lipids. These are manufactured by hydrolyzing LCTs and MCTs together and then randomly reesterifying the hydrolyzed fatty-acid chains.[142] The resulting triglycerides consist of a glycerol backbone with variable-length fatty-acid chains in the same molecule.[143] The structured lipids may become preferred fat sources because they offer the advantage of enhanced absorption and EFA content.

Large amounts of linoleic acid, an ω-6 polyunsaturated fatty acid (PUFA) and a precursor of arachidonic acid, have been implicated in immune suppression.[144,145] When ω-3 PUFAs are substituted, there is a reduction in prostaglandin E_2, which is known to be immunosuppressive. In addition, the ω-3 PUFAs appear to modulate release of certain cytokines, such as interleukin 1 and tumor necrosis factor.[146] Fish oil is the best-known and richest source of ω-3 PUFAs. Parenteral and enteral infusion of fish oil in animals has demonstrated improved survival and reduction of the inflammatory response to endotoxins.[147-149] In a double-blind prospective randomized controlled trial of burn patients receiving enteral feedings with a variety of lipid-based formulas, the solution that contained fish oil as 50% of the fat source, specifically eicosapentaenoic acid (EPA) and docosahexaenoic acid (DHA), was associated with the highest survival rate.[150]

Combinations of Nutrients

Many of these nutrients have been added to commercially available enteral formulas in varying amounts with the intention of improving immune and metabolic functions, thus enhancing patient outcome while meeting nutritional requirements. In a blinded prospective controlled trial, Daly and colleagues randomized 85 patients undergoing surgery for upper gastrointestinal malignancies to receive either a standard tube feeding (Osmolite HN) or a specialty formula enriched with arginine, RNA, and fish oil (Impact).[151] Patients who received the special formula had improved immune response and nitrogen balance, a 70% reduction in infectious and wound complications, and a 22% reduction in hospital length of stay. Although the formulas were not isonitrogenous and nitrogen balance studies were conducted only in the first 20 patients, no correlation was observed between immune response and mean daily nitrogen balance in the standard-diet group. This suggests that immune response was independent of nitrogen balance. Although the difference was not statistically significant, patients who received the standard formula tended to be slightly older and to have more extensive surgery.

Cerra and colleagues conducted a prospective blinded trial to evaluate the use of Impact in intensive care unit patients.[152] Eleven patients were randomized to receive Impact and 10 others received Osmolite HN. The two groups received the same numbers of calories and amounts of nitrogen. No significant differences were noted in nitrogen balance or nutrition assessment parameters between the two groups; however, the group fed the Impact showed a significant improvement in immune function parameters, whereas the control group demonstrated no improvement or progressive suppression of immune function tests. The authors concluded that it was the specific nutrients in Impact, independent of nitrogen balance, that improved immune function. Because this was a small study, the authors were unable to demonstrate any significant difference in clinical outcomes.

Similar outcome results have been reported in other clinical trials. Daly and colleagues, in a blinded prospective randomized controlled study of 60 patients who underwent major abdominal surgery for upper gastrointestinal cancer, noted a 27% reduction in length of stay and a 77% reduction in infections and wound complications in patients receiving Impact as compared with another "trauma formula."[153] They utilized the same study design as in their earlier trial, the differences being that the diets were isocaloric and isonitrogenous. In a large multicenter double-blind prospective randomized trial, 326 critically ill intensive care unit patients received either Impact or Osmolite HN as a tube feeding.[154] The patients were stratified as having sepsis or systemic inflammatory response syndrome. Extensive subgroup analysis of the data was performed. There was a 36% reduction in length of stay and a 60% lower infection rate in the septic patients who were fed early. For the patients who received at least 821 ml per day of Impact, the median length of stay was reduced by 8 days. There were 62% fewer antibiotic days during the late feeding period. There was no difference in mortality between the two groups.

Attempts have been made to perform meta-analysis to address whether enteral nutrition with immune-enhancing properties benefits critically ill patients.[155] An analysis of 13 randomized controlled trials comparing patients receiving standard enteral nutrition with patients receiving Impact or Immune Aid showed there was no effect on mortality. However, there were significant reductions in infection rate, ventilator days, and length of stay in the group that received the immune-enhancing products. There was a positive effect seen in all the studies, with the greatest benefit in the surgical population.

In another study, Galban and colleagues evaluated an immune-enhancing diet to determine whether early enteral feeding in septic patients improves clinical outcomes when compared with a high-protein enteral formula.[156] The study was a prospective randomized multicenter trial. The immune-enhancing enteral nutrition formula resulted in a significant reduction in the mortality rate and infection rate. The reductions were greatest for patients with less severe illness.

Recently, a summit on immune-enhancing enteral therapy was held to develop a consensus on the use of these products.[157] The focus was on surgical, critically injured, and critically ill patients. The recommendations from the summit were that patients undergoing elective gastrointestinal surgery with moderate to severe malnutrition and patients with blunt penetrating torso trauma should receive early enteral nutrition with an immune-enhancing formula. There were other groups of patients, i.e., elective surgery for aortic reconstruction, head and neck surgery, severe head injury burns, and ventilator-dependent patients, who may benefit from these formulas, although there were insufficient data to conclusively recommend them.

Many of these studies suggest promising therapeutic effects for these nutrients. These products and the nutrients they contain may be considered useful and suitable for various types

of critical illnesses. Data are beginning to emerge to show efficacy in certain patient populations.

Diabetes

Several enteral formulas have been developed for patients with abnormal glucose tolerance, and in particular for patients with diabetes mellitus. Historically, diet therapy, alone or in combination with insulin or oral hypoglycemic agents, has been the cornerstone of treatment for diabetes mellitus (see Chapter 37). Many of the special enteral formulas have been designed to reflect the guidelines of the American Diabetes Association for macronutrients: approximately 10% to 20% protein, 30% fat (one third saturated, one third polyunsaturated, and one third monounsaturated), 55% to 60% carbohydrate (principally complex), and 20 to 35 g of dietary fiber.[158]

Some of these products have been formulated to contain very high levels of fat, as much as 40% to 50% of the calories (principally monounsaturated fatty acids) to assist with blood sugar control. The formulas were designed with a higher fat content in order to prevent rapid gastric emptying and erratic blood sugar elevations. Improved blood sugar control has been observed when these products have been compared with standard enteral formulas.[159,160] The subjects in these studies were not hospitalized, and they were allowed to consume the formulas by mouth. Thus, it is not clear that the same effect would be observed if the formulas were delivered by tube. Unfortunately, the composition, and the carbohydrate content in particular, was not controlled in these trials. The high fat content of this formula could delay gastric emptying in patients with gastroparesis.

Fiber has been added to these formulas in an attempt to delay gastric emptying, alter intestinal transit time, and increase insulin sensitivity. The response varies with the type and amount of fiber added (see Chapter 13). Soluble fibers such as pectin and guar have been associated with decreased postprandial glycemic response and decreased insulin response in some patients with diabetes;[161] however, these soluble fibers tend to be very viscous and, so, are not routinely added to enteral formulas. Most commercially prepared formulas contain soy polysaccharide, a soluble fiber that is readily available, inexpensive, and easily suspended in liquid. Some manufacturers have added a combination of fiber sources, such as oat, soy, pectin, gum arabic, and hydrolyzed guar, to provide a combination of soluble and insoluble fibers. Exactly how much is necessary to achieve adequate blood sugar control is also a matter of debate. It appears that the amount required may be as much as 50 g per day,[162] and most enteral formulas do not provide this much fiber.

There are very few controlled trials of these specialty formulas, and none of them has been able to demonstrate significant differences in clinical outcomes. Such products may, however, be useful and suitable for patients with abnormal glucose tolerance who cannot be managed with standard formulas.

Human Immunodeficiency Virus Infection

Malnutrition, as evidenced by progressive weight loss and wasting, has been associated with human immunodeficiency virus (HIV) and acquired immunodeficiency syndrome (AIDS) (see Chapter 36). Malnutrition among persons living with HIV/AIDS has been associated with a poor prognosis and prolonged hospitalization.[163,164] The causes of malnutrition include malabsorption, decreased intake, and increased requirements. Various nutrients have been combined in enteral formulas for their pharmacologic value or their use in malabsorption.

Chlebowski and coworkers conducted a prospective randomized trial comparing the use of a standard enteral formula (Ensure) with a special formula designed for persons with HIV or AIDS (Advera).[165] This peptide-based formula contains a blend of fats, canola oil, medium chain triglycerides (MCTs), and sardine oil and is fortified with beta-carotene and soy polysaccharide. All patients consumed an oral diet but received an average intake of 500 ml per day of one of these supplements. Patients fed the Advera had fewer hospitalizations and gained more weight over the 6-month study period. Although the patients were evenly matched according the nutritional and clinical parameters, more patients in the Advera group had contracted HIV through intravenous drug use. It is important to note that the patients were not severely malnourished; they were not in the advanced stages of the disease and showed no signs of severe malabsorption. The data show some promise for Advera as an adjunct in treatment of this disease; however, the limitations of this study with regard to patient selection and numbers preclude any definitive statements on the use of this product in patients with HIV or AIDS. Additional studies will be required to expand these observations and explore potential mechanisms of action.

Dipeptides Versus Single Amino Acids

Use of peptides of varying lengths versus single AAs as the protein source in enteral formulas is still a matter of debate (see Chapter 7). The controversy centers on which form best enhances absorption of and tolerance for enteral feedings. Protein digestion and absorption are relatively efficient and occur throughout the entire small intestine, but mainly in the jejunum and ileum. There are separate noncompeting carrier transport systems for AAs and small peptides in the gastrointestinal tract. Absorption of AAs from solutions containing di- and tripeptides differs both quantitatively and qualitatively from solutions containing free AAs.[166-170]

Most comparisons of the absorption of free AAs and peptide-based diets have studied animals. There are some data to suggest that peptide-based diets are associated with improved absorption, lower mortality, and decreased incidence of gut bacterial translocation as compared with AA-based diets. In most cases, animals fed a standard chow diet had the best responses.[171-174]

Peptide-based diets have been proposed for use in patients with marginally functional gastrointestinal tracts who otherwise would require total parenteral nutrition.[175] Peptides have been shown to be superior to free AAs as the nitrogen source in enteral nutrition during starvation.[176] These formulas have been shown to stimulate water and electrolyte absorption;[177,178] however, Rees and colleagues found no differences in nitrogen assimilation in patients with gastrectomy, ileostomy, or steator-

rhea when enteral diets containing medium-chain protein hydrolysates or whole protein were given.[179] McIntyre and colleagues found that patients with ileostomies who had between 60 and 150 cm of small intestine absorbed whole or partially hydrolyzed protein equally well.[180]

A number of studies have examined protein absorption and the incidence of diarrhea in critically ill patients. It appears that the form of protein can influence absorption rates in critically ill patients and that peptides appear to be absorbed better than intact protein, which in turn may be absorbed better than AAs;[181,182] however, it is important to note that the studies did not control for medication use or pseudomembranous colitis.

In a prospective study of 12 intensive care patients after abdominal surgery it was concluded that enteral formulas containing small peptides were more effective in restoring plasma amino acid and protein levels than an equivalent diet that contained whole proteins.[183] In another comparison of tolerance and nutritional outcome, however, between a peptide and a standard enteral formula in critically ill hypoalbuminemic patients, the peptide formula offered no advantage over the standard enteral formula.[184]

The use of peptide-based formulas remains controversial.[185] Most of the clinical studies did not control for the presence of pseudomembranous colitis, use of medications containing sorbitol, and disorders of pancreatic or intestinal lipase. Formulas that contain intact protein should be used whenever possible. Peptide-based diets may improve absorption and decrease gut bacterial translocation in certain disease states better than AA-based diets do. In certain clinical conditions such as malabsorption and critical illness, peptide-based diets may be absorbed better than intact protein.

Critical Evaluation of Nutrition Research

Critical evaluation of the literature is important to evaluate new products, services, techniques, and procedures that will ultimately result in better patient care and outcomes. As economic and health care resources become scarce, this becomes even more important. The literature must be reviewed with a "critical eye" and "dissected" carefully (Box 20-1).

Clinical research can be difficult and costly to perform. Nutrition studies often do not show clear clinical outcomes supported by careful designs and methods. Longer studies with larger samples are generally needed. Unfortunately, because of the required sample size in an inherently varied study population, it may not be possible to demonstrate the type of results we would like to see. It may be necessary to conduct multicenter trials to obtain a sample of appropriate size. The situation is further complicated by the fact that one single nutrient may not be responsible for various proposed beneficial effects. Rather, a unique combination of nutrients may be most beneficial.

The importance of study design to the demonstration of efficacy cannot be overemphasized (see Chapter 46). The prospective double-blind controlled trial is the gold standard. Appropriate patient selection is crucial. Although most of these studies do not demonstrate efficacy, there are data to show that these formulas are safe and may be useful and suitable for the care of patients.

Evaluating Research Publications

GENERAL
1. Is the study of value to my knowledge, interest, or practice?
2. Will this article change my practice?
3. Is the research important to the field? Does it address an important question?
4. Does this paper make a significant contribution to the literature?

TITLE AND AUTHORSHIP
1. Is the title clear and informative? Does it convey the major findings of the paper?
2. Are the authors well known in the field? Are they employed by industry? Is there potential for a conflict of interest?
3. How was the study funded?

ABSTRACT/INTRODUCTION
1. Is the abstract well written? Does it summarize the purpose, design, results, conclusions, and applications of the study?
2. Do the authors state the purpose of the study in the introduction to the paper? Is the hypothesis clearly stated?

MATERIALS AND METHODS
1. Does the study design address the objectives? Did the authors adequately describe the study end points?
2. Are the materials and methods described in a clear, straightforward manner? Are the methods appropriate and accurate? Is a detailed description of the entry and rejection criteria presented? Could this study be reproduced from the description of the methods?
3. Is the sample size adequate to achieve statistical analysis?
4. Have the patients been selected appropriately and well matched?
5. Did the authors obtain informed consent?
6. Were the control and experimental treatment regimens, including placebos, adequately described?
7. Is the control protocol identical to the treatment? Was the timing of each treatment group identical?
8. Was the study randomized and blinded?
9. Was the study conducted for a reasonable length of time?

DATA ANALYSIS
1. Were the appropriate and relevant outcome variables evaluated?
2. Was the appropriate statistical analysis applied? Were appropriate p values used to determine statistical significance?
3. Were all the patients included in the statistical analysis?
4. Were any data eliminated from analysis?
5. Did the authors have to do subgroup analysis to achieve statistical significance?

RESULTS
1. Are the results clear, concise, and appropriately analyzed?
2. Do the results follow the same order described in the materials and methods section?
3. Were there any treatment complications?
4. Are the tables and figures accurate and appropriate? Do they add to the paper? Do all the numbers add up?
5. Do the data support the conclusions?

DISCUSSION
1. Is the discussion section relevant to the findings?
2. Did the authors accurately interpret their results relevant to other papers?
3. Were all possible interpretations of the results considered?
4. Did the authors state clear and reasonable applications of their results?
5. Are the references current, appropriate, and complete?

Conclusion

There have been many enteral and parenteral formulas developed for individuals with specific metabolic derangements. The rationale for the design of these formulas is based on physiologic and medical principles. There is an increasing amount of data to show that these formulas are safe and suitable for use in various disease states. When selecting these formulas it is important to consider the specific disease process and choose a formula appropriate for that condition. Future research will be required to document efficacy of specialized formulas in specific patient populations.

REFERENCES

1. Matarese LE: Rationale and efficacy of specialized enteral nutrition, *NCP* 9(2): 58-64, 1995.
2. *Federal Register*, 61:231, November 29, 1996.
3. Feinstein EI: Total parenteral nutrition support of patients with acute renal failure, *NCP* 3(1):9-13, 1988.
4. Coles GA: Body composition in chronic renal failure, *QJ Med* 41:25-47, 1972.
5. Kopple JD, Swendseid ME: Protein and amino acid metabolism in uremic patients undergoing maintenance hemodialysis, *Kidney Int Suppl* 2:64-72, 1975.
6. Blumenkrantz MJ, Kopple JD: Incidence of nutritional abnormalities in uremic patients entering dialysis therapy, *Kidney Int* 10:514, 1976 (abstract).
7. Rose WC: Amino acid requirements of man, *Fed Proc* 8:546-552, 1949.
8. Mirtallo J, Kudsk K, Ebbert M: Nutritional support of patients with renal disease, *Clin Pharm* 3:253-263, 1984.
9. Giordano C: Use of exogenous and endogenous urea for protein synthesis in normal and uremic subjects, *J Lab Clin Med* 62:231-246, 1963.
10. Giovannetti S, Maggiore Q: A low nitrogen diet with protein of high biological value for severe chronic uremia, *Lancet* 1:1000-1003, 1964.
11. Wilmore DW, Dudrick SJ: Treatment of acute renal failure with intravenous essential L-amino acids, *Arch Surg* 99:669-673, 1969.
12. Dudrick SJ, Steiger E, Long JM: Renal failure in surgical patients. Treatment with intravenous essential amino acids and hypertonic glucose, *Surgery* 68:180-186, 1970.
13. Abel RM, Abbott WM, Fischer JE: Acute renal failure. Treatment without dialysis by total parenteral nutrition, *Arch Surg* 103:513-514, 1971.
14. Abbott WM, Abel RM, Fischer JE: Treatment of acute renal insufficiency after aortoiliac surgery, *Arch Surg* 103:590-594, 1971.
15. Abel RM, Beck CH, Abbott WM, et al: Improved survival from acute renal failure after treatment with intravenous essential L-amino acids and glucose. Results of a prospective, double-blind study, *N Engl J Med* 288:695-699, 1973.
16. Varcoe AR, Halliday D, Carson ER, et al: Anabolic role of urea in renal failure, *Am J Clin Nutr* 31:1601-1607, 1978.
17. Ell S, Flynn M, Richards P, Halliday D: Metabolic studies with keto acid diets, *Am J Clin Nutr* 31:1776-1783, 1978.
18. Long C, Jeevanandam M, Kinney JM: Metabolism and recycling of urea in man, *Am J Clin Nutr* 31:1367-1382, 1978.
19. Richards P: Nutritional potential of nitrogen recycling in man, *Am J Clin Nutr* 25:615-625, 1972.
20. Freund J, Atamian S, Fischer JE: Comparative study of parenteral nutrition in renal failure using essential and nonessential amino acid–containing solutions, *Surg Gynecol Obstet* 151:652-656, 1980.
21. Feinstein EI, Blumenkrantz MJ, Healy M, et al: Clinical and metabolic responses to parenteral nutrition in acute renal failure. A controlled, double-blind study, *Medicine* 60:124-137, 1981.
22. Feinstein EI, Kopple JD, Silberman H, Massry SG: Total parenteral nutrition with high or low nitrogen intakes in patients with acute renal failure, *Kidney Int* 26:319-323, 1983.
23. Mirtallo JM, Schneider PJ, Mavko K, et al: A comparison of essential and general amino acid infusions in the nutritional support of patients with compromised renal function, *J Parenter Enteral Nutr* 6:109-113, 1982.
24. Kopple JD, Swendseid ME: Nitrogen balance and plasma amino acid levels in uremic patients fed an essential amino acid diet, *Am J Clin Nutr* 27:806-812, 1974.

25. Sofio CA, Nicora RW, Osborn TW, Amen RJ: Oral essential amino acids in the management of acute and chronic renal failure, *J Parenter Enteral Nutr* 3:506, 1979 (abstract).

26. Attman PO, Bucht H, Isaksson B, Uddebom G: Nitrogen balance studies with amino acid supplemented low-protein diet in uremia, *Am J Clin Nutr* 32:2033-2039, 1979.

27. Maschio G, Oldrizzi L, Tessitore N, et al: Effects of dietary protein and phosphorus restriction on the progression of early renal failure, *Kidney Int* 22:371-376, 1982.

28. Maschio G, Oldrizzi L, Tessitore N, et al: Early dietary protein and phosphorus restriction is effective in delaying progression of chronic renal failure, *Kidney Int* 24(suppl 16):S273-S277, 1983.

29. Ihle BU, Becker GJ, Whitworth JA, et al: The effect of protein restriction on the progression of renal insufficiency, *N Engl J Med* 321:1773-1777, 1989.

30. Oldrizzi L, Rugiu C, Maschio G: Different protein diets in renal failure: a self-controlled study, *Am J Nephrol* 9:184-189, 1989.

31. Brouhard BH, LaGrone L: Effect of dietary protein restriction on functional renal reserve in diabetic neuropathy, *Am J Med* 89:427-431, 1990.

32. Locatelli F, Alberti D, Grazini G, et al: Prospective, randomized multicentre trial of effect of protein restriction on progression of chronic renal insufficiency, *Lancet* 337:1299-1304, 1991.

33. ASPEN Board of Directors: Guidelines for the use of parenteral and enteral nutrition in adult and pediatric patients, *J Parenter Enteral Nutr* 17:1SA-52SA, 1993.

34. Mendenhall CL, Anderson S, Weesner RE, et al: Protein-calorie malnutrition associated with alcoholic hepatitis, *Am J Med* 76:211-222, 1984.

35. Fischer JE: Branched-chain-enriched amino acid solutions in patients with liver failure: an early example of nutritional pharmacology, *J Parenter Enteral Nutr* 14:249S-256S, 1990.

36. Fischer JE, Funovics JM, Aguirre A, et al: The role of plasma amino acids in hepatic encephalopathy, *Surgery* 78:276-290, 1975.

37. Fischer JE, Baldessarini R: False neurotransmitters and hepatic failure, *Lancet* 2:75-80, 1971.

38. Fischer JE, James JH: Treatment of hepatic coma and hepatorenal syndrome: Mechanism of action of L-dopa and aramine, *Am J Surg* 123:222-230, 1972.

39. Talbot JM: Guidelines for the scientific review of enteral food products for special medical purposes, *J Parenter Enteral Nutr* 15(3):99S-174S, 1991.

40. Brennan MF, Cerra F, Daly JM, et al: Report of a research workshop: branched-chain amino acids in stress and injury, *J Parenter Enteral Nutr* 10:446-452, 1986.

41. Schafer K, Winther MB, Ukida M, et al: Influence of an orally administered protein mixture enriched in branched chain amino acids on the chronic hepatic encephalopathy (CHE) of patients with liver cirrhosis, *Z Gastroenterol* 19:356-362, 1981.

42. Eriksson LS, Persson A, Wahren J: Branched-chain amino acids in the treatment of chronic hepatic encephalopathy, *Gut* 23:801-806, 1982.

43. McGhee A, Henderson JM, Millikan WJ Jr, et al: Comparison of the effects of Hepatic-Aid and a casein modular diet on encephalopathy, plasma amino acids, and nitrogen balance in cirrhotic patients, *Ann Surg* 197:288-293, 1983.

44. Horst D, Grace ND, Conn HO, et al: Comparison of dietary protein with an oral, branched chain-enriched amino acid supplement in chronic portal-systemic encephalopathy: a randomized controlled trial, *Hepatology* 4:279-287, 1984.

45. Marchesini G, Dioguardi FS, Bianchi GP, et al: Long-term oral branched-chain amino acid treatment in chronic hepatic encephalopathy. A randomized double-blind casein-controlled trial, *J Hepatol* 11:92-101, 1990.

46. Cabre E, Gonzalez-Huix F, Abad-Lacruz A, et al: Effect of total enteral nutrition on the short-term outcome of severely malnourished cirrhotics: a randomized controlled trial, *Gastroenterology* 98:715-720, 1990.

47. Smith J, Horowitz J, Henderson JM, Heymsfield S: Enteral hyperalimentation in undernourished patients with cirrhosis and ascites, *Am J Clin Nutr* 35:56-72, 1982.

48. Calvey H, Davis M, Williams R: Controlled trial of nutritional supplementation, with and without branched chain amino acid enrichment, in treatment of acute alcoholic hepatitis, *J Hepatol* 1:141-151, 1985.

49. Erikkson LS, Conn HO: Branched-chain amino acids in the management of hepatic encephalopathy: an analysis of variants, *Hepatology* 10:228-246, 1989.

50. Rossi-Fanelli F, Riggio O, Cangiano C, et al: Branched-chain amino acids vs lactulose in the treatment of hepatic coma: a controlled study, *Dig Dis Sci* 27:929-935, 1982.

51. Wahren J, Denis J, Desurmont P, et al: Is intravenous administration of branched chain amino acids effective in the treatment of hepatic encephalopathy? A multicenter study, *Hepatology* 3:475-480, 1983.

52. Cerra FB, Cheung NK, Fischer JE, et al: Disease-specific amino acid infusion (FO80) in hepatic encephalopathy: a prospective, randomized, double-blind, controlled trial, *J Parenter Enteral Nutr* 9:288-295, 1985.

53. Naylor CD, O'Rourke K, Detsky AS, Baker JP: Parenteral nutrition with branched-chain amino acids in hepatic encephalopathy: a meta-analysis, *Gastroenterology* 97:1003-1042, 1989.

54. Fan, ST; Lo, CM; Lai, EC, et al: Perioperive nutritional support in patients undergoing hepatectomy for hepatocelluar carcinoma, *New Eng J Med* 331(23):1547-1552, 1994.

55. Openbrier DR, Irwin MM, Rodgers RM, et al: Nutritional status and lung function in patients with emphysema and chronic bronchitis, *Chest* 83:17-22, 1983.

56. Hunter AMB, Carey MA, Larsh HW: The nutritional status of patients with chronic obstructive pulmonary disease, *Am Rev Respir Dis* 124:376-381, 1981.

57. Driver AG, LeBrun M: Iatrogenic malnutrition in patients receiving ventilatory support, *JAMA* 244:2195-2196, 1980.

58. Driver AG, McAlevy MT, Smith JL: Nutritional assessment of patients with chronic obstructive pulmonary disease and acute respiratory failure, *Chest* 82:568-571, 1982.

59. Arora NS, Rochester DF: Respiratory muscle strength and maximal voluntary ventilation in undernourished patients, *Am Rev Respir Dis* 126:5-8, 1982.

60. Arora NS, Rochester DF: Effect of body weight and muscularity on human diaphragm muscle mass, thickness, and area, *J Appl Physiol* 52:64-70, 1982.

61. Jeejeebhoy K: Bulk or bounce: The object of nutritional support, *J Parenter Enteral Nutr* 12:539-549, 1988.

62. Donahoe M, Rogers RM: Nutritional assessment and support in chronic obstructive pulmonary disease, *Clin Chest Med* 11:487-504, 1990.

63. Doekel RC, Zwillich CW, Scoogin CH, et al: Clinical semistarvation: depression of hypoxic ventilatory response, *N Engl J Med* 295:358-361, 1976.

64. Schwartz DB: Pulmonary failure. In Gottschlich MM, Matarese LF, Shronts EP (eds):*Nutrition support dietetics core curriculum*, Silver Spring, MD, 1993, ASPEN, pp 251-260.

65. Edelman NH, Rucker RB, Peavy HH: NIH Workshop Summary: nutrition and the respiratory system: chronic obstructive pulmonary disease (COPD), *Am Rev Respir Dis* 134:347-352, 1986.

66. Kelly SM, Rosa A, Field S, et al: Inspiratory muscle strength and body composition in patients receiving total parenteral nutrition therapy, *Am Rev Respir Dis* 130:33-37, 1984.

67. Larca L, Greenbaum DM: Effectiveness of intensive nutritional regimes in patients who fail to wean from mechanical ventilation, *Crit Care Med* 10:297-300, 1982.

68. Askanazi J, Elwyn DH, Silverberg PA, et al: Respiratory distress secondary to a high carbohydrate load: a case report, *Surgery* 87:596-598, 1980.

69. Covelli HD, Black JW, Olsen MS, Beekman JF: Respiratory failure precipitated by high carbohydrate loads, *Ann Intern Med* 95:579-581, 1981.

70. Ireton-Jones CS, Turner WW: The use of respiratory quotient to determine the efficacy of nutrition support regimens, *J Am Diet Assoc* 87:180-183, 1987.

71. MacFie J, Homfield HHM, King RF, Hill GL: Effect of the energy source on changes in energy expenditure and respiratory quotient during total parenteral nutrition, *J Parenter Enteral Nutr* 7:1-5, 1983.

72. Bartlett RH, Dechert RE, Mault JR, Clark SF: Metabolic studies in chest trauma, *J Thorac Cardiovasc Surg* 87:503-508, 1984.

73. Askanazi J, Rosenbaum SH, Hyman AI, et al: Respiratory changes induced by the large glucose loads of total parenteral nutrition, *JAMA* 243:1444-1447, 1980.

74. Brown RO, Heizer WD: Nutrition and respiratory disease, *Clin Pharm* 3:152-161, 1984.

75. Deitel M, Williams VP, Rice TW: Nutrition and the patient requiring mechanical ventilatory support, *J Am Coll Nutr* 2:25-32, 1983.

76. Askanazi J, Nordenstrom J, Rosenbaum SH, et al: Nutrition for the patient with respiratory failure: glucose vs fat, *Anesthesiology* 54:373-377, 1981.

77. Angelillo VA, Bedi S, Durfee D, et al: Effects of low and high carbohydrate feedings in ambulatory patients with chronic obstructive pulmonary disease and chronic hypercapnia, *Ann Intern Med* 103:883-885, 1985.

78. Goldstein SA, Thomashow B, Askanazi J: Functional changes during nutritional repletion in patients with lung disease, *Clin Chest Med* 7(1):141-151, 1986.

79. Goldstein SA, Askanazi J, Elwyn DH, et al: Submaximal exercise in emphysema and malnutrition at two levels of carbohydrate and fat intake, *J Appl Physiol* 67:1048-1055, 1989.

80. Al-Saady NM, Blakemore CM, Bennett ED: High fat, low carbohydrate, enteral feeding lowers $Paco_2$ and reduces the period of ventilation in artificially ventilated patients, *Intensive Care Med* 15:290-295, 1989.

81. Silberman H, Silberman AW: Parenteral nutrition, biochemistry, and respiratory gas exchange, *J Parenter Enteral Nutr* 10:151-154, 1986.

82. Talpers SS, Romberger DJ, Bunce SB, Pingleton SK: Nutritionally associated increased carbon dioxide production. Excess total calories vs high proportion of carbohydrate calories, *Chest* 102:551-555, 1992.

83. Cerra FB: Hypermetabolism, organ failure, and metabolic support, *Surgery* 101:1-14, 1987.

84. Brennan MF, Cerra F, Daly JM, et al: Report of a research workshop: branched-chain amino acids in stress and injury, *J Parenter Enteral Nut r*10:446-452, 1986.

85. Buse MG, Reid SS: Leucine: a possible regulator of protein turnover in muscle, *J Clin Invest* 56:1250-1261, 1975.

86. Cerra FB, Shronts EP, Konstantinides NN, et al: Enteral feeding in sepsis: a prospective, randomized, double-blind trial, *Surgery* 98:632-639, 1985.

87. Cerra FB, Mazuski J, Chute E, et al: Branched chain metabolic support: a prospective, randomized, double-blind trial in surgical stress, *Ann Surg* 199:286-291, 1984.

88. Bower RH, Muggia-Sullam M, Vallgren S, et al: Branched-chain amino acid–enriched solutions in the septic patient. A randomized, prospective trial, *Ann Surg* 203:13-20, 1986.

89. Chiarla C, Siegel J, Kidd S, et al: Inhibition of post-traumatic septic proteolysis and ureagenesis and stimulation of hepatic acute-phase protein production by branched-chain amino acid TPN, *J Trauma* 28:1145-1172, 1988.

90. Kuhl DA, Brown RO, Vehe KL, et al: Use of selected visceral protein measurements in the comparison of branched-chain amino acids with standard amino acids in parenteral nutrition support of injured patients, *Surgery* 107:503-510, 1990.

91. Yu, YM, Wagner DA, Walesrewski JC, et al: A kinetic study of leucine metabolism in severely burned patients: comparison between a conventional and branched-chain amino acid-enriched nutritional therapy, *Ann Surg* 207;421-429, 1988.

92. Freund H, Hoover HC, Atamian S, et al: Infusion of the branched chain amino acids in postoperative patients. Anticatabolic properties, *Ann Surg* 190:18-23, 1979.

93. Lenssen P, Cheney C, Aker S, et al: Intravenous branched chain amino acid trial in marrow transplant recipients, *J Parenter Enteral Nutr* 11:112-118, 1987.

94. von Meyenfeldt MF, Soeters PB, Vente JP, et al: Effect of branched chain amino acid enrichment of total parenteral nutrition of nitrogen sparing and clinical outcome of sepsis and trauma: a prospective randomized double blind trial, *Br J Surg* 77:924-929, 1990.

95. Brennan MF, Cerra F, Daly JM, et al: Report of a research workshop: branched-chain amino acids in stress and injury, *J Parenter Enteral Nutr* 10:446-452, 1986.

96. Lacey JM, Wilmore DW: Is glutamine a conditionally essential amino acid? *Nutr Rev* 48(8):297-309, 1990.

97. Souba WW, Smith RJ, Wilmore DW: Glutamine metabolism by the intestinal tract, *J Parenter Enteral Nutr* 9(5):608-617, 1985.

98. Smith RJ: Glutamine metabolism and its physiologic importance, *J Parenter Enteral Nutr* 14(suppl 4):40S-44S, 1990.

99. Lochs H, Hubl W: Metabolic basis for selecting glutamine-containing substrates for parenteral nutrition, *J Parenter Enteral Nutr* 14(suppl):114S-117S, 1990.

100. Tamada H, Nezu R, Matsuo Y, et al: Alanyl glutamine-enriched total parenteral nutrition restores intestinal adaptation after either proximal or distal massive resection in rats, *J Parenter Enteral Nutr* 17:236-242, 1993.

101. Gardemann A, Watanabe Y, Grobe V, et al: Increases in intestinal glucose absorption and hepatic glucose uptake elicited by luminal but not vascular glutamine in the jointly perfused small intestine and liver of the rat, *Biochem J* 283:795-765, 1992.

102. Rhoads JM, Keku EO, Quinn J, et al: L-Glutamine stimulates jejunal sodium and chloride absorption in pig rotavirus enteritis, *Gastroenterology* 100:683-691, 1991.

103. Grant JP, Snyder PJ: Use of L-glutamine in total parenteral nutrition, *J Surg Res* 44:506-513, 1988.

104. Klimberg VS, Salloum RM, Kasper M, et al: Oral glutamine accelerates healing of the small intestine and improves outcome after whole abdominal radiation, *Arch Surg* 125:1040-1045, 1990.

105. Alverdy JC: Effects of glutamine-supplemented diets on immunology of the gut, *J Parenter Enteral Nutr* 14:109S-113S, 1990.

106. Rombeau JL: A review of the effects of glutamine-enriched diets on experimentally induced enterocolitis, *J Parenter Enteral Nutr* 14:100S-105S, 1990.

107. O'Dwyer ST, Smith RJ, Hwang TL, Wilmore DW: Maintenance of small bowel mucosa with glutamine-enriched parenteral nutrition, *J Parenter Enteral Nutr* 13:579-585, 1989.

108. Fox AD, Kripke SA, De Paula J, et al: Effect of glutamine-supplemented enteral diet on methotrexate-induced enterocolitis, *J Parenter Enteral Nutr* 12:325-331, 1988.

109. Salloum RM, Souba WW, Klimberg VS, et al: Glutamine is superior to glutamate in supporting gut metabolism, stimulating intestinal glutaminase activity, and preventing bacterial translocation, *Surg Forum* 40:6-8, 1989.

110. Bryne TA, Morrissey TB, Nattakom TV, et al: Growth hormone, glutamine, and a modified diet enhance nutrient absorption in patients with severe short bowel syndrome, *J Parenter Enteral Nutr* 19(4):296-302, 1995.

111. Ziegler TR, Young LS, Benfell K, et al: Clinical and metabolic efficacy of glutamine-supplemented parenteral nutrition after bone marrow transplantation. A randomized, double-blind, controlled study, *Ann Intern Med* 116:821-828, 1992.

112. Schloerb PR, Amare M: Total parenteral nutrition with glutamine in bone marrow transplantation and other clinical applications (a randomized, double-blind study), *J Parenter Enteral Nutr* 17:407-413, 1993.

113. Weber FL, Veach GL: The importance of small intestine in gut ammonia production in the fasting dog, *Gastroenterology* 77:235-240, 1979.

114. Kuhn KS, Stehle P, Furst P: Glutamine content of protein and peptide-based enteral products, *J Parenter Enteral Nutr* 20(4):292-295, 1996.

115. Swails W, Bell SJ, Borlase BC, et al: Glutamine content of whole proteins: implications for enteral formulas, *NCP* 7:77-80, 1992.

116. Barbul A, Wasserkrug HL, Yoshimura N, et al: High arginine levels in intravenous hyperalimentation abrogate post-traumatic immune suppression, *J Surg Res* 36:620-624, 1984.

117. Barbul A, Rettura G, Levenson SM, Seifter E: Wound healing and thymtropic effects of arginine: a pituitary mechanism of action, *Am J Clin Nutr* 37:786-794, 1983.

118. Sitren HS, Fisher H: Nitrogen retention in rats fed on diets enriched with arginine and glycine. I. Improved N retention after trauma, *Br J Nutr* 37:195-208, 1977.

119. Nirgiotis JG, Hennessey PJ, Andrassy RJ: The effects of an arginine-free enteral diet on wound healing and immune function in the postsurgical rat, *J Pediatr Surg* 26:936-941, 1991.

120. Saito H, Trocki O, Wang SL, et al: Metabolic and immune effects of dietary arginine supplementation after burn, *Arch Surg* 122:784-789, 1987.

121. Barbul A, Rettura G, Levenson SM, Seifter E: Arginine: thymotropic and wound healing promoting agent, *Surg Forum* 28:101-103, 1977.

122. Barbul A, Sisto DA, Wasserkrug HL, Efron G: Arginine stimulates lymphocyte immune response in healthy human beings, *Surgery* 90:244-251, 1981.

123. Daly JM, Reynolds JV, Thom A, et al: Immune and metabolic effects of arginine in the surgical patient, *Ann Surg* 208:512-523, 1988.

124. Alexander JW, Gottschlich MM: Nutritional immunomodulation in burn patients, *Crit Care Med* 18(2):S149-153, 1990.

125. Kirk SJ, Hurson M, Regan MC, et al: Arginine stimulates wound healing and immune function in elderly human beings, *Surgery* 114(2):155-160, 1993.

126. Kulkarni AD, Fanslow WC, Drath DB, et al: Influence of dietary nucleotide restriction on bacterial sepsis and phagocytic function in mice, *Arch Surg* 121:169-172, 1986.

127. Fanslow WC, Kulkarni AD, Van Buren CT, et al: Effect of nucleotide restriction and supplementation on resistance to experimental murine candidiasis, *J Parenter Enteral Nutr* 12(1):49-52, 1988.

128. Van Buren CT, Kulkarni AD, Schandle VB, Rudolph FB: The influence of dietary nucleotides on cell-mediated immunity, *Transplantation* 36(3):350-352, 1983.

129. Rudolph FB, Kulkarni AD, Schandel VB, Van Buren CT: Involvement of dietary nucleotides in T lymphocyte function, *Adv Exp Med Biol* 165B:175-178, 1984.

130. Kulkarni Ad, Schandle VB, Rudolph FB, Van Buren CT: Suppression of delayed type hypersensitivity (DHT) to SRBC in mice fed nucleotide-free diet, *Fed Proc* 41:589, 1982.

131. Van Buren CT, Kulkarni AD, Fanslow WC, Rudolph FB: Dietary nucleotides, a requirement of helper/inducer T-lymphocytes, *Transplantation* 40(5):694-697, 1985.

132. Kulkarni AD, Fanslow WC, Drath DB, et al: Influence of dietary nucleotide restriction on bacterial sepsis and phagocytic function in mice, *Arch Surg* 121:169-172, 1986.

133. Kulkarni AD, Fanslow WC, Rudolph FB, Van Buren CT: Effect of dietary nucleotides on response to bacterial infections, *J Parenter Enteral Nutr* 10(2):169-171, 1986.

134. Van Buren CT, Rudolph FB, Kulkarni A, et al: Reversal of immunosuppression induced by a protein-free diet: comparison of nucleotides, fish oil and arginine, *Crit Care Med* 18(2)114S-117S, 1990.

135. Sobrado J, Moldawer LL, Pompeselli JJ, et al: Lipid emulsions and reticuloendothelial system function in healthy and burned guinea pigs, *Am J Clin Nutr* 42:855-863, 1985.

136. Hamawy KJ, Moldawer LL, Georgieff M, et al: The effect of lipid emulsions on reticuloendothelial system function in the injured animal, *J Parenter Enteral Nutr* 9(5):559-565, 1985.

137. Lauser ME, Saba TM: Neutrophil-mediated lung location of bacteria: a mechanism for pulmonary injury, *Surgery* 90:473-481, 1981.

138. Seidner DL, Mascioli EA, Istfan NW, et al: Effects of long-chain triglyceride emulsions on reticuloendothelial system in humans, *J Parenter Enteral Nutr* 13:614-619, 1989.

139. Guisard D, Debry G: Metabolic effects of medium-chain triglyceride emulsion injected intravenously in man, *Horm Metab Res* 4:509, 1972.

140. Bach AC, Babayan VK: Medium-chain triglycerides. An Update, *Am J Clin Nutr* 36:950-962, 1982.

141. Jensen GL, Mascioli EA, Seidner DL, et al: Parenteral infusion of medium chain triglycerides and reticuloendothelial system function in man, *Am J Clin Nutr* 47:786, 1988.

142. Babayan VK: Medium-chain triglycerides and structured lipids, *Lipids* 22:417-420, 1987.

143. Mascioli EA, Bistrian BR, Babayan VK, Blackburn GL: Medium-chain triglycerides and structured lipids as unique nonglucose energy sources in hyperalimentation, *Lipids* 22:421-423, 1987.

144. Kinsella JE: Lipids, membrane receptors, and enzymes: effects of dietary fatty acids, *J Parenter Enteral Nutr* 14(suppl):200S-217S, 1990.

145. Kinsella JE, Lokesh B, Broughton S, Whelan J: Dietary polyunsaturated fatty acids and eicosanoids: potential effects on the modulation of inflammatory and immune cells: an overview, *Nutrition* 6:24-44, 1990.

146. Endres S, Ghorbani R, Kelley VE, et al: The effect of dietary supplementation with n-3 polyunsaturated fatty acids on the synthesis of interleukin 1 and tumor necrosis factor by mononuclear cells, *N Engl J Med* 320(5):265-271, 1989.

147. Mascioli EA, Leader L, Flores F, et al: Enhanced survival to endotoxin in guinea pigs fed IV fish oil emulsion, *Lipids* 23:623-625, 1988.

148. Mascioli EA, Iwasa Y, Trimbo S, et al: Endotoxin challenge after menhaden oil diet: effects on survival of guinea pigs, *Am J Clin Nutr* 49:277-282, 1989.

149. Trocki O, Heyd T, Waymack P, Alexander JW: Effects of fish oil on postburn metabolism and immunity, *J Parenter Enteral Nutr* 11(6):521-528, 1987.

150. Gottschlich MM, Jenkins M, Warden GD, et al: Differential effects of three enteral dietary regimens on selected outcome variables in burn patients, *J Parenter Enteral Nutr* 14:225-236, 1990.

151. Daly JM, Lieberman MD, Goldfine J, et al: Enteral nutrition with supplemental arginine, RNA, and omega-3 fatty acids in patients after operation: immunologic, metabolic, and clinical outcome, *Surgery* 112(1):56-67, 1992.

152. Cerra FB, Lehman S, Konstantinides N, et al: Effect of enteral nutrient on in vitro tests of immune function in ICU patients: a preliminary report, *Nutrition* 6(1):84-87, 1990.

153. Daly JM, Weintraub FN, Shou J, et al: Enteral nutrition during multimodality therapy in upper gastrointestinal cancer patients, *Ann Surg* 221(4):327-338, 1995.

154. Bower RH, Cerra FB, Bershadsky B, et al: Early enteral administration of a formula (Impact) supplemented with arginine, nucleotides, and fish oil in intensive care unit patients: results of a multicenter, prospective, randomized, clinical trial, *Crit Care Med* 23(3):436-449, 1995.

155. Beale RJ, Bryg DJ, Bihari DJ. Immunonutrition in the critically ill: a systematic review of clinical outcome, *Crit Care Med* 27(12):2799-2805, 1999.

156. Galban C, Montejo CJ, Mesejo A, et al: An immune-enhancing enteral diet reduces mortality rate and episodes of bacteremia in septic intensive care unit patients, *Crit Care Med* 28(3):643-648, 2000.

157. Proceedings from Summit on Immune-Enhancing Enteral Therapy, *J Parenter Enteral Nutr* 25(2):S1-S63, 2001.

158. American Diabetes Association: Nutritional recommendations and principles for people with diabetes mellitus, *Diabetes Care* 17:519-522, 1994.

159. Peters AL, Davidson MB, Isaac RM: Lack of glucose elevation after simulated tube feeding with a low-carbohydrate, high fat enteral formula in patients with type 1 diabetes, *Am J Med* 87:178-182, 1989.

160. Peters AL, Davidson MB: Effects of various enteral feeding products on postprandial blood glucose response in patients with type 1 diabetes, *J Parenter Enteral Nutr* 16:69-74, 1992.

161. Jenkins DJ, Goff DV, Leeds AR, et al: Unabsorbed carbohydrate and diabetes: decreased postprandial hyperglycemia, *Lancet* 2:172-174, 1976.

162. Anderson JW, Gustafson NJ, Bryant CA, Tietyen-Clark J: Dietary fiber and diabetes: a comprehensive review and practical application, *J Am Diet Assoc* 87(9):1189-1197, 1987.

163. Chlebowski RT, Grosvenor MB, Bernard NH, et al: Nutritional status, gastrointestinal dysfunction and survival in patients with AIDS, *Am J Gastroenterology* 84:1288-1293, 1989.

164. Kotler DP, Tierney AR, Wang J, Pierson RN: Magnitude of body-cell-mass depletion and the timing of death from wasting in AIDS, *Am J Clin Nutr* 50:444-447, 1989.

165. Chlebowski RT, Beall G, Grosvenor M, et al: Long-term effects of early nutritional support with new enterotropic peptide-based formula vs. standard enteral formula in HIV-infected patients: randomized prospective trial, *Nutrition* 9(6):507-512, 1993.

166. Adibi SA, Morse EL: Intestinal transport of dipeptides in man: relative importance of hydrolysis and intact absorption, *J Clin Invest* 50:2266-2275, 1971.

167. Silk DBA, Perrett D, Clark ML: Intestinal transport of two dipeptides containing the same two neutral amino acids in man, *Clin Sci Molec Med* 45:291, 1973.

168. Adibi SA, Fogel MR, Agrawal RM: Comparison of free amino acid and dipeptide absorption in the jejunum of sprue patients, *Gastroenterology* 15:494-501, 1974.

169. Silk DBA, Kumar PJ, Perrett D, et al: Amino acid and peptide absorption in patients with coeliac disease and dermatitis herpetiformis, *Gut* 15:1-8, 1974.

170. Keohane P, Brown B, Grimble G, Silk DBA: The peptide nitrogen source of elemental diets: comparisons of absorptive properties of five partial enzymic hydrolysates of whole protein, *J Parenter Enteral Nutr* 5:568, 1981.

171. Alverdy JC, Aoys E, Moss GS: Total parenteral nutrition promotes bacterial translocation from the gut, *Surgery* 104:185-190, 1988.

172. Zaloga GP: Physiologic effects of peptide-based enteral formulas, *NCP* 5:231-237, 1990.

173. Trocki O, Mochizuki H, Dominioni L, Alexander JW: Intact protein versus free amino acids in the nutritional support of thermally injured animals, *J Parenter Enteral Nutr* 10:139-145, 1986.

174. Brinson RR, Pitts VL, Taylor AE: Intestinal absorption of peptide enteral formulas in hypoproteninemic (volume expanded) rats: a paired analysis, *Crit Care Med* 17(7):657-660, 1989.

175. Heimburger DC: Peptides in clinical practice, *NCP* 5:225-226, 1990.

176. Vazquez JA, Morse EL, Adibi A: Effect of starvation on amino acid and peptide transport hydrolysis in humans, *Am J Physiol* 249 (5 Pt 1): G563-566, 1985.

177. Silk DBA, Fairclough PD, Clark ML, et al: Use of peptide rather than free amino acid nitrogen source in chemically defined elemental diets, *J Parenter Enteral Nutr* 4(6):548-553, 1980.

178. Keohane PP, Silk DBA: Peptides and free amino acids. In Rombeau JL, Caldwell MD (eds): *Clinical nutrition. Enteral and tube feeding*, Philadelphia, 1984, WB Saunders, pp 44-59.

179. Rees RG, Payne-James JJ, Grimble GK, Silk DBA: Requirement of peptides versus whole protein in patients with impaired gastrointestinal function: a double-blind controlled trial, *J Parenter Enteral Nutr* 12 (suppl):12S, 1988.

180. McIntyre PB, Fitchew M, Lennard-Jones JE: Patients with a high ileostomy do not need a special diet, *Gastroenterology* 91:25-33, 1986.

181. Brinson R, Kolts B: Diarrhea associated with severe hypoalbuminemia: a comparison of a peptide-based chemically defined and standard enteral alimentation, *Crit Care Med* 16(2):130-136, 1988.

182. Meredith JW, Ditescheim JA, Zaloga GP: Visceral protein levels in trauma patients are greater with peptide diet than with intact protein diet, *J Trauma* 30(7):825-829, 1990.

183. Ziegler F, Oliver JM, Cynober L, et al: Efficiency of enteral nitrogen support in surgical patients: small peptides v non-degraded proteins, *Gut* 31(11):1277-1283, 1990.

184. Mowatt-Larssen CA, Brown RO, Wojtysiak SL, Kudsk KA: Comparison of tolerance and nutritional outcome between a peptide and a standard enteral formula in critically ill, hypoalbuminemic patients, *J Parenter Enteral Nutr* 16(1):20-24, 1992.

185. Grimble GK, Silk DB: The nitrogen source of elemental diets—an unresolved issue? *NCP* 5(6):227-230, 1990 (review).

Early and Perioperative Nutrition Support

21

Michele M. Gottschlich, PhD, RD, LD, CNSD

STRESSFUL conditions such as surgery, trauma, burns, and sepsis are characterized by hypermetabolism, frequently in association with significant erosion of critical protein stores, impaired immune function, and delayed recuperation. Consequently, the goals of nutrition support in these patient populations are to provide adequate and appropriate amounts of calories, protein, and essential nutrients to meet the increased and altered demands and to attenuate the cascade of catabolic events associated with the metabolic response to stress. The clinician is therefore faced with serious decisions about what, how, and when to feed these patients. This chapter reviews evidence that suggests that provision of enteral stimulation, early implementation time for nutrition support, and gut-specific components of the feeding program represent important decisions in critical care because of their potent effects on small intestine mass and function, nutritional status, immunocompetence, wound healing, and outcome. Attention is directed toward the indications and contraindications for early or perioperative (pre-, post-, and intraoperative) enteral feedings, with considerable emphasis given to the use of nasogastric, nasoduodenal, nasojejunal, and jejunostomy routes of support. Parenteral techniques for early and perioperative support are briefly examined.

The Role of the Gastrointestinal Tract

Traditional teaching considers the gut quiescent after operation or during critical illness. Consequently, efforts were directed at preserving priority organ function, which did not include the gastrointestinal (GI) tract. In the past, digestion, absorption, and secretion were thought to be the only significant functions of the gut. (A concise review of these processes can be found in Chapter 31.) Motility is another important function. The gut provides transport of nutrients, exposure of nutrients to absorptive mucosa, and prevention of stasis and bacterial overgrowth. The GI tract is also a metabolically active organ. Studies have shown that the gut is a central organ of amino acid metabolism, a role that may become more pronounced during critical illness. The most convincing evidence for this is the elucidation of glutamine kinetics by Souba and Wilmore and their respective colleagues.[1-3]

It is now evident that the GI tract also plays protective roles: It acts as a mechanical barrier and is important in immune function.[4-11] Deitch[10] was the first to postulate that viable intraluminal bacteria and endotoxins could pass through the gut epithelial layer into the blood or lymph, a process now referred to as *bacterial translocation* (Fig. 21-1). Under normal conditions these microbes and microbial products are confined to the intestinal lumen by processes that depend on GI barrier permeability, food ingestion, blood flow, defecation, and interactions between the gut-associated lymphoid tissue and the systemic immune system. In critically ill patients, barrier function can be disrupted by a variety of insults originating from the illness or injury, sepsis, or the treatment.[2,9-19] Whereas one would never doubt, for example, the seriousness of a major burn injury to the skin in terms of its effect on infection risk, a breach in the gut's integrity might not be recognized as a risk factor for infection because it cannot be seen; nevertheless it can be similarly vital. Although still controversial,[20-22] it is hypothesized that when the gut mucosal barrier is compromised, bacteria enter the systemic circulation, which can precipitate cytokine production, activation of the complement and coagulation cascades, and reprioritization of hepatic synthesis from constituent proteins to acute-phase reactants, producing altered immune function and inflammatory responses. The cytokines also stimulate production of neuromediators, which in turn prompt the peripheral endocrine organs to produce large quantities of cortisol, catecholamines, and glucagon, which mediate hypermetabolism (Fig. 21-2).[23,24] This can have devastating consequences for the host, including evidence suggesting that gut-derived bacteria can lead to nosocomial pneumonia, sepsis, and multisystem organ failure.[10,13,14,17,25-28]

The Route of Feeding—Parenteral Versus Enteral

In recent years, a great deal of attention has been given to the route of alimentation and how it may affect metabolic and immune responses. As new knowledge is acquired about the effects of surgery, injury, and illness, it is becoming increasingly clear that the gut plays a central role in the pathophysiologic response.[12,25,29] The constant turnover and the high rate of metabolic activity in the intestinal mucosa make it particularly vulnerable to the effects of starvation or luminal nutrient deprivation, ischemia, critical illness, and injury. Thus, supporting the health of the GI tract should be a major goal of nutrition support.

Many clinical studies[18,24,30-39] and animal models[40-46] comparing the efficacy of enteral and parenteral feeding have shown that enteral nutrition is associated with improved outcome variables. For example, Kudsk and coworkers[40] demonstrated that rats consuming protein-deficient diets for 2 weeks and then refed by the enteral route (using either an oral or intragastric diet) had a significantly higher survival rate after intraperitoneal challenge of *Escherichia coli* and hemoglobin as compared with

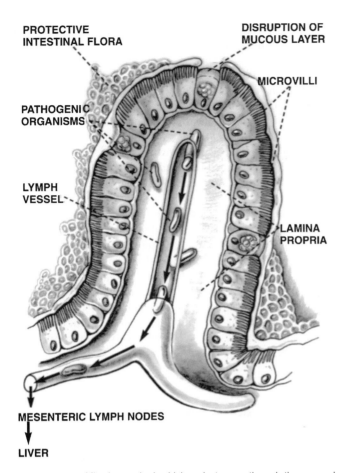

FIGURE 21-1 Microbes and microbial products pass through the mucosal surface of the intestine and enter the systemic circulation.

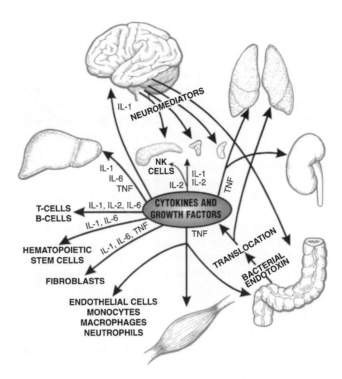

FIGURE 21-2 Schema for the development of the hypermetabolic response. (Adapted with permission from Alexander JW, Gottschlich MM: Nutritional immunomodulation in burn patients, *Crit Care Med* 18:S149–S153, 1990.)

animals repleted with the same nutrient solution administered intravenously.

Alverdy and colleagues[42] performed an interesting study of rats fed a normal chow diet, an oral parenteral nutrition (PN) solution, or intravenous PN. The animals fed a standard oral diet exhibited no translocation. Those fed PN, regardless of route, exhibited translocation of bacteria from the intestine to mesenteric lymph nodes. The rates of translocation in the enterally and parenterally fed animals—33% and 66%, respectively—once again demonstrated that the gut is the preferred route of feeding. The PN diets were devoid of fiber or glutamine, both nutrients that seem to protect intestinal epithelial cells, and this may have promoted bacterial translocation from the gut. As an alternative hypothesis, cecal bacterial counts revealed overgrowth of gram-negative aerobes in both PN groups, but only the parenterally fed group had diminished secretory immunoglobulin (s-IgA) levels in the bile. Bacterial overgrowth and diminished humoral immunity may also explain why the group fed intravenously exhibited the greatest translocation.

Kudsk and associates[30,34,37] have documented a significantly lower incidence of septic morbidity (i.e., pneumonias, intraabdominal abscess, line sepsis) in trauma patients fed enterally than in subjects randomized to receive PN. In an attempt to describe the immunosuppressive effects of PN, Herndon and colleagues[35] characterized a syndrome of decreased natural

killer cell activity, depressed helper-suppressor T-cell ratio, and increased mortality in patients with burns more extensive than 50% who were randomized to receive PN plus enteral support or an enteral diet alone. They concluded that the highest rates of mortality and immunosuppression were associated with the least enteral intake.

There are a number of reasons why enteral feeding may be optimal for resistance to infection. Parenteral feedings have been associated with disruption of gut microflora[9,45] and impaired neutrophil function,[47] and it may facilitate bacterial translocation.[9,42,44,45,48] Lower helper-suppressor T-cell ratios,[35] reduced phytohemagglutinin- and concanavalin A–induced blastogenic response,[45] enhanced production of tumor necrosis factor,[24] decreased levels of secretory IgA (the principal defense against attachment of intestinal bacteria to mucosal cells),[5,6,42] and a higher incidence of sepsis, even with meticulous catheter care[30,31,33,34,39,49] have also been demonstrated with intravenous alimentation as compared with enteral feeding.

It is recognized that enteral nutrition is the best single method of maintaining GI mass and function.[23,36,41,50-56] Bowel rest, as associated with delayed enteral nutrition, elemental diets, or PN, also results in drastic reductions in gut hormones such as enteroglucagon, gastrin, and gastric inhibitor polypeptide.[44,57-60] Fasting, even if it is short lived, likewise is associated with decreased enzyme (e.g., disaccharidase) activity.[51,61] Decreased levels of gut hormones and digestive enzymes can impair host absorption capacity for nutrients.

Eating food stimulates growth of enterocytes and thus decreases intestinal hypoplasia. The trophic effects of luminal nutrition are well documented, even when relatively small amounts of nutrients are provided.[62] What stimulates enterocytes to grow is not a single nutrient. Rather, food (or enteral formula), in and of itself, stimulates blood flow to the GI tract, which may help preserve gut barrier function. Enteral nutrition also stimulates secretion of mucus, which acts as a barrier, and it stimulates secretion of bile salts, which can help neutralize endotoxins. Enteral feeding stimulates defecation. This may seem obvious, but it is very important in purging the gut of bacteria and toxins. Consequently, a healthy GI tract acts as a barrier to pathogens and thus may limit translocation of bacteria, endotoxins, or other active substances into the lymph or portal circulation. For these reasons, enteral alimentation is the preferred feeding route. Moreover, there is increasing experimental evidence that the earlier the feedings can be started, the greater are the systemic advantages for critically ill patients. Furthermore, early enteral feeding does not appear to have adverse effects on the blood flow or oxygen balance of the intestine.[56,63,64]

Early Feeding

What is *early feeding?* Time frames used in various studies underscore numerous differences in the definition of early feeding. Immediate feeding may involve enteral, parenteral, or a combination feeding approach and may be further characterized according to implementation time (Table 21-1). The Performance Improvement Program at the Shriners Hospital for Children in Cincinnati defines *early feeding* as the initiation of tube feeding within 24 hours after traumatic injury. It is also specified in the nutrition improvement plan that patients take nothing by mouth for no longer than 8 hours on operative days. The exact timing of early feeding that provides clinical benefits has not been established, although the sooner it is implemented, the more apparent are the improvements in outcome variables.

Early Parenteral Feeding

Early feeding can be accomplished parenterally.[31,67,74,82,88,90,96,97] It can begin as soon as central venous access is obtained. This route for early feeding, however, has considerable disadvantages, including higher mechanical, infectious, and metabolic complications as compared with enteral support. For example, although Rapp[88] and Young[96] and their respective colleagues reported some beneficial effects from early PN, they noted that septic complications such as pneumonia developed in a large percentage of these patients.

TABLE 21-1

Differentiation of Various Definitions of "Early" or "Immediate" Feeding Implementation Time

Reference	Model	Feeding Route	Implementation Time
Andrassy et al.[65]	Abdominal surgery patients	Needle catheter jejunostomy	Postoperative day 1
Berseth[66]	Preterm infants	Orogastric	Postnatal day 3 to 5
Brownlee et al.[67]	Preterm infants	PN	36 hr postpartum
Chiarelli et al.[68]	Burn patients	Nasogastric	Within 4 hr after burn
Domioni et al.[69]	Burned guinea pigs	Gastric	2 hr after burn
Engelhardt & Clark[70]	Pediatric burn patients	Nasoduodenal	12 hr after burn
Eyer et al.[71]	Blunt trauma patients	Nasoduodenal	Within 24 hr after ICU admission
Gianotti et al.[54]	Burned guinea pigs	Gastric	1 hr after burn
Gottschlich et al.[72]	Pediatric burn patients	Nasoduodenal	Within 48 hr after burn
Grahm et al.[73]	Head-injured patients	Nasojejunal	Within 36 hr of admission
Hadley et al.[74]	Head-injured patients	Nasogastric or PN	Within 48 hr of admission
Hansbrough et al.[75]	Adult burn patients	Nasogastric	Within 24 hr of admission
Hasse et al.[76]	Liver transplant patients	Nasojejunal	12 hr postop
Inoue et al.[77]	Burned guinea pigs	Gastric	2 hr after burn
Jenkins et al.[78]	Adult burn patients	Nasoduodenal	8 hr after burn
Jenkins et al.[79]	Burn patients	Nasoduodenal	12 hr after burn
Kaufman et al.[80]	Adult burn patients	Oral or nasogastric	Within 24 hr after burn
Kirby et al.[81]	Brain-injured patients	Gastrojejunal	Within 5 days of injury
Kolacinski[82]	Drug poisoning patients	PN	After 24 hr of conservative treatment
McArdle et al.[83,84]	Burn patients	Nasoduodenal	2 to 4 days after burn
McDonald et al.[85]	Burn patients	Nasogastric	1 hr of admission and 6 hr after burn
Mochizuki et al.[53,86]	Burned guinea pigs	Gastrostomy	2 hr after burn
Moore et al.[31]	Abdominal trauma patients	Needle catheter jejunostomy or PN	12 hr postop
Moore et al.[39]	Abdominal trauma patients	Needle catheter jejunostomy	18 hr postop
Ostertag et al.[87]	Very low birth-weight infants	Nasogastric gavage	Postnatal day 1
Rapp et al.[88]	Head-injured patients	PN	Within 48 hr of admission
Riley et al.[89]	Abdominal surgery patients	Nasojejunal or jejunostomy	Recovery room
Sacks et al.[90]	Head-injured patients	PN	Within 24 hr of admission
Saito et al.[41]	Burned guinea pigs	Gastrostomy	2 hr after burn
Schroeder et al.[91]	Bowel resection patients	Nasojejunal	Postop day 1
Slagle and Cross[92]	Very low birth-weight infants	Gastric gavage	Postnatal day 1, postnatal day 8
Trocki et al.[93]	Pediatric burn patients	Nasogastric	As soon as the patient met stabilization criteria
Wood et al.[94]	Burned rats	Gastrostomy	2 hr after burn
Zaloga et al.[95]	Abdominal surgery rats	Gastroduodenal	Immediately postop

Early Enteral Feeding

The benefits of immediate enteral support are obvious and obscure (Table 21-2). Obvious reasons include the ability to satisfy nutritional requirements immediately and avoidance of mechanical, infectious, and metabolic complications associated with PN (see Chapter 19). It should be recognized that enteral nutrition has its own set of complications (see Chapter 17), although these are regarded as less serious. Compared with parenteral feeding, early enteral is a cost-effective method of nutrition support.[98-100] The average daily cost of PN may be as much as 4 to 5 times that of enteral nutrition.[98,100] Furthermore, using the gut to feed has promoted bowel mucosal integrity and improved tube feeding tolerance.

Clinically, the transition to enteral nutrition support after a period of fasting or PN is often accompanied by diarrhea and malabsorption, and it has been suggested that this may be related to some degree to mucosal atrophy as a result of bowel inactivity.[101] By impairing the patient's ability to tolerate enteral feeding, this diarrheal state may further limit enteral intake and promote mucosal suppression. Therefore it is easy to visualize a potential cycle in which starvation or PN, by causing mucosal atrophy, predisposes to malabsorption and diarrhea and thus impairs the patient's ability to tolerate enteral feedings. This is not to suggest that there is no role for parenteral nutrition as a supplement to enteral alimentation in hypermetabolic patients with intractable diarrhea; however, it is believed that at least some volume of tube feeding (even as little as 5 to 10 ml per hour) should be administered via the enteral route, even during bouts of malabsorption.

More surprisingly, tube feeding instituted early after operation or injury improves wound healing;[91,95] reduces length of hospital stay;[73] decreases rates of viral infection,[76] sepsis,[30,31,39,73,79] and bacterial translocation;[19,48,54,77,102] and suppresses the intensity of the injury response.[24,41,53,54,56,68,69,86] For example, Zaloga and colleagues[95] report that rats fed enterally immediately after abdominal surgery demonstrated increased wound strength 5 days later. Early feeding was also associated with less weight loss.

EARLY NASOGASTRIC FEEDING. A number of clinical studies have shown that a nasogastric tube can be a safe and effective route for early feeding.[68,75,80,85,93] It seems that if the patient receives enteral support before gastric edema develops, the incidence of ileus is minimized or avoided. For example, McDonald's group[85] has reported beginning nasogastric feeding within 1 hour of admission and within 6 hours of injury in 106 consecutive patients whose burns averaged 40% of body surface area. Enteral feedings were administered as bolus gastric feedings every 2 hours. At the end of each 2-hour period, before the next bolus feeding, the gastric-residual was aspirated and its volume recorded. This early feeding protocol was tolerated well. None of the patients had clinical evidence of aspiration pneumonia, and 82% absorbed at least a portion of their tube feeding on the day of injury. The percentage of patients who could tolerate their bolus nasogastric tube feeding increased daily until day 4, when it reached 95%. The most common complication, vomiting, occurred in 15% of patients.

Diarrhea is usually the limiting factor in using the GI tract as a route of nutrition in critically ill patients. The fact that none of McDonald's patients developed diarrhea severe enough to require cessation or modification of enteral feeding suggests that immediate feeding may improve nutrient absorption by limiting or preventing mucosal atrophy.[85]

Previous work from our unit[72] prospectively examined factors associated with diarrhea in 50 burn patients. A high degree of correlation between antibiotics and malabsorption existed. A significant relationship was also reported between delayed feeding and diarrhea. Implementation of tube feeding within 48 hours after the burn injury was associated with decreased incidence of diarrhea. Early feeding is optimal, presumably because intraluminal nutrients help maintain the integrity of the mucosal epithelium, thus sustaining normal and efficient digestive and absorptive processes.

Reduction in hypermetabolic response. Numerous animal studies conducted in Alexander's laboratory,[23,41,53,54,56,69,86] such as one by Mochizuki and coworkers[53] have demonstrated that immediate (defined as within 2 hours) postburn gastrostomy tube feeding prevents the hypermetabolic response observed in control animals not fed for 24 to 72 hours after the burn injury. Resting energy expenditure was lowest in animals fed early. This reduction in hypermetabolism was associated with significantly lower levels of serum cortisol and glucagon and reduced excretion of catecholamines in the urine. In addition, with delayed feeding animals lost nearly 50% of the mucosal weight of the jejunum, whereas immediate tube feeding prevented loss of mucosal mass. These findings were confirmed by electron microscopy. Figure 21-3, *A* shows normal, control guinea pig intestinal villi: There are tall projections that are reasonably close together, and the tips are healthy. Figure 21-3, *B* demonstrates what happens to the intestinal villi of guinea pigs who sustained a burn injury but were not fed for 24 hours. After only 24 hours of injury, the villi are markedly shrunken, with larger spaces between them, and erosions of the tips are observed. When the animals were fed enterally immediately after the burn injury, the villi were much closer together, the tips normal, and the height maintained (Fig. 21-3, *C*). After 2 weeks, animals fed early were in a markedly better nutritional state than those whose feeding was delayed, as evidenced by less weight loss and positive nitrogen balance. Early feeding was also associated with decreased incidence of diarrhea.

In a follow-up study by Saito, Alexander, and colleagues,[41] it was established that immediate parenteral support was not as effective as immediate enteral nutrition. The average nitrogen balance, for example, was significantly better in the group fed intragastrically than in the intravenous group. Animals fed enterally failed to demonstrate increased secretion of catabolic hormones such as plasma cortisol, plasma glucagon, and

TABLE 21-2

Benefits of Early Enteral Support

Absolute Benefits	Relative Benefits
Satisfies nutrient needs	Improves wound healing
Avoids PN-related complications	Reduces hospital stay
Cost effective	Decreases incidence of infection, sepsis,
Promotes bowel mucosal integrity	and bacterial translocation
Improves tube-feeding tolerance	Suppresses the hypermetabolic response

urinary vanillylmandelic acid. The enteral feeding group also showed enhanced mucosal weight and thickness.

More recently, Gianotti, Alexander, and colleagues[54] studied guinea pigs that received gavage with radioisotope-labeled *Escherichia coli* 18 hours after burn injury. Half of the animals received enteral feeding by gastrostomy immediately after injury; control animals received lactated Ringer's solution. Gianotti and colleagues showed that the amount of bacteria escaping from the gut lumen after burn injury paralleled serum

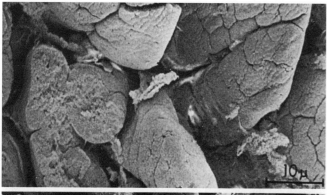
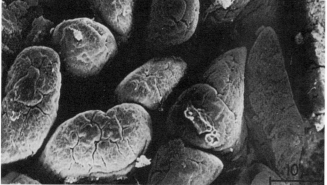
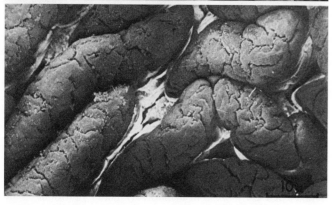

FIGURE 21-3 Mucosal villus appearance of jejunum taken by scanning electron microscope at the same power (x1500). (*A*) Jejunal mucosa of preburn group. Villi were predominantly tongue shaped with small spaces between individual villi. (*B*) Jejunal mucosa of the fasted, lactated Ringer's group after 24 hours postburn. Villi were a mixture of tongue and narrow finger-shaped. (*C*) Jejunal mucosa of early-fed group 24 hours postburn. Villi were predominantly tongue-shaped with some broad ridges. (Reproduced with permission from Mochizuki H, Trocki O, Dominioni L, et al: Mechanism of prevention of postburn hypermetabolism and catabolism by early enteral feeding, *Ann Surg* 200:297–310, 1984.)

levels of catabolic hormones (cortisol and vanillylmandelic acid) and the measured resting energy expenditure. Their guinea pig model also demonstrated that early enteral feeding effectively supported higher mucosal and body weights in the animals and minimized bacterial translocation.

Clinical work by Chiarelli and colleagues,[68] by Jenkins and colleagues,[78,79] and by McArdle and colleagues[83,84] supports Alexander's findings. Chiarelli[68] studied 20 patients with burns ranging from 25% to 60% of body surface area. Nasogastric tube feedings were implemented within 4 hours after injury in the early-feeding group. Patients who were fed early had lower plasma glucagon concentrations and lower urinary catecholamine excretion, suggesting a reduced injury response. The group fed early also achieved positive nitrogen balance faster than patients who were not fed until 48 hours after hospital admission. Once again the incidence of complications related to early gastric feeding were minimal.

CLINICAL STUDIES OF EARLY INTESTINAL FEEDING. It appears that alert patients with a functional GI tract generally tolerate nasogastric tube feedings quite well. On one hand, proper attention to monitoring of gastric residual and gut function are essential for success and risk management. On the other hand, many critically ill patients are not alert or may present with posttraumatic, septic, or surgical ileus, for which nasogastric tube feedings are generally contraindicated. Standard surgical teaching in the past held that the entire GI tract was nonfunctional after injury or operation because it was unavailable for absorption of nutrients and was nonpropulsive. Recent physiologic and clinical studies refute this teaching. Although it is true that the stomach may be intolerant of oral intake for a minimum of 1 or 2 days and the colon undergoes a period of ileus approximating 3 to 5 days, small bowel motility and absorptive capability usually remain intact.[103-106] Therefore insertion of a nasoenteric feeding tube into the third portion of the duodenum or upper jejunum can provide a means for safely delivering early enteral nutrition to patients with poor gastric emptying.[70,73,79,99,107-110]

Grahm and colleagues[73] found early alimentation via the nasojejunal route to be beneficial in 32 head-injured patients. Within 36 hours of injury, the early group received postpyloric nutrition equal to their measured energy expenditure. The control group were fed gastrically when bowel sounds returned. No differences existed in age, sex, or Glasgow Coma Scale score; however, the incidence of infection and days of ICU hospitalization were significantly reduced with early enteral feeding.

At our institution, fluoroscopic placement of a nasoduodenal feeding tube is routine for patients whose burns extend over more than 25% of body surface area. Once tube placement is confirmed, continuous infusion of full-strength product is begun immediately with a tube-feeding pump. Most patients tolerate an initial hourly rate of half of their calculated caloric needs. Feedings are then advanced 5 ml per hour in children and 10 ml per hour in older children and adults until individual caloric goals are achieved. Thus during periods of gastric ileus this protocol makes it possible to deliver the desired nutrient needs without delay via the intestine. Gastric decompression is maintained via a nasogastric tube connected to suction until active bowel sounds return.

Utilizing the aforementioned clinical guidelines, we conducted a pilot study from 1986 to 1989 designed to evaluate the feasibility and safety of immediate nutrition support after thermal injury and to examine its effect on the hypermetabolic response.[79] Patients were randomly assigned to one or two groups: early feeding (i.e., nasoduodenal tube feeding begun within 12 hours of injury) and control (nutrition support instituted 72 hours after injury). Both groups received the same tube-feeding product.

Eighteen patients who had burns over more than 30% of body surface area were evaluated. There were no significant differences between the groups on the variables of age, total burn area, or percentage of full-thickness burns. The groups also had similar resting energy expenditure, calorie intake, protein intake, and duration of tube-feeding support. Both groups maintained their weight throughout the study period.

There were no significant differences in the hormones measured. Serum cortisol remained within normal limits for both groups throughout the study period. Glucagon levels were elevated for both groups throughout the 4-week period. Serum albumin and total protein were significantly higher in postburn week 1 in the early-fed group. Both visceral proteins remained higher in the early group throughout the rest of the study period but did not achieve statistical significance except for total protein in postburn week 4.

There were 14 infectious complications in the control group and 7 in the group fed early. The control group required a mean of 9.4 days of systemic antibiotic therapy, compared with 2.8 days in the early-fed group. There were no differences in length of hospital stay, number of operative procedures, deaths, or complications possibly related to nutrition support. Both groups experienced a high incidence of hyperglycemia requiring insulin therapy. Constipation was the next most frequent symptom. Diarrhea, gastric residual, and electrolyte imbalance were noted infrequently. No patient in either group suffered aspiration.

Although we were pleased that this initial clinical study[79] suggested that early feeding can be accomplished in the presence of gastric ileus, we were unable to reproduce Alexander's findings in the burned guinea pig model of decreased metabolic rate, decreased catabolic hormones, and improved immune status with immediate enteral support.[41,53,54,77,86] We tentatively attributed the discrepancies between animal and clinical work to the fact that it had been standard practice to give patients nothing by mouth before and during operative procedures. Because the patients in this study were scheduled for burn wound excision on one day, followed by overnight stabilization and grafting on the second day, in effect, they received minimal enteral support for 48 hours each time they underwent skin grafting. These periods of negligible enteral support might in part have negated any reduction of the hypermetabolic response realized from immediate feeding. Consequently, we conducted a follow-up study of early feeding in which duodenal tube feeding was continued during operative procedures in an attempt to control this extraneous variable.

The effectiveness of early enteral feeding was prospectively studied in pediatric patients who had burns in excess of 25% total body surface area.[111] Seventy-seven patients were randomized to two groups: early (tube feeding begun within 24 hours of injury) versus control (enteral support delayed at least 48 hours postburn). Patients continued their tube-feeding regimen during operative procedures. Nutrient intake was measured daily, indirect calorimetry was performed biweekly, and weekly blood and urine samples were obtained for the assay of cortisol, glucagon, insulin, epinephrine, norepinephrine, dopamine, albumin, transferrin, prealbumin, retinol-binding protein glucose, nitrogen balance, and 3-methylhistidine.

Patient demographics and select outcomes are summarized in Table 21-3. Three protocol violations occurred and two patients transferred to another hospital; these patients were dropped from the study. No patient in either group experienced tube-feeding aspiration. No differences were evident in infection, diarrhea, hospital length of stay, or mortality outcomes. A higher incidence of reportable adverse events coincided with early feeding (22% versus 8%), but this was not statistically significant (Tables 21-3 and 21-4). One control patient and four early patients, respectively, developed bowel necrosis. The delayed feeding group demonstrated a significant caloric deficit during postburn week (PBW) 1 ($p < 0.0001$) and PBW 2 ($p < 0.04$). Serum insulin was higher in the early fed group during PBW 1 ($p < 0.09$) and PBW 2 ($p < 0.03$). No other differences in study outcome variables were noted. This study suggests that provision of enteral nutrients shortly after burn injury reduces caloric deficits and may stimulate insulin secretion. These data, however, do not necessarily reaffirm the safety of early enteral feeding, nor do they associate earlier feeding with a direct improvement in nutritional status or a reduction in hypermetabolism, infection, or hospital stay.

The attenuation of the hypermetabolic response with early feeding has been questioned by others as well.[71,73,94,112] For example, Eyer and associates[71] studied 52 blunt trauma patients randomized to receive early nasoenteric feeding (initiated 31 ± 13 hours after injury) or late nutrition (82 ± 11 hours). These investigators failed to demonstrate any difference in metabolic responses (e.g., plasma lactate, total urinary nitrogen, catecholamines, cortisol) or clinical outcome variables (e.g., intensive care unit days, ventilator days, organ system failure, specific infections, mortality). It is conceivable that enteral feeding was not introduced early enough in the treated group to elicit an effect. In Alexander's successful animal model[41,53,54,77,86] and Chiarelli's clinical work[68] the treated groups were fed within 2 and 4 hours, respectively.

JEJUNOSTOMY FEEDINGS. Jejunostomy feedings—the standard surgical jejunostomy,[113] the percutaneous endoscopic gastrojejunostomy advocated more recently,[81] and the needle catheter jejunostomy[30,31,39,65] are for early feeding, particularly for patients with facial trauma or disease of the upper aerodigestive tract that precludes nasoenteral tube placement.

Early postoperative and postinjury enteral nutrition using needle catheter jejunostomy has proved safe and efficacious with a variety of monomeric and polymeric formulas in a number of different patient groups who underwent emergency or elective operation for a variety of upper GI, colon, and retroperitoneal problems.[30,31,39,65,113-115] Furthermore, studies performed by Moore, Moore, and Jones[31,39] clearly demonstrated that the practice of implementing immediate jejunostomy feeding instead of PN significantly reduces complications after major abdominal trauma. From the higher rate of infection,

TABLE 21-3
Patient Demographics and Select Outcomes

Group n = 72	Age	% Burn	% Third	Inhalation Injury	TF Start Time (Hrs. postburn)	# of Patients with Adverse Event	Length of Stay	Death
Early n=36	8.9 ± 0.7	51.1 ± 3.2	43.0 ± 3.8	20	15.6 ± 1.0 (range 4.5-29)	8	53.3 ± 6.0	4
Control n = 36	9.6 ± 0.8	53.2 ± 3.4	45.5 ± 4.3	23	48.5 ± 0.4 (range 48-60.5)	3	54.8 ± 4.6	3
$p<0.001$	NS	NS	NS	NS	0.0001		NS	NS

TABLE 21-4
Characterization of Adverse Events (n = 11 patients)

Group	Demographic Data	Outcome	Relationship to Adverse Events*
1. Control	57% burn, inhalation injury	ARDS, expired	Remotely
2. Control	90.5% burn, inhalation injury	ARDS, expired	Remotely
3. Control	87.5% burn, inhalation injury	Bowel necrosis, expired	Possibly
4. Early	49.5% burn, inhalation injury	Catheter tip sheared	Unrelated
5. Early	70% burn	Acute renal failure, ARDS, multisystem organ failure, expired	Remotely
6. Early	88% burn, inhalation injury	Bowel necrosis, renal failure, multisystem organ failure, expired	Possibly
7. Early	45.5% burn, inhalation injury	Thrombophlebitis of foot	Unrelated
8. Early	70% burn, inhalation injury	Bowel necrosis, renal failure, ARDS, endocarditis, expired	Possibly
9. Early	63.5% burn	Cultured skin lab infection error, laparotomy, sepsis, multisystem organ failure	Remotely
10. Early	68% burn	Bowel necrosis, expired	Possibly
11. Early	75% burn, inhalation injury	Bowel necrosis	Possibly

*Relationship rating
Unrelated: An event for which sufficient information exists to indicate that the etiology is unrelated to the investigation.
Remotely: An event for which insufficient information exists to indicate a temporal relationship between the event and the investigation.
Possibly: An event that follows a reasonable temporal sequence with the investigation, but that could readily have been produced by a number of other factors.
Probably: An event that follows a reasonable temporal sequence with the investigation; that follows a known or expected response pattern to the investigation; that is confirmed by stopping or reducing the dosage of the investigational product; and that could not be reasonably explained by the known characteristics of the subject's clinical state.
Definitely: An event that follows a reasonable temporal sequence from administration of the investigational product or in which the investigational product level has been established in body fluids or tissues; that follows a known or expected response pattern to the suspected investigational product; and that is confirmed by improvement on stopping or reducing the dosage of the investigational product, and reappearance of the event on repeated exposure (rechallenge).

especially pneumonia, among the PN group the authors conclude that delaying enteral nutrition likely results in translocation of gut bacteria, which then contaminate impaired lungs.[31]

Perioperative Nutrition Support

More than 65 years have elapsed since the relationship between preoperative weight loss and increased postoperative mortality was first documented.[116] The objective of perioperative alimentation is to maintain or correct nutritional status before, during, and after surgery, in an effort to minimize malnutrition-induced complications. In addition to improved nutrition, other desirable features particularly associated with enteral perioperative support are the ability to minimize changes in gut microflora, impaired gut function, and disruption of the integrity of the mucosal barrier typically associated with disuse. The indications and contraindications of preoperative, postoperative, and intraoperative nutrition therapy are examined next. It is important that these methods be employed without incurring unjustified expense or undue risk of complications.

Preoperative Nutritional Repletion

In the preoperative period, enteral and parenteral nutrition support has been used in patients who are candidates for immediate surgery but who present with severe malnutrition, and for patients whose condition dictates that a major surgical procedure be delayed. A controlled clinical trial of the latter population has not been performed because it would be unethical to induce iatrogenic malnutrition in patients who cannot immediately undergo operation. Instead, clinical judgment and intuition explain the widespread use (and obvious value) of providing nonvolitional nutrition support to patients who are expected to experience a substantial period of preoperative starvation.[117,118]

Many clinical trials have attempted to define the efficacy of preoperative enteral or parenteral nutrition when prompt surgery is possible but not emergent. These investigations have been critically reviewed elsewhere,[117,119-122] and the efficacy of delaying surgery to allow aggressive preoperative feeding remains to be established. Many studies that report improved nutrition status or outcome[29,123-134] or no evidence thereof[135-138] contain shortcomings: Nutrition regimens were often inadequate or the period of repletion too short; complications were various and often not related to malnutrition; criteria used to assess malnutrition or morbidity were insufficiently strict; too few patients were entered in the trial or nonrandomized controls were used; and well-nourished patients were often considered when interpreting the results.

Analysis of the many published reports reveals that three well-designed randomized controlled trials employing preoperative PN[49,139,140] and two using enteral feeding[141,142] demonstrated significant improvement in morbidity in malnourished patients. Bellantone and coworkers[140] prospectively randomized patients with GI diseases who were to undergo resection to receive either a standard hospital diet or preoperative PN for 7 days or more. When only malnourished patients were considered, those who received preoperative PN had a lower incidence of postoperative sepsis (21% versus 53%) than their counterparts did who did not receive PN. In the subgroup of malnourished patients with gastric cancer, septic complications occurred in 100% of the patients in the control group and in only 16.7% of the study group. Postoperative mortality was similar in both groups.

A Veterans' Administration multicenter prospective trial addressed the issue of efficacy of preoperative nutrition support when immediate surgery is an option. In this study[49] patients with mild to severe malnutrition who required major elective GI surgery were randomized to receive PN for 7 to 15 days before surgery and 3 days after operation *or* no PN until at least 3 days postoperatively. The results of the investigation failed to demonstrate clinical benefit of preoperative PN for mildly or moderately malnourished patients, and more infectious complications occurred in the PN-treated group. In contrast, severely malnourished patients who received preoperative PN had fewer noninfectious complications and no more infectious complications. The incidence of mortality was similar for the treatment and control groups.

Judging from the studies of preoperative PN, its efficacy in reducing complications in patients who are candidates for immediate operation seems to be limited to those who have severe preexisting nutritional deficits. Furthermore it is unlikely that giving PN for less than 1 week in the preoperative period would be effective in reducing postoperative complications.

Studies of the effects of prophylactic enteral feedings on outcome include an investigation by Shukla and coworkers,[141] which demonstrated that 10 days of a preoperative polymeric diet decreased the complication rate, length of hospital stay, and mortality of patients after surgery for a variety of diseases. More recently, Foschi and colleagues[142] demonstrated that preoperative enteral support after percutaneous transhepatic biliary drainage for obstructive jaundice was beneficial. The tube-fed patients had reduced rates of anastomotic disruptions, organ failure, and death.

Postoperative Feeding

In the postoperative period it is becoming increasingly popular to use early and more aggressive nutrition support to reduce nutritional deficits that ordinarily develop during the period of starvation that typically follows surgery before return of gut function. How long postoperative starvation can be tolerated before complications develop is not known; however, it undoubtedly is influenced by the patient's preexisting nutritional state, extent of the surgical insult, and nature and degree of intercurrent illness or stress. If the period is expected to exceed 1 week, early postoperative nutrition support may be beneficial for mildly (and perhaps even adequately) nourished persons. Institution of nutrition support as early as possible after surgery is judicious with severely malnourished patients, and it should be continued for all patients who require preoperative feedings. The optimal route for early postoperative feeding requires consideration.

Although gastric dysfunction usually prevents immediate oral or gastric feeding after operation, postpyloric access to the GI tract provides a means for delivering nutrients in lieu of evidence that small intestinal digestive, absorptive, and motility capabilities are considered normal shortly after surgery.[104-106,143] Increasing evidence indicates that the basis for suspending enteral feeding postoperatively is not well founded.[107] Studies suggest that early postoperative enteral support is a safe practice and it decreases complications, prevents postoperative ileus, and enhances recovery.[30-33,39,83,84,91,95,106,114,115,144-150] Hoover and colleagues[145] and Moore and Jones[39] report a more positive nitrogen balance in patients who received immediate postoperative jejunal feedings.

Schroeder and coworkers[91] conducted a randomized prospective trial to evaluate the effects of immediate postoperative nasojejunal tube feedings after small bowel resection. This study demonstrated improved wound healing in the enterally fed group as measured by hydroxyproline accumulation on implanted Gore-Tex tubes. Others likewise reported improved wound healing with early postoperative nutrition support.[95,104,147,151]

Significant benefits of postoperative enteral over parenteral feedings have been shown. Moore and colleagues[31] demonstrated that infectious complications, namely pneumonias, were significantly reduced in enterally supported trauma patients fed by needle catheter jejunostomy immediately after emergency celiotomy. There were fewer abscesses in the enteral group as well, but the difference was not statistically significant.

A meta-analysis[33] of eight prospectively randomized controlled trials compared 118 enterally versus 112 parenterally fed patients whose nutrition support was begun within 8 to 72 hours after surgery. Although no significant difference was demonstrated in mortality rate, length of stay, or cost, the number of infections was significantly greater in the PN group.

If enteral intervention is not feasible, parenteral nutrition is an option for patients who require aggressive postsurgical feeding. Studies by Collins,[152] Delany,[147] and Yamada[153] and their respective coworkers suggest that the use of PN in the immediate postoperative period significantly reduces complications and deaths after major abdominal surgery, whereas Woolfson and Smith[154] were unable to demonstrate any benefit from the use of PN.

Other issues of perioperative enteral feeding pertain to the point, if any, at which it should be discontinued before surgery as well as the appropriate interval after surgery before initiation of postoperative nutrition support. The issue is whether these relatively short periods of inadequate intake have significant effects on recovery because periods of fasting are an obstacle to adequate nutrition and predispose the patient to impaired gut and immune function.

There is a growing realization that overnight fasting is probably unnecessary before elective surgery. Several reports indicate that administration of oral fluids or gastric tube feeding 1 to 2 hours before surgery is safe.[155-157] Data on the optimal time for resumption of postoperative feedings are scant, although it has been shown that delaying alimentation for 3 days or more can have negative clinical ramifications as compared with early postsurgical nutrition support.[104,147]

Intraoperative Nutrition Support

Acknowledging the benefits of preoperative, postoperative, and early nutrition support, a question we recently addressed was whether enteral feeding could be continued intraoperatively without complications.[107,108,158] One investigation[107] studied 80 thermally injured patients, all of whom received (through duodenal feeding tubes placed under fluoroscopy) isocaloric nutrition support calculated to meet measured energy needs. Forty patients received enteral support throughout 161 surgical procedures, and 40 patients randomly matched for age and percentage of burn, had tube feedings withheld during 129 procedures. No patients in either group experienced aspiration. The unfed group, however, demonstrated a significant caloric deficit and an increased incidence of wound infection and required more albumin supplementation to maintain serum levels at a minimum of 2.5 g/dl. A subsequent study[158] followed 15 pediatric burn patients receiving continuous nasoduodenal feeding during 91 operative (primarily excision and grafting) procedures. No differences were detected in the pH of gastric drainage measured before and during surgery, nor was there any intraoperative diarrhea or aspiration. This study provides further support of the safety of delivering enteral nutrition support during the perioperative period.

CANDIDATES FOR EARLY OR PERIOPERATIVE FEEDING. The indications for early or perioperative feeding vary widely and are based on the success that different investigators observed after various procedures. In the preoperative period, surgery should probably be delayed whenever possible and nutrition support given to malnourished patients in adequate amounts for 7 days or more. There are also several groups of critically ill immunocompromised patients who could benefit from early postinjury, postoperative, or intraoperative feeding, assuming that relatively long-term nutrition support is indicated—as for polytrauma, severe head injury, burns, mechanical ventilatory support, preoperative malnutrition, anorexia due to cancer, radiation or chemotherapy, and major surgery such as gastric or intestinal resection, organ transplantation, and aortic or hepatobiliary procedures. There seems to be little disagreement that nutrition support should usually be delivered enterally. In most patients a nasoduodenal or nasojejunal tube can be passed or surgical jejunostomy conducted intraoperatively, and feedings can be started immediately after injury or operation. If enteral support is contraindicated, the decision to initiate parenteral nutrition must recognize the somewhat higher cost and complication rate associated with this form of therapy.

CONTRAINDICATIONS OF ENTERAL INTERVENTION. There are a number of absolute and relative contraindications for early enteral feeding. It is absolutely contraindicated when it is not possible, as may occur with conditions such as small or large bowel obstruction, major GI bleed, severe hypovolemia, or hypoperfusion or when aggressive nutrition support is not desired by the patient or legal guardian. Intrinsic small bowel disease, such as regional enteritis or radiation enteritis, may be a contraindication to surgical jejunostomy because of the risk of leakage or fistula formation. Intrinsic disease, however, does not necessarily restrict early feeding by the nasoenteral route. Other relative contraindications include severe short-bowel syndrome and cardiorespiratory insufficiency, when any degree of abdominal distention can impair borderline hemodynamics.

POTENTIAL COMPLICATIONS. A detailed discussion of the complications associated with enteral nutrition and PN is beyond the scope of this review, and the reader is referred to Chapters 17 and 19. Although enteral support is preferred to parenteral, its success depends on the commitment of the clinician. More feeding interruptions typically occur with enteral nutrition than with PN. Whenever enteral feedings are temporarily interrupted, it is imperative to flush the tube thoroughly to prevent clogging. Flushing the tube before and after administration of medication also reduces the risk of obstruction.

Diligent monitoring of tube position and other potential complications is critical to ensure the success and safety of the enteral nutrition program. For example, in an effort to be able to detect dislodgment of a nasal feeding tube, it is recommended that an initial measurement from the nares to the end of the tube be taken at insertion and repeated at frequent intervals. Coughing, vomiting, or vigorous suctioning can displace small-bore tubes. Whenever malposition is suspected, tube feeding should be temporarily discontinued and tube position verified by roentgenogram.

Patients with artificial airways and diminished cough or gag reflexes are at risk for pulmonary aspiration. Certainly, intestinal feeding with concomitant gastric decompression helps prevent reflux aspiration. It is nevertheless a risk and it can result in immediate respiratory distress or be quite insidious. The diagnosis may not be made until symptoms or radiographic changes develop. Because of the seriousness of aspiration, the measures previously outlined are essential for monitoring patients at high risk. Intubation, even with a cuffed tube, does not completely protect the airway from aspiration. If reflux aspiration is suspected, tube feeding should be suspended and vigorous tracheal suctioning instituted. Bronchoscopy, ventilatory support, or both may be necessary. Antibiotic therapy is indicated if clinical signs of infection are evident.

Diarrhea may also be a complication of tube feeding; however, early feeding is associated with reduced risk. Diarrhea should first be treated with antidiarrheal medications rather than product dilution. Other less common GI complications are constipation and abdominal distention. Constipation can be alleviated by ensuring adequate fluid intake, administering bulking agents, and encouraging physical activity. Monitoring gastric residual, stool frequency, bowel sounds, and abdominal girth helps to identify patients with elimination problems or abdominal distention and to prevent more serious complications such as aspiration.

Metabolic complications include hyperglycemia, electrolyte imbalance, dehydration, and hypercapnia. Hyperglycemia is usually the result of excessive calorie administration or sepsis. Elevated serum glucose levels can usually be adequately controlled by exogenous insulin, administered by sliding scale or continuous infusion. It is almost never necessary to discontinue or decrease enteral support to control hyperglycemia.

Serum electrolytes should be monitored to assist in the detection of disturbances commonly observed in patients receiving tube feedings. Hypernatremia most often develops as a result of dehydration and can be treated successfully by rehydration with hypotonic solutions. Diarrhea, administration of insulin, or diuretics can result in hypokalemia, requiring potassium supplementation. In addition to serum electrolyte changes, blood urea nitrogen and hematocrit are indicators of protein intolerance or dehydration. Increasing fluids should correct these problems.

Increased carbon dioxide production can develop with the delivery of excessive calories. Patients often exhibit an increased respiratory quotient and accelerated alveolar and minute ventilation. Enteral support should be monitored to maintain the respiratory quotient within a range of 0.80 to 0.95, particularly when attempting to wean from ventilatory support. Adjusting intake on the basis of measured caloric needs should prevent overfeeding and potential pulmonary complications.

Optimal Formulations

In addition to the optimal route and proper procedures for the initiation and monitoring of nutrition support, the composition of feeding substrate also requires consideration. In many cases, standard commercial products are acceptable for early and feeding. Because metabolic aberrations or gastrointestinal intolerance is sometimes observed clinically, considerable research has been devoted to several specific nutrients to see whether they might improve product tolerance, maximize gut function, and serve as major fuels for the intestinal tract (namely glutamine, fiber, and short-chain fatty acids).

Glutamine

Recent reports have emphasized the critical role of glutamine in the regulation of muscle protein balance[159,160] as well as supporting immune[161-167] and intestinal function.[1,3,161,167-171] It is an important oxidative fuel for rapidly dividing cells, such as enterocytes, colonocytes, macrophages, and lymphocytes. It is taken up by cells of the intestine at a rate equivalent to that of glucose uptake. Adequate glutamine appears to be essential for the maintenance of normal GI structure and function, including gut-associated lymphatic tissue and secretory immunoglobulin A (s-IgA)[167]; this may help limit bacterial translocation.[161,164,168,171]

Glutamine supplementation of enteral and parenteral diets enhances GI health. Enteral administration of glutamine can prevent development of radiation enteritis and promote intestinal rescue once radiation enteritis is well established.[3] These models also demonstrate significant improvement in survival rate for animals receiving glutamine. Other studies suggest that the provision of enteral glutamine prevents deterioration of gut permeability and bacterial translocation and improves nitrogen

balance and survival.[102,168,172,173] Enteral glutamine is tolerated well without evidence of clinical toxicity or generation of toxic metabolites.[174,175]

Provision of glutamine by PN has likewise been performed safely in both humans and animals without evidence of toxicity or untoward biochemical effects.[169,174] Administration of glutamine-enriched PN attenuates intestinal hypoplasia and promotes nitrogen retention.[3,168,169,171] In addition, glutamine-supplemented PN improves intestinal immune function more than standard PN by maintaining s-IgA synthesis and preventing bacterial translocation to mesenteric lymph nodes.[161] Clinical trials of the efficacy of intravenous glutamine are under way.

Fiber

Sources of dietary fiber can be divided into two categories: insoluble and soluble in the GI tract. Insoluble fibers rich in soy polysaccharide or cellulose and lignin (hydrophilic fibers in wheat bran, psyllium seed, and ispaghula husk) have been shown to increase fecal mass by holding water.[170,176] They are also believed to help normalize bowel function[166,170,177] and structure,[177,178] suppress bacterial translocation,[178-181] and help regulate GI transit time.[170,176,177,182]

Soluble fibers such as pectin, mucilages, and gums are fermented rapidly and completely in the cecum by anaerobic microflora and represent important substrates for maintaining colonic structure and function. Studies have shown that soluble fiber can prevent atrophy of the ileal and colonic mucosa,[170,182-184] stimulate mucosal proliferation,[170,182] slow intestinal transit time,[185] and provide fuel for colonic bacteria by generating short-chain fatty acids.[170,176,182]

Short-Chain Fatty Acids

Short-chain fatty acids (SCFAs) likewise appear to have important effects on the gut. These effects can be derived from the administration of SCFAs as such, or from the formation of SCFAs in the GI tract of animals by bacterial fermentation of dietary fiber polysaccharides. Rombeau and colleagues[183,185,186] have contributed a great deal to our understanding of SCFA metabolism.

Among their various properties, SCFAs provide calories to the host, are readily absorbed by the GI mucosa, and serve as the principal source of fuel for the colon.[170] Studies have shown SCFAs to enhance intestinal blood flow, stimulate mucosal proliferation, stimulate pancreatic enzymes, and increase sodium and water absorption in the colon.[170,187-190] Short-chain fatty acids may have merit in the prevention of gut mucosal atrophy. Koruda and colleagues have shown that after massive small bowel resection in the rat, supplementation with SCFA significantly reduced the mucosal atrophy associated with parenteral nutrition.[189] Taken together, the stimulatory effects of glutamine, fiber, and SCFAs on the intestinal mucosa suggest that these compounds may be of further clinical use in the prevention of bacterial translocation across a weakened gut wall. Their inclusion in nutrition support regimens may prove important in the future.

Conclusion

In conclusion, enteral nutrition support appears to be preferable to parenteral feeding. Furthermore, many favor a policy of immediate enteral nutrition, although data are still emerging and there is no consensus from experts regarding its safety and efficacy. Studies are needed to establish precise feeding times that maximize clinical benefit while minimizing morbidity. However, it is clear that feeding into the intestine can begin much earlier than it traditionally has. *Early* postinjury and intraoperative enteral support are measures that theoretically can help minimize gut mucosal atrophy and some of the other negative effects associated with delayed enteral feeding. Why enteral treatment strategies maintain gut mass and function and improve resistance to infection better than parenteral feedings is not completely understood.

Besides the advantages offered by early intraluminal nutrition over delayed enteral or parenteral feeding, the specific composition of the feeding regimen may exert further remarkable benefits. In fact, some of the most exciting scientific advances of this decade involve the recognition of the importance of how gut and immune function can be altered by certain nutrients. The effects of supplementation of enteral and parenteral formulations with key gut nutrients (such as glutamine, fiber, or SCFAs) will continue to be important areas of investigation.

Aggressive and tissue-specific nutrition support appears to be a valuable tool in critical care medicine. Proper selection of route of administration and implementation time and the availability of gut fuels in medical and dietary foods are more involved in the treatment of various clinical conditions than was realized heretofore. If the optimistic preliminary results on the use of early and perioperative feeding and gut-specific nutrition support are confirmed by continued research over the next few years, these techniques will no doubt have significant effects on patient outcome for this and future generations.

REFERENCES

1. Souba WW, Smith RJ, Wilmore DW: Glutamine metabolism by the intestinal tract, *J Parenter Enteral Nutr* 9(5):608–617,1985.
2. Wilmore DW, Smith RJ, O'Dwyer ST, et al: The gut: a central organ after surgical stress, *Surgery* 104(5):917–923, 1988.
3. Souba WW, Klimberg VS, Plumley DA, et al: The role of glutamine in maintaining a healthy gut and supporting the metabolic response to injury and infection, *J Surg Res* 48(4):383–391,1990.
4. Phillips MC, Olson LR: The immunologic role of the gastrointestinal tract, *Crit Care Nurs Clin North Am* 5(1):107–120, 1993.
5. Lankamp-Henken B, Glezer JA, Kudsk KA: Immunologic structure and function of the gastrointestinal tract, *Nutr Clin Pract* 7(3):100–108, 1992.
6. Alverdy J, Chi HS, Sheldon GF: The effect of parenteral nutrition on gastrointestinal immunity. The importance of enteral stimulation, *Ann Surg* 202(6):681–684, 1985.
7. Maddaus MA, Wells CL, Platt JL, et al: Effect of T cell modulation on the translocation of bacteria from the gut and mesenteric lymph node, *Ann Surg* 207(4):387–398, 1988.
8. Strober W, James SP: The immunologic basis of inflammatory bowel disease, *J Clin Immunol* 6(6):415–432, 1986.
9. Bengmark S: Econutrition and health maintenance—a new concept to prevent GI inflammation, ulceration and sepsis, *Clin Nutr* 15:1–10, 1996.
10. Deitch EA: Does the gut protect injured patients in the ICU? *Perspect Crit Care* 1:1–24, 1988.
11. Johnson CD, Kudsk DA: Nutritional and intestinal mucosal immunity, *Clin Nutr* 18(6):337–344, 1999.
12. Fink M: Why the GI tract is pivotal in trauma, sepsis, and multiple organ failure, *J Crit Illness* 6:253–274, 1991.
13. Deitch EA, Winterton J, Li M, Berg R: The gut as a portal of entry for bacteremia. Role of protein malnutrition, *Ann Surg* 205(6):681–692, 1987.
14. Deitch EA: Multiple organ failure. Pathophysiology and potential future therapy, *Ann Surg* 216(2):117–134, 1992.
15. Ryan CM, Yarmush ML, Burke JF, Tomkins RG: Increased gut permeability early after burns correlates with the extent of burn injury, *Crit Care Med* 20(11):1508–1512, 1992.
16. Alexander JW, Boyce ST, Babcock GF, et al: The process of microbial translocation, *Ann Surg* 212(4):496–512, 1990.
17. LeVoyer T, Cioffi WG, Pratt L, et al: Alterations in intestinal permeability after thermal injury, *Arch Surg* 127(1):26–30, 1992.
18. Kueppers PM, Miller TA, Chen CYK, et al: Effect of total parenteral nutrition plus morphine on bacterial translocation in rats, *Ann Surg* 217(3):286–292, 1993.
19. Peng YZ, Yuan ZQ, Xiao GX: Effects of early enteral feeding on the prevention of enterogenic infection in severely burned patients, *Burns* 27(2):145–149, 2001.
20. Fink MP: Effect of critical illness on microbial translocation and gastrointestinal mucosa permeability, *Semin Respir Infect* 9(4):256–260, 1994.
21. Moore FA, Moore EE: Evolving concepts in the pathogenesis of postinjury multiple organ failure, *Surg Clin North Am* 75(2):257–277, 1995.
22. Lipman TO: Bacterial translocation and enteral nutrition in humans. An outsider looks in, *J Parenter Enteral Nutr* 19(2):156–165, 1995.
23. Alexander JW, Gottschlich MM: Nutritional immunomodulation in burn patients, *Crit Care Med* 18(2 suppl):S149–S153, 1990.
24. Fong Y, Marano MA, Barber A, et al: Total parenteral nutrition and bowel rest modify the metabolic response to endotoxin in humans, *Ann Surg* 210(4):449–456, 1989.
25. Border JR, Hassett J, LaDuca J, et al: The gut origin septic states in blunt multiple trauma (ISS = 40) in the ICU, *Ann Surg* 206(4):427–448, 1987.
26. Carrico CJ, Meakins JL, Marshall JC, et al: Multi-organ failure syndrome, *Arch Surg* 121(2):196–208, 1986.
27. Marshall JC, Christou NV, Horn R, Meakins JL: The microbiology of multiple organ failure. The proximal gastrointestinal tract as an occult reservoir of pathogens, *Arch Surg* 123(3):309–315, 1988.
28. Heyland D, Mandell LA: Gastric colonization by gram-negative bacilli and nosocomial pneumonia in the intensive care unit patient: evidence for causation, *Chest* 101(1):187–193, 1992.
29. Rombeau JL, Barot LR, Williamson CE, Mullen JL: Preoperative total parenteral nutrition and surgical outcome in patients with inflammatory bowel disease, *Am J Surg* 143(1):139–143, 1982.
30. Kudsk KA, Croce MA, Fabian TC, et al: Enteral versus parenteral feeding: effects on septic morbidity after blunt and penetrating abdominal trauma, *Ann Surg* 215(5):503–513, 1992.
31. Moore FA, Moore EE, Jones TN, et al: TEN vs TPN following major abdominal trauma—reduced septic morbidity, *J Trauma* 29(7):916–923, 1989.
32. Bower RH, Talamini MA, Sax HC, et al: Postoperative enteral vs. parenteral nutrition: a randomized controlled trial, *Arch Surg* 121(9):1040–1045, 1986.
33. Moore FA, Feliciano DV, Andrassy RJ, et al: Early enteral feeding, compared with parenteral, reduces postoperative septic complications. The results of a meta-analysis, *Ann Surg* 216(2):172–183, 1992.
34. Kudsk KA: Gut mucosal nutritional support–enteral nutrition as primary therapy after multiple system trauma, *Gut* 35(1 suppl):S52–S54, 1994.
35. Herndon DN, Barrow RE, Stein M, et al: Increased mortality with intravenous supplemental feeding in severely burned patients, *J Burn Care Rehabil* 10(4):309–313, 1989.
36. Suchner V, Senftleben U, Eckart T, et al: Enteral versus parenteral nutrition: effects on gastrointestinal function and metabolism, *Nutrition* 12(1):13–22, 1996.
37. Kudsk KA, Minard G, Wojtysiak SL, et al: Visceral protein response to enteral versus parenteral nutrition and sepsis in patients with trauma, *Surgery* 116(3):516–523, 1994.
38. Peterson VM, Moore EE, Jones TN, et al: Total enteral nutrition vs. total parenteral nutrition after major torso injury: attenuation of hepatic protein reprioritization, *Surgery* 104(2):199–207, 1988.
39. Moore EE, Jones TN: Benefits of immediate jejunostomy feeding after major abdominal trauma: a prospective, randomized trial, *J Trauma* 26(10):874–881, 1986.
40. Kudsk KA, Carpenter G, Petersen S, Sheldon GF: Effect of enteral and parenteral feeding in malnourished rats with *E. coli*–hemoglobin adjuvant peritonitis, *J Surg Res* 31(2):105–110, 1981.
41. Saito H, Trocki O, Alexander JW, et al: The effect of route of nutrient administration on the nutritional state, catabolic hormone secretion, and gut mucosal integrity after burn injury, *J Parenter Enteral Nutr* 11(1):1–7, 1987.
42. Alverdy JC, Aoys E, Moss GS: Total parenteral nutrition promotes bacterial translocation from the gut, *Surgery* 104(2):185–190, 1988.

43. Delany HM, John J, Tek EL, et al: Contrasting effects of identical nutrients given parenterally or enterally after 70% hepatectomy, *J Surg* 167:135–144, 1994.

44. Pappo I, Polacheck I, Zmora O, et al: Altered gut barrier function to *Candida* during parenteral nutrition, *Nutrition* 10(2):151–154, 1994.

45. Mainous M, Xu D, Lu Q, et al: Oral-TPN-induced bacterial translocation and impaired immune defenses are reversed by refeeding, *Surgery* 110(2):277–284, 1991.

46. Waters B, Kudsk KA, Jarvi EJ, et al: Effect of route of nutrition on recovery of hepatic organic anion clearance after fasting, *Surgery* 115(3):370–374. 1994.

47. Meyer J, Yurt RW, Duhaney R, et al: Differential neutrophil activation before and after endotoxin infusion in enterally versus parenterally fed volunteers, *Surg Gynecol Obstet* 167(6):501–509, 1988.

48. Braga M, Gianotti L, Costantini E, et al: Impact of enteral nutrition on intestinal bacterial translocation and mortality in burned mice, *Clin Nutr* 13:256–261, 1994.

49. The Veterans Affairs total parenteral nutrition cooperative study group: Perioperative total parenteral nutrition in surgical patients, *N Engl J Med* 325(8):525–532, 1991.

50. Johnson LR, Copeland EM, Dudrick SJ, et al: Structural and hormonal alterations in the gastrointestinal tract of parenterally fed rats, *Gastroenterology* 68(5 Pt 1):1177–1183, 1975.

51. Levine GM, Deren JJ, Steiger E, Zinno R: Role of oral intake in maintenance of gut mass and disaccharide activity, *Gastroenterology* 67(5):975–982, 1974.

52. Jackson WD, Grand RJ: The human intestinal response to enteral nutrients: a review, *J Am Coll Nutr* 10(5):500–509, 1991.

53. Mochizuki H, Trocki O, Dominioni L, et al: Mechanism of prevention of postburn hypermetabolism and catabolism by early enteral feeding, *Ann Surg* 200(3):297–310, 1984.

54. Gianotti L, Nelson JL, Alexander JW, et al: Post-injury hypermetabolic response and magnitude of translocation: prevention by early enteral nutrition, *Nutrition* 10(3):225–231, 1994.

55. Hosoda N, Nishi M, Nakagawa M, et al: Structural and functional alteration in the gut of parenterally or enterally fed rats, *J Surg Res* 47:129–133, 1989.

56. Inoue S, Lukes S, Alexander JW, et al: Increased gut blood flow with early enteral feeding in burned guinea pigs, *J Burn Care Rehabil* 10(4):300–308, 1989.

57. Haskel Y, Xu D, Deitch E: Elemental diet-induced bacterial translocation can be hormonally modulated, *Ann Surg* 217(6):634–643, 1993.

58. Evers BM, Izukura M, Townsend CM, et al: Differential effects of gut hormones on pancreatic and intestinal growth during administration of an elemental diet, *Ann Surg* 211(5):630–638, 1990.

59. Majumdar APN: Effects of fasting and refeeding on antral, duodenal and serum gastrin levels and on colonic thymidine kinase activity in rats, *Hormone Res* 19(2):127–134, 1984.

60. Lucas A, Bloom SR, Aynsley-Green A: Gut hormones and "minimal enteral feeding," *Acta Paediatr Scand* 75(5):719–723, 1986.

61. Kotler DP, Kral JG, Bjorntorp P: Refeeding after a fast in rats: effects on small intestinal enzymes, *Am J Clin Nutr* 36(3):457–462, 1982.

62. Zaloga GP, Ward Black KW, Prielipp R: Effect of rate of enteral nutrient supply on gut mass, *J Parenter Enteral Nutr* 16(1):39–42, 1992.

63. Roberts PR, Black KW, Zaloga GP: Enteral nutrition blunts decrease in mesenteric blood flow (MBF) during high dose phenylephrine administration, *Crit Care Med* 27:135S, 1999.

64. Andel H, Rab M, Andel D, et al: Impact of early high caloric duodenal feeding on the oxygen balance of the splanchnic region after severe burn injury, *Burns* 27(4):389–393, 2001.

65. Andrassy RJ, Page CP, Patterson RS: Early postoperative jejunal feeding: does nitrogen source affect utilization? *Nutrition* 2:317–321, 1986.

66. Berseth CL: Effect of early feeding on maturation of the preterm infant's small intestine, *J Pediatr* 120(6):947–953, 1992.

67. Brownlee KG, Kelly EJ, Ng PC, et al: Early or late parenteral nutrition for the sick preterm infant? *Arch Dis Child* 69(3):281–283, 1993.

68. Chiarelli A, Enzi G, Casadei A, et al: Very early nutrition supplementation in burned patients, *Am J Clin Nutr* 51(6):1035–1039, 1990.

69. Dominioni L, Trocki O, Mochizuki H, et al: Prevention of severe postburn hypermetabolism and catabolism by immediate intragastric feeding, *J Burn Care Rehabil* 5(2):106–112, 1984.

70. Engelhardt VJ, Clark SM: Early enteral feeding of a severely burned pediatric patient, *J Burn Care Rehabil* 15(3):293–297, 1994.

71. Eyer SD, Micon LT, Konstantinides FN, et al: Early enteral feeding does not attenuate metabolic response after blunt trauma, *J Trauma* 34(5):639–644, 1993.

72. Gottschlich MM, Warden GD, Michel M, et al: Diarrhea in tube-fed burn patients: Incidence, etiology, nutritional impact, and prevention, *J Parenter Enteral Nutr* 12(4):338–345, 1988.

73. Grahm TW, Zadrozny DB, Harrington T: The benefits of early jejunal hyperalimentation in the head-injured patient, *Neurosurgery* 25(5):729–735, 1989.

74. Hadley MN, Grahm TW, Harrington T, et al: Nutritional support and neurotrauma: a critical review of early nutrition in forty-five acute head injury patients, *Neurosurgery* 19(3):367–373, 1986.

75. Hansbrough WB, Hansbrough JF: Success of immediate intragastric feeding of patients with burns, *J Burn Care Rehabil* 14(5):512–516, 1993.

76. Hasse JM, Blue LS, Liepa GU, et al: Early enteral nutrition support in patients undergoing liver transplantation, *J Parenter Enteral Nutr* 19(6):437–443, 1995.

77. Inoue S, Epstein MD, Alexander JW, et al: Prevention of yeast translocation across the gut by a single enteral feeding after burn injury, *J Parenter Enteral Nutr* 13(6):565–571, 1989.

78. Jenkins M, Gottschlich MM, Alexander JW, Warden GD: Enteral alimentation in the early postburn phase. In Blackburn GL, Bell SJ, Mullen JL (eds): *Nutritional Medicine: A Case Management Approach,* Philadelphia, 1989, WB Saunders, pp 1–5.

79. Jenkins M, Gottschlich M, Alexander JW, Warden GD: Effect of immediate enteral feeding on the hypermetabolic response following severe burn injury, *J Parenter Enteral Nutr* 13(1 suppl):12S, 1989.

80. Kaufman T, Hirshowitz B, Moscona R, Brooks GJ: Early enteral nutrition for mass burn injury: the revised egg-rich diet, *Burns* 12:260–263, 1986.

81. Kirby DF, Clifton GL, Turner H, et al: Early enteral nutrition after brain injury by percutaneous endoscopic gastrojejunostomy, *J Parenter Enteral Nutr* 15(3):298–302, 1991.

82. Kolacinski Z: Early parenteral nutrition in patients unconscious because of acute drug poisoning, *J Parenter Enteral Nutr* 17(1):25–29, 1993.

83. McArdle AH, Palmason C, Brown RA, et al: Early enteral feeding of patients with major burns: prevention of catabolism, *Ann Plast Surg* 13(5):396–401, 1984.

84. McArdle AH, Palmason C, Brown RA, et al: Protection from catabolism in major burns: a new formula for the immediate enteral feeding of burn patients, *J Burn Care Rehabil* 4(1):245–250, 1983.

85. McDonald WS, Sharp CW, Deitch EA: Immediate enteral feeding in burn patients is safe and effective, *Ann Surg* 213(2):177–183, 1991.

86. Mochizuki H, Trocki O, Dominioni L, Alexander JW: Reduction of postburn hypermetabolism by early enteral feeding, *Curr Surg* 42(2):121–125, 1985.

87. Ostertag SG, LaGamma EF, Reisen CE, Ferrentino FL: Early enteral feeding does not affect the incidence of necrotizing enterocolitis, *Pediatrics* 77:275–280, 1986.

88. Rapp RP, Young B, Twyman D, et al: The favorable effect of early parenteral feeding on survival of head-injured patients, *J Neurosurg* 58(6):906–912, 1983.

89. Riley HK, White JL, Jarrett PA, et al: Immediate postoperative enteral nutrition, *Surg Forum* 31:103–105, 1980.

90. Sacks GS, Brown RO, Teague D, et al: Early nutrition support modifies immune function in patients sustaining severe head injury, *J Parenter Enteral Nutr* 19(5):387–392, 1995.

91. Schroeder D, Gillanders L, Mahr K, Hill GL: Effects of immediate postoperative enteral nutrition on body composition, muscle function, and wound healing, *J Parenter Enteral Nutr* 15(4):376–383, 1991.

92. Slagle TA, Gross SJ: Effect of early low-volume enteral substrate on subsequent feeding tolerance in very low birth weight infants, *J Pediatrics* 113(3):526–531, 1988.

93. Trocki O, Michelini JA, Robbins ST, Eichelberger MR: Evaluation of early enteral feeding in children less than 3 years old with smaller (8—25 per cent) TBSA, *Burns* 21(1):17–23, 1995.

94. Wood RH, Caldwell FT Jr, Bowser-Wallace BH: The effect of early feeding on postburn hypermetabolism, *J Trauma* 28(2):177–183, 1988 (abstract).

95. Zaloga GP, Bortenschlager L, Black KW, Prielipp R: Immediate postoperative enteral feeding decreases weight loss and improves wound healing after abdominal surgery in rats, *Crit Care Med* 20(1):115–118, 1992.

96. Young B, Ott L, Twyman D, et al: The effect of nutritional support on outcome from severe head injury, *J Neurosurg* 67(5):668–676, 1987.

97. Kudsk KA, Mowatt-Larssen C, Bukar J, et al: Effect of recombinant human insulin-like growth factor I and early total parenteral nutrition on immune depression following severe head injury, *Arch Surg* 129(1):66–71, 1994.

98. Reilly JJ, Hull SF, Albert N, et al: Economic impact of malnutrition: a model system for hospitalized patients, *J Parenter Enteral Nutr* 12(4):371–376, 1988.
99. Chellis MJ, Sanders SV, Webster H, et al: Early enteral feeding in the pediatric intensive care unit, *J Parenter Enteral Nutr* 20(1):71–73, 1996.
100. Braga M, Gianotti L, Gentillini O, et al: Early postoperataive enteral nutrition improves gut oxygenation and reduces costs compared with total parenteral nutrition, *Crit Care Med* 29(2):242–248, 2001.
101. Playford RJ, Woodman AC, Clark P, et al: Effect of luminal growth factor preservation on intestinal growth, *Lancet* 341(8849):843–848, 1993.
102. Zapata-Sirvent RL, Hansbrough JF, O'Hara MM, et al: Bacterial translocation in burned mice after administration of various diets including fiber- and glutamine-enriched enteral formulas, *Crit Care Med* 22(4):690–696, 1994.
103. Page C: Early postoperative feeding: pathophysiology, safety and utility, *Contemp Surg* 32S:14–20, 1988.
104. Moss G, Greenstein A, Levy S, Bierenbaum A: Maintenance of GI function after bowel surgery and immediate enteral full nutrition. I. Doubling of canine colorectal anastomotic bursting pressure and intestinal wound mature collagen content, *J Parenter Enteral Nutr* 4:535–538, 1980.
105. Tinckler LF: Surgery and intestinal motility, *Br J Surg* 52:140–150, 1965.
106. Glucksman DL, Kalser MH, Warren WD: Small intestinal absorption in the immediate postoperative period, *Surgery* 60(5):1020–1025, 1966.
107. Jenkins ME, Gottschlich MM, Warden GD: Enteral feeding during operative procedures in thermal injuries, *J Burn Care Rehabil* 15(2):199–205, 1994.
108. Fischer CG, Jenkins MM, Gottschlich MM, Warden GD: Perioperative enteral nutrition in the pediatric burn patient. In *Proceedings of the International Anesthesiology Research Society Clinical Congress,* Honolulu, March 1995.
109. Kravitz M, Woodruff J, Petersen S, Warden GD: The use of the Dobhoff tube to provide additional nutritional support in thermally injured patients, *J Burn Care Rehabil* 3(4):226–228, 1982.
110. Grant JP, Curtas MS, Kelvin FM: Fluoroscopic placement of nasojejunal feeding tubes with immediate feeding using a nonelemental diet, *J Parenter Enteral Nutr* 7(3):299–303, 1983.
111. Gottschlich MM, Jenkins ME, Mayes T, Khoury J, Warden GD: An evaluation of the effects of early versus delayed enteral support on feeding tolerance and clinical, nutritional and hormonal outcomes following burns, *J Burn Care Rehabil,* in press.
112. Wolfe RR, Durkot MJ, Clarke CC, et al: Effect of food intake on hypermetabolic response to burn injury in guinea pigs, *J Nutr* 110(7):1310–1312, 1980.
113. Khoury TL, Borlase BC, Forse RA, et al: Early enteral feeding via a jejunostomy: a safe technique in critically ill patients. In Borlase BC, Bell SJ, Blackburn GL, Forse RA (eds): *Enteral nutrition,* New York, 1994, Chapman and Hall, pp 142–151.
114. Andrassy RJ, DuBois T, Page CP, et al: Early postoperative nutritional enhancement utilizing enteral branched-chain amino acids by way of a needle catheter jejunostomy, *Am J Surg* 150(6):730–734, 1985.
115. Jones TN, Moore EE, Moore FA: Early postoperative feeding. In Borlase BC, Bell SJ, Blackburn GL, Forse RA (eds): *Enteral nutrition,* New York, 1994, Chapman and Hall, 19pp 78–106.
116. Studley HO: Percentage of weight loss: a basic indicator of surgical risk in patients with chronic peptic ulcer, *JAMA* 106:458–460, 1936.
117. ASPEN Board of Directors: Guidelines for the use of parenteral and enteral nutrition in adult and pediatric patients, *J Parenter Enteral Nutr* 17(4 suppl):1SA–4SA, 1993.
118. Buzby GP: Perioperative nutritional support, *J Parenter Enteral Nutr* 14(5 suppl):197S–199S, 1990.
119. Detsky AS, Baker JP, O'Rourke K, Goel V: Perioperative parenteral nutrition: a meta-analysis, *Ann Intern Med* 107(2):195–203, 1987.
120. Chwals WJ, Blackburn GL: Perioperative nutritional support in the cancer patient, *Surg Clin North Am* 66(6):1137–1165, 1986.
121. Campos AC, Meguid MM: A critical appraisal of the usefulness of perioperative nutritional support, *Am J Clin Nutr* 55(1):117–130, 1992.
122. Maxfield D, Geehan D, Van Way CW: Perioperative nutrition support*, Nutr Clin Pract* 16(2):69–73, 2001.
123. Daly JM, Redmond HP, Gallagher H: Perioperative nutrition in cancer patients, *J Parenter Enteral Nutr* 16(6 suppl):100S–105S, 1992.
124. Smale BF, Mullen JL, Buzby GP, Rosato EF: The efficacy of nutritional assessment and support in cancer surgery, *Cancer* 47(10):2375–2381, 1981.
125. Muller JM, Keller HW, Brenner U, et al: Indications and effects of preoperative parenteral nutrition, *World J Surg* 10(1):53–63, 1986.
126. Holter AR, Fischer JE: The effects of perioperative hyperalimentation on complications in patients with carcinoma and weight loss, *J Surg Res* 23(1):31–34, 1977.
127. Moghissi K, Hornshaw J, Teasdale PR, Dawes EA: Parenteral nutrition in carcinoma of the esophagus treated by surgery: nitrogen balance and clinical studies, *Br J Surg* 64(2):125–128, 1977.
128. Gouma DJ, von Meyenfeldt MF, Rouflart M, Soeters PB: Preoperative total parenteral nutrition (TPN) in severe Crohn's disease, *Surgery* 103(6):648–652, 1988.
129. Otaki M: Surgical treatment of patients with cardiac cachexia: an analysis of factors affecting operative mortality, *Chest* 105(5):1347–1351, 1994.
130. Smith RC, Hartemink R: Improvement of nutritional measures during preoperative parenteral nutrition in patients selected by the Prognostic Nutritional Index: a randomized controlled trial, *J Parenter Enteral Nutr* 12(6):587–591, 1988.
131. Starker PM, LaSala PA, Askanazi J, et al: The influence of preoperative total parenteral nutrition upon morbidity and mortality, *Surg Gynecol Obstet* 162(6):569–574, 1986.
132. Daly JM, Massar E, Giacco G, et al: Parenteral nutrition in esophageal cancer patients, *Ann Surg* 196(2):203–208, 1982.
133. Mullen JL, Buzby GP, Mathews DC, et al: Reduction of operative morbidity and mortality by combined preoperative and postoperative nutritional support, *Ann Surg* 192(5):604–613, 1980.
134. Heatley RV, Williams RHP, Lewis MH: Pre-operative intravenous feeding: a controlled trial, *Postgrad Med J* 55(646):541–545, 1979.
135. Schildt B, Groth O, Larsson J, et al: Failure of preoperative TPN to improve nutritional status in gastric carcinoma, *J Parenter Enteral Nutr* 5:360, 1981.
136. Thompson BR, Julian TB, Stremple JF: Perioperative total parenteral nutrition in patients with gastrointestinal cancer, *J Surg Res* 30(5):497–500, 1981.
137. Lim STK, Choa RG, Lam KM, et al: Total parenteral nutrition versus gastrostomy in the preoperative preparation of patients with carcinoma of the esophagus, *Br J Surg* 68(2):69–72, 1981.
138. Steffers C, Fromm D: Is preoperative parenteral nutrition necessary for patients with predominantly ileal Crohn's disease? *Arch Surg* 127(10):1210–1212, 1992.
139. Bellantone R, Doglietto GB, Bossola M, et al: Preoperative parenteral nutrition in malnourished high-risk surgical patients, *Nutrition* 6(2):168–170, 1990.
140. Bellantone R, Doglietto GB, Bossola M, et al: Preoperative parenteral nutrition in the high risk surgical patient, *J Parenter Enteral Nutr* 12(2):195–197, 1988.
141. Shukla HS, Rao RR, Banu N, et al: Enteral hyperalimentation in malnourished surgical patients, *Indian J Med Res* 80(Sept.):339–346, 1984.
142. Foschi D, Cavagna G, Callioni F, et al: Hyperalimentation of jaundiced patients on percutaneous transhepatic biliary drainage, *Br J Surg* 73(9):716–719, 1986.
143. Hulten L, Andersson H, Bosaeus I, et al: Enteral alimentation in the early postoperative course, *J Parenter Enteral Nutr* 4(5):455–459, 1980.
144. Daly JM, Bonau R, Stofberg P, et al: Immediate postoperative jejunostomy feeding: clinical and metabolic results in a prospective trial, *Am J Surg* 153(2):198–206, 1987.
145. Hoover HC, Ryan JA, Anderson EJ, Fischer JE: Nutritional benefits of immediate postoperative jejunal feeding of an elemental diet, *Am J Surg* 139(1):153–159, 1980.
146. Sagar S, Harland P, Shields R: Early postoperative feeding with elemental diet, *BMJ* 1(6159):293–295, 1979.
147. Delany HM, Demetriou AA, Teh E, Levenson SM: Effect of early postoperative nutritional support on skin wound and colon anastomosis healing, *J Parenter Enteral Nutr* 14(4):357–361, 1990.
148. Eagon JC, Alpers D: Gut rest versus early feeding after elective abdominal surgery, *Nutrition* 13(2):155–156, 1997.
149. Bickel A, Shtamler B, Mizrahi S: Early oral feeding following removal of nasogastric tube in gastrointestinal operations: a randomized prospective study, *Arch Surg* 127(3):287–289, 1992.
150. Mayes T, Gottschlich MM, Warden GD: Nutrition intervention in pediatric patients with thermal injuries who require laparotomy, *J Burn Care Rehabil* Sep-Oct 21(5):451–456, 2000.
151. Ward MW, Danzi M, Lewin MR, Clark CG: The effects of subclinical malnutrition and refeeding on the healing of experimental colonic anastomoses, *Br J Surg* 69(6):308–310, 1982.
152. Collins JP, Oxby CB, Hill GL: Intravenous amino acids and intravenous hyperalimentation as protein sparing therapy after major surgery. A controlled clinical trial, *Lancet* 1(8068):788–791, 1978.

153. Yamada N, Koyama H, Hioki K, et al: Effect of postoperative total parenteral nutrition (TPN) as an adjunct to gastrectomy for advanced gastric carcinoma, *Br J Surg* 70(5):267–274, 1983.

154. Woolfson AMJ, Smith JAR: Elective nutritional support after major surgery: a prospective randomized trial, *Clin Nutr* 8:15–21, 1989.

155. Maltby JR, Sutherland AD, Sade JP, Shaffer EA: Preoperative oral fluids: is a five hour fast justified prior to elective surgery? *Anesth Analg* 65(11):1112–1116, 1986.

156. Pearson KS, From RP, Symreng T, Kealey GP: Continuous enteral feeding and short fasting periods enhance perioperative nutrition in patients with burns, *J Burn Care Rehabil* 13(4):477–481, 1992.

157. Splinter WM, Steward SA, Muir JG: The effect of preoperative apple juice on gastric content, thirst, and hunger in children, *Can J Anaesth* 36(1):55–58, 1989.

158. Jenkins M, Gottschlich M, Fischer C, Warden G: Perioperative enteral nutrition in the pediatric burn patient, *Proc Am Burn Assoc* 26:237, 1994.

159. Jepson MM, Bates PC, Broadbent P, et al: Relationship between glutamine concentration and protein synthesis in rat skeletal muscle, *Am J Physiol* 255(2 Pt 1):E166–172, 1988.

160. Vinnars E, Hammarqvist F, Von Der Decken A, Wernerman J: Role of glutamine and its analogs in post-traumatic muscle protein and amino acid metabolism, *J Parenter Enteral Nutr* 14(4 suppl):125S–129S, 1990.

161. Burke DJ, Alverdy JC, Aoys E, Moss GS: Glutamine supplemented total parenteral nutrition improves gut immune function, *Arch Surg* 124(12):1396–1399, 1989.

162. Newsholme EA, Newsholme P, Curi R: A role for muscle in the immune system and its importance in surgery, trauma, sepsis and burns, *Nutrition* 4:261, 1988.

163. Ogle CK, Ogle JD, Mao J-X, et al: Effect of glutamine on phagocytosis and bacterial killing by normal and pediatric burn patient neutrophils, *J Parenter Enteral Nutr* 18(2):128–133, 1994.

164. Ardawi MS, Newsholme EA: Glutamine metabolism in lymphocytes of the rat, *Biochem J* 212(3):835–842, 1983.

165. Calden PC: Glutamine and the immune system, *Clin Nutr* 13:2, 1994.

166. Juretic A, Spagnoli GC, Horigtt J: Glutamine requirements in the generation of lymphokine-activated killer cells, *Clin Nutr* 13:42–49, 1994.

167. Alverdy JC: Effects of glutamine supplemented diets on immunology of the gut, *J Parenter Enteral Nutr* 14(4 suppl):109S–113S, 1990.

168. van der Hulst RR, van Kreel BK, von Meyenfelt MF, et al: Glutamine and the preservation of gut integrity, *Lancet* 341(8857):1363–1365, 1993.

169. Grant JP, Snyder PJ: Use of L-glutamine in total parenteral nutrition, *J Surg Res* 44(5):506–513, 1988.

170. Evans MA, Shronts EP: Intestinal fuels: glutamine, short-chain fatty acids, and dietary fiber, *J Am Diet Assoc* 92(10):1239–1249, 1992.

171. Hwang TL, O'Dwyer ST, Smith RJ, Wilmore DW: Preservation of small bowel mucosa using glutamine-enriched parenteral nutrition, *Surg Forum* 37:56–58, 1986.

172. Fox AD, Kripke SA, De Paula J, et al: Effect of a glutamine-supplemented enteral diet on methotrexate-induced enterocolitis, *J Parenter Enteral Nutr* 12(4):325–331, 1988.

173. Fox AD, De Paula JA, Kripke SA, et al: Glutamine-supplemented elemental diets reduce endotoxemia in a lethal model of enterocolitis, *Surg Forum* 39:46–48, 1988.

174. Korein J: Oral L-glutamine well tolerated, *N Engl J Med* 301(19):1066, 1979.

175. Ziegler TR, Benfell K, Smith RJ, et al: Safety and metabolic effects of L-glutamine administration in humans, *J Parenter Enteral Nutr* 14(4 suppl):137S–146S, 1990.

176. Scheppach W, Burghardt W, Bartram P, Kasper H: Addition of dietary fiber to liquid formula diets: the pros and cons, *J Parenter Enteral Nutr* 14(2):204–209, 1990.

177. Frankenfield DC, Beyer PL: Soy-polysaccharide fiber: effect on diarrhea in tube-fed head-injured patients, *Am J Clin Nutr* 50(3):533–538, 1989.

178. Ryan GP, Dudrick SJ, Copeland EM, Johnson LR: Effects of various diets on colonic growth in rats, *Gastroenterology* 77(4 Pt 1):658–663, 1979.

179. Goodlad RA, Wright NA: Effects of addition of kaolin or cellulose to an elemental diet on intestinal cell proliferation in the mouse, *Br J Nutr* 50(1):91–98, 1983.

180. Deitch EA, Xu D, Qi L, Berg R: Elemental diet-induced immune suppression is caused by both bacterial and dietary factors, *J Parenter Enteral Nutr* 17(4):332–336, 1993.

181. Spaeth G, Specian RD, Berg RD, Deitch EA: Bulk prevents bacterial translocation induced by the oral administration of total parenteral nutrition solution, *J Parenter Enteral Nutr* 14(5):442–447, 1990.

182. Palacio JC, Rombeau JL: Dietary fiber: A brief review and potential application to enteral nutrition, *Nutr Clin Pract* 5(3):99–106, 1990.

183. Silk DBA: Fibre and enteral nutrition, *Gut* 30(2):246–264, 1989.

184. Koruda MJ, Rolandelli RH, Settle RG, et al: The effect of a pectin-supplemented elemental diet on intestinal adaptation to massive bowel resection, *J Parenter Enteral Nutr* 10(4):343–350, 1986.

185. Meier R, Beglinger C, Schneider H, et al: Effect of a liquid diet with and without soluble fiber supplementation on intestinal transit and cholecystokinin release in volunteers, *J Parenter Enteral Nutr* 17(3):231–235, 1993.

186. Rolandelli RH, Saul SH, Settle RG, et al: Comparison of parenteral nutrition and enteral feeding with pectin in experimental colitis in the rat, *Am J Clin Nutr* 47(4):715–721, 1988.

187. Rolandelli RH, Koruda MJ, Settle RG, Rombeau JL: Effects of intraluminal short-chain fatty acids on healing of colonic anastomosis in the rat, *Surgery* 100(2):198–204, 1986.

188. Friedel D, Levine GM: Effect of short-chain fatty acids on colonic function and structure, *J Parenter Enteral Nutr* 16(1):1–4, 1992.

189. Koruda MJ, Rolandelli RH, Bliss DZ, et al: Parenteral nutrition supplemented with short-chain fatty acids: effect on the small bowel mucosa in normal rats, *Am J Clin Nutr* 51(4):685–689, 1990.

190. Lynch JW, Miles JM, Bailey JW: Effects of the short-chain triglyceride triacetin on intestinal mucosa and metabolic substrates in rats, *J Parenter Enteral Nutr* 18(3):208–213, 1994

Combined and Transitional Feeding Modalities

22

Reneé Piazza-Barnett, MEd, RD, CNSD

COMBINED feeding is a technique for providing nutrition support to patients, principally those who are critically ill. It involves simultaneous feeding of parenteral nutrition (PN), enteral nutrition (EN) administered through a feeding tube, and oral nutrition. It combines a dependable means of delivering calories, protein, fluid, and micronutrients (including acid-base management) by PN with the physiologic benefits of EN and oral nutrition. Recipients of combined feeding are initially too sick to take all nutrition and metabolic support by the enteral or oral route. Thus combined feeding offers the advantages of all three feeding modalities. As time passes, the rate of PN decreases and that of EN or oral intake increases. After 7 to 10 days, most patients can successfully make the transition to full EN or an oral diet.

Very little research has been conducted in the area of combined and transitional feeding. Thus techniques for administering combined feeding and strategies for transitioning from one feeding modality to another are based largely on clinical bias rather than on information derived from randomized prospective trials. Institutional differences in combined and transitional feeding techniques are unavoidable given variations in patient populations. The combined and transitional feeding techniques presented in this chapter represent the practice of the Nutrition Support Team (NST) at The Cleveland Clinic Foundation (CCF) in Cleveland, Ohio and the Nutrition Support Service and the Enteral Nutrition Service at the Deaconess Hospital in Boston, Massachusetts. Due to the number of critically ill patients at these institutions, physicians tend to have a conservative approach to combined and transitional feedings.

This chapter discusses the benefits of using a combined approach to feeding, how to determine who should receive combined feeding, when and how to administer it, how to transition patients from one feeding modality to another once the acute phase of illness has abated, and special considerations for discharge planning.

Clinical Benefits and Limitations of Feeding Routes

Parenteral Nutrition

There is little question that the development of PN has revolutionized patient care, particularly in the critically ill population. The delivery of nutrients intravenously ensures that patients

who are not able to receive or tolerate enteral or oral feeding due to a compromised bowel are being adequately fed. In addition, PN provides a vehicle for readily correcting fluid, electrolyte, micronutrient, and acid-base disturbances. In this manner, PN can provide nutrition as well as metabolic support when the enteral or oral route is not available or when its use is limited.

Parenteral nutrition, however, is not without limitations. The intravenous administration of nutrition is not a physiologic means of providing nutrients; there is no first-pass effect whereby the liver is the first recipient of all nutrients. There also is no stimulation of pancreatic or biliary enzymes with parenteral nutrition. Thus the risk for developing gallbladder disease is increased in patients receiving long-term total PN.[1] Moreover, the lack of stimulation to the gastrointestinal (GI) tract has been shown to cause bowel atrophy and to increase the risk of bacterial translocation.[2] Another limitation of PN is the risk of mechanical and infectious complications (see Chapter 19).

A final limitation of PN is cost. The price paid by pharmacy for the dextrose and amino acids contained in 1 L of maximally concentrated PN (i.e., 210 g dextrose and 70 g amino acids, when using 70% dextrose and 10% amino acids) is approximately three times the hospital cost of 1 L of a standard polymeric enteral formula. The additional expenses encountered when compounding (i.e., equipment for mixing, additives, labor) and administering (i.e., bag, tubing, central line) parenteral formulas make it much more costly than EN.

Enteral/Oral Nutrition

One of the most frequently cited benefits of EN and oral nutrition is that it has been shown to preserve intestinal mucosal integrity. Presumably, maintenance of the gut's mucosal barrier function and intestinal immunocompetence helps to prevent bacterial translocation.[2,3] In recent years, a substantial body of clinical[4-7] and experimental[2,8-11] research has emerged that suggests that the route of nutrient administration may significantly influence the immune and metabolic responses to injury and sepsis (see Chapter 21).

Combined Feeding

Combined feeding captures the advantages of parenteral, enteral, and oral nutrition and has few limitations or drawbacks. It may also assist in a more rapid transition to the enteral or oral route. Patients who are already candidates for PN and cannot fulfill their nutrition needs via the enteral or

Acknowledgment: A special thank you is extended to Wendy Swails Bollinger, RD, CNSD, and Stacey Bell, DSc, RD, who contributed to the first edition chapter.

oral route owing to GI compromise are guaranteed to get the remainder of their macro- and micronutrient and fluid requirements with the addition of PN. Even if patients can tolerate only 10 to 20 ml/hr of EN, experimental evidence suggests that providing a mere 20% of total calories as EN (and the remainder as PN) may decrease the rate of bacterial translocation to mesenteric lymph nodes and completely reverse PN-associated peritoneal macrophage suppression.[11]

Candidates for Combined Feeding

Two scenarios can render a patient a candidate for combined feeding. The first scenario involves a patient who is unable to be advanced to full EN. This frequently occurs due to increased residuals with intragastric feedings. Other reasons could be nausea, abdominal pain and distention, or diarrhea with advancement of the EN. Decreasing or stopping the rate of the infusion while attempting postpyloric feeding tube placement will result in diminished efficacy of feeding. The initiation of PN provides a dependable means of delivering calories, protein, and fluid while continuing to attempt EN.

Patients with weight loss less than 10% of usual body weight and whose degree of inflammation is mild may not need PN initiated if EN or an oral diet is expected to meet their nutritional needs within 1 week.[12] Patients with moderate to severe malnutrition or catabolism who will be unable to meet their needs enterally or orally for 5 or more days should be started on PN. The PN may be used to provide the balance of their nutritional requirements until their goal enteral rate can be achieved or an oral diet initiated and tolerated.

The second scenario involves a patient who has been on PN who appears to be having a return of GI function. It is prudent to continue PN until it is proven that the patient can tolerate EN or an oral diet. Although there may be several days that the patient is receiving both parenteral and enteral/oral nutrition, the PN should be decreased as the EN is advanced or oral intake increases. More specific details regarding adjusting the rates of PN and EN will be discussed in the section on transitional feedings.

In both scenarios the patient is usually unable to be fully supported by the enteral or oral route owing to temporary impairment of GI function. Although these scenarios can occur in any unit in the hospital and in a variety of diseases, the majority of patients who are likely to require and benefit from simultaneous administration of PN and EN are those who are critically ill. In order for patients to receive combined feeding they must already be deemed candidates for PN and EN. This implies that candidates for PN will require parenteral support for at least 5 to 7 days.

Due to the potential for small bowel necrosis, EN should be instituted cautiously in patients who require vasopressors or inotropic drugs for blood pressure support or who suffer from shock or known bowel ischemia.[13-15] Such patients may not be candidates for combined feeding. Other clinical settings that may preclude enteral feeding are discussed elsewhere (see Chapter 17).

Administration of Combined Feeding

WHEN TO INITIATE COMBINED FEEDING. Parenteral nutrition can generally be started as soon as venous access has been established. If the patient has just undergone surgery and has received excessive amounts of replacement fluids, it may be prudent to withhold PN for 1 or 2 days, until the patient's hemodynamic and fluid status have stabilized. Enteral nutrition can be initiated as soon as it is established that the patient's GI tract can be used and some type of feeding tube, either temporary or permanent, has been placed. Most patients experience gastric ileus for 3 days or more after abdominal surgery or during sepsis, thus precluding immediate institution of intragastric feeding.[16] In contrast, small bowel motility is minimally affected by acute metabolic stress. Thus patients with a nasoduodenal, nasojejunal, or surgical jejunostomy feeding tube can generally receive EN at a slow rate as soon as the tube is placed. For such patients, this often means that feeding can begin in the recovery room.

Both animal and clinical studies have shown that with respect to wound healing and infectious complications, nutrition support is better begun early (i.e., within 24 hours of insult) than delayed (see Chapter 21). Several studies have reported improvement in abdominal and colonic wound healing in animals receiving early (within 24 hours of injury or surgery) as compared with those that received delayed (within 72 hours) enteral nutrition.[17-19] Although this finding has been largely demonstrated in animal models, a recent prospective clinical trial showed similar results.[20]

In addition to improving wound healing, instituting early EN has been shown to reduce infectious complications in burn,[7,21] trauma,[22] and head injury patients,[23] compared with EN delayed 3 to 5 days after an injury. These studies suggest that for the benefits of EN to be recognized, feeds should ideally be initiated within the first 24 hours of injury.

Techniques for Combined Feeding

SELECTION OF PARENTERAL ACCESS. Parenteral nutrition can be delivered via a central or peripheral vein. The route of administration depends on the anticipated length of therapy, nutritional requirements, available intravenous access, and fluid status. Central PN is usually indicated in patients requiring longer parenteral support who have increased nutritional requirements and/or a restriction on fluid intake. Peripheral PN may be appropriate for patients requiring nutrition support for less than 2 weeks who are not markedly catabolic or fluid restricted and have good peripheral access.[24]

Patients requiring short-term PN (i.e., several days to 3 to 4 weeks) are candidates for temporary venous access via the subclavian, internal, or external jugular vein.[24,25] These temporary catheters do not require surgery, may be inserted at the bedside, and are generally used in the hospital only. How many lumens the catheter has depends on what it is to be used for in addition to nutrition support. If the patient requires a number of medications or blood products, a catheter with more than one lumen may be needed.

If it is anticipated that the patient will need PN for an extended period (at least 1 to 3 months), insertion of a permanent central catheter with one to three lumens is indicated.[24,25] There are generally two classes of permanent catheters: tunneled catheters and implantable venous access disks (ports).[25] Tunneled catheters (Hickman, Broviac, Groshong) are inserted into the central venous system and exit the skin via a subcutaneous tunnel. Implantable venous access disks are placed subcutaneously, thus eliminating the external portion of the catheter. These devices are accessed using a special needle, produce minimal disruption of body image, and are thought to protect against ascending organisms.[26] The choice of an external catheter or an implantable venous access disk generally depends on what the catheter will be used for and the patient's preference.

In addition to the aforementioned types of central lines, there is also a type of catheter, known as the *peripherally inserted central catheter (PICC)*. These long Silastic catheters are inserted peripherally, usually through the basilic or cephalic vein near the antecubital fossa. The tip must lie in the superior vena cava in order to deliver a hypertonic dextrose solution.[27] Some institutions prefer PICC lines for home PN, especially if the anticipated duration of therapy is less than a month. Another indication for a PICC line would be poor peripheral access in a patient requiring short-term PN. Complications of PICC lines include accidental dislodgment of the catheter[28] and venous thrombosis.[29]

SELECTION OF ENTERAL ACCESS. The type of enteral access selected depends upon the anticipated duration of therapy, adequacy of gastric function, lower esophageal sphincter competence, and the risk of aspiration. See Figure 22-1 for details regarding the determination of appropriate enteral access. If short-term EN is needed (4 to 6 weeks or less), a nasogastric or nasoenteric (nasoduodenal or nasojejunal) feeding tube may be used. A gastrostomy or jejunostomy should be used if the duration of EN is anticipated to be greater than 6 weeks. These may be placed endoscopically or surgically. Gastrostomy tubes are often preferred because they permit intermittent bolus feedings and may eliminate the need for an administration set and pump. These tubes are indicated when gastric emptying is normal, a gag reflex is present, and esophageal reflux is absent.

Candidates for jejunal feedings include those at risk of aspiration and patients with severe esophageal reflux, obstruction, stricture, fistulas, or ileus of the upper GI tract. Jejunal feedings have been found to decrease the risk of abdominal distention, nausea, vomiting, and pulmonary aspiration.[13,30,31] Another type of jejunal feeding is the insertion of a small tube through a percutaneous endoscopic gastrostomy (PEG) into the jejunum, referred to as a jejunal extension tube (JET). This type of feeding tube is known as a JET-PEG. The tubes may be used for jejunal feedings and simultaneous gastric decompression.

SELECTION OF ENTERAL FORMULAS. Selection of a formula is based on several factors. A patient with a normally functioning GI tract without a preexisting medical condition that affects nutrient metabolism may tolerate a standard polymeric formula. If digestive capability and absorptive capacity are impaired, a predigested formula should be used. The patient's ability to handle fluid volume should also be considered, and in some instances a calorically dense formula may be necessary. Finally, the patient may have a preexisting medical condition that would necessitate the use of a disease-specific formula. Generally speaking, enteral formulas can be grouped into three main categories: polymeric (concentrated, high protein, and fiber enriched), predigested (elemental and peptide based), and disease specific (products for lung, liver, and kidney disease, and those that enhance immune function).

When selecting an enteral formula for combined or transitional feeding, most patients with a normally functioning GI tract can be started on a polymeric formula. The osmolality of these products can range from approximately 270 to 800 mOsm/kg water. Hypertonic formulas can frequently be initiated at full strength because the osmolality of enteral formulas has few discernible effects on GI tolerance in gastric or duodenal tube feedings.[32] Predigested formulas are indicated in patients with compromised GI tracts because hydrolyzed nutrients require less active digestion than do intact components. Low-fat defined formulas have been used in the treatment of inflammatory bowel disease and pancreatitis with some success and are sometimes used as starter regimens in patients who have not received enteral or oral nutrition for extended periods.[32]

Stage I (Predigested) Formulas. Predigested formulas contain macronutrients, most notably protein, that have been partially hydrolyzed. Instead of intact protein sources such as casein or soy protein isolate (the two most common sources of protein in polymeric formulas), the protein in predigested formulas is either peptides or free amino acids. In addition, these formulas, particularly free amino acid based, are generally lower in fat than polymeric formulas.

Patients expected to have significant impairment of GI function (i.e., those undergoing extensive bowel surgery; those who have long been NPO); and those with specific diseases (i.e., acquired immunodeficiency syndrome, pancreatitis) that are frequently accompanied by fat intolerance may benefit from initially receiving a predigested formula. The easily absorbed nutrients and low fat content of predigested formulas are ideal for patients with known or suspected impairment of bowel function. Such formulas help to avoid "stressing" the already compromised intestine's digestive and absorptive capacity and may subsequently decrease the incidence of GI intolerance and maximize nutrient absorption. Several studies of critically ill patients report a lower incidence of diarrhea among those who received peptide-based formulas than in those who received whole-protein formulas.[33,34]

The use of low-fat predigested formulas may also benefit patients at risk for aspiration who are being fed intragastrically for two reasons. First, because dietary fat delays gastric emptying [35] and decreases lower esophageal sphincter pressure,[36] the risk of aspiration may be greater for patients receiving higher-fat (i.e., polymeric) formulas. Second, given the inflammatory and immunosuppressant effects of the eicosanoids arising from ω-6 fatty acid metabolism, [37] the aspiration of an enteral formula rich in ω-6 fatty acids may predispose a patient to worsening inflammation and possibly sepsis. Of note, although peptide-based formulas are higher in total fat content than free amino acid–based formulas, the additional fat in these products generally comes from medium-chain triglycerides rather than the potentially harmful ω-6 fatty acids. A study done at Deaconess Hospital in Boston showed no appreciable differences in tolerance or compliance with nutrient goals in critically ill patients receiving defined-formula diets that contained either amino acids or peptides as the protein source.[38]

Predigested formulas are three to five times more expensive than polymeric formulas. Thus once the acute phase of illness has subsided and gut function is believed to have improved, attempts should be made to transition gradually to a less expensive polymeric formula.

Stage II (Polymeric) Formulas. Polymeric formulas contain intact macronutrients (carbohydrate, protein, fat) and therefore

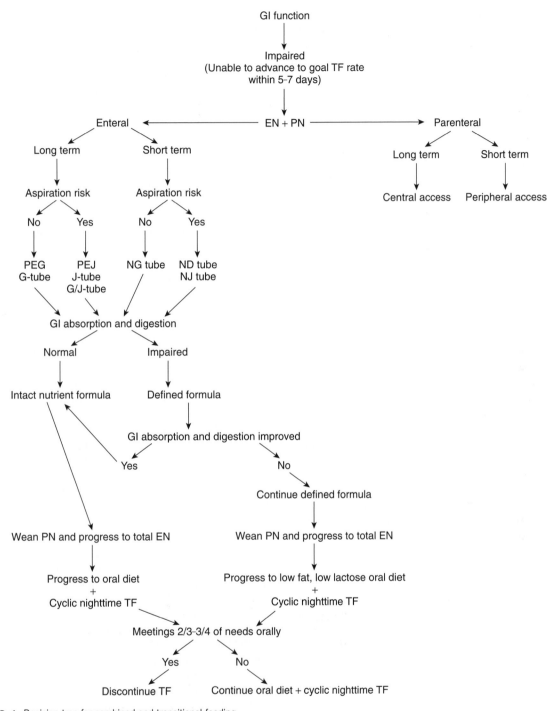

FIGURE 22-1 Decision tree for combined and transitional feeding.

require normal digestive and absorptive capability. As a result, patients who have normal GI function, have been NPO for a short time, or have demonstrated tolerance for a predigested formula administered at goal rate most likely will tolerate a polymeric formula.

Traditionally, clinicians believed that regardless of bowel function all patients being fed into the small bowel had to receive a predigested formula because the digestive processes of the stomach were being bypassed. Recently, however, a prospective randomized trial showed no difference in the GI tolerance of patients undergoing routine abdominal surgery

who received a free amino acid–based diet compared with those receiving a polymeric formula via a feeding jejunostomy.[39] It is important to note, however, that these patients were not critically ill and had minimal GI dysfunction.

Initial Diet Advancement During Combined Feedings

Central PN may be intitiated at 50% the goal caloric requirements and 100% goal protein requirements. If tolerated, calories may be advanced to full on the second day of PN. Exceptions would be a patient who is at risk of developing refeeding syndrome or who is experiencing difficulties with glycemic control or electrolyte management. These patients may take 3 to 4 days to reach their caloric goal. In contrast, peripheral parenteral nutrition may often be initiated at full caloric goal due to its lower dextrose concentration. Although EN can start simultaneously, it is typically started at such a slow rate that its nutrition contribution is negligible.

Because a large portion of the patients who require combined feeding are critically ill, they often exhibit signs of delayed gastric emptying and do not tolerate intragastric EN. This is undoubtedly related to the transient impairment of gut function that frequently accompanies critical illness. In view of this, it may be prudent to start patients receiving combined feeding on EN that is infused beyond the ligament of Treitz. Further recommendations regarding enteral formula advancement will be discussed in Making the Transition from Parenteral Nutrition to Enteral Nutrition.

Trouble-Shooting Problems Associated with Combined Feeding

HYPERGLYCEMIA. There is an association between elevated blood glucose levels and the development of infectious complications. Therefore the goal should be to keep patients' blood sugar levels at or less than 200 mg/dl. The total amount of carbohydrate being administered (from parenteral and enteral sources) should be monitored carefully and ideally should not exceed 4.0 mg/kg/min, the optimal rate of glucose utilization in stressed patients.[40] Because the goal of combined feeding is to transition the patient completely over to EN or an oral diet, every effort should be made to maintain the enteral infusion rate. Thus if total carbohydrate infusion exceeds 4.0 mg/kg/min, the amount of dextrose delivered parenterally, rather than the enteral infusion rate, should be decreased. It is generally easier to reduce the carbohydrate content of parenteral formulas than of enteral ones, owing to the modular nature of the parenteral solution and the fixed macronutrient percentages inherent in commercially available enteral products.

Another reason for the development of hyperglycemia in patients receiving combined feeding is inappropriate insulin delivery. The route of insulin administration should correspond with the primary route of feeding. In patients receiving the majority of their dextrose from PN, Regular insulin should be provided in the PN bag. At The Cleveland Clinic Foundation, blood sugar levels more than 200 mg/dl necessitate the addition of regular insulin in 10-unit increments and monitoring blood sugar levels every 2 to 4 hours until the level is less than 200 mg/dl.[41] The frequency of monitoring can usually be decreased to every 6 hours as blood sugars remain controlled. As the enteral infusion rate is increased, and the patient begins to receive a greater proportion of calories enterally rather than parenterally, the amount of insulin delivered via PN should be decreased and subcutaneous insulin injections should be started. Daytime hyperglycemia resulting from enteral or oral intake must not be managed with insulin in the PN, or nighttime hypoglycemia may result.

DIARRHEA. Diarrhea is typically defined as stool output greater than 500 ml over 24 hours or more than three stools per day.[42] It occurs in up to 30% of all patients receiving EN.[43] Because the enteral infusion rate is increased gradually (i.e.,

10 ml/hr every 12 to 24 hours) during combined feeding, it affords the bowel ample time to adapt to the infusion of nutrients. Thus formula osmolality is rarely the cause of diarrhea. But medications with high osmolalities (i.e., cimetidine, theophylline, elixirs containing sorbitol) administered through the feeding tube are a major cause of diarrhea.[44] Such medications also irritate the GI tract, particularly when they are "bolused" undiluted down the feeding tube. As long as the patient is receiving combined feeding, it is best to administer all medications intravenously when possible. If the diarrhea persists, the enteral infusion rate may be decreased, or if fat malabsorption is suspected the enteral formula should be switched to a low-fat formula or one rich in medium-chain triglycerides. Fiber-containing formulas may help some patients with diarrhea by increasing intestinal transit time and by supplying the colon with fermentable fiber, which produces short-chain fatty acids, the primary fuel of the colon.[45] Finally, some antibiotics may effect opportunistic proliferation of pathogenic organisms normally suppressed by competitive organisms in the GI tract. *Clostridium difficile,* the organism most often associated with antibiotic-related diarrhea, accounts for 10% to 25% of all cases.[46] If the stool culture is negative for *C. difficile,* antidiarrheal medications may be provided to the patient.

HIGH GASTRIC RESIDUALS. Regurgitation occurs when the enteral formula is not absorbed and consequently accumulates and backs up in the GI tract. Major causes of delayed gastric emptying are sepsis, hyperglycemia, diabetic gastroparesis, postoperative gastric ileus, electrolyte imbalance, and anticholinergic and narcotic drugs. If the patient is being fed intragastrically, the head of the bed should be raised 30 degrees or more and gastric residuals should be monitored every 4 to 6 hours. Generally, if the residuals exceed 200 ml, it is prudent to hold the feeds for at least 1 hour and then start them at the last tolerated infusion rate.[30] Selection of a very low-fat diet (less than 10% of total calories) or administration of intravenous metoclopramide (gastric stimulant) may be useful in patients with continually elevated gastric residuals. Aspiration may occur as a complication of regurgitation. In addition to the preceding recommendations for decreasing gastric residuals, the risk of aspiration may be lessened by using a JET-PEG and feeding transpylorically while decompressing the stomach.

FEEDING TUBE OBSTRUCTION. Feeding tube obstruction may occur due to formula coagulation, obstruction by pill fragments, tube kinking, and precipitation by incompatible medications. It is preferable to dislodge the obstruction rather than replace the tube. In order to minimize the risk of feeding tube obstruction: (1) provide medications in the form of elixirs, rather than pills, if they are to be delivered via the feeding tube; (2) flush the tube with water or saline before and after medication administration; and (3) flush the tube with water or saline after gastric residuals are checked.[47]

Transitional Feeding
Making the Transition from Parenteral Nutrition to Enteral Nutrition

Formula selection when transitioning from PN to EN depends on the digestive and absorptive capabilities of the GI tract (Fig. 22-2). Standard polymeric formulas may be used for patients

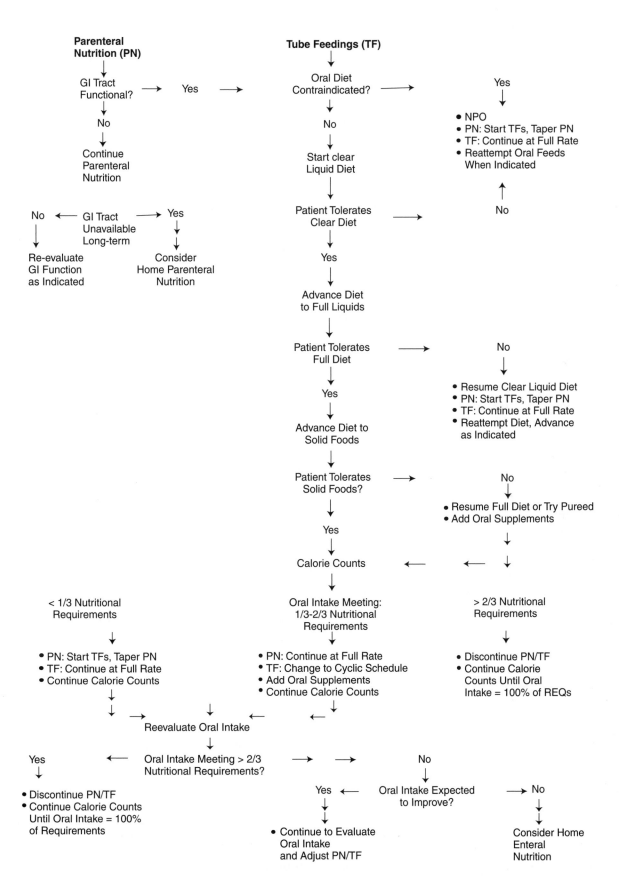

FIGURE 22-2 Transitional feedings. (Reprinted with permission from Matarese LE: *Nutrition support handbook,* Cleveland, OH, 1997, The Cleveland Clinic Foundation, p 96.)

TABLE 22-1
Dual Feeding Schedule and Dosing

Optimal Schedule	Parenteral Diet	Enteral Diet
Day 1	100% of nutrient requirements*	10 ml/hr
Day 2	Decrease infusion rate by 10-20 ml/hr	20-30 ml/hr†
Day 3	Decrease infusion rate by 10-20 ml/hr	30-40 ml/hr†
Day 4	Decrease infusion rate by 10-20 ml/hr	40-50 ml/hr†
Day 5	Stop parenteral nutrition‡; continue intravenous infusion of fluid and electrolytes if necessary	Continue to increase enteral diet by 10 ml/hr every 12-24 hr until goal rate is reached; then mix in additives as needed

*Only possible if patient does not require fluid restriction or is not at risk for refeeding syndrome or electrolyte abnormalities.
†Advance enteral infusion rate only if tolerated.
‡If possible, leave central line in place until certain that patient can tolerate goal tube-feeding rate.

who have the capacity to digest and absorb nutrients. Those patients with impaired digestion and absorption should receive a predigested formula. How long it takes for a patient to advance from PN to EN depends on his or her clinical status. If a patient experiences signs and symptoms of GI intolerance (i.e., abdominal distention, nausea, vomiting, diarrhea) as the tube feeds are advanced, it may be necessary to hold the EN at 10 to 20 ml/hr for several days or weeks until the intestine adapts.

In contrast, patients whose GI insult or dysfunction is minimal should be able to transition from PN to EN within a week. Enteral nutrition may be started full strength at 25 to 50 ml/hr and advanced in 10- to 25-ml/hr increments every 12 to 24 hours until the goal rate is obtained. After tolerance to EN is demonstrated, PN should be tapered by approximately the same amount of calories, protein, and fluid that are being provided by the EN. Parenteral nutrition can usually be discontinued when the patient is receiving about 75% of his or her requirements via EN,[48] unless the patient has significant urine, stool, or drain output that requires supplementation with intravenous fluid and electrolytes. After discontinuation of PN, the enteral infusion rate should continue to increase by 10 to 25 ml/hr every 12 to 24 hours until the patient reaches the goal rate. Once the patient's goal rate has been reached, additional additives such as protein modules can be mixed into the enteral formula (Table 22-1). This approach may help to decrease the incidence of GI overload and failure of enteral technique often associated with more aggressive approaches to initial feeding of patients with transient gut dysfunction. If possible, intravenous access should be left in place, even after PN is stopped, until it has been established that the patient can tolerate the goal enteral feeding rate.

Transition to bolus, intermittent, or cyclic EN is best done after tolerance to continuous feeding is demonstrated. Bolusing of the EN involves the rapid delivery (20 minutes or less) of 240 to 400 ml of formula several times a day. A syringe is used to infuse the feeding into the stomach. This method is more frequently used in home care or with rehabilitation patients to allow them to return to normal activities of daily living. Because bolus feedings can sometimes result in nausea, diarrhea, vomiting, distention, cramps, or aspiration, intolerance can be managed by changing to an intermittent delivery or providing continuously via a cycle. With intermittent feedings,

TABLE 22-2
Guidelines for Transition from a Predigested to a Polymeric Formula

Day	Guideline
1	¾ defined formula + ¼ polymeric formula*
2	½ defined formula + ½ polymeric formula
3	¼ defined formula + ¾ polymeric formula
4	Full-strength polymeric formula
5	Full-strength polymeric formula plus admixtures (i.e., protein module)

*Assuming patient was receiving 1500 ml of a defined formula per day; on day 1, patient would receive 1125 ml (¾ or 75%) of defined formula blended with 375 ml (¼ or 25%) of polymeric formula.

up to 400 ml of formula is delivered into the stomach over a 20- to 30-minute period several times per day by gravity drip or an infusion pump. Cyclic feedings are usually given continuously via an infusion pump over 10 to 12 hours so as to allow the patient mobility when not hooked up to the feeding. Patients who are unable to tolerate large fluid volumes at an increased rate (i.e., patients with congestive heart failure, impaired renal function, or the elderly) may need to be switched to a more calorically dense formula.

Making the Transition from Predigested to Polymeric Enteral Formulas
Some patients receiving combined feeding may initially require a predigested formula owing to transient impairment of gut function related to acute illness or surgery. Once these patients have successfully been transitioned from PN to EN and have demonstrated that they are able to tolerate receiving their full nutrient needs from the predigested formula, it is time to consider transitioning to a polymeric formula. Deaconess Hospital in Boston has developed a novel method for transitioning a patient from a predigested to a polymeric formula (Table 22-2).[49] Although some patients may tolerate being switched directly from a predigested to a polymeric formula, others, particularly those who have long been fed a predigested formula, may exhibit signs of intolerance (i.e., abdominal distention, diarrhea). For such patients, the transitioning method shown in Table 22-2 affords the gut a chance to adapt to the intact protein source and increased fat content of the polymeric formula.

TABLE 22-3

Criteria for Readiness for Transition from Tube to Oral Feeding*

Readiness Criterion	Original Medical Problem Stabilized or Resolved	Nutritional Status Documented as Good	Oral Motor Skills Appropriate	Swallowing Ability Present	Gut Function Adequate
Indicator	Physician judgement	<10% weight loss since admission with nutrition reserves present as judged by anthropometry and/or creatinine height index	Absence of oral motor dysfunction as judged by an occupational or speech/language pathologist	Satisfactory results of videofluoroscopic swallowing study and/or swallowing observed to be normal	Demonstrates tolerance of enteral feeding administered at goal rate
Overcoming barriers	Continue medical treatment	Increase volume of enteral feedings to build reserves	Treat oral motor dysfunction to allow safe oral feeding	Correct tendency toward silent aspiration; provide foods of appropriate consistency	Initiate calorie counts; provide diet appropriate for digestive and absorptive capacity; supplement with nocturnal cyclic tube feedings

*Adapted from Schauster H, Dwyer J: Transition from tube feedings to feedings by mouth in children: Preventing eating dysfunction, *J Am Diet Assoc;* 96: 277–281, 1996.

There are several reasons for making the transition to a polymeric diet. First, polymeric formulas are generally less expensive and require less preparation than some of the predigested formulas. This is relevant for patients fed at home. More important, however, the nutrient composition of polymeric formulas more closely approximates that of an oral diet. Thus, the transition to a polymeric diet helps to prepare the patient for the eventual transition from EN to an oral diet.

Making the Transition from Enteral Nutrition to an Oral Diet

The first step in facilitating a smooth transition from EN to an oral diet is to assess the patient's readiness for making the transition. Table 22-3 lists some criteria for this decision process.[50] Once it has been determined that the patient is indeed ready to start oral feeding, the next step is to implement a feeding plan tailored to meet the patient's nutritional and clinical requirements.

Patients with normal GI function who are not mechanically ventilated and who are tolerating a polymeric formula can generally eat solid foods if these are introduced gradually over 1 to 2 days. Patients usually first receive a clear liquid diet in the morning, and, if that is tolerated, advance to a full liquid diet by afternoon. As soon as the patient has tolerated full liquids for 24 hours, the diet may be advanced to solid food. Although this is the usual diet progression, some patients may be able to proceed directly from clear liquids to solids.

In contrast, patients with impaired GI function (because of extensive bowel resection, malabsorption, or prolonged EN or PN) may require more time to transition to solid foods. Clear liquids are indicated initially for these patients but may have to be diluted to half strength or provided as the sugar-free (i.e., low-calorie) counterpart owing to their hyperosmolarity (Table 22-4).[51] Once patients can tolerate clear liquids, they can be advanced to a low-fat, low-lactose, full-liquid diet (Box 22-1). Patients who have not consumed products containing lactose for more than a month and those who have undergone significant GI surgery are often unable to tolerate the lactose products that are typically provided in a full-liquid diet (i.e., milk, pudding, frappés). For such patients, low-lactose or

TABLE 22-4

Osmolality of Clear Liquids

Item	Mean Osmolality (mOsm/kg)
Cranberry juice	836
Apple juice	705
Orange juice	601
Low-calorie cranberry juice	287
Flavored ice (i.e., Italian ice)	1064
Jell-O	735
Low-calorie Jell-O	57
Cola	714
Diet cola	43
Ginger ale	565
Diet ginger ale	53

Adapted from Bell SJ, Anderson FL, Bistrian BR, et al: Osmolality of beverages commonly provided on clear and full liquid menu, *Nutr Clin Prac* 2:241-244, 1987.

BOX 22-1

Suggestions for Low-Fat, Low-Lactose Full-Liquid Diet for Patients with Gastrointestinal Dysfunction

- All items offered on clear liquid menu (dilute to half strength if patient exhibits signs of intolerance)
- Low-lactose skim milk
- Cream of wheat, cream of rice, farina (if milk is required, use low-lactose skim milk)
- Carnation Instant Breakfast (CIB) made with low-lactose skim milk and additional LactAid drops (to digest lactose in CIB powder)
- Sherbet
- Shakes made by mixing fruit juices and sherbet*
- Yogurt (without fruit) containing active bacterial cultures*
- Commercially available low-fat, low-lactose oral supplements

*Introduce gradually to assess tolerance.

lactose-free products are indicated. In addition, these patients, particularly those with known fat malabsorption or intolerance secondary to disease or surgery, often do better with a low-fat diet. As the patient is gradually transitioned to solid food, it is

TABLE 22-5

Guidelines for Initiating Cyclic Nighttime Feedings

Day	Guideline
1	Cycle tube feeding over 18 hr (i.e., 18:00-12:00)
2	Decrease cycle to 12 hr (i.e., 20:00-08:00)
3	Decrease cycle to 8 or 10 hr (i.e., 20:00-06:00)

usually possible to liberalize the lactose and fat restrictions without causing undesirable repercussions.

Another group of patients who may need more time to make the transition from EN to an oral diet are those who have difficulty swallowing because of a tracheostomy, prolonged intubation, or a neurologic impairment. A swallowing evaluation by the speech therapist will help to determine whether the patient is ready to begin eating and, if so, what types of foods (i.e., thin liquids, thickened liquids, pureed) will be tolerated best. Such patients may initially require help with eating. In addition, they should be monitored while eating for signs of dysphagia, aspiration, and swallowing discomfort.

Regardless of whether the patient's transition period is short or long, assessment of caloric intake (i.e., calorie counts) should begin when a full-liquid diet is ordered. Then, for patients who can tolerate an oral diet, the volume of the EN should be decreased accordingly and given only at night. Although this is controversial, many clinicians believe that nocturnal cycling of the EN may help to improve the patient's appetite. At the very least, nocturnal cyclic EN allows the patient to move about more during the day. An example of how cyclic nighttime feedings can be initiated and progressed is shown in Table 22-5.[52]

Once the patient can consume two thirds to three quarters of his or her calorie and protein needs by mouth [52] and at least 1000 ml of fluid for 3 consecutive days, the EN may be stopped. If oral intake is slow to improve, it may be necessary to employ the use of oral supplements. The nasogastric or transnasally placed postpyloric tube should be removed. If the patient has a permanent access tube, it should be capped and flushed with at least 30 ml of warm water daily to preserve patency. Permanent feeding tubes should be left in place until the next outpatient visit, at which time a nutrition support clinician can reassess the patient's nutritional status before the tube is removed.

Making the Transition from Parenteral Nutrition to an Oral Diet

The guidelines presented above for initiating oral feeding of patients, with or without GI dysfunction, can also be applied to the transition from PN to an oral diet. Patients receiving PN often complain of anorexia that interferes with their ability to resume normal oral intake. Although the mechanisms underlying the development of PN-induced anorexia remain controversial, several theories exist. It has been suggested that the feeling of satiety that some patients experience when receiving PN may be related to an elevated serum insulin level that is similar to that of the postprandial state.[53] Other investigators suggest that the anorexia associated with PN may be related to delayed gastric emptying rather than satiety or an existing disease.[54] This finding, coupled with the fact that elevated

blood glucose levels have been shown to delay gastric emptying,[55,56] suggests that maintaining good blood glucose control is essential during attempts to transition from PN to an oral diet. Otherwise, gastric emptying may be further delayed and elevated serum insulin levels may induce feelings of satiety.

Although gastric emptying and serum insulin levels undoubtedly play a role in reducing food intake during PN, Meguid and colleagues suggest that spontaneous food intake during PN is regulated by a more complex series of mechanisms. Experimental evidence suggests that meal size and meal number are controlled by two different neurotransmitters, dopamine and serotonin, respectively, that are secreted in two separate areas of the hypothalamus.[57] During eating, dopamine levels increase in proportion to meal size.[58] This rise in dopamine levels during oral intake is thought to be related to increased plasma glucose levels and to positive stimuli from the mouth and the nose.[59] During the parenteral infusion of nutrients, the oronasal stimuli are lacking and dopamine release is blunted. Dopamine release is also controlled by the liver. When the liver senses absorbed nutrients in the blood, it signals the brain to reduce dopamine release.[59] Taken together, these two factors help to further explain the reduction in oral intake often associated with PN.

These findings suggest that, as with EN, it may be beneficial to cycle the PN at night to help increase the patient's appetite during the day. Cycling the PN allows the liver to mobilize stored glycogen and may decrease the incidence of fatty liver and promote better nitrogen accretion.[59] Parenteral nutrition solutions may be concentrated and the total volume infused reduced as the patient begins oral intake to prevent fluid overload. To avoid abrupt fluctuations in blood glucose and insulin levels induced by cyclic PN, the solution is generally infused at 50% of the goal rate for the first hour and tapered in the same manner 1 hour before cessation.[59] Calorie counting should begin once the patient begins a full-liquid diet, and as intake of fluids, calories, and protein increases, the PN formula should be adjusted accordingly. Once the patient is able to consume two thirds to three quarters of the protein and calorie needs by mouth[52] and drink at least 1000 ml of fluid per day for 3 consecutive days, PN may be discontinued. If the patient is tolerating an oral diet but is simply unable to eat enough to meet nutrient requirements (even with oral supplements), cyclic nocturnal EN should be considered.

Discharge Planning

Some patients may be medically stable and ready for discharge from the hospital but have yet to complete their diet transition; the discharge process should not be delayed for such patients. Continuation of nutrition support and advancement to an oral diet (following the aforementioned plans) can readily be accomplished at home or in a long-term care facility.

The transition to home or to a long-term care facility for a patient requiring continued nutrition support can be facilitated provided a few simple steps are taken before discharge from the hospital. The first step is to ensure that the patient has the appropriate feeding access for continuation of nutrition support after discharge. Next the nutrition support clinician and the patient need to coordinate a reasonable and convenient plan for administering nutrition support at home. Patients with gastrostomy tubes who go home on EN may prefer to administer their formula via the bolus or intermittent gravity-flow method as opposed to the continual nocturnal cycle. In contrast, because patients being fed into the small bowel rarely tolerate bolus or gravity-drip feedings, they will likely need to continue nocturnal cyclic feedings. If a formula change is indicated, ideally, patients should be switched to the appropriate formula before discharge to ensure tolerance. Once the administration method, feeding schedule, and the type and amount of formula needed have been determined, the home care agency or long-term care facility should be informed of the patient's upcoming discharge.

Preparing a patient for discharge home from The CCF on PN requires a thorough evaluation by a multidisciplinary team. Persons involved in the screening process who evaluate the appropriateness of home PN therapy include physicians, NST dietitians, NST pharmacist, NST nurses, NST social worker, a case manager, and a psychiatrist. In general, patients must be stable, without major organ failure, able to perform all tasks necessary (or have a designated caregiver), and have a reasonable life expectancy and quality of life. Placement of a long-term venous access device is required in patients leaving the hospital on home PN. Once the fluid, energy, and protein requirements are determined and the patient is stable on the PN formula, cycling of the daily infusion in a stepwise fashion should begin with the goal of providing the PN for only part of the day. As the PN formula is being adjusted and cycled, patient and family teaching is initiated. The patient is ready for discharge once the formula is stable, the PN is cycled and tolerated, fluid and electrolytes have been adjusted, and the patient or family member can perform all procedures independently and feels ready to go home.

The complete feeding regimen, whether PN or EN, should be documented by the nutrition support clinician in the patient's medical record, along with a statement that home nutrition support is medically necessary (which is required for third-party reimbursement). In addition, patients going home should be provided with a copy of their feeding regimen and instructions on how to complete the transition to an oral diet, if appropriate. The final essential step in the discharge process is to ensure that some system for ongoing patient follow-up is in place.

Conclusion

Combined feeding is clearly an effective means of providing nutrition to a variety of patients, but those who most often need combined feeding and will most likely benefit from it are the critically ill. Traditionally, critically ill patients were fed principally via the parenteral route, owing to frequent disturbances in GI function that were believed to preclude the use of EN. More recently, clinicians have come to recognize the importance of EN for maintaining gut mucosal integrity and immunocompetence. In addition, we now know that the gut is a potential source of sepsis when the intestinal barrier is disrupted. In view of these findings, maintaining gut function and integrity through EN (even small amounts) during critical illness may be essential for minimizing septic complications and organ failure. Thus the simultaneous use of PN and oral

nutrition provides dependable nutrition support while delivering the benefits of enteral feeding without the side effects related to tolerance.

With the exception of clinical conditions that absolutely preclude the administration of EN, most patients who are candidates for PN should be able to receive EN at the same time (Fig. 22-2). Candidates for combined feeding tend to fall into one of two categories: patients who have been receiving or are expected to receive PN for more than 5 to 7 days, and patients who have been or are expected to be unable to advance to their goal enteral feeding rate within 5 to 7 days. The one thing that these two categories of patients have in common is that they are initially unable to be fully supported via the enteral route. Most often the limiting factor is a temporary impairment of GI function. In view of this, GI tolerance during combined feeding is often best if the EN is delivered distal to the pylorus. Upon initiation of combined feeding, most of the calories, micronutrients, and fluids are given by vein, and EN is infused at a slow rate (10 to 20 ml/hr). As the patient convalesces and the enteral infusion rate is gradually increased, the rate of the parenteral nutrition is decreased and eventually stopped. Patients who are tolerating all of their nutrient needs via EN may begin the transition to an oral diet. If after discharge the patient continues to require EN, the formula should ideally be provided overnight with daytime oral intake if appropriate.

REFERENCES

1. Roslyn JJ, Pitt A, Mann LL, et al: Gallbladder disease in patients on long-term parenteral nutrition, *Gastroenterology* 84:148-154, 1983.
2. Saito H, Trocki O, Alexander JW, et al: The effect of route of nutrient administration on the nutritional state, catabolic hormone secretion, and gut mucosal integrity after burn injury, *J Parenter Enteral Nutr* 11:1-7, 1987.
3. Alverdy J, Chi HS, Sheldon GF: The effect of parenteral nutrition on gastrointestinal immunity. The importance of enteral stimulation, *Ann Surg* 202:681-684, 1985.
4. Moore FA, Moore EE, Jones TN, et al: TEN versus TPN following major abdominal trauma-reduced septic morbidity, *J Trauma* 29:916-923, 1989.
5. Moore FA, Feliciano DV, Andrassy RJ, et al: Early enteral feeding, compared with parenteral, reduces postoperative septic complications. The results of a meta-analysis, *Ann Surg* 216:172-183, 1992.
6. Kudsk KA, Croce MA, Fabian TC, et al: Enteral versus parenteral feeding. Effects on septic morbidity after blunt and penetrating abdominal trauma, *Ann Surg* 215:503-513, 1992.
7. Chiarelli A, Enzi G, Casadei A, et al: Very early nutrition supplementation in burned patients, *Am J Clin Nutr* 51:1035-1039, 1990.
8. Mochizuki H, Trocki O, Dominioni L, et al: Mechanism of prevention of postburn hypermetabolism and catabolism by early enteral feeding, *Ann Surg* 200:297-310, 1984.
9. Kudsk KA, Stone JM, Carpenter G, Sheldon GF: Enteral and parenteral feeding influences mortality after hemoglobin B E. coli peritonitis in normal rats, *J Trauma* 23:605-609, 1983.
10. Kudsk KA, Carpenter BA, Peterson S, Sheldon GF: Effect of enteral and parenteral feeding in malnourished rats with E. coli–hemoglobin adjuvant peritonitis, *J Surg Res* 31:105-110, 1981.
11. Shou J, Lappin J, Minnard EA, Daly JM: Total parenteral nutrition, bacterial translocation, and host immune function, *Am J Surg* 167:145-150, 1994.
12. Steiger E et al: Patient selection. In Matarese LE (ed): *Nutrition support handbook*, Cleveland, OH, 1997, The Cleveland Clinic Foundation, pp 9-11.
13. Kudsk KA, Minard G: Enteral nutrition. In Zaloga GP (ed): *Nutrition in critical care*, St Louis, 1994, Mosby, pp 331-360.
14. Smith-Choban P, Max MH: Feeding jejunostomy: A small bowel stress test? *Am J Surg* 155:112-117, 1988.
15. Khoury TL, Borlase BC, Forse RA, et al: Early enteral feeding via a jejunostomy: a safe technique in critically ill patients. In Borlase BC, Bell SJ, Blackburn GL, Forse RA (eds): *Enteral nutrition*, New York, 1994, Chapman and Hall, pp 142-151.

16. Rombeau JL: Enteral nutrition and critical illness. In Borlase BC, Bell SJ, Blackburn GL, Forse RA (eds): *Enteral nutrition,* New York, 1994, Chapman and Hall, pp 25-36.

17. Moss G, Greenstein A, Levy S, et al: Maintenance of GI function after bowel surgery and immediate enteral full nutrition. I. Doubling of canine colorectal anastomotic bursting pressure and intestinal wound mature collagen content, *J Parenter Enteral Nutr* 4:535-538, 1980.

18. Delany HM, Demetrio AA, Teh E, Levenson SM: Effect of early postoperative nutritional support on skin wound and colon anastomosis healing, *J Parenter Enteral Nutr* 14:357-361, 1990.

19. Zaloga GP, Bortenschlager L, Black KW, Prielipp R: Immediate postoperative enteral feeding decreases weight loss and improves wound healing after abdominal surgery in rats, *Crit Care Med* 20:115-118, 1992.

20. Schroeder D, Gillanders L, Mahr K, Hill GL: Effects of immediate postoperative enteral nutrition on body composition, muscle function, and wound healing, *J Parenter Enteral Nutr* 15:376-383, 1991.

21. Jenkins M, Gottschlich M, Warden GD: Enteral feeding during operative procedures in thermal injuries, *J Burn Care Rehabil* 15:199-205, 1994.

22. Moore EE, Jones TN: Benefits of immediate jejunostomy feeding after major abdominal trauma—a prospective, randomized study, *J Trauma* 26:874-881, 1986.

23. Grahm TW, Zadrozny DB, Harrington T: The benefits of early jejunal hyperalimentation in the head-injured patient, *Neurosurgery* 25:729-735, 1989.

24. Skipper A, Marian MJ: Parenteral nutrition. In Gottschlich MM, Matarese LE, Shronts EP (eds): Nutrition support dietetics core curriculum, ed 2, Silver Spring, MD, 1994, *Am J Parenter Enteral Nutr,* pp 105-117.

25. Labow CA: Venous access device options, *Surg Oncol Clin North Am* 4:473-478, 1995.

26. Orr M: Vascular access device selection for parenteral nutrition, *Nutr Clin Pract* 14: 172-177, 1999.

27. Thompson SE: Insertion of peripherally inserted central catheters for the administration of total parenteral nutrition, *Nutr Clin Pract* 14:191-193, 1993.

28. Alkimyary A, Fernandez C, Picard M, et al: Safety and efficacy of total parenteral nutrition delivered via a peripherally inserted central venous catheter, *Nutr Clin Pract* 11:199-203, 1996.

29. Allen AW, Megargell JL, Brown DB, et al: Venous thrombosis associated with the placement of peripherally inserted central catheters, *JVIR* 11:1309-1314, 2000.

30. Russell M, Cromer M, Grant J: Complications of enteral nutrition therapy. In Gottschlich MM (ed): *The science and practice of nutrition support, a core-based curriculum,* Dubuque, IA, Kendall/Hunt Publishing Company, 2001, pp 189-210.

31. Klodell CT, Carroll M, Carrillo E, et al: Routine intragastric feeding following traumatic brain injury is safe and well tolerated, *Am J Surg* 179:168-171, 2000.

32. DeChicco RS, Matarese LE: Selection of nutrition support regimens, *Nutr Clin Pract* 7:239-245, 1992.

33. Brinson RR, Kolts BE: Diarrhea associated with severe hypoalbuminemia: a comparison of a peptide-based chemically defined diet and standard enteral alimentation, *Crit Care Med* 16:130-136, 1988.

34. Brinson RR, Pitts WM: Enteral nutrition in the critically ill patient: role of hypoalbuminemia, *Crit Care Med* 17:367-370, 1989.

35. Cooke AR: Localization of receptors inhibiting gastric emptying in the gut, *Gastroenterology* 72:875-880, 1977.

36. Kroop HS, Long WB, Alavi A, et al: Effect of water and fat on gastric emptying of solid meals, *Gastroenterology* 77:997-1000, 1979.

37. Kinsella JE, Lokesh B., Broughton S, Whelan J: Dietary polyunsaturated fatty acid and eicosanoids: potential effects on the modulation of inflammatory and immune cells: an overview, *Nutrition* 6:24-45, 1990.

38. Borlase BC, Bell SJ, Lewis EJ, et al: Tolerance to enteral tube feeding diets in hypoalbuminemic critically ill, geriatric patients, *Surg Gynecol Obstet* 174:181-188, 1992.

39. Ford EG, Hull SF, Jenning M, Andrassy RJ: Clinical comparison of tolerance to elemental or polymeric enteral feedings in the postoperative patient, *J Am Coll Nutr* 11:11-16, 1992.

40. Burke JF, Wolfe RR, Mullany CJ, et al: Glucose requirements following burn injury: parameters of optimal glucose infusion and possible hepatic and respiratory abnormalities following excessive glucose intake, *Ann Surg* 190:274-285, 1979.

41. Steiger E et al: Recognition and management of complications. In Matarese LE (ed): *Nutrition support handbook,* Cleveland, OH, 1997, The Cleveland Clinic Foundation, pp 73-80.

42. Thomas S: Gastrointestinal complications: diarrhea and high gastric residuals. In Borlase BC, Bell SJ, Blackburn GL, Forse RA (eds): *Enteral nutrition,* New York, 1994, Chapman and Hall, pp 188-192.

43. DeChicco RS, Hamilton C, Piazza-Barnett R: Enteral and parenteral nutrition support. In Niedert KC (ed): *Nutrition care of the older adult.* Consultant Dietitians in Health Care Facilities and The American Dietetic Association, Chicago, 1998, pp 133-151.

44. Edes TE, Walk BE, Austin JL: Diarrhea in tube-fed patients: feeding formula not necessarily the cause, *Am J Med* 88:91-93, 1990.

45. Collier P, Kudsk KA, Glazer J, et al: Fiber-containing formula and needle catheter jejunostomies: a clinical evaluation, *Nutr Clin Pract* 9:101-108, 1994.

46. Piazza-Barnett R, Matarese, LE: Enteral nutrition in adult medical/surgical oncology. In McCallum PD, Polisena CG (eds): *The clinical guide to oncology nutrition,* Oncology Nutrition Dietetic Practice Group and The American Dietetic Association, Chicago, pp 106-118, 2000.

47. Hamaoui E, Kodsi R: Complications of enteral feeding and their prevention. In Rombeau JL, Rolandelli RH (eds): *Enteral and tube feeding,* Philadelphia, 1997, WB Saunders, pp 554-574.

48. Steiger E et al: Transitional feedings. In Matarese LE (ed): *Nutrition support handbook,* Cleveland, OH, 1997, The Cleveland Clinic Foundation, pp 93-96.

49. Trujillo EB: Transitional feeding strategies for discharge. In Borlase BC, Bell SJ, Blackburn GL, Forse RA (eds): *Enteral nutrition,* New York, 1994, Chapman and Hall, pp 199-205.

50. Schauster H, Dwyer J: Transition from tube feedings to feedings by mouth in children: Preventing eating dysfunction, *J Am Diet Assoc* 96:277-281, 1996.

51. Bell SJ, Anderson FL, Bistrian BR, et al: Osmolality of beverages commonly provided on clear and full liquid menu, *Nutr Clin Pract* 2:241-244, 1987.

52. Zibrida JM, Carlson SJ: Transitional feeding. In Gottschlich MM, Matarese LE, Shronts EP (eds): *Nutrition support dietetics core curriculum,* ed 2, Silver Spring, MD, 1994, American Society for Parenteral and Enteral Nutrition, pp 105-117.

53. Vanderweele DA: Insulin is a prandial satiety hormone, *Physiol Behav* 56:619-622, 1994.

54. De Myttenaere SB, Gil KM, Heymsfield SB, et al: Gastric emptying in humans: influence of different regimes of parenteral nutrition, *Am J Clin Nutr* 60:244-248, 1994.

55. MacGregor IL, Gueller R, Watts HD, Meyer JH: The effect of acute hyperglycemia on gastric emptying in man, *Gastroenterology* 70:190-196, 1976.

56. Nompleggi D, Bell SJ, Blackburn GL, Bistrian BR: Overview of gastrointestinal disorders due to diabetes mellitus: emphasis on nutritional support, *J Parenter Enteral Nutr* 13:84-91, 1989.

57. Meguid MM, Yang ZJ, Koseki M: Eating induced LHA-dopamine rise correlates with meal size in normal and bulbectomized rats, *Brain Res Bull* 36:487-490, 1995.

58. Yang ZJ, Oler A, Meguid MM, et al: Liver plays an inhibitory role on hypothalamic dopamine release during eating and TPN, *Surg Forum* 45:166-169, 1995.

59. Benotti PN, Bothe A Jr, Miller JDB, et al: Cyclic hyperalimentation, *Comp Therapy* 2:27-36, 1976.

Carol Ireton-Jones, PhD, RD, LD, CNSD, FACN

HOME nutrition support is an important component of the expanding sector of home health care. The push to move people quickly through costly acute care systems and on to alternative care sites, especially their homes, will result in more and more people receiving home care, including nutrition support. In 1992 it was estimated that 152,000 patients were receiving enteral nutrition support at home and 40,000 were receiving home parenteral nutrition (HPN).[1] Data from Britain report a population of 2000 to 2500 home enteral nutrition (HEN) and 200 HPN patients.[2] Rollins reported estimates of HPN usage from data management organizations indicating that 36,000 patients were receiving HPN; however, by 1997 the estimate was 35,000 HPN patients with a predicted continuing decline of 1000 HPN patients per year.[3] There are no current figures for the number of people receiving home nutrition support.

The expansion of nutrition support in the home can be attributed to a number of factors.[4] Advances in technology now allow safe, effective administration of nutrition support outside hospitals. Recognition by third-party payers of the relative costs of home care as compared with hospital care as well as the continuing compression of hospital length of stay has expanded insurance coverage options for home nutrition support. There is an increased emphasis on using the GI tract when possible and therefore using enteral nutrition support as well as enteral feeding for conditions previously associated with parenteral nutrition.[3] Nutrition support, especially enteral nutrition, is widely used in long-term care, hospice, and other alternative sites.

Patient surveys indicate that patients prefer home infusion therapy to hospital therapy; thus quality of life is an important advantage of home therapy.[5] Patients receiving home infusion therapy, including home nutrition support, rank being at home with friends and family as the most important aspect of home therapy. In addition, many home patients can return to work or at least to activities of daily living.

Application of Home Nutrition Support

The key to an optimal nutrition outcome and therefore medical outcome for a patient on home nutrition support is providing appropriate and cost-effective nutrition support. A nutrition assessment by a registered dietitian determines nutritional status using medical, nutrition, and medication histories; phys-

ical examination; anthropometry; and laboratory data.[6] Next, energy requirements are estimated from energy equations or indirect calorimetry. A nutrition assessment defines the patient's needs according to nutritional status, therapy goals, and the proposed modality of nutrition support.[6] The choice of the route depends on gastrointestinal (GI) tract function and the patient's ability to eat (Fig. 23-1). Enteral feeding should be used if the gut is functional. Parenteral nutrition is indicated when absorption or function of the GI tract is not sufficient to meet nutrition needs.[7] The appropriate feeding regimen should be individualized for each patient based on realistic therapy goals that may or may not include recovery or return to normal functioning.

An assessment of the home should be made to determine if the patient is truly a candidate for home care given the complexity of home enteral or parenteral nutrition support. Some patients have nutrition support initiated in their homes without being previously hospitalized. Ensuring that an appropriate home environment and care partner are available, as well as proper access has been achieved, is extremely important in these cases. Both HEN and HPN can be well tolerated at home as long-term nutrition support.[3, 8]

Home Enteral Nutrition

Indications

HEN has a variety of clinical indications. The American Society for Parenteral and Enteral Nutrition (ASPEN) has published standards and guidelines for appropriate use of enteral nutrition support for home and long-term care.[9-11] HEN may be used in specific disease states such as cancer, inflammatory bowel disease, acute and progressive neurologic conditions, failure to thrive, and inborn errors of metabolism.[12-16]

In addition to medical diagnosis, a number of other factors should be considered before initiating HEN. Box 23-1 describes some of these important concepts. Ethical implications must also be reviewed before the initiation of HEN. A

BOX 23-1

Selection Criteria for Home Enteral Nutrition

Adequate nutritional intake not possible by modification of oral diet
Medical condition stable
Patient or family consents to therapy
Patient or family able to perform techniques correctly
Safe and adequate home environment
Supplies and home care follow-up available

Acknowledgment: A special thank you is extended to Jody Weckwerth, RD, CNSD, who contributed to the first edition chapter, and to Marianne Duda, MS, RD, LD, CNSD, who reviewed the second edition chapter.

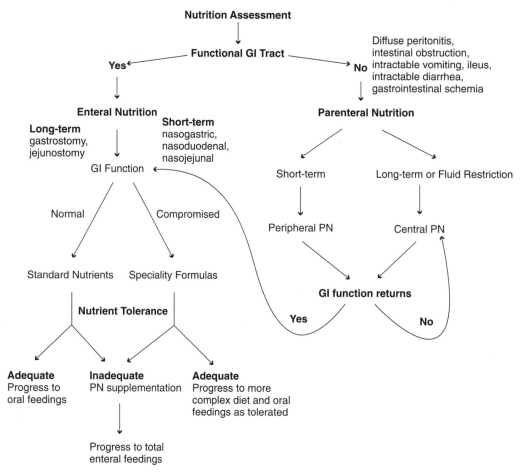

FIGURE 23-1 Route of administration of specialized nutrition support. *GI*, gastrointestinal; *PN*, parenteral nutrition. (Adapted from ASPEN: Clinical pathways and algorithms for delivery of parenteral and enteral nutrition support in adults), *J Parenter Enteral Nutr* 26:8, 2002. Reprinted with permission from *JPEN*.

frank discussion with the patient and/or family of the benefits and burdens of HEN is necessary because it allows participation in the decision-making process. Occasionally this discussion may result in a decision to forgo or delay therapy.[17,18] Ultimately, however, thoroughly informed patients and families adjust better once they are home because they know what to expect.

Formulating the Nutrition Care Plan

ACCESS. When HEN is deemed appropriate, a home nutrition care plan must be developed. Access, formula, and administration technique are addressed. Whenever possible, the potential need for long-term enteral nutrition support should be anticipated before placement of an enteral access device. The patient's diagnosis, level of responsiveness, GI function, long-term nutrition goals, cost, and reimbursement, and personal preference should be considered in the choice of enteral access as should the advantages and disadvantages of various devices (Table 23-1).

Nasogastric and nasointestinal tubes have traditionally been used for short-term (less than 4 weeks) nutrition support. However, nasal tubes can be used much longer, more than 4 years in some instances.[14] For long-term nasoenteric feedings,

the tube should be changed periodically to decrease the risk of nasopharyngeal erosion and tube disintegration. Medicare reimbursement allows one new nasal tube per month. It has been recommended that children have their silicone nasal tubes changed monthly and polyvinyl chloride tubes weekly.[15] Some patients can be taught to place their own nasogastric tubes daily. This enhances acceptance of the enteral therapy, especially by children and adolescents.

Techniques for percutaneous or laparoscopic placement of gastrostomy tubes have made direct gastric access an option, even for patients in whom open procedures are contraindicated. Complications of percutaneous endoscopic gastrostomy (PEG) placement can occur, but the advantages of PEG tubes often outweigh the risks.[19,20] It has been suggested that using PEG for very frail elderly patients is associated with a poor outcome and needs further study.[21]

For children and active adult patients, the low-profile gastrostomy tube design can provide access with minimal effect on body image. Low-profile tubes allow for nearly normal activity with little risk of dislodgment. These access devices are designed as replacements for existing gastrostomy sites but have also been placed at initial laparotomy. Accurate measurement of the stoma tract is essential to securing good fit and

TABLE 23-1
Enteral Access Devices

Type of Tube	Description	Advantages	Disadvantages
Nasogastric			
Adult	No. 8-14 French (F) 36-45 in	Low-risk placement Easy removal	Placement difficult to verify outside hospital Easily dislodged with vomiting or coughing
Pediatric	No. 5-8 F, 20-36 in	Allows for short-term feeding Can be used to verify tolerance before abdominal tube placement Can be inserted and removed daily for active patients	Some discomfort for patient Poor patient body image Difficult to aspirate residual
Nasointestinal	No. 8-12 F, 42-45 in	Low-risk placement Easy removal Allows for short-term feedings	As for nasogastric tube Bolus feedings poorly tolerated
Percutaneous endoscopic gastrostomy	No. 14-22 F	Placed without general anesthesia Body image improved over nasal tube Allows for aspiration of residuals Usable within hours of placement	Requires invasive procedure Removal may require endoscopy Skin irritation or infection may occur Risk of aspiration with bolus feedings and poor gag reflex
Surgical gastrostomy	No. 14-30 F	Body image improved over nasal tube Allows for aspiration of residuals	Placement requires surgical procedure Skin irritation or infection may occur Risk of aspiration with bolus feedings and poor gag reflex
Low-profile gastrostomy	No. 14-24 F, 0.8-4.5 cm	Improved body image Allows for active patient Allows for aspiration of residuals	More costly than regular replacement tubes Size and length must be measured accurately or discomfort and leakage may occur
Surgical jejunostomy	No. 12-24 F	Allows for access below obstructions or fistulae Body image improved over nasal tube	Placement requires surgical procedure Bolus feedings poorly tolerated Difficult to replace Skin irritation or infection may occur

avoiding leakage. Low-profile tubes are more expensive than conventional gastrostomy replacements and therefore might be prohibitive for some patients.[22]

Jejunostomy tubes are the preferred enteral access for patients with gastric dysmotility or obstruction or fistula of the stomach or duodenum. One of the principal disadvantages of jejunal access for home or long-term care is that feedings delivered by syringe or rapid-gravity drip are not well tolerated. Many patients with jejunal access may thus require continuous drip feedings or frequent small-volume intermittent feedings. This can greatly reduce their sense of control over their nutrition support therapy, participation in accustomed activities, and their satisfaction. Though some patients may tolerate jejunal bolus feedings, they are in the minority. Jejunal access is also recommended for patients who are at a high risk for aspiration and whose gag reflex is poor. Gastric feedings can cause relaxation of the lower esophageal sphincter and a corresponding increase in reflux and aspiration.[23] For these patients, jejunostomy access can minimize the potential for respiratory complications. For patients with gastric access who experience aspiration or delayed emptying, gastrojejunal tubes are available. Dual-lumen tubes allow for simultaneous jejunal feeding and gastric decompression.

FORMULA SELECTION. The wide variety of commercial enteral formulas makes it possible to tailor the nutritional regimen to the patient's needs. Factors that determine the formula of choice in an acute care setting may not apply to home or long-term care. Thus the selection of an appropriate formula for long-term use should take into account patients' long-term nutrient requirements, fluid needs, GI tolerance, access site, and medical condition as well as their ability or a care partner's ability to prepare and administer the feeding. Routine reassessment is recommended, and factors such as osmolality, fiber content, and calorie density should be considered. Enteral formulas are reviewed in Chapters 15 and 20.

At home, cost and availability of enteral formula are primary concerns. Patients or care partners must be able to prepare their formula simply and independently. They must have adequate storage for their supply of formula. The form of packaging can also affect the choice of formula for home care. For example, "ready-to-hang" closed systems can decrease the risk of bacterial contamination and may be easier to use if patients have difficulty opening cans, but they may not be as practical for patients on intermittent feeding. Formula, cost, availability, ease of use, and storage issues can affect quality of life and compliance, and ultimately, the success of HEN.

ADMINISTRATION TECHNIQUE. Three options for administration of enteral nutrition in the home care setting are continuous infusion, intermittent gravity-drip infusion, and bolus infusion feedings. *Continuous infusion* is defined as a controlled delivery of formula at a constant rate using an infusion pump. Whenever possible, the rate of infusion during home continuous feedings should be increased to allow a 10- to 14-hour infusion schedule (usually overnight), which facilitates activity during the day. The continuous method is preferred for patients with small bowel access because it minimizes complications such as cramping, bloating, and diarrhea. Although feedings may be administered continuously without an infusion pump, accuracy is more difficult and close monitoring must be maintained to detect inadvertent changes in infusion rate. A need for close monitoring may prohibit nighttime feeding.

Intermittent gravity-drip infusion delivers set volumes of formula at intervals throughout the day. Individual tolerance is widely variable, but most home feedings take 20 to 60 minutes. Feeding volumes of 250 to 500 ml are customary; a few patients tolerate as much as 750 ml per feeding.[24] Gravity-drip infusion may be preferred over continuous infusion in the home setting because it eliminates the need for an infusion pump.

Bolus infusion delivers a large volume of formula over a short time. Like gravity-drip, bolus infusion is intermittent with three to six (or more) feedings per day. Volumes are similar but the rate is much faster. Bolus infusion is most often accomplished with a syringe. The principal advantages of this method are the inexpensive simple equipment, the speed in which feedings can be completed, and the similarity to regular meals. The disadvantage is increased risk of regurgitation, aspiration, and GI intolerance. Bolus feedings are rarely recommended for small bowel infusion.

Most enteral patients utilize bolus or intermittent feedings; however, some may require a pump. This is often initiated after a failure of the other two methods of administration due to the extra cost of infusion pumps. Sound clinical judgment is necessary to determine when a trial of gravity infusion is reasonable and when it would be inappropriate because of the patient's medical condition.

The patient and family should be encouraged to help decide which infusion method they will use at home. They should also help design the home regimen, taking into account work schedules, family activities, and other commitments. Providing feedings in a "mealtime" pattern can enhance socialization and a positive attitude of the patient. The feeding schedule and medication regimen should be adjusted to the regular home routine. Allowing the patient and family to create their own schedules may enhance acceptance of home enteral therapy.[25,26]

Reimbursement

Reimbursement of home enteral feedings can be quite challenging. Third party payer (insurance company) contracts vary related to enteral feeding coverage at home. Many reimburse for enteral feeding supplies and services using a range of a daily, or per diem, rate. The enteral feeding product is not always covered and if covered is usually reimbursed at a rate at or less than average wholesale price. Reimbursement availability also plays a role in selection of administration technique. Owing to the extra cost of infusion pumps, some third party payers may require proof of intolerance to bolus or gravity infusion before they approve reimbursement for a pump.

Medicare reimbursement of enteral feedings is based on strict guidelines set forth by the Centers for Medicare & Medicaid Services (CMS), formerly the Healthcare Financing Administration. There are two main criteria that must be met for Medicare to reimburse for home enteral feeding. First the patient must meet the criteria of permanence, meaning that the patient will require enteral feeding at home for a long and indefinite period of at least 90 days or lifetime, and second, the patient must have a impaired functional capacity either anatomically or due to a motility disorder. If a patient requires a pump-assisted feeding, or a specialized formula, additional documentation is required to obtain reimbursement from Medicare. For surgically or percutaneously endoscopically placed gastric or jejunal feeding tubes, Medicare covers one feeding device every 3 months. A skilled home nutrition support clinician can assist the patient, referral source, and home care provider in ensuring that appropriate documentation is provided so that Medicare reimbursement or reimbursement by a third party payer is obtained.

Additionally, many payers do not reimburse for clinical management for enteral patients other than an initial teaching visit. Clinicians generally agree that some home enteral patients require more intensive clinical management such as those patients receiving jejnunal feedings with specialty formulas for pancreatitis; however, negotiations for reimbursement of clinician fees for patient management usually must be negotiated outside of the usual contractual agreements.

Preparing Patient and Family

EDUCATION. As soon as a patient is identified as a potential candidate for HEN, training should commence. The longer the patient is included in performing the techniques of HEN, the easier the transition to home will be; however, due to shorter hospital stays, many patients receive only partial instruction in the hospital, which is continued at home.[27-30] Patient education should cover the feeding tube, formula, supplies, monitoring, and potential complications whether the patient receives this information in the hospital prior to discharge or when HEN is initiated in the home. Table 23-2 lists the steps of educating HEN patients. Standardized teaching plans and educational materials can greatly facilitate patient education. A number of excellent materials are available for HEN.[31] At minimum, the following information should be provided to the patient in writing and documented in the medical record:

- Site and brand of tube and length of tube remaining outside the body
- Type of formula and its concentration
- Total daily formula volume
- Method and rate of administration
- Feeding frequency schedule (times)
- Volume and times for tube flushes
- Dose and times for medications
- Guidelines for oral intake

Detailed information and recommendations provided to home care agencies allow for education to continue in the patient's own home. Figure 23-2 depicts a nutrition care plan summary designed to facilitate communication between hospital and home care clinicians. Adequate patient and care partner education as well as regular follow-up will help to avoid readmission from complications.

SUPPLIES. Along with education and training, the coordinators of HEN support are responsible for helping the patient obtain necessary supplies and equipment. Options include home nutrition support companies, durable medical equipment (DME) supply companies, hospital-based home care agencies, and local pharmacies. Factors in choosing a supplier are the anticipated duration of therapy, need for clinical monitoring, complexity of the equipment, convenience, reliability, and the patient's finances or third-party coverage.

Patients who require HEN for less than 2 weeks may be able to take enough supplies home with them from the hospital so that arrangements with another vendor will not be necessary.

TABLE 23-2

Home Enteral Education Checklist

Patient Outcome	Intervention
A. Patient will state understanding of feeding therapy and equipment.	1. Provide educational materials. 2. Discuss reason for enteral nutrition. 3. Show and discuss function of equipment. 4. Identify brand and size of patient's feeding tube and record. 5. Record and explain feeding schedule, rate of delivery, and total volume required. 6. Have patient state reason for therapy and function of equipment.
B. Patient will demonstrate checking of tube placement.	Instruct and observe in: 1. Demonstration of tube placement check (residual check or tube marking)
C. Patient will demonstrate correct procedure for feeding administration.	Instruct and observe in: 1. Hand washing 2. Formula preparation 3. Equipment setup 4. Patient position for feeding 5. Priming of tubing 6. Connection to feeding tube 7. Rate control with flow regulator or pump
D. Patient will demonstrate correct procedure for discontinuation of administration.	Instruct and observe in: 1. Stopping pump or clamping set 2. Disconnecting tubing from feeding tube 3. Flushing tube 4. Clamping of feeding tube 5. Positioning of tube when off feedings 6. Care and storage of feeding equipment
E. Patient will demonstrate medication administration through feeding tube.	Instruct and observe in: 1. Crushing of meds or liquid preparations 2. Meds to not use in feeding tube 3. Dosage and time of meds 4. Tube flushing before and after each med 5. Potential side effects and/or drug-nutrient interactions
F. Patient will demonstrate correct tube site care.	Instruct and observe in: 1. Dressing removal 2. Cleansing of skin 3. Removal of crusts with diluted hydrogen peroxide 4. Observing for signs of irritation or infection 5. Applying clean dressing 6. Retaping procedure
G. Patient will state potential complications and interventions.	Explain procedure and actions to take for: 1. Tube dislodgment 2. Tube clogging 3. Intolerance to enteral feedings: diarrhea, nausea, vomiting, constipation, bloating 4. Weight changes 5. Method for recording oral and tube intake 6. Procedure for contacting home health nurse, dietitian, or physician

Local pharmacies or discount stores can also provide formula and simple equipment such as syringes and site care needs, sometimes at lower cost than full-service home care companies. This option is particularly good for patients whose primary insurance coverage is Medicare and whose HEN therapy is expected to be short term (deemed by the physician to be required for fewer than 90 days). Because Medicare does not reimburse for short-term HEN, the patient and family may save money by purchasing their formula and disposable supplies directly from a pharmacy or discount store.

Although most HEN patients could benefit from a full-service home infusion provider, many patients receive HEN supplies and formula from a DME company. Rarely is clinical monitoring provided by a DME company because in most cases, the company provides only supplies. Home nutrition support companies provide the benefits of consistency and product availability, 24-hour support, home delivery, monitoring of progress by trained health care professionals, follow-up reports to the referring physician, and expertise in billing and obtaining reimbursement. For companies that are accredited, standards must be maintained that can help ensure high-quality service to HEN patients.[32]

MONITORING AND COMPLICATIONS. The recommended frequency and intensity of monitoring of patients on home enteral nutrition support vary a great deal depending on the patient's medical condition, tolerance, and ability for self-care. If the

MAYO CLINIC ▬▬▬▬ HOSPITAL ▬

Enteral Nutrition Dismissal Summary

☐ Saint Marys
☐ Methodist
☐ Mayo Clinic (outpatient)

Date _____ Referral to _____

Referral from _____ _____

Phone (507) _____ _____

Hospital _____

_____
Number and Name (above)

Age _____ Height _____ cm _____ inches Oral intake _____

Weight: Current _____ kg _____ pounds Goals _____

Goal _____ kg _____ pounds _____

Formula _____ Manufacturer _____

Volume per day _____ provides _____ kcal per day

Concentration _____ _____ grams protein per day

If this product is unavailable, _____ can be used.

Infusion Method and Schedule:

____ Intermittent: Infuse _____ ml over _____ minutes _____ times per day

____ Continuous: Infuse _____ ml/hour for _____ hours from _____ to _____

Feeding Tube Type: _____ Size _____

____ Nasogastric ____ Percutaneous gastrostomy ____ Gastrostomy ____ Jejunostomy ____ Other _____

Water Flushes: Volume per day _____ ml _____ ml water per flush _____ flushes per day

Vitamin/mineral supplementation _____

Recommend that weight be monitored _____ times per week

Recommend that electrolytes (Na, K, Cl, HCO_3), pH, blood glucose, albumin, creatinine, AST and alkaline phosphatase be monitored every

_____ day(s) until stable and every _____ thereafter

Enteral nutrition administration instructions have been given to _____

Enteral nutrition equipment and supplies and follow-up are being arranged by _____, Registered Dietitian,
Mayo Clinic, W-18, Rochester, MN 55905. Telephone: (507) 284-4990.

Additional information:

MEDICAL RECORD COPY

FIGURE 23-2 Nutrition care plan summary. (Reprinted with permission of Mayo Foundation for Medical Education and Research, Rochester, MN.)

referring physician or nutrition support team will not be following the patient, it is important to determine if the HEN provider has nutrition support clinicians on staff to monitor HEN patients prior to referral. Periodic follow-up and laboratory monitoring are useful to determine progress. Patients with electrolyte or glucose fluctuations, hypoalbuminemia, or complex disease processes should be assessed at regular intervals.[33,34] Vitamin and mineral deficiencies can occur if the enteral feeding is inadequate or the disease process changes or progresses. Some HEN patients may require daily follow-up initially (usually telephonically), then weekly, and later monthly. Stable, long-term HEN patients require follow-up only once or twice per year.[35]

Rehospitalization is rarely necessary for complications of HEN, according to data from the Oley Foundation. For example, in their report, rehospitalization rates for patients with a primary diagnosis of neoplasm were just 0.36 admission per patient per year for HEN-related problems. Readmission rates for HEN-unrelated problems were higher: 2.58 admissions per patient per year; however, because of the nature of HEN complications it is often difficult to determine whether a particular complication is a direct result of HEN therapy or is due to an

underlying medical condition.[1] When HEN patients and families are prepared in advance for problems that might occur, the complications of HEN therapy can be addressed before they become serious enough to require expensive interventions such as emergency department care or hospitalization.

A thorough discussion of the management of complications of enteral nutrition can be found in Chapter 17. The complications seen more frequently in home care settings are discussed in the following text and in Table 23-3. Mechanical problems such as tube clogging can usually be prevented by appropriate medication administration and by proper flushing. Medication dosing forms and administration technique should be reviewed to ensure compatibility with enteral feedings.[36] Flushing tubes before, between, and after administration of medications results in fewer clogs than flushing only *after* the medication is given.[37] Water flushes should also be given at 4- to 8-hour intervals throughout a continuous infusion and before and after each intermittent feeding. Smaller tubes may have to be flushed every 2 hours. Patients receiving fiber-enhanced, high-calorie or high protein formulas may require more frequent flushing.

Once a tube has clogged, usual recommendations are to clear it with warm water, soda pop, or pancreatic enzyme (in

Home Enteral Nutrition Complications

Complication	Possible Causes	Prevention and Interventions
Mechanical		Clean site, cover with dressing.
Accidental removal of abdominal tube		Replace tube as soon as possible (tract will close in a few hours).
Coughing, choking, gagging with nasal tube	Displacement of tube	Confirm tube placement.
		Remove tube if symptoms persist.
Clogged tube	Inadequate flushing	Aspirate tube contents with empty syringe.
	Small tube diameter	Flush repeatedly with warm water.
	Medications sticking to tube	Flush with pancreatic enzymes/bicarbonate.
		Gently manipulate length of tube with fingertips.
Tube site irritation or infection	Composition of tube	Pull tube up until internal balloon is against stomach wall; anchor.
	Sensitive skin	
	Leakage of gastric contents due to migration of balloon away from stomach wall	Clean site once or twice daily.
	Inadequate cleaning techniques	Do not repeatedly use strong solutions such as hydrogen peroxide, povidone/iodine (Betadine), or alcohol.
	Overly aggressive cleaning techniques	Use topical antibiotics for infections.
Gastrointestinal		
Diarrhea	Antibiotic therapy or diarrhea-inducing medications	Identify medications with sorbitol, magnesium, or laxatives.
	Formula too cold	Administer at room temperature.
	Bacterial contamination	Use clean technique for preparation and administration.
		Limit reuse of feeding sets and bags.
		Check formula expiration date.
	Infusion rate too rapid	Decrease rate of infusion.
	Osmolality of formula too high	Temporarily dilute hypertonic formula.
		Change to formula with lower osmolality.
Constipation	Low-residue diet	Add fiber or change to fiber-containing formula.
	Inadequate fluid intake	Increase fluids.
	Low-residue diet	Add fiber or change to fiber-containing formula.
	Inactivity	Add stool softeners or laxatives.
	Medications	
Nausea, vomiting	Too rapid infusion rate	Decrease rate or volume of infusion.
	Gastric outlet obstruction	Add prokinetic medications.
	Volume too large	Change to intestinal access.
	Gastroparesis	
Distention, gas, bloating, cramping	Too rapid infusion rate	Decrease rate of infusion.
	Temporary adjustment to feedings	Clear all air before connecting set to tube; keep tube clamped when not in use.
	Air in tubing	Add prokinetic medications.
	Inactivity	Change to formula with lower fat content.
	Gastroparesis	
Other		
Aspiration	Inappropriate oral intake	Assess safety of swallow before allowing oral feeding.
	Feeding while lying flat	Elevate head of bed during and for 1 hour after feedings.
	Feeding volume too large	Decrease rate or volume of feeding.
		Change to intestinal access.
Dehydration	Inadequate fluid intake	Increase fluid intake.
	Excessive fluid loss via diarrhea, vomiting, or gastric drainage	Treat diarrhea.
		Replace GI losses.
		Use H_2 blocker to decrease gastric output.

that order).[38, 39] Carbonated beverages, coffee, cranberry juice, or a solution of meat tenderizer dissolved in water have also been suggested for declogging the tube. These liquids are usually ineffective and show no significant advantage over early detection and flushing with warm water. These substances may actually result in erosion or chemical damage to the integrity of the tube's interior lumen, resulting in further clogging. The preferred method for opening a long-standing clogged tube is use of pancreatic enzyme and bicarbonate dissolved in water. (A prescription for pancreatic enzyme may be included as part of the discharge orders for an "as needed" use.) If attempts to open an obstructed tube at home fail, patients

must go to their physician's office or the local hospital to have the tube cleared or replaced. Mechanical methods of opening a tube with a stylus or brush run the risk of puncturing the tube and/or the patient's GI tract, and at the very least should be performed only by experienced practitioners. If clogging occurs repeatedly, medication dosing forms, flushing techniques, and tube care should be reviewed. Replacement with a larger lumen tube can be helpful in some cases. Patients who have an established gastrostomy tract can be taught to replace their own tubes. Home care nurses can also assist with this replacement.

The GI complications of HEN are numerous and prevalent: diarrhea, constipation, nausea, vomiting, distention, bloating, and cramping. Although some patients have none of these side effects, as many as 70% of home patients experience them at one time or another.[27] Adequate education and careful monitoring can usually enable complications to be corrected at home without rehospitalization.[35]

In particular, diarrhea from contaminated feedings can be minimized with proper technique. Rates of bacterial contamination have been found to be higher in the home setting than in the hospital, perhaps because of the reuse of feeding containers and tubing.[40-43] Feeding sets are often rinsed and reused at home, to save money. Mixing or diluting formula can also increase the risk of contamination.[44] Because the type and number of manipulations of the feeding system are associated with the risk of contamination, a hang time as long as the entire infusion time can be recommended.[45] Diarrhea in a tube-fed patient cannot always be attributed to the enteral feedings. Factors such as underlying disease process, antibiotic treatment, hypoalbuminemia, medications with sorbitol or other elixirs added to the feeding, and even the varying definition of diarrhea all affect the incidence of this well-known complication.[46, 47]

Whatever the complications of HEN, they should be addressed by health care personnel. Patients should have access to assistance 24 hours per day and should be informed clearly of whom to call when complications arise. Whenever possible, routine problems should be addressed in the home setting; however, routine problems have the potential to become emergencies. Patients should be trained to identify which situations call for immediate attention and where to obtain assistance: HEN provider, clinic, hospital, or emergency department.

Home Parenteral Nutrition

Indications

GI length and function form the basis for the decision to initiate parenteral nutrition (PN). Further, diagnosis and prognosis as well as possible complications from oral or enteral feeding regimens and contraindications to these feedings should be considered. Diagnoses associated with home PN or HPN include intestinal failure from Crohn's disease and short-bowel syndrome (of any length in the presence of life-threatening malnutrition) that usually becomes a long-term or lifetime therapy.[9,48-50] HPN may be indicated when there is a short-term loss of GI function due to complications associated with a diagnosis or the effects of treatments such as radiation enteritis secondary to cancer treatment. Other patients for whom HPN may be considered are those who refuse enteral feedings or who have a temporary or permanent failure of enteral feedings. Although disease state, GI function, and nutrition status figure into the determination of the nutrition support regimen to be utilized at home, prognosis may also be a factor.[33] HPN has been successfully utilized in patients with inoperable malignant bowel obstruction, especially those with primary tumors of the GI tract, by improving quality of life although not affecting the overall expected outcome.[51]

Formulating the Nutrition Care Plan

Nutrition assessment is a vital task in developing a home nutrition care plan for a patient receiving HPN. Energy needs may increase or decrease after the patient is home because of changes in activity, recovery from injury or illness, or exacerbation of disease processes. Management of the HPN (or HEN) patient should include ongoing analysis of energy needs to avoid the consequences of over- or underfeeding. Like energy requirements, protein requirements may change over the course of HPN. It is important to monitor home nutrition support patients to ensure that nutrition status is maintained or enhanced by the home support regimen. Assessment of children's growth patterns helps clinicians assess adequacy of nutrient and energy intake. When appropriate, the nutrition care plan should include progression to an enteral or oral diet. Close monitoring and expertise by the home infusion provider's nutrition support clinicians working in concert with the prescribing physician is required to ensure a smooth and successful transition from HPN.

Access

Once the decision has been made to initiate parenteral nutrition, the type of intravenous access must be determined. If HPN therapy is to last more than a few weeks, establishment of a secure central venous access avoids hospital readmission or interruption in therapy related to loss or displacement of the access catheter.[52] Table 23-4 lists the venous catheters most often used for HPN. A long-term access device such as an implanted port or a tunneled catheter is most secure and easiest for the patient or care partner to manage. For intermediate-length therapy, a peripherally inserted central catheter (PICC) is another option that obviates surgical placement of a long-term device. A PICC line is inserted in a vein in the antecubital area and advanced through the upper arm into the subclavian vein. Although radiographic confirmation of placement is required before infusion of a hypertonic HPN solution, PICC insertion into the superior vena cava can be done in the home by an experienced nurse. It has been estimated that more than 212,000 venous ports, 103,000 tunneled right atrial catheters, and 668,000 PICCs are inserted in the United States each year.[53]

Most patients receiving HPN are administered hypertonic solutions via a centrally placed catheter, although parenteral nutrition support utilizing the peripheral route (peripheral parenteral nutrition, PPN) may also be given at home. PPN is the administration of amino acids, no greater than a 10% dextrose solution, and maintenance electrolytes via a peripheral vein as a temporary measure for maintaining nutritional status in patients who would otherwise undergo a short period of starvation. Therefore PPN is usually considered as a transitional therapy that must be evaluated on a patient-by-patient basis for clinical efficacy, applicability, and reimbursement. Central venous access is the most often used method of providing HPN because it allows for infusion of hypertonic solutions at varying volumes with options for prescription changes.

Determining the HPN Solution

At discharge the HPN prescription is verified and final adjustments to the solution are made. Seven classes of nutrients make up the typical HPN regimen: protein, in the form of crystalline amino acids; fats, as lipid emulsion; carbohydrate, provided as dextrose; electrolytes; trace elements; vitamins; and free water.[52] Development of the HPN formulation starts with the

TABLE 23-4

Venous Catheters for HPN

Catheter Type	Description	Utilization for PN
Peripheral	Canal placed in a peripheral vessel, most commonly a vein in the forearm	Peripheral parenteral nutrition only (maximum final concentration of dextrose 10%) Short-term therapy only (<2 wk)
Peripherally inserted central venous catheters	Central catheter inserted by direct venipuncture using a percutaneous approach into the subclavian, jugular, or femoral vein with the tip lying in the distal superior or inferior vena cava	Short- or long-term parenteral nutrition
Tunneled catheter	Central catheter inserted percutaneously into the subclavian, jugular, or femoral vein with the tip ending in the distal superior or inferior vena cava. The end of the catheter is tunneled in the subcutaneous tissue and exits on the chest wall.	Long-term parenteral nutrition
Implanted ports	Central catheter with a totally implantable chamber. The catheter is inserted into the subclavian or jugular vein.	Long-term parenteral nutrition; usually initially inserted for chemotherapy and subsequently used for nutrition therapy

determination of calorie and protein requirements to provide for macronutrient content. Total calories including those from protein are considered as the basis for the HPN formulation. First, protein requirements are subtracted from the total calories required. For example, if a patient requires 2000 calories daily and 100 g of protein, then 400 kcal would be subtracted from total kcal because amino acids have approximately 4 kcal/g. Most patients receive between 20% and 30% of total calories from fat emulsion; therefore, using the 2000 kcal example, the patient would require 400 to 600 kcal from fat (as fat emulsion). Finally, carbohydrate (dextrose) would be provided in amounts to make up the balance of calories. Sterile water is added to meet calculated fluid requirements as well as appropriate electrolytes, vitamins, and trace elements. An HPN solution is usually calculated to provide 3 to 7 days of nutrition support unlike PN provided in the hospital that can be changed daily. Therefore a careful evaluation of the patient's metabolic status is important to ensure that complications do not occur. Some home infusion companies have the ability to customize HPN solutions to meet very specific patient needs for macro- and micronutrients, which may not be available from a hospital pharmacy. Chapters 18 and 20 provide more detailed information on PN formulations.

Nutrients

PROTEIN. Protein requirements for normal children and adults are based on the Recommended Dietary Allowances (RDA; see Chapter 7) and vary according to disease state and the amount of physiologic stress each disease can cause.[54] Protein in HPN solutions takes the form of various crystalline amino acid formulations. Individualized amino acid preparations are available, such as branched-chain–enhanced formulas or specialty compounded formulations such as the amino acid formulation for maple-syrup urine disease. Taurine-supplemented amino acid formulas are used for pediatric patients and usually are not recommended for patients older than 5 years; however, preliminary data suggest that one such amino acid formula had a positive effect on nitrogen balance in pediatric patients older than 5 years and on trauma patients.[55]

Because of the trend for earlier hospital discharge, more acutely ill patients will be seen in alternative care sites. These patients may require a higher protein formula initially, which may be decreased as they recover. Most parameters for assessing protein adequacy and tolerance are available in home care, including blood urea nitrogen, creatinine, liver function tests, and indices of one or more serum proteins, such as albumin. A 24-hour urine collection for measuring urine urea nitrogen is possible in home care but is not a practical way of assessing adequacy of protein intake. Subjective measures such as progression of wound healing and repletion of body cell mass, as measured by increasing functional status, are useful.

CARBOHYDRATE. Carbohydrate is an important energy source for the body and (as dextrose) is the chief calorie source in most PN solutions used in the hospital and at home. Dextrose concentration in an HPN formula depends on route of administration, total calorie-nitrogen ratio, glucose tolerance, and fluid requirements. The "acuity" of patients receiving HPN is increasing and practitioners need to be aware of the consequences of excessive dextrose infusion. Patients with normal insulin response can tolerate glucose infusions of up to 7 mg/kg/min (calculated over a 24-hour period). However, stressed patients have decreased glucose tolerance, and it may be advisable to limit glucose to 5 mg/kg/min.[56,57] Because most HPN patients receive infusions over 10- to 12-hour periods, evaluating of glucose administration in mg per kg per minute is not applicable because this has not been studied for infusions of less than 24 hours. Monitoring of blood glucose levels will indicate tolerance to the dextrose component of the HPN formula. Beginning highly concentrated glucose infusions slowly and judiciously adding insulin to the solution when necessary can enhance glucose tolerance. Nonprotein calories provided from fat should substitute for a percentage of the dextrose calories when glucose intolerance is noted or the disease state warrants such as preexisting diabetes or poor blood glucose control prior to hospital discharge.

FAT. Intravenous fat emulsions can be provided as a calorie source specifically for the purpose of preventing essential fatty acid deficiency (EFAD). When at least 5% of the total calorie intake takes the form of long-chain triglycerides (linoleic acid), EFAD is prevented.[58,59] Fat (lipid) is the most concentrated source of energy for the body. Lipids can be infused as "piggy-backed" solutions to a dextrose-based HPN solution or mixed in a three-in-one solution; or given as a completely separate infusion. Solutions in which the fats are mixed with the HPN solution are known as three-in-one, all-in-one, or TNAs (total nutrient admixtures). Before infusing a TNA solution, the patient or care partner should examine the solution for streaks, oil, and color change. Key considerations in using a TNA solution for HPN are:

1. Their stability is usually shorter lived (7 days refrigerated) than that of most standard HPN solutions (i.e., glucose-based parenteral nutrition, 30 days refrigerated).
2. A TNA solution requires a 1.2-μm in-line filter, whereas dextrose-based HPN solutions require a 0.22-μm filter.
3. "Cracking" or "oiling out" may occur when the fat emulsion separates, forming droplets of free fat.[60]

Some patients receive fat every day as a calorie source, especially if their fluid is restricted or they need more calories. Although mixed fuel systems can be useful for certain populations, parenteral lipid regimens do have shortcomings. Intravenous lipid emulsions may have deleterious effects on the immune system, such as inhibiting in vitro neutrophil chemotaxis and migration and blocking the reticuloendothelial system. The overall effect on outcome remains controversial.[61] In addition, carbohydrate is more efficient than fat at protein sparing.[61,62] It is generally recommended that 20% to 35%, but not more than 60%, of kcal in an HPN solution be provided as fat emulsions. Dietary fat of 30% of total calories may be a useful guideline for HPN when a total nutrient admixture is being provided. Further research is needed to determine the safety and efficacy of high-fat parenteral or enteral regimens because current research suggests they might be detrimental to recovery.[62,63]

There are lipid emulsions currently used in Europe and under review in the United States that consist of alternative types of fats such as medium-chain triglycerides, structured lipds, and monounsatured lipids. Federal and governmental agencies in the United States must approve any new intravenous fat emulsion before providers can purchase it for distribution.

OTHER NUTRIENTS. Electrolytes are salts and minerals the body needs to sustain metabolism and to support many enzyme reactions. Electrolytes including sodium, potassium, chloride, calcium, magnesium, phosphate, and acetate, among others, are present in varying concentrations in PN formulas. Chapter 10 reviews electrolyte considerations. Each HPN formula is tailored to the patient's specific electrolyte needs as determined by clinical and laboratory evaluations and overall product stability. Monitoring fluid and electrolyte balance is extremely important and provides guidance for determining the appropriate electrolyte regimen.

Vitamins and trace elements (micronutrients) are necessary to maintain normal nutrition status. When a patient is found to be deficient in a specific vitamin or mineral, additions to the HPN solution can be provided as individual components.[64] Parenteral multivitamins should be administered to malnourished patients and to normally nourished ones, to prevent depletion of vitamin stores. The absence of parenteral vitamins

in any HPN order should be investigated.[61] The U.S. Food and Drug Administration (FDA) is requiring manufacturers to implement the intravenous multivitamin formulation changes put forth in August 1985 Federal Register.[65] The parenteral vitamin formulation includes the following changes: increase of B_1 (thiamine) from 3 mg to 6 mg, increase of B_6 (pyridoxine) from 4 mg to 6 mg, increase of C (ascorbic acid) from 100 mg to 200 mg, increase of folic acid from 400 mcg to 600 μg and the addition of vitamin K at 150 μg. Vitamin K had previously been provided to HPN patients as either a weekly intramuscular injection of 10 mg or a weekly addition of 10 mg to the HPN bag. For HPN patients receiving concomitant anticoagulation therapy, periodic monitoring of prothrombin/INR response by the patient's physician is essential in determining the appropriate dosage of anticoagulant therapy.

Vitamin and trace element needs may change over time related to disease processes for long-term HPN patients. Additionally, vitamin and trace element shortages may occur due to supply and manufacturing issues that can affect adequacy of micronutrient status. Therefore monitoring of vitamin and trace element status should be included in the routine monitoring plan of HPN patients.

ADMINISTRATION TECHNIQUE. PN is infused continuously over 24 hours in the hospital but at home is usually infused for 10 to 16 hours overnight. Most HPN patients prefer cyclic infusion and generally choose evening or nighttime for their infusion. This frees the patient from the pump during the day, promoting independence and a normal lifestyle.

To make the transition from a continuous infusion to a cyclic one the patient must tolerate a larger fluid load and must metabolize nutrients, especially glucose, more rapidly.[66] Most patients tolerate cyclic or intermittent infusions readily, but coexisting diseases such as diabetes (generally addressed with insulin), renal disease, or cardiac disease may require adjustments to the cycle or, in some cases, continuous infusion. Cyclic administration does not constantly tax the digestive and endocrine systems and is less likely to result in accumulation of fat in the liver. This fat accumulation is sometimes the result of continuous PN because the liver is not given the chance to perform its filtering function adequately.

Preparing Patient and Family

Transferring a patient on parenteral nutrition from the hospital to the home or initiating therapy at home requires integrating the therapy into the patient's lifestyle and ensuring that the therapy is safely administered and adequately monitored (Box 23-2). The home care nurse usually performs a home assessment, ideally before the patient's discharge to home, but often at the nurse's initial home visit. The home environment must be inspected for electrical and sanitary conditions and the care partner's ability to assist the HPN patient (Box 23-3). When a patient is discharged from the hospital, a coordinated effort among the hospital staff, usually consisting of the multidisciplinary nutrition support team if available, discharge planners or case managers, and the home care provider staff, helps to facilitate a seamless transition.[67] When a patient has PN therapy initiated at home, often the coordination of care is done primarily by the home infusion provider in coordination with the physician's office staff. When PN is started in the home, the home infusion provider must be aware of the potential for complications, especially refeeding syndrome; therefore, it is best to choose a provider with extensive experience in nutrition support therapy at home.[68]

EDUCATION. Education of the HPN patient should begin in the hospital. As the lengths of hospital stay continue to decrease, the opportunity to teach all aspects of HPN before discharge has likewise decreased. Patient education of HPN patients during the hospital stay now focuses on the skills that are most needed on discharge: site care, use of the infusion pump, infusion schedule (although that may change once the patient is home), and trouble shooting. Written materials should also be provided. Patients who initiate HPN in the home may initially require more frequent nursing visits to ensure that ade-

quate education and skills have been achieved. Agencies such as the Oley Foundation and the American Society for Parenteral and Enteral Nutrition also offer materials for patient education.

The nurse is present for the first home infusion of HPN to teach and observe the patient's technique and to serve as a backup should the patient be unable to perform the procedures independently.[69] The nurse calls the patient or returns the following morning to review how to disconnect the HPN and to evaluate how the first infusion went. This nursing support continues until the patient or care partner demonstrates competency and comfort in managing the complexities of therapy. Every patient must have a support system in place in case he or she becomes too ill or otherwise unable to manage the care. Many patients are able to provide self-care and manage all aspects of HPN. When the patient is unable to provide self-care, a care partner is utilized.

Monitoring and Complications

Clinical pathways and other monitoring guidelines have been developed to ensure that the most appropriate, yet cost-effective patient management occurs at home.[70] Pediatric and adult patients have differing psychosocial and monitoring requirements, especially related to initiating or resuming an oral diet. Pediatric patients should be managed by home care clinicians with expertise in this area. Home nutrition support monitoring guidelines for pediatric patients are not specifically covered in this chapter. Fluid and electrolyte abnormalities are common in the first days of HPN, whereas hyperglycemia is the most frequent metabolic complication related to cyclic infusions of parenteral nutrition.[60] Serum glucose levels that are consistently greater than 250 mg/dl require addition of insulin to the HPN solution. Hypoglycemia can occur, but it can be avoided by incrementally adjusting to the usual hourly rate over 1 hour at the beginning of the cycle and tapering off over the last hour at the end of the cycle. Postinfusion hypoglycemia can be avoided by extending the taper-down period or by having the patient eat carbohydrate, simple or complex, if absorption is possible.

Fluid or volume intolerance can also affect infusion time and require prolongation of the infusion period or reduction of the total volume of solution. Symptoms such as nocturnal dypsnea, chest fullness, and edema may indicate fluid or volume intolerance. The patient should be alerted to report these symptoms. Box 23-4 provides monitoring parameters for HPN.

The most common and serious complication of long-term HPN is related neither to the solution nor to the metabolic response but to the catheter. Catheter-associated sepsis is usually caused by *Staphylococcus epidermidis, S. aureus,* or *Candida* species.[71] Treatment, determined by the physician, may include the use of anti-infective agents or removal of the catheter. The incidence of catheter sepsis can be significantly decreased with proper catheter care. Immunosuppressed patients may be at increased risk for catheter and other infectious complications; however, Singer and colleagues successfully used HPN in patients with AIDS but did not observe an increased incidence of catheter sepsis compared with that of the overall population receiving HPN.[72]

Due to the challenges of obtaining accurate data outside the hospital setting, there are only a few published studies of

Monitoring Guidelines for HPN

CLINICAL PARAMETERS
Daily temperature
Daily blood glucose 1 hr after infusion discontinued
Intake and output, in cases of large GI losses or fluid imbalances
Weekly weight

LABORATORY PARAMETERS
Baseline
    Chemical profile: electrolytes, CO_2, creatinine, calcium, total protein, triglyceride, BUN, phosphorus, glucose, albumin, magnesium
    Liver function tests: total bilirubin, alkaline phosphatase, LDH, SGOT (AST), SGPT (ALT), prothrombin time, complete blood count
Optional Baseline (depends on underlying disease)
    Zinc, B_{12}, iron studies, copper
Monitoring
    Chemical profile-electrolytes, CO_2, creatinine, calcium, total protein, triglyceride, BUN, phosphorus, glucose, albumin, magnesium; iron studies, complete blood count
Frequency
    1-2 times/wk for 1-2 wk until stable; then once/2 wk for 6 wks; then monthly until mo 6; then quarterly until 1 yr
    After 1 yr, lab results drawn q 6 mo
    Iron studies (at 3 mo, then q 6 mo)
    Complete blood count (1, 2, 3, 6, 12 mo, then q 6 mo)

Adapted from Ireton-Jones CS, Hennessy K, Howard D, et al: Multidisciplinary clinical care of the home parenteral nutrition patient, *Infusion* 1(8):21-30, 1995.

catheter infection data from home care settings. Catheter-related infection data are reported as an incidence ratio (number of infections per 1000 catheter days). Tokars and colleagues evaluated rates of bloodstream infections among 827 patients receiving home infusion therapy for 1 year through central catheters and found an occurrence rate of 0.99/1000 catheter days.[73] In addition, these authors evaluated the risk factors for catheter infections with bone marrow transplant being highly associated with the risk of a bloodstream infection followed by receipt of parenteral nutrition, receipt of therapy outside the home, use of a multilumen catheter, and previous bloodstream infection. The Mayo Clinic reported a median rate of catheter infections of 2.65 per 1000 days from 20 years of data collected for 225 patients receiving HPN.[74] Another recently reported study of data from 2314 HPN patients collected over 1 year showed a suspected catheter related infection rate of 0.71/1000 catheter days.[75] These data continue to underscore the importance of thorough teaching of the patient at home to ensure compliance to proper procedures when catheters are accessed.

Psychosocial aspects of long-term parenteral nutrition therapy have been evaluated related to quality of life.[76] Some people have been receiving HPN for a year or many years, and these individuals have returned to their work and recreational activities. Availability of portable equipment, decreased infusion times, and awareness of HPN and HEN throughout the United States and many parts of the world have made travel easier.[77] Another component of care that has been enhanced is the creation of a support group designed for people on home nutrition support and their families and care partners. The Oley Foundation was started in 1985 by a long-term HPN patient

and his doctor. It has grown into an important component of many long-term nutrition support patients' lives.

Long-term complications such as the incidence of metabolic bone disease, liver failure, and micronutrient deficiencies have been identified.[78, 79] Careful attention to monitoring parameters for short-term and long-term patients as well as comprehensive patient education and compliance monitoring are essential components for successful HPN management.

Reimbursement

An understanding of reimbursement mechanisms and consideration of the patient's financial situation are essential for successful HPN and HEN programs. Even though HEN is less expensive than HPN, the costs of either therapy can be significant. Reddy and Malone reviewed the costs of HPN and HEN from Medicare charge estimates. In 1996 the average annual cost for HPN intravenous solutions and pump was $56,683 for a single patient; for HEN, the annual cost for a single patient was $10,733 for tube-feeding product and pump. These amounts did not include costs for labs, nursing visits, or miscellaneous items.[80]

Medicare coverage for HPN requires specific and significant deficits of digestion or absorption. There are two main criteria, including permanence (patient will require therapy for 90 days or greater—the same requirement for enteral nutrition) and malabsorption of nutrients (defined as a condition involving the small intestine or its exocrine glands, which impairs absorption) or a motility disorder, that impairs the ability of nutrients to be transported through the gastrointestinal tract. There are specific definitions and documentation requirements to verify the reason for the malabsorption. If documentation is inaccurate or insufficient, Medicare will not provide reimbursement; therefore, it is essential that careful attention be paid to obtaining the correct diagnosis and reason for the HPN therapy. A nutrition support clinician can be extremely helpful in working with the physician and the home infusion provider to obtain appropriate documentation as well as ensure that enteral feeding, if appropriate, has been adequately tried before HPN is initiated.

Third-party coverage for home nutrition support varies with private carriers and state Medicaid programs. A detailed discussion of reimbursement criteria for home nutrition support can be found in Chapter 45. Helping home nutrition support patients with financial concerns can improve their compliance, acceptance of the therapy, and overall quality of life.

Transitioning Home Nutrition Support

Adjusting to the transition from HPN to HEN or to oral intake requires careful monitoring (see Chapter 22). Often an HPN patient makes the transition to HEN as a slow progression to ensure tolerance, especially if malabsorption or GI disease is a factor in the medical diagnosis. Parenteral access should be maintained until there is reasonable assurance that adequate enteral or oral intake can be sustained. Sometimes a patient goes directly from HPN to an oral diet. A registered dietitian is necessary not only to monitor the transition but also provide suggestions for oral intake and to monitor the adequacy of oral feeding. The transition from enteral to oral intake is usually a gradual one with enteral access being maintained until oral intake is known to be adequate.

In some cases, owing to terminal illness, a patient may transition off both HEN and HPN without establishing adequate oral intake. Debate continues about whether nutrition and hydration are necessary or whether they are extraordinary forms of therapy that may be terminated by patients or their surrogates. HPN has been shown to be palliative and to facilitate compassionate home care for certain patients with inoperable malignant bowel obstruction.[80] When the decision is made to terminate feedings, clinicians are often concerned about the effects that no nutrition support will have on a terminal patient. McCann and colleagues studied 27 patients in a comfort care unit who received food and water intake inadequate to sustain basal nutritional requirements.[81] No patients received artificial nutrition or hydration, and 63% of them experienced no hunger; 34% initially expressed hunger but eventually lost their appetites. Most of the patients (87%) felt no pain. Those who experienced pain attributed it to the disease process for which they were admitted. These authors suggest that care partners, patients, and families need to know that loss of a normal appetite is common in dying patients and does not contribute substantially to their suffering.

Conclusion

As the move toward shorter lengths of stay in acute care settings continues, the use of parenteral and enteral nutrition therapy in home care and alternative sites will likely increase. Reimbursement policies dictate efficient use of the therapies, with positive clinical outcomes becoming the principal goal. Advancing technology, refinement of techniques, standardized monitoring, and access to the expertise provided by skilled nutrition support clinicians will contribute to the overall outcomes as well as the enhancement of the quality of life of persons who receive long-term nutrition support.

REFERENCES

1. The Oley Foundation: *North American home parenteral and enteral nutrition patient registry annual report,* Albany, NY, 1994, The Oley Foundation, pp 1-23.
2. Elia M: Home enteral nutrition: General aspects and a comparison between the United States and Britain, *Nutrition* 10:115-123, 1994.
3. Rollins CJ: Home care issues with multivitamin therapy, *Nutr Clin Prac* 16;S12-S16, 2000.
4. Arno PS, Bonuck KA, Padgug R: The economic impact of high-technology home care, *Hastings Cent Rep* 24:S15-S19, 1994.
5. Patients give home IV two thumbs up newslines, *Infusion* 1(8):5-6, 1984.
6. Ireton-Jones CS, Hasse JM: Comprehensive nutritional assessment: the dietitian's contribution to the team effort, *Nutrition* 8(2):75-81, 1992.
7. Sax HC, Hasselgren P-O: Indications. In Fischer JE (ed): *Total parenteral nutrition,* Boston, 1991, Little, Brown, pp 3-11.
8. Schneider AM, Raina C, Pugliese P, et al: Outcome or patients treated with home enteral nutrition, *J Parenter Enteral Nutr* 26 (4):203-209, 2001.
9. ASPEN Board of Directors: Guidelines for the use of parenteral and enteral nutrition in adult and pediatric patients, *J Parenter Enteral Nutr* 17(suppl):1SA-52SA, 1993.
10. ASPEN Board of Directors: Standards for home nutrition support, *Nutr Clin Pract* 14:151-162, 1999.
11. ASPEN Board of Directors: Standards for nutrition support for residents of long-term care facilities, *Nutr Clin Pract* 4:148-153, 1989.
12. Howard L: Home parenteral and enteral nutrition in cancer patients, *Cancer* 72:3531-3541, 1993.
13. Hirakawa H, Fukuda Y, Tanida N, et al: Home elemental enteral hyperalimentation (HEEH) for the maintenance of remission in patients with Crohn's disease, *Gastroenterology* 28:379-384, 1993.
14. Henderson CT, Trumbore LS, Mobarhan S, et al: Prolonged tube feeding in long-term care: Nutritional status and clinical outcomes, *J Am Coll Nutr* 11:309-325, 1992.
15. Holden CE, Puntis JWL, Charlton CPL, Booth IW: Nasogastric feeding at home: acceptability and safety, *Arch Dis Child* 66:148-151, 1991.
16. Goldberg T, Slonim AE: Nutrition therapy for hepatic glycogen storage diseases, *J Am Diet Assoc* 93:1423-1430, 1993.
17. American Dietetic Association: Position of the American Dietetic Association: issues in feeding the terminally ill adult, *J Am Diet Assoc* 92:996-1005, 1992.
18. American Dietetic Association: Position of the American Dietetic Association: legal and ethical issues in feeding permanently unconscious patients, *J Am Diet Assoc* 95:231-234, 1995.
19. Larson DE, Burton DD, Schroeder KW, DiMagno EP: Percutaneous endoscopic gastrostomy. Indications, success, complications and mortality in 314 consecutive patients, *Gastroenterology* 93:48-52, 1987.
20. Hull MA, Rawlings J, Murray FE, et al: Audit of outcome of long-term enteral nutrition by percutaneous endoscopic gastrostomy, *Lancet* 341:869-872, 1993.
21. Raha SK, Woodhouse KW: The use of percutaneous endoscopic gastrostomy (PEG) in 161 consecutive elderly patients, *Age Ageing* 23:162-163, 1994.
22. Haas-Beckert B, Heyman MB: Comparison of two skin-level gastrostomy feeding tubes for infants and children, *Pediatr Nurs* 19:351-354, 364, 1993.
23. Coben RM, Weintraub A, DiMarino AJ, Cohen SA: Gastroesophageal reflux during gastrostomy feeding, *Gastroenterology* 106:13-18, 1994.
24. Heitkemper ME, Martin DL, Hansen BC: Rate and volume of intermittent enteral feeding, *J Parenter Enteral Nutr* 5:125-129, 1981.
25. Shuster MH, Mancino JM: Ensuring successful tube feeding in the geriatric population, *Geriatric Nurs* 15:67-81, 1994.
26. Michaelis CA, Warzak WJ, Stanek K, Van Riper C: Parental and professional perceptions of problems associated with long-term pediatric home tube feeding, *J Am Diet Assoc* 92:1235-1238, 1992.
27. Weckwerth JA, Liffrig TL, Starkson SP, Nelson JK: Home enteral nutrition: outcomes and patient perspectives. (Unpublished).
28. Park RHR, Galloway A, Russell RI, et al: Home sweet HEN guide to home enteral nutrition, *Br J Clin Pract* 46:105-110, 1992.
29. Young CK, White S: Preparing patients for tube feeding at home, *Am J Nurs* 92:46-53, 1992.
30. Allison SP, Micklewright A, Rawlings J, Hull M: Organisation and evaluation of home enteral nutrition services, *Clin Nutr* 12:S38-S43, 1993.
31. Evans MA, Czopek S: Home nutrition support materials, *Nutr Clin Pract* 10:37-39, 1995.
32. Joint Commission on Accreditation of Healthcare Organizations: *Accreditation manual for home care, 1995,* Oakbrook Terrace, IL, 1994, JCAHO.
33. American Dietetic Association: Position of the American Dietetic Association: nutrition monitoring of the home parenteral and enteral patient, *J Am Diet Assoc* 94:664-666, 1994.
34. McWhirter JP, Hambling CE, Pennington CR: The nutritional status of patients receiving home enteral feedings, *Clin Nutr* 13:207-211, 1994.
35. Nelson JK, Palumbo PJ, O'Brien PC: Home enteral nutrition: observations of a newly established program, *Nutr Clin Pract* 1:193-199, 1986.
36. Estoup M: Approaches and limitations of medication delivery in patients with enteral feeding tubes, *Crit Care Nurs* 14:68-72, 77-79, 1994.
37. Scanlan M, Frisch S: Nasoduodenal feeding tubes: prevention of occlusion, *J Neurosci Nurs* 24:256-259, 1992.
38. Metheny N, Eisenberg P, McSweeney M: Effect of feeding tube properties and three irrigants on clogging rates, *Nurs Res* 37:165-169, 1988.
39. Marcuard SP, Stegall KS: Unclogging feeding tubes with pancreatic enzyme, *J Parenter Enteral Nutr* 14:198-200, 1994.
40. Patchell CJ, Anderton A, MacDonald A, et al: Bacterial contamination of enteral feeds, *Arch Dis Child* 70:327-330, 1994.
41. Ole S, Kamiya A, Hironga K, Koshiro A: Microbial contamination of enteral feeding solution and its prevention, *Am J Infect Control* 21:34-38, 1993.
42. Anderton A, Nwoguh CE, McKune I, et al: A comparative study of the numbers of bacteria present in enteral feeds prepared and administered in hospital and the home, *J Hosp Infect* 23:43-49, 1993.

43. Grunow JE, Christenson JC, Moutos D: Contamination of enteral nutrition systems during prolonged intermittent use, *J Parenter Enteral Nutr* 13:23-25, 1989.

44. Freedland CP, Roller RD, Wolfe BM, Flynn NM: Microbial contamination of continuous drip feedings, *J Parenter Enteral Nutr* 13:18-22, 1989.

45. Anderton A: Bacterial contamination of enteral feeds and feeding systems, *Clin Nutr* 12(suppl):S16-S32, 1993.

46. Heimburger DC, Sockwell DG, Geels WJ: Diarrhea with enteral feeding: prospective reappraisal of putative causes, *Nutrition* 10:392-396, 1994.

47. Bliss DZ, Guenter PA, Settle RG: Defining and reporting diarrhea in tube-fed patients—what a mess! *Am J Clin Nutr* 55:753-759, 1992.

48. Ireton-Jones C, DeLegge M: Home parenteral nutrition management, *Support Line* 21(2):20-25, 1999.

49. Gouttebel MC, Saint Aubert B, Astre C, Joyeaux H: Total parenteral nutrition needs in different types of short-bowel syndrome, *Dig Dis Sci* 31(7):718-723, 1986.

50. Adams A: Venous access devices: case studies for appropriate access devices, *Infusion* 1(8):11-14, 1995.

51. August DA, Thom D, Fischer RL, et al: Home parenteral nutrition for patients with inoperable malignant bowel obstruction, *J Parenter Enteral Nutr* 15(3):323-327, 1991.

52. Bower RH: Home parenteral nutrition. In Fisher JE (ed): *Total parenteral nutrition*, Boston, 1991, Little, Brown, pp 367-387.

53. Frost and Sullivan. US Catheter Market, 1995.

54. Williamson J: Physiologic stress: trauma, sepsis, burns, and surgery. In Mahan LK, Arlin MT (eds): *Food, nutrition and diet therapy,* Philadelphia, 1992, WB Saunders, p 496.

55. Geggel HS, Ament ME, Heckenlively JR, et al: Nutritional requirement for taurine in patients receiving long-term parenteral nutrition, *N Engl J Med* 312(5):142-146, 1985.

56. Burke JF, Wolfe RR, Mullany CJ, et al: Glucose requirements following burn injury, *Ann Surg* 190(3):274-285, 1979.

57. Wolfe RR, O'Donnell TF, Stone MD, et al: Investigation of factors determining the optimal glucose infusion rate in total parenteral nutrition, *Metabolism* 29:892-900, 1980.

58. Meguid MM, Muscaritoli M: Current uses of total parenteral nutrition, *Am Family Phys* 47(2):383-394, 1993.

59. McClave SA, Short AF, Mattingly DB, et al: Total parenteral nutrition: conquering the complexities, *Postgrad Med* 88(1):235-248, 1990.

60. Ireton-Jones CS, Hennessy K, Howard D, et al: Multidisciplinary clinical care of the home parenteral nutrition patient, *Infusion* 1(8):21-30, 1995.

61. Gottschlich MM: Selection of optimal lipid sources in enteral and parenteral nutrition, *Nutr Clin Pract* 7:152-165, 1992.

62. Long JM, Wilmore DW, Mason AD, et al: Effect of carbohydrate and fat intake on nitrogen excretion during total intravenous feeding, *Ann Surg* 185:417-422, 1997.

63. Wretlind A: Development of fat emulsions, *J Parenter Enteral Nutr* 5(3):230-235, 1981.

64. Driscoll DF: Parenteral vitamin requirements: etiology of selected nutrient imbalances, *Newslines* 3(4):1-3, 1994.

65. U.S. Department of Health and Human Services, Federal Register 65: Number 77, April 20, 2000.

66. Maini B, Blackburn GL, Bistrian BR, et al: Cyclic hyperalimentation: an optimal technique for preservation of visceral protein, *J Surg Res* 20:515-525, 1976.

67. Anthony PS, Ireton-Jones C: Dietitians in home care: a new challenge, *Support Line* 16(6):1-8, 1994.

68. Crocker KS, Ricciardi C, DiIeso M: Initiating total parenteral nutrition at home, *Nutr Clin Pract* 14:124-130, 1999.

69. Orr ME: Nutritional support in home care, *Nurs Clin North Am* 24(2):437-445, 1989.

70. Ireton-Jones CS, Hennessy K, Howard D, et al: Multidisciplinary clinical care of the home parenteral nutrition patient, *Infusion* 1(8):21-30, 1995.

71. Buchman AL, Moukarzel A, Goodson B, et al: Catheter-related infections associated with home parenteral nutrition and predictive factors for the need for catheter removal in their treatment, *J Parenter Enteral Nutr* 18:297-302, 1994.

72. Singer P, Rothkopf MM, Kvetan V, et al: Risks and benefits of home parenteral nutrition in the acquired immunodeficiency syndrome, *J Parenter Enteral Nutr* 15(1):75-79, 1991.

73. Tokars JI, Cookson ST, McArthur MA, et al: Prospective evaluation of risk factors for bloodstream infections in patients receiving home infusion therapy, *Ann Intern Med* 131(5): 340-347, 1999.

74. Scolapio JS, Flemming R, Kelly DG, et al: Survival of home parenteral nutrition treated patients: 20 years of experience at the Mayo Clinic, *Mayo Clin Proc* 74:217-223, 1999.

75. Ireton-Jones C, DeLegge M, Hamilton K: Home parenteral nutrition registry, 1999. Patient demographics and outcomes (Abstract.), *Nutr Clin Pract* 16(2):117, 2001.

76. Smith CE: Quality of life in long-term parenteral nutrition patients and their family caregivers, *J Parenter Enteral Nutr* 17(6):501-506, 1993.

77. Steiger, E, Ireton-Jones C: The evolution of home parenteral nutrition in the United States, *Nutr Clin Pract.* 16(4):236-239, 2001.

78. Buchman AL, Sohol M, Brown M, et al: Verbal and visual memory improve after choline supplementation in long-term total parenteral nutrition: a pilot study, *J Parenter Enteral Nutr* 25: 30-35, 2001.

79. Seidner DL, Licata A: Parenteral nutrition-associated metabolic bone disease: pathophysiology, evaluation, and treatment, *Nutr Clin Pract* 15:163-170, 2000.

80. Reddy P, Malone M: Cost and outcomes analysis of home parenteral and enteral nutrition, *J Parenter Enteral Nutr* 22(6):302-310, 1998.

81. McCann RM, Hall WJ, Groth-Juncker A: Comfort care for terminally ill patients, *JAMA* 272(16):1263-1266, 1994.

General Pharmacologic Issues

Carol J. Rollins, MS, RD, CNSD, Pharm D, BCNSP

BROADLY defined, *pharmacology* is the study of chemicals (drugs) that affect living organisms. Pharmacologic questions and problems involve some aspect of a medication, anything from physical properties to biologic functions. Both parenteral nutrition (PN) and enteral nutrition (EN) are affected by pharmacologic issues. Occasionally, clearly established protocols address pharmacologic issues related to specialized nutrition support therapy. More frequently, however, multiple approaches to PN and EN therapy have been developed in various facilities because definitive research is lacking, available research provides conflicting results, products with similar nutritional composition differ in chemical properties that affect stability and compatibility, and there are several ways of achieving the desired result. Understanding the general principles of pharmacologic issues related to PN and EN allows the nutrition support practitioner to address them more effectively. This chapter, therefore, focuses on general principles and provides some examples to illustrate pharmacologic issues that may affect safe and efficacious provision of PN and EN therapy.

Types of Incompatibility

Any inappropriate or undesirable effect of the interaction of two or more substances represents incompatibility between them. Interactions that produce direct physical or chemical effects such as precipitation or gelation are common examples. An interaction that alters the response to either the formula or a medication, rather than causing obvious physical or chemical changes, is also a form of incompatibility, although it is frequently called *intolerance* or a *side effect*. Based on the specific results and/or mechanisms involved, incompatibility associated with PN or EN therapy can be divided into five types (Table 24-1). This approach, which emphasizes understanding the mechanisms underlying the incompatibility rather than simply listing the results of incompatibility, was first described to dietitians as part of a presentation on compatibility of medications with enteral feeding, but it applies equally to PN incompatibility.[1] Application of the five types of incompatibility to specialized nutrition support practice requires a basic understanding of the pharmacologic concepts, but does not require training per se.

Physical Incompatibility

Physical incompatibility is manifested in an undesirable physical change when substances are combined. The change is frequently evident on visual inspection, although some changes are too subtle to be observed by the naked eye or are obscured in opaque substances. Observation of flow characteristics can also reveal physical incompatibility when at least one of the substances is a liquid. Both PN and EN formulas are complex liquid compounds, each component of which has potential to

---

TABLE 24-1

Types of Incompatibility with Nutrition Support

Type of Incompatibility and Definition	Examples	
	PN	**EN**
Physical: Physical change in the formula or medication	Precipitation: separation of oil from IV lipids	Curdling: altered viscosity or consistency
Pharmaceutical: Alteration of a dosage form so that medication delivery is unsafe or inappropriate	None	Crushing of sustained-release, enteric-coated, sublingual, or buccal dosage forms
Pharmacologic: Intolerance to PN or EN therapy resulting from a medication's mechanism of action		Nausea due to stimulation of the CTZ by chemotherapy or morphine
Interference with a medication's action by a component of PN or EN therapy	Warfarin resistance due to vitamin K in pediatric MVI or phytonadione added to a PN formula	Warfarin (Coumadin) resistance due to vitamin K in an EN formula
Physiologic: Altered tolerance to specialized nutrition support due to nonpharmacologic responses to medications	Phlebitis due to an irritating medication given by Y-site infusion with peripheral PN	Diarrhea due to a hyperosmotic or sorbitol-containing medication given with an EN formula
Pharmacokinetic: Altered absorption, distribution, metabolism, or elimination of a medication due to a nutrient	Altered peak and trough levels of a medication added to PN	Decreased tetracycline absorption when given with an EN formula containing calcium
Altered absorption, distribution, metabolism, or elimination of a nutrient due to a medication	Vitamin A loss to PN container; thiamine loss due to sodium bisulfite in amino acid solutions	Altered vitamin D metabolism and/or altered calcium absorption due to phenytoin

CTZ, Chemoreceptor trigger zone; *EN,* enteral nutrition; *IV,* intravenous; *PN,* parenteral nutrition.

interact in a direct physicochemical manner with any other one and with other substances that physically contact the formula, including medications. Precipitation is the most common physical incompatibility associated with PN; curdling is more often associated with EN. Other examples of physical changes include flocculation, phase separation, and altered consistency or viscosity (thinning, thickening, coagulation, or gelling). Variables that affect physical incompatibility include pH, cation-anion interaction, concentration and chemical complexity of individual components, temperature, time, and order of mixing.

Physical incompatibility is a major concern with PN formulas. The typical order for PN contains 10 to 15 (or more) components, including macronutrients, electrolytes, minerals, and vitamins. Various preservatives, stabilizers, and solubilizers are also present in each PN formula.

Interaction of PN components can have positive and negative effects. Such interactions may not be totally predictable by standard chemical solubility rules, and minor changes in the PN formula's content or temperature or how long components are together can alter the interaction. Exposure to light may even alter stability and interaction among PN components. For example, decomposition of ascorbic acid is accelerated with light exposure. The oxalate formed can subsequently interact with calcium in the PN to form insoluble calcium oxalate.[2-4] Each addition to a PN formula must, therefore, be evaluated for compatibility with every other PN component and with the mixture. For example, if a PN order includes a medication, an individual amino acid additive (e.g., L-cysteine, glutamine), or vitamins in addition to a standard multivitamin preparation, the pharmacist must be certain that nothing in the product will precipitate with or adversely alter the interaction among amino acids, calcium, magnesium, phosphate, acetate, insulin, vitamins, and any other components of the formula for the period from preparation to completion of infusion. Products to be coinfused via a single venous access device with the PN formula must also be evaluated for possible physical incompatibility. A product may be acceptable for coinfusion with PN but not for direct mixing into the PN formula because of differences in dilution, contact time, and completeness of mixing. Risks of toxicity and infection can also affect the choice of coinfusion or direct mixing with the PN formula. Intravenous infusion of components that are physically incompatible can have grave consequences such as pulmonary deposition of crystals or even death.[5,6]

Calcium-phosphate precipitation and "three-in-one" or total nutrient admixture (TNA) destabilization are among the most complex physical incompatibilities among PN components. Many factors are involved in both incompatibilities. Because of their complexity and critical importance in PN therapy, these issues are addressed separately.

When PN therapy is ordered, adequate venous access is generally established to allow administration of the PN formula separately from all other intravenous treatments. Limited venous access in some patients, however, requires PN to be either withheld or administered with another therapy. Inadequate venous access can be a problem with critically ill neonates and children and with adults who are receiving multiple intravenous therapies with poor compatibility profiles relative to other medications. The most appropriate approach to inadequate venous access is generally determined by policies and procedures of the health care facility and available information on compatibility. Published information on medication compatibility with PN formulas must be carefully evaluated for differences between the formula cited and the one being provided to the patient. Some tested formulas lack components routinely included in PN formulas such as calcium, trace elements, or vitamins, whereas others differ only in the brand or concentration of amino acids.[7-9] Even seemingly minor differences warrant evaluation for compatibility: medication concentration, amino acid stock solution, preservative content of additives, and the PN formulation tested, including final concentrations of dextrose, amino acids, lipid emulsion, electrolytes, vitamins, trace elements, heparin, insulin, and other additives. For example, a medication may be compatible with standard adult amino acid formulas but not with pediatric formulas, or with a calcium concentration of 4.7 mEq/L of PN (a typical adult dose) but not with 20 mEq/L. Likewise, 100 mg of ascorbic acid from an injectable multivitamin preparation in the PN formula might be compatible, whereas 1000 mg would adversely affect other PN components. Trace elements can have a stabilizing effect in one instance and a destabilizing effect in another. The order in which a multitrace element solution or individual trace elements are added can also affect physical reactions. For instance, green discoloration from a copper-cimetidine metal complex can occur when these components are added sequentially, but it does not when the components are adequately separated.[10,11]

The most problematic PN components in relation to compatibility with medications are trace elements, calcium, magnesium, and heparin. Medications likely to interact with electrolytes and those incompatible with pH values less than 5 or greater than 7 generally are not suitable for direct admixture with PN formula and Y-site administration via the PN tubing. Table 24-2 lists medications considered compatible and incompatible with PN formulations typically used by the Nutrition Support Team at the Arizona Health Sciences Center, Tucson. All other medications must be checked for compatibility with a pharmacist or treated as incompatible. Medications classified as incompatible may exhibit physical incompatibility or any other type of incompatibility that makes Y-site administration of the medication unacceptable. Different formulas and different preparation and storage procedures can alter compatibility; thus, medications listed as compatible in Table 24-2 may not be compatible in all facilities that provide PN. Final decisions on compatibility must be made by a health care professional who is familiar with the specific composition of the PN formula with which the medication is to be combined. Policies and procedures of the health care facility must also be considered because Y-site administration via the same vascular access as PN or direct addition to PN may be prohibited.

Pediatric PN Therapy

Children, especially critically ill neonates and infants, present special PN challenges. Several issues are unique or of heightened concern to pediatrics.

TABLE 24-2

Medication Compatibility for Coinfusion with Parenteral Nutrition (PN) Including Dextrose-Based (2 + 1) and Fat-Based (3-in-1 or TNA) Formulations[a]

Compatible with PN[b]	Incompatible with PN[c]
ANTIINFECTIVES Aminoglycosides: amikacin, gentamicin, kanamycin, netilmicin, tobramycin Aztreonam Cephalosporins: cefazolin,[d] cefonicid, cefoperizone, cefotaxime, cefotetan, cefoxitin, ceftazidime, ceftriaxone, ceftrizoxime, cefuroxime Chloramphenicol Clindamycin Fluconazole Penicillins: azlocillin, carbenicillin, mezlocillin, nafcillin, oxacillin, piperacillin, piperacillin-tazobactam (Zosyn), ticarcillin, ticarcillin-clavulanate (Timentin), (not ampicillin, ampicillin-sulbactam;[e] possible problems with penicillin GK) Vancomycin (should not Y-site when heparin is admixed in PN)	**ANTIINFECTIVES** Acyclovir Amphotericin (all formulations) Ampicillin[e] Ampicillin-sulbactam (Augmentin)[e] Ganciclovir Imipenem-cilastatin (Primaxin)[g] Metronidazole (Flagyl)[g] Minocycline Quinolones: ciprofloxacin, ofloxacin[e] Tetracyclines[e] Trimethoprim-sulfamethoxazole (Bactrim, Septra)[f]
MEDICATIONS FOR PAIN CONTROL Fentanyl Meperidine (Demerol) Morphine (compatible at 1 mg/ml; *not* compatible at 15 mg/ml)	**OTHER MEDICATIONS:** Diazepam (Valium) Immunoglobulins (IVIG) Midazolam (Versed) Phenytoin (Dilantin) Sodium bicarbonate
HISTAMINE-2 ANTAGONISTS (H₂ BLOCKERS) Cimetidine (Tagamet) Famotidine (Pepcid) Ranitidine (Zantac)	**COMPATIBLE WITH 2+1 FORMULATIONS; FAT-BASED FORMULATIONS DISRUPTED[h]** Droperidol Haloperidol (Haldol) Heparin (100 units/ml) Lorazepam (Ativan) Morphine (15 mg/ml) Ondansetron (Zofran) Pentobarbitol Phenobarbitol
OTHER MEDICATIONS Cyclosporin A[g] Digoxin Diphenhydramine (Benadryl) Dobutamine Hydrocortisone Insulin, regular Lidocaine Mesna Nitroprusside Norepinephrine Nitroglycerine Octreotide[e] Propofol Tacrolimus; FK-506	

Rollins Associates, Copyright 2001.

[a] Coinfusion of medications with PN is *not* the standard of practice. The standard of practice is for PN formulations to be administered via venous access, or one lumen of a multiple lumen device, which is dedicated solely to PN administration. Coinfusion of medications with PN should be used only when other access cannot be obtained and only when the risks associated with dual use of PN access are justified. The extent of prior use of the venous access device (maintenance fluid versus multiple therapies), the insertion site (subclavian versus femoral), conditions of placement (operating room versus emergency room), catheter material (silicone elastic versus nonsilastic materials), and the catheter type (permanent versus temporary, nontunneled) may influence the risks associated with coinfusion of a medication with a PN formulation.

[b] Compatibility is only for *coinfusion* via Y-site injection or a double-lumen device attached at the catheter hub. Mixing in a volumetric infusion device (Buretrol) or admixture in PN is *not* evaluated. Compatibility is for individual medications only and may change if another medication is coinfused or admixed in the PN formulation. Compatibility for most of the medications listed is based only on physical compatibility, not chemical stability (see footnote "e" below).

[c] The recommended procedure for administering incompatible medications is to stop the PN, flush the line with 0.9% NaCl (then D₅W for medications incompatible with NaCl) before and after administering the medication, then restart the PN. Risk of reactive hypoglycemia may be associated with stopping the PN infusion without tapering down over 30 to 60 minutes. Disrupting or opening the PN administration system may increase risk of infection.

[d] Most studies report that cefazolin is compatible with PN formulations. Small amounts of precipitate were reported in two dextrose-based formulations in one study.[8] Use a 0.2 mm in-line filter between the Y-site and the venous catheter. Stop the infusion immediately if evidence of precipitate and report this to the Doctor of Pharmacy on-call for PN.

[e] Studies based strictly on physical compatibility (precipitation, lipid emulsion disruption) suggest compatibility; however, problems with chemical stability (inactivation or loss of activity of the medication) have been documented or have a high likelihood of occurring. Octreotide can be administered via Y-site, but loss of activity occurs if admixed in PN.

[f] Treat as incompatible although compatibility has been reported under certain conditions.

[g] Acceptable in PN formulations containing Intralipid fat emulsion, but not with some formulations containing Liposyn III emulsion.[9] Intralipid is used at University Medical Center (UMC). Small amounts of precipitate were reported after 4 hours with dextrose-based PN formulations.[8] If Y-site administration of cyclosporin A with PN is necessary, use the Y-site that is closest to the catheter hub.

[h] Immediate disruption with oiling out was reported with most of the medications during accelerated life testing.[9] It is uncertain if the emulsion disruption occurs rapidly enough to create problems in clinical practice; however, it is safest to consider these medications incompatible with fat-based PN formulations.

Special Pediatric Amino Acid Solutions

Special pediatric amino acid solutions are designed to achieve a normal 2-hour postprandial amino acid pattern in the bloodstream of neonates and infants. The concentrations of several amino acids in the pediatric solution differ somewhat from those in standard adult amino acid solutions. The major differences are the inclusion of taurine in the pediatric solution and the recommendation for the addition of 0.4 g of L-cysteine per 10 g of amino acids during compounding of PN formulas. The L-cysteine is stable in solution for only about 24 hours. Pediatric amino acid solutions tend to be marginally acceptable for use in PN formulas containing lipid emulsion and lipids should not be admixed when the pH has been reduced by the addition of L-cysteine. Limited data are available on compatibility of medications with PN formulas containing pediatric amino acid solutions.

Inadequate Venous Access and Fluid Limitations

Few critically ill pediatric patients have adequate venous access to allow use of one line or port exclusively for PN; thus, coinfusion of medications with PN is common. In addition, because of the risk of fluid overload, PN formula is used as the diluent for medications. This is accomplished with a volumetric infusion chamber such as a Buretrol, which is rigged between the PN bag and the infusion pump. Such chambers hold a small volume of PN to which a dose of medication is added. For example, PN formula in the volume to be infused over an hour is added to the volumetric infusion chamber, and then the dose of a medication to be administered over an hour is added. Data are limited on Y-site administration of medications with PN formulas compounded using pediatric amino acid solutions. Data on compatibility of medications prepared in volumetric infusion chambers with PN formula as the diluent are even more limited. Caution is therefore advised when extrapolating data for Y-site administration of drugs with PN formulas containing standard amino acid solutions to coinfusion with pediatric PN using a volumetric infusion chamber.

Calcium Phosphate Precipitation

Children have greater calcium and phosphate requirements than adults. Neonates and infants have the highest requirements, especially those born prematurely. The PN formulas prepared for these patients, therefore, typically contain calcium and phosphate at the upper limits of solubility. (See Calcium and Phosphate in Parenteral Nutrition for a more complete discussion of solubility.) Fluid limitations may require relatively slow administration rates, which can increase the risk of calcium phosphate precipitation in the infusion pump chamber or tubing.[12]

Toxicity of "Inactive" Ingredients

Ingredients considered inert when given to normal adults may be toxic to neonates and infants, especially those born prematurely. These patients have varying degrees of renal, hepatic, and enzyme system immaturity that prevent effective detoxification or elimination of certain chemicals. For example, normal detoxification of the preservative benzyl alcohol is impaired for the first several weeks of life. Limited capacity for conjugation of benzoic acid with glycine results in accumulation of benzoic acid. A potentially fatal syndrome consisting of multiorgan failure, severe metabolic acidosis, and gasping respirations may then occur.[13] Cumulative doses of benzyl alcohol exceeding 99 mg/kg in preterm neonates are associated with this gasping syndrome. Thus, products containing benzyl alcohol or benzoic acid should not generally be given to neonates. Solubilizing agents such as propylene glycol and emulsifiers such as the polysorbates have also been associated with toxicity in neonates and small infants.[14,15] Likewise, formation of toxic hydroperoxides from intravenous lipid emulsion repackaged in plastic containers can be a greater risk for this population.[16] Attention to all packaging products and components of PN additives is therefore necessary when working with pediatric PN.

Physical Incompatibility with Enteral Nutrition Formulas

Physical incompatibility can be a major problem when medications (including electrolyte preparations) are administered with EN formulas. The consequence of physical incompatibility with EN formulas is typically clogged feeding tubes. While not life threatening, obstructed tubes can reduce nutrient intake. Several studies evaluated the physical compatibility of various liquid medication preparations with EN formulas.[17-22] Unfortunately, none evaluated pediatric formulas or flow through pediatric feeding tubes. Table 24-3 summarizes the incompatibility of pharmaceutical preparations with EN formulas noted in at least one study.

Results of published studies on compatibility of drugs with EN formulas suggest that both can affect compatibility. The most important properties for pharmaceutical preparations are pH and the base component (sugar–water–based syrups, alcohol-based elixirs, or oil-based preparations).[17-19] The form of protein (intact, hydrolyzed, or free amino acid) is the most critical property of EN formulas.[18-20] Nitrogen content, fiber content, and dilution of the EN formula do not appear to affect compatibility with drug preparations.[17-21]

Cutie and colleagues reported acidic pharmaceutical preparations, especially syrups, caused the greatest problem during compatibility testing with three intact protein EN formulas (Ensure, Ensure Plus, and Osmolite).[17] The same results were reported when high-nitrogen versions of the three EN formulas were tested.[18] Of the incompatible preparations in these studies for which pH could be measured, more than 80% (nine of 11) had a pH of 4 or less. Three of four pharmaceutical syrups with a pH of 4 or less (75%) produced immediate clumping of the EN formula and increases in particle size and viscosity that could not be prevented by slow addition and stirring or dilution of the product. Two of five acidic elixirs (40%) were incompatible; the remaining three were compatible when added slowly while the EN formula was stirred rapidly. Both oil-based products tested were also incompatible.

In addition to the three high-nitrogen EN formulas, the study by Altman and Cutie included a hydrolyzed protein formula (Vital).[18] The hydrolyzed formula was much less incompatible with acidic pharmaceutical preparations but not with oil-based ones. Only three of 53 preparations were incompatible with

TABLE 24-3

Pharmaceutical Preparations Physically Incompatible with Selected EN Formulas

| | | Protein Form of the Formula | | |
| | | Intact protein | | Hydrolyzed protein |
Pharmaceutical Preparation	pH	No fiber	Fiber	
Bentyl	4.5	I	—	C
Chlorpromazine 100 mg/ml	NA	I	I	C
Cibalith-S syrup	4-5	I	—	C
Dimetane elixir	<4	I	I	C
Dimetapp elixir	<4	I	I	C
Feosol elixir	<4	I	I	C
Fleet Phosphosoda	5.0	I	I	C
Gevrabon liquid vitamins	NA	I	I	C
Kaon (K + gluconate) liquid	6.0	I	—	C
KCl liquid (Barre)	5-6	I	—	I
Klovess syrup	<4	I	—	C
Mandelamine suspension	Oil	I	—	I
MCT Oil	Oil	I	—	I
Mellaril solution 100 mg/ml	<4	I	—	C
Mellaril concentrate 30 mg/ml	NA	I	I	C
Mylanta II	7.5	I	—	C
Neo-Calglucon syrup	4	I	I	C
Paregoric elixir	4.5	I	I	C
Reglan syrup	NA	C	I	C
Riopan	7.5	I	—	C
Robitussin expectorant	<4	I	I	C
Sudafed syrup	<4	I	I	C
Tagamet (cimetidine)	5.5	I	—	C
Thorazine concentrate	<4	I	—	C
Zinc sulfate 220 mg	NA	I	I	C

Compiled and adapted from Cutie AJ, Altman E, Lenkel L: Compatibility of enteral products with commonly employed drug additives, *J Parenter Enteral Nutr* 7: 186-191, 1983; Altman E, Cutie AJ: Compatibility of enteral products with commonly employed drug additives, *Nutr Support Serv* 1:8-17, 1984; Fagerman KE, Ballov AE: Drug compatibilities with enteral leading solutions co-administered by lube, *Nutr Support Serv* 8:31-32, 1988; Burns PE, McCall L, Wirsching R: Physical compatibility of enteral formulas with various common medications, *J Am Diet Assoc* 88:1094-1096, 1988.

C, Compatible; *I*, incompatible; *NA*, not available.

Vital, including both oil-based products tested (mandelamine suspension and medium-chain triglyceride oil) plus a moderately acidic liquid potassium chloride preparation. Fagerman and Ballou also reported less incompatibility with Vital than with intact protein formulas (Osmolite and Osmolite HN).[19] Not one of the 16 pharmaceutical preparations tested in this study was incompatible with the hydrolyzed protein formula, whereas nearly 40% were incompatible with both intact protein formulas.

Likewise, not one of 39 medications that Burns and coworkers tested was incompatible with the free amino acid formula Vivonex EN.[20] Nearly one third of the medications were incompatible with both the fiber-added intact protein formula (Enrich) and the low-residue intact protein formula (TwoCal HN).

Caution is advised when applying information from the published compatibility studies to specialized nutrition support practice. Fewer than 100 pharmaceutical preparations and only 13 EN formulas (none of which were designed for pediatric patients) were included in the studies. Approximately 30% of the pharmaceutical preparations tested were incompatible with

at least one EN formula. Given the hundreds of available pharmaceutical preparations, many more preparations are likely to be incompatible with EN formulas. In addition, nonmedicinal ("inert") ingredients in the pharmaceutical preparations tested may have changed, and many of the EN formulas used in these studies have undergone revisions since the studies were completed. The protein source for nine of 11 intact protein formulas used in these studies was a combination of sodium and calcium caseinates plus soy protein isolates. Two formulas contained only sodium and calcium caseinates as protein sources. Formulas using different sources of intact protein such as nonfat milk or lactalbumin may react differently with the pharmaceutical preparations. Limited data does, in fact, suggest that intact casein and soy proteins are more likely to cause clumping and precipitate formation with pharmaceutical preparations than is whey protein.[23] Vital contains partially hydrolyzed whey, meat, and soy protein. Hydrolyzed protein formulas that differ from Vital in the source of hydrolyzed proteins or in the percentages of free amino acids, short peptides, and oligopeptides may also react differently with drugs. Vivonex EN contains free amino acids, which may react differently than partially hydrolyzed protein in some cases. In short, compatibility testing in vitro with the formula the patient receives is advisable before *any* pharmaceutical preparation is mixed with an EN formula.

Methods of Avoiding Physical Incompatibility

Physical incompatibility between PN or EN formulas and drugs can be avoided by not mixing the two. This includes flushing the intravenous tubing or feeding tube with an appropriate fluid (0.9% sodium chloride for intravenous tubing, water for feeding tubes) before and after each dose of medication. Altering the PN formula to omit an incompatible component or changing the EN formula to a hydrolyzed or free amino acid formula may be effective in avoiding physical incompatibility. Changing the medication, if possible, may also avoid physical incompatibility. Medication changes can include reducing the dose, if this is therapeutically acceptable; using an alternate dosage form such as an opened capsule rather than an acidic syrup for administration via a feeding tube; using an alternate route of administration (e.g., rectal, sublingual, intramuscular, transdermal); or switching to a therapeutically equivalent medication that is compatible with the PN or EN formula. Table 24-4 summarizes methods of avoiding incompatibilities with specialized nutritional formulas.[24]

Therapeutic Equivalents

Therapeutically equivalent medications—ones that produce the same clinical results—can be chemically distinct entities. Many health care facilities and providers include one or two therapeutically equivalent medications in their formularies. Physicians must justify use of a nonformulary medication. Seldom, if ever, is compatibility with PN or EN formulas considered in the selection of a medication for a formulary. Examples include penicillin and erythromycin used to treat "strep throat," ibuprofen and naproxen for muscle aches, loperamide (Imodium) and diphenoxylate (Lomotil) for diarrhea, promethazine (Phenergan) and prochlorperazine (Compazine)

From Thomson CA, Rollins CJ: Enteral feeding and medication incompatibilities, *Support Line* 8: 9-11, 1991.

TABLE 24-4

Avoiding Incompatibilities Between Medications and Enteral Formulas

Action to Be Taken	Type of Incompatibility				
	Physical	Pharmaceutical	Pharmacologic	Physiologic	Pharmacokinetic
Do not mix medication with enteral formula	✓				✓
Try another enteral formula	✓			✓	✓
Use an alternate dosage form	✓	✓		✓	✓
Use an alternate route for administration	✓	✓		✓	✓
Use a therapeutic equivalent	✓	✓	✓	✓	✓
Check dosing for appropriateness	✓		✓	✓	✓
Use adjunct medication to treat adverse effect			✓	✓	
Dilute medication				✓	

for postoperative nausea and vomiting, and ondansetron (Zofran) and granisetron (Kytril) for vomiting secondary to cancer chemotherapy.

Dosage Forms

A *dosage form* is a drug or combination plus nonmedicinal (inert) ingredients called *excipients*. The excipients stabilize the medication or render it appropriate for administration. For example, an oral liquid medication may contain alcohol as a solubilizing agent and sweeteners for palatability. Likewise, lactose is often added to dilute an active ingredient so it is suitable for tablet formulation. Starch is used as a binder that allows the active ingredient, when compressed into a tablet, to "hold together." Pure crystals of a medication rarely stay compressed in a tablet without a binder. Talc and magnesium stearate are often used to improve flow characteristics of medication granules before they are formed into tablets and to prevent formed tablets from sticking to dies or molds. Different excipients may be needed to formulate a given drug in different forms (e.g., tablet, capsule, suspension, or solution) and to produce a given dosage form from different medications. Because excipients are considered inert or therapeutically inactive, manufacturers are not required to list them as ingredients. In addition, excipients can be changed without notifying customers or health care professionals, although the manufacturer may be required to prove bioequivalence to the Food and Drug Administration (FDA) when excipients are changed. Common dosage forms include tablets, capsules, granules, suspensions, syrups, elixirs, solutions, suppositories, transdermal patches, creams, and ointments.

Some dosage forms contain subgroups designed for specific applications, for example, coated tablets. Enteric-coated tablets are specifically designed to withstand stomach acid and to dissolve only in the higher-pH environment of the small bowel. Medications that are destroyed by acid or that irritate the stomach are usually enteric coated. Sublingual and buccal tablets contain relatively small doses of medication designed for rapid release. Drugs taken thus are absorbed directly into the bloodstream, so medications that are highly metabolized by the liver can be given in much smaller quantities than if swallowed and absorbed through the small bowel into the portal circulation. A sublingual or buccal dose given via a feeding tube generally provides insufficient medication by the time it

reaches the bloodstream. Slow-release or sustained-action tablets contain several doses of medication that are released sequentially over a long time. Slow release of medication from a tablet can be accomplished by using a special wax-matrix or membrane system or multiple layers that dissolve sequentially. Capsules can also release a drug slowly if they contain pellets or beads with different dissolution times.

Dosage Forms That Should Not Be Crushed

Crushing an enteric-coated tablet for administration via a gastric feeding tube delivers the medication to an inappropriate site. An acid-labile medication will not be protected from stomach acid resulting in destruction of the medication or the stomach will not be protected from an irritating medication and the risk of nausea, vomiting, or gastric erosion increases. Crushing a sustained-release product also creates pharmaceutical incompatibility because all doses of the medication are released immediately (causing an "overdose"), rather than gradually over several (generally 12 to 24) hours. Pharmaceutical incompatibility is a concern principally when solid dosage forms of medications must be administered through a feeding tube.

Lists of medications that should not be altered are routinely published and updated.[25] Abbreviations and manufacturer-specific terms can also be used to identify associated dosage forms that should not be altered. The abbreviations are typically added to medication names, such as SR (sustained or slow release). Special forms of drugs must be evaluated individually by a pharmacist to determine if the medication can safely be altered. Although crushing is rarely acceptable, minor alteration of the dosage form of some enteric-coated or slow-release preparations may be acceptable. Facilities that routinely administer medications via feeding tubes should consider developing a formulary-specific list of those that must not be altered and alternatives for administration via feeding tubes.

Enteric-Coated and Slow-Release Dosage Forms

The technology used to create an enteric-coated or slow-release capsule determines the acceptability of opening it to deliver the contents via a feeding tube. Capsules containing many small enteric-coated beads, such as erythromycin can generally be opened and the entire contents administered via the feeding tube. The tube openings must be large enough to accommodate the intact beads without clogging because crushing or dissolving the beads would destroy the enteric coating. Gastrostomy tubes are usually the only tubes large enough to accommodate the intact beads. When an enteric-coated medication is delivered via tube into the small bowel, destruction of the enteric coating may be acceptable because stomach acid has already been bypassed. Slow-release capsules containing many small beads may also be acceptable for administration via a feeding tube if the intact beads can pass through the tube openings without clogging the tube. With a slow-release capsule, the actual capsule serves only to hold together the correct combination of beads. Proper dosing is ensured as long as the beads remain intact (not crushed or dissolved) for administration and the complete contents of the capsule, minus the capsule itself, are delivered as a single dose.

Administration of Intravenous Dosage Forms via the Gastrointestinal Tract

The intravenous form of medication is sometimes considered an attractive alternative for feeding tube administration when an oral liquid form is not available or when sweeteners or dyes are thought to contribute to gastrointestinal (GI) intolerance. In general, administration of intravenous dosage forms via the GI tract can result in underdosing medication. Most intravenous dosage forms are not designed to withstand conditions in the GI tract, especially gastric acidity and digestive enzymes. Solutions for intravenous administration may form insoluble precipitates in an acid environment or may be rapidly degraded so that very little active medication reaches the blood. Electrolyte preparations designed for intravenous administration, however, do appear to be effective when administered via the GI tract. (See Incompatibility [Intolerance] with Enteral Nutrition under the Physiologic Incompatibility section that discusses GI intolerance associated with sweeteners and dyes.)

Methods of Avoiding Pharmaceutical Incompatibility

Selecting an alternate dosage form (e.g., morphine elixir rather than sustained-release morphine tablets) sometimes avoids pharmaceutical incompatibility. Different formulations of a drug may exhibit different tolerances for crushing. Erythromycin, for example, is available in four tablet formulations. Tablets of erythromycin base and erythromycin stearate are not acceptable for crushing and administering through a gastric tube because they are acid labile and require enteric coating to maintain activity. Erythromycin ethylsuccinate tablets can be crushed if necessary, because they are relatively stable in acid. Erythromycin estolate tablets, the most acid stable of the four erythromycin tablet formulations, can be crushed and administered intragastrically without losing therapeutic activity. Other approaches to pharmaceutical incompatibility include selecting an alternate route of administration (e.g., topical application of nitroglycerin ointment or transdermal patch rather than sublingual nitroglycerin tablets) or using a therapeutic equivalent (e.g., isosorbide dinitrate rather than sublingual nitroglycerin). The pharmacist is generally consulted when pharmaceutical incompatibility is a problem; however, the dietitian or nurse may need to alert the

pharmacist to the problem if a multidisciplinary nutrition support service does not monitor EN patients.

Pharmacologic Incompatibility

Pharmacologic effects, those related to the mechanism of a drug's action, tend to be predictable in most patients, but secondary pharmacologic effects occasionally are undesirable. This is clearly seen with the nonselective β-adrenergic antagonist (β-blocker) propranolol. Used for its ability to decrease heart rate and contractile force by blocking β-receptors in the heart, propranolol also affects β-receptors in smooth muscle of the lungs to cause undesirable bronchoconstriction. Although such undesirable drug effects are frequently called *side effects* or *intolerance*, when they interfere with PN or EN therapy they are also a form of incompatibility. Pharmacologic incompatibility refers to intolerances to PN and/or EN therapy that occur as a result of a medication's mechanism of action or to interference with a medication's mechanism of action by a component of PN or EN therapy. The most common pharmacologic incompatibility involves EN therapy with medications that act on GI motility or on the chemoreceptor trigger zone (CTZ).

Gastrointestinal Tract Pharmacology

The GI tract is a complex system composed of longitudinal and circular muscle layers and secretory cells responsive to a variety of neurotransmitters, polypeptides, and hormones. Both the sympathetic and parasympathetic divisions of the autonomic nervous system innervate the GI tract, providing links to the brain and spinal cord. The two divisions provide opposing effects in the GI tract, but intrinsic innervation of the GI tract also modulates responses, as do certain GI hormones. Medications may therefore exert effects directly on the GI tract or through central nervous system–mediated responses.

Norepinephrine is the primary neurotransmitter of the sympathetic system at the effector organs, such as smooth muscle in the GI tract. Both α-adrenergic and β-adrenergic receptors are involved in regulation of tone and motility in the GI tract, whereas α-receptors control GI sphincter response. The general response to adrenergic stimulation (norepinephrine release at the receptor) is decreased peristalsis and tone in the GI tract lumen and constriction of sphincters. Substances that prevent reuptake of norepinephrine into storage vesicles prolong the response. Alpha- or β-antagonists block the response to norepinephrine, resulting in unregulated parasympathetic response. Adrenergic effects in the GI tract tend to be transient, however, and may not be clinically significant.

Acetylcholine is the primary neurotransmitter associated with the parasympathetic system. The general response to parasympathetic (cholinergic) stimulation in the GI tract is increased peristalsis, increased secretory activity from gastric and pancreatic glands, and relaxation of sphincters. Substances that mimic the action of acetylcholine (e.g., succinylcholine) or prevent acetylcholine breakdown by cholinesterase enzymes (e.g., physostigmine) prolong parasympathetic effects. Blocking of acetylcholine receptors in the GI tract by substances such as atropine or scopolamine results in unregulated sympathetic response (e.g., decreased peristalsis and tone in the lumen and constriction of sphincters). However, not all substances act equally throughout the GI tract. Some have a more powerful effect in a particular segment (e.g., stomach, small bowel, or colon.)

In addition to sympathetic and parasympathetic innervation, the GI tract contains intrinsic neurons whose cell bodies are located in the wall of the GI tract. Ganglia (clusters of cell bodies) and bundles of neuronal processes connecting the ganglia lie between the longitudinal and circular muscle layers forming the myenteric (Auerbach's) plexus and in the submucosa forming the submucosal (Meissner's) plexus. Sympathetic and parasympathetic fibers are also located in these plexuses. Smooth muscle cells and secretory cells of the GI tract are innervated by excitatory or inhibitory effector neurons of the intrinsic system. Intrinsic excitatory neurons release acetylcholine as a neurotransmitter. Transmitters for inhibitory neurons and interneurons include various polypeptides, such as vasoactive intestinal peptide (VIP), substance P, and some GI hormones. Postganglionic sympathetic neurons and intrinsic sensory neurons also affect the intrinsic excitatory and inhibitory neurons. In addition, preganglionic parasympathetic fibers form synapses with intrinsic neurons. The net effect is modulation of parasympathetic activity by integration of information from the other systems. Thus, GI tract control is complex and subject to the effects of many transmitter substances. Any medication that stimulates or inhibits the autonomic nervous system or intrinsic GI system can influence GI function.

Medications That Affect Gastrointestinal Motility

Medications that cause increased GI motility by virtue of their pharmacology include metoclopramide (Reglan), cisapride (Propulsid), and erythromycin. Such drugs may decrease tolerance to EN therapy by causing abdominal cramping or diarrhea. Opiates (morphine and morphinelike compounds) decrease GI motility. The resting tone of smooth muscles in the GI tract increases with these compounds, resulting in both delayed gastric emptying and decreased peristaltic movement. Anticholinergic agents (cholinergic blocking agents) decrease GI motility by blocking the acetylcholine stimulation of GI motility. Anticholinergic agents include the belladonna alkaloids (e.g., atropine and scopolamine), and benztropine mesylate (Cogentin) and trihexyphenidyl (Artane) which are used to treat Parkinson's disease. Amitriptyline, a tricyclic antidepressant, and diphenhydramine (Benadryl), an antihistamine, also possess significant anticholinergic activity. Medications that decrease GI motility may result in poor gastric emptying, constipation, or fecal impaction, which in turn may prevent adequate delivery of nutrients in tube feedings.

Medications That Affect the Chemoreceptor Trigger Zone

Medications that affect the chemoreceptor trigger zone (CTZ) can affect tolerance to EN therapy by inducing or suppressing vomiting. The CTZ consists of a group of cells on the floor of the fourth ventricle of the brain. This area contains dopamine receptors and is thus responsive to medications that stimulate or block dopamine activity. Medications that stimulate dopamine activity at the CTZ tend to induce vomiting; cisplatin, an antineoplastic agent, is highly emetogenic, for example. Other anti-

neoplastic agents associated with severe vomiting secondary to stimulation of the CTZ are doxorubicin (Adriamycin), mechlorethamine (Mustargen), cyclophosphamide (Cytoxan, Endoxan), chlorambucil (Leukeran), melphalan (Alkeran, L-PAM), dacarbazine (DTIC), and dactinomycin (Actinomycin-D, Cosmegen). Opiates such as morphine also stimulate the CTZ.

Dopamine-blocking agents can suppress vomiting initiated in the CTZ, and thus have the potential to improve tolerance to EN therapy. Metoclopramide (Reglan) is frequently used as an antiemetic for its dopamine-blocking effect. Phenothiazines also exert antiemetic effect by blocking dopamine receptors in the CTZ. Ondansetron (Zofran) and granisetron (Kytril) are effective antiemetic agents for patients receiving chemotherapy, but they act by blocking 5-hydroxytryptamine (serotonin type 3 or 5-HT3) receptors rather than dopamine receptors.

Glucocorticoids

Pharmacologic effects of glucocorticoids—hydrocortisone, prednisone, prednisolone, and dexamethasone—include decreased peripheral utilization of glucose, promotion of gluconeogenesis (through both peripheral and hepatic action), and accelerated synthesis of glucose from pyruvate in hepatic mitochondria. The net result of these pharmacologic effects tends to be hyperglycemia with insulin resistance. The hyperglycemia may be severe enough to prevent adequate caloric provision via PN or EN therapy. Thus, glucocorticoids exhibit a type of pharmacologic incompatibility with specialized nutrition support based on altered metabolism.

Broad-Spectrum Antibiotics

Intolerance to EN therapy frequently is secondary to *Clostridium difficile* diarrhea induced by broad-spectrum antibiotics. By killing normal GI flora through pharmacologic actions on bacterial cell wall synthesis, protein synthesis, cell membrane stability, or interference with bacterial ribosomal functions, these antibiotics allow unrestricted growth of resistant bacteria and fungi in the GI tract. Sporulating organisms such as *C. difficile* survive antibiotic exposure as spores and then flourish in the vegetative state after antibiotic concentrations in the colon decrease.[26] Antibiotics most often implicated in *C. difficile*-induced colitis include clindamycin, cephalosporins, ampicillin, and amoxicillin.[26-28] Other antibiotics have also been associated with diarrhea in tube-fed patients, although nonpharmacologic actions may be involved in some cases.[29-31]

Antagonism of Vitamin K with Warfarin

Antagonism of warfarin sodium (Coumadin) by vitamin K is the most significant pharmacologic incompatibility in which a component of specialized nutrition therapy interferes with a pharmacologic action. Warfarin blocks formation of active vitamin K-dependent clotting factors (factors II, VII, IX, and X) in the coagulation cascade. Anticoagulation with warfarin generally occurs with vitamin K intake of 300 to 500 µg per day from the typical Western diet.[32] The recommended dietary intake (RDI) for vitamin K is only 45 to 80 µg per day for adults.[33] In adults, however, a single parenteral or oral dose of vitamin K as small as 2.5 mg rapidly reverses or substantially decreases the anticoagulant effect of warfarin for several days.

Doses of vitamin K smaller than 2.5 mg can inhibit anticoagulation by warfarin, especially when taken daily. Relatively large doses of warfarin can overcome anticoagulation inhibition induced by vitamin K, but this increases the risk of severe bleeding if the vitamin K is discontinued.

The vitamin K in either PN or EN formulas can interfere with warfarin anticoagulation. The vitamin K content of PN formulas is provided in a multivitamin preparation and/or phytonadione (vitamin K-1, AquaMEPHYTON) added to the formulas. Adult parenteral multivitamin preparations previously did not contain vitamin K and did not interfere with warfarin therapy. Because many facilities included phytonadione in standard PN orders, however, problems did occur when standard PN orders were written for a patient receiving warfarin. Typical PN formulas contained 1 mg phytonadione per liter of formula per day, 2 mg phytonadione per total daily volume of formula, or 10 mg phytonadione once per week. Alternatively a weekly 10-mg dose could be given by subcutaneous or intramuscular injection.

The FDA has published notice that the conditions for marketing an effective adult parenteral multivitamin drug product published in the *Federal Register* of September 17, 1984 (49 FR 36446) are being amended.[34] Manufacturers have until 2004 to fully implement the new requirements. Once fully implemented, parenteral adult multivitamin preparations will contain 150 µg of vitamin K (phylloquinone) per unit dose. Some parenteral adult multivitamin preparations are now appearing with the new formulation. The change in vitamin K and other changes to the adult parenteral multivitamin formulation are based on data presented and discussed at a 1985 public workshop sponsored by the FDA and American Medical Association. Label changes are also to occur. Under the precaution section on the label, a paragraph is to be added in bold type advising caution for administration of the product to patients on warfarin sodium-type anticoagulant therapy and stating that periodic monitoring of prothrombin time is essential.

Pediatric parenteral multivitamin preparations contain 200 µg of vitamin K in a standard 5-ml daily dose. This dose is inadequate to reverse anticoagulation in adults but requires periodic monitoring of prothrombin time. This dose can significantly interfere with warfarin anticoagulation in pediatric patients. To avoid pharmacologic incompatibility between pediatric PN formulas and warfarin, therefore, it may be necessary to omit the pediatric multivitamin preparation. This action, however, raises the potential for serious complications, even death, from vitamin deficiency.[35-37] An oral multivitamin supplement without vitamin K should be provided if the injectable pediatric multivitamin preparation is to be omitted and GI function is adequate to ensure vitamin absorption. For patients with inadequate oral absorption, an appropriate quantity of an adult injectable multivitamin preparation without vitamin K could be used while this product is still available. Once the adult formulation is changed to include 150 µg of vitamin K per unit dose, the product may still provide a reasonable option for pediatric patients with inadequate oral absorption because this is less vitamin K than is contained in the pediatric formulation, especially when less than the full adult unit dose may be appropriate for a pediatric patient. The potential contribution of intravenous lipid emulsion to warfarin sodium resistance should also be considered.[38]

Many reports of interference between warfarin anticoagulation and EN formulas can be found in the literature.[39-49] Incompatibility between warfarin therapy and vitamin K in EN formulas must be managed through formula selection, since vitamin K comes in the formula from the manufacturer. The vitamin K content of many EN formulas was reduced after the initial reports of warfarin resistance; however, over a sixfold variation still exists in vitamin K content of the various EN formulas (Table 24-5).[48,49] Changing from a low-vitamin K formula to one with more vitamin K could inhibit warfarin anticoagulation, whereas changing from high to low vitamin K content could result in excessive anticoagulation and bleeding. When evaluating EN formulas for inclusion in a formulary, the vitamin K content should be considered with respect to the patient population most likely to receive the formula. For critically ill trauma patients, for example, an EN formula with moderate to high vitamin K content may be desirable. These patients rarely receive warfarin but frequently receive multiple antibiotics, which reduce normal GI flora, thus increasing the risk of inadequate vitamin K production by the remaining flora. Cardiac care unit patients, on the other hand, frequently receive warfarin therapy and their fluids are often restricted as well. Thus, a low vitamin K content may be desirable for a nutrient-dense formula selected for use in the cardiac care unit. There is also some evidence that warfarin may bind to a filterable component (most likely protein) in enteral formulas. In

TABLE 24-5

Vitamin K Content of Selected Enteral Formulas

Formula	Manufacturer	Vitamin K (mg/1000 kcal)
Respalor	Mead Johnson	37
Ensure Plus	Ross	38
Pediasure	Ross	38
Vivonex T.E.N.	Novartis	40
Osmolite	Ross	41
NovaSource 2.0	Novartis	42
Nepro	Ross	43
TwoCal HN	Ross	43
Vivonex Plus	Novartis	44
Boost Plus	Mead Johnson	45
Crucial	Nestle	50
Glytrol	Nestle	50
Nutren 1.0	Nestle	50
Peptamen VHP	Nestle	50
Replete	Nestle	50
Perative	Ross	54
Vital HN	Ross	54
Glucerna	Ross	57
Pulmocare	Ross	57
Jevity	Ross	58
Complete	Novartis	62.7
IsoSource HN	Novartis	66.7
DiabetiSource	Novartis	67
Impact	Novartis	67
Ensure	Ross	80
Isocal HN	Mead Johnson	100
Choice dm	Mead Johnson	120
Deliver 2.0	Ross	125
Isocal	Mead Johnson	125
Boost	Mead Johnson	127
Boost High Protein	Mead Johnson	238

this instance, separating warfarin administration from formula administration, by at least an hour before and after, may avoid the loss of warfarin activity.[50]

Methods of Avoiding Pharmacologic Incompatibility

Methods that can be used to avoid pharmacologic incompatibility include use of a therapeutic equivalent, if available, and medicating to prevent or treat the undesired effect. For example, a dopamine antagonist (blocking agent) such as metoclopramide (Reglan) can be used as part of the protocol for antineoplastic agents that stimulate the CTZ. Medication for adverse effects may include a stimulant laxative to overcome constipation associated with morphine. Avoiding excess medication is another way of preventing some pharmacologic incompatibilities because pharmacologic effects are often dose dependent. A morphine dose of 5 mg every 6 hours, for example, is expected to be less constipating than 5 mg per hour in continuous infusion.

Physiologic Incompatibility

Physiologic responses to medications are exemplified by fluid shifts secondary to osmotic activity and irritant reactions such as inflammation. No receptor stimulation or inhibition, or other mechanism by which a specific medication acts, is involved. Although the responses are not pharmacologic, they can produce physiologic incompatibility.

Incompatibility (Intolerance) with Parenteral Nutrition

Medications rarely exhibit physiologic incompatibility or intolerance with PN therapy administered via a central venous catheter but are frequently a problem with peripheral PN therapy. Medications associated with a high incidence of phlebitis (venous inflammation) should be considered physiologically inappropriate for Y-site administration with peripheral PN therapy, regardless of whether they are physically compatible with PN formulas. For example, nafcillin is physically compatible with PN formulas but produces significant venous irritation when administered via a peripheral vein. Nafcillin is thus inappropriate for Y-site administration with peripheral PN because of physiologic intolerance. Supplemental intravenous potassium chloride doses are also very irritating to peripheral veins when mixed in the typical concentration of 10 mEq per 50 ml of 5% dextrose in water or 0.9% saline. Therefore, at least a relative physiologic incompatibility exists for Y-site administration of potassium chloride with peripheral PN. Dobutamine and erythromycin also cause significant venous irritation when infused via peripheral veins, thus increasing the risk of venous irritation or damage if coinfused with peripheral PN therapy.

Incompatibility (Intolerance) with Enteral Nutrition

Many medications exhibit physiologic incompatibility with EN therapy. Intolerance is typically manifested by nausea, vomiting, diarrhea, abdominal pain, cramping, or bloating. The osmolality of medications and electrolyte solutions has been implicated as a principal factor in physiologic incompatibility

with EN therapy.[51-53] Intolerance to excipients used in the formulation of liquid and solid dosage forms and GI tract irritation have also been implicated.[14, 54-66] The osmolality of liquid dosage forms frequently exceeds 3000 mOsm/kg (Table 24-6). In addition, many liquid dosage forms were developed for pediatric dosing, so adults may need 10 to 40 ml per dose. Very small volumes of hyperosmolar medications generally cause minimal GI intolerance, especially when administered into the stomach, where gastric fluid dilutes them. Large volumes or formulas of extremely high osmolality administered intragastrically, however, are likely to cause GI intolerance because dilution to 300 mOsm/kg does not occur before dumping into the duodenum. Hyperosmolar fluid in the small bowel, whether dumped from the stomach or delivered directly by a feeding tube, can result in an influx of fluid and, consequently, diarrhea.

Intravenous dosage forms contain no sorbitol or other sweeteners, dyes, or fillers (e.g., lactose) that could contribute to GI intolerance, but osmolality can still be very high secondary to the solvent system, stabilizers, or preservatives. As expected with electrolyte formulations, the osmolality is high, regardless of the intended route of administration. Although administration via the GI tract is acceptable for electrolyte solutions, for most intravenous medications it is inappropriate. (See Pharmaceutical Incompatibility, which discusses administration of intravenous dosage forms via the GI tract.)

Dilution Volume for Hyperosmolar Medications

Dilution of a hyperosmolar medication to approximately 300 mOsm/kg reduces the risk of medication-induced diarrhea. The volume of water required to achieve the desired osmolality can be calculated from the following equation:

$$[(\text{medication osmolality/desired osmolality}) \times \text{medication volume in ml}]$$
$$- \text{medication volume in ml} = \text{volume of water}$$

Calculation for a 10-mg dose of metoclopramide using a 1 mg/ml concentration of syrup with an osmolality of 8350 mOsm/kg:

$$[(8350 \text{ mOsm/kg}/300 \text{ mOsm/kg}) \times 10 \text{ ml}] - 10 \text{ ml} = 268 \text{ ml}$$

Thus, the 10-ml dose of metoclopramide must be diluted with 268 ml of water to reduce the osmolality to approximately 300 mOsm/kg.

To calculate a 40-mEq dose of potassium chloride using a 10% liquid preparation with an osmolality of 3000 mOsm/kg, the volume of liquid potassium chloride must first be calculated. The 10% preparation contains 10 g potassium chloride per 100 ml. The milliequivalent weight of potassium chloride is 74.5 mg/mEq. Thus, each ml of 10% potassium chloride equals 1.34 mEq potassium chloride, and 40 mEq potassium chloride equals 30 ml. The volume of water for dilution can then be calculated as follows:

$$[(3000 \text{ mOsm/kg}/300 \text{ mOsm/kg}) \times 30 \text{ ml}] - 30 \text{ ml} = 270 \text{ ml}$$

The 40-mEq potassium chloride dose must be diluted with 270 ml of water to reduce the osmolality to approximately 300 mOsm/kg. By dividing the 40-mEq (30-ml) dose into three 10-ml doses (13.4 mEq per dose), dilution with the typical

TABLE 24-6

Average Osmolality Values of Commercially Available Drug Solutions and Suspensions

Product	Manufacturer	Average Osmolality (mOsm/kg)
Acetaminophen elixir, 65 mg/ml	Roxane	5400
Acetaminophen with codeine elixir	Wyeth	4700
Amantadine hydrochloride solution, 10 mg/ml	Du Pont	3900
Aminophylline liquid, 21 mg/ml	Fisons	450
Amoxicillin suspension, 50 mg/ml	Squibb	2250
Ampicillin suspension, 50 mg/ml	Squibb	2250
Ampicillin suspension, 100 mg/ml	Bristol	1850
Belladonna alkaloids elixir	Robins	1050
Calcium glubionate syrup, 0.36 g/ml	Sandoz	2550
Cascara Sagrada Aromatic Fluid extract	Roxane	1000
Cephalexin suspension, 50 mg/ml	Dista	1950
Chloral hydrate syrup, 50 mg/ml	Pharmaceutical Associates	4400
Cimetidine solution, 60 mg/ml	Smith Kline & French	5550
Co-trimoxazole suspension	Burroughs Wellcome	2200
Dexamethasone elixir, 0.1 mg/ml	Organon	3350
Dexamethasone solution, 1 mg/ml	Roxane	3100
Dextromethorphan hydrobromide syrup, 2 mg/ml	Parke-Davis	5950
Digoxin elixir, 50 μg/ml	Burroughs Wellcome	1350
Diphenhydramine hydrochloride elixir, 2.5 mg/ml	Roxane	850
Diphenoxylate hydrochloride – atropine sulfate suspension	Roxane	8800
Docusate sodium syrup, 3.3 mg/ml	Pharmaceutical Associates	4700
Docusate sodium syrup, 3.3 mg/ml	Roxane	3900
Erythromycin ethylsuccinate suspension, 40 mg/ml	Abbott	1750
Ferrous Sulfate liquid, 60 mg/ml	Roxane	4700
Fluphenazine hydrochloride elixir, 0.5 mg/ml	Squibb	1750
Furosemide solution, 10 mg/ml	Hoechst-Roussel	2050
Kaolin–pectin suspension	Roxane	900
Haloperidol concentrate, 2 mg/ml	McNeil	500
Hydroxyzine hydrochloride syrup. 2 mg/ml	Roerig	4450
Lactulose syrup, 0.67 g/ml	Roerig	3600
Lithium citrate syrup, 1.6 inEq/ml	Roxane	6850
Magnesium citrate solution	Medalist	1000
Methyldopa suspension, 50 mg/ml	Merck Sharp & Dohme	2050
Metoclopramide hydrochloride syrup, 1 mg/ml	Robins	8350
Milk of magnesia suspension	Pharmaceutical Associates	1250
Multivitamin liquid	Upjohn	5700
Nystatin suspension, 100,000 units/ml	Squibb	3300
Paregoric tincture	Roxane	1350
Phenytoin sodium suspension, 6 mg/ml	Parke-Davis	2000
Phenytoin sodium suspension, 25 mg/ml	Parke-Davis	1500
Potassium–sodium citrate solution	Willen	2700
Potassium chloride liquid, 10%	Adria	3000
Potassium chloride liquid, 10%	Roxane	3300
Potassium chloride liquid, 10%	Roxane	4350
Potassium chloride liquid, 10%	Roxane	3550
Potassium iodide saturated solution, 1 g/ml	Upsher Smith	10,950
Primidone suspension, 50 mg/ml	Ayerst	450
Prochlorperaziné syrup, 1 mg/ml	Glaxo SmithKline	3250
Promethazine hydrochloride syrup, 1.25 mg/ml	Wyeth	3500
Pyrantel parnoate suspension, 50 mg/ml	PFI Pharmaceutics	4350
Pyridostigmine bromide syrup, 12 mg/ml	Roche	3800
Sodium citrate liquid	Willen	2050
Sodium phosphate liquid, 0.5 g/ml	Fleet	7250
Theophylline solution, 5.33 mg/ml	Berlex	800
Theophylline solution, 5.33 mg/ml	Pharmaceutical Associates	600
Thiabendazole suspension, 100 mg/ml	Merck Sharp & Dohme	2150
Thioridazine suspension, 20 mg/ml	Sandoz	2050
Trace element injection	LyphoMed	500

100 ml of water per dose would reduce the osmolality to about 275 mOsm/kg.

Sorbitol

Most flavored medications contain either sugar or sorbitol, both of which contribute to high osmolality. Sorbitol is a hyperosmotic laxative commonly used with activated charcoal and sodium polystyrene sulfonate (Kayexalate) for its purgative effect. The cumulative daily dose of sorbitol from liquid dosage forms can easily equal the usual purgative dose of 20 to 50 g. Sorbitol doses of 20 g are reported to cause severe cramping and diarrhea in the majority of people, and doses of 5 to 10 g cause bloating and flatulence in a substantial portion of people.[54] Published data on the sorbitol content of liquid dosage forms demonstrate that the sorbitol content of a given medication varies by manufacturer.[55] Obtaining manufacturer-specific information may be difficult, however, because some manufacturers consider sorbitol content proprietary information. As an inert excipient, sorbitol is not required to be listed as an ingredient and is frequently omitted from pharmacy references even when the manufacturer discloses sorbitol content in the package information.[55] In addition, as an inert ingredient, sorbitol content can be changed without notifying patients or health care professionals. To the extent that information can be obtained, therefore, current manufacturers' data for the product in use should always be used in preference to that published previously.

Lactose

Lactose is another excipient that occasionally causes symptoms that are misinterpreted as EN intolerance. Although lactose intolerance is well known to result in watery diarrhea and bloating, the lactose content of most individual dosage forms of medication is too small to result in significant problems. Patients who are very sensitive to lactose and take many medications containing lactose, however, can develop symptoms of lactose intolerance. Solid dosage forms, including tablets and capsules, are more likely than liquid forms to contain lactose.

Gluten

Celiac sprue (gluten-induced enteropathy) is associated with symptoms that could be mistaken for EN intolerance, including abdominal pain, bloating, and diarrhea. Excipients containing gluten (e.g., wheat flour or corn starch) can cause GI symptoms in EN patients who have severe celiac sprue. A list of gluten-free pharmaceutical preparations for a specific manufacturer can sometimes be obtained through the manufacturer. As for any excipients, however, the gluten content of medications can change without notification of the public or health care community. A new list of gluten-free products must, therefore, be obtained regularly to be sure the information is current.

Gastrointestinal Tract Irritants

Medications that irritate the GI tract and result in pain, cramping, bloating, and diarrhea can interfere with EN therapy. Oral iron preparations are typical of medications that irritate the GI tract. Aspirin and nonsteroidal antiinflammatory agents such as ibuprofen, naproxen, indomethacin (Indocin), and ketorolac tromethamine (Toradol) are also associated with GI irritation.

In addition, pharmacologic effects on prostaglandin synthesis or release and platelet aggregation may contribute to the risk of GI bleeding with these agents. Dyes are another group of excipients used in medications or added to EN formulas that may result in adverse reactions.[14, 65] Occasionally, reactions to dyes include GI symptoms that could be interpreted as EN intolerance. At other times, dye may produce systemic toxicity.[66] The dye content of selected pediatric antibiotic preparations has been published, but, except for tartrazine, dye content is proprietary information that can be changed without notation on the label.[65]

Methods of Avoiding Physiologic Incompatibility

Physiologic incompatibility or intolerance can be avoided by several methods. Dilution of highly osmolar medications to an osmolality of 300 mOsm/kg before it is administered prevents influx of fluid into the GI tract but may require too much fluid to be practical in some cases. Dividing the dose into two to four smaller doses may be effective for some hyperosmolar medications and electrolyte solutions. For example, 40 mEq of potassium chloride can be divided into four doses of 10 mEq given at 1- to 2-hour intervals. Addition of about 70 ml of water per 10-mEq dose could then reduce the osmolality from 3000 mOsm/kg to about 300 mOsm/kg. Diluting irritating medications or dividing them into smaller doses also tends to reduce symptoms of intolerance due to GI irritation. Administration of an antacid before or after medication may occasionally be recommended to reduce GI irritation, but caution must be used to avoid potential medication interactions and clogging of the feeding tube. Medications known to cause GI intolerance in a patient should be avoided if possible. An alternative dosage form (e.g., a capsule rather than syrup) may frequently avoid physiologic intolerance. An intravenous dosage form of lower osmolality, however, may not be appropriate for administration via feeding tube. Therapeutic alternatives or alternate routes of administration are also effective ways of avoiding physiologic incompatibility when they can be employed. When diarrhea does occur because of physiologic intolerance, appropriate treatment may allow continued tube feeding.

Pharmacokinetic Incompatibility

Pharmacokinetics is the branch of pharmacy that deals with absorption, distribution, metabolism, and elimination of medications. Pharmacokinetic incompatibility refers to alteration of at least one of these parameters of a medication as a result of specialized nutrition support or alteration of the parameter(s) for a nutrient in a specialized nutrition formula as a result of a medication. Consequences of such incompatibilities can range from inconsequential to life threatening.

Absorption

A drug is said to have been absorbed when it has passed from the site of administration into the bloodstream or lymphatic system. To be effective beyond the immediate site of administration, any drug given by any except the intravenous route must be absorbed. Intravenous administration bypasses the absorptive process by delivering a medication or nutrient directly into the blood. Alterations of absorption relative to specialized nutrition support thus relate principally to EN therapy and administration of medications via the feeding tube. Altered bioavailability can involve any route of administration, however, including the intravenous one. The term *bioavailability* is used to describe the percentage or fraction of an administered dose that reaches the blood or another site of measurement. Absorption is an important component of bioavailability, but chemical instability, photodegradation, sorption, enzymatic degradation, and hepatic metabolism also contribute to differences between the quantity of medication or nutrient initially added to the nutrition formula and the quantity that reaches the blood or tissue.

Chemical Instability

Chemical instability of additives to PN and EN formulations results in delivery of less than the desired amount of nutrient or medication. The instability is detected only through specific testing in vitro before the formula is administered. In vivo monitoring of a chemically unstable nutrient or medication mimics the results noted with reduced absorption; thus, it may be referred to as an *apparent alteration of absorption*. Vitamin and medication additives are of particular concern with respect to chemical instability. The most important factors that affect chemical instability for PN and EN additives include pH, time, and temperature. The final pH of most PN formulas is slightly acidic, so vitamins or medications that are inactivated in an acid environment tend to lose activity when added to a PN formula. Increased acidity, as with the addition of L-cysteine to neonatal PN formulations, can increase both the extent and the rate of activity loss. In general, losses tend to increase as time in the acidic environment increases. Increasing temperature usually increases the rate of loss as well. Preservatives in individual components of PN formulas can also affect additive stability. Thiamine stability, for example, is reduced in the presence of sodium bisulfite, an antioxidant used in some amino acid solutions.[67]

Photodegradation

Exposure to light can cause oxidation, hydrolysis, and loss of activity in photosensitive vitamins and medications. Cyanocobalamin, folic acid, phytonadione, pyridoxine, riboflavin, thiamine, and vitamin A are all subject to photodegradation. Degradation of ascorbic acid, and subsequent oxalate formation, may also be accelerated by exposure to light.[2-4] Losses increase with exposure time and light intensity. Because fluorescent light is more intense than that produced by standard incandescent bulbs, it can increase loss of light-sensitive vitamins and medications.[67,68] Photodegradation is seldom a problem with EN formulas because light does not penetrate these formulas. The opacity of PN formulas that include lipid emulsion can also be protective of light-sensitive vitamins and medications.

Sorption (Adsorption)

Sorption, or adsorption, results in altered bioavailability secondary to loss of medication into or onto the surface of a container. High lipid solubility increases the risk of adsorption, the degree of loss depending on the storage container. Glass containers are least adsorptive. Polyvinyl chloride containers uti-

lizing diethylheptaphthalate (DEHP) appear to cause the greatest adsorptive losses. Vitamin A losses from containers with DEHP can be substantial.[69] Adsorptive losses of insulin vary with the PN formula and its storage container. Feeding tubes and administration sets are potential sources of adsorptive losses with EN therapy. In vitro studies of phenytoin and carbamazepine have observed loss of medication after administration through a feeding tube.[70,71] Diluting these medications before administration reduced losses, as did irrigating the tube after administration.

Mechanisms of Absorption

Four distinct mechanisms of absorption exist. Passive absorption, or diffusion, relies on a concentration gradient. The rate of absorption increases with concentration gradient. Substances absorbed via passive diffusion must generally be small, nonionized, or lipid-soluble. Passive diffusion is the principal mechanism for absorption of most water-soluble nutrients and medications. Facilitated absorption relies on both a concentration gradient and a carrier mechanism that is not energy dependent. The rate of absorption is initially proportional to the concentration gradient, but it reaches a maximum as all carrier molecules are saturated. Fructose depends on facilitated absorption, and some water-soluble medications appear to utilize this mechanism. Active absorption requires energy in the form of adenosine triphosphate to move substances against a concentration gradient. Glucose, galactose, and amino acids, plus a few medications whose chemical structures mimic these substances, depend on active absorption. Competition between nutrients and medications for the same active absorption sites can result in undesired effects. For example, the effectiveness of levodopa in Parkinson's disease and methyldopa in hypertension is reduced if patients eat a high-protein diet because of competition for the same active absorption sites. Pinocytosis or phagocytosis, in which the cell engulfs a particle or organism, also requires energy. This mechanism has limited importance for absorption of nutrients and medications, although fats, oil-based medications, and proteins are occasionally so absorbed.

Many factors affect absorption, including dissolution rate, site of medication or nutrient delivery, the absorptive environment, and transit time through the GI tract. Solid dosage forms must dissolve because solutes rather than solids are generally absorbed. Medications administered through a feeding tube are often in liquid form, which requires no dissolution, or in suspensions or finely crushed tablets, which may dissolve more rapidly than intact tablets. This could alter the rate or extent of absorption, especially when the variable of gastric emptying is eliminated by delivering the drug directly into the small bowel.

Site of Delivery

The site of delivery influences the absorptive environment and chemical stability of medications and nutrients in the GI tract. Relatively little absorption occurs in the stomach as compared with the small bowel, which has a much larger absorptive surface area. In addition, the higher pH of the small bowel increases the amount of nonionized (absorbable) solute for weak bases, which includes most medications. Intragastric feeding may delay, reduce, or enhance absorption of medication, depending on formula and medication characteristics.

Altered absorption is very likely when medications that are designed to be taken on an empty stomach are administered with intragastric feedings. Any EN formula characteristic that decreases gastric emptying, such as high osmolality, high viscosity, or high fat content, can be expected to slow absorption of medication. This is especially true for medications that do not dissolve until they reach the small intestine, such as enteric-coated products. If a medication is unstable in acids, the amount of medication absorbed may also be reduced. For example, absorption of digoxin and the acid-labile penicillins (ampicillin, cloxacillin, dicloxacillin, penicillin G, penicillin V) is reduced when gastric emptying is delayed. On the other hand, if an acid environment is conducive to activation or dissolution of a medication, delayed gastric emptying may enhance absorption, whereas delivering it into the small bowel can severely reduce absorption. Ketoconazole, for example, is expected to have considerably poorer absorption when delivered into the small bowel than when delivered into the stomach because it requires an acidic environment for dissolution and conversion to the hydrochloride salt that can be absorbed. Griseofulvin also benefits from delayed gastric emptying because it is acid stable but poorly soluble and thus has more time to dissolve.

Few studies have compared intragastric to intraduodenal or intrajejunal administration of medications. Magnusson compared oral and intrajejunal dosing of digoxin to determine the effect of administration site on metabolic inactivation.[72] Oral intake resulted in significantly greater excretion of hydrolytic metabolites (2.9% versus 0.6%) and nonextractable metabolites (11.4% versus 4.7%) than intrajejunal administration. Significantly more nonmetabolized digoxin was recovered after intrajejunal administration (96.3% versus 90.8%). This suggests a need for dose reduction if digoxin is administered via a feeding tube into the small bowel rather than into the stomach. Ciprofloxacin also appears to be better absorbed in the small bowel than in the stomach. Yuk and colleagues compared results of ciprofloxacin administered via nasogastric tube, gastrostomy, or nasoduodenal tube.[73] Absorption nearly doubled in the four patients dosed via nasoduodenal tube compared with the three patients dosed into the stomach.

Method of Nutrient Delivery

The method of EN formula delivery can also influence absorption of medications. When Semple and colleagues compared oral administration of hydralazine solution with administration via a feeding tube, they found that the rate of nutrient administration affected absorption and/or metabolism.[74] The maximum serum concentration of hydralazine was higher with slow infusion of EN formula than with bolus EN feeding. The EN formula itself did not appear to affect absorption, since eating a standard breakfast produced results similar to those of bolus EN formula, whereas results during fasting were similar to those of slow formula infusion. Bhargava and colleagues also noted no effect of EN formula or food on absorption of sustained-release theophylline.[75] EN formula *has* been reported to interfere with absorption of phenytoin and carbamazepine.[76-85]

Phenytoin and Enteral Nutrition

In 1982, Bauer published the first report of an interaction between phenytoin and EN therapy that resulted in subthera-

peutic phenytoin concentrations.[76] Multiple studies and reports have since addressed this phenomenon.[77-83] The best way to administer phenytoin to a patient receiving continuous EN formula remains unclear, however, since published findings often conflict. Holding the feeding formula for 2 hours before and 2 hours after the phenytoin dose has been suggested as a way of avoiding the interaction.[76] Others have found this method ineffective.[77,78] Changing from a protein hydrolysate formula to a meat-based (blenderized) or elemental EN formula has been reported to improve phenytoin management.[78,79] Some investigators suggest using phenytoin capsules rather than suspension, although others disagree.[80-82] Regardless of what method is selected for managing the phenytoin interaction with EN formula, it appears that close serum phenytoin monitoring and appropriate dose adjustments are required to ensure therapeutic drug levels.

Distribution, Metabolism, Excretion

Distribution, metabolism, and excretion are affected by several variables, including modification of a delivery pathway, competition for common mechanisms, and stimulation or inhibition of enzymes involved in metabolism. *Distribution* is moving a substance from the blood to its desired site of action in the body. Medications and nutrients may occasionally compete for sites on transport proteins such as albumin or for surface receptors that determine transport into a cell. Such competition creates the potential for altered distribution of a medication or nutrient. Folic acid and phenytoin appear to compete for transport proteins owing to their structural similarity.[86] Too much folic acid in the diet can thus compromise the efficacy of phenytoin for seizure control.

Altered metabolism is a concern when nutrients and medications share metabolic pathways or are capable of inhibiting or stimulating such pathways. High-protein diets have been reported to accelerate hepatic metabolism of certain medications, and a protein-poor diet can decrease renal clearance of medications.[87] Enteral formulas are expected to affect metabolism and clearance much as whole foods do, although little research has been done. Deficiency or excess of vitamins that serve as cofactors in enzyme systems may affect enzyme-dependent metabolism or clearance of medications. For instance, pyridoxine serves as a cofactor for dopa decarboxylase, an enzyme involved in metabolism of levodopa and methyldopa. Excess pyridoxine can accelerate metabolism of these medications and decrease their effectiveness. Phenytoin, on the other hand, stimulates hepatic microsomal enzymes, which increase metabolism of all substances that are biotransformed by these enzymes, including vitamin D.

Altered pharmacokinetic parameters must be considered when evaluating the feasibility of adding a medication directly to a specialized nutrition formula. This is generally more important with PN than with EN therapy. Most PN is provided as a continuous infusion or as an overnight infusion (cyclic PN). Medications added to a PN formula are thus given by continuous infusion over 24 hours (or the specified cycle time). Pharmacokinetic parameters such as maximum serum concentration (peak) and minimum serum concentration (trough) are different for continuous infusion and intermittent infusion of a medication. Distribution, metabolism, and elimination can also change with the administration method. The net result of such changes may be decreased efficacy or increased toxicity of the medication. For example, lower serum peak and higher serum trough levels of aminoglycoside antibiotics (gentamicin, tobramycin, amikacin) are associated with continuous infusion. Lower peaks may reduce efficacy, and higher trough levels increase the risk of renal toxicity and ototoxicity. Other medications are equally efficacious and no more toxic when administered by continuous, rather than intermittent, infusion. Continuous infusion is an acceptable way of giving clindamycin and H_2-receptor-blocking agents (cimetidine, ranitidine, famotidine), for instance. Because of pharmacokinetic alterations, medications listed in Table 24-2 as appropriate for Y-site administration may not be so for direct addition to the PN formula.

Avoiding Pharmacokinetic Incompatibility

Problems related to binding of medication with a component of enteral formula can be avoided by not mixing the two. Changing to a formula with different nutrient sources may help. Different protein sources, and the degree of protein hydrolysis in particular, affect interactions with medications. Sometimes an alternate dosage form or different salt of the medication avoids interactions. Using an alternate route of administration may avoid incompatibilities that affect absorption, but they are less likely to affect incompatibilities related to distribution, metabolism, or elimination. A therapeutic equivalent may avoid certain pharmacokinetic incompatibilities, especially when food affects absorption of one medication but not the therapeutic equivalent. Appropriate dosing limits the risk of incompatibilities in some cases.

Delivering Medication via Feeding Tube

Despite potential incompatibilities, administration of medications via feeding tube is common in patients receiving EN therapy. General guidelines for administration of medications via gastrostomy or nasoenteric feeding tube are presented in Box 24-1. Jejunal feeding tubes require additional caution because their small lumens, especially those of needle catheter jejunostomy tubes, are more likely to clog. These tubes should be used to administer medications only when specifically approved by a physician or authorized person familiar with the characteristics of the tube and the medication. Crushed tablets should not be administered via needle catheter jejunostomy. Pediatric patients fed with very small-bore tubes are also at high risk for tube occlusion. Small-bore tubes are even more likely to clog when fluid restriction leads to inadequate flush volumes. The volumes suggested in Box 24-1 may be excessive for neonates, infants, and very small children. Flush volume calculations for these patients should be based on tube diameter and length. The flush volume must be adequate to fully clear medications from the tube, or tube occlusion will occur.

It is difficult to give medications via a feeding tube when a patient is also undergoing gastric suction or decompression. Special jejunal tubes are available that have a gastric port. Other patients may have both a nasogastric tube and a tube for small bowel feeding. Care must be taken to ensure that medications are delivered via the proper tube. Delayed gastric emp-

---

BOX 24-1

General Guidelines for Medication Administration via Feeding Tube

1. Administer medications orally whenever possible. Consider alternate routes such as sublingual or transdermal when available.
2. When medications must be administered via feeding tube, use an oral liquid dosage form whenever possible.
   a. Elixirs and suspensions are preferable to syrups when the syrup is acidic.
   b. Dilute viscous liquids with water before administration.
   c. Dilute hypertonic or GI irritant medications with at least 30 ml of water before administration.
   d. Consider dividing the dose of hypertonic medications into three or four daily doses administered at least an hour apart when this is therapeutically acceptable.
   e. Be sure that the dosage or dosing schedule does not need to be adjusted when changing from one dosage form to another (e.g., from a tablet to a suspension).
3. Crush tablets to a fine powder and mix with at least 30 ml warm water.
   a. Be sure the tablet is acceptable for crushing. Check with a pharmacist if in doubt.
   b. Hard gelatin capsules can be opened at the seam and the powder mixed with water. Capsules containing beads should be opened only with the approval of a pharmacist.
   c. Soft gelatin capsules can be punctured at one end with a needle to form a small hole from which the contents can be squeezed and mixed with water for administration. Because medication is lost with this method, when partial or variable dose delivery is unacceptable (e.g., digoxin), the capsule should be dissolved in warm water for administration via the tube. This approach is more accurate but much slower than the needle puncture method.
   d. Use only water for mixing and flushing.
4. Do not mix medications directly into the enteral formula. Nutrients typically present in a formula, such as sodium chloride, vitamins, or trace elements, may be exceptions, depending on the formulation of the product. When adding a medication to EN formula, do so slowly while stirring the formula.
5. Administer each medication separately. Do not mix medications because this increases the risk of incompatibility.
6. When one medication follows another, flush the tube with at least 5 ml of water between each medication.
7. Flush the feeding tube with at least 10 to 20 ml of warm water before and after administering medication via nasogastric tubes. It may take 20 to 30 ml of water to clear a tube in the small bowel.
8. Pull the prepared medication into a 30- to 60-ml catheter tip or Luer tip syringe, as appropriate for the tube connector. Allow the medication to flow by gravity into the tube (with a gentle push of the plunger, if necessary). Excessive pressure can damage the feeding tube.
9. Restart the feeding at the appropriate time if feedings were stopped to administer medications. Feedings may be stopped for varying periods before and after medication administration when required for proper absorption of a medication.
10. Assess the patient for desired therapeutic response to medications. Response to EN therapy should also be evaluated periodically, especially when the feedings are stopped for significant periods to give medication.

---

tying can reduce the rate or degree of absorption of medication delivered into the stomach of some patients who require gastric suction or decompression. In addition, suction or decompression must be stopped for a while after gastric delivery; otherwise, the medication will be suctioned away before it reaches the small bowel and is absorbed. The medication can also be lost when a small bowel tube used for medications migrates into the stomach or retrograde peristalsis propels enteral formula into the stomach.

Calcium and Phosphate in Parenteral Nutrition

Calcium and phosphorus are essential for many body processes, such as cardiac function, muscle activity, nerve conduction, and enzymatic reactions. When calcium and phosphorus intake are inadequate, normal serum concentrations are maintained at the expense of bone demineralization. Over time, pathologic fractures can result from demineralization of bone. Most EN formulas contain adequate calcium and phosphorus at least to meet RDIs. Unfortunately, provision of calcium and phosphorus in PN formulas is limited by solubility. Patients who have the least bone mineral content or require the most (e.g., infants, especially premature ones; children; and frail elderly women) are at greatest risk for calcium and phosphorus deficiency, especially when fluids are also restricted.

Factors Related to pH

Calcium Phosphate Solubility

Solubility of calcium phosphate is critical for PN formulations. Deaths related to calcium phosphate precipitation have been reported in hospitalized patients receiving PN.[6] The solubility of calcium phosphate depends on the balance between pH and concentrations of calcium and phosphate. The effect of pH on phosphate is critical to the solubility of calcium phosphate. Increasing pH increases dibasic phosphate (HPO_4^{-2}), which when bound with calcium as dibasic calcium phosphate is very insoluble (30 mg/dl). The net result is precipitation of calcium phosphate at relatively low concentrations of calcium and phosphate. Monobasic calcium phosphate, which predominates at low pH values, is much more soluble (1800 mg/dl).[88,89] This allows higher concentrations of calcium and phosphate to be present without precipitating when the pH is acidic. In some cases, precipitation of calcium phosphate may be reversed by lowering the pH. This is the rationale for instilling 0.1 N hydrochloric acid into a central venous catheter when calcium phosphate occlusion is suspected.

Several factors in addition to pH and calcium and phosphate concentrations affect calcium phosphate solubility in PN formulations. Some are related to pH; others to concentration.

Amino Acid Solution

The amino acid solution selected for PN preparation is at the core of pH-related factors. Commercial amino acid solutions range in pH from 4.5 to 7. The final pH of a PN formulation tends to be very near that of the selected amino acid solution. The higher the pH of the selected amino acid solution is, the greater is the risk of calcium phosphate precipitation at a given concentration of calcium and phosphate.

Final Concentration of Amino Acids

The final concentration of amino acids is also important to calcium phosphate solubility. Low amino acid concentrations, especially final concentration below 2%, reduce calcium phosphate solubility.[90] Low levels of titratable acidity associated with low final amino acid concentrations may allow the pH to increase, thus increasing the proportion of dibasic phosphate available for combining with calcium. Low final concentrations of amino acids reduce the amount of calcium and phosphate in soluble complexes with amino acids. This leaves more calcium and phosphate available to complex with one another.

Additive pH

Individual amino acids and other additives to PN formulas also have the potential to alter pH. For instance, adding L-cysteine HCl to neonatal PN decreases its pH and increases calcium phosphate solubility. Dextrose also has the potential to decrease pH, especially when the final mixture has a high dextrose and a low amino acid concentration. In addition, the increased viscosity associated with high dextrose concentrations may reduce calcium phosphate precipitation by minimizing particle movement and collisions.[91] Infusion of lipid emulsion via Y-site administration has been reported to increase the risk of calcium phosphate precipitation because it also increases the pH.[88] Other reports suggest only minimal increases in pH as the proportion of lipid emulsion is increased in PN formulas.[92] To alter the pH of a PN formula, an additive must be significantly higher or lower on the pH scale than the amino acid solution used to prepare it. In addition, the additive must be used in a quantity sufficient to overcome the buffering capacity of the amino acid solution.

Factors Related to Concentration

Order of Addition

Adding calcium salts to PN formulas before phosphate salts are added reduces calcium phosphate solubility. The mechanism of this phenomenon is not well documented, but it may be related to the proportion of unbound dibasic phosphate present when the calcium is added. A local concentration effect is also likely when the additives are injected into the PN formula. Phosphate solutions used as additives to PN are approximately 10 times more concentrated, volume for volume, than the calcium gluconate solution. Injecting the more concentrated phosphate solution into the PN formula first allows dilution before the phosphate is exposed to calcium.

Calcium and Phosphate Concentrations

The total concentration of calcium salts and phosphate salts, the particular calcium salt, temperature, and time are clearly concentration-related variables that affect calcium phosphate solubility. The calcium phosphate solubility product serves as a guide to the total concentration of calcium and phosphate that can be added to a PN formula.

CALCULATION OF A CALCIUM PHOSPHATE PRODUCT. *Solubility product* is the term used in chemistry to describe a constant calculated by multiplying the concentrations of the various ions in a saturated solution of electrolytes by one another. The product is calculated for a given temperature and in a specific solvent, such as water. The product of specific electrolyte concentrations, such as calcium and phosphate, can be calculated for a solution to determine if the solubility product has been exceeded, in which case the solution is supersaturated and precipitation would eventually occur. Thus, the solubility product predicts what concentrations of the specified electrolytes can be safely combined without precipitating.

Determining a safe calcium phosphate product for PN formulas is complicated by the many factors affecting calcium phosphate solubility and by the intrinsic complexity of PN formulations. The various methods used to express calcium and phosphate concentrations in PN formulations also contribute to confusion about safe calcium phosphate products for use in clinical practice. These electrolytes may be ordered in milligram quantities of the elemental electrolyte (e.g., milligrams of calcium), milligrams of the electrolyte salt (e.g., calcium gluconate), milliequivalents of electrolyte (e.g., calcium), milliequivalents of ion associated with the electrolyte (e.g., potassium as phosphate), or millimoles of electrolyte (e.g., millimoles of phosphate). The concentration of electrolyte must also be included on the order, generally as the amount per liter or the amount per total volume of PN formula. Nutrition support practitioners must be careful to use the correct units for the calcium phosphate product designated as safe in their health care facility.

The calcium phosphate product for a PN formula can be calculated from one of the following equations:

$$\text{calcium mEq/L} \times (\text{phosphate mM/L} \times 1.8) = \text{calcium phosphate product}$$

$$\text{calcium mM/L} \times \text{phosphate mM/L} = \text{calcium phosphate product}$$

A product less than 300 is considered safe with the first equation, whereas with the second equation the upper limit of the safe range is 75.[93,94] The safe values serve only as guidelines to what calcium and phosphate concentrations in PN formulas generally are not associated with precipitation. The calcium and phosphate concentrations suggested as safe according to these equations are not absolutes because many factors affect the product at which precipitation occurs. Some health care facilities may, therefore, select "safe" values that are appropriate to the specific products they prepare but are different from the values suggested for the previous equations. Equations that use different units of volume for ingredients may be used in some facilities. The relationship between milligrams, milliequivalents, and millimoles makes it possible to convert values and develop several other equations from the two previously presented. For example, equation 1 can be converted to the following equations and approximately equivalent safe values:

$$\text{calcium mEq/L} \times \text{potassium as phosphate mEq/L} < 250$$

$$\text{calcium mEq/L} \times \text{sodium as phosphate mEq/L} < 225$$

$$\text{calcium mEq/L} \times \text{phosphate mM/L} < 150$$

$$\text{calcium mM/L} \times \text{potassium as phosphate mEq/L} < 125$$

$$\text{calcium mM/L} \times \text{phosphate mM/L} < 75$$

(as in equation 2)

As an alternative to calculating a calcium phosphate product, published graphs of calcium phosphate solubility can be used as a guide for addition of these electrolytes to PN formulas.[7,88] The phosphate content of all additives, including medications and PN components (e.g., amino acid solution and lipid emulsion), should be considered when calculating total phosphate concentration. Clindamycin phosphate, for instance, could contribute to calcium phosphate precipitation with an otherwise "safe" calcium phosphate product. The intrinsic phosphate content of amino acid solutions is accounted for in solubility graphs developed for specific amino acid solutions.

Calcium Salt

The calcium salt selected for use in PN formulas affects the extent of calcium dissociation, which is an important determinant of calcium phosphate solubility. Calcium phosphate forms only when free calcium binds with free phosphate. So calcium phosphate precipitation cannot occur when calcium remains bound to its anion (usually gluconate) or phosphate remains bound to its cation (sodium or potassium). Calcium gluconate is the preferred calcium salt for PN formulas because it dissociates less readily than calcium chloride or calcium acetate. If calcium chloride or calcium acetate are used in PN formulas, calcium phosphate precipitation may occur at an otherwise "safe" calcium phosphate product.

Temperature

Temperature has a concentration-related effect on calcium phosphate solubility. As temperature increases, dissociation of calcium and phosphate from their respective salts also increases. Thus, there are more opportunities for free (ionized) calcium and phosphate molecules to collide, and the net result is increased binding of the molecules to form calcium phosphate. Precipitation occurs once a critical calcium phosphate concentration is reached. Temperature is a clinically relevant factor, especially when incubators or heat lamps or heating blankets are in use. Calcium phosphate deposition in a central venous catheter has even been associated with increased body temperature.[95,96] Use of in-line filters for administration of PN cannot prevent such precipitate formation; strict adherence to protocols for addition of calcium and phosphate to PN formulations remains the best defense against precipitate formation.

Time Since Preparation

Dissociation of calcium and phosphate from their respective salts occurs slowly in the absence of a catalyst such as heat. Over time, however, dissociation may be sufficient for calcium phosphate formation to exceed its solubility. In addition, the concentration of calcium and phosphate in the PN formula may increase over time as a result of water loss through the container. This concentration-related effect of time is seen clinically as calcium phosphate precipitation several hours to days after the PN formula has been prepared. Delayed precipitation is more common than immediate precipitation, unless the calcium phosphate product far exceeds the safe value. Thus, pushing the calcium phosphate product to the safe limit is more risky for PN formulas used in the home, where several days' PN formula is made at one time.

Total Nutrient Admixtures

Three-in-one, all-in-one, and *total nutrient admixture* (TNA) are terms used to describe PN formulations in which lipid emulsion is included with other PN components in a single container. Intravenous lipid emulsion is an intricate system consisting of soybean oil triglycerides, and safflower oil in some cases, dispersed in an aqueous phase. The dispersion is stabilized by egg phospholipid as the emulsifier. The hydrophobic, nonpolar fatty acid section of the emulsifier aligns with the triglycerides. The hydrophilic, polar section containing phosphate aligns with the aqueous phase of the emulsion. The result is chylomicron-like lipid particles with an inner core of triglycerides protected by a mechanical barrier of phospholipid emulsifier. The phosphate section of the emulsifier protruding from the surface imparts a negative surface charge, or zeta potential, to the lipid particles. Electrostatic repulsion maintains the dispersion of lipid particles in the aqueous phase.

As manufactured, intravenous lipid emulsions carry a zeta potential of about −30 to −40 millivolts (mV).[96-99] Instability begins to occur when the zeta potential rises above about −30 mV, and flocculation at around −14 mV.[100] Thus, anything that decreases the surface charge has the potential of destabilizing the lipid emulsion. Admixture of lipid emulsion to other PN components creates an extremely complex aqueous phase. At this point, the lipid emulsion no longer behaves as a predictable colloid dispersion. Because of their complexity and unpredictability, instability is a major concern with TNA formulas.

Destabilization of Emulsions

CREAMING. Instability, or destabilization, of emulsions is described by the terms *creaming* and *cracking*. Creaming is a reversible stage of instability in which two emulsions of different densities form. The cream layer contains a higher concentration of the dispersed or internal (oil) phase and larger droplets than the original TNA, but the oil remains emulsified. With the greater emulsified oil content the cream layer rises to the surface. In the other layer the concentration of dispersed lipid particles is lower than in the original TNA, but droplets remain emulsified and their size is relatively unchanged. Close observation is generally required to discern creaming because the only visible difference between layers may be that the cream layer is slightly whiter. A TNA with mild creaming is considered safe for use after the creaming is reversed by gentle agitation. If creaming reappears fairly soon—within an hour or two—aggregation of the emulsified lipid particles may have advanced to the point where the particles are too large to remain dispersed. Such a TNA is unstable and should not be administered to a patient.

CRACKING. Cracking, also called *oiling out* or *breaking* of the emulsion, represents an irreversible stage of instability in which oil droplets separate from the emulsion. The initial sign of cracking may be loss of the uniformly opaque appearance that characterizes stable TNA formulas. A subtle cottage cheese–like appearance occurs, with areas of different degrees of whiteness. Small pockets of this instability increase in size and develop oil streaks or globules as time passes. Close observation of the TNA is necessary to discern the early stage of cracking. Often cracking progresses to an amber or clear oil layer on the surface of the TNA before it is noted. Administration of the TNA should be stopped immediately when there is any sign of cracking because life-threatening oil embolization could occur.[101] Anyone responsible for administering a TNA formula, including nurses, home care patients, and caregivers for home care patients, should be trained to recognize signs of TNA instability.

Instability of Total Nutrient Admixtures

Many factors affect TNA stability. The contribution of any single factor to TNA destabilization, however, is difficult to judge. In the clinical setting, known destabilizing factors are generally controlled within desired (stable) ranges. As a consequence, instability appears to result from the interaction between factors rather than from a single factor outside an acceptable range. Interactions resulting in TNA instability are complex and are not fully understood; thus, complete control of destabilization may be difficult. Fortunately, TNA instability appears to occur infrequently when factors known to cause it are controlled.[102] Adherence to appropriate mixing protocols and additive restrictions, however, is essential for minimizing TNA instability.

Effect of pH

A major factor associated with TNA destabilization is pH. The pH of intravenous lipid emulsion is adjusted to approximately 8, and a pH range of 5 to 10 is considered stable.[103,104] The pH of TNA formulas is generally in the range of 5.4 to 6.5, the exact value being determined largely by the amino acid component of the PN formula. Amino acid solutions that keep the TNA's pH below 6.3 seem to produce more unstable formulas than solutions that produce a higher pH.[89] In general, amino acid solutions with pH values in the low 5 range should be used with caution for TNA preparation. The importance of pH for TNA preparation is demonstrated by the availability of Aminosyn and Aminosyn II amino acid solutions. For a given concentration of amino acid solution, these products are nearly identical, except for pH. Standard Aminosyn solutions have a pH of approximately 5.3, whereas Aminosyn II solutions, which are recommended for TNA preparation, have a pH range of 6 to 6.5.

Destabilization of TNA formulas in a low pH may be explained by phospholipid instability as pH decreases. The negative surface charge on the emulsifier is reduced when the pH drops below 5 to 5.5, and at a pH of approximately 2.5, it is neutralized.[103,105,106] As the pH becomes more acidic, more hydrogen ions are available to bind the negatively charged hydrophilic portion of the phospholipid emulsifier. The resulting decrease in zeta potential reduces electrostatic repulsion and allows aggregation of lipid particles. Below pH 5 instability may be further aggravated by denaturation of the emulsifier.[107] The mechanical barrier between oil and water phases becomes less effective as denaturation proceeds. With reduced zeta potential and an ineffective mechanical barrier, coalescence and eventually cracking of the emulsion occur.

Changes in the electrical charge of amino acids may also contribute to TNA instability as pH decreases. Crystalline amino acids generally are present as dipolar ions (zwitterions) in neutral aqueous solutions. At a given pH, called the *isoelectric point*, an amino acid molecule has no net charge. Most individual amino acids in the solutions used for PN preparation have an isoelectric point between pH 5.4 and 6, many near 6. Above the isoelectric point the net charge is negative; thus, most amino acids in a PN formula with a pH above 6 are negatively charged. Below the isoelectric point the net charge is positive. The net charge becomes progressively more positive as the pH of a PN formula decreases below 6 because more individual amino acids become positively charged. Instability can occur in TNA formulas as the pH decreases and electrostatic repulsion is neutralized.[108] The incorporation of amino acids into the oil-water interface of dispersed lipid particles can also change as the net charge develops on amino acids. This, however, can stabilize the emulsion by strengthening the mechanical barrier between oil and water layers, at least until the pH drops to the point at which the phospholipid emulsifier deteriorates.[107]

Final Concentrations of Amino Acids and Dextrose

Low final amino acid concentrations are associated with TNA instability. The buffering capacity conferred by the amino acid solution is reduced when the final concentration of amino acids is low.[97] PN formulas with poor buffering capacity are subject to greater fluctuations in pH. Fortunately, most TNA components have a pH greater than 5.5 or are added in quantities too small to affect pH. The major exception is dextrose monohydrate solution. The pH of dextrose solution averages about 4, and the volume added to TNA formulas is relatively large. Thus, dextrose can decrease the pH of a TNA formula that has inadequate buffering capacity. Low final amino acid concentrations coupled with relatively high final dextrose concentrations pose the greatest risk of pH changes. High final amino acid concentrations coupled with relatively high final dextrose concentrations, however, may make a more stable formula than when the dextrose concentration is low. With adequate buffering capacity from amino acids, the higher viscosity associated with higher dextrose concentrations appears to provide more TNA stability than lower dextrose concentrations.[91]

Sequence of Admixture

The low pH of dextrose accounts for the role order of mixing plays in TNA destabilization. Adding lipid emulsion directly to dextrose solution can result in rapid destabilization of the emulsion because of the low pH of dextrose. Therefore, dextrose solution and lipid emulsion should never be mixed directly unless amino acid solution is added concurrently. Manufacturers of automated compounding machines generally provide guidelines for the order of mixing that are tailored to the exact sequence of delivery and flushing from each position on the machine. The sequence commonly used for preparing TNA formulas, with or without an automated compounder, is dextrose solution, amino acid solution, then lipid emulsion.

Final Concentration of Lipid

The final concentration of lipids in TNA formulas affects destabilization. High-lipid concentration formulas tend to be more stable than low-concentration ones probably because of a dilutional effect on the phospholipid emulsifier when the final concentration of lipid emulsion is low. Facilities that use TNA formulas should establish a lower limit for the final concentration of lipid below which the lipid emulsion must be administered as a separate infusion. What concentration is selected depends on the brand of lipid emulsion and amino acid solution used for TNA preparation and on all other factors that affect TNA stability. At the Arizona Health Sciences Center in Tucson, 2.5% final concentration of lipid has been established as the lower limit for typical TNA formulas. Final concentrations as low as 2% have been accepted for some TNA formulas, based on information provided by the manufacturers of the amino acid solution, the lipid emulsion, and the automated compounder used for TNA preparation. Upper limits for the final concentration of lipid are usually controlled by the greatest acceptable percentage of calories provided as fat, rather than by stability issues.

Electrolyte Concentrations

Electrolyte concentrations of TNA formulas are critical. Cations are capable of neutralizing the zeta potential of the phospholipid emulsifier. Trivalent cations are most disruptive to lipid stability but are seldom a problem in clinical practice, with the exception of parenteral iron. Do not add iron preparations, even in small doses, to TNA formulas.[106] Divalent cations are the greatest clinical concern, but no cation in a TNA should be ignored. Facilities that use TNA formulas should establish upper limits for divalent cations in the formulas. Limits on monovalent cations should also be considered. At the Arizona Health Sciences Center, Tucson, the maximum concentration of magnesium plus calcium in a TNA formula has been set at 30 mEq/L. Relatively small quantities of trace elements are normally included in parenteral nutrition (PN) formulations. The upper limit for divalent cations must be reassessed if increased quantities of trace elements are required. Limits for calcium, magnesium, and trace elements in TNA formulas reported in the literature must be carefully evaluated before being adopted by another health care facility, since small changes in TNA components, such as a different brand of amino acid solution, can alter the limits of stability.

Storage Conditions and Time

Storage conditions and time also affect TNA destabilization. Formulas that contain lipid emulsion are generally stored at refrigerator temperatures, although their stability may be no greater than at room temperature. Temperatures above standard room temperature may contribute to TNA destabilization. Freezing a TNA formula is also likely to result in a cracked emulsion secondary to disruption of the phospholipid barrier by ice crystals. Risk of destabilization increases with the time between preparation and infusion. A formula that is stable at 48 hours may be cracked by 96 hours because aggregation and flocculation of lipid particles appear to be continuous processes. Because of this, TNA formulas prepared for home care patients may need to meet more conservative guidelines for final amino acid and lipid concentrations or electrolyte additives than TNA formulas prepared for use within 24 to 36 hours.

Other Additives

Additives to TNA formulas must be carefully evaluated. Electrical charge and pH are especially important. Medications or nutrients that are stable in dextrose-based PN formulas may destabilize TNA formulas. In simulated Y-site administration, several medications reported as compatible with dextrose-amino acid formulation were found to disrupt preparations containing lipid emulsion (see Table 24-2).[8,9] Ascorbic acid and iron dextran are examples of nutrients that may destabilize TNA formulas. The complexities of TNA formulas require careful attention to all aspects of PN preparation and administration. The decision to use TNA formulas must be made with the understanding that limitations are imposed and established guidelines followed. Health care professionals knowledgeable in the complexities and limitations of TNA formulas should participate in all decisions related to TNA use.

Filters Used with Total Nutrient Admixture Formulations

In addition to stability issues, TNA formulations raise issues related to filtration during PN administration. Dextrose-based PN formulations can be safely passed through 0.22-μm filters. The lipid particles in TNA formulations, however, are too large to pass through such small filters. To prevent disruption of the lipid particles, a filter of at least 1.2 μm must be used if PN administration policies require an in-line filter. A 5-μm filter is also acceptable for filtration of a TNA.

Conclusion

Safe and efficacious provision of PN and EN therapy is influenced by many pharmacologic issues. Both PN and EN formulas are complex mixtures of many different components capable of creating physiologic responses and physicochemical interactions. Pharmaceutical dosage forms are also capable of various physicochemical interactions and physiologic responses, in addition to the pharmacologic responses for which they are administered. The specific design of the dosage form, the active medicinal ingredient, and excipient characteristics contribute to the interactions and responses associated with medications. When PN or EN formulas and medications are administered to the same patient, several types of undesirable effects or incompatibilities can occur as a result of the complexity of each therapy. The consequences of such incompatibilities range from inconveniences to life-threatening conditions. Avoiding or minimizing the incompatibilities is, thus, a goal of nutrition support practitioners. Unfortunately, those well-designed studies of practical pharmacologic issues of specialized nutrition support that have been conducted are often limited in scope. Research results must frequently be extrapolated to PN or EN formulas of different composition than those studied or to different medication doses. Such extrapolations must be done cautiously because seemingly minor changes in formula or medication can result in unanticipated problems. Professionals familiar with available PN and EN formulas, characteristics of potential additive or coadministered products, and the patient population the health care facility serves must be involved in determining the limitations and guidelines because there are few absolutes.

REFERENCES

1. Rollins CJ: Medications and enteral feeding: are they compatible? Presented at the Arizona Dietetic Association Annual Meeting, Tempe, AZ, June 16, 1989.
2. Gupta VD: Stability of vitamins in total parenteral nutrient solutions, *Am J Hosp Pharm* 43:2132, 1986 (letter).
3. Allwood MC: Response to letter: Gupta VD: Stability of vitamins in total parenteral nutrient solutions [*Am J Hosp Pharm* 43:2132, 1986], *Am J Hosp Pharm* 43:2138, 1986.
4. Louie N: Response to letter: Gupta VD: Stability of vitamins in total parenteral nutrient solutions [*Am J Hosp Pharm* 43:2132, 1986], *Am J Hosp Pharm* 43:2138, 2143, 1986.
5. Knowles JB, Cusson G, Smith M, et al: Pulmonary deposition of calcium phosphate crystals as a complication of home total parenteral nutrition, *J Parenter Enteral Nutr* 13(2):209-213, 1989.
6. Lumpkin MM: Safety alert: hazards of precipitation associated with parenteral nutrition, *Am J Hosp Pharm* 51:1427-1428, 1994.
7. Trissel LA: *Handbook on injectable drugs,* ed 10, Bethesda, MD, 1998, American Society of Hospital Pharmacists.
8. Trissel LA, Gilbert DL, Martinez JF, et al: Compatibility of parenteral nutrient solutions with selected drugs during simulated Y-site administration, *Am J Health Syst Pharm* 54(26):1295-1300, 1997.
9. Trissel LA, Gilbert DL, Martinez JF, et al: Compatibility of medications with 3-in-1 parenteral nutrition admixtures, *J Parenter Enteral Nutr* 23(2):67-74, 1999.
10. Greenway FT, Brown LM, Dabrowski JC, et al: Copper (II) complexes of the antiulcer drug cimetidine, *J Am Chem Soc* 102(26):7782-7784, 1980.
11. Mitrano FP, Baptista RJ: Stability of cimetidine and copper sulfate in a TPN solution. DICP, *Ann Pharmacother* 23:429-430, 1989.
12. Pomerance HH, Rader RE: Crystal formation: a new complication of total parenteral nutrition, *Pediatrics* 52(6):864-866, 1973.
13. Gershanik J, Boecler B, Ensley H, et al: The gasping syndrome and benzyl alcohol poisoning, *N Engl J Med* 307(22):1384-1388, 1982.
14. American Academy of Pediatrics Committee on Drugs: "Inactive" ingredients in pharmaceutical products, *Pediatrics* 76(4):635-643, 1985.
15. Balisteri WF, Farrell MK, Bove KE: Lessons from the E-Ferol tragedy, *Pediatrics* 78(3):503-506, 1986.
16. Helback HJ, Moltehnik KA, Ames BN: Toxic hydroperoxides in intravenous lipid emulsions used in preterm infants, *Pediatrics* 91(1):83-87, 1993.
17. Cutie AJ, Altman E, Lenkel L: Compatibility of enteral products with commonly employed drug additives, *J Parenter Enteral Nutr* 7(2):186-191, 1983.
18. Altman E, Cutie AJ: Compatibility of enteral products with commonly employed drug additives, *Nutr Support Serv* 4:8-17, 1984.
19. Fagerman KE, Ballou AE: Drug compatibilities with enteral feeding solutions co-administered by tube, *Nutr Support Serv* 8:31-32, 1988.
20. Burns PE, McCall L, Wirsching R: Physical compatibility of enteral formulas with various common medications, *J Am Diet Assoc* 88(9):1094-1096, 1988.
21. Holtz L, Milton J, Sturek JK: Compatibility of medications with enteral feedings, *J Parenter Enteral Nutr* 11(2):183-186, 1987.
22. Strom JG, Miller SW: Stability of drugs with enteral nutrient formulas, *Drug Intell Clin Pharm* 24:130-134, 1990.
23. Rollins CJ: Tube feeding formula and medication characteristics contributing to undesirable interactions, *J Parenter Enteral Nutr* 23(1):S13, 1999 (abstract).
24. Thomson CA, Rollins CJ: Enteral feeding and medication incompatibilities, *Support Line* 8:9-11, 1991.
25. Mitchell JF: Oral dosage forms that should not be crushed: 2000 update, *Hosp Pharm* 35(5):553-567, 2000.
26. Bartlett JG: *Clostridium difficile*: clinical considerations, *Rev Infect Dis* 12(suppl 2):243S-251S, 1990.
27. Kelly CP, Pothoulakis C, LaMont JT: *Clostridium difficile* colitis, *N Engl J Med* 330(4):257-262, 1994.
28. Silva J, Fekety R, Werk C, et al: Inciting and etiologic agents of colitis, *Rev Infect Dis* (suppl 1):214S-221S, 1984.
29. Kohn CL, Keithley JK: Techniques for evaluating and managing diarrhea in the tube-fed patient, *Nutr Clin Pract* 2(6):250-257, 1987.
30. Keohane PP, Attrill H, Love M, Frost P, et al: Relation between osmolality of diet and gastrointestinal side effects in enteral nutrition, *Br Med J* 288:678-680, 1984.
31. Heimburger DC: Diarrhea with enteral feeding. Will the real cause please stand up? *Am J Med* 88:89-90, 1990.
32. National Research Council: *Recommended dietary allowances,* ed 10, Washington, DC, 1989, National Academy Press.
33. Olson JA: Recommended dietary intake of vitamin K (RDI) in humans, *Am J Clin Nutr* 45:687-692, 1987.
34. Food and Drug Administration. Parenteral multivitamin products; drugs for human use; drug efficacy study implementation; amendment (21 CFR 5.7), *Federal Register* 65(77):21200-21201, 2000.
35. Anonymous: Deaths associated with thiamine-deficient total parenteral nutrition, *MMWR Morb Mortal Wkly Rep* 38:43-46, 1989.
36. Anonymous: Lactic acidosis traced to thiamine deficiency related to nationwide shortage of multivitamins for total parenteral nutrition, *MMWR Morb Mortal Wkly Rep* 46:523-528, 1997.
37. Velez RJ, Myers B, Guber MS: Severe acute metabolic acidosis (acute beriberi): an avoidable complication of total parenteral nutrition, *J Parenter Enteral Nutr* 9(2):216-219, 1985.

38. Lutomski DM, Palascak JE, Bower RH: Warfarin resistance associated with intravenous lipid administration, *J Parenter Enteral Nutr* 11(3):316-318, 1987.

39. Watson AJM, Pegg M, Green JRB: Enteral feeds may antagonize warfarin, *Br Med J* 288:557, 1984.

40. Parr MD, Record KE, Griffith GL, et al: Effect of enteral nutrition on warfarin therapy, *Clin Pharm* 1:274-276, 1982.

41. Landau J, Moulda RF: Warfarin resistance caused by vitamin K in intestinal feeds, *Med J Aust* 2:283(2):263-264, 1982 (letter).

42. Gimmon Z: Oral anticoagulation therapy in patients who require nutritional support, *J Parenter Enteral Nutr* 11(1):102-103, 1987 (letter).

43. Westfall LK: An unrecognized case of warfarin resistance, *Drug Intell Clin Pharm* 15:131, 1981.

44. Lader E, Yang L, Clarke A: Warfarin dosage and vitamin K in Osmolite, *Ann Intern Med* 93(2):373-374, 1980 (letter).

45. O'Reilly RA, Rytand DA: "Resistance" to warfarin due to unrecognized vitamin K supplementation, *N Engl J Med* 303(3):160-161, 1980 (letter).

46. Howard PA, Hannaman KN: Warfarin resistance linked to enteral nutrition products, *J Am Diet Assoc* 85(6):713-714, 1985.

47. Petretich DA: Reversal of Osmolite-warfarin interaction by changing warfarin administration time, *Clin Pharm* 9:93, 1990 (letter.)

48. Lee M, Schwartz RN, Sharifi R: Warfarin resistance and vitamin K, *Ann Intern Med* 94(1):140-141, 1981 (letter).

49. Kutsup JJ: Update on vitamin K content of enteral products, *Am J Hosp Pharm* 41:1762, 1984 (letter).

50. Penrod LE, Allen JB, Cabacungan LR. Warfarin resistance and enteral feedings: 2 case reports and a supporting in vitro study, *Arch Phys Med Rehabil* 82:1270-1271, 2001.

51. Niemec PW, Vanderveen TW, Morrison JL, Hohenwarter MW: Gastrointestinal disorders caused by medication and electrolyte solution osmolality during enteral nutrition, *J Parenter Enteral Nutr* 7(4):387-389, 1983.

52. White KC, Harkavy KL: Hypertonic formula resulting from added oral medications, *Am J Dis Child* 136:931-933, 1982.

53. Dickerson RN, Melnik G: Osmolality of oral drug solutions and suspensions, *Am J Hosp Pharm* 45:832-834, 1988.

54. Hyams JS: Sorbitol intolerance. An unappreciated cause of functional gastrointestinal complaints, *Gastroenterology* 84(1):30-33, 1983.

55. Johnston KR, Govel LA, Andritz MH: Gastrointestinal effects of sorbitol as an additive in liquid medications, *Am J Med* 97:185-191, 1994.

56. Edes TE, Walk BE, Austin JL: Diarrhea in tube-fed patients: feeding formula not necessarily the cause, *Am J Med* 88:91-93, 1990.

57. Hill DB, Henderson LM, McClain CJ: Osmotic diarrhea induced by sugar-free theophylline solution in critically ill patients, *J Parenter Enteral Nutr* 15(3):332-336, 1991.

58. Greenwood J, Brown G: Sorbitol-induced diarrhea in a tube-fed patient, *Can J Hosp Pharm* 44(6):297-300, 1991.

59. Charney EB, Bodurtha JN: Intractable diarrhea associated with the use of sorbitol, *J Pediatr* 98(1):157-158, 1981.

60. Lutomski DM, Gora ML, Wright SM, Martin JE: Sorbitol content of selected oral liquids, *Ann Pharmacother* 27:269-273, 1993.

61. Miller SJ, Oliver AD: Sorbitol content of selected sugar-free medications, *Hosp Pharm* 28(8):741-744, 755, 1993.

62. Crowe SJP, Falini NP: Gluten in pharmaceutical products, *Am J Health Syst Pharm* 58:396-401, 2001.

63. Hill EM, Flaitz CM, Frost GR: Sweetener content of common pediatric oral liquid medications, *Am J Hosp Pharm* 41:135-142, 1988.

64. Veerman MW: Excipients in valproic acid syrup may cause diarrhea: a case report. DICP, *Ann Pharmacother* 24:832-833, 1990.

65. Kumar A, Weatherly MR, Beaman DC: Sweeteners, flavorings, and dyes in antibiotic preparations, *Pediatrics* 87(3):352-360, 1991.

66. Maloney JP, Halbower AC, Balasubramaniam VB, et al: Systemic absorption of food dye in patients with sepsis, *N Engl J Med* 343(14):1047-1048, 2000 (letter).

67. Smith JL, Canham JE, Wells PA: Effect of phototherapy light, sodium bisulfite, and pH on vitamin stability in total parenteral nutrition admixtures, *J Parenter Enteral Nutr* 12(4):394-402, 1988.

68. Newton DW: Physiochemical determinants of incompatibility and instability in injectable drug solutions and admixtures, *Am J Hosp Pharm* 35:1213-1222, 1978.

69. Howard L, Chu R, Feman S, et al: Vitamin A deficiency from long-term parenteral nutrition, *Ann Intern Med* 93(4):576-577, 1980.

70. Cacek AT, DeVito JM, Koonce JR: In vitro evaluation of nasogastric administration methods for phenytoin, *Am J Hosp Pharm* 43:689-692, 1986.

71. Clark-Schmidt AL, Garnett WR, Lowe DR, Karnes HT: Loss of carbamazepine suspension through nasogastric feeding tubes, *Am J Hosp Pharm* 47:2034-2037, 1990.

72. Magnusson JO: Metabolism of digoxin after oral and intrajejunal administration, *Br J Pharm* 16:741-742, 1983.

73. Yuk JH, Nightingale CH, Quintiliani R, et al: Absorption of ciprofloxacin administered through a nasogastric or nasoduodenal tube in volunteers and patients receiving enteral nutrition, *Diag Microbiol Infect Dis* 13:99-102, 1990.

74. Semple HA, Koo W, Tam YK, et al: Interactions between hydralazine and oral nutrients in humans, *Ther Drug Monitor* 13(4):304-308, 1991.

75. Bhargava VO, Schaaf LJ, Berlinger WG, Jungnickel PW: Effect of an enteral nutrient formula on sustained-release theophylline absorption, *Ther Drug Monitor* 11(5):515-519, 1989.

76. Bauer LA: Interference of oral phenytoin absorption by continuous infusion nasogastric feedings, *Neurology* 32:570-572, 1982.

77. Ozuna J, Friel P: Effect of enteral tube feeding on serum phenytoin levels, *J Neurosurg Nurs* 16(6):289-291, 1984.

78. Maynard GA, Jones KM, Guidry JR: Phenytoin absorption from tube feedings, *Arch Intern Med* 147:1821-1823, 1987.

79. Marvel ME, Bertino JS: Comparative effects of an elemental and a complex enteral feeding formulation on the absorption of phenytoin suspension, *J Parenter Enteral Nutr* 15(3):316-318, 1991.

80. Nishimura LY, Armstrong EP, Plezia PM, Iacono RP: Influence of enteral feedings on phenytoin sodium absorption from capsules, *Drug Intell Clin Pharm* 22:130-133, 1988.

81. Fitzsimmons WE, Garnett WR, Krueger KA: Comment: phenytoin and enteral feedings, *Drug Intell Clin Pharm* 22:920, 1988 (letter).

82. Gilbert S, Hatton J, Magnuson B: How to minimize interaction between phenytoin and enteral feedings: two approaches, *Nutr Clin Pract* 11(1):28-31, 1996.

83. Sakad JJ, Graves RH, Sharp WP: Interaction of oral phenytoin with enteral feedings, *J Parenter Enteral Nutr* 10(3):322-323, 1986.

84. Kassam RM, Friesen E, Locock RA: In vitro recovery of carbamazepine from Ensure, *J Parenter Enteral Nutr* 13(3):272-276, 1989.

85. Bass J, Miles MV, Tennison MB, et al: Effects of enteral tube feeding on the absorption and pharmacokinetic profile of carbamazepine suspension, *Epilepsia* 30(3):364-369, 1989.

86. Berg MJ, Stumbo PJ, Chenard CA, et al: Folic acid improves phenytoin pharmacokinetics, *J Am Diet Assoc* 95(3):352-356, 1995.

87. Williams L, Davis JA, Lowenthal DT: The influence of food on the absorption and metabolism of drugs, *Med Clin North Am* 77:815-829, 1993.

88. Eggert LD, Rusho WJ, MacKay MW, Chan GM: Calcium and phosphorus compatibility in parenteral nutrition solutions for neonates, *Am J Hosp Pharm* 39:49-53, 1982.

89. Bettner FS, Stennett DJ: Effects of pH, temperature, concentration, and time on particle counts in lipid-containing total parenteral nutrition admixtures, *J Parenter Enteral Nutr* 10(4):375-380, 1986.

90. Poole RL, Rupp CA, Kerner JA: Calcium and phosphorus in neonatal parenteral nutrition solutions, *J Parenter Enteral Nutr* 7(4):358-360, 1983.

91. Driscoll DF: Total nutrient admixtures: theory and practice, *Nutr Clin Pract* 10(3):114-118, 1995.

92. Parry VA, Harrie KR, McIntosh-Lowe NL: Effect of various nutrient ratios on the emulsion stability of total nutrient admixtures, *Am J Hosp Pharm* 43:3017-3022, 1986.

93. Baumgartner TG: Calcium. In Baumgartner TG (ed): *Clinical guide to parenteral micronutrition,* ed 2, USA, 1991, Fujisawa, pp 1-51.

94. Mierzwa MW: Stability and compatibility in preparing TPN solutions. In Lebenthal E (ed): *Total parenteral nutrition: indications, utilization, complications, and pathophysiological considerations.* New York, 1986, Raven, pp 219-244.

95. Stennett DJ, Gerwick WH, Egging PK, et al: Precipitate analysis from an indwelling total parenteral nutrition catheter, *J Parenter Enteral Nutr* 12(1):88-92, 1988.

96. Robinson LA, Wright BT: Central venous catheter occlusion caused by body-heat-mediated calcium phosphate precipitation, *Am J Hosp Pharm* 39:120-121, 1982.

97. Brown R, Quercia RA, Sigman R: Total nutrient admixture: a review, *J Parenter Enteral Nutr* 10(6):650-658, 1986.

98. Barnett MI. Physical stability of all in one admixtures: factors affecting fat droplets, *Nutrition* 5(5):348-349, 1989.

99. Gimble GK, Silk DBA: Administration of fat emulsions with nutritional mixtures from the three-liter delivery system in TPN: efficacy and safety, *Nutr Support Serv* 7:14-16, 1987.

100. Knutsen OH: Stability of intralipid fat emulsion in amino acid solutions, *Crit Care Med* 14(7):638-641, 1986.
101. Leveen HH, Giordano P, Spletzer J: The mechanism of removal of intravenous injected fat. Its relationship to toxicity, *Arch Surg* 83:311-321, 1961.
102. Rollins CJ: Stability of three-in-one TPN solutions, *J Parenter Enteral Nutr* 16(3):296-297, 1992 (response to letter).
103. Driscoll DF, Baptista RJ, Bistrian BR, Blackburn GL: Practical considerations regarding the use of total nutrient admixtures, *Am J Hosp Pharm* 43:416-419, 1986.
104. Johnson GC, Anderson JD: Compounding considerations. In Teasley-Strausburg KM, Cerra FB, Lehmann S, Shronts EP (eds): *Nutrition support handbook: a compendium of products with guidelines for usage.* Cincinnati, 1992, Harvey Whitney, pp 133-146.
105. Barat AC, Harrie K, Jacob M, et al: Effect of amino acid solutions on total nutrient admixture stability, *J Parenter Enteral Nutr* 11(4):384-388, 1987.
106. Mitrano FP, Baptista RJ: Stability of total nutrient admixtures as affected by micronutrients and medications, *Nutr Support Serv* 7:21-24, 1987.
107. Black CD, Popovich NG: A study of intravenous emulsion compatibility: effects of dextrose, amino acids, and selected electrolytes, *Drug Intell Clin Pharm* 15:184-193, 1981.
108. Takamura A, Ishii F, Noro S, et al: Study of intravenous hyperalimentation: effect of selected amino acids on the stability of intravenous fat emulsions, *J Pharm Sci* 73(1):91-94, 1984.
109. Vaughan LM, Small C, Plunkett V: Incompatibility of iron dextran and a total nutrient admixture, *Am J Hosp Pharm* 47:1745-1746, 1990.

Pregnancy 25

Maureen MacBurney, MBA, MS, RD, LD
Laura E. Matarese, MS, RD, LD, FADA, CNSD

I T is well known that maternal nutrition during pregnancy has a tremendous effect on fetal outcome and infant mortality.[1-3] This is of particular importance when considering the infant's risk of long-term health problems such as hypertension, obesity, and cardiovascular disease.[4] When normal oral intake is not possible, nutrition intervention is required. There are no documented untoward outcomes related to this nutrition intervention when appropriate protocols are followed, although complications with intravenous feeding have been cited[5,6] (Chapter 19). When considering parenteral or enteral feeding for a pregnant woman, the clinician and the patient must carefully consider the potential for complications, particularly when short-term intervention is likely and benefits may be questionable. The following factors need to be considered for the initiation of specialized nutrition support in pregnancy: (1) maternal disease state or stress, (2) low prepregnancy weight for height, (3) inadequate weight gain or weight loss, (4) risk of undernutrition to the fetus and mother. These factors must be assessed based on their interaction and impact upon each other.[7] Nutrition assessment and the identification of appropriate candidates for parenteral nutrition are essential for the best clinical outcome and cost-effectiveness.[8]

Metabolic and Physiologic Changes

During pregnancy, several metabolic and physiologic changes occur. These changes affect the assessment of nutritional status, nutrient requirements, and methods of feeding. Normal hormonal changes associated with pregnancy lead to alterations in carbohydrate, fat, and protein metabolism. A teleologic increase in estrogen and progesterone levels occurs during the first trimester, resulting in an anabolic state with increased glycogen and fat stores.[9] Plasma glucose levels decrease, insulin secretion increases, and maternal tissues become more insulin resistant favoring glucose delivery to the fetus.[10] In addition, urea production and excretion are reduced during the third trimester, which leads to increased nitrogen retention and tissue synthesis.

Plasma volume increases approximately 50% during pregnancy, resulting in a dilutional decrease in hemoglobin levels, blood glucose values, serum albumin, other serum proteins, and water-soluble vitamins.[11] The decline in serum albumin contributes to a tendency for extracellular fluid accumulation during pregnancy.[12] Serum concentrations of fat soluble vitamins, triglycerides, cholesterol, and free fatty acids increase.[13-14] This increase in plasma blood volume also results in a higher glomerular filtration rate. This may result in increased renal excretion of some nutrients.

Changes in cardiovascular and pulmonary function also occur,[14] and cardiac output increases during pregnancy. In most cases blood pressure decreases in the first two trimesters because of peripheral vasodilation, with a return to normal during the third trimester. Maternal oxygen requirements increase, but gas exchange in the lung is more efficient.

Gastrointestinal (GI) function also changes during pregnancy.[15] Nausea and vomiting often occur in the first trimester, which may be prolonged in some cases. When appetite does return, cravings or aversions for certain foods, as well as pica, may increase. Increased progesterone levels result in decreased GI motility, which aids in nutrient absorption and contributes to regurgitation, gastric acid reflux, and constipation.

Nutrition Assessment

Assessment of nutritional status is essential to identify those patients who are at nutritional risk and may require nutrition intervention. Maternal nutritional status, both current and preconception, and insufficient weight gain during pregnancy affect birth weight and fetal outcome.[16] Adverse effects of maternal malnutrition on the growing fetus can be related to several factors including inadequate blood volume, reduced maternal nutrient stores, decreased maternal-fetal exchange, and abnormal placental development. Poor maternal nutritional status in the first trimester may cause premature births and increase perinatal mortality and congenital malformations in the central nervous system. Third trimester malnutrition causes delivery of a low-birth weight infant, increasing the risk of neonatal death, or complications associated with premature neonates.

Maternal Weight Gain

The mother's prepregnancy height and weight affect the infant's outcome. In 1990 the Institute of Medicine (IOM) recommended that maternal nutritional status be assessed using body mass index (BMI)[17] (Table 25-1). Low prepregnancy weight for height and inadequate weight gain are two of the most significant nutritional risk factors for the development of a low-birth-weight infant. Maternal body mass may, however, be more predictive of birth weight than absolute weight gain during pregnancy because the risk for producing a low-birth-weight infant diminishes as prepregnancy BMI increases. Therefore, a prepregnancy BMI greater than 29 is more predictive of healthy birth weight than gestational weight gain. Alternatively, women who have a low BMI should focus on gaining enough weight to enhance birth weight.[16,18-20] These women may be at particular risk if feeding problems or complications arise during the pregnancy because of

TABLE 25-1

Recommended Total Weight Gain Ranges for Pregnant Women, by Prepregnancy Body Mass Index

Weight for Height (BMI)	Recommended Total Gain (kg/lb)
Low (BMI < 19.8)	12.5-18/28-40
Normal (BMI of 19.8-26)	11.5-18/25-35
High (BMI > 26-29)	7.0-11.5/15-25
Obese (BMI > 29)	≥ 6/15

Adapted with permission from *Nutrition during pregnancy*, Copyright 1990 by the National Academy of Sciences. Courtesy of the National Academy Press, Washington, DC.

TABLE 25-2

Distribution of Weight Gain During Pregnancy (kg)

3.4-3.86	Fetus
3.4	Fat and protein stores
1.8	Blood
1.22	Tissue fluids
0.9	Uterus
0.8	Amniotic fluid
0.68	Placenta and umbilical cord
0.45	Breast tissue
12.7-13.2	Total weight gain

chronic or acute illness, inflammatory bowel disease, or hyperemesis gravidarum.

Good pregnancy outcome occurs within a wide range of maternal weight gains.[16,21] Weight gain reflects increases in extracellular fluid and blood volume; amniotic fluid; maternal fat accretion; and the products of conception, the fetus and placenta (Table 25-2). Low weight gain during pregnancy is related to neonatal morbidity. Neonatal morbidity and mortality rates decrease as birth weight increases, to an optimum of 3 to 4 kg.[16-18] Alternatively, excessive weight gain is associated with higher birth weights and increased rates of hypertension and preeclampsia, cesarean delivery, labor abnormalities, "postdatism," and meconium staining.[20,22-24]

The IOM recommends weight gain be based on the prepregnancy BMI (see Table 25-1). These recommendations have been supported in a subsequent study by Parker and Abrams[21] in which weight gain in 6690 pregnancies was examined, including those resulting in low or high birth weight for gestational age and cesarean deliveries. They demonstrated that women who had weight gains outside the IOM guidelines were at greater risk for poor pregnancy outcome. Those with lower prenatal weight gain were at increased risk for small-for-gestational-age infants and higher weight gain was associated with the risk of large-for-gestational-age infants and cesarean delivery.[21] A recent review of the literature on weight gain and birth outcome since the IOM recommendations did not find any evidence that these recommendations are harmful to mothers or infants.[23-24]

Biochemical Assessment

Biochemical indices for nonpregnant women frequently are not applicable to pregnant women; therefore, interpretation of laboratory data requires knowledge of the normal physiologic changes of pregnancy. Misinterpretation of laboratory data may result in a misdiagnosis of malnutrition or an inappropriate nutrition intervention.[13]

Serum albumin concentration, frequently used in nutrition assessment profiles, falls rapidly during the first trimester and continues to decline more gradually until weeks 24 to 28. Little change occurs after this time. The total decline in serum albumin is approximately 1 g/100 ml. The initial drop represents a decrease in the total circulating albumin, which then rises again with the expansion of blood volume. Ultimately the total circulating albumin concentration is close to the concentrations in the nonpregnant state; however, this is not reflected in the serum albumin concentration.[13-14]

Total iron-binding capacity (TIBC) and transferrin levels gradually increase throughout gestation, peaking during the last trimester. This occurs even with iron therapy, although the increase is then less pronounced. Elevated TIBC and transferrin levels should not be mistaken for iron deficiency. Depressed TIBC and transferrin levels may be due to disease, including infection or inflammatory bowel disease. Patients with a TIBC of less than 350 g/100 ml and transferrin saturation of less than 20% should be evaluated for anemia.[25,26] Iron deficiency anemia is common in pregnancy. A marked increase in the maternal blood supply during pregnancy greatly increases the demand for iron. Hemoglobin and hematocrit levels decline during the first and second trimesters, then rise again during the third trimester. Acceptable cutoff levels are 11, 10.5, and 11 g/100 ml, in the first, second, and third trimesters, respectively.[27] Depletion of iron stores during pregnancy is reflected by serum ferritin levels. Because this can occur without significant changes in hemoglobin or hematocrit levels, it is recommended that ferritin levels be checked during the first prenatal visit in the first or second trimester. Checking the ferritin level during the third trimester is not recommended because it may not accurately reflect iron stores during this period.[28-29]

Fasting blood glucose levels decrease steadily from the first trimester. Pregnant women also demonstrate impaired glucose tolerance postprandially and in response to oral glucose challenge.[30] Changes in renal function can cause glucosuria in nondiabetic pregnant patients even with normal concentrations of blood glucose; therefore, urinary glucose should not be used to assess glucose tolerance.[31]

Hyperlipidemia is characteristic in pregnancy. Serum triglycerides may be 250% to 400% above normal. Cholesterol and phospholipid levels may increase from 25% to as high as 180%. These increases begin to rise progressively from the end of the first trimester, reaching maximum at term. Complications from hyperlipidemia in pregnancy are rare and do not appear to affect long-term maternal health.[32,33]

Nutritional Goals and Prescription

The nutritional goals for these patients are to achieve a normal rate of weight gain and positive nitrogen balance, to provide safe and effective vitamin and mineral therapy, and to avoid metabolic and septic complications. Patients should be transitioned from parenteral to enteral feeding and from enteral feeding to oral nutrition as soon as feasible.

Energy

The recommended dietary allowance (RDA) for calories for normal women during pregnancy is an additional 300 kcal per day during the second and third trimesters.[34] This recommendation was based on the calculated average additional total calorie requirement of pregnancy (80,000 kcal) for a healthy, well-nourished woman. The additional calories are required for maternal fat deposition, uterine and mammary tissue growth, fetal development, and an increase in basal metabolic rate (BMR). In studies from developed countries, the change in BMR contributes most to the total energy cost of pregnancy;[35-40] however, the increase in BMR does not occur linearly throughout the pregnancy and variability is high. The most significant increases occurred during the second half of pregnancy in all of the studies. Additional calories may be needed to meet metabolic demands associated with stress and trauma (see Chapters 35, 39, and 42). The total recommended weight gain depends on the BMI (see Table 25-1).

Carbohydrate

Carbohydrate has the greatest effect on blood glucose levels compared with fat and protein.[41] The carbohydrate content of most enteral formulas is in the form of complex carbohydrates such as maltodextrin and corn starch. These are generally well tolerated by pregnant women. Dextrose, the energy source most often used in parenteral nutrition, is also tolerated well by pregnant women; however, glucose should be limited to 5 mg/kg per minute per day. Strict glucose control of no greater than 120 mg/dl should be maintained during the parenteral nutrition infusion to allow normal fetal growth and prevent complications due to hyperglycemia.[42,43] Elevated blood sugar levels can occur with diabetes mellitus or metabolic stress. Elevated blood sugars are transferred to the fetus with resultant fetal hyperglycemia and hyperinsulinemia. Poor maternal glycemic control is associated with an increased risk of stillbirth, fetal macrosomia, and increased rates of cesarean deliveries and neonatal metabolic abnormalities.[44-47] If blood sugar control becomes difficult to achieve, it may be necessary to replace dextrose calories with fat calories.

Conversely, inadequate amounts of carbohydrate can result in increased ketone production, which has been shown to be deleterious to the growing fetus.[48, 49] The developing fetus can metabolize ketone bodies to some extent, but the potential risks are a concern, and care should be given to provide adequate amounts of carbohydrate.

Fat

Fatty acids are essential for fetal development and prostaglandin synthesis. The requirement for essential fatty acids increases in pregnancy to 4.5% of total calories.[50] Fat emulsions are generally administered as a source of calories and essential fatty acids. Early concerns regarding the infusion of fat emulsion have been alleviated with the use of soy and safflower oil emulsions because no complications have been documented with their use.[51] Intravenous fat emulsions should contain both linoleic and linolenic acids. Fat emulsion may be given weekly to meet essential fatty acid requirements. When fat emulsion is used as a regular calorie source, it should not exceed 30% of total calories. Jensen recommends limiting fat emulsion to

1g/kg of ideal body weight infused over at least 12 hours to avoid immune dysfunction and possible hypertriglyceridemia.[52]

Protein

Additional protein is required to support the synthesis of maternal and fetal tissues. The 1989 RDAs recommends an additional 10 g of protein per day. Protein requirements by trimester are increased by 1.3, 6.1, and 10.7 g per day during the first, second, and third trimesters, respectively.[34] Additional protein may be required for stress, trauma, or extraordinary losses (see Chapters 35, 39, and 42). Amino acids cross the placenta by active transport. Thus, there may be competition for transport if the amino acids are present in excessive or deficient amounts in the parenteral nutrition solution.[53] The most appropriate amino acid profile for the developing fetus has not been determined. Parenteral nutrition solutions with a balance of essential and nonessential amino acids should be used because the fetus lacks developed metabolic pathways. Total protein intake should not exceed 1.3 g/kg per day in a normal pregnant adult and 2 g/kg per day in a severely stressed pregnant woman.

Vitamins

Data on vitamin metabolism in pregnancy are scarce and are influenced by recent dietary intake, vitamin intake, age, parity, season of the year, smoking, socioeconomic status, drug-nutrient interactions, and disease state. Maintenance of health for both the mother and the growing fetus during the course of pregnancy requires an adequate supply of vitamins.

Levels of water-soluble vitamins tend to decrease in pregnancy.[54] In general, requirements are increased to support the growth of the fetus. *Thiamin* is increased to support maternal and fetal growth and because of the increased energy intake. There are several reports of the occurrence of Wernicke's encephalopathy associated with the infusion of dextrose without vitamin supplementation.[55] The increased energy intake during pregnancy also results in increased *niacin* requirements. *Riboflavin* and *pyridoxine* requirements are increased to support increased tissue synthesis. The recommended allowance for *vitamin B$_{12}$* is increased for safety but may not be required. Additional *folate* is required for rapidly growing tissue and for prevention of megaloblastic anemia, which occurs most frequently in pregnant women. Concerns about fetal neural tube defect and macrocytic anemia have promoted recommendations for folic acid supplementation before conception and through the twelfth week of gestation.[56] Women with high-risk pregnancies, low serum or red blood cell folate levels at the start of pregnancy, chronic hemolytic states or malabsorption, multigravidas, and those taking anticonvulsant drugs are at particular risk. There is no increased requirement for *biotin* because a decline in blood levels is not associated with poor outcome.[34] An additional 10 mg/day of *ascorbic acid* is recommended for pregnant women. Low plasma levels of ascorbic acid have been associated with preeclampsia and premature rupture of the amniotic membranes.[57]

Blood levels of fat-soluble vitamins increase during pregnancy in association with elevated lipid components. Deficiency of *vitamin K* may occur with fat malabsorption, prolonged antibiotic therapy, and parenteral nutrition without vitamin K supplementation; however, no increase in vitamin K

TABLE 25-3

Daily Vitamin Requirements in Normal Pregnancy Compared with Standard Parenteral Vitamin Injection

	DRI	MVI-12
Vitamin A	800 μg retinol equivalent	3300 USP units (retinol)
Vitamin D	200 IU (5 μg cholecalciferol)	200 USP units
Vitamin E (α-TE)	10 mg	10 USP units
Vitamin K	65 μg	150 μg
Ascorbic acid	70 mg	200 mg
Thiamin	1.4 mg	6 mg
Riboflavin	1.4 mg	3.6 mg
Pyridoxine	1.9 mg	6 mg
Niacin	18 mg	40 mg
Pantothenic acid	4-7 mg*	15 mg
Biotin	30-100 μg*	60 μg
Folic acid	600 μg	600 μg
Vitamin B_{12}	2.6 μg	5 μg

*Estimated safe and adequate daily dietary intakes for nonpregnant adults.

intake is recommended during pregnancy. Recommendations for *vitamin A* have not been increased because maternal stores can easily meet the needs of the growing fetus. Rather teratogenicity is a concern with excessive intakes of vitamin A. Several case reports of adverse outcome have been associated with daily ingestion of 25,000 IU.[58] Increased cranial neural crest defect has been associated with intakes as low as 10,000 IU per day.[59] Intakes greater than 8000 IU per day as retinol or retinol esters should be avoided because vitamin A may be associated with spontaneous abortions and birth defects. The requirement for *vitamin D* is increased in women older than 24 years because of the increased calcium requirement and for deposition in the fetus. An intake no greater than twice the RDA is recommended because of the potential for toxic effects on the fetus.[60] The requirements for *vitamin E* are believed to be increased during pregnancy. Vitamin E deficiency has been associated with spontaneous abortions in experimental animals. The current parenteral multivitamin (Table 25-3) meets or exceeds the established vitamin requirements for pregnancy after conversion from oral to parenteral dosing.[61]

Minerals and Trace Elements

Serum *calcium* levels decline 2% to 10% below prepregnancy values. When this occurs in conjunction with a decline in serum proteins it may reflect a decline in bound calcium secondary to hemodilution. Fetal calcium requirements will peak during the third trimester with the formation of teeth and skeletal growth. Calcium supplementation has been associated with a reduction in pregnancy-induced hypertension[62] and reduced risk of preterm delivery.[63] Serum *magnesium* drops from 7% to 12% below prepregnancy values. The RDA for magnesium in pregnancy includes an increase to meet the needs of maternal and fetal growth. Magnesium supplementation during pregnancy has been linked to reduced incidence of preeclampsia and intrauterine growth retardation. Serum *phosphate* levels decline during gestation; however, increases maybe be observed near term.[13, 14, ,64,65]

Iron is necessary for additional erythrocyte production and growth of the placenta and fetus during pregnancy. To ensure that an adequate amount is absorbed through the GI tract, a total intake of 30 mg/day of iron is required. This is generally supplied in the form of ferrous salts. The recommended amount of intravenous elemental iron is 3 mg/day.[28] Iron is not routinely added to parenteral nutrition solutions. There is concern over the use of intravenous iron because of the potential for anaphylaxis, and test doses should always be given. Most women with normal iron stores do not require supplementation during the first trimester.[28] However, several authors have used intravenous iron-dextran to correct anemia during the second or third trimester.[66, 67] Iron dextran should not be added to parenteral nutrition formulations containing fat emulsion.[68,69]

Blood levels of *zinc* begin to decline in the first trimester and continue throughout gestation. They decline to 20% to 35% below prepregnancy levels independent of supplementation.[70] Zinc deficiency has been associated with congenital abnormalities, impaired fetal growth, and maternal complications. Zinc requirements will increase if the patient has GI diseases, causing increased losses or malabsorption, acute infections, or trauma.[34,71] Zinc supplementation in women with low prepregnancy weights and low plasma zinc levels has been shown to increase infant birth weight.[72] Plasma zinc levels should be maintained at least 50 g/L.

Copper levels increase during pregnancy in conjunction with increasing levels of ceruloplasmin. They may increase up to four times prepregnancy levels.[13] Because low serum copper levels have been associated with placental insufficiency and intrauterine death, copper levels should be maintained at least at the nonpregnant levels.[73] *Iodine* is also required during pregnancy.[34, 74] Maternal iodine deficiency has been associated with infant cretinism.[75] Patients will receive some iodine if a povidone-iodine solution is used for care of the catheter exit site. When parenteral nutrition is required for less than 2 weeks, iodine supplementation is not necessary. If parenteral nutrition is required for a longer time, iodine will have to be added because currently available multiple trace element injections do not contain it.

Although the importance of trace elements for fetal development is not fully understood, recommendations have been established (Table 25-4).[34] The American Medical Association nutrition advisory group has established guidelines for trace element preparations for parenteral use.[76]

Enteral Nutrition

Enteral feedings either with oral supplements or nonvolitional tube feeding may be used when oral intake is inadequate, but the GI tract is functional. Enteral nutrition has been provided during pregnancy for hyperemesis gravidarum[77-79] and trauma[80] with positive outcomes. For patients with gastroparesis or hyperemesis gravidarum, there is a theoretic advantage to placing the feeding tube beyond the stomach in order to minimize the risk of aspiration and regurgitation. Gulley and colleagues reported a decreased incidence of nausea when the patients were fed intragastrically as opposed to postpylorically and there were no reports of aspiration.[78] It is important to weigh the benefits of enteral nutrition for patients with hyperemesis against the risks of pulmonary aspiration and tube dislodgement. Enteral feedings have been provided through PEG tubes when long-term feeding is required.[81,82] Long-term

TABLE 25-4

Daily Mineral and Trace Element Requirements in Normal Pregnancy Compared with Standard Trace Element Injection

	DRI	Parenteral Dose
Calcium	1300 mg (≤ 18 years old)	9.6-12.5 mEq
	1000 mg (≥19 years old)	
Phosphorus	1250 mg (≤18 years old)	30-45 mmol
	700 mg (≥19 years old)	
Magnesium	15 mEq (≤18 years old)	10-15 mEq
	12.9 mEq (19-30 years old)	
	13 mEq (31-50 years old)	
Zinc	15 mg	2.55-3.0 mg
Copper	1.5-3.0 mg	0.5-1.5 mg
Manganese	2.0-5.0 mg	0.15-0.8 mg
Iodine	175 µg	50 µg
Selenium	65 µg	20-40 µg
Iron	10 + 30-60 mg supplement	3-6 mg
Chromium	0.05-0.2 mg	10-15 µg

enteral feedings have also been provided to pregnant women with insulin-dependent diabetes.[83]

In general, the macronutrient composition of most enteral formulas is adequate to support the growth of the fetus and sustain the nutritional status of the mother. Use of disease-specific formulas should be used with caution because they may not contain a full complement of nutrients or have elevated levels of others. The micronutrient composition of the enteral formula should be compared to the dietary reference intakes for pregnancy to ensure that all requirements for vitamins, minerals, and trace elements are met.

Parenteral Nutrition

Parenteral nutrition is recommended for pregnant patients who are unable to eat by mouth or who do not tolerate tube feedings. The use of parenteral nutrition in pregnancy is rare, but it does occur and has been used successfully in many cases.[84-86] Parenteral nutrition should be considered only when all attempts at enteral nutrition have failed. The goals for parenteral nutrition support include: (1) achievement of normal rate of weight gain, (2) achievement of positive nitrogen balance, (3) providing safe and effective vitamin and mineral therapy, and (4) avoiding metabolic and septic complications. The indications for parenteral nutrition during pregnancy include gastroparesis, pancreatitis, cholecystitis, GI obstruction or ileus, inflammatory bowel disease, esophageal disease, and hyperemesis gravidarum. Early intervention in hyperemesis may not be indicated. Nausea and vomiting seen in early pregnancy has been associated with a decreased risk of miscarriage and fetal mortality,[87] and hyperemesis may be treated successfully with more conservative interventions of hydration and vitamins.[88] However, when hyperemesis is persistent, aggressive intervention may be necessary because these women are at higher risk for nutritional deficiencies. In all conditions, enteral nutrition should be considered before parenteral nutrition is initiated.

Because of the relatively short duration of parenteral nutrition in pregnancy, peripheral inserted central catheters (PICC) are often used. When placement is adequate, that is, in central

circulation, central concentrations of total parenteral nutrition may be used. Although most of the use of parenteral nutrition in pregnancy has been via the central route, peripheral parenteral nutrition has been used for short periods as a bridge to enteral nutrition.[89]

There have also been reports of pregnant women receiving long-term home parenteral nutrition from conception to delivery.[90-94] These patients are of particular concern because the data regarding the intravenous nutrient requirements for the mother and the growing fetus are limited. Care should be taken to provide all of the known nutrients required, with careful monitoring of potential complications.

Medications

Other additives such as heparin and insulin are often included in parenteral nutrition solutions. Heparin is used in parenteral nutrition solutions in very small doses, generally 1 U/ml parenteral nutrition volume (1000 to 3000 U per day). At this dose, no effect on coagulation appears to occur. Insulin can be added to control blood sugar. Regular human insulin is considered safe for use in pregnancy. H_2 antagonists are also compatible with parenteral nutrition formulations. The compatibility and teratogenicity of any medication should be considered before it is added to parenteral nutrition solutions.[95]

Monitoring

All potential complications associated with infusion of parenteral nutrition apply also to pregnant women (see Chapter 19). In addition, it is imperative to monitor maternal weight gain. Fetal sonograms may provide information on fetal growth and development. Women receiving long-term parenteral nutrition during pregnancy should be monitored for potential nutritional deficiencies based on the medical and nutritional history. Careful assessment of nutritional status should be ongoing and include micronutrient and macronutrient status.

Conclusion

Nutrition support during pregnancy constitutes a special situation in which nutrition is necessary for both the mother and the growing fetus. There is a tremendous responsibility to provide the best possible nutritional care in order to decrease the morbidity and mortality for each of these lives.

REFERENCES

1. Susser M: Prenatal nutrition, birth weight, and psychological development: an overview of experiments, quasi-experiments, and natural experiments in the past decade, *Am J Clin Nutr* 34(suppl 4):784-803, 1981.
2. Falkner F: Maternal nutrition and fetal growth, *Am J Clin Nutr* 34(suppl 4):676-774, 1981.
3. Metcalf J: Maternal nutrition and fetal outcome, *Am J Clin Nutr* 34(suppl 4):708-721, 1981.
4. Barker DJP: Fetal origins of coronary heart disease, *Br Med J* 311:171-174, 1995.
5. Caruso A, DeCarolis S, Ferranzzani S, et al: Pregnancy outcome and total parenteral nutrition in malnourished pregnant women, *Fetal Diagn Ther* 13(3):136-140, 1998.
6. Russo-Stieglitz KE, Levine AB, Wagner BA, Armenti VT: Pregnancy outcome in patients requiring parenteral nutrition, *J Maternal Fetal Med* 8(4):164-167, 1999.

7. Lee RV, Rodgers BD, Young, Eddy E, Cardinal J: Total parenteral nutrition during pregnancy, *Obstet Gynecol* 68(4):563-571, 1986.

8. MacBurney M, Wilmore DW: Parenteral nutrition in pregnancy. In Rombeau J, Caldwell M (eds): *Parenteral nutrition,* Philadelphia, 1993, WB Saunders, pp 696-715.

9. Whitehead RG: Pregnancy and lactation. In Shils ME, Young VR (eds): *Modern nutrition in health and disease,* 7th ed, Philadelphia, 1988, Lea & Febiger, pp 931-943.

10. Winick M: *Nutrition, pregnancy, and early infancy,* Baltimore, 1989, Williams & Wilkins.

11. King JC, Weininger J: Pregnancy and lactation. In Brown ML (ed): *Present knowledge in nutrition,* 6th ed, Washington, DC, 1990, Nutrition Foundation, pp 314-319.

12. Robertson EG, Cheyne GA: Plasma biochemistry in relation to oedema of pregnancy, *J Obstet Gynecol Br Common* 79(9):769-776, 1972.

13. National Research Council: *Laboratory indices of nutritional status in pregnancy,* Washington, DC, 1989, National Academy of Sciences.

14. Hytten FE: Nutrition. In Hytten FE, Chamberlain G (eds): *Clinical physiology in obstetrics,* Oxford, England, 1980, Blackwell Scientific Publications, pp 163-192.

15. Fagen C: Nutrition during pregnancy and lactation. In Mahan LK, Escott-Stump S (eds): *Krause's food, nutrition, & diet therapy,* Philadelphia, 2000, WB Saunders, pp 167-195.

16. Kramer MS: Intrauterine growth and gestational duration determinants, *Pediatrics* 80(4):502-511, 1987.

17. Institute of Medicine (US) Subcommittee on Nutritional Status and Weight Gain During Pregnancy: *Part 1: Weight gain,* Washington, DC, 1990, National Academy Press, pp 9-10.

18. Kramer MS: Determinants of low birth weight: methodological assessment and meta-analysis, *Bull WHO* 65(5):663-737, 1987.

19. Abrams B, Laros RK: Prepregnancy weight, weight gain, and birth weight, *Am J Obstet Gynecol* 154(3):503-509, 1986.

20. Wolfe HM, Gross TL: Obesity in pregnancy, *Clin Obstet Gynecol* 37(3):596-604, 1994.

21. Parker JD, Abrams B: Prenatal weight gain advice: an examination of the recent prenatal weight gain recommendations of the Institute of Medicine, *Obstet Gynecol* 79(5 Pt 1):664-669, 1992.

22. Shepard MJ, Hellenbrand KG, Bracken MB: Proportional weight gain and the complications of pregnancy, labor, and delivery in healthy women of normal prepregnant stature, *Am J Obstet Gynecol* 155(5):947-954, 1986.

23. Abrams B: Weight gain and energy intake during pregnancy, *Clin Obstet Gynecol* 37(3):515-524, 1994.

24. Abrams B, Altman SL, Pickett KE: Pregnancy weight gain: still controversial, *Am J Clin Nutr* 71(5 suppl):1233S-1241S, 2000.

25. Carr MC: The diagnosis of iron deficiency in pregnancy, *Obstet Gynecol* 43(1):15-21, 1974.

26. Pitkin RM: Vitamins and minerals in pregnancy, *Clin Perinatol* 2(2):221-232, 1975.

27. CDC Criteria for anemia in children and childbearing-aged women, *MMWR Morb Mortal Wkly Rep* 38:400-404, 1989.

28. Institute of Medicine (US) Subcommittee on Nutritional Status and Weight Gain During Pregnancy: *Part II: Nutrient supplements,* Washington, DC, 1990, National Academy Press, p 274.

29. Earl R, Wotek CE (eds): Iron deficiency anemia: recommended guidelines for the prevention, detection and management among U.S. children and women of childbearing age, Washington D.C, 1993, National Academy Press, pp 11-25.

30. Lind T, Bellewicz WZ, Brown G: A serial study of changes occurring in the oral glucose tolerance test in pregnancy, *J Obstet Gynaecol Br Common* 80(2):1033-1039, 1973.

31. Davison JM, Hytten FE: The effect of pregnancy on the renal handling of glucose, *Br J Obstet Gynecol* 82(5):374-381, 1975.

32. Herrera E, Gomez-Coronado D, Lasuncion MA: Lipid metabolism in pregnancy, *Biol Neonate* 51(2):70-77, 1987.

33. Biezenski JJ: Maternal lipid metabolism, *Obstet Gynecol Annu* 3(0):203-233, 1974.

34. Food and Nutrition Board: *Recommended dietary allowances,* ed 10, Washington, DC, 1989, National Academy of Sciences.

35. Durnin JVGA, McKillop FM, Grant S, Fitzgerald G: Energy requirements of pregnancy in Scotland, *Lancet* 2(8564):897-900, 1987.

36. van Raaij JMA, Vermaat-Miedema SH, Schonk CM, et al: Energy requirements of pregnancy in the Netherlands, *Lancet* 2(8565):953-955, 1987.

37. van Raaij JMA, Schonk CM, Vermaat-Miedema SH, et al: Body fat mass and basal metabolism rate in Dutch women before, during, and after pregnancy: a reappraisal of energy cost of pregnancy, *Am J Clin Nutr* 49(5):765-772, 1989.

38. Goldberg GR, Prentice AM, Coward WA, et al: Longitudinal assessment of energy expenditure by the doubly labeled water method, *Am J Clin Nutr* 57(4):494-505, 1993.

39. Forsum E, Sadurskis A, Wager J: Resting metabolic rate and body composition of healthy Swedish women during pregnancy, *Am J Clin Nutr* 47(6):942-947, 1988.

40. Kopp-Hoolihan LE, van Load MD, Wong WW, et al: Longitudinal assessment of energy balance in well-nourished pregnant women, *Am J Clin Nutr* 69(4):697-704, 1999.

41. Phelps RL, Metzger BE, Freinkel N: Carbohydrate metabolism in pregnancy. Diurnal profiles of plasma glucose, insulin, free fatty acids, triglycerides, cholesterol, and individual amino acids in late normal pregnancy, *Am J Obstet Gynecol* 140(7):730-736, 1981.

42. Rayburn W, Wolk R, Mercer N, Roberts J: Parenteral nutrition in obstetrics and gynecology, *Obstet Gynecol Surv* 41(4):200-214, 1986.

43. Moore TR: Diabetes in pregnancy. In Creasy RK, Resnick R (eds). *Maternal-fetal medicine,* 4th ed, Philadelphia, 1999, WB Saunders, p 969.

44. Jacobson JD, Cousins L: A population-based study of maternal and perinatal outcome in patients with gestational diabetes, *Am J Obstet Gynecol* 161(4):981-986, 1989.

45. Gabbe SG, Mestman JG, Freeman RK, et al: Management and outcome of class A diabetes mellitus, *Am J Obstet Gynecol* 127(5):465-469, 1977.

46. Dandrow RV, O'Sullivan JB: Obstetric hazards of gestational diabetes, *Am J Obstet Gynecol* 96(8):1144-1147, 1966.

47. Miller JM Jr: A reappraisal of "tight control" in diabetic pregnancies, *Am J Obstet Gynecol* 147(2):158-162, 1983.

48. Weigensberg M, Sobel R, Garcia-Palmer F, Freinkel N: Temporal differences in vulnerability to fuel mediated teratogenesis, *Diabetes* 37(suppl 1):85A, 1988.

49. Churchill JA, Berendes HN, Nemore J: Neuropsychological deficits in children of diabetic mothers. A report from the Collaborative Study of Cerebral Palsy, *Am J Obstet Gynecol* 105(2):257-268, 1969.

50. Crawford MA: Estimation of essential fatty acid requirements in pregnancy and lactation, *Prog Fd Nutr Sci* 4(5):75-80, 1980.

51. Greenspoon JS, Safarik RH, Hayashi JT, et al: Parenteral nutrition during pregnancy. Lack of association with idiopathic preterm labor or preeclampsia, *J Reprod Med* 39(2):89-91, 1994.

52. Jensen GL, Mascioli EA, Seidner DL, et al: Parenteral infusion of long-and medium-chain triglycerides and reticuloendothelial system function in man, *J Parenter Enteral Nutr* 14(5):467-471, 1990.

53. Hay WW: Fetal requirements and placental transfer of nitrogenous compounds. In Polin RA, Fox WW (eds): *Fetal and neonatal physiology,* Philadelphia, PA, 1988, WB Saunders, pp 619-635.

54. Pitkin RM: Assessment of nutritional status of the mother, fetus, and newborn, *Am J Clin Nutr* 34:(suppl 4):658-668, 1981.

55. Wood P, Murray A, Sinha B, et al: Wernicke's encephalopathy induced by hyperemesis gravidarum. Case reports, *Br J Obstet Gynecol* 90(6):583-586, 1983.

56. MRC Vitamin Study Research Group: Prevention of neural tube defects: result of the medical research council vitamins study, *Lancet* 338(8760):131-137, 1991.

57. Casanueva E, Polo E, Tejero E, et al: Premature rupture of amniotic membranes as functional assessment of vitamin C status during pregnancy, *Ann NY Acad Sci* 678:369-370, 1993.

58. Rosa FW, Wilk AL, Kelsey FO, et al: Vitamin A congeners, *Teratology* 33(3):355-364, 1986.

59. Rothman KJ, Moore LL, Singer MR, et al: Teratogenicity of high vitamin A intake, *N Engl J Med* 333(21):1369-1373, 1995.

60. Little G, Frigoletto F (eds): *Guidelines for perinatal care,* ed 2, Washington, DC, 1988, American Academy of Pediatrics, American College of Obstetricians and Gynecologists.

61. AMA Nutrition Advisory Group: Multivitamin preparations for parenteral use, *J Parenter Enteral Nutr* 3(4):258-262, 1979.

62. Belizan JM, Villar J, Repke J: The relationship between calcium intake and pregnancy-induced hypertension: up-to-date evidence, *Am J Obstet Gynecol* 158(4):898-902, 1988.

63. Murtaugh MA, Weingart J: Individual nutrient effects on length of gestation and pregnancy outcome, *Semin Perinatal* 19(3):197-210, 1995.

64. Scott J, DiSaia P, Hammond C, Spellacy W (eds): *Danforth's obstetrics and gynecology,* ed 6, Philadelphia, 1990, JB Lippincott.

65. Institute of Medicine, Food and Nutrition Board. *Dietary reference intakes for calcium, phosphorus, magnesium, vitamin D and fluoride,* Washington, DC, 1997, National Academy Press.

66. Oluboyede O, Ogunbode O, Ayeni O: Iron deficiency anemia during pregnancy: a comparative trial of treatment by iron-poly complex Ferastral given intramuscularly and iron dextran by total dose infusion, *E Afr Med J* 57(9):626-633, 1980.

67. Sood SK, Ramachandran K, Rani K, et al: WHO sponsored collaborative studies on nutritional anemia in India. The effect of parenteral iron administration in the control of anemia of pregnancy, *Br J Nutr* 42(3):399-406, 1979.

68. Burns DL, Mascioli EA, Bistrian BR: Effect of iron-supplemented total parenteral nutrition in patients with iron deficiency anemia, *Nutrition* 12(6):411-415, 1996.

69. Driscoll DF, Bhargara HN, Li L, et al: Physicochemical stability of total nutrient admixtures, *Am J Health Syst Pharm* 52(6):623-634, 1995.

70. Hambridge KM, Krebs NF, Jacobs MA, et al: Zinc nutritional status during pregnancy: a longitudinal study, *Am J Clin Nutr* 37(3):429-442, 1983.

71. King JC: Determinants of maternal zinc status during pregnancy, *Am J Clin Nutr* 71(5 suppl):1334S-1343S, 2000.

72. Goldenberg RL, Tamura T, Neggers Y, et al: The effect of zinc supplementation on pregnancy outcome, *JAMA* 274(6):463-468, 1995.

73. O'Leary JA: Serum copper levels as a measure of placental function, *Am J Obstet Gynecol* 105(4):636-637, 1969.

74. Elnagar B, Eltom A, Wide L, et al: Iodine status, thyroid function and pregnancy: study of Swedish and Sudanese women, *Eur J Clin Nutr* 52(5):351-355, 1998.

75. Cao XY, Jiang XM, Dou ZH et al: Timing of vulnerability of the brain to iodine deficiency in endemic cretinism, *N Engl J Med* 331(26):1739-1744, 1994.

76. AMA Nutrition Advisory Group: AMA Guidelines for essential trace element preparations for parenteral use, *J Parenter Enteral Nutr* 3(4):263-267, 1979.

77. Boyce RA: Enteral nutrition in hyperemesis gravidarum: a new development, *J Am Diet Assoc* 92(6):733-736, 1992.

78. Gulley RM, Pleog NV, Gulley JM: Treatment of hyperemesis gravidarum with nasogastric feeding, *Nutr Clin Pract* 8(1):33-35, 1993.

79. Barclay BA: Experience with enteral nutrition in the treatment of hyperemesis gravidarum, *Nutr Clin Pract* 5(4):153-155, 1990.

80. Landye ST: Successful enteral support of a pregnant comatose patient: a case study, *J Am Diet Assoc* 88(6):718-720, 1988.

81. Koh ML, Lipkin EW: Nutrition support of a pregnant comatose patient via percutaneous endoscopic gastrostomy, *J Parenter Enteral Nutr* 17(4):384-387, 1993.

82. Godil A, Chen YK: Percutaneous endoscopic gastrostomy for nutrition support in pregnancy associated with hyperemesis gravidarum and anorexia nervosa, *J Parenter Enteral Nutr* 22(4):238, 1998.

83. Smith CV, Rufleth P, Phelan JP, et al: Long-term enteral hyperalimentation in the pregnant women with insulin-dependent diabetes: a report of two cases, *Am J Obstet Gynecol* 141(2):180-183, 1981.

84. Kirby DF, Fiorenza V, Craig RM: Intravenous nutritional support during pregnancy, *J Parenter Enteral Nutr* 12(6):72-80, 1988.

85. Wolk RA, Rayburn WF: Parenteral nutrition in obstetric patients, *Nutr Clin Prac* 5(4):139-152, 1990.

86. Levine MG, Esser D: Total parenteral nutrition for the treatment of severe hyperemesis gravidarum: maternal nutritional effects and fetal outcome, *Obstet Gynecol* 72(1):102-107, 1988.

87. Weigel RM, Weigel MM: Nausea and vomiting of early pregnancy and pregnancy outcome, *Br J Obstet Gynaecol* 96(11):1312-1318, 1989.

88. van Stuijvenberg ME, Schabort I, Labadarios D: The nutritional status and treatment of patients with hyperemesis gravidarum, *Am J Obstet Gynecol* 172(5):1585-1591, 1995.

89. Watson LA, Bommarito AA, Marshall JF: Total peripheral parenteral nutrition in pregnancy, *J Parenter Enteral Nutr* 14(5):485-489, 1990.

90. Nugent FW, Rajala M, O'Shea R, et al: Total parenteral nutrition in pregnancy: conception to delivery, *J Parenter Enteral Nutr* 11(4):535-427, 1987.

91. Breen KJ, McDonald IA, Panelli D, et al: Planned pregnancy in a patient who was receiving home parenteral nutrition, *Med J Australia* 146(4):215-217, 1987.

92. Mughal MM, Shaffer JL, Turner M, et al: Nutritional management of pregnancy in patients on home parenteral nutrition, *Br J Obstet Gynaecol* 94(1):44-49, 1987.

93. Tresadern JC, Falconer GF, Turnberg LA, et al: Maintenance of pregnancy in a home parenteral nutrition patient, *J Parenter Enteral Nutr* 8(2):199-202, 1984.

94. Brown MC: Pregnancy in a patient on home parenteral nutrition, *Br Med J Clin Res Ed* 286(6370):1060-1061, 1983.

95. Trissel LA, et al: Compatibility of medications with 3-in-1 parenteral nutrition admixtures, *J Parenter Enteral Nutr* 23(2):67-74, 1999.

Neonates 26

Diane M. Anderson, PhD, RD, CSP, FADA

THE neonatal period—defined as the first 28 days of life—is a critical interval during which nutrition can affect the infant's growth and development.[1,2] Term infants are born between 37 and 42 weeks' gestation, and premature infants before 37 weeks' gestation.[3] At birth, newborns are abruptly thrust from the intrauterine environment that met their physiologic and nutritional needs and must adapt to an environment in which they must rely on their own ability to assimilate nutrition and control physiologic functions. For a healthy term infant, this can be a smooth transition, but sick term infants and preterm infants have many difficulties to overcome.

Breast-feeding provides optimal nutrition for healthy term infants, but sick term infants and premature infants frequently require alternative methods and parenteral nutrition (PN). Premature infants have increased nutrient needs that differ from those of term infants because of smaller body nutrient stores, immature physiologic systems, increased incidence of illness, and the potential for rapid growth.

Nutrition management in the newborn intensive care unit (NICU) is a dynamic process for high-risk infants who exhibit various clinical problems, and the nutritional goal remains to promote optimal growth and development. Although the neonatal period is defined as the first month of life, premature infants reside in the NICU or hospital until approximately their term due date. These infants' continuing development changes how nutrition is delivered and their nutrient requirements. Several reviews on monitoring and assessing the needs of healthy breast-fed or formula-fed term infants are available.[4,5]

Assessment of Nutritional Status

Upon admission to the NICU, each infant is evaluated by gestational age, intrauterine growth, maternal history, and clinical condition to anticipate nutrient needs and to determine the initial method of feeding. Daily nutrition monitoring is indicated for this group of infants because of the constant changes in clinical conditions, developmental capabilities, and nutrient demands. Nutrition assessment, including dietary parameters, anthropometric measurements, and biochemical parameters, is reviewed under monitoring.

Infant Classification

At birth, infants are classified by their growth in utero.[6] Birth weight is plotted against gestational age on an intrauterine growth grid. Infants can be small for gestational age (birth weight below the 10th percentile for gestational age), appropri-ate for gestational age (birth weight between the 10th and 90th percentiles), or large for gestational age (birth weight above the 90th percentile for gestational age). This classification can help anticipate clinical problems or nutrient demands.

For example, small-for-dates infants are at increased risk for hypoglycemia because of decreased glycogen stores, impaired gluconeogenesis, and increased basal metabolic rate. Large-for-dates infants are also at risk for hypoglycemia related to insulin overproduction. Monitoring of blood glucose and early nutrition is warranted to prevent hypoglycemia.[7]

Maternal History

The mother's history can warn of the possibility of early clinical problems for her infant, have implications for infant growth, or raise concerns with the use of her milk. The infant of a mother who received magnesium sulfate during labor and delivery often has an elevated serum magnesium level.[7] This elevation can lead to decreased gut motility, hypotonia, and poor suck.[7] Magnesium should be omitted from parenteral fluids until serum magnesium levels are normal.

An infant who is small for dates because the mother developed preeclampsia has a good chance of catch-up growth.[6] This insult is of late onset as compared with, say, exposure to a virus early in gestation, which affects a longer period of critical growth and development.

Breast-feeding is contraindicated for any mother who uses cocaine[8] because the drug is transferred in the milk and can produce neonatal hypertension and seizures.[8] In the United States, a mother who has tested positive for the human immunodeficiency virus (HIV) antibody should not breast-feed, lest the virus be transferred to the infant in the milk.[4]

Apgar Scores

Apgar scores are assigned at 1 and 5 minutes after birth. They reflect the infant's status at birth and the response to resuscitation.[9] The score consists of five signs: heart rate, respiratory effort, muscle tone, reflex irritability, and color. Each sign is worth 2 points, for a maximum total score of 10. A score of 6 or less at 5 minutes is considered low and has been considered a risk factor for necrotizing enterocolitis (NEC).[10] If additional signs of hypoxia are noted, such as hematuria and proteinuria, consideration should be given to postponing enteral feeding.

Medical Problems

The infant's clinical condition dictates when feedings can begin. Specific problems are discussed in the section on contraindications.

Clinical Signs of Deficiency

Premature infants are at risk for nutritional deficiencies because they have poor nutrient stores with limited nutritional intake, a need to grow rapidly, and often are ill. Clinical signs of nutrient deficiency were described in a recent review.[11]

Specific Nutrient Requirements

Table 26-1 lists nutrient guidelines for breast-fed, healthy term infants and for enterally fed premature infants. Illness and surgery can change these guidelines. PN guidelines are listed in Table 26-2. These recommendations vary among individual infants according to growth in utero, gestational age, day of life, and clinical condition. Nutrient needs may be increased for tissue repair or decreased to prevent nutrient toxicity with selective illnesses.

Term Infants

The adequate intakes recommendations are used for the 0 to 6 month old infants' dietary references intakes (DRI).[12-15] These nutrient guidelines are based on the average intake per day of breast-fed infants 0 to 6 months of age.[12-15, 18] The infants were test weighed before and after breast-feeding to quantify volume intake, which averaged 780 ml/day. For a breast-fed infant who

TABLE 26-1
Neonatal Enteral Nutrient Guidelines

Nutrient	Breast-Fed Term[12-15]	Premature[16,17]
Energy	108 kcal/kg*	105-130 kcal/kg/day
Protein	2.2 g/kg*	3.0-4.0 g/kg/day
Vitamin A	400 µg/day	210-450 µg/kg/day
Vitamin D	5.0 µg/day	3.75-10 µg/kg/day
Vitamin E	4.0 mg/day	6-12 mg/kg/day
Vitamin K	2.0 µg/day	8-10 µg/kg/day
Vitamin C	40 mg/day	18-24 mg/kg/day
Thiamin	0.2 mg/day	0.18-0.24 mg/kg/day
Riboflavin	0.3 mg/day	0.25-0.36 mg/kg/day
Niacin	2.0 mg/day	3.6-4.8 mg/kg/day
Vitamin B$_6$	0.1 mg/day	0.15-0.2 mg/kg/day
Folate	65 µg/day	25-50 µg/kg/day
Vitamin B$_{12}$	0.4 µg/day	0.3 µg/kg/day
Calcium	210 mg/day	120-230 mg/kg/day
Phosphorus	100 mg/day	60-140 mg/kg/day
Magnesium	30 mg/day	7.9-15 mg/kg/day
Iron	0.27 mg/day	2.0-4.0 mg/kg/day
Zinc	2.0 mg/day	1 mg/kg/day
Iodine	110 µg/day	30-60 µg/kg/day
Selenium	15 µg/day	1.3-3.0 µg/kg/day
Biotin	5 µg/day	3.6-6.0 µg/kg/day
Pantothenic Acid	1.7 µg/day	1.2-1.7 µg/kg/day
Choline	125 mg/day	14.4-28 mg/kg/day
Copper	0.2 mg/day	0.12-0.15 mg/kg/day
Manganese	0.003 mg/day	7.5 µg/kg/day
Chromium	0.2 µg/day	0.1-0.5 µg/kg/day
Molybdenum	2.0 µg/day	0.3 µg/kg/day
Sodium	5.2 mEq/day*	2.0-3.0 mEq/kg/day
Chloride	5.1 mEq/day*	2.0-3.0 mEq/kg/day
Potassium	12.8 mEq/day*	2.0-3.0 mEq/kg/day

*Guideline levels taken from the National Research Council, Food and Nutrition Board: *Recommended dietary allowances*, ed 10, Washington, DC, 1989, National Academy Press.

nurses from a healthy mother, weight gain of 20 to 30 g per day after the first 2 weeks of life is defined as appropriate.[5] Several useful texts are available to aid in the management of lactation and breast-feeding.[21,22]

Limited information is available on nutritional needs of ill term infants, but the DRIs are used as a starting point. The infant's clinical status and rate of weight gain can guide assessment of the nutrition provided.

Premature Infants

Nutrient guidelines for the premature infant are based on the growth and body composition of the healthy fetus of the same gestational age without inducing metabolic complications for the infant.[23] Ziegler's reference fetus is one example.[24] Regression analysis was applied to the body composition of 22 fetuses to construct fetal nutrient accretion rates. Nutrient losses via the skin, urine, and stool were factored into these fetal accretion rates.[16] In general, premature infants' nutrient needs are greater than those of the term infant.[17,23] This is because premature infants are born before many nutrient stores are established, they grow rapidly and absorb nutrients less efficiently, and illness can further increase their needs for specific nutrients.

Special Nutrient Requirements
CALCIUM AND PHOSPHORUS. Calcium and phosphorus intakes are major issues with premature infants.[25, 26] Osteopenia of prematurity (inadequate bone mineralization) will occur if infants are not provided sufficient calcium and phosphorus or have excessive losses in association with diuretic therapy. Premature infants develop this disease because of increased mineral requirements, decreased mineral intake, and increased urinary losses. Infants fed long-term PN or unfortified human milk are at high risk for osteopenia. Adequate volume intakes of human milk which is fortified with human milk fortifiers and/or use of premature infant formula by the premature infant can be

TABLE 26-2
Parenteral Guidelines for the Neonate[16,17,19,20]

Nutrient	Daily Amount (per kg)	
	Preterm	Term
Energy (kcal)	80-110	80-110
Glucose (mg/kg/min)	5-12	7-14
Lipid (g)	0.5-3.0	0.5-4.0
Amino Acids (g)	2.5-3.8	1.5-3.0
Sodium (mEq)	2.0-3.0	2.0-4.0
Potassium (mEq)	2.0-3.0	2.0-4.0
Chloride (mEq)	2.0-3.0	2.0-4.0
Calcium (mg)	60-100	60-90
Magnesium (mg)	3-7.2	4.3-7.2
Phosphorus (mg)	43-70	47-70
Zinc (µg)	400	250
Copper (µg)	20	20
Manganese (µg)	1.0	1.0
Chromium (µg)	0.05-0.2	0.05-0.2
Molybdenum (µg)	0.25	0.25
Selenium (µg)	1.5-2.0	1.5-2.0
Iodine (µg)	1.0	1.0

helpful in preventing osteopenia and treating the infant who has developed this diease.[23] Biochemically this disease is noted by an elevation in serum alkaline phosphatase activity levels, decreased serum phosphorus concentrations, and variable serum calcium levels.[25,26] The diagnosis is made by radiograph of the wrist.[25]

IRON. Infants are born with iron stores, but these are depleted by the time their birth weight doubles.[4,23] Premature infants require iron supplementation sooner and in larger doses than term infants. Iron can be introduced for term infants either as iron and vitamin C fortified foods or iron drops for breast-fed infants or as iron-fortified formula.[27] For the exclusively breast-fed infant, supplementation should begin by 6 months of age. When to introduce iron to the premature infant's diet is not clear; a range of 2 weeks to 2 months of age has been suggested.[23] Premature infants have decreased stores of vitamin E, and have developed hemolytic anemia when excessive iron was provided with a formula high in polyunsaturated fatty acids (PUFA).[23] Today, the human milk fortifiers and premature infant formulas have an appropriate vitamin E to PUFA ratio and contain iron at an acceptable level so that hemolytic anemia should not occur with their use.[23] An iron-fortified premature-infant formula (15 mg/L) can increase the plasma ferritin level and prevent iron deficiency anemia.[28] For premature infants receiving recombinant erythropoietin therapy, 6 mg/kg of iron is recommended.[23] However a recent report suggests that this therapy does not prevent the need for early transfusions and perhaps should not be a routine therapy in the NICU.[29]

Enteral Nutrition

Milk Selection Review

HUMAN MILK. Human milk is adequate for term neonates. Vitamin D supplements are recommended for infants of dark skin or those not exposed to sunlight. Vitamin D and iron can be provided as a multivitamin with iron.[4,5,30] The additional vitamins are neither necessary nor harmful. Fluoride supplementation is not indicated before age 6 months.[5,31]

Human milk is also the choice for premature infants. Human milk must be fortified for premature infants, whose nutrient requirements are increased. Two forms of supplementation are available in the United States. One form is a powder and is available as Enfamil Human Milk Fortifier (EHMF) made by Mead Johnson Nutritionals and as Similac Human Milk Fortifier (SHMF) made by Ross Products Division. Both fortifiers are added as 1 packet of fortifier to 25 ml of milk to yield approximately a 24 kcal/oz milk. The other form is a liquid, Similac Natural Care by Ross Products Division, which is added in equal volumes to human milk to yield approximately 22 kcal/oz milk. Currently, only the EHMF product contains iron, which provides 2 mg/kg of iron at an intake of 150 ml/kg of fortified human milk. A liquid iron supplement can be provided to those premature infants receiving the other fortifiers. In addition, hyponatremia may develop when human milk is used because of its low sodium content.[32] Liquid sodium chloride can be added as indicated by the presence of hyponatremia. The EHMF product has been reformulated but has not been studied. The SHMF has recently been developed

and was compared with the original EHMF.[33] The SHMF product resulted in better gains in weight and length and head circumference growth. Higher serum alkaline phosphatase levels were reported, which may reflect better linear growth because serum phosphorus levels were normal. Less emesis was also reported with the new SHMF. The reformulated and new fortifiers contain fat as medium-chain triglycerides (MCTs); have decreased amounts of carbohydrate, which lowers the osmolality; and increased protein and sodium content. The zinc concentration is greater in the SHMF.

A recent study examined the use of varied amounts of human milk fortifier, based on the infants' serum urea nitrogen levels.[34] Daily nitrogen intake and weight gain increased in response to such supplementation as compared with those fed a standard dosing regimen. This method needs to be explored further as a means of individualizing the nutritional management of premature infants. Protein supplements added to fortified human milk for the premature infant is under investigation.[35]

When the mother has a greater milk volume production than her infant's intake and the premature infant is not growing, the use of fortified hind milk can increase energy intake and the infant's weight gain.[36] This practice can be considered for infants who are not growing after fortified milk volume has been increased to maximum tolerance and the feeding method has been evaluated. For example, continuous infusion of human milk can result in precipitation of the powdered human milk fortifier and separation of the milk fat, which effects can be eliminated by switching to intermittent gavage feedings.[23] When continuous human milk infusion must be used, the shortest length of feeding tube should be used, and the syringe pump should be in an upright position to facilitate milk fat delivery to the infant instead of adhering to the tube and syringe.

STANDARD INFANT FORMULAS. Standard infant formulas are designed to mimic the composition of human milk and are acceptable alternatives for term infants. Iron-fortified formulas are recommended over low-iron ones by The American Academy of Pediatrics.[37] No additional nutrient supplementation is needed. Standard iron-fortified infant formulas have traditionally been given to premature infants as they become ready for discharge. Before being discharged, premature infants should demonstrate adequate weight gain while consuming milk that will be fed at home. Larger premature infants may be able to consume adequate term formula at discharge to support adequate growth. Preterm discharge formulas are available to support the growth of the smaller premature infant.

PREMATURE INFANT FORMULAS. Special formulas are designed for premature infants who do not receive human milk during the early neonatal period. As compared with standard formulas, premature formulas are more nutrient dense, and the nutrients are more readily digested and absorbed.[23] Preterm infants produce less lactase than term babies, and these formulas provide less lactose because they contain a mixture of glucose polymers and lactose. MCTs constitute part of the fat to compensate for premature infants' compromised ability to assimilate fat. Preterm infants have decreased levels of bile salts and pancreatic lipase.[23] A protein source that is mostly whey instead of casein is used to provide more cysteine and less phenylalanine and tyrosine. Because of the premature infant's low hepatic enzyme concentrations, methionine cannot be converted effectively to cysteine, and phenylalanine and tyrosine cannot be readily oxidized.[16,23] Metabolic acidosis is also more common when the premature infant consumes a predominantly casein formula.[16]

PREMATURE DISCHARGE FORMULAS. Nutrient enriched follow-up formulas are products designed for premature infants at discharge. Nutrient content is between the high of premature formulas and that contained in standard infant formulas. The nutrient sources also represent a transition product between preterm and term formulas. The formula contains glucose polymers, lactose, and long- and medium-chain triglycerides like those in preterm formula. In one investigation, preterm infants with a birth weight less than 1800 g were fed either standard infant formula or premature discharge formula until 1 year of corrected age.[38] Improved growth was reported for infants with a birth weight less than 1250 g who were fed the premature discharge formula. Weight, length, and head circumference were noted to be larger as was the growth rate for these infants as compared with those fed the standard infant formula. At 2 and 3 months of corrected age, infants fed the premature discharge formula consumed similar energy intakes, but smaller milk volumes, and higher protein intakes. At 9 and 12 months of corrected age, the infants fed the premature discharge formula had higher serum prealbumin and retinol binding protein levels.

In another study using a similar product in England, improved growth in weight and length was noted at 9 and 18 months with premature infants fed a premature discharge formula versus a standard infant formula.[39] However, no differences were noted in head circumferences or developmental testing at 9 or 18 months of age. Using this preterm discharge formula with small-for-gestational age, term infants for the first 9 months of life, resulted in increased gain in weight and length at 9 and 18 months as compared with infants fed the standard formula.[40]

It has been suggested that these formulas can be provided to preterm infants through the first year of life.[23,38,41] These formulas should be considered for those who have a birth weight less than 1250 g, cannot consume adequate milk volume for growth, or have a history of osteopenia or history of poor nutrient intake during hospitalization.

SOY FORMULAS. Soy-based formulas are indicated for infants who are lactose intolerant, have demonstrated IgE-mediated allergy to cow's milk protein, or have galactosemia.[42] Human milk and soy formula may be used for infants of vegetarian mothers. Soy formulas are lactose free and thus are appropriate for infants with galactosemia. The absence of lactose is helpful for the management of diarrhea and secondary temporary decreased lactase, but many infants can continue their diets of human milk or standard formula during diarrhea.[42] The soy protein concentration is higher than in term formula, and L-methionine is added so that the biologic value of soy formula is similar to that of the cow's milk protein formula. The vegetable fat blends are similar to those in standard infant formulas.

An infant who is intolerant to cow's milk protein is frequently sensitive to soy protein as well, and a hydrolyzed protein product is indicated. Soy formulas are not recommended for premature infants who weigh less than 1800 g. The amino acid composition is not appropriate for premature infants because lower serum proteins are noted with this formula as compared with standard infant formula. The phytates in the soy formulas will bind phosphorus and can lead to osteopenia.[42] Additionally, the aluminum contained in soy formulas may contribute to osteopenia by its inhibition of calcium absorption. Further, reduced growth has been demonstrated by preterm infants fed soy formulas.

SPECIAL FORMULAS. Several casein hydrolysate formulas are available, including Alimentum (Ross Products Division, Abbott Laboratories, Columbus, Ohio), Nutramigen (Mead Johnson Nutritionals, Evansville, IN) and Pregestimil (Mead Johnson Nutritionals, Evansville, IN). Alimentum and Pregestimil are semielemental infant formulas. They contain glucose polymers, hydrolyzed casein, and MCTs.[41,43] Alimentum does contain some sucrose, and both formulas contain long-chain fatty acids. These formulas are used for infants who do not tolerate standard, premature, or soy formulas. Indications may include diarrhea, gastrointestinal surgery, and pancreatic or hepatic disorders. These formulas do not meet the nutritional needs of premature infants. Once full-volume feeding has been achieved with Pregestimil or Alimentum, a more nutritionally appropriate premature infant formula may be introduced. Recently, a descriptive report suggests that the premature infant formula may be tolerated by infants who have undergone gastrointestinal resection and enterostomy placement.[44]

Nutramigen (Mead Johnson Nutritionals, Evansville, IN) is used for cow's milk protein–intolerant term infants.[41] This formula is composed of hydrolyzed protein, glucose polymers, and long-chain fatty acids. Alimentum and Pregestimil may also be provided to the infant with cow's milk protein intolerance.

Neocate (SHS North America, Gaithersburg, MD) is indicated for the infant with severe protein allergy and who does not tolerate a casein hydrolysate formula.[45,46] This formula is comprised of free amino acids, glucose polymers, long chain fatty acids, and a small amount of MCTs.

Portagen (Mead Johnson Nutritionals, Evansville, IN) is indicated for infants with fat malabsorption, because it has a higher concentration of MCTs than most other formulas.[41] It is also helpful when chylothorax occurs because Portagen limits the amount of long-chain triglycerides absorbed into the lymphatic system.[41] This formula has been associated with essential fatty acid deficiency.[41,47] The linoleic concentration of Portagen is 3.5% of its calories, which meets the American Academy of Pediatrics' Recommendation but is not always adequate for infants with cholestatis.[41]

Feeding Management

GUT PRIMING FOR PRETERM INFANTS. Gut priming consists of providing small volumes of enteral feedings to stimulate gut development, but does not provide a major source of nutrient intake.[48] Feeding intolerance is common with premature infants. The idea is that early, small feedings may facilitate progression of enteral feeding. Benefits of gut priming are more rapid progression of feedings because of improved tolerance, decreased cholestatic jaundice, quicker resolution of hyperbilirubinemia with phototherapy, increased nutrient intake, increased nutrient retention, enhanced gut development as a result of increased gastrin production, and a more mature gut motility pattern.[48-50] Although investigators reported no increased incidence of NEC in association with early small-volume feedings, the study samples were too small to provide adequate power to state this claim.[51] Introduction of enteral feedings is a concern with high-risk neonates because of the association of feeding and the development of NEC.[52] The exact cause of NEC is not known, but it is believed to result from the combination of three factors.[52] The first factor is a hypoxic insult to the gut that makes it more permeable and thus more vulnerable to invasion of bacteria.[10] The other factors are bacterial invasion of the intestinal wall and nutrients for bacterial growth in the form of enteral feedings. The feeding volume, feeding rate, and use of hypertonic feedings may also play a role.[52]

The method of gut priming is not standardized. Each investigator has used a different feeding volume, rate of advancement, and choice of milk or formula. Feeding volumes have ranged from 2.5 to 24 ml/kg per day.[50] It is not known whether it is better to prime the gut by providing a constant volume for a while or to continue to advance feedings as tolerated.[48,49] Early feeding should be initiated in the NICU with the premature infant.[50,53]

CONTRAINDICATIONS FOR FEEDING. There are many barriers to feeding the sick neonate. The main concern is the risk of NEC. The use of umbilical artery catheters (UACs) has been associated with the development of NEC, and, generally feeds have not been started while an UAC was in place.[52] A recent report demonstrated that feeding with a low UAC in place, instead of waiting until the catheter was removed, resulted in improved feeding tolerance as demonstrated by more rapid feeding advancement.[54] Also, the group fed early required fewer evaluations for sepsis, which could render the infant's status NPO (nothing by mouth).[54] The "delayed-fed" group received more PN and needed more percutaneous venous catheters.[53] Additional studies have demonstrated that feeds can be initiated with the UAC in place.[55,56]

Conditions that alter mesenteric blood flow and might cause a hypoxic insult to the intestine are an indication to withhold feedings.[10,57] Such conditions include clinically significant persistent patent ductus arteriosus requiring indomethacin treatment, hypotension requiring volume expanders, and cardiac malformations (until surgical correction is accomplished). Infants whose indirect bilirubin level is near their exchange transfusion level are not fed because NEC is associated with exchange transfusions.[58]

Infants who appear septic are unstable, and they should not be fed until their conditions stabilize and NEC is ruled out. Both NEC and sepsis can present in similar fashion. Presenting symptoms include temperature instability, apnea and bradycardia, lethargy, abdominal distention, gastric residuals, bilious vomiting, occult or frank blood in stools, acidosis, and disseminated intravascular coagulation.[10]

FEEDING SCHEDULE. The goal is to progress feedings in increments that should be tolerated and that do not contribute to development of NEC. Human milk is the preferred milk of choice because of the decreased incidence of NEC and sepsis associated with its use instead of infant formula.[49] Hypertonic feedings should not be given to premature infants because they have been associated with development of NEC.[52] Fortified human milk and most infant formulas are isotonic.

Volume increments of 10 to 20 ml/kg per day have been suggested for infants who weigh less than 1500 g.[23,59,60] More rapid increases have been associated with the development of

NEC.[60] A recent investigation examined volume advancements of 15 or 35 ml/kg per day of feeds and did not note a difference in the incidence of NEC.[61] However, the optimal rate of volume advancement remains unknown.[62]

METHODS. Sick and premature infants are difficult to feed. Each infant's circumstances dictate what method can safely be used.

Tube. Tube feedings are indicated for infants who cannot coordinate sucking, swallowing, and breathing or who require ventilatory intubation. Premature infants cannot coordinate sucking, swallowing, and breathing until approximately 32 to 34 weeks' gestation of age.[23] Respiratory distress syndrome places the infant at risk for aspirating milk and developing pneumonia. Supplemental tube feedings are required until breast-feeding or bottle-feeding can be established. Both nasogastric and orogastric tube feedings are used in the nursery.[23] Continuous infusion and bolus feeds have been used with equal success, depending on the particulars of each case.[23,53] In a recent report, premature infants who received bolus feedings experienced improved feeding tolerance and weight gain compared with the premature infants fed by continuous infusion.[49] After intestinal resection, incremental continuous feeding infusions have been suggested.[63] Providing a pacifier with tube feedings (nonnutritive sucking) may help develop the sucking reflex and may facilitate oral feeding.[64]

Transpyloric feedings are used for infants with delayed gastric emptying and those at risk for feeding aspiration.[23,64] Feedings that bypass the stomach may decrease the risk of milk reflux and subsequent aspiration.[23] This feeding route requires continuous infusion of nutrients rather than boluses.[23] Transpyloric feedings have been associated with perforation, NEC, fat malabsorption, diarrhea, and bleeding.[64] This method does benefit infants who cannot tolerate gastric feedings.

Neurologically impaired infants may not be able to feed effectively from the breast or bottle. Such infants often suffer from absence of the gag reflex, a hypoactive state of consciousness, or poor coordination of sucking and swallowing.[64] Many of these infants may require a gastrostomy tube. Gastrostomy tubes are also used for infants with gastrointestinal anomalies such as esophagotracheal fistula or esophageal atresia until surgical correction has been completed.

Breast. Support is imperative for mothers who plan to breast-feed their high-risk infants. These mothers often experience stress related to concern for their infants' welfare. Mothers will have to express milk until the infant is ready to nurse, and they will need instruction on milk expression, storage, transport, and their own diet.

Before the infant can nurse, the mother can practice kangaroo care, which involves placing the infant on the mother's chest for skin-to-skin contact. Kangaroo care has been linked to increased duration of breast-feeding.[65] It is also helpful for fathers to do kangaroo care to enhance the bonding process. Initial breast-feeding sessions may be limited to one to three times per day, to prevent young, premature, or sick term infants from tiring and expending too much energy.

Bottle. Bottle-feedings are given to term infants who are stable and to stable, premature infants who are at least 32 to 34 weeks' gestational age. Bottle-feedings are often introduced one to three times per day and increased in number as the infant demonstrates the ability to consume the feedings without problems. Premature and ill term infants tire easily and must learn how to feed.[64] The use of pacing, which is removing the bottle from the mouth during a feed, allows the infant time to breath and is helpful.[64] Infants born at less than 30 weeks' gestation have more difficulty with accomplishing bottle-feeding than the older infant, when feedings are attempted at approximately 34 weeks' gestation.[66]

Parenteral Nutrition

Indications

PN is provided to infants who have impaired gastrointestinal function, compromised cardiac and/or respiratory status, or inadequate enteral intake. Gastrointestinal anomalies such as gastroschisis and omphalocele require that the infant receive PN until surgical correction is completed and bowel function established. Infants who develop NEC require PN with nasogastric suction and antibiotic therapy to allow the diseased bowel to rest.[10] During this period, surgical intervention to remove necrotic bowel may or may not be performed. Short-gut syndrome is one complication of this surgery that results in long-term PN use.[67] NEC remains a major cause of morbidity and mortality for hospitalized neonates.[10]

Cardiac anomalies that decrease the infant's mesenteric blood flow increase the risk of developing NEC.[10] These conditions can include a clinically significant persistent patent ductus arteriosus, coarctation of the aorta, and other cardiac malformations. Enteral feedings are not initiated until the problem has been medically treated or surgically corrected. If surgical correction will take place at a later date, trophic feedings or slow introduction of feedings may take place.[68]

The premature infant may be dependent on PN to supplement enteral feeding because of the immaturity of the gastrointestinal tract. Gastric capacity is limited, gastric emptying is delayed, gastrointestinal motility is decreased, and digestion and absorption of nutrients are immature. Feeding intolerance is common and, with the risk of NEC, feedings are advanced slowly. The exact cause of NEC is not known, but a rapid feeding rate may be a factor.[60,62] Premature infants frequently suffer from respiratory distress syndrome and feedings can slowly be advanced with PN supplementation.[69]

Currently, very young infants supported by extracorporeal membrane oxygenation therapy are not fed through the gastrointestinal tract because of decreased gut motility and the risk for NEC.[70] These infants are clinically unstable, and the general practice has been to delay enteral feedings until extracorporeal oxygenation therapy is discontinued. PN including lipids should be advanced as tolerated.[71] Concerns have been raised that lipids will interfere with membrane lung function, but research is needed to clarify this concern.[71,72] Lipids should be given to at least prevent essential fatty acid deficiency.[68,71] Extracorporeal membrane oxygenation therapy oxygenates the blood while allowing the infant's lungs to rest and heal. This therapy is used when conventional ventilatory management has failed for the following conditions: meconium aspiration syndrome, respiratory distress syndrome, idiopathic pulmonary hypertension of the newborn, pneumonia, sepsis, asphyxia, and congenital diaphragmatic hernia.[73]

Nutrient Initiation and Progression

Traditionally, only dextrose solutions were given on the first day of life, to prevent dehydration and hypoglycemia. Additional nutrients were not given because of the belief that illness would prevent utilization of nutrients and because attaining venous access was difficult.[74] Presently, giving PN containing protein within the first 24 hours of life has been shown to be tolerated by preterm infants, to promote positive nitrogen balance, and to increase protein synthesis.[75,76]

Fluid and Electrolytes

Fluid and electrolyte management is a process of continuing evaluation and modification.[77] Intakes, outputs, daily weights, and laboratory indices aid in this assessment. Postnatal diuresis decreases total body water, and fluid shifts from the extracellular to the intracellular compartment.[78] This diuresis is reflected in initial weight loss. The term infant may lose as much as 5% to 10% of birth weight during the first week of life, and the premature infant, 10% to 20%.[78] Healthy term infants should regain birth weight by age 8 to 14 days, but small premature infants may take 15 to 22 days.[21,79] Regaining birth weight depends on birth weight, illness, and nutrition management.

Initial fluids are begun at the rate of 60 to 70 ml/kg body weight for term infants and 80 to 100 ml/kg for premature infants.[77,78] The amount is advanced by 10 to 20 ml/kg per day, based on the infant's fluid and electrolyte status. Premature infants have increased insensible fluid losses because their surface area to body mass ratio is high and their immature skin provides little protection against fluid loss.[78] Fluid requirements increase with radiant warming and phototherapy; humidified incubators decrease insensible fluid losses and fluid requirements.[78] For infants with renal failure, congestive heart failure, patent ductus arteriosus, meningitis, bronchopulmonary dysplasia, or after an operation fluids may need to be restricted.[77,78] Excess fluid administration has been associated with the development of patent ductus arteriosus, NEC, intraventricular hemorrhage, and death.[77,80] The infant should be assessed at least daily to determine whether fluid volume can be advanced and the correct amounts of electrolytes have been provided.

Addition of sodium, potassium, and chloride to the PN solution depends on the infant's electrolyte status. Hyponatremia in the first week of life is usually due to fluid overload and should be corrected by fluid restriction.[81] Hyperkalemia is common with extremely low-birth-weight infants, and should be avoided.[77] Potassium should not be added to intravenous fluids until urine output is established and serum potassium levels are normal. Excessively high serum potassium levels may be treated with insulin and glucose infusions.[77]

Premature infants' renal function and hormonal control are underdeveloped, which complicates fluid and electrolyte therapy.[23] Premature infants have difficulty concentrating urine, excreting a large fluid load, and maintaining normal serum and urine electrolyte concentrations.[78]

Glucose

Intravenous glucose is first given at rates of 4 to 6 mg/kg per minute and advanced by 1 to 2 mg/kg per minute to a maximum of 12 mg/kg per minute to promote glucose homeostasis.[23] The volume of fluids required by the neonate and the type of intravenous line placement dictate the glucose concentration that can be provided. For example, premature infants who need large volumes of fluid to replace excessive insensible losses require lower dextrose concentrations to prevent hyperglycemia from glucose overload. With a peripheral line, 12.5% dextrose is the maximum concentration recommended; greater concentrations can lead to venous infiltration.[23]

Glucose metabolism is often impaired in premature infants, especially extremely low-birth-weight infants who weighed less than 1000 g.[7] Hyperglycemia is common during the first week of life while the infant is receiving intravenous nutrition.[82] It is defined as a blood glucose value greater than 125 mg/dl or plasma glucose greater than 150 mg/dl.[83] Three factors are implicated in the cause of hyperglycemia:[83] (1) low levels of insulin secretion in response to serum glucose, (2) failure of hepatic glucose release to decrease with intravenous glucose infusion, and/or (3) peripheral insulin resistance. This insulin resistance may be explained by stress-induced release of catecholamines, which inhibit glucose use and insulin release.[7] Respiratory illness, sepsis, surgery, and other metabolic problems increase catecholamine release.[83] The use of intravenous lipids has also been associated with hyperglycemia.[23] However, in these reports, lipids were infused at a rate of 0.25 to 0.5 g/kg per hour, which is faster than present recommendations.[23,84,85] It was suggested that the rise in serum free fatty acids may enhance plasma glucose levels by decreasing insulin activity, decreasing the rate of glycolysis, or increasing gluconeogenesis.[84]

Hyperglycemia may lead to osmotic fluid shifts in the brain and cause intracranial hemorrhage, and may result in glycosuria with increased fluid and electrolyte losses.[7] The standard treatment for hyperglycemia is to decrease the glucose load.[7,83] The addition of amino acids to intravenous nutrition fluids will enhance glucose intolerance.[75,76] With persistent hyperglycemia, inadequate caloric intake, and poor weight gain, continuous insulin infusion can be helpful.[23] The insulin drip should be placed on its own pump, but it can be infused with the parenteral fluids via a three-way stopcock.[7] There is no standard insulin dosage, but a range of 0.001 to 0.01 U/kg per minute has been suggested.[7] Each infant's therapy must be individualized in response to frequent blood and urine glucose measurements.[7]

Hypoglycemia is defined as a blood glucose value less than 40 mg/dl.[7] Frequently it occurs in an infant who suffers from intrauterine growth retardation or has a diabetic mother or whose intravenous fluids were inappropriately decreased or discontinued. The goal of therapy is to provide an increased glucose load.

Protein
Preterm infants provided protein at the rate of 1.5 g/kg per day for the first 3 days of life maintain normal plasma amino acid levels and have improved glucose tolerance, nitrogen balance, and protein anabolism.[75,76,83] Protein can be initiated at 1 to 2 g/kg the first day of life and be advanced as tolerated.[82] Although the protein guidelines range from 2.5 to 3.8 g/kg per day for preterm infants, 3 g/kg per day replicates fetal nitrogen accretion.[17,23,86] Protein intake of 1.8 g/kg per day equals the nitrogen accretion of a breast-fed term infant, and the guideline of 2.3 to 2.7 g/kg per day should allow for individual variation among term infants.[19]

Premature infants do not effectively synthesize cysteine, tyrosine, or taurine. The pediatric solutions Trophamine (McGaw Laboratories, Irvine, California) and Aminosyn PF (Abbott Laboratories, Chicago, Illinois) contain higher levels of taurine and tyrosine than the adult formulations. Cysteine is available as a cysteine hydrochloride additive. Because this compound is easily oxidized, it is added to the PN solution during preparation.[87] The pH of the solution is decreased by this additive, which facilitates addition of calcium and phosphorus.[23] Metabolic acidosis can occur with the cysteine additive; however, it can be corrected by decreasing or discontinuing the supplement.[87]

Lipids
Intravenous lipids are given to provide essential fatty acids and energy. Lipids are initiated and advanced at 0.5 to 1.0 g/kg per day to a maximum of 3 g/kg per day.[23] An intake of 0.5 to 1 g of fat per kilogram of body weight meets the infant's essential fatty acids requirement.[82] Lipids can be started on the first day of life.[56,88] A 24-hour infusion is recommended at the rate of 0.15 g/kg per hour to promote triglyceride and free fatty acid clearance.[23] Lipid emulsions of 20% are preferred over the 10% emulsions, as in some cases serum triglycerides, cholesterol, and phospholipid levels have been shown to be elevated with infusion of 10% lipids.[87,89,90] These elevations are thought to be due to the increased amount of phospholipids delivered per gram of fat in the 10% emulsion, which form phospholipid liposomes.[87,89] The liposomes may prevent removal of triglycerides from plasma.[87,89]

Hyperbilirubinemia has been a contraindication to the use of intravenous lipids because the free fatty acids compete with bilirubin for binding to albumin.[90] If unconjugated bilirubin is displaced by free fatty acids on albumin, bilirubin can enter brain cells and cause bilirubin encephalopathy. At infusions of less than 3.25 g/kg, the blood level of free fatty acids generated are generally acceptable and serum bilirubin levels are not increased.[90] When serum bilirubin levels are near exchange transfusion levels, lipids should not be provided.[23] Because the tolerance for lipids declines with decreasing gestational age, retarded intrauterine growth, or sepsis, serum triglycerides need to be monitored.[90] The lipid infusion dose may need to be limited in these conditions.[90]

Neonates' serum carnitine levels decrease when carnitine-free parenteral fluids are given, even though the carnitine precursors (lysine and methionine) are provided.[90] Carnitine supplementation has not been recommended during the neonatal period because of conflicting reports of its effectiveness in increasing fatty acid oxidation.[90] In fact, increased protein oxidation and decreased weight gain have been reported in low-birth-weight infants who received 49 mg/kg carnitine supplementation;[91] however, after 1 month of carnitine-free PN, carnitine supplementation has been shown to be helpful.[92] A recent report examined the use of carnitine supplementation during the first 2 weeks of life and found that serum and urine carnitine levels and ketone levels increased.[93] Improved weight gain, increased lipid tolerance, and increased erythrocyte carnitine levels were found with infants whose birth weight was greater than 1000 g.[93] Additional guidelines are needed to determine an optimal dosing schedule and method of administration, but a dose of 8 mg/kg has been suggested.[90]

Minerals

Guidelines for mineral intake are listed in Table 26-2. The levels for calcium, phosphorus, and magnesium are based on a volume intake of 120 to 150 ml/kg and a protein concentration of 2.5%.[20] Smaller fluid volumes and acid loads from the protein might result in mineral precipitation.[23]

Trace element guidelines vary from the initiation of trace elements with PN to providing zinc for only the first 2 weeks of therapy.[23] In practice, trace minerals are usually begun with the initiation of PN because trace minerals are added as a multitrace supplement. Molybdenum is provided once the infant has received solely PN for a month.[20] When the infant suffers from renal failure, selenium and chromium should be deleted from therapy to prevent toxicity because these elements are excreted via the kidneys.[20] Likewise, copper and manganese should be omitted from therapy when the infant develops cholestatic jaundice to prevent toxicity because both elements are excreted in bile.[20] No specific direct bilirubin level is currently recommended at which to discontinue these two minerals.

Vitamins

Recommendations for vitamins are listed in Table 26-3.[20] These guidelines are designed to provide vitamins at required levels without inducing toxicity from excessive vitamin intake or emulsifier administration.[20]

Line Selection

Venous access is a problem with sick neonates. Percutaneous venous catheters (PCVC) have become popular. They avoid frequent replacement of dislodged peripheral lines and the associated stress to the infant.[94] These lines can be threaded from a peripheral site to a central one, to allow the use of solutions with greater nutrient density. PCVC placement does not require anesthesia as Broviac placement does, so the risks and costs of intravenous nutrition are decreased. Like other central PCVCs, these lines are associated with increased risk of infection, but it may be no greater than for small infants who receive prolonged PN via perpherial lines.[94,95] PCVCs have replaced Broviac catheters except when placement of a PCVC has

failed. Central line placement is indicated for infants whose fluids are restricted (and so, are energy restricted) or who have limited vascular access or are expected to need long-term PN.[94]

Umbilical arterial and often venous catheters are placed in sick newborns shortly after birth to provide direct access for blood gas measurements.[95] These catheters are available with double and triple lumen, which allow for blood sampling and multiple infusions. Many utilize this site for PN, and solutions of high osmolality can be used. Providing a large glucose load via the umbilical catheter can, however, be a problem if the umbilical artery line must be removed quickly because of vascular complications. A high dextrose concentration cannot be provided peripherally, and the decreased glucose load would place the neonate at risk for hypoglycemia. UACs should be removed as soon as the infant is stable.[95] Complications include limb ischemia, thrombosis, infection, blood loss, vascular trauma, and death.[95]

A peripheral line is often used to provide nutrition because most infants start enteral feedings or trophic feedings as soon as they are stable.[23] Nutrition adequate to support growth can be provided via peripheral lines for many premature infants.[23]

Transitional Feeding

The transition to full enteral feedings is the usual progression of nutrition in the NICU. In fact, in the early neonatal period both parenteral and enteral modes are advanced simultaneously as the infant exhibits tolerance of fluid volume and enteral feedings. For the infant who is solely fed by PN, initial enteral feedings may be small and parenteral fluids are not decreased until the infant demonstrates tolerance of enteral feedings. Parenteral nutrient intake can be decreased by either a decrease in volume intake and/or nutrient concentrations.

Monitoring

Dietary

INTAKE. Because the infants in the NICU are constantly changing in their clinical and nutrient status, the infant's nutritional intake is assessed daily (see Tables 26-1, 26-2, and 26-3). The daily volume and energy intake per kilogram of body weight are helpful markers for assessing dietary manipulations. Intake of all nutrients in PN is calculated because all nutrient concentrations can be manipulated.

A premature infant fed fortified human milk supplemented with iron or iron-fortified premature infant formula will meet nutrient guidelines when an energy intake of 120 kcal/kg is achieved. For a preterm infant fed a formula not designed for premature infants, vitamin or mineral supplementation may be indicated. However, an infant who requires a special formula may not tolerate these supplements because of their high osmolality. Such infants should be switched to a "premature" product as soon as that is feasible. Slow transition can be helpful by mixing the special formula in incremental proportions with the premature formula.

TOLERANCE. Feeding tolerance is monitored to pick up early signs of feeding intolerance, sepsis, or NEC so that appropriate changes can be made. Systemic signs of illness include apnea and bradycardia, temperature instability, and changes in white blood cell count.

TABLE 26-3		

Parenteral Multivitamin Injection (MVI) Guidelines[20]

	Preterm*	Term
Dosage	2 ml/kg	5 ml/d
Vitamin C	32 mg	80 mg
Vitamin A	280 μg	700 μg
Vitamin D	4.0 μg	10 μg
Thiamin	0.48 mg	1.2 mg
Riboflavin	0.56 mg	1.4 mg
Vitamin B$_6$	0.4 mg	1 mg
Niacin	6.8 mg	17 mg
Pantothenic Acid	2.0 mg	5 mg
Vitamin E	2.8 mg	7 mg
Biotin	8.0 μg	20 μg
Folate	56 μg	140 μg
Vitamin B$_{12}$	0.4 μg	1 μg
Vitamin K	80 μg	200 μg

*Maximum intake not to exceed daily term dose.

Vomiting can be a sign of overfeeding, gastrointestinal obstruction, gastroesophageal reflux, allergy, illness, or swallowed air. Gastric residuals are checked before each bolus tube feeding and with vital signs during continuous infusions. Generally, 50% of a bolus feeding volume and 100% of the continuous infusion rate are acceptable.[96] Increased residual may be due to large feeding volume, increased calorie density, poor gastrointestinal motility, NEC, or intestinal obstruction.[96] The composition of the residual is important. Mucus is common and reflects lung disease. Residual consisting of undigested formula may suggest the need to decrease the volume of milk. Residuals containing bile may be seen with transpyloric feeding, but with gastric feedings, they are cause for greater concern. Bile in the stomach can indicate slow intestinal motility, blockage, or pyloric incompetence.

Abdominal girth may be measured every nursing shift, but the abdominal tonicity is noted throughout the day to detect illness that presents as abdominal distention and/or tenderness.[49]

Occult or gross blood in the stool should always be noted and evaluated. It could be due to illness, NEC, feeding tube irritation of the intestine, anal fissure, or blood swallowed during delivery.[96]

METHOD OF FEEDING. Advancing to the most "physiologic" feeding method should be evaluated in relation to the infant's clinical condition and development. Introduction of enteral feeds should always be considered. Breast-feeding or bottle-feeding should be introduced as soon as the infant is physiologically and developmentally ready.

RESTARTING FEEDS AFTER NOTHING-BY-MOUTH STATUS. There are no absolute rules for initiating feeds after an infant has "been NPO." The reason for NPO status, the underlying medical problems, the feeding schedule, or the point of interruption influence the decision. If the infant was rendered NPO by respiratory distress rather than gastrointestinal problems, feedings can often be resumed at the original volume and strength; however, if aspiration is a major concern, transpyloric feedings may prove helpful.[23]

For an infant who has persistent and significant residual and whose girth increases with no signs of systemic illness, a change in feeding volume, rate, or strength may be helpful. Premature infants often have difficulty tolerating feedings, and changes in feeding plans must accommodate the infant.

Anthropometric Measurements

WEIGHT. Weight should be recorded daily at the same time because of circadian changes. Changes in weight must be assessed in relation to fluid and electrolyte balance, equipment attached to the infant, and caloric intake. After the initial period of weight loss, term infants should gain 20 to 30 g per day and preterm infants 10 to 35 g per day, or 10 to 20 g/kg per day.[97] For the very low-birth-weight infant (< 1500 g), a daily extrauterine weight chart is helpful to track weight patterns (Fig. 26-1).[98] Charts for weekly changes in length, head circumference, and midarm circumference are also available.[98] Weight, length, and head circumference can be plotted for preterm and term infants on the Babson Chart (Fig. 26-2).[99] Additional charts are available for infants.[100-102]

LENGTH. The crown-to-heel measurement should be obtained with a length board and two people to obtain accurate

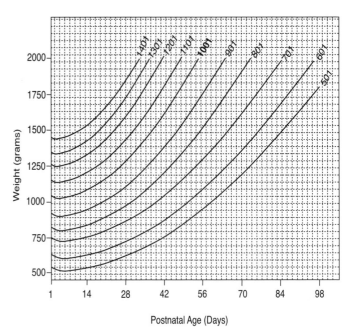

FIGURE 26-1 Daily neonatal weight chart. (Ehrenkranz RA, Younes N, Lemons JA, et al: Longitudinal growth of hospitalized very low birth weight infants. Reproduced with permission from *Pediatrics* 104:283, 1999.)

measurements.[97] Weekly gains of 0.8 to 1.1 cm for preterm infants and 0.9 to 0.75 cm for term infants are suggested.

HEAD CIRCUMFERENCE. A disposable paper tape can be used to obtain a weekly measurement. A goal of 0.7 to 1.1 cm is suggested for preterm infants, and 0.5 cm for term infants.[97] The head circumference of infants with hydrocephalus is measured more frequently.

SKINFOLD THICKNESS AND MIDARM CIRCUMFERENCE. Standards for neonatal skinfold thickness and midarm circumference are limited.[98,103,104] As a clinical tool, these parameters generally are not helpful, but they aid in interpretation of composition of growth with feeding studies.

Biochemical Parameters

Biochemical parameters used for assessment are divided according to category of nutrition therapy. Before the decision is made to obtain blood for analysis, it should be determined that the test can be used to guide nutrition therapy. A sufficient volume of blood and a site from which to draw it are not always easy to obtain in a tiny preemie. Neonatal laboratory values are listed.[105]

FLUIDS AND ELECTROLYTES. During the initial period of stabilization of high-risk neonates, daily electrolytes, glucose, blood urea nitrogen, serum creatinine, and acid-base balance require assessment. Often, these values may have to be determined every 8 to 12 hours until blood electrolyte levels have stabilized. Urine electrolytes or glucose can be determined when the infant suffers from hyperglycemia or hyponatremia to determine the correct therapy. Serum calcium and ionized calcium are measured to detect hypocalcemia, which may require treatment.[7] Serum calcium decreases during the first 24 hours of life because the infant no longer receives the continuous placental calcium infusion, serum parathyroid hormone levels have decreased, and serum calcitonin levels are elevated.[7]

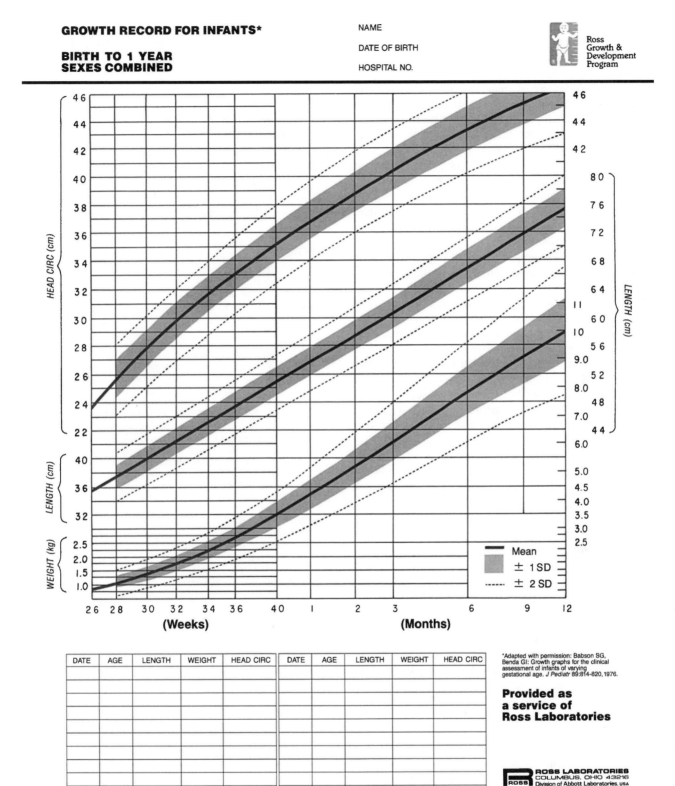

FIGURE 26-2 Growth chart for clinical assessment. (From Ross Laboratories, Columbus, Ohio. Adapted with permission from Babson SG, Benda GI: Growth graphs for the clinical assessment of infants of varying gestational age, *J Pediatr* 89:814-820, 1976.)

PARENTERAL NUTRITION. The laboratory tests used for fluid and electrolyte therapy are repeated daily until values are stable; subsequently, they are performed twice a week.[106] Monitoring of blood urea nitrogen can help detect protein or fluid overload, inadequate intake, or catabolism.[78] An elevated serum creatinine can indicate impaired renal function and the need to limit protein intake. The serum triglyceride value should be kept under 150 mg/dl and should be measured with increases in lipid intakes.[23] When the infant appears septic, a triglyceride level may be helpful to determine tolerance. Infants receiving dexamethasone therapy often experience elevations in their triglyceride levels.[107]

With parenteral therapy of more than 2 weeks' duration, serum direct bilirubin should be determined to observe for development of cholestasis, and serum alanine aminotransferase (ALT, serum glutamic-pyruvic transaminase) should be determined for hepatic function.[106] Additionally, vitamin and trace mineral evaluation may be indicated with long-term PN past the neonatal period, especially for infants with ostomy output.[106]

Standards are available for serum proteins, prealbumin, and retinol-binding protein.[105] Serum protein levels are influenced by the infant's hepatic development, vitamin A, and zinc status, and the presence of stress or infection.[16] Assays for vitamins and minerals should be completed when a specific nutrient deficiency is suspected or additional supplementation is being considered.[105]

ENTERAL FEEDINGS. Biochemical assessment has not been well defined during enteral feeding.[105] Serum electrolyte determination is indicated for infants with a history of serum electrolyte abnormalities until they are stable. Hyponatremia commonly occurs in preterm infants fed human milk, which contains little sodium. Hematocrit and hemoglobin status are monitored from birth in the NICU, but decreased levels are generally a reflection of blood drawing, not of a nutrient deficiency. Blood transfusions are used as indicated (see Iron for iron supplementation).

Osteopenia occurs in premature infants receiving prolonged PN or enteral feedings without sufficient calcium and phosphorus[25,26] (e.g., "nonpremature" infant formulas and nonfortified human milk). Serum calcium, phosphorus, and alkaline phosphatase values can be useful in the diagnosis of osteopenia.

Criteria and Planning for Discharge

Criteria

Allowing parents and grandparents unlimited visitation in the NICU can enhance their bonding with, knowledge of, and confidence with a premature infant.[108] An infant is ready for discharge when the infant is able to feed well enough to grow and to maintain body temperature and when a caretaker is ready to provide appropriate care for this high-risk infant. To prepare parents for discharge, rooming in with the infant affords a supervised environment where they can develop confidence and skills for caring for the infant.

Planning

The nursery staff often have a checklist of activities to be completed with the parents before the infant is discharged to review neonatal knowledge and skills.[109] Breast-feeding and formula preparation are two important skills. For the bottle-fed infant, feeding frequency, volume, and the need to continue increasing feeding volume should be reviewed. Before discharge a breast-feeding mother should be able effectively to put her infant to breast and should have a resource person to contact about future concerns. Vitamin and mineral supplementation should be reviewed as needed. Nutrition follow-up can be provided by the public health department, the developmental follow-up

clinic, or the private physician's office. Infants who qualify should be enrolled into the Women, Infant, and Children's Supplemental Feeding Program.

Conclusion

The first goal of neonatal nutrition is to initiate enteral feedings and parenteral fluids (if needed) as soon as possible. The second goal is to advance feedings and parenteral intake as tolerated to meet the infant's nutritional needs. Early nutrition not only affects immediate growth in the NICU but also growth and development later in childhood. Finally, the parents should be prepared to manage their infant's nutrition effectively at home.

REFERENCES

1. Guyer B, Freedman MA, Strobino DM, et al: Annual summary of vital statistics: trends in the health of Americans during the 20th century, *Pediatrics* 106:1307-1317, 2000.
2. Lucas A, Morley R, Cole TJ: Randomised trial of early diet in preterm babies and later intelligence quotient, *Br Med J* 317:1481-1487, 1998.
3. American Academy of Pediatrics, American College of Obstetricians and Gynecologists: *Guidelines for perinatal care,* ed 4, Evanston, 1997, American Academy of Pediatrics.
4. Committee on Nutrition, American Academy of Pediatrics: Breastfeeding. In Kleinman RE (ed): *Pediatric nutrition handbook,* ed 4, Elk Grove, IL, 1998, American Academy of Pediatrics, pp 3-20.
5. Fomon SJ: *Nutrition for normal infants,* St Louis, 1993, Mosby.
6. Southgate WM, Pittard WB: Classification and physical examination of the newborn infant. In Klaus MH, Fanaroff AA (eds): *Care of the high-risk neonate,* ed 5, Philadelphia, 2001, WB Saunders, pp 100-129.
7. Kliegman RM: Problems in metabolic adaptation: glucose, calcium and magnesium. In Klaus MH, Fanaroff AA (eds): *Care of the high-risk neonate,* ed 5, Philadelphia, 2001, WB Saunders, pp 301-323.
8. Committee on Drugs, American Academy of Pediatrics: The transfer of drugs and other chemical into human milk, *Pediatrics* 108:776-789, 2001.
9. Niermeyer S, Keenan W: Resuscitation of the newborn infant. In Klaus MH, Fanaroff AA (eds): *Care of the high-risk neonate,* ed 5, Philadelphia, 2001, WB Saunders, pp 23-34.
10. Wilson-Costello D, Kliegman RM, Fanaroff AA: Necrotizing enterocolitis. In Klaus MH, Fanaroff AA (ed): *Care of the high-risk neonate,* ed 5, Philadelphia, 2001, WB Saunders, pp 186-194.
11. Keller G: Clinical assessment. In Groh-Wargo S, Thompson M, Cox JH (eds): *Nutritional care for high-risk newborns,* rev ed 3, Chicago, 2000, Precept Press, pp 23-34.
12. Institute of Medicine: *Dietary reference intakes for calcium, phosphorus, magnesium, vitamin D, and fluoride,* Food and Nutrition Board, Washington, DC, 1997, National Academy Press.
13. Institute of Medicine: *Dietary reference intakes for thiamin, riboflavin, niacin, vitamin B6, folate, vitamin B12, pantothenic acid, biotin, and choline,* Food and Nutrition Board, Washington, DC, 1998, National Academy Press.
14. Institute of Medicine: *Dietary reference intakes for vitamin C, vitamin E, selenium, and carotenoids,* Food and Nutrition Board, Washington, DC, 2000, National Academy Press.
15. Institute of Medicine: *Dietary reference intakes for vitamin A, vitamin K, arsenic, boron, chromium, copper, iodine, iron, molybdenun, nickel, silicon, vanadium, and zinc,* Food and Nutrition Board, Washington, DC, 2001, National Academy Press.
16. Micheli JL, Fawer CL, Schutz Y: Protein requirement of the extremely low-birthweight preterm infant. In Ziegler EE, Lucas A, Moro GE (eds): *Nutrition of the very low birthweight infant,* Vevey, Switzerland, 1999, Nestec, Ltd, pp 155-178.
17. Hansen JW: Appendix. Table A.1. In Tsang RC, Lucas A, Uauy R, Zlotkin S (eds): *Nutritional needs of the preterm infant,* Baltimore, 1993, Williams & Wilkins, pp 288-289.
18. National Research Council, Food and Nutrition Board: *Recommended dietary allowances,* ed 10, Washington, DC, 1989, National Academy Press.
19. Zlotkin SH: Intravenous nitrogen intake requirements in full-term newborns undergoing surgery, *Pediatrics* 73:493-496, 1984.

20. Greene HL, Hambidge M, Schanler R, Tsang RC: Guidelines for the use of vitamins, trace elements, calcium, magnesium and phosphorus in infants and children receiving total parenteral nutrition. Report of the Subcommittee on Pediatric Parenteral Nutrient Requirements from the Committee on Clinical Practice Issues of The American Society for Clinical Nutrition, *Am J Clin Nutr* 48:1324-1342, 1988.

21. Neifert MR: Clinical aspects of lactation: promoting breastfeeding success, *Clin Perinatol* 26:281-306, 1999.

22. Lawrence RA: *Breastfeeding: a guide for the medical profession,* ed 5, St Louis, 1999, CV Mosby.

23. Committee on Nutrition, American Academy of Pediatrics: Nutritional needs of preterm infants. In Kleinman RE (ed): *Pediatric nutrition handbook,* ed 4, Elk Grove, IL, 1998, American Academy of Pediatrics, pp 55-88.

24. Ziegler EE, O'Donnell AM, Nelson SE, Fomon SJ: Body composition of the reference fetus, *Growth* 40:329-341, 1976.

25. Koo WWK, Steichen JJ: Osteopenia and rickets of prematurity. In Polin RA, Fox WW (eds): *Fetal and neonatal physiology,* ed 2, Philadelphia, 1998, WB Saunders, pp 2335-2349.

26. Rigo J, De Curtis M, Pieltain C, et al: Bone mineral metabolism in the micropremie, *Clin Perinatol* 27:147-170, 2000.

27. Griffin I J, Abrams SA: Iron and breastfeeding, *Pediatr Clin North Am* 48:401-413, 2001.

28. Hall RT, Wheeler RE, Benson J, et al: Feeding iron-fortified premature formula during initial hospitalization to infants less than 1800 grams birth weight, *Pediatrics* 92:409- 414, 1993.

29. Olhs RK, Ehrenkranz RA, Wright LL, et al: Effects of early erythropoietin therapy on the transfusion requirements of preterm infants below 1250 grams birth weight: a multicenter, randomized, controlled trial, *Pediatrics* 108:934-942, 2001.

30. Greer FR: Do breastfeed infants need supplemental vitamins? *Pediatr Clin North Am* 48:415-423, 2001.

31. Committee on Nutrition, American Academy of Pediatrics: Nutrition and oral health. In Kleinman RE (ed): *Pediatric nutrition handbook,* ed 4, Elk Grove, IL, 1998, American Academy of Pediatrics, pp 523-524.

32. Baumgart S, Costarino AT: Water and electrolyte metabolism of the micropremie, *Clin Perinatol* 27:131-146, 2000.

33. Reis BB, Hall RT, Schanler RJ, et al: Enhanced growth of preterm infants fed a new powdered human milk fortifier: a randomized, controlled trial. *Pediatrics* 106:581-588, 2000.

34. Moro GE, Minoli I: Fortification of human milk. In Ziegler EE, Lucas A, Moro GE (eds): *Nutrition of the very low birthweight infant,* Vevey, Switzerland, 1999, Nestec, Ltd, pp 81-94.

35. Carlson SJ, Johnson KJ, Gress GA, et al: Higher protein intake improves growth of VLBW infants fed fortified breast milk, *Pediatr Res* 54:278A, 1999.

36. Valentine CJ, Hurst NM, Schanler RJ: Hindmilk improves weight gain in low-birth weight infants fed human milk, *J Pediatr Gastroenterol Nutri* 18:474-477, 1994.

37. Committee on Nutrition. American Academy Pediatrics: Iron fortification of infant formulas (RE9865), *Pediatrics* 104:119-123, 1999.

38. Carver JD, Wu PYK, Hall RT, et al: Growth of preterm infants fed nutrient-enriched or term formula after hospital discharge, *Pediatrics* 107;683-689, 2001.

39. Lucas A, Fewtrell MS, Morley R, et al: Randomized trial of nutrient-enriched formula versus standard formula for postdischarge preterm infants, *Pediatrics* 108:703-711, 2001.

40. Fewtrell MS, Morley R, Abbott RA, et al: Catch-up growth in small-for-gestational-age term infants: a randomized trial, *Am J Clin Nutr* 74:516-523, 2001.

41. *Enfamil Family Pediatric Products Handbook,* Evansville, IL, 1999, Mead Johnson Nutritionals.

42. Committee on Nutrition. American Academy of Pediatrics: Soy protein-based formulas: Recommendations for use in infant feeding, *Pediatrics* 101:148-153, 1998.

43. *Pediatric Nutritionals Product Guide,* Columbus, 2001, Ross Laboratories.

44. Puangco MA, Schanler RJ: Comparing alternatives to an extensive hydrolyzed protein formula in feeding premature infants following gastrointestinal resection and enterostomy placement, *Nutr Clin Pract* 16:296-301, 2001.

45. Neocate, Gaithersburg, MD, 1998, SHS North America.

46. Vanderhoof JA, Murray ND, Kaufman SS, et al: Intolerance to protein hydrolysate infant formulas: an underrecognized cause of gastrointestinal symptoms in infants, *J Pediatr* 131:741-744, 1997.

47. Kaufman SS, Scrivner DJ, Murray ND, et al: Influence of Portagen and Pregestimil on essential fatty acid status in infantile liver disease, *Pediatrics* 89:151-154, 1992.

48. Berseth CL: Minimal enteral feedings, *Clin Perinatol* 22:195-206, 1995.

49. Schanler RJ, Shulman RJ, Lau C, et al: Feeding strategies for premature infants: randomized trial of gastrointestinal priming and tube-feeding method, *Pediatrics* 103:434-439, 1999.

50. Ziegler EE: Trophic feeds. In Ziegler EE, Lucas A, Moro GE (eds): *Nutrition of the very low birthweight infant,* Vevey, Switzerland, 1999, Nestec, Ltd, pp 233-244

51. Tyson JE, Kennedy KA: Minimal enteral nutrition for promoting feeding tolerance and preventing morbidity in parenterally fed infants (Cochrane Review). In *The Cochrane Library,* Issue 3, Oxford, 2001, Update Software, www.nichd.nih.gov/cochrane.htm

52. Kliegman RM: Pathophysiology and epidemiology of necrotizing enterocolitis. In Polin RA, Fox WW (eds): *Fetal and neonatal physiology,* ed 2, Philadelphia, 1998, WB Saunders, pp 1425-1432.

53. Newell SJ: Enteral feeding of the micropremie, *Clin Perinatol* 27:221-234, 2000.

54. Davey AM, Wagner CL, Cox C, Kendig JW: Feeding premature infants while low umbilical artery catheters are in place: a prospective, randomized trial, *J Pediatr* 124:795-799, 1994.

55. Dunn L, Hulman S, Weiner J, Kliegman R: Beneficial effect of early hypocaloric enteral feeding on neonatal gastrointestinal function: preliminary report of a randomized trial, *J Pediatr* 112:622-629, 1988.

56. Wilson DC, Cairns P, Halliday HL, et al: Randomised controlled trial of an aggressive nutritional regimen in sick very low birthweight infants, *Arch Dis Child* 77:F4-F11, 1997.

57. Thureen PJ. Early aggressive nutrition in the neonate, *Pediatr Rev* 20:e45-e55, 2000. Retrieved from http://pedsinreview.aapjournals.org/cgi/content/full/20/9/e45.

58. Maisels MJ: Neonatal hyperbilirubinemia. In Klaus MH, Fanaroff AA (eds): *Care of the high-risk neonate,* ed 5, Philadelphia, 2001, WB Saunders, pp 324-362.

59. McKeown RE, Marsh TD, Amarnath U, et al: Role of delayed feeding and of feeding increments in necrotizing enterocolitis, *J Pediatr* 121:764-770, 1992.

60. Anderson DM, Kliegman RM: The relationship of neonatal alimentation practices to the occurrence of endemic necrotizing enterocolitis, *Am J Perinatol* 8:62-67, 1991.

61. Rayyis SF, Ambalavanan N, Wright L, et al: Randomized trial of "slow" versus "fast" feed advancements on the incidence of necrotizing enterocolitis in very low birth weight infants, *J Pediatr* 134:293-297, 1999.

62. Kennedy KA, Tyson JE, Chammanvanakij S: Rapid versus slow rate of advancement of feedings for promoting growth and preventing necrotizing enterocolitis in parenterally fed low-birth-weight infants (Cochrane Review). In *The Cochrane Library,* Issue 3, Oxford, 2001, Update Software, www.nichd.nih.gov/cochrane.htm

63. Parker P, Stroop S, Greene H: A controlled comparison of continuous versus intermittent feeding in the treatment of infants with intestinal disease, *J Pediatr* 99:360-364, 1981.

64. Wessel JJ: Feeding methodologies. In Groh-Wargo S, Thompson M, Cox JH (eds): *Nutritional care for high-risk newborns,* rev ed 3, Chicago, 2000, Precept Press, pp 321-330.

65. Schanler RJ: The use of human milk for premature infants, *Pediatr Clin North Am* 48:207-219, 2001.

66. Lau C, Schanler RJ: Oral feeding in premature infants: advantage of a self-paced milk flow, *Acta Paediatr* 89:453-459, 2000.

67. Wessel JJ: Short bowel syndrome. In Groh-Wargo S, Thompson M, Cox JH (eds): *Nutritional care for high-risk newborns,* rev ed 3, Chicago, 2000, Precept Press, pp 3469-487.

68. Wessell JJ: Cardiology. In Samour PQ, Helm KK, Lang CE (eds): *Handbook of pediatric nutrition,* ed 2, Gaithersburg, MD, 1999, Aspen Publishers, pp 413-424.

69. Martin RJ, Sosenko RS, Bancalari E: Respiratory problems. In Klaus MH, Fanaroff AA (eds): *Care of the high-risk neonate,* ed 5, Philadelphia, 2001, WB Saunders, pp 243-276.

70. Shew SB, Keshen TH, Jahoor F, et al: The determinants of protein catabolism in neonates on extracorporeal membrane oxygenation, *J Pediatr Surg.* 34:1086-1090, 1999.

71. Short BL: Clinical management of the neonatal ECMO patient. In Arensman RM, Cornish JD (eds): *Extracorporeal life support,* Boston, 1993, Blackwell, pp 195-206.

72. Buck ML, Ksenich RA, Wooldridge P: Effect of infusing fat emulsion into extracorporeal membrane oxygenation circuits, *Pharmacotherapy* 17:1292-1295, 1997.

73. Carlo WA: Assisted ventilation. In Klaus MH, Fanaroff AA (eds): *Care of the high-risk neonate,* ed 5, Philadelphia, 2001, WB Saunders, pp 277-300.

74. Ziegler EE: Protein in premature feeding, Nutrition 10:69-71, 1994.

75. Rivera A, Bell EF, Bier DM: Effect of intravenous amino acids on protein metabolism of preterm infants during the first three days of life, *Pediatr Res* 33:106-111, 1993.

76. Rivera A, Bell EF, Stegink LS, Ziegler EE: Plasma amino acid profiles during the first three days of life in infants with respiratory distress syndrome: effect of parenteral amino acid supplementation, *J Pediatr* 115:465-468, 1989.

77. Baumgart S, Costarino AT: Water and electrolyte metabolism of the micropremie, *Clin Perinatol* 27;131-146, 2000.

78. Bell EF, Oh W: Fluid and electrolyte management. In Avery GB, Fletcher MA, MacDonald MG (eds): *Neonatology: pathophysiology and management of the newborn,* ed 5, Philadelphia, 1999, JB Lippincott, pp 345-361.

79. Ehrenkranz RA: Growth outcomes of very low birth weight infants in the newborn intensive care unit, *Clin Perinatol* 27:325-345, 2000.

80. Bell EF, Acarregui MJ: Restricted versus liberal water intake for preventing morbidity and mortality in preterm infants (Cochrane Review). In *The Cochrane Library,* Issue 4, Oxford, 1998, Update Software, www.nichd.nih.gov/cochrane.htm

81. Modi N: Hyponatraemia in the newborn, *Arch Dis Child Fetal Neonatal Ed* 78:F81-F84, 1998.

82. Thureen PJ, Hay WW: Intravenous nutrition and postnatal growth of the micropremie, *Clin Perinatol* 27:197-219, 2000.

83. Farrag HM, Cowett RM: Glucose homeostasis in the micropremie, *Clin Perinatol* 27:1-22, 2000.

84. Vileisis RA, Cowett RM, Oh W: Glycemic response to lipid infusion in the premature neonate, *J Pediatr* 100:108-112, 1982.

85. Savich RD, Finley DL, Ogata ES: Intravenous lipid and amino acids briskly increase plasma glucose concentrations in small premature infants, *Am J Perinatol* 5:201-205, 1988.

86. Zlotkin SH, Bryan MH, Anderson GH: Intravenous nitrogen and energy intakes required to duplicate in utero nitrogen accretion in prematurely born human infants, *J Pediatr* 99:115-120, 1981.

87. Mitton SG: Amino acids and lipid in total parenteral nutrition for the newborn, *J Pediatr Gastroenterol Nutr* 18:25-31, 1994.

88. Murdock N, Crighton A, Nelson LM, et al: Low birthweight infants and total parenteral nutrition immediately after birth. II. Randomised study of biochemical tolerance of intravenous glucose, amino acids, and lipid, *Arch Dis Child* 73: F8-F12, 1995.

89. Haumont D, Deckelbaum RJ, Richelle M, et al: Plasma lipid and plasma lipoprotein concentrations in low birth weight infants given parenteral nutrition with twenty or ten percent lipid emulsion, *J Pediatr* 115:787-793, 1989.

90. Putet G: Lipid metabolism of the micropremie, *Clin Perinatol* 27:57-70, 2000.

91. Sulkers EJ, Lafeber HN, Degenhart HJ, et al: Effects of high carnitine supplementation on substrate utilization in low-birth-weight infants receiving total parenteral nutrition, *Am J Clin Nutr* 52:889-894, 1990.

92. Christensen ML, Helms RA, Mauer EC, Storm MC: Plasma carnitine concentration and lipid metabolism in infants receiving parenteral nutrition, *J Pediatr* 115:794-798, 1989.

93. Bonner CM, DeBrie KL, Hug G, et al: Effects of parenteral L-carnitine supplementation on fat metabolism and nutrition in premature neonates, *J Pediatr* 126:287-292, 1995.

94. Parellanda JA, Moise AA, Hegemier S: Percutaneous central catheters and peripheral intravenous catheters have similar infection rates in very low birth weight infants, *J Perinatol* 19:251-254, 1999.

95. Lefrak L, Lund CH: Nursing practice in the neonatal intensive care unit. In Klaus MH, Fanaroff AA (ed): *Care of the high-risk neonate,* ed 5, Philadelphia, 2001, WB Saunders, pp 223-242.

96. Keller G: Clinical assessment. In Groh-Wargo S, Thompson M, Cox JH (eds): *Nutritional care for high-risk newborns,* rev ed 3, Chicago, 2000, Precept Press, pp 23-34.

97. Catrine K: Anthropometric assessment. In Groh-Wargo S, Thompson M, Cox JH (eds): *Nutritional care for high-risk newborns,* rev ed 3, Chicago, 2000, Precept Press, pp 11-22.

98. Ehrenkranz RA, Younes N, Lemons JA, et al: Longitudinal growth of hospitalized very low birth weight infants, *Pediatrics* 104:280-289, 1999.

99. Babson SG, Benda GI: Growth graphs for the clinical assessment of infants of varying gestational age, *J Pediatr* 89:814-820, 1976.

100. Shaffer SG, Quimiro CL, Anderson JV, et al: Postnatal weight changes in low birth weight infants, *Pediatrics* 79:702-705, 1987.

101. Wright K, Dawson JP, Fallis D, et al: New postnatal grids for very low birth weight infants, *Pediatrics* 91:922-926, 1993.

102. Ogden CL, Kuczmarski RJ, Flegal KM, et al: Centers for disease control and prevention 2000 growth charts for the United States: improvements to the 1977 national center for health statistics version, *Pediatrics* 109:45-60, 2002.

103. Vaucher YE, Harrison GG, Udall JN, Morrow G: Skinfold thickness in North American infants 24-41 weeks gestation, *Hum Biol* 56:713-731, 1984.

104. Sasanow SR, Georgieff MK, Pereira GR: Mid-arm circumference and midarm/head circumference ratios: standard curves for anthropometric assessment of the neonatal nutritional status, *J Pediatr* 109:311-315, 1986.

105. Moyer-Mileur L: Laboratory assessment. In Groh-Wargo S, Thompson M, Cox JH (eds): *Nutritional care for high-risk newborns,* rev ed, Chicago, 1994, Precept Press, pp 34-40.

106. Anderson D, Pittard WB: Parenteral nutrition for neonates. In Baker RD, Baker SS, Davis AM (eds): *Pediatric parenteral nutrition,* New York, 1997, Chapman & Hall, pp 301-314.

107. Sentipal-Walerius J, Dollberg S, Mimouni F, et al: Effect of pulsed dexamethasone therapy on tolerance of intravenously administered lipids in extremely low birth weight infants, *J Pediatr* 134:229-232, 1999.

108. Klaus MH, Kennell JH: Care of the parents. In Klaus MH, Fanaroff AA (eds): *Care of the high-risk neonate,* ed 5, Philadelphia, 2001, WB Saunders, pp 195-222.

109. Committee on Fetus and Newborn, American Academy of Pediatrics: Hospital discharge of the high-risk neonate-proposed guidelines, *Pediatrics* 102:411-417, 1998.

Anne M. Davis, MS, RD, CNSD

Randi Stanko-Kline, RD, CNSD

NUTRITION support for children has different requirements for enteral formulas, tubes, lines, amino acid solutions, and administration techniques than that for adults. Infants and children have lower energy and nutrient reserves, which places them at earlier risk for nutritional deficiency and malnutrition. Because of the demands of growth, they require more nutrients, on a per-kilogram basis, than do adults. This chapter discusses growth and development needs of term infants and children and related issues. Special emphasis includes conditions such as pediatric formulas, oral-motor concerns, and transitional feeding as it affects nutrition support.

Pediatric Nutrition Assessment

Growth

Growth is most rapid during infancy. Infants usually double their birth weight by age 6 months and triple it by 12 months (Table 27-1). It is known that acute and chronic disease, sickness, or injury itself can adversely affect growth, development, and body composition.[1] It is also thought that inadequate provisions of some nutrients early in life will have an impact on potential development. For example, infants with iron deficiency have been found to have a lower intellectual achievement at 5 years of age compared with their infant counterparts without iron deficiency.[2,3] Inadequate nutrition in low-birth-weight infants also has an impact on developmental scores later in infancy. Preterm infants with prolonged caloric deprivation (greater than 4 weeks) have been shown to result in smaller head size and lower motor developmental scores at 1 year of corrected age.[4]

TABLE 27-1

Growth Velocity of Normal Infants and Children

Age	Weight (g/day)	Length (cm/mo)	Head Circumference (cm/wk)
<3 mo	25-35	2.6-3.5	0.5
3-6 mo	15-21	1.6-2.5	0.5
6-12 mo	10-13	1.2-1.7	0.5
1-3 yr	4-10	0.7-1.1	
4-6 yr	5-8	0.5-0.8	
7-10 yr	5-12	0.4-0.6	

Adapted from Fomon SJ, Haschke F, et al: Body composition of reference children from birth to age 10 years, *Am J Clin Nutr* 35: 1169, 1982. Reproduced with permission of the *American Journal of Clinical Nutrition*, American Society for Clinical Nutrition.

Development

Eating and feeding are learned skills and therefore a component of development. Feeding disorders are quite common among pediatric recipients of nutrition support (parenteral and enteral). Development of normal eating behaviors may be neglected or overlooked in children on nutrition support. A child may receive nothing by mouth (NPO) and lack appropriate oral stimulation during critical development phases (age 6 to 12 months). This ignored stage hinders the transition to oral feeding. Nonnutritive sucking (sucking on a pacifier) and oral motor programs (sensory stimulation) that encourage mouthing of fingers and toys may counteract the development of negative oral sensitivity.[5] Infants, who have been intubated repeatedly, often develop oral hypersensitivity and defensive oral behaviors (learned gagging, choking, vomiting). In addition, children fed enterally or parenterally may have never learned or may have forgotten the association with hunger, oral feeding, and satiety. For a child who has never eaten during the first year of life, flavor, texture, odor, and extreme temperatures can be overwhelming.[6,7] It is important to involve a pediatric occupational therapist and speech therapist with children receiving long-term nutrition support that precludes oral intake.[8,9] Pediatric feeding disorder teams (i.e., behavioral psychologist, occupational therapist, speech therapist, dietitian) are extremely helpful for clinicians and families.

Screening

All children admitted to the hospital should receive a nutrition assessment.[10] It is estimated that 30% to 50% of all pediatric patients admitted to a U.S. hospital are malnourished.[11,12] Nutrition screening, unlike assessment, identifies children at-risk for malnutrition, not those children who currently are undernourished. Routine screening of nutritional risk has been hindered by lack of a validated nutritional screening tool. A prospective study in France showed that the factors that are most predictive of weight loss in children during a hospital stay included poor food intake, pain, and severity of disease. The combination of these factors was the best predictor of whether patients were at risk of nutritional depletion.[13]

Assessment

A nutrition assessment includes data collection and evaluation of clinical, anthropometric, laboratory, and dietary information (Table 27-2). Nutrition assessment is especially important for children because undernutrition is the single most important cause of growth retardation. Severe malnutrition during critical phases of growth can result in suboptimal organ growth or function (Fig. 27-1).[14]

TABLE 27-2

Nutrition Assessment Guidelines in Pediatrics

	Clinical	Anthropometric	Laboratory	Dietary
Screening	Dental and medical exams	Weight, length/height, head circumference, growth percentiles	Hemoglobin, hematocrit, albumin, total protein, total lymphocyte count, blood urea nitrogen	Typical intake pattern including vitamin and mineral supplement use
Detailed		Triceps skinfolds, midarm muscle circumference, bone age, growth velocity	Transferrin, prealbumin, retinol-binding protein, specific vitamin, mineral, and trace element levels	Calorie and nutrient intake from all sources (oral, enteral, parenteral)

From Routes to deliver nutrition support in pediatric patients. In Guidelines for the use of parenteral and enteral nutrition in adult and pediatric patients, *J Parenter Enteral Nutr* 17:4(suppl)32SA, 1993.

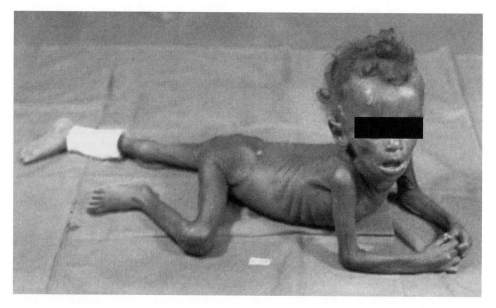

FIGURE 27-1   Child with marasmic kwashiorkor. Note pedal edema is present. (From Brunser O, Carrazza FR, Gracey M, et al (eds): *Clinical nutrition of the young child,* New York, 1991, Raven Press, p 143.)

Dietary and feeding parameters that are of specific importance to pediatrics include formula changes and preparation, breastfeeding practice, and previous serial measurements of growth. Other necessary considerations surround daily caloric and protein intake, stool pattern, and feeding milestones such as introduction to solid food, texture progression, breast milk–formula transition, and feeding skills.[15] Growth is assessed from anthropometric data. Premature infants' growth should be "corrected" for gestational age; weight should be corrected until the child is 24 months of age, length until 36 months of age, and head circumference until 18 months of age.[16]

The new Centers for Disease Control and Prevention (CDC) clinical growth charts, released in May 2000, are the most representative standard for infants and children in the United States. The new charts are based on a different reference population, but they appear similar to the charts that have been used. The 1977 charts consisted of 14 charts based on age, gender, weight-for-age, length-for-age, height-for-age, head circumference, weight-for-length, and weight-for-height. The new charts

have 16 charts including body mass index (BMI)-for-age for boys and girls aged 2 to 20 years. Nationally representative data comes from anthropometric measurements collected during a series of National Health and Examination Surveys (NHANES I to III) conducted by the National Center for Health Statistics from 1971 to 1994. Supplementary data were used to fill in the void of data from birth to 2 months. Very low-birth-weight (VLBW) infants were excluded from the reference data because literature shows that these infants grow differently than non-VLBW infants. A decision was made to exclude the HANES III weight data for children 6 years and older to avoid the influence of an increase in body weight that occurred between the previous national surveys and the HANES III survey. A required feature of a reference is that it is stable over time. Without this exclusion, the 85th and 95th percentile curves would have been higher and fewer children and adolescents would have been classified as overweight or at risk of overweight. These charts are racially and ethnically diverse and representative of breastfed and formula-fed infants. The clinical growth charts can be downloaded or printed from the

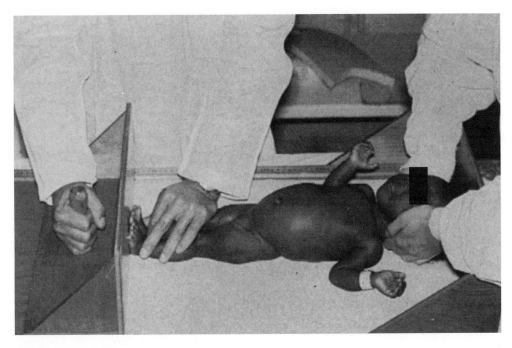

FIGURE 27-2 Technique of and design for measurement of recumbent length. (From Brunser O, Carrazza FR, Gracey M, et al (eds): *Clinical nutrition of the young child,* New York, 1991, Raven Press, p 35.)

website http://www.cdc.gov/growthcharts. Other growth charts are available for specific conditions such as Down syndrome and Turner's syndrome.

Weight-for-age is a valuable indicator of underweight. Underweight-for-age indicates acute malnutrition. Standard weight, height, head circumference, or weight-for-height is the 50th percentile for age and gender. A deficit in height- or length-for-age usually indicates stunting and essentially measures long-term growth faltering. It is important to determine whether the cause is chronic undernutrition or constitutional short stature (Fig. 27-2). Weight-for-height assesses body weight in proportion to height and distinguishes wasting from dwarfism.[17] Head circumference reflects brain growth, is used to screen for potential developmental or neurologic disabilities, and it is the last anthropometric parameter to be affected by nutritional status. (Fig. 27-3). Growth changes can also be assessed by using triceps skinfold thickness, midarm muscle circumference, bone age, and Z scores. (A Z score denotes standard deviation units from the median and is used to interpret weight-for-age, height-for-age, and weight-for-height data.[18]) Severity of malnutrition is calculated by using percent standard for weight-for-age, height-for-age, or weight-for-height (Table 27-3).[19,20]

Tanner stages of growth are also used to assess nutritional status during the adolescence growth spurt. Tanner's stages of sexual development or maturation (from 1, preadolescence, to 5, maturity) use a clinical rating scale (development and maturation of breasts, labia majora, hair, and skin for girls and testes, penis, hair, and skin for boys) to evaluate development. Body mass index (BMI) (weight in kilograms/height in meter^2) is used to evaluate obesity in children and adolescents.[21] BMI-for-age is the only indicator that allows one to plot a measure of weight and height with age on the same chart. It can be used as a tool to screen (not diagnose) for overweight or risk of over-

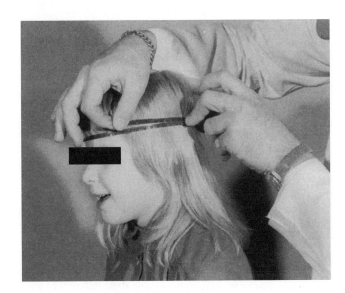

FIGURE 27-3 Head circumference measurement. (From Brunser O, Carrazza FR, Gracey M, et al (eds): *Clinical nutrition of the young child,* New York, 1991, Raven Press, p 36.)

weight in children. It correlates with clinical risk factors for cardiovascular disease, including hyperlipidemia, elevated insulin, and high blood pressure. BMI has not been validated to date as a tool to assess for undernutrition.

Biochemical assessment should include screening for iron deficiency anemia. Hypochloremia secondary to chronic diuretic therapy can cause poor appetite and growth failure.[22] Thus, it is important to assess for potential drug-nutrient interactions. When drugs such as anticonvulsants, diuretics, antibiotics, bronchodilators, and chemotherapy are given over long periods of

TABLE 27-3
Assessment of Malnutrition

Waterflow Classification		
Grade of malnutrition	Weight/Height (% of standard)	Height/Age (% of standard)
0 degree	>90	>95
First degree (mild)	81-90	90-95
Second degree (moderate)	70-80	85-89
Third degree (severe)	<70	<85

Gomez Criteria	
Degree of malnutrition	Weight/Age (% of standard)
First degree (mild)	75-85
Second degree (moderate)	64-74
Third degree (severe)	<64

CALCULATING PERCENT OF STANDARD:
Appropriate to use for weight, height/age, weight/height

$$\% \text{ standard} = \frac{\text{actual measure}}{\text{expected measure (50th percentile for age)}}$$

Example: 6-month-old boy: length, 66 cm; weight, 6.2 kg; IBW/Length, 7.5 kg; head circumference, 43 cm

Length/age: 25th percentile; 97% of standard
Weight/age: 5th percentile; 79% of standard
Weight/length: 5th percentile; 83% of standard

Assessment: First-degree malnutrition based on: % standard wt/age and wt/length

From Boston Children's Hospital: *Pediatric nutrition handbook,* Boston, 1993, Boston Children's Hospital, pp 10-11.
IBW, Ideal body weight.

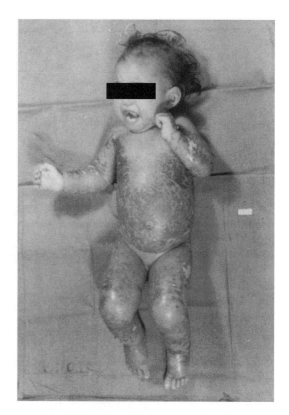

FIGURE 27-4   Child with kwashiorkor who exhibits the apathy and irritability associated with the disease. Note flaky-paint dermatosis over the trunk and limbs. (From Brunser O, Carrazza FR, Gracey M, et al (eds): *Clinical nutrition of the young child,* New York, 1991, Raven Press, p 144.)

time for chronic conditions, infants and children are at particular risk for biochemical abnormalities. Metabolic acidosis also causes growth failure. If a child who is provided sufficient calories and protein fails to grow properly, a micronutrient (possibly zinc) deficiency should be suspected. If the child was premature (i.e., born before 37 weeks' gestation), tissue stores may be inadequate.[23,24] Normal laboratory values for various biochemical parameters—albumin, vitamin levels, phosphorus, trace elements, and alkaline phosphatase—are different from adult values and vary with the age of the child. A depressed alkaline phosphatase level may also indicate zinc deficiency.

Reassessment

Changes in clinical status and shifting needs of growth and development in pediatrics demands periodic nutritional reassessment. Reassessment determines whether or not preestablished goals are being met or additional nutrition problems or risks have developed. For example, a 2-month-old term infant was started on tube feedings to provide 110 kcal/kg per day at a weight of 3.70 kg. Seven days later the infant is still receiving the same tube feeding and has a weight of 4.10 kg. The same tube feeding after 7 days is now providing 99 kcal/kg per day. A reassessment indicates that growth velocity has achieved an average weight gain of 57 g per day. In order to maintain the same growth velocity, the tube feeding caloric delivery needs to be increased. Reassessment is an ongoing

process in pediatrics. A nutrition care plan is developed to design goals, implement the goals, follow response, and record outcomes of nutrition therapy. Recurrent evaluation of goals creates the process of reassessment and drives modification of the nutrition care plan. Goals need to be identified in measurable behavioral or quantitative terms and directly related to the usefulness of nutrition interventions.

Indications for Nutrition Support

Guidelines for timely and appropriate intervention with special nutrition support should be based on the child's clinical condition. Normally, well-nourished children who are not eating enough should be given special nutrition support after 5 to 7 days of suboptimal nutrient intake. For term neonates, nutrition support should be initiated within 3 to 5 days.[10] Therefore, organized hospital nutrition screening programs and caloric intake records are a clinical necessity. Malnourished children who are not eating enough, and some children who are overtly hypermetabolic, should be given specialized nutrition support sooner.[10] When the nutrition intervention begins depends on the disease process and clinical status (Box 27-1, Fig. 27-4).

Enteral nutrition is the preferred method of support unless a specific contraindication exists, such as bowel obstruction (Box 27-2). The enteral route is preferable to parenteral nutrition for many reasons. Nutrients supplied enterally to the

BOX 27-1

Nutrition Support in the Pediatric Intensive Care Unit

WITHIN 1 TO 5 DAYS OF ADMISSION
1. Optimize intravenous fluid support with 10% dextrose in water (protein-sparing) 0.34 kcal/ml.
2. Promptly initiate enteral/oral feeds to prevent gut atrophy (trophic feeding).
3. Absence of bowel sounds *does not* eliminate use of enteral/oral feeds.
4. Unless the delivery of PN/PPN is given for > 3 to 5 days, there is very little nutritional benefit.

PEDIATRIC NUTRITION ASSESSMENT
Assess nutritional status to determine if well nourished or malnourished (see Table 27-3). Complete a pediatric nutrition assessment within 1 to 5 days of PICU admission.

INTERVENTION

Malnourished	Timing of Intervention*
< 1 yr	24 hr
1-5 yr	48 hr
5-18 yr	72 hr

Well-Nourished	Timing of Intervention*
< 1 yr (term)	3-5 days
1-5 yr	5-7 days
5-18 yr	5-7 days

*Depending on clinical condition and hemodynamic stability

PEDIATRIC NUTRITION SUPPORT

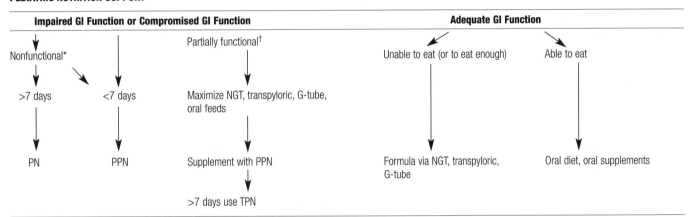

GI, Gastrointestinal, *NG-T,* nasogastric tube, *PPN,* peripheral parenteral nutrition; *PN,* total parenteral nutrition.
* Nonfunctional GI access:
• Paralytic ileus only
• Chronic intractable vomiting
• Small bowel ischemia
• Necrotizing enterocolitis
• Severe acute pancreatitis
• Surgical intestinal disorders (gastroschisis, omphalocele, multiple intestinal atresia, tracheoesophageal atresia/fistula, malrotation/volvulus, diaphragmatic hernia) only until enteral route is accessed
† Partially functional GI access:
• Increased nutrient requirement due to disease state or excessive losses that cannot be met after enteral support is maximized.
• Risk of aspiration/reflux when transpyloric feeds cannot be accessed
• Burns, multisystem organ failure
• Malabsorption, chronic intractable diarrhea with dehydration; short-gut; villous atrophy)
• Start nutrition support immediately when:
• Low-birth-weight/premature infants in PICU with immature GI function
• Weight loss of >5%-10% of usual body weight or a decrease in two growth channels (standard deviations) within 1-4 weeks
• Weight-for-height ratio < 5th percentile *or* child gains no weight for 3 months
• GI tract dysfunction (may be due to short length [congenital or secondary to disease] or motility disorders)

gastrointestinal (GI) tract offer benefits that parenteral support does not. Enteral nutrition prevents possible gut atrophy and may stimulate maturation and prevent breakdown of the GI barrier.[25] Enteral nutrition is the primary mode of nutrition rehabilitation today. Infants and children who stand to benefit are those with failure to thrive secondary to conditions such as congenital heart disease, cystic fibrosis and chronic lung disease, cancer, renal failure, metabolic disorders, trauma and burns, inflammatory bowel disease, cerebral palsy, and gastroesophageal reflux.[26-29]

When GI and medical problems of children preclude or severely limit use of the GI tract for nutrition support, parenteral nutrition is indicated (Box 27-3). Nevertheless, even small amounts of enteral nutrition can benefit the GI tract and should be used when possible.[30,31] Very little nutritional benefit is derived from parenteral nutrition used for 3 days or less.[32] Parenteral nutrition (PN) was first used successfully to feed a malnourished infant in 1944. Parenteral nutrition has been life saving, especially for infants with conditions such as intestinal atresia and small bowel ischemia.

Nutritional Requirements

A quantitative and qualitative evaluation of nutrient needs should precede initiation of any specialized nutrition support.[10] Nutrient needs are greatly influenced by the child's age (gestational age), gender, intrauterine growth status, body surface area, weight, appropriateness of previous growth pattern, specific disease state(s), initial nutritional status, and anticipated duration of inadequate oral intake. Developmental needs unique to the infant or child must be taken into consideration when formulating nutrient goals (Box 27-4, Table 27-4). Many different

---

BOX 27-2

General Indications for Enteral Nutrition in Pediatrics

Impaired nutrient ingestion
  Neurologic disorders
  Acquired immunodeficiency syndrome
  Facial trauma
  Rhabdomyosarcoma of the nasopharynx
  Oral or esophageal injury
  Congenital anomalies
  Handicapping conditions
  Respiratory impairment
Inability to take full nutrient needs by mouth
  Increased metabolic needs
  Anorexia from chronic disease
  Psychosocial disorder
  Impaired energy consumption (< 50%-60% of RDA plus total feeding time > 4 to 6 hr/day)
Impaired digestion, absorption, or metabolism: inborn errors of metabolism
Impaired growth/development: severe and deteriorating wasting and/or depressed linear growth

---

BOX 27-3

Indications for Parenteral Nutrition in Pediatrics

Paralytic ileus
Necrotizing enterocolitis
Severe acute pancreatitis
Gastroschisis
Malrotation/volvulus
Severe inflammatory bowel disease
Omphalocele
Short-gut syndrome
Congenital malformation
Intestinal atresia
Chronic idiopathic intestinal pseudoobstruction
Severe Hirschsprung's disease
Microvillus inclusion disease
Small bowel ischemia
Severe motility/absorptive/secretory disorders
Gardner's syndrome
Hypermetabolism with limited enteral tolerance and/or access
  Sepsis
  Multisystem organ failure
  Multiple or major trauma
  Malignancy, bone marrow transplantation
  Severe burns

BOX 27-4

Guidelines to Ensure Adequacy of Nutrition Support

Identify macronutrient needs: calories, protein, carbohydrate, fat
Monitor nutrient distribution:

Carbohydrate	35%-65% of total calories
Protein	5%-16% of total calories (<25% in severe stress); for infants do not exceed 5 g/kg/day
Fat	30%-55% of total calories

Identify risks for micronutrient deficiencies (refeeding syndrome, prematurity, short gut, cystic fibrosis); supplement as needed.
Determine fluid needs. If fluid is restricted, formulas and solutions can be concentrated.
Evaluate osmolality and renal solute load (enteral) or osmolarity (PPN). Monitor hydration status closely.
Consider the need for fat, carbohydrate, or protein modulation, depending on disease and clinical condition.
Evaluate vitamin, mineral, and electrolyte provisions, especially when using adult formulas or solutions (vitamin D, calcium, phosphorus).
Add dietary fiber to long-term enteral feedings (0.66 to 1.0 g/kg, up to 45 g/day).
Monitor growth (weight, height, head circumference) and nutrient intake regularly to prevent patient from *outgrowing* calorie supply.

TABLE 27-4

Suggestions for Estimating Calorie Requirements in Children with Developmental Disabilities

Clinical Condition	Calorie Recommendation
Down syndrome (boys aged 5-12 yr)	16.1 kcal/cm height (40.9 kcal/in)
Down syndrome (girls aged 5-12 yr)	14.3 kcal/cm height (36.3 kcal/in)
Prader-Willi syndrome	10-11 kcal/cm height for maintenance (26.7 kcal/in)
	8.5 kcal/cm height for weight loss (21.6 kcal/in)
Myelomeningocele (spina bifida)	9-11 kcal/cm height for maintenance (25.0 kcal/in)
	7 kcal/cm height for weight loss (17.78 kcal/in)
Cerebral palsy (age 5-11 yr)	13.9 kcal/cm height with mild to moderate activity (35.3 kcal/in)
	11.1 kcal/cm height with severe physical restrictions (28.2 kcal/in)

Adapted from Ekvall SW, Bandini L, Ekvall V: Obesity. In Ekvall SW (ed): *Pediatric nutrition in chronic diseases and developmental disorders*, New York, 1993, Oxford University Press, p 168. Used with permission from Rokusek C, Heinricks E, eds: *Nutrition and feeding for the developmentally disabled. A how to manual*, Vermillion, SD, 1985, South Dakota University Affiliated Facility Center for Developmentally Disabled.

tables and methods are available to calculate calorie and protein requirements of infants and children (Tables 27-5, 27-6). Overfeeding can be considered a type of malnutrition, so objective measurements of actual calorie needs (indirect calorimetry) and of nitrogen requirements (urinary nitrogen assay) are more accurate and should be used if available.[10,33,34] The Harris-Benedict equation should be used only to calculate calorie requirements for postpubescent adolescents because it does not include a factor for growth. Various pediatric basal metabolic rate tables plus activity and stress factors can be used to set goals for normal growth for age. New dietary reference intakes (DRIs) are being established for energy needs to replace the 1989 recommended dietary allowances (RDAs). It should be noted that DRIs are quantitative reference values of estimates of nutrient intakes for healthy people in the United States and Canada. DRIs include estimated average requirement (EAR), recommended dietary allowance (RDA), adequate intake (AI), and tolerable upper level intake (UL). DRI reports may be found at http://www.nap.edu. Information gaps on nutrient needs of infants and children, nutrient-to-nutrient interactions, and studies to detect adverse effects of chronic high intakes of nutrients still remain. Much of the infant data available is based on the nutrient content of human milk. Other problems encountered when using DRIs to calculate energy needs in this population include individual variablilty with respect to body size, disease state(s), and genetic susceptibility. When either growth or nutritional status is suboptimal, catch-up requirements should be provided.[35] For children who have failed to thrive, long-term catch-up growth depends on provision of calories and protein in excess of normal requirements.[36] Catch-up calorie needs are calculated as the product of the ideal body weight for age (50th percentile) and the DRI calorie recommendation for weight for age. This calorie-per-kilogram figure is then divided by the actual body weight (Box 27-5).

Fluid requirements are an important consideration in nutrition support to prevent either dehydration or overhydration (Table 27-7). Factors that decrease fluid requirements include heat shields, thermal blankets, double-walled incubators, renal oliguria, mist tents, and warm, humidified air via an endotracheal tube. Factors that increase fluid requirements in infants and children include fever, diarrhea, vomiting, respiratory distress, hyperventilation, phototherapy, glycosuria, radiant warmers, conventional single-walled incubators, hypermetabolism, renal tubule defects, diuretic therapy, fistulas, stomas, and increased fiber intake. Fluid and hydration status needs to be evaluated daily. Infants are unable to signal (verbalize) thirst. In addition, an infant's normal body composition is much higher in water than that of an adult.

Compendium of Pediatric Formulations (Enteral Feedings)

The choice of an enteral or parenteral formula should be individualized and should take into consideration such factors as nutritional requirements, fluid requirements, age, disease state, clinical condition, GI function, route of delivery, growth,

---

TABLE 27-5

Basal Energy Metabolism of Infants and Children

Age 1 wk 10 mo		Age 11-36 mo			Age 3-16 yr		
Metabolic rate		Metabolic rate (kcal/hr)			Metabolic rate (kcal/hr)		
Weight (kg)	Male or female (kcal/hr)	Weight (kg)	Male	Female	Weight (kg)	Male	Female
3.5	8.4	9.0	22.0	21.2	15	35.8	33.3
4.0	9.5	9.5	22.8	22.0	20	39.7	37.4
4.5	10.5	10.0	23.6	22.8	25	43.6	41.5
5.0	11.6	10.5	24.4	23.6	30	47.5	45.5
5.5	12.7	11.0	25.2	24.4	35	51.3	49.6
6.0	13.8	11.5	26.0	25.2	40	55.2	53.7
6.5	14.9	12.0	26.8	26.0	45	59.1	57.8
7.0	16.0	12.5	27.6	26.9	50	63.0	61.9
7.5	17.1	13.0	28.4	27.7	55	66.9	66.0
8.0	18.2	13.5	29.2	28.5	60	70.8	70.0
8.5	19.3	14.0	30.0	29.3	65	74.7	74.0
9.0	20.4	14.5	30.8	30.1	70	78.6	78.1
9.5	21.4	15.0	31.6	30.9	75	82.5	82.2
10.0	22.5	15.5	32.4	31.7			
10.5	23.6	16.0	33.2	32.6			
11.0	24.7	16.5	34.0	33.4			

From Altman PL, Dittner DS (eds): *Metabolism*, Bethesda, MD, 1968, Federation of American Societies for Experimental Biology.

estimated energy requirements (kcal/day) = resting energy expenditure × activity factor × stress factor

Activity Factors		Stress Factors			
Paralyzed	1.0	Surgery	1.2-1.2	Burn	1.5-2.5
Confined to bed	1.1	Infection	1.2-1.6	Starvation	0.70
Ambulatory	1.2-1.3	Trauma	1.1-1.8	Growth failure	1.5-2.0

From Nutrient requirements. In Page CP, Hardin TC, Melnik G (eds): *Nutritional assessment and support – a primer*, ed 2, Baltimore, 1994, Williams & Wilkins, p 32.

TABLE 27-6
Suggested Daily Amounts of Nutrients for Maintenance Pediatric Parenteral Nutrition Solutions

Nutrient	Infants/Toddlers	Children	Adolescents
Calories	80-130	60-90	30-75
Dextrose (g/kg)	10-30	8-28	5-20
Protein (g/kg)	1.5-3.0	1.0-2.5	0.8-2.0
Fat (g/kg)	0.5-4.0	1.0-3.0	1.0-3.0
Sodium (mEq/kg)	2-4	2-4	60-150 mEq/day
Potassium (mEq/kg)	2-4	2-4	70-180 mEq/day
Chloride (mEq/kg)	2-4	2-4	60-150 mEq/day
Magnesium (mEq/kg) (125 mg = 1 mEq)	0.25-1.0	0.25-1.0	8-32 mEq/day
Calcium (mEq/kg) (20 mg = 1 mEq)	0.45-4.0	0.45-3.15	10-40 mEq/day
Phosphorus (mmol/kg) (31 mg = 1 mmol)	0.5-2.0	0.5-2.0	9-30 mmol/day
Zinc (μg/kg)	50-250	50 up to 5 mg	5 mg/day
Copper (μg/kg)	20	20	300 μg/day
Chromium (μg/kg)	0.20	0.20	10-15 μg/day
Manganese (μg/kg)	1.0	1.0	10-15 μg/day
Selenium (μg/kg)	2.0	2.0	30-60 μg/day
Molybdenum (μg/kg)	0.25	0.25	20-120 μg/day
Iodide (μg/kg)	1.0	1.0	150 μg/day
Pediatric MVI*(ml/day)	3.3 (1-3 kg)	5.0 (3-39 kg)	Adult MVI (≥40 kg)
Iron (μg/kg)	100	1.0 mg/day	1-3 mg/day

Adapted from American Academy of Pediatrics, Committee on Nutrition: *Pediatric nutrition handbook*, ed 4, Elk Grove Village, IL, 1998, American Academy of Pediatrics, pp 290-299.
MVI, Multivitamin infusion.
*Contains vitamins A, D, E, B₁, B₂, B₆, B₁₂, C, K, folic acid, biotin, and dexapanthenol in amounts based on the current Food and Drug Administration recommendations for pediatric intravenous vitamins and from the AMA Nutrition Advisory Group.

BOX 27-5
Calculating Catch-Up Growth Requirements

UPPER LIMIT GOAL

$$\text{kcal/kg/day} = \frac{\text{RDA (kcal) for weight age} \times \text{ideal body weight for age}}{\text{actual weight}}$$

$$\text{protein/kg/day} = \frac{\text{*RDA (g) protein for weight age} \times \text{ideal body weight for age}}{\text{actual weight}}$$

LOWER LIMIT GOAL

$$\text{kcal/kg/day} = \frac{\text{RDA (kcal) for weight age} \times \text{ideal body weight for height}}{\text{actual weight}}$$

$$\text{protein/kg/day} = \frac{\text{RDA (g) protein for weight age} \times \text{ideal body weight for height}}{\text{actual weight}}$$

*Not to exceed 5-6 g protein/kg/day

RDA, Recommended daily allowance.

tolerance, cost, and convenience. Generally, formulas are grouped according to the patient's age: premature infants, term infants, children age 1 to 10 years, and children older than 10 years (see Table 15-2). Premature infant formulas are discussed in Chapter 26.

TABLE 27-7
Fluid Requirements in Infants and Children

Body Weight (kg)	Daily Baseline Fluid Requirement*
1-10	100 ml/kg
11-20	1000 ml + 50 ml/kg for each kg >10 kg
>20	1500 ml + 20 ml/kg for each kg >20 kg

From Fluid and electrolytes. In Johnson KB (ed): *The Harriet Lane handbook*, St. Louis, 1996, Mosby, pp 216-217.
* Increase by 12% for each degree by which body temperature >37.5°C.
Holiday-Segar Method: Estimates calorie expenditure from weight alone and assumes that for each 100 calories metabolized 100 ml of water is required. (This method is not appropriate for neonates <14 days or for conditions associated with abnormal losses.)

Term Infants

For term infants who have normal GI function, the feeding of choice for the first year of life is breast milk. Considered the "gold standard" nutrition for neonates, human milk has a unique combination of nutrients, enzymes, hormones, and immunologic components. When breast milk is the sole nutrient, supplementation is needed after age 6 months because the infant's need for iron exceeds the quantity available in breast milk. Human milk production can be divided into three stages: (1) colostrum (approximately the first 7 days postpartum), (2) transitional milk (approximately 7 days to 2 weeks postpartum), and (3) mature milk. The composition of breast milk is difficult to measure because many variables affect the tests: time of milk collection, stage of lactation, whether fore or hind milk is collected, and biologic variables among women (Table 27-8). As milk matures, the concentrations of total proteins, immunoglobulins, and fat-soluble vitamins decrease while those of lactose, fat, and water-soluble vitamins increase. These changes are thought to represent the changing nutritional needs of the growing infant. The feeding of breast milk is associated with decreased morbidity, respiratory infections, diarrhea, and otitis media.[37,38] It is common practice for breast milk to be used for tube feedings, and when it is used for continuous tube feedings, nutrient losses due to separation of the fat in breast milk and adherence to the tubing must be taken into account.[39,40] It is estimated that 20% of fat from breast milk adheres to the tubing, thus decreasing the number of calories delivered. When the tubing is flushed with water, the infant may receive a fat bolus. On the other hand, adherence of fat to tubing and potential delivery of fat boluses are not associated with intermittent breast milk tube feedings.[41,42] One method to combat the separation and rise of the human milk fat component within the syringe during continuous feedings is to tilt the pump at an angle of 25 to 40 degrees.[41]

Breast Milk Substitutes

The alternative to breast milk is commercially prepared infant formulas (Table 27-9), which are available in ready-to-feed, liquid concentrate, and powder forms. Powder formulas are generally the least expensive and ready-to-feed ones, the most expensive (e.g., Enfamil, Good Nature, Gerber, Good Start, Parent Choice, Similac). All infant formulas contain adequate iron with the exception of cow's milk–based formula labeled as

TABLE 27-8

Comparison of Human Breast Milk with Two Iron-Supplemented Commercial Infant Formulas

Nutrient	Content per Liter		
	Human milk	Enfamil	Similac
Calories	680	680	680
Protein (g)	10.5	15.2	14.5
% of total kcal	6	9	9
Source	Human milk	Reduced minerals and nonfat cow's milk	Nonfat cow's milk
Carbohydrate (g)	72	70	72.3
% of total kcal	42	41	43
Source	Lactose	Lactose	Lactose
Fat (g)	39	38	36.5
% of total kcal	52	50	48
Source	Human milk	Palm olein, soy, coconut, and sunflower oils	Soy and coconut oils
Polyunsaturated (g)	4.8	10.5	13
Saturated (g)	17.4	19.1	16
Monounsaturated (g)	14.9	5.4	6
Linoleic acid (mg)	3971	7500	8790
Cholesterol (mg)	133.2	<11	11
Minerals			
Calcium (mg)	280	470	493
Phosphorus (mg)	140	320	380
Magnesium (mg)	35	53	41
Iron (mg)	0.3	12.8	12
Zinc (mg)	1.2	5.3	5.1
Manganese (μg)	6	106	34
Copper (μg)	252	540	610
Iodine (μg)	110	69	94.6
Selenium (μg)	15	12	15
Chromium (μg)	50	4.8	
Molybdenum (μg)		12	
Fluoride (μg)	16	Varies	Varies
Sodium (mEq)	7.8	8	8
Potassium (mEq)	13.4	18.7	18.1
Chloride (mEq)	11.9	12.1	12.2
Vitamins			
A (IU)	2230	2100	2030
D (IU)	20	430	410
E (IU)	2.3 mg	21	20
K (μg)	2.1	58	54
Thiamine (μg)	210	530	680
Riboflavin (μg)	350	1060	1010
B_1 (μg)	205	430	410
B_2 (μg)	0.5	1.6	1.7
Niacin (μg)	1500	8500	7100
Folic acid (μg)	50	106	100
Pantothenic acid (μg)	1800	3200	3040
Biotin (μg)	4	15.6	30
Ascorbic acid (mg)	40	55	60
Choline (mg)	92	106	108
Inositol (mg)	149	32	32
Water (ml)	880	910	900
Renal solute load (mOsm/L)	75.1	100	96.3
Osmolality (mOsm/kg H_2O)	290	300	300

Adapted from *Composition of feedings for infants and young children in the hospital,* Columbus, Ohio, 1995, Ross Laboratories. Used with permission of Ross Products Division, Abbott Laboratories, Columbus, OH 43216. From Feeding for Infants and Children. © 1995 Ross Products Division, Abbott Laboratories.

TABLE 27-9

Daily Fluoride Supplementation*

Age	Fluoride Concentration in Local Water Supply, ppm		
	< 0.3	0.3-0.6	>0.6
6 mo to 3 yr	0.25 mg	0.00 mg	0.00 mg
3-6 yr	0.50 mg	0.25 mg	0.00 mg
6-16 yr	1.00 mg	0.50 mg	0.00 mg

Adapted from American Academy of Pediatrics: Nutrition and oral health. In Pediatric Nutrition handbook, ed 4, Elk Grove Village, IL, 1998, American Academy of Pediatrics, p 525.
* Must know fluoride concentration in patient's drinking water before prescribing fluoride supplements.

low-iron. Indications for a low-iron formula are virtually non-existent.[43] Infant formulas vary in protein, carbohydrate, fat, vitamin, and mineral content.

MINERALS. A new line of infant formula has been designed to support the needs of growing premature infants after discharge from the hospital (e.g., Enfamil 22 and NeoSure). It has higher caloric density (22 kcal per ounce instead of the standard 20) and contains more protein, vitamins, and minerals (especially calcium, phosphorus, and zinc) than standard term infant formulas. Fluoride is present neither in infant formula nor human milk. The fluoride content of primary drinking water should be known. Supplementation, if indicated, should begin at 6 months of age (see Table 27-9).

PROTEIN. Standard infant formula contains cow's milk protein, predominantly either whey or casein. Breast milk contains more whey than casein. Soy-based formula is made from soy protein isolates to which methionine is added to make the protein quality equivalent to that of casein. Soy formulas are used for infants with cow's milk protein intolerance, lactase deficiency, or galactosemia (e.g., Alsoy, Gerber Soy, Isomil, Prosobee). Approximately 20% to 50% of children who are allergic to cow's milk protein are also allergic to soy protein.[44] Hydrolyzed protein formula is therefore indicated (e.g., Alimentum, Elecare, Nutramigen, Pregestimil). Hydrolyzed protein infant formulas are not all hypoallergenic. To be labeled "hypoallergenic," formula (extensively hydrolyzed or free amino acid-based) must not provoke reactions in 90% of infants or children with confirmed cow's milk protein allergy (e.g., Elecare, Pediatric Vivonex, Neocate, Neocate One+).[45] Hydrolyzed protein formula can be fed to infants with protein intolerance, pancreatic insufficiency, or another disorder of digestion, absorption, or metabolism.

CARBOHYDRATE. The main carbohydrate source in breast milk and standard infant formulas is lactose. Soy protein and hydrolyzed protein formulas are lactose free but contain one or more of the following carbohydrate sources: corn syrup solids, sucrose, glucose polymers, and hydrolyzed corn starch. A cow's milk-based lactose-free formula is also available (e.g., Lactofree, Similac Lactose Free). New advancements include the addition of fructo-oligosaccharide added to formula for a prebiotic effect.

FAT. The ideal source(s) of fat for the sick or injured child is not known. It is known that medium-chain triglyceride (MCT) oil is important in the management of steatorrhea, chylothorax, chylous ascites, ileal resection, and intestinal lymphangiectasia. Infant formulas contain varying amounts of MCT oil (e.g., Lipisorb, Portagen, Pregestimil). Infants receiving formula containing 86% of its fat source as MCT oil must be closely monitored because essential fatty acid deficiency can develop with long-term use.[46,47] New fatty acids, docosahexaenoic acid and arachidonic acid, are currently being considered by the FDA to be added in the U.S. to infant formula. These fatty acids are found in breast milk but not in cow's milk.

Other specific metabolic formulas (more than 81 of them) are not discussed in detail here. All infant formulas are prepared to a standard of 20 calories per ounce. They contain vitamins and minerals in accordance with the recommendations of the American Academy of Pediatrics and the Infant Formula Act of 1980.[48,49] Daily vitamin and mineral needs are met by 25 to 32 oz of 20-kcal-per-ounce formula. The osmolality of standard formula ranges from 150 to 380 mOsm/kg. The American Academy of Pediatrics recommends that the osmolality of infant formula be less than 460 mOsm/kg.[48] Follow-up formulas are designed for toddlers who receive an inadequate quantity of solid foods (specifically protein and minerals).

Children Age 1 to 10 Years

A caloric density of 30 kcal per ounce (1.0 kcal/ml) is needed for this age group. Adult formulas are not appropriate for the child. They contain too much protein, sodium, potassium, chloride, and magnesium. Adult formulas do not provide sufficient iron, zinc, calcium, phosphorus, and vitamin D for the growing child.[50-52] Typically, standard pediatric formulas designed for children age 10 or younger are both lactose free and gluten free and supply 100% of the RDAs for vitamins and minerals in a volume of 950 to 1100 ml. Newer predigested formulas have recently been developed (Table 27-10) for children in this age group whose digestion and absorption are impaired. Blenderized feedings (commercially prepared or baby food mixed with milk or juice) are also used for children. Careful

TABLE 27-10

Selection of Pediatric Enteral Formulas (Excluding Formulas for Inborn Errors of Metabolism)

Clinical Condition	Formula Description	Examples
INFANCY		
Discharged premature infant	Breast milk or formula supplemented with additional calories, calcium, and phosphorus	Supplemented breast milk with modules, formula, human milk fortifier,* Similac Natural Care, or Similac NeoCare
Term infant	Breast milk; 60:40 whey-casein formulas with lactose	Breast milk, Good Nature, Enfamil with iron, Similac with iron, Good Start, Gerber, store brand
Primary or secondary lactose intolerance	Lactose-free cow's milk formula	Lactofree
Cow's milk protein sensitivity or lactose-intolerance galactosemia	Lactose-free soy protein isolate formula	Prosobee, Isomil, Isomil DF, Soyalac, I-Soyalac, Gerber Soy, Isomil SF, Store brand
Renal or cardiac disease	Low electrolyte/renal solute load formula	Similac PM 60:40, Enfamil with iron, or modular nutrients with infant formula to meet needs
Steatorrhea associated with bile acid deficiency, ileal resection, or lymphatic anomalies	Formula with medium-chain triglyceride (MCT) oil	Portagen, Pregestimil, Alimentum
Cow's milk protein and soy protein sensitivity, abnormal nutrient digestion, absorption, and transport; intractable diarrhea or protein-calorie malnutrition	Hydrolyzed casein, lactose, and sucrose formula	Nutramigen (normal absorption); Alimentum, Pregestimil,* Neocate,* Pediatric Vivonex *Hypoallergenic
AGE 1-10 YR		
Tube feeding or oral supplement	Complete nutrition in 950-1100 ml, 1.0 kcal/ml, gluten- and lactose-free, isotonic	Kindercal, Pediasure, Pediasure with Fiber, Nutren Junior, Nutren Junior with fiber
Compromised gastrointestinal or pancreatic function, cow's milk protein and soy protein sensitivity, intractable diarrhea or protein-calorie malnutrition	Predigested formula with free amino acids or small peptides and MCT oil	Vivonex Pediatric, Neocate One Plus, Peptamen Junior, EleCare
Steatorrhea or liver disease	Formula with major source of fat from MCT oil	Lipisorb
AGE OVER 10 YR		
	For children with handicaps or neurologic impairment: weight age should be >10 yr	Use adult formula
MODULAR NUTRIENTS		
Carbohydrate	Added to infant or pediatric formulas to increase calories	Moducal, Sumacal, Polycose, Product 80056, LC Corpak, PC Corpak, Pro-Phree
Protein	Added to infant or pediatric formulas to increase protein (calories)	Elementra, Alterna, Casec, Promod, Propac, Pro-Mix RDP
Fat	Added to infant or pediatric formulas to increase calories	Microlipid, Lipomul, MCT oil, high-MCT powder

MCT, Medium-chain triglyceride.
* These supplements are not available retail.

and regular monitoring of osmolality, viscosity, sanitation, and nutrient and fluid adequacy or excess is in order.[53]

Children Older Than 10 Years

Typically, adult formulas are used for this age group. The indications are the same as for adults (see Chapter 15). Often children who are small compared with their age continue on pediatric formulas for additional minerals suited for their body size.

Alterations of Infant Formula

The caloric density of standard infant formula is 20 kcal per ounce (0.67 kcal/ml), similar to that of breast milk. Infants who have higher than normal energy or nutrient requirements but may not be able to tolerate a large volume of formula or who require fluid restriction need "hypercaloric" formula. The caloric density can be increased in two ways: (1) adding less water to a powder or liquid concentrate form or (2) adding

single nutrients such as fat, carbohydrate, protein, or a combination to the existing formula (Boxes 27-6 and 27-7). Daily increases in caloric density are usually tolerated in 2 to 4 kcal per ounce increments. Increasing caloric density by concentrating formula ensures that nutrients are distributed properly. When single nutrients are added to formula, calorie and nutrient distribution should be calculated. The recommended macronutrient composition of an infant's diet calls for 35% to 65% of total calories from carbohydrate, 7% to 16% from protein, and 30% to 55% of total calories from fat.[54] Fat intake greater than 60% of total calories can induce ketosis, and protein intakes less than 6% of total calories can result in protein deficiency.[55] For example, if 10 carbohydrate calories per ounce is added to a limited volume of 20-kcal per ounce infant formula, the final formula may be deficient in protein, vitamins, and minerals. Azotemia and negative water balance can result from protein intake greater than 16% of total calories. Protein intake should not exceed 5 g/kg per day.

BOX 27-6

Increasing the Calorie Density of Infant Formula

USING FORMULA CONCENTRATION:

Advantages	Disadvantages
Provide adequate protein, vitamins, minerals in limited amounts	May exceed renal concentrating ability
Nutrients are properly balanced	Hypervitaminosis

USING NUTRIENT MODULES:

Advantages	Disadvantages
Provide additional energy as needed to promote growth	May exceed capacity of gut to absorb and utilize nutrient sources
	May fail to meet nutrient needs if formulated improperly

DECISION TREE

Will ready-to-feed formula meet all needs?
NO ✓
Are protein goals met?
↓
Determine concentration of selected formula needed to meet the protein goal with a given formula intake.
↓
Are energy goals met?
↓
NO ✓
Add modules to provide desired calorie concentration in a given volume. Calculate nutrient distribution.
↓
Are vitamin/mineral needs met?
NO ✓
Calculate doses of needed supplements.
↓
Are fluid needs met?
Standard 20 kcal/oz infant formula is ~ 90% free water
Standard 24 kcal/oz infant formula is ~ 88% free water
Standard 27 kcal/oz infant formula is ~ 87% free water
Standard 30 kcal/oz infant formula is ~ 84% free water

BOX 27-7

Example for Increasing the Calorie Density of Infant Formula

START
20 kcal/oz Standard infant formula (0.67 kcal/ml)

STEP 1
Add 4 kcal/oz. (0.13 kcal/ml) by formula concentration
(One 13 oz can of liquid infant formula concentrate plus 8 oz water)
24 kcal/oz (0.8 kcal/ml)

STEP 2
Add 4 kcal/oz. (0.13 kcal/ml) by carbohydrate
(3 tablespoons of powdered Polycose per 500 ml [16.6 oz.])
28 kcal/oz (0.93 kcal/ml)

STEP 3
Add 4 kcal/oz. (0.13 kcal/ml) of fat
(15 ml [1 tablespoon] Microlipid per 500 ml [16.6 oz.])
32 kcal/oz (1.06 kcal/ml)

STEP 4
Add 4 kcal/oz. (0.13 kcal/ml) by formula concentration
(One 13-oz can of liquid infant formula concentrate plus 5.5 oz water)

FINISH
36 kcal/oz (1.2 kcal/ml)

NUTRIENT GUIDELINES

Carbohydrate	35%-65% of total kcal
Protein	7%-16% of total kcal
Fat	30%-55% of total kcal

FINAL FORMULA

36 kcal/oz	(1.2 kcal/ml)
Base formula, 28 kcal/oz	(7% as protein)
Carbohydrate, 4 kcal/oz	(45% as carbohydrate)
Fat, 4 kcal/oz	(48% as fat)
Estimated renal solute load	135 mOsm/L
Estimated osmolality	498 mOsm/kg water
Estimated free water	80.5%

Infant formula can safely be concentrated to 30 kcal per ounce. Because concentrated infant formula contains less water, careful attention must be paid to available free water. When water intake is inadequate, the capacity of the kidneys to concentrate and excrete renal solute may be exceeded and the infant may become dehydrated. The renal solute load (RSL) of infant formula is estimated as follows:

$$RSL \text{ (mOsm)} = [\text{protein (g)} \times 4] + [\text{Na (mEq)} + \text{K (mEq)} + \text{Cl (mEq)}]$$

Previously, potential renal solute load (PRSL) was calculated only for low-birth-weight infants because of their potential immature renal development. The American Academy of Pediatrics now recommends that PRSL be used for all infant formulas. The PRSL of infant formula is estimated as follows:

$$PRSL \text{ (mOsm)} = (\text{protein (g)}/0.175) + [\text{Na (mEq)} + \text{K (mEq)} + \text{Cl (mEq)} + (\text{P (mg)})/31]$$

Carbohydrate and fat as single nutrient additives do not add to the renal solute load of formula. Infant formula rendered hypercaloric by the addition of single nutrients is beneficial for infants who require increased energy, such as in those with renal, hepatic, or metabolic disorders, whose fluid, protein, or electrolyte intake may be restricted (Table 27-11).

Specific Pediatric Parenteral Feedings

In general, the same carbohydrate and fat substrates are used in pediatric parenteral solutions as in adult solutions. Specialized pediatric amino acid solutions are available (Trophamine, McGaw Inc, Irvine, CA, and Aminosyn-PF, Abbott Laboratories, North Chicago, IL). These solutions contain higher concentrations of tyrosine and histidine than standard amino acid solutions, which are thought to be essential amino acids for infants, and added taurine, thought to be essential for neonates. Studies comparing Trophamine and Aminosyn-PF have shown similar weight gain, nitrogen balance, and nitrogen retention.[56] Trophamine has been associated with a lower incidence of cholestasis.[57] In one study, Trophamine showed improved nitrogen retention in critically ill children (median age 15 months).[57] Trophamine has also been found to be stable as a total nutrient admixture and to allow greater quantities of

calcium and phosphorus to be added in solution because of its lower pH.[58] Provision of adequate calcium and phosphorus is difficult in small-volume pediatric PN feedings, so patients are at risk for metabolic bone disease.[59]

Defining the optimal amino acid requirements of infants who are dependent on parenteral nutrition has yet to be determined. While it appears that ingested phenylalanine and methionine are converted to tyrosine and cysteine, respectively, this conversion does not occur in parenterally administered phenylalanine and methionine.[60] Some amino acids are either not stable (cysteine and glutamine) or insoluble (tyrosine) in parenteral solution. Although soluble dipeptides have been shown to be safe in adults, pediatric safety data are lacking. Data on amino acid requirements in growth versus response to stress are also deficient.

It has also been suggested that preterm and term infants lack sufficient hepatic cystathionase to convert methionine to cysteine.[61] Cysteine hydrochloride is available as an additive to parenteral nutrition solutions. The addition of cysteine will increase calcium and phosphorus solubility by lowering the pH of the final solution. This can be beneficial in pediatric patients who have higher calcium and phosphorus needs or fluid restrictions (i.e., metabolic bone disease, post–bone marrow transplant, cardiac conditions). However, because of the lowered pH, adjustments may need to be made to the solution to avoid metabolic acidosis and zinc loss.[62,63]

Twenty percent fat emulsion or higher is preferred over 10% because it has a lower phospholipid to triglyceride ratio. Phospholipid is thought to inhibit lipoprotein lipase, an enzyme needed for intravenous lipid clearance. Other countries are starting to use modified parenteral fat preparations in pediatrics. Typically, long-chain triglycerides (LCTs) are used in parenteral fat products. Recently, structured lipids such as MCTs have been combined with LCT to show an improved nitrogen balance in postsurgical patients.[64] The potential advantage of use in pediatrics would be for conditions in which endogenous lipoprotein lipase levels are low, as in patients with sepsis or trauma. Further studies are needed to evaluate the use of structured lipids in pediatrics. Eicosapentaenoic acid (EPA) and docosahexaenoic acid (DHA) are essential for brain development but are not available in soybean-based intravenous fat products.

Routes and Administration of Nutrition Support

Enteral

Delivery routes for enteral nutrition support include nasogastric, orogastric, nasoduodenal, nasojejunal, gastrostomy (surgical and percutaneous endoscopic gastrostomy [PEG]), and jejunostomy feedings (GJ tube, surgical placement, or needle catheter). Indications, advantages, and disadvantages are discussed in Chapter 14. Specific to infants and children, soft, small-bore tubes should be used with nasal feedings (No. 5, 6, and 8 French). Transpyloric feedings are recommended for children with gastroesophageal reflux, delayed gastric emptying, or critical illness, or with respiratory compromise that places them at risk for aspiration.[65]

Newer PEGs allow feeding immediately after placement. Enteral feeds are generally started with full-strength isotonic formula. Feedings can be started and advanced as continuous

TABLE 27-11

Powdered Infant Formula Information

Formula	Weight (g) per Scoop	Calories per Scoop	Displacement Volume (ml) per Scoop
EnfaCare*	9.80	48.5	6.10
Enfamil w/Fe*	8.50	44.0	6.10
Enfamil AR*	8.70	44.0	6.10
Nutramigen*	9.08	44.0	6.30
Pregestimil*	8.80	44.0	6.10
Prosobee*	8.80	44.0	6.10
Isomil†	8.70	44.6	6.20
Similac Neosure†	9.6	49.4	7.40
Similac w/Fe†	8.50	44.4	6.20
Neocate‡	4.75	20.0	3.75

* Mead Johnson Nutritionals, Evanston, IL.
† Ross Products Division of Abbott Laboratories, Columbus, OH.
‡ Scientific Hospital Supplies Inc., Gaithersburg, MD.

24-hour, bolus or intermittent, continuous cyclic, or a combination of any of the methods previously mentioned (Table 27-12). Generally, slow, continuous enteral infusions are tolerated well as initial feedings than bolus feedings. Continuous feedings have been associated with superior nutrient absorption and less aspiration than bolus feedings.[66-68] Because of cost, lack of third-party payment, and need for increased mobility, feedings are often intermittent. To prevent diarrhea and cramping (dumping syndrome), infusion of intermittent feeds should not exceed more than 30 ml per minute.[69] Cycled tube feedings are widely used for pediatric enteral support. They offer infusion of a larger volume overnight than intermittent feeding and allow "time off" during the day for the child to attend school, develop an appetite to eat by mouth, or practice oral-motor feeding exercises to learn to eat. It is not uncommon for a child's first meal or sign of hunger to appear 4 to 8 hours after the cyclic tube feeding is discontinued. Cyclic continuous infusion is also clinically beneficial in preventing hypoglycemia in children with glycogen storage disease.

Parenteral

Parenteral nutrition solutions can be administered via standard peripheral intravenous catheters where the osmolarity of the solution should not exceed 900 mOsm/L.[70] For solutions with higher osmolarity, central access is needed. Broviac or Hickman right atrial catheters are placed for long-term access in the subclavian or internal jugular vein and advanced toward the right atrium. Specific catheters (percutaneous inserted central catheter [PICC] lines) can be introduced distally and percutaneously into the subclavian vein.

Assessment and correction of metabolic abnormalities should be done before initiating parenteral nutrition. Usually, infants can be started at dextrose 7 to 8 mg/kg per minute, 50% of protein needs, and lipid 0.5 to 1.0 g/kg. Parenteral nutrition longer than 4 weeks should provide intravenous lipid at the rate of 0.5 to 1.0 g/kg per day (3% to 5% of total calories), to prevent essential fatty acid deficiency.[71] Depending on the clinical status, children usually tolerate incremental daily dextrose advances of 2 to 3 mg/kg per minute (5% dextrose per day) and

of lipid 0.5 to 1.0 g/kg. Solution goals include dextrose 30 g/kg per day (11 to 21 mg/kg per minute per day), protein 3.0 g/kg per day, and lipid 2.5 to 3.0 g/kg per day (see Table 27-8). Higher glucose loads (>26 mg/kg per minute) should be avoided because they may contribute to the fatty infiltration of the liver.[72] Final macronutrient distribution goals are the same as those for enteral feedings. Long-term PN (longer than 4 weeks) requires the addition of selenium and molybdenum to the trace elements.

Cyclic PN is also indicated for long-term PN as a method of simplifying PN management and minimizing adverse effects such as liver complications.[73-74] Cycling generally involves a gradual increase in the infusion rate during the night and a decrease in the amount of time the patient is off parenteral nutrition during the day. Before initiation of cyclic PN, the infant or child must have (1) stable electrolytes and metabolic status, (2) at least 2 to 4 days of documented weight gain on continuous PN, and (3) a well-positioned central venous catheter.[75] Cycling of pediatric PN should be done slowly over 3 to 7 days. The following calculation illustrates cyclic rates.

1. $$\frac{\text{Total volume}}{\text{Total infusion hours} - 1} = \frac{\text{(X) infusion rate for second hour}}{\text{through the hour before the last hour}}$$

2. $$\frac{\text{Total volume} - [(\text{X})(\text{total hours} - 2)]}{2} = \text{rate for first and last hour}$$

Example: To determine cycling rate for 850 ml cycled over 20 hours:

1. $$\frac{850 \text{ ml}}{20 \text{ hours} - 1} = 45 \text{ ml/hr for second through the 19th hour}$$

2. $$\frac{850 \text{ ml} - (45 \times 18)}{2} = 20 \text{ ml/hr for the first and 20th hour}$$

Rates should be judiciously tapered to the maximum infusion rate and down until discontinuation to prevent complications from hyperglycemia or rebound hypoglycemia. Urine and blood glucose should be monitored daily while cycling PN.

TABLE 27-12

Suggestions for Initiation and Advancement of Continuous, Bolus, and Cyclic Tube Feedings

Age	Initial Infusion	Advances	Goal
CONTINUOUS FEEDINGS			
<12 mo	1-2 ml/kg/hr	1-2 ml/kg every 2-8 hr	6 ml/kg/hr
1-6 yr	1 ml/kg/hr	1 ml/kg every 2-8 hr	4-5 ml/kg/hr
>6 yr	25 ml/hr	25 ml/hr every 2-8 hr	100-150 ml/hr
BOLUS FEEDINGS			
<12 mo	10-60 ml/2-3 hr	10-60 ml/feeding	90-180 ml/4-5 hr
1-6 yr	30-90 ml/2-3 hr	30-90 ml/feeding	150-300 ml/4-5 hr
>6 yr	60-120 ml/2-3 hr	60-90 ml/feeding	240-480 ml/4-5 hr
CYCLIC FEEDINGS			
<12 mo	1-2 ml/kg/hr	1-2 ml/kg/2 hr	60-90 ml/hr 12-18 hr/days
1-6 yr	1 ml/kg/hr	1 ml/kg/hr/2 hr	75-125 ml/hr 8-16 hr/days
>6 yr	25 ml/hr	25 ml/hr/2 hr	100-175 ml/hr 8-16 hr/days

Abnormal glucose tolerance with cycled PN may not be from a high dextrose infusion over a condensed amount of time but a decreased capacity to release insulin.[76]

Transitional and Dual Feeding

The transition from parenteral to enteral feedings requires consideration of individual requirements. Small volume feedings are gradually advanced (see Table 27-12). As enteral feedings reach 50% of goal nutrient requirements, parenteral nutrition may begin to be decreased (often 1 ml increase for 1 ml decrease). When enteral feedings are providing 75% of goal requirements and absorption is adequate, parenteral nutrition can be discontinued. Total fluid intake should be monitored during the transition period for overhydration with overlapping fluid administration.

During the transition from pediatric parenteral feedings to oral feedings, the methodical approach is often abandoned. Commonly, the goal is successfully achieved when the infant or child takes any food or beverage of preference by mouth. Therefore, combination feeding is commonplace in pediatrics.

Before a child begins the transition from enteral feedings to oral feedings, the following measures are in order: (1) reevaluation of the original reason for enteral feedings—the child may not be ready if there has been no change in the medical condition; (2) evaluation of the quality of oral motor skills, swallowing capability, and feeding safety; and (3) evaluation of the parents' readiness, support, and attitudes toward oral feeding.[77] Enteral feedings, whether they are continuous, bolus, or cyclic, may be discontinued in many ways. Spacing feeding allows time for the child to develop an appetite and for caregivers to organize regular meal and snack times. Simultaneously, decreasing parenteral caloric intake by 25% (every week to every month) is often successful. Food diaries (for calories and fluid) are helpful to evaluate appropriateness of timing of tube feeding decrements.

Complications and Monitoring

Infectious Complications

Catheter-related sepsis is a major complication of PN. Fever alone is not an indication for removing the central line. Other sources of infection should be investigated. Signs of sepsis in the neonate include lethargy, hyperbilirubinemia, temperature instability, and intolerance to parenteral substrates (hyperglycemia, hypertriglyceridemia) of previously tolerated solutions.[75] Infections from enteral feeds are usually secondary to contaminated improperly handled formula or aspiration pneumonia. Contamination is more common in altered formulas (i.e., those that contain modular additives).[53] Nonsterile (breast milk and blenderized) feedings should not be left at room temperature for infusions of more than 4 hours' duration.

Mechanical Complications

Malposition of a central line can be signaled by a rapid drop in serum glucose level or sudden onset of circulatory or respiratory compromise. Pneumothorax and brachial plexus injury are common complications of percutaneous subclavian line insertion in infants and children. Thrombophlebitis can occur in peripheral veins infused with hypertonic solutions or solutions rich in calcium.[73] Catheter occlusion caused by lipid material from PN has been successfully cleared with ethanol after urokinase has failed to clear these occlusions. Mechanical complications of enteral feedings in children are similar to those adults experience (see Chapter 17). Problems specific to pediatrics include nasopharyngeal erosions, otitis media, sinusitis, esophagitis, and gastric irritation associated with the use of large-diameter tubes. These problems can be prevented by careful tube positioning (sometimes under fluoroscopy); small-bore, soft feeding tubes; and expert tube placement.[33] Another common problem is tube occlusion. The tube should be irrigated after each feeding, or every 8 hours when feedings are administered by continuous infusion.[33] Risk of tube occlusion is lessened when liquid forms of all medications and nutrients are administered through the tube followed by a water flush. Cranberry juice, water, carbonated beverages, pancreatic enzymes, and papain are often used to declog feeding tubes.[78-80] Caution should be exercised with pediatric patients because papain (meat tenderizer) can alter GI pH and function, and cranberry juice can have a hyperosmotic effect on GI tolerance.

Gastrointestinal Complications

Because parenteral nutrition bypasses the GI tract altogether, it poses its own set of problems such as gut atrophy and possible bacterial translocation from breakdown of the gut's barrier function.[25] Liver disease is the major GI complication associated with PN. On histologic examination of the liver, cholestasis, hepatocellular necrosis, and cirrhosis may be found.[81] Elevated liver function tests can occur after 2 weeks of PN. The treatment for PN-associated cholestasis includes (1) discontinuation of therapy, if possible; (2) if that is not possible, cyclic PN and low-dose enteral feedings; (3) decreasing total calories, protein (to maintenance amounts) and lipid (to provide no more than 50% of total calories).[82] GI complications of enteral feeding include nausea, vomiting, diarrhea, and constipation. Vomiting can result from improper tube placement, medications, too rapid infusion of formula or hyperosmolality, and decreased GI motility. Vomiting or reflux can be treated with proper positioning, administration of prokinetic medications, and decreasing the rate of infusion. Constipation can be relieved by increasing fiber, fluids, and activity, and occasionally by adding stool softeners. When diarrhea is present, infections and hyperosmotic medications and formulas should be considered first. Formulas that contain fiber may help. For short-gut syndrome, pectin or medications that slow GI motility or bind bile salts may be beneficial.

Metabolic and Nutritional Complications

The most common metabolic complications are overhydration and underhydration. Overhydration occurs during the transition from PN to enteral feeding and when volume from other fluid sources (intravenous lines or water flushes) are not carefully monitored. Dehydration can occur when prolonged hyperglycemia is not addressed, when inadequate fluids are provided enterally or parenterally, or when fluid requirements are increased or the renal solute load is increased. Other complications include hypoglycemia; electrolyte imbalances (refeeding syndrome); inadequate weight gain; and deficiencies of vitamins, minerals, and trace elements. Hypoglycemia can occur on abrupt cessation of PN or tube feeding. Infants on cyclic feedings may be at risk for hypoglycemia when nutrition support is interrupted for more than 6 to 8 hours. Children with severe malnutrition should have daily electrolyte and mineral monitoring to watch for refeeding syndrome. This term is used to describe metabolic disturbances that occur when malnourished patients are rapidly refed. Often, intravenous supplementation of potassium, 2 to 4 mEq/kg per day, and of phosphorus, 0.2 to 0.5 mmol/kg over 6 hours (or 1 to 2 mmol/kg per day), is required to treat severe hypophosphatemia and hypokalemia from refeeding syndrome. Whenever intravenous phosphorus is given, serum (or ionized) calcium levels should be monitored. Zinc deficiency may develop in children with prolonged diarrhea or excessive ostomy drainage. When a patient being fed appropriate calories and protein stops gaining weight, zinc status should be evaluated. Other trace element and mineral deficiencies can result in growth failure.[83]

Propofol is a lipid-based sedative that provides 1.1 kcal/ml. It is being used routinely in critical care units because it has rapid onset and quick recovery. Infusion of propofol or any other lipid-based drug must be closely monitored when given with enteral or parenteral nutrition to avoid the pitfalls of overfeeding and hypertriglyceridemia.[84] Cyclosporine has also been associated with elevated serum cholesterol and triglycerides in patients undergoing bone marrow or renal transplantation. Carnitine is needed for optimal oxidation of fatty acids. PN currently used contains no carnitine but does contain precursors for endogenous production. Unfortunately, infants and children on PN have decreased plasma and tissue carnitine levels. Carnitine may be supplemented at 10 mg/kg per day after 2 to 4 weeks of PN, using either oral or intravenous L-carnitine. Carnitine deficiency may be associated with abnormal oxidation of long-chain fatty acids and progressive hepatic dysfunction.

Cholestasis can be seen in infants on PN for more than 2 weeks. The earliest abnormality noted is an elevated serum γ-glutamyltransferase (GGT) or bile acid level. Hepatomegaly with mild elevation of serum transaminases in the absence of cholestasis may result from hepatic accumulation of lipid or glycogen due to either excess carbohydrate calories or an imbalanced nonnitrogen calorie to nitrogen ratio. Fatty infiltration of the liver can be a result of excessive caloric intake and is readily reversible by decreasing the total caloric infusion. Abnormal liver function tests are common to long-term PN patients. Children with chronic intestinal conditions that are complicated by infection and bacterial overgrowth are susceptible to hepatic complications. In most children, elevated liver enzymes improve with the initiation of partial enteral nutrition. Only a small percentage of children go on to develop chronic liver disease with poor growth, cirrhosis, and hepatic failure.

Monitoring

Proper management of pediatric nutrition support entails routine and careful monitoring of growth parameters; energy; macronutrient and micronutrient provisions (with routine adjustments to promote growth); and metabolic, mechanical, and GI parameters (Table 27-13). Frequent monitoring helps avoid complications of nutrition support. Other important parameters to monitor are input and output, temperature, vital signs, stool frequency and consistency, evidence of edema,

and gastric residuals. Baseline collection of monitoring parameters is essential to determine tolerance and adequacy of therapy and individual substrates. In long-term (> 4 weeks) PN without enteral feeding, carnitine, choline, and aluminum should be monitored. Choline deficiency is thought to be associated with hepatic dysfunction.[85] Current PN solutions are contaminated with aluminum and can accumulate in bone after 3 weeks of PN in infants. Accumulation of aluminum can result in metabolic bone disease, encephalopathy, and may induce cholestasis.[86] Toxic effects are directly proportional to tissue aluminum load. Intravenous calcium, phosphorus, and albumin solutions have high aluminum levels (>500 μg/L). Crystalline amino acids, sterile water, and dextrose have low levels (< 50 μg/L). Aluminum intake safety limit is 2.0 μg/kg per day (Table 27-14). Manganese deposition can result from long-term PN, especially in the basal ganglia.[87]

Home Pediatric Nutrition Support

Long-term parenteral nutrition at home is now commonplace for GI failure. To date, there are no published cost-utility appraisals of home parenteral nutrition in pediatrics. Children who are considered for home nutrition support should be

TABLE 27-13
Monitoring Guidelines for Pediatric Nutrition Support

Parameter	Monitoring Interval	
	Initially	*Later/At home*
GROWTH		
Weight	Daily	Weekly to monthly
Height/length	Weekly	Monthly
Head circumference	Weekly	Monthly
Body composition	Monthly	As indicated
LABORATORY*		
Electrolytes	Daily to weekly	Weekly to monthly
BUN/creatinine	Weekly	Monthly
Acid-base status	Until stable	Monthly
Minerals	2x/wk	Weekly to monthly
Albumin/prealbumin	Weekly	Weekly to monthly
Glucose	Daily	Weekly to monthly
Triglycerides	4 hrs after dose increase	As indicated
CBC w/differential	Weekly	Weekly to monthly
Iron (total)/ferritin	As indicated	As indicated
Trace elements	Monthly	2x/yr
Platelet count	Weekly	As indicated
Liver function tests	Weekly	Weekly to monthly
Folate/vitamin B12	As indicated	As indicated
Fat-soluble vitamins	As indicated	1-2x/yr
Carnitine	As indicated	1-2x/yr
Blood cultures	As indicated	As indicated
URINALYSIS		
Glucose	Daily	Weekly to monthly
CLINICAL OBSERVATIONS		
Activity, temperature, etc.	Daily	Daily

Adapted from American Academy of Pediatrics. Parenteral nutrition. In *Pediatric nutrition handbook*, ed 4, Elk Grove Village, IL, 1998, American Academy of Pediatrics, p. 289.
*For metabolically unstable patients, values need to be checked more frequently.

TABLE 27-14

Average Aluminum Content of Parenteral Nutrition Products

Product	Average Aluminum Content (mcg/L)
Pediatric trace elements	130-3000
Potassium phosphate	9800
Sodium phosphate	13,000
10% calcium gluconate	4400
6.5% amino acids	120
12.5% amino acids	121
20% lipid emulsion	20-180
Water-soluble vitamins	12
Fat-soluble vitamins	360

Adapted from Popinska K, Kierkus J, Lyszkowska M, et al: Aluminum contamination of parenteral nutrition additives, amino acid solutions, and lipid emulsions, *Nutrition* 15: 683-686, 1999.

carefully evaluated and monitored by multidisciplinary pediatric nutrition support professionals.[33] The home nutrition support program should be tailored to meet family and individual lifestyle needs of the household (see Chapter 23). For home pediatric PN patients, it is important to evaluate the number and quantity of trace elements provided in available trace element packages, because home care company–dosing protocols vary. Selecting a home care company should include seeking out specialty trained health care professionals sensitive to the needs and special conditions of children and the pediatric products and supplies availability. Developmental needs should continue to be addressed and served by pediatric occupational therapists, physical therapists, speech therapists, and psychologists. Families must learn to master technical skills before discharge on home PN. Such skills include (1) using aseptic technique, (2) adding medications to the PN solution, (3) administering PN through the central venous line, (4) operating the infusion pump, (5) heparin-locking the line, and (6) performing dressing changes.

Periods of pediatric multivitamin product shortages have occurred. Because MVI-Pediatric is reserved for hospitalized low-birth-weight infants, an equivalent dose of MVI-12 up to a maximum dose of 5 ml/day should be used for home patients. MVI-12 contains no vitamin K. Term infants and children should be supplemented with 200 µg/day of vitamin K, which can be given as a weekly dose. Supplementation of vitamin D should also be considered in order to provide 160 IU/kg of body weight up to 400 IU vitamin D per day. The shortage of MVI-Pediatric has resulted in clinical deficiency states, especially of thiamine. Periodic updates on guidelines to administer multivitamins in pediatrics during a shortage are supplied by the American Society for Parenteral and Enteral Nutrition (ASPEN) (http://www.clinnutr.org).

Special Conditions

The goals of nutrition support are to sustain normal growth and development, promote catch-up growth in malnourished children, and improve the clinical outcome when possible. ASPEN provides clinical guidelines for several clinical conditions. Data are lacking on specialized nutrition support for pediatric pancreatitis and perioperative care.[88]

Practice Guidelines

CANCER AND BONE MARROW TRANSPLANTATION

1. Nutrition support and oral dietary interventions should be instituted to ensure adequate growth, development, and nutrient requirements to those infants and children who cannot meet their needs orally.[89-92]
2. Nutrition support is not indicated for children with advanced cancer who are debilitated and unresponsive to therapy.[93]

CHRONIC RENAL FAILURE

1. Children with acute renal failure receiving continuous renal replacement therapies should be provided with nutrition support to promote positive nitrogen balance and growth and meet their energy needs.[94]
2. With polyuric, salt-wasting renal disease, children should be supplemented with fluid and sodium.[95]

INBORN ERRORS OF METABOLISM

1. Aggressive medical management and nutrition support during times of catabolic stress are indicated to prevent metabolic decompensation, severe neurologic complications, and death.

LIVER DISEASE

1. Preoperative and postoperative nutrition support is frequently indicated for children with end-stage chronic liver disease undergoing liver transplantation.
2. MCTs should be given to promote growth.
3. Children with chronic cholestatic liver disease require vitamin A, D, E, and K supplementation and monitoring.

CYSTIC FIBROSIS

1. When a weight-for-height index is less than 90%, enteral support is indicated.
2. Infants and children with cystic fibrosis (CF) and exocrine pancreatic insufficiency require pancreatic enzyme replacement therapy and a water-miscible multivitamin specifically designed for CF.
3. A formula whose fat source is in large part MCT oil is beneficial for decreasing the quantity of enzyme dosing, which can cause a feeling of fullness. For cycled continuous overnight tube feedings, we administer 75% of the calculated enzyme dose at the beginning of the feeding and the remaining 25% at the end. Pancreatic enzyme replacement is impractical, and compliance is poor, when enzyme administration is recommended at the midpoint of the tube feeding infusion (i.e., in the middle of the night). For bolus feedings, the calculated enzyme dose is given just before the administration of each bolus feeding. Whenever possible, use of enteric-coated microspheres is recommended. Enzymes should not be added to the formula because the microsphere coating dissolves when pH is above 5.75. Powdered forms of pancreatic enzymes are not very efficacious and are inactivated by pH below 4.0. When using small diameter tubes (No. 5 or 6 French are used), the microspheres do not pass through the tubes. If the infant can swallow, the microspheres should be given by mouth in strained baby fruit. If an infant is intubated or otherwise unable to swallow, powdered pancreatic enzymes are used. They should not be added directly to the formula. High-protein foods inactivate the enzyme. When using powdered enzyme it is prudent to also administer H_2 receptor antagonist with gastric feeds because the lipase is inactivated in a pH below 4.0. A

high-carbohydrate elemental formula should be fed with caution because the incidence of cystic fibrosis related–diabetes (CFRD) is rising.

4. Serum fat-soluble vitamins A, D, E, and K levels should be monitored annually.

INFLAMMATORY BOWEL DISEASE

1. Enteral nutrition should be given to children with growth retardation.
2. Enteral nutrition should be used as an adjunct to medical therapy in children with Crohn's disease who are unable to maintain their nutritional status with oral intake.[96]
3. PN support is indicated for children with Crohn's disease who have bowel obstruction.

CRITICAL CARE

1. Transpyloric feedings should be used to minimize the risk of gastroesophageal reflux and aspiration.
2. Elevated liver function values are common in critically ill persons receiving PN, and they usually return to normal after enteral nutrition is resumed. PN solutions should not be used to replace GI losses.
3. To avoid overfeeding, use indirect calorimetry to measure energy expenditure. If it is not feasible or available, energy calculation should be based on published calculations or nomograms.[97]

NEUROLOGIC IMPAIRMENT

1. Nutrient requirements for children with developmental disabilities are extremely variable and should be customized to their level of disability and current nutritional deficits.

DIABETES

1. Blood glucose levels should be maintained between 100 and 200 mg/dl in the hospital setting.
2. When PN is indicated, intravenous insulin may be started with 0.1 U of Regular human insulin for each gram of dextrose in the PN solution.

CHRONIC INTRACTABLE DIARRHEA

1. Continuous enteral nutrition support should be attempted first because enteral nutrients are the major stimulus for mucosal repair.

SHORT BOWEL SYNDROME

1. Infants and children with short bowel syndrome (SBS) are at nutritional risk. PN should be started soon after surgery.
2. Continuous enteral feedings should be initiated as soon as possible.

PSEUDO-OBSTRUCTION

1. Continuous enteral nutrition with access placed above the isolated dysmotile segment should be considered.[98]

Conclusion

Nutrition support for infants and children is a challenge and an opportunity. The test is to meet the requirements for growth and for alterations in metabolism secondary to illness. The prospect of providing adequate and appropriate nutrition support for children in the hospital and home has permitted the survival, growth, and development of many infants and children who would have otherwise not survived. Decisions about pediatric nutrition support are complex and change constantly. As technology continues to advance, each child (and family) needs to be individually considered. Future directions look toward further infant formula advances to mimic human milk and to prevent PN-induced cholestasis. Imitation of human milk involves more than replication of its composition. Developmental, medical, and intellectual outcomes are now being studied to look at growth quality, incidence of infection, and sleep patterns, to name a few.[99]

REFERENCES

1. Widdowson EM: Growth and body composition in childhood. In Brunser O, Carrazza FR, Gracey M (eds): *Clinical nutrition of the young child,* New York, 1991, Raven, pp 1-14.
2. Lozoff B, Jimenez E, Wolf AW: Long term developmental outcomes of infants with iron deficiency, *N Engl J Med* 325:687-694, 1991.
3. Walter T, DeAndraca I, Chadud P, Perales CG: Iron deficiency anemia: adverse effects on psychomotor development, *Pediatrics* 84:7-17, 1989.
4. Georgieff MK, Hoffman JS, Pereira GR, Bernbaum J, Hoffman-Williamson M: Effect of neonatal caloric deprivation on head growth and 1-year developmental status in preterm infants, *J Pediatr* 107:581-587, 1985.
5. Measel CP, Anderson GC: Non-nutritive sucking during tube feedings: effect on clinical course in premature infants, *J Obstet Gynecol Nurs* 8:265-272, 1979.
6. Illingwith RS, Lister J: The critical or sensitive period with special reference to certain feeding problems in infants and children, *J Pediatr* 65(6):839-848, 1964.
7. Blackman JA, Nelson CLA: Rapid introduction of oral feeding to tube fed patients, *J Dev Behav Pediatr* 8:63-67, 1987.
8. Bayzyk S: Factors associated with transition to oral feedings in infants fed by nasogastric tubes, *Am J Occup Ther* 44(2):1070-1078, 1990.
9. Manikam R, Perman JA: Pediatric feeding disorders, *J Clin Gastroenterol* 30:34-46, 2000.
10. American Society for Parenteral and Enteral Nutrition: Standards for nutrition support: hospitalized pediatric patients, *Nutr Clin Pract* 4:33-37, 1989.
11. Merritt RJ, Suskind RM: Nutritional survey of hospitalized pediatric patients, *Am J Clin Nutr* 32:1320, 1979.
12. Parsons HG, Francoeur TE, Howland P, et al: The nutritional status of hospitalized children, *Am J Clin Nutr* 33:1140-1146, 1980.
13. Sermet-Gaudelus I, Piosson-Salomon AS, Colomb V, et al: Simple pediatric nutritional risk score to identify children at risk of malnutrition, *Am J Clin Nutr* 72:64-70, 2000.
14. Suskind RM, Varna RN: Assessment of nutritional status of children, *Pediatr Rev* 5(7):195-202, 1984.
15. Queen PM, Boatright SL, McNamara MM, Henry RR: Nutritional assessment of pediatric patients, *Nutr Support Serv* 3(5):23-34, 1983.
16. Brandt I: Growth dynamics of low birth weight infants with emphasis on the perinatal period. In Falkner F, Tanner JM (eds): *Human growth,* vol II, *Postnatal growth,* New York, 1978, Plenum.
17. WHO Working Group. Use and interpretation of anthropometric indicators of nutritional status, *Bull World Health Organ* 64:924-941, 1986.
18. Krick J: Using the Z score as a descriptor of discrete changes in growth, *Nutr Support Serv* 6:14-21, 1986.
19. Waterlow JC: Classification and definition of protein-energy malnutrition. In Beaton GH, Bengoa JM (eds): *Nutrition in preventive medicine: the major deficiency syndromes, epidemiology and approaches to control,* (62): 530-55, Geneva, 1976, WHO.
20. Gomez F, Galvan RR, Frenk S: Mortality in second- and third-degree malnutrition, *J Trop Pediatr* 2:77, 1956.
21. Rosner B, Prineas R, Loggie J, Daniels SR: Percentiles for body mass index in U.S. children 5 to 17 years of age, *J Pediatr* 132:211-222, 1998.
22. Perlman JM, Moore V, Siegel MJ, Dawson J: Is chloride depletion an important contributing factor of death in infants with bronchopulmonary dysplasia? *Pediatrics* 77:212-216, 1986.
23. Hambidge KM: Zinc deficiency in the weanling—how important? *Acta Paediatr Scand* 223(suppl):52-58, 1986.
24. Walravens PA, Hambidge KM, Koepfer DM: Zinc supplementation in infants with a nutritional pattern of failure to thrive: a double-blind, controlled study, *Pediatrics* 83:532-538, 1989.
25. Seidman EG: Gastrointestinal benefits of enteral feeds. In Baker SS, Baker RD, Davis A (eds): *Pediatric enteral nutrition,* New York, 1994, Chapman and Hall, pp 46-67.

26. Claris-Appiani A, Ardissino GL, Dacco V, et al: Catch-up growth in children with chronic renal failure treated with long-term enteral nutrition, *J Parenter Enteral Nutr* 19(3):175-178, 1995.

27. Shepard RW, Ho HTL, Thomas BJ, et al: Effects of long-term nutritional rehabilitation in cystic fibrosis: controlled studies of effects in nutritional growth retardation, body protein turnover, and course of pulmonary disease, *J Pediatr* 109:788-794, 1986.

28. Schwarz SM, Gewitz MH, See CC, et al: Enteral nutrition in infants with congenital heart disease and growth failure, *Pediatrics* 86:368-373, 1990.

29. Kurzner SI, Garg M, Baustita D, et al: Growth failure in bronchopulmonary dysplasia: elevated metabolic rates and pulmonary mechanics, *J Pediatr* 112:73-80, 1988.

30. Berseth CL: Effect of early feeding on the maturation of the preterm infant's small intestine, *J Pediatr* 120:947-953, 1992.

31. Slagle TA, Gross SJ: Effect of early low-volume enteral substrate on subsequent feeding tolerance in very low birth weight infants, *J Pediatr* 113:526-531, 1988.

32. American Society for Parenteral and Enteral Nutrition: Use of parenteral nutrition in the hospitalized adult patient, *J Parenter Enteral Nutr* 10:441-445, 1986.

33. American Society for Parenteral and Enteral Nutrition: Rationale for pediatric nutrition support guidelines. In Guidelines for the use of parenteral and enteral nutrition in adult and pediatric patients, *J Parenter Enteral Nutr* 17(suppl 4):27SA, 1993.

34. Thomson MA, Bucol S, Quirk P, Sheperd RW: Measured versus predicted resting energy expenditure in infants: a need for reappraisal, *J Pediatr* 126:21-27, 1995.

35. Peterson KE, Washington J, Rathburn JM: Team management of failure to thrive, *J Am Diet Assoc* 84:810-815, 1984.

36. Fjeld CR, Schoeller DA, Brown KH: Body composition of children recovering from severe protein-energy malnutrition at two rates of catch-up growth, *Am J Clin Nutr* 50:1266-1275, 1989.

37. Cunningham AS: Morbidity in breast-fed and artificially fed infants, *J Pediatr* 95:685, 1979.

38. Saarinen UM: Prolonged breast feeding as prophylaxis for recurrent otitis media, *Acta Paediatr Scand* 71:567-571, 1982.

39. Stocks RJ, Davies DP, Allen F, Sewell D: Loss of breast milk nutrients during tube feeding, *Arch Dis Child* 60:164, 1985.

40. Lavine M, Clark RM: The effect of short term refrigeration and addition of breast milk fortifier on the delivery of lipids during tube feeding, *J Pediatr Gastroenterol Nutr* 8:496-499, 1989.

41. Narayanan I, Singh B, Harvey D: Fat loss during feedings of human milk, *Arch Dis Child* 59:475-477, 1984.

42. Greer FR, McCormick A, Loaker J: Changes in fat concentration of human milk during delivery by intermittent bolus and continuous mechanical pump infusion, *J Pediatr* 105:745-749, 1984.

43. American Academy of Pediatrics, Committee on Nutrition: Iron fortification of infant formulas, *Pediatrics* 104:119-123, 1999.

44. Whitington PF, Gibson R: Soy protein intolerance: four patients with concomitant cow's milk intolerance, *Pediatrics* 59:730-732, 1977.

45. American Academy of Pediatrics, Committee on Nutrition: Hypoallergenic infant formulas, *Pediatrics* 106:346-349, 2000.

46. Kaufman SS, Scriver DJ, Murray ND, et al: Influence of Portagen and Pregestimil on essential fatty acid status in infantile liver disease, *Pediatrics* 89:151-154, 1992.

47. Kaufman SS, Murray ND, Wood RP, et al: Nutritional support for the infant with extra-hepatic biliary atresia, *J Pediatr* 110:679-686, 1987.

48. American Academy of Pediatrics, Committee on Nutrition: Commentary on breast feeding and infant formulas, including proposed standards for formulas, *Pediatrics* 57:278-285, 1976.

49. United States Congress: Infant Formula Act of 1980. Public Law 96-359, Sept. 26, 1980.

50. Braunschweig CL, Wesley JR, Clark SF, Mercer N: Rationale and guidelines for parenteral and enteral transition feeding of the 3 to 30 kg child, *J Am Diet Assoc* 88:479-482, 1988.

51. Dorf A: Tube feeding the young child: current practices and concerns of pediatric nutritionists, *J Am Diet Assoc* 89:1658-1660, 1989.

52. Brammer EM: Shortcomings of current formulae for long term enteral feeding in pediatrics, *Nutr Clin Pract* 5:160-162, 1990.

53. Patchell CJ, Anderton A, MacDonald A, et al: Bacterial contamination of enteral feeds, *Arch Dis Child* 70:327-330, 1994.

54. Fomon SJ, Ziegler EE, O'Donnell AM: Infant feeding in health and disease. In Fomon SJ (ed): *Infant nutrition,* ed 2, Philadelphia, 1974, WB Saunders, pp 472-519.

55. Marian M: Pediatric nutrition support, *Nutr Clin Pract* 8:199-209, 1993.

56. Heird WC, Dell RB, Helms RA, et al: Amino acid mixture designed to maintain normal plasma amino acid patterns of infants and children requiring parenteral nutrition, *Pediatrics* 80:401-408, 1987.

57. Steinhorn D, Konstantinides F: Supplemental branched-chain amino acid improves nitrogen retention during acute critical-illness in children, *Crit Care Med* 22:A211, 1994 (abstract).

58. Bullock L, Fitzgerald JF, Walter WV: Emulsion stability of total nutrient admixtures containing a pediatric amino acid formulation, *J Parenter Enteral Nutr* 16:64-68, 1992.

59. Klein GL, Horst RL, Norman AW, et al: Reduced serum levels of 1-alpha, 25 dihydroxyvitamin D during long term total parenteral nutrition, *Ann Intern Med* 94:638-643, 1981.

60. Heird WC: Amino acids in pediatric and neonatal nutrition, *Curr Opin Clin Nutr Metab Care* 1:73-78, 1998.

61. Zlotkin SH, Anderson H: The development of cystathionase activity during the first year of life, *Pediatr Res* 16:65-68, 1982.

62. Laine L, Shulman RJ, Pitre D, et al: Cysteine usage increases the need for acetate in neonates who receive total parenteral nutrition, *Am J Clin Nutr* 54:565-567, 1991.

63. Zlotkin SH: Nutrient interactions with total parenteral nutrition: effect of histidine and cysteine intake on urinary zinc excretion, *J Pediatr* 114(5):859-864, 1989.

64. Lai H, Chen W. Effects of medium-chain and long-chain triacylglycerols in pediatric surgical patients, *Nutrition* 16:401-406, 2000.

65. Coben RM, Weintraub A, Di Marino AJ, Cohen S: Gastroesophageal reflux during gastrostomy feeding, *Gastroenterology* 106:13-18, 1994.

66. Parker P, Stroop S, Greene H: A controlled comparison of continuous versus intermittent feeding in the treatment of infants with intestinal disease, *J Pediatr* 99:360-364, 1981.

67. Parathyras AJ, Kassak LA: Tolerance, nutritional adequacy and cost-effectiveness in continuous drip versus bolus and/or intermittent feeding techniques, *Nutr Support Serv* 3(5):56-62, 1983.

68. Leider A, Sullivan L, Mullen MA: Intermittent tube feeding: pros and cons, *Nutr Support Serv* 4:59-61, 1984.

69. Heitkemper ME, Martin DL, Hansen BC, et al: Rate and volume of intermittent enteral feeding, *J Parenter Enteral Nutr* 5:125-129, 1981.

70. American Academy of Pediatrics, Committee on Nutrition: Parenteral nutrition. In *Pediatric nutrition handbook,* Elk Grove Village, IL, 1993, American Academy of Pediatrics, pp 154-166.

71. Friedman Z, Danon A, Stahlman MT, Oates JA: Rapid onset of essential fatty acid deficiency in the newborn, *Pediatrics* 58:640-649, 1976.

72. American Academy of Pediatrics, Committee on Nutrition: Parenteral nutrition. In *Pediatric nutrition handbook,* Elk Grove Village, IL, 1998, American Academy of Pediatrics, pp 285-306.

73. Collier S, Crouch J, Hendricks K, Caballero B: Use of cyclic parenteral nutrition in infants less than 6 months of age, *Nutr Clin Pract* 9:65-68, 1994.

74. Faubion WC, Baker WL, Iott BA, et al: Cyclic TPN for hospitalized pediatric patients, *Nutr Support Serv* 1:24-25, 1981.

75. Kerner JA (ed): *Manual of pediatric parenteral nutrition,* New York, 1983 Wiley, pp 307-311.

76. Lienhardt A, Rakoambinina B, Colomb V, et al: Insulin secretion and sensitivity in children on cyclic total parenteral nutrition, *J Parenter Enteral Nutr* 22:382-386, 1998.

77. Tuchman DN, Walter RS (eds): *Disorders of feeding and swallowing in infants and children,* San Diego, 1994, Singular Publishing Group, pp 77-114.

78. Marcuard SP, Perkins AM. Clogging of feeding tubes, *J Parenter Enteral Nutr* 12:403-405, 1988.

79. Marcuard SP, Stegall KS: Unclogging feeding tubes with pancreatic enzymes, *J Parenter Enteral Nutr* 14:198-200, 1990.

80. Nicholson LJ: Declogging small-bore feeding tubes, *J Parenter Enteral Nutr* 11:594-597, 1987.

81. Whitington PF: Cholestasis associated with total parenteral nutrition in infants, *Hepatology* 5:693-696, 1985.

82. Sandler RH, Kleinman RE: Cholestasis associated with parenteral nutrition. In Walker WA, Drurie PR, Hamilton JR, et al. (eds): *Pediatric gastrointestinal disease,* vol 2, Philadelphia, 1991, BC Decker, p 1069.

83. Greene HL, Hambidge KM, Schanler R, Tsang RC: Guidelines for the use of vitamins, trace elements, calcium, magnesium and phosphorus in infants and children receiving total parenteral nutrition: report of the Subcommittee on Clinical Practice Issues of the American Society for Clinical Nutrition, *Am J Clin Nutr* 48:1324-1342, 1988.

84. Lowrey TS, Dunlap AW, Brown RO, et al: Pharmacologic influence on nutrition support therapy: use of propofol in a patient receiving combined enteral and parenteral nutrition support, *Nutr Clin Pract* 11:147-149, 1996.

85. Misra S, Ahn C, Ament ME, et al: Plasma choline concentrations in children requiring long-term home parenteral nutrition: a case control study, *J Parenter Enteral Nutr* 23:305-308, 1999.

86. Popinska K, Kierkus J, Lyszkowska M, et al: Aluminum contamination of parenteral additives, amino acid solutions, and lipid emulsions, *Nutrition* 15:683-686, 1999.

87. Suita S, Masumoto K, Yamanouchi T, et al: Complications in neonates with short bowel syndrome and long-term parenteral nutrition, *J Parenter Enteral Nutr* (suppl 5):S106-S109, 1999.

88. American Society for Parenteral and Enteral Nutrition: Nutrition support for infants and children with specific diseases and conditions. In Guidelines for the use of parenteral and enteral nutrition in adult and pediatric patients, *J Parenter Enteral Nutr* 17(suppl 4):39SA-49SA, 1993.

89. Pencharz PB: Aggressive oral, enteral or parenteral nutrition: prescriptive decisions in children with cancer, *Int J Cancer Suppl* 11:73-75, 1998.

90. Skolin I, Axelsson K, Ghannad P, et al: Nutrient intakes and weight development in children during chemotherapy for malignant disease, *Oral Oncol* 33:364-368, 1997.

91. Pietsch JB, Ford C, Whitlock JA: Nasogastric tube feedings in children with high-risk cancer: a pilot study, *Hematol Oncol* 21:111-114, 1999.

92. Novy MA, Saavedra JM: Nutrition therapy for the pediatric cancer patient, *Top Clin Nutr* 12:16-25, 1997.

93. Torelli GF, Campos AD, Meguid MM: Use of TPN in terminally ill cancer patients, *Nutrition* 15:665-667, 1999.

94. Reed E, Roy L, Gaskin K, et al: Nutrition intervention and growth in children with chronic renal failure, *J Renal Nutr* 8:122-126, 1998.

95. Sedman AS, Parekh RS, DeVee JL, et al: Cost effective management of children with polyuric renal failure, *J Am Soc Neph* 7:1398, 1996(abstract #A0763).

96. Heuschkel RB, Menache CC, Megerian JT, Baird AE: Enteral nutrition and corticosteroids in the treatment of acute Crohn's disease in children, *J Pediatr Gastroenterol Nutr* 31:8-15, 2000.

97. Coss-Bu JA, Jefferson LS, Walding D, et al: Resting energy expenditure and nitrogen balance in critically ill pediatric patients on mechanical ventilation, *Nutrition* 14:649-652, 1998.

98. Heneyke S, Smith VV, Spitz L, Milla PJ: Chronic intestinal pseudo-obstruction in children: treatment and long-term follow-up of 44 patients, *Arch Dis Child* 81:21-27, 1999.

99. August DA: Outcomes research in nutrition support: background, methods and practical applications. In Ireton-Jones CS, Gottschlich M, Bell S (eds): *Practice-oriented nutrition research,* Gaithersburg, MD, 1998, Aspen Publishers, p 132.

Ruth E. Johnston, MS, RD, LD, CDE
Ronni Chernoff, PhD, RD, FADA

THE terms *elderly* and *senior citizen* are used to denote any person older than 65 years; the term preferred by this age group is *older adult*. In earlier decades, everyone aged 65 or over was categorized as *old*. Because of the change in life expectancy, many of those over age 65 have a greater likelihood of living into their 80s or 90s. For this reason, this population segment has grown significantly. Today, new stratifications are becoming more necessary and familiar, with terms such as *young old, old,* and *old old*. Some specialty geriatric programs are using 75 years as the minimum age limit because of the large numbers of persons aged 65 to 74 years.

Demographics of the U.S. Elderly Population

According to the 2000 U.S. census, over 34 million Americans are older than 65 years. This population group will grow increasingly large as the baby boom generation, those born between 1946 and 1964, ages and as the estimated life expectancy increases. Based on data from the Social Security Administration, it is projected that more than 50 million Americans will be aged 65 and older by the year 2020. For these reasons, we focus on the unique differences in nutrition support needs of the geriatric population in this chapter.

Body Composition Changes in the Elderly

Several changes in body composition occur with aging (see Chapter 3). Lean muscle mass decreases from about 45% at age 30, to approximately 27% of body weight at age 70 years. Skeletal muscle, smooth muscle, and body organs all experience this loss. At the same time, there is a proportional increase in total body fat from about 14% at age 30 to approximately 30%, and it is redistributed throughout the body. Total body water also decreases to about 53% of total body weight, which parallels the loss of lean body mass.

Bone density decreases with age. Two types of osteoporosis affect elders: postmenopausal (usually between ages 51 and 75 years) and senile (usually after age 70). Postmenopausal osteoporosis, also known as *primary* or type 1, alters trabecular bone and is six times more prevalent in women than in men. Senile osteoporosis, also known as *involutional* or *type 2 osteoporosis,* is attributed to age-related changes in vitamin D synthesis. Senile osteoporosis alters both trabecular and cortical bone density and is twice as prevalent in women as in men. Women can be affected concurrently with both types of bone density loss.[1] Because of negative bone balance of the vertebral column and general osteoporosis, humans shrink in stature by approximately 1 cm per decade after the age of 20 years.[2]

Nutrition Assessment

There are several levels of assessing nutritional status in older adults. The first level, screening for the risk of malnutrition related to existing factors, was addressed by The Nutrition Screening Initiative (NSI), a collaboration of the American Academy of Family Physicians, the American Dietetic Association, and the National Council of the Aging. Members of the Technical Review Committee developed a nutrition checklist, "Determine Your Nutritional Health" (Fig. 28-1) for early screening. This tool focuses on the major nutritional risk factors of elderly people: inadequate food intake, poverty, social isolation, dependency and disability, acute and chronic diseases or conditions, chronic medication use, oral health, and advanced age. Those deemed at moderate or high risk should be referred to a registered dietitian for evaluation because this instrument is not an *assessment* tool. It can, however, be the initial step toward identifying older Americans at risk for malnutrition.

Anthropometrics

A clinician who plans to use anthropometrics routinely for nutrition assessment of the elderly must be aware of the variability of results (see Chapter 3). Much variance has been noted among trained clinicians when they take and retake anthropometric measurements.[3] It is best if the same technician or clinician obtains the anthropometric measurements and performs routine validity testing.

The ideal way to obtain height is direct measurement. Unfortunately, this is not possible with many elderly patients because of bone and joint disease, neurologic conditions such as stroke or balance disorders, paralysis, limb loss, frailty, or functional dependence. If a geriatric patient is unable to stand upright, height can be measured in a recumbent position with a nonstretchable measuring tape. Another alternative is to use knee height calipers and to extrapolate height by using the appropriate equation for gender and race.[4] Another option is to use "segmental measurements" that use physically prominent markers (e.g., hip crest, scapular) to measure length; this may be a reasonable alternative for patients with contractures. Frame size can be determined by one of two methods: wrist circumference or elbow breadth measurement.[4] If a patient has a large or small frame size, the desired body weight can be increased or decreased accordingly by 10%.

The Warning Signs of poor nutritional health are often overlooked. Use this checklist to find out if you or someone you know is at nutritional risk.

Read the statements below. Circle the number in the yes column for those that apply to you or someone you know. For each yes answer, score the number in the box. Total your nutritional score.

DETERMINE YOUR NUTRITIONAL HEALTH

	YES
I have an illness or condition that made me change the kind and/or amount of food I eat.	2
I eat fewer than 2 meals per day.	3
I eat few fruits or vegetables, or milk products.	2
I have 3 or more drinks of beer, liquor or wine almost every day.	2
I have tooth or mouth problems that make it hard for me to eat.	2
I don't always have enough money to buy the food I need.	4
I eat alone most of the time.	1
I take 3 or more different prescribed or over-the-counter drugs a day.	1
Without wanting to, I have lost or gained 10 pounds in the last 6 months.	2
I am not always physically able to shop, cook and/or feed myself.	2
	TOTAL

Total Your Nutritional Score. If it's ---

0-2   **Good!** Recheck your nutritional score in 6 months.

3-5   **You are at moderate nutritional risk.** See what can be done to improve your eating habits and lifestyle. Your office on aging, senior nutrition program, senior citizens center or health department can help. Recheck your nutritional score in 3 months.

6 or more **You are at high nutritional risk.** Bring this checklist the next time you see your doctor, dietitian or other qualified health or social service professional. Talk with them about any problems you may have. Ask for help to improve your nutritional health.

These materials developed and distributed by the Nutrition Screening Initiative, a project of:

AMERICAN ACADEMY OF FAMILY PHYSICIANS

THE AMERICAN DIETETIC ASSOCIATION
NATIONAL COUNCIL ON THE AGING, INC.
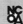

Remember that warning signs suggest risk, but do not represent diagnosis of any condition. Turn the page to learn more about the Warning Signs of poor nutritional health.

FIGURE 28-1   "Determine your nutritional health" checklist. *Continued on next page.* (Reprinted with permission of the Nutrition Screening Initiative, a project of the American Academy of Family Physicians, the American Dietetic Association and the National Council on Aging, Inc., and funded in part by a grant from Ross Products Division, Abbott Laboratories, Inc.)

The Nutrition Checklist is based on the Warning Signs described below. Use the word **DETERMINE** to remind you of the Warning Signs.

Disease

Any disease, illness or chronic condition which causes you to change the way you eat, or makes it hard for you to eat, puts your nutritional health at risk. Four out of five adults have chronic diseases that are affected by diet. Confusion or memory loss that keeps getting worse is estimated to affect one out of five or more of older adults. This can make it hard to remember what, when or if you've eaten. Feeling sad or depressed, which happens to about one in eight older adults, can cause big changes in appetite, digestion, energy level, weight and well-being.

Eating Poorly

Eating too little and eating too much both lead to poor health. Eating the same foods day after day or not eating fruit, vegetables, and milk products daily will also cause poor nutritional health. One in five adults skip meals daily. Only 13% of adults eat the minimum amount of fruit and vegetables needed. One in four older adults drink too much alcohol. Many health problems become worse if you drink more than one or two alcoholic beverages per day.

Tooth Loss/ Mouth Pain

A healthy mouth, teeth and gums are needed to eat. Missing, loose or rotten teeth or dentures which don't fit well or cause mouth sores make it hard to eat.

Economic Hardship

As many as 40% of older Americans have incomes of less than $6,000 per year. Having less--or choosing to spend less--than $25-30 per week for food makes it very hard to get the foods you need to stay healthy.

Reduced Social Contact

One-third of all older people live alone. Being with people daily has a positive effect on morale, well-being and eating.

Multiple Medicines

Many older Americans must take medicines for health problems. Almost half of older Americans take multiple medicines daily. Growing old may change the way we respond to drugs. The more medicines you take, the greater the chance for side effects such as increased or decreased appetite, change in taste, constipation, weakness, drowsiness, diarrhea, nausea, and others. Vitamins or minerals when taken in large doses act like drugs and can cause harm. Alert your doctor to everything you take.

Involuntary Weight Loss/Gain

Losing or gaining a lot of weight when you are not trying to do so is an important warning sign that must not be ignored. Being overweight or underweight also increases your chance of poor health.

Needs Assistance in Self Care

Although most older people are able to eat, one of every five have trouble walking, shopping, buying and cooking food, especially as they get older.

Elder Years Above Age 80

Most older people lead full and productive lives. But as age increases, risk of frailty and health problems increase. Checking your nutritional health regularly makes good sense.

The Nutrition Screening Initiative • 2626 **Pennsylvania Avenue, NW** • **Suite 301** • **Washington, DC 20037**
The Nutrition Screening Initiative is funded in part by a grant from Ross Laboratories, a division of Abbott Laboratories.

FIGURE 28-1 *Continued.*

If at all possible, weighing should be done on an upright balance beam scale, although for bedfast persons, bed scales are available. Wheelchair patients can be weighed on special scales while seated (the weight of the wheelchair is then subtracted from the total weight obtained). Using the same scale consistently over time allows more accurate weight determination. Ideally, scales should be calibrated regularly to maintain validity of the results.

Body mass index (BMI) is determined by dividing the patient's weight in kilograms by the height in meters squared. According to the NSI guidelines, a BMI value below 22 may indicate illness or malnutrition; a value over 27 indicates obesity.

Skinfold measurements provide useful information on both muscle mass and body fat stores. Fat distribution is different in elderly men and women; therefore, different skinfold measurements are recommended. In men, truncal measurements such as suprailiac and subscapular skinfold more accurately reflect fat stores. Skinfold measurements of the extremities, biceps and triceps, as well as midarm muscle circumference, are better predictors of fat stores in women. In elderly patients, hydration status can complicate body composition assessment; however, skinfold measurements are affected less by hydration than is weight. Using one, or preferably several, skinfold or circumference measurements along with laboratory indices such as albumin or prealbumin can be helpful in evaluating body composition.

Laboratory Values

Albumin is a reliable indicator of visceral protein stores in the geriatric population in the absence of liver disease, renal disease, cancer, prolonged bed rest, or infection. Normal levels range between 3.5 and 5 g/dl but may vary depending on the local laboratory standards. A difference of up to 11 g/L may occur with different laboratory techniques. In a previously ambulatory elderly patient, the albumin concentration may drop by up to 5 g/dl after only 8 hours of bed rest.[5] It takes about 20 days for loss of protein stores to be reflected in the serum albumin level in an individual without the conditions listed above (see Chapter 4).

Serum albumin levels less than 2.8 g/dl are associated with the beginning stages of generalized edema. If nutrition therapy is initiated for a malnourished patient, the albumin level may initially decline before it begins to increase. This is typical of the refeeding syndrome and its associated shifts in extracellular and intracellular fluids.

Transferrin, which has a half-life of approximately 9 days, may seem to be a better choice than albumin; however, iron stores in body tissues increase with age, which causes the serum transferrin levels to fall. A healthy older person may have transferrin levels that appear to be depressed while an elderly patient with protein calorie malnutrition and depleted iron stores might have a normal transferrin level. The transferrin can also be affected negatively by acute hepatitis, estrogen, and poor nutrient intake.

Another biochemical measure of visceral protein stores is prealbumin, which has a 2-day half-life. The disadvantage of this test is that it may cost more than albumin measures. Normal levels for prealbumin are between 18 and 40 mg/dl, and the screening level for risk of malnutrition is less than 11 mg/dl.

The total lymphocyte count can be used as a predictor of malnutrition. A normal count is more than 1500 cells per cubic millimeter. Except in cases of immune deficiency and diseases such as cancer, a depressed count could indicate malnutrition or illness.

It is important to be aware that reference values for nutrition assessment measures have not been derived from or validated on populations of elderly people, and although they provide some framework for evaluating nutritional patency, they are not definitive and should not be used as such.

Evaluation of Oral Intake

The most notable change in nutrition requirements for the elderly is a decrease in energy or calorie needs. This is related both to the reduced energy expenditure and the decrease in lean muscle mass. This reduced lean muscle mass may be associated with decreased activity levels. Fewer calories are required because of a reduction in the basal energy rate associated with diminished active metabolic mass.

One might expect elders to have a lower protein requirement because of the reduced lean muscle mass; however, when caloric intake decreases, the amount of nitrogen retained by the body also decreases. It is important to provide enough protein to produce a positive nitrogen balance unless more protein is needed to repair or replace damaged tissue. For healthy geriatric patients, 1.0 g/kg of actual body weight appears to be adequate.[6,7] If the patient has healing pressure ulcers or surgical wounds, for example, more protein—up to 1.5 g/kg or more—may be appropriate. Except for those who have hepatic or renal disease, geriatric patients can tolerate higher protein intake without deterioration of kidney function, although it is important that these patients maintain adequate hydration. Bedfast or immobilized patients such as institutionalized elderly need more protein to achieve positive nitrogen balance. Immobility contributes directly to negative nitrogen balance. Strength training can help the frail elderly enhance protein turnover and encourage replenishment of muscle mass losses. No guidelines have been established for strength training in older persons; however, ongoing and future research in this area should provide insight for guidance.

The recommendation for carbohydrate intake is the same for elders as for younger adults. However, the ability to metabolize glucose declines with age. The acceptable fasting blood sugar level of 140 mg/dl for those older than 65, the acceptable standard for many years,[8] was changed in recent years to be the same level as that of younger adults. The consequences of this remain to be seen; nevertheless, the elderly should be encouraged to eat complex carbohydrates, not only because of their lower glucose tolerance but also because of their need for fiber. Constipation, a major gastrointestinal complaint of the elderly, can be managed by increasing fluids and fiber intake and encouraging ambulation. Constipation can be aggravated by polypharmacy, decreased fluid intake, and inactivity. Older patients often avoid eating fresh fruits and vegetables because they can be difficult to chew and are expensive when out of season. Whole grain breads and cereals are examples of fiber-rich complex carbohydrates that geriatric patients should eat routinely. Recommended daily dietary fiber intake is 25 to 35 g.[9] Bulk-forming laxatives are recommended for ambulatory elderly patients, whereas hyperosmotic laxatives are better for bedridden patients.

Recommendations for fat intake in the elderly vary. Fat provides energy, essential fatty acids, and fat-soluble vitamins. Limiting fat in the diet can reduce total calories without restricting other nutrients; however a dramatic reduction of lipids can result in a calorie deficit. Changing the type of fat in the diet of older Americans is controversial. Quality of life and health maintenance are high priorities for some older persons. Modifying the diet too much could restrict the intake of important nutrients. Fat restriction may not need to be tightly controlled because some studies indicate that, after age 65, systolic hypertension may be a more significant risk factor than cholesterol level for progression of heart disease. A cholesterol level over 250 mg/dl is nevertheless reason for further evaluation.

Except for vitamin D, vitamin B_{12}, vitamin B_6, folate, and riboflavin, there is no evidence of age-related changes in vitamin recommendations (Table 28-1). Reasons for the changes of these nutrients vary. As people age they may reduce (1) their intake of vitamin D–fortified dairy products because of lactose intolerance and (2) their exposure to sunlight. Immobile and institutionalized geriatric patients spend less time outdoors, and many who do go outside use sunscreen. Other factors that contribute to the risk of vitamin D deficiency include the reduction with age of the vitamin D precursor in the skin (7-dehydrocholesterol) and reduced efficiency of the kidneys in converting vitamin D to its active form. Therefore increasing exposure to sunlight and a daily supplement of 400 IU vitamin D daily are recommended.[10]

Many geriatric patients are at high risk for vitamin B_{12} deficiency. Major sources of this vitamin are red meat and organ meats, which persons who are trying to reduce dietary fat and cholesterol typically omit from their diet. Also, the cost of meat can be prohibitive for persons living on a fixed income, and chewing meat can be difficult with poor dentition. With aging there is also risk of decreased gastric acid production and a tenfold increase in the risk of achlorhydria. Intrinsic factor production also declines with a reduction of gastric acid, which is necessary for release of vitamin B_{12} from its protein carrier, its binding to intrinsic factor, and its subsequent absorption.

With a higher percentage of fat stores in elders there is greater risk of vitamin A toxicity than of deficiency in the geriatric patient. Those who take over-the-counter vitamin supplements should monitor their vitamin A intake. Symptoms of vitamin A toxicity include night sweats, vertigo, dry and fissured skin and lips, bone pain, abdominal pain, and vomiting.

Vitamin K deficiency is uncommon but can be induced by anticoagulants, antibiotics, or sulfa drugs. Vitamin E deficiency is extremely rare but can be related to genetic diseases or malabsorption syndromes.

Except for iron, most mineral requirements do not change with age; iron stores increase with age and menstrual blood loss in women ceases. Because of the prevalence of osteoporosis in the elderly, some clinicians believe that increasing calcium intake is warranted, but more studies are needed. Other mineral requirements remain the same, although deficiencies can be due to inadequate dietary intake or disease processes.

TABLE 28-1

Nutrient Requirements for Older Adults[6,7,10,11]

Major Nutrients	Changes With Age
Calories/energy	Needs decrease about one third from age 30
Protein	Needs are higher than RDA; 1+ g/kg BW/day 20% total calories
Carbohydrates	Needs remain the same 50%-60% total calories
Fat	Needs remain the same 20%-30% total calories
Water/fluid	1-2 L/day

Sufficient Data on RDAs	Comments
Vitamin A	No new data for change; RDA may be too high Males, 1000 µg RE Females, 800 µg RE
Vitamin D	RDA probably too low for elderly Males/females, 5 µg/day Recommend low dose supplement: 10 µg/day
Vitamin E	No new data for change Males, 10 mg α-tocopherol Females, 8 mg α-tocopherol
Thiamine	No new data for change Males, 1.2 mg/day Females, 1 mg/day
Riboflavin	RDA probably too low for elderly Males, 1.4 mg/day Females, 1.2 mg/day Recommend resuming previous RDAs: 1.7 mg/day for men and 1.3 mg/day for women
Vitamin B_6	RDA probably too low for elderly Males, 2 mg/day Females, 1.6 mg/day Recommend resuming previous RDA: 2.2 mg/day for men and 2 mg/day for women
Vitamin B_{12}	RDA probably too low for elderly Males, 2 µg/day Females, 1.6 µg/day Recommend resuming previous RDA: 3 µg/day for men and women
Folate	Probably too low; recommend 400 µg/day Males, 200 µg/day Females, 180 µg/day
Vitamin C	No data for change Males/females 60 mg/day

Insufficient Data	
Vitamin K	
Niacin	
Pantothenic acid	
Biotin	

BW, Body weight; *RDA*, recommended daily allowance; *RE*, retinol equivalent.

Hydration is extremely important in the elderly. Inadequate intake of water can lead to dehydration, the symptoms of which include sunken eyes, swollen tongue, increased body temperature, decreased blood pressure, nausea, vomiting, confusion, electrolyte imbalances, and decreased urine output. The two main stimuli for thirst are cellular dehydration and hypovolemia. With aging, thirst sensitivity decreases, especially in persons with high serum sodium and osmolality levels. In the frail elderly, loss of thirst sensation can lead to severe dehydration and mental confusion. The recommended fluid intake is 1 ml of fluid per kilocalorie ingested or 30 ml of fluid per kilogram of body weight.[9] The minimum level, regardless of weight, is 1500 ml per day. Severely dehydrated patients who experience vomiting and diarrhea may need 2 to 4 L of water per day.[9] Overhydrated patients may exhibit hyponatremia, depression, weakness, confusion, and anorexia. The two most common causes of water toxicity are decreased renal capacity secondary to acute or chronic reduced renal blood flow and hyponatremia caused by antidiuretic hormone.[9]

Loss or alteration of taste and smell with aging can affect dietary intake.[12] In addition to physical disabilities, social factors play a role in decreased dietary intake. Lifestyle changes after loss of a spouse and subsequent social isolation can lead to decreased intake and lack of variety in the diet. Entire food groups may be lacking in the diet and, therefore, certain nutrients may also be inadequate; ill-fitting dentures, or incomplete dentition can adversely affect dietary intake. Many of the eating problems encountered in the elderly are related to problems or conditions in the mouth. A thorough examination of teeth, lips, mouth, and tongue is indicated.[13,14] Many older adults of limited income must often choose between food and medicine when money is short. Some feeding programs for the elderly, including home delivered meals and common site feeding locations, are financially stressed also and can help only so many people.

While healthy geriatric patients may not require dietary supplementation, the needs of the frail elderly client should be assessed individually. Carbohydrate and protein supplements are available that can be added to a patient's diet with little change in flavor or texture. For those on limited incomes, dry milk powder or powdered instant breakfast products can be used, although it is important to assess the patient for lactose intolerance. Vitamin supplements are available in pills, capsules, and liquid forms to replace depleted vitamins and minerals. High-calorie and high-protein snack foods can be added to the diet—peanut butter sandwiches, cheese and crackers, whole milk, and ice cream—if the patient needs to increase oral intake.

For some patients, commercially available liquid formulas may be indicated. Those who might benefit from these products are cancer patients, long-term care patients, and functionally compromised homebound individuals. Special products are available for patients with diabetes, renal failure, chronic obstructive pulmonary disease, immune diseases, lactose intolerance, or gluten intolerance.

Indications for Nutrition Support

The three groups for whom nutrition support is indicated include those who cannot eat, those who refuse to eat, and those whose increased calorie and protein needs cannot be met by consuming their usual diet. Many things prevent patients from eating: oral or esophageal obstruction; dysphagia; chronic diseases such as Parkinson's, Huntington's, and multiple sclerosis; coma; and stroke. Polytrauma such as occurs in a motor vehicle accident or thermal injury (burns) can limit the patient's ability to consume the amount of calories, protein, fluid, and other nutrients needed when requirements have increased dramatically because of the physiologic insult and need to make significant amounts of new tissue.

Patients who will not eat may be depressed or anorexic, possibly as a side effect of medication. Dementia can be a precipitating factor in decreased intake in elderly persons who forget to eat. Functionally dependent elders often need help getting to the grocery store, purchasing foods, and preparing meals. Some geriatric patients recovering from an acute or chronic condition can be limited by walkers, canes, or wheelchairs. Assessing a patient's capabilities in activities of daily living (e.g., feeding self and toileting) and in instrumental activities of daily living (e.g., shopping, food preparation, transportation) is essential when creating nutrition care plans. Subjective or clinical identification of malnutrition in the elderly can be difficult because several signs of malnutrition—dry hair, reduced skin turgor, decreased subcutaneous fat, and decreased muscle tone—are also associated with normal physiologic aging.[13]

Anorexia of aging, a chronic state of decreased appetite, and therefore of decreased nutrient intake, can occur both with aging and in association with diseases common to elders.[15] In elderly people failure to thrive is defined as a combination of malnutrition, depression, and confusion, either delirium or dementia.[16] Loss of appetite is a common symptom of depression regardless of the patient's age. Clinicians caring for geriatric patients should know that depression can have organic, nonpsychogenic causes, such as medications, electrolyte disorders, hormone imbalances, and brain diseases.[17] Confusion can lead to decreased nutritional intake, which accelerates the process of protein calorie malnutrition. Often, causes of confusion in the elderly—polypharmacy, electrolyte imbalance, and infections such as urinary tract infections—are reversible.

A patient may also develop symptoms of failure to thrive associated with dehydration, pressure sores, slow wound healing, or the trauma of a surgical procedure. Weight may be maintained by decreased energy requirements secondary to reduced energy expenditure. Until a trigger event occurs, specific nutritional deficiencies may not be apparent, such as deficits in tissue stores of water-soluble vitamins. When an elderly patient incurs a stressful insult, his physical condition often declines quickly. Geriatric patients respond more slowly to nutrition therapy and take longer to recover. This puts them at a higher risk for infections because of a depressed immune response or malnutrition-induced anemia.[2] Nutrition therapy can improve indices such as weight, serum albumin, and vitamin and mineral levels, but not necessarily indices of immune function.[13]

Enteral Feedings

Although it is preferable to replenish nutrient deficits with food or oral supplements, some geriatric patients cannot meet their needs in this way, such as those who have dysphagia, oral lesions, esophageal obstruction, malabsorption, or gastric or bowel resection. Contraindications to enteral feeds for the elderly can include terminal illness or the patient's refusal of consent.

Short-term tube feedings can be accomplished by placement of a nasogastric tube, provided the patient can tolerate the size and material of the tube.[18] For a frail elderly person with a chronic condition, placement of a gastrostomy tube may be considered. Percutaneous endoscopic gastrostomy (PEG) or percutaneous endoscopic jejunostomy (PEJ) tubes are often recommended for patients who become agitated, who self-extubate, who have had gastric resection, or who have gastrointestinal obstructions.

Chronic underfeeding of geriatric patients can result in decreased gut absorption. This can be reversed with nutrition therapy. Dilute solutions or predigested formulas may be indicated. Certain chronic conditions may require special products. In choosing the formula, the clinician should consider the protein, calorie, fluid, volume, vitamin, and mineral needs of the patient; estimated duration of tube feeding; expense; and product availability.

The decision to feed intermittently or continuously should be made according to the patient's needs and tolerances. If continuous feeding during the day interferes with the patient's therapy or lifestyle, nocturnal feedings should be considered. It will be important to keep the head of the bed elevated to avoid aspiration during enteral feeding.

Complications of enteral feeding for the elderly can include aspiration, bloating, diarrhea, constipation, clogged tubes, tube migration, and self-extubation (see Chapter 17). Diarrhea, the most common gastrointestinal complication of enteral feedings, can be due to the volume, dilution, or osmolality of the formula; to *Clostridium difficile;* or to medications such as antibiotics. Choosing a formula with soluble fiber and reducing either the rate of feeding or dilution of the formula have been helpful in resolving complaints of diarrhea.

Fluid requirements for enteral feeds are estimated to be 1 ml of water per kilocalorie of formula. Most enteral formulas are suspensions of nutrient components with fluid being displaced by the solids; therefore, 1 L of tube feeding formula actually contains only 750 ml of fluid. Therefore, a compensatory addition of water or other fluid, 25% of the total volume, becomes necessary to meet elderly patients' fluid needs and to prevent dehydration. Water can be used as a feeding tube flush several times a day, typically 50 to 100 ml each time a feeding is given or once each nursing shift. If the patient has some oral intake, fluid requirements may be met with juices, gelatins, or other foods that are liquid at room temperature. Many chronically ill elderly patients may be habitually underfed because of infusion of volumes of formula inadequate to meet their protein, energy, vitamin, and mineral needs. It is important that the clinician be aware of the nutrient demands of individual patients and of the volumes of tube feeding that are ordered and actually provided to the patient.

Parenteral Nutrition

Indications for parenteral nutrition are the same for the elderly as for other adults: a nonfunctional gastrointestinal tract and extended nutrition support for which enteral or oral feeding is not appropriate. Contraindications include terminal illness, no expected improvement in quality of life, and lack of patient or family consent.

Fat emulsions may be indicated for an elderly patient when fluid must be restricted or the patient is glucose intolerant. The clearance rate of lipids in older adults needs further research. Older patients who recently had a myocardial infarction or who have uncontrolled hyperlipidemia, gallbladder disease, or a history of pancreatitis, are at high risk for complications if given fat emulsions.[18,19] Monitoring triglyceride levels of geriatric patients before giving lipids and after the first infusion is important. If serum triglyceride levels exceed 500 mg/dl after the first lipid infusion, the risk of exacerbating or causing acute pancreatitis is increased.[20] Tolerance for fat emulsions is also decreased in elderly patients with infections.[21] Limiting fat to 1.2 g/kg body weight per day given over 16 to 24 hours is recommended for geriatric patients.[21] Because glucose tolerance declines with age, monitoring glucose levels during administration of parenteral nutrition is critical and insulin may be added cautiously as needed.

The fragile elderly may have thin skin, which makes venous access another concern. Catheter infections are a major risk that without proper management and care can lead to increased morbidity and mortality. This problem is exacerbated in geriatric patients, who take longer than younger adults to recover from illness, infection, or injury.

Ethical Considerations

Obtaining informed consent for nutrition support from a geriatric patient can be a challenge (see Chapter 44). The practitioner must be certain that the patient or next of kin has the needed information and understands it well enough to make an educated decision. One study found that comprehension of elderly patients is positively correlated to social support, reading comprehension, intelligence, and mental status.[22] Although more research is needed in this area, the best instrument now available for evaluating potential for comprehension is the Mini Mental State Exam (MMSE).[22]

Planning ahead with an advance directive can eliminate agonizing on-the-spot decisions for family members. Many factors should be considered, including the patient's desires, estimated duration of nutrition support, the nutritional benefits and how they will be measured, when support shall be discontinued, expected improvement in quality or quantity of life, prognosis, and the expense to the family and the facility. Because laws vary from state to state and policies differ among institutions, it is important for the practitioner to know the local laws and policies.

Conclusion

Two major considerations for nutrition support of the elderly are maintenance of proper hydration and provision of adequate fiber for maintenance of usual elimination patterns. Choosing an appropriate formula is just as important, if not more so, in older as in younger adults. An illness or injury to a geriatric patient may be superimposed on long-term chronic illnesses. This can increase the time it takes for an elderly patient to respond or to rebound from nutritional deficiency. Patience and willingness to try a variety of therapeutic methods are helpful when working with debilitated or frail, malnourished elderly clients.

REFERENCES

1. Musculoskeletal disorders: metabolic bone disease. In Abrams WB, Beers MH, Berkow R, Fletcher AJ (eds): *The Merck manual of geriatrics,* ed 2, Whitehouse Station, NJ, 1995, Merck & Co., pp 897-916.

2. Lipschitz D: Nutrition and aging. In Evans JG, Williams TF (eds): *Oxford textbook of geriatric medicine,* Oxford, 1992, Oxford University Press, p 870.

3. Sullivan DH, Patch GA, Baden AL, Lipschitz DA: An approach to assessing the reliability of anthropometrics in elderly patients, *J Am Geriatr Soc* 37:607, 1989.

4. Chumlea WC, Roche AF, Mukherjee D: Techniques for nutritional anthropometric assessment. In *Nutritional assessment of the elderly through anthropometry,* Columbus, OH, 1988, The Ross Medical Nutritional System, p 4.

5. Sullivan DH: What do the serum proteins tell us about our elderly patients? *J Gerontology* 56A(2):M71B-M74, 2001.

6. Carter WJ: Macronutrient requirements for the elderly person. In Chernoff R (ed): *Geriatric nutrition: the health professional's handbook,* ed 2, Gaithersburg, MD, 1999, Aspen Publishing, pp 13-26.

7. Campbell WW, Trappe TA, Wolfe RR, et al: The recommended dietary allowance for protein may not be adequate for older people to maintain skeletal muscle, *J Gerontol Med Sci* 56A(6):373-380, 2001.

8. Metabolic and endocrine disorders: diabetes mellitus and other disorders of carbohydrate metabolism. In Abrams WB, Beers MH, Berkow R, Fletcher AJ (eds): *The Merck manual of geriatrics,* ed 2, Whitehouse Station, NJ, 1995, Merck & Co., pp 997-1022.

9. Chernoff R: Thirst and fluid requirements, *Nutr Rev* 52(8):S3-S5, 1994.

10. Russell RM, Suter PM: Vitamin requirements of the elderly: an update, *Am J Clin Nutr* 58:4-14, 1993.

11. Suter PM: Vitamin requirements. In Chernoff R (ed): *Geriatric nutrition: the health professional's handbook,* ed 2, Gaithersburg, MD, 1999, Aspen Publishing, pp 27-62.

12. Roils BJ: Appetite and satiety in the elderly, *Nutr Rev* 52(8): S9-S10, 1994.

13. Mitchell CO, Chernoff R: Nutritional assessment of the elderly. In Chernoff R (ed): *Geriatric nutrition: the health professional's handbook,* ed 2, Gaithersburg, MD, 1999, Aspen Publishing, pp 382-415.

14. Martin WE: Oral health in the elderly. In Chernoff R (ed): *Geriatric nutrition: the health professional's handbook,* ed 2, Gaithersburg, MD, 1999, Aspen Publishing, pp 107-169.

15. Morley JE, Silver AJ: Anorexia in the elderly, *Neurobiol Aging* 9:9-16, 1988.

16. Groom DD: Eldercare. A diagnostic model for failure to thrive, *J Gerontol Nurs* 19(6):12-16, 1993.

17. Field WE: Physical causes of depression, *J Psychosoc Nurs* 23(10):6-11, 1985.

18. Mason JB, Russell RM: Parenteral nutrition in the elderly. In Rombeau JL, Caldwell MD (eds): *Clinical nutrition, parenteral nutrition,* ed 2, Philadelphia, 1993, WB Saunders, p 737.

19. Sullivan DH: Nutritional support for elderly patients. In Morley JE, Glick Z, Rubenstein LZ (eds): *Geriatric nutrition: a comprehensive review,* New York, 1990, Raven, pp 343-361.

20. Lashner B, Kirsner J, Hanauer S: Acute pancreatitis associated with high-concentration lipid emulsion during total parenteral nutrition therapy for Crohn's disease, *Gastroenterology* 90:1039-1041, 1986.

21. Dahn M, Kirkpatrick J, Blaiser R: Alterations in the metabolism of exogenous lipid associated with sepsis, *J Parenter Enteral Nutr* 8:169-173, 1984.

22. Krynski MD, Tymchuk A J, Ouslander JG: How informed can consent be? New light on comprehension among elderly people making decisions about enteral tube feeding, *Gerontologist* 34(1):36-43, 1994.

Neurologic Impairments 29

Carmen S. Brunner, RD, LD

NEUROLOGIC impairments comprise myriad diseases and conditions that require nutrition intervention. Crises such as traumatic brain injury, spinal cord disruption, sudden hemiparesis, or autoimmune-mediated disruption of nerve transmission affect the patient's ability to procure, and sometimes to utilize nutrition resources. Such insults can elicit metabolic responses that alter gut function and induce rapid tissue degradation. Other neurologic diseases cause gradual, subtle changes in mobility, mental processing, and ability to function. Symptoms of dysphagia may go unnoticed until aspiration pneumonia develops. The clinician is challenged to formulate nutrition care plans that sustain lean muscle mass, preserve neurologic function, and ameliorate metabolic abnormalities. In this chapter we examine some of the more common neurologic impairments from the standpoint of nutrition intervention and discuss metabolic alterations, monitoring of parameters, and route of nutrition support.

Traumatic Brain Injury

The brain, the center of the nervous system, controls not only many of the body's regulatory centers for homeostasis but also the essence of the person. Brain injury threatens the total being. Seventy percent of fatal accidents involve head injuries. Two thirds of head-injured patients die before they reach the hospital. Of those admitted, half die.[1] A majority of these patients are men younger than 35 years.[2] Head injuries account for 40 times as many cases of permanent injury per year as do spinal cord injuries.[3] Aggressive nutrition intervention is warranted to support these patients and minimize the damaging effects of the initial insult and the subsequent hypermetabolic and hypercatabolic responses.[4]

Traumatic brain injury (TBI) is any insult to the brain from trauma. With closed head injuries the protective barrier remains intact but secondary brain injury can result from increased intracranial pressure (ICP). Because of its snug fit in the skull, the brain cannot shift much. Hemorrhage, cerebral edema, or hypoxia from trauma can rapidly increase volume and ICP. Extreme ICP can cause the brain to herniate through the foramen magnum, which can be fatal. Occasionally, craniotomy is needed to remove necrotic tissue and reduce pressure.[5] Goal ICP is less than 20 mm Hg, but this is difficult to attain when head injury is severe.[6] Signs of increased ICP include nonreactive pupils and pupil dilation, decreased level of consciousness (LOC), and motor posturing (decorticate, decerebrate, flaccid).[7]

Management of Increased Intracranial Pressure

Management of increased ICP may include induced hyperventilation to reduce cerebral blood flow, positioning to increase venous drainage, placement of catheters to drain cerebrospinal fluid (CSF), inducing hypothermia, sedation, and drug therapy.[7] Medications used to reduce ICP include osmotic diuretics, loop diuretics, carbonic anhydrase inhibitors, mannitol, corticosteroids, and barbiturates.[8,9] Mannitol, an osmotic diuretic, draws fluid from the brain. Mannitol can cause profound electrolyte disturbances and can compound acute renal failure.[7] Steroids have been administered to treat increased ICP,[10-12] but this approach is controversial. They are known to prolong and intensify amino acid alterations and to increase urine urea nitrogen (UUN) loss.[13] Steroid therapies have also been recognized to enhance the effect of the catabolic response.[12] Sundberg reviewed studies on the effects of steroids on acute brain trauma. In three studies the survival rate increased among the patients in vegetative coma or otherwise severely obtunded. Seven studies found no benefit from steroid use, whereas two others identified a subgroup of patients with early improved Glasgow Coma Scale (GCS) for whom steroids improved long-term outcome. In addition to increased nitrogen loss, acute adverse effects of steroids include gastrointestinal bleeding, hyperglycemia, pneumonia, hyponatremia, and increased infectious complications.[8]

With head injury, pentobarbital is used to control ICP if initial therapy is insufficient.[7] Barbiturates administered to TBI patients reduced nitrogen excretion 40%, improved nitrogen balance,[14] and reduced energy expenditure to 86% of the predicted basal value.[15] It has been proposed that patients in acute phase of TBI be given a combination of barbiturates and propranolol to decrease metabolic rate and nitrogen wasting during the first 2 weeks after injury.[16] Barbiturates indirectly decrease gastrointestinal motility and promote large gastric residual in patients fed enterally.[7] This has been circumvented by endoscopically placing nasojejunal tubes and successfully feeding the patient in pentobarbital coma.[17]

Another drug widely used along with the treatment for intracranial pressure is propofol (Diprivan, Stuart Pharmaceuticals, Wilmington, DE). It is a sedative that is delivered in a lipid emulsion as a continuous infusion because of its brief duration and rapid onset. The lipid content of propofol is

A special thank you is extended to Diane Hester, MS, RD, CNSD, and June Kjelde, MS, RD, LD, who contributed to the first edition chapter.

0.1 g fat/ml, which translates to 1.1 kcal/ml.[18-20] Because it can contribute a significant number of calories to the nutrition support regimen, it is critical to monitor the amount of the drug administered and make adjustments as necessary. Because of this, hypertriglyceridemia may pose a risk, and it is suggested to regularly monitor serum triglyceride levels on patients receiving propofol.[19] One study suggests a baseline level and follow-up blood draws 2 to 3 times per week.[20]

In 1995, the Brain Trauma Foundation published guidelines for the treatment of severe head injury that presented a critical pathway to be used as a guide in determining the course of treatment for ICP. It was developed through evidence-based committee consensus and uses an algorithm for possible treatment options. It also includes recommendations for nutrition support of the brain-injured patient, which are discussed later in this chapter.[12]

Hypermetabolism of Head Injury

Severe head injury is characterized by moderate to severe hypermetabolism after the first few days following trauma (Table 29-1).[13,21-30] This state may persist 4 to 6 weeks after injury.[27] Metabolic changes are generally attributed to hypothalamus and pituitary gland malfunctions resulting from mechanical jarring. Hypermetabolic changes of TBI include increased cortisol, glucagon, catecholamines, and cellular products (e.g., cytokines) in the blood, urine, and CSF.[32] Individual responses vary, but most patients have some degree of hypermetabolic response (see Table 29-1). Of note, elevated glucose levels are found to be inversely related to the GCS and outcome.[33]

The GCS, the standard tool for evaluating severity of head injury and LOC, categorizes responses to verbal and pain stimuli (Table 29-2).[2,34] It is used to track improvement or deterioration in the patient's condition.[2] A GCS score of 3 to 8 is considered severe; in one study, a GCS less than 8 was associated with mortality of 50%.[35] Patients who have lower GCS scores tend to have a more prolonged gastric ileus and are less likely to tolerate enteral feedings immediately after injury, while those with a higher GCS score tolerate gastric feeds earlier.[9]

Head-injured patients are often young, well-nourished males with no history of nutrition problems.[4] Severe brain injury may induce hypermetabolic and hypercatabolic responses,[36] leading to weight loss,[4,37,38] decreased cell body mass,[39] and prolonged recovery.[40] The goal of nutrition and metabolic therapy is to preserve neurologic function, minimize the loss of lean body mass, and facilitate return of maximum function.[41]

Early Nutrition Assessment

In the first 2 weeks after injury, it is difficult to ascertain nutrition needs because the metabolic response can mask developing nutrition deficiencies.[4] Hepatic transport proteins and weight can change drastically with fluid status, sepsis, and shock.[7] Monitoring UUN loss, serial weight changes, serial prealbumin levels, and indirect calorimetry helps determine whether nutrition is adequate.[31]

Energy Assessment

In TBI, the range of energy expenditure has been reported as 75% to 250% of the basal energy expenditure (BEE) (average 140%). Expected energy utilization varies with clinical course (Box 29-1).[21,22,42] Patients with posturing response to pain have the greatest energy needs; those who are clinically brain dead or in barbiturate coma expend the least energy.[15,21,25,27] A recent preliminary study reported that energy utilization decreased 22% beyond 19 days after injury.[39] Other conditions also affect energy requirements in head injury (Box 29-2).

TABLE 29-1

Metabolic Changes in Response to Brain Injury[4,31]

Increase	Decrease	Alteration
Oxygen consumption	Immunocompetence	Fluid balance
Carbon dioxide production	Vascular resistance	Electrolytes
UUN loss	Body weight	Amino acids in plasma
Cardiac output	Serum albumin	
Liver function tests	Thyroxine-binding protein	
Serum fibrinogen	Thyroxine retinol-binding prealbumin	
C-reactive protein	Muscle mass	
Lactic acid in blood	Serum zinc	
Blood glucose		
Urinary zinc		
Urinary calcium		
Blood calcium		

TABLE 29-2

Glasgow Coma Scale

Response	Score
EYES	
Open:	
Spontaneously	4
To verbal command	3
To pain	2
No response	1
BEST MOTOR RESPONSE	
To Verbal Command:	
Obeys	6
To Painful Stimulus:	
Localizes pain	5
Flexion-withdrawal	4
Flexion-abnormal	3
Extension	2
No response	1
BEST VERBAL RESPONSE	
Oriented and converses	5
Disoriented and converses	4
Inappropriate words	3
Incomprehensible sounds	2
No response	1
Total	3-15

From Teasdale G, Jennett B: Assessment of coma and impaired consciousness: a practical scale, *Lancet* 2:81–84, 1974.

BOX 29-1

Determinants of Energy Expenditure in Brain-Injured Patients[4,31,32]

Severity of head injury
Secondary infections
Catecholamine response
Spontaneous muscle activity
Use of barbiturate, sedative, paralyzing, or propranolol therapy

Seizures
Elevated temperature from brain injury
Nutrient infusion (thermogenesis)
Other injuries

BOX 29-2

Guidelines for Predicting Energy Expenditure in Closed Brain Injury Patients*

Fever/sepsis	Increase calories 7.2% over standard estimates for every 1° F of body temperature above normal
Seizures/posturing	Increase 20%-30% over standard estimates, depending on frequency (maximum 3500-4000 total calories)
Nonsedated coma	140% basal energy expenditure (per Harris-Benedict)
Pentobarbital coma	100%-120% basal energy expenditure (per Harris-Benedict)
Afebrile non-ICU patients	120%-130% basal energy expenditure (per Harris-Benedict)
Standard head injury range	140%-200% basal energy expenditure (per Harris-Benedict)

*Indirect calorimetry is the best indicator of nutrition needs after a patient experiences a major medical change (energy expenditure measured as nonprotein calories).
From Harper RA, Magnuson B, Loan T: Nutrition support for traumatic brain injury, *Support Line* XVII(4):12-17, 1995.

Indirect Calorimetry

In view of the wide reported range in energy expenditure, indirect calorimetry is recommended[4,7,9,35] because it quantifies oxygen consumption and carbon dioxide production as determinants of energy use.[43] Quantification helps prevent underfeeding or overfeeding with variations in the patient's clinical course.[31] Short-term (2-hour) indirect calorimetry reliably reflects 24-hour metabolic utilization in clinically stable, sedated, ventilated patients who comply with ventilation. The metabolic rate of a patient with body temperature fluctuations who is clinically unstable may vary as much as 25% in the course of a day, and the patient may benefit from ongoing measurement.[39]

If indirect calorimetry is not available, the Harris-Benedict equation can be used to estimate energy needs in TBI (BEE × 140%; see Box 29-2).[21,26,44,46] Adjustments may be made for sedation and the clinical status of the patient.[22,32,45] The 2000 guidelines from the Brain Trauma Foundation recommend 100% of the resting energy expenditure (REE) for paralyzed patients.[46] In a recent study, REE was used without stress factors to avoid overfeeding.[10]

Protein Assessment

TBI increases catecholamine release and autonomic nervous system response manifested by hypercatabolism and hyperme-

tabolism.[4] This, in turn, dramatically increases nitrogen excretion and produces an abnormal plasma amino acid pattern.[41] Conversion of protein as an energy source increases threefold to fourfold.[31] Hypercatabolic TBI patients show signs of muscle wasting, biochemical alterations, and weight loss.[4] In a study of TBI patients, 75% of weight loss was fat-free body mass.[39] Nonsupplemented TBI patients can lose up to 10% of lean body mass in a week, 25% in 2 weeks, and 30% to 40% in 3 weeks, which can increase morbidity and mortality.[45] Average UUN excretion in TBI patients is similar to that observed in burned or severely stressed patients.[9,31] Although UUN loss is expected to peak in 10 days, it can continue for some time.[4] Studies indicate that even provision of excess calories and protein may not meet the metabolic demands of TBI and reverse negative nitrogen balance until the catabolic phase has passed.[47]

Researchers in TBI have explored the role of other factors in tissue degradation. The magnitude of loss of protein stores is not related to the severity of brain injury.[4] Immobilization increases UUN in healthy adults but is thought to play only a minor role in TBI patients.[41] Steroids such as dexamethasone, used to reduce ICP, induce greater nitrogen excretion, somatic protein mobilization, and total urinary nitrogen loss.[48]

Periodic measurement of urinary nitrogen excretion is recommended to assess protein status. A goal of +2 to +4 nitrogen balance is optimal for wound healing but unrealistic in early treatment of the TBI population.[31] Clinicians rarely achieve positive nitrogen balance, but providing nutrients improves nitrogen retention. Protein needs of head-injured patients range from 1.5 to 2.0 g/kg but have been reported to be as high as 2.5 g/kg.[7,31] After the acute phase, approximately 2.2 g of protein per kilogram of usual body weight, with adequate kilocalories, may be required to achieve positive nitrogen balance.[29,47,49] For obese patients (weight at least 125% of IBW), an adjusted body weight may be used to estimate needs.[31]

Fluid Management

Neurosurgeons still disagree about the role of fluid in cerebral edema and neurologic deterioration. Results of studies conducted in patients and animals indicate that large volumes of isotonic or hypertonic intravenous fluids, with or without glucose, have no effect on ICP, neurologic outcome, brain edema, or serum hyperosmolarity.[50] Fluid-related disorders can nevertheless accompany head injury. Diabetes insipidus results when the pituitary stalk has been damaged. The resulting high-volume, hypernatremic urine output is treated with adequate fluid replacement and medications.[2] The syndrome of inappropriate antidiuretic hormone (SIADH), caused by hypothalamic damage, results in hyponatremia and concentrated urine. Hyponatremia can aggravate cerebral edema, depress neurologic function, or precipitate seizures. Treatment involves restricting free water with occasional use of diuretics.[11]

Micronutrient Needs

Because protein and energy needs increase with TBI, it is assumed that micronutrient requirements must be increased as well, even though no additional requirements are known at this time. The dietary reference intakes (DRIs) are based on healthy adults and do not account for the increased needs from such injuries but may provide at least a starting point for estimation. Supplementation with vitamins and minerals is needed if the nutrition regimen falls below the DRIs.[31] McClain and colleagues found alterations in trace elements during the acute phase of head injury.[51] Zinc deficiency,[10] increased urinary zinc, reduced iron concentration, and elevated serum copper have been reported.[52] It is recommended to supplement 10 to 12 mg zinc daily in the head-injured patient.[9,53] Excess urinary zinc is associated with hypermetabolism, poor wound healing, and depressed immune function. In metabolic management of TBI patients, serum sodium may be kept slightly elevated while other electrolytes are maintained within normal limits. It has been reported that serum phosphorus, potassium, and magnesium may need aggressive intravenous or oral replacement because they can fall sharply with the initiation of feeding.[31]

Nutrition Support

Nutrition support is a high priority for head-injured patients[54] and should start as soon as the patient is hemodynamically stable.[7] Some studies have indicated that parenteral nutrition (PN) demonstrated improved survival and neurologic outcome for head-injured patients as compared with enteral support.[38,40] In one of these studies, however, calorie intake and protein intake were much greater in the PN group than in those who received enteral support because of tube feeding intolerance.[40] Borzotta and colleagues reported that PN and enteral support were equally effective when nutrition support was based on measured energy expenditure and nitrogen excretion.[24] Similarly, Hadley and coworkers found no difference in morbidity and mortality in patients on parenteral or enteral support;[45] however, a recent study found that enteral feedings promoted intestinal mucosal health, more rapid improvement in nutritional status, and better tolerance than PN. Parenteral support was associated with unfavorable changes in pancreatic enzymes and impaired liver function.[10]

In some conditions traditional nutrition parameters (e.g., weight fluctuations, albumin, and transferrin) are monitored throughout the course of treatment to study the efficacy of nutrition support; however, within the first 2 weeks of TBI, these parameters do not reflect nutritional status, because of fluid and electrolyte imbalances. Despite aggressive nutrition support, albumin continues to decrease until 2 weeks after injury.[4,52] Exogenous albumin has been administered in an attempt to correct hypoalbuminemia and fluid balance after severe head injuries. Although studies are inconclusive, some evidence indicates that albumin may reduce the incidence of major complications.[4]

Enteral Support

Severely head-injured patients often require EN or PN support. When it is clinically feasible, enteral nutrition (EN) should be used because it offers significant economic and physiologic benefits and fewer severe complications.[10,55] It has been suggested that it may improve immune status as compared with PN.[4] Investigators have proposed that enteral nutrients are more effective for maintaining intestinal integrity and decreasing bacterial translocation and risk of infection.[56] Although some report that a percutaneous endoscopic gastrostomy (PEG) can be used as a safe and reliable method of nutrition support

---

BOX 29-3

Contributing Factors to Enteral Feeding Intolerance in Brain-Injured Patients[7,61]

Inhibition of gut function through the brain-gut link
Reduced lower esophageal sphincter pressure
Increased gastroesophageal reflux
Hypoalbuminemia
Prolonged ileus
Gastroparesis
Use of medications (e.g., neuromuscular blockers, paralytic agents, other drugs that reduce gastric motility)
Immobility

---

for head-injured patients,[55,57,58] other studies indicate that 20% to 50% of TBI patients in acute phase do not tolerate enteral feeding.[32] The causes of enteral feeding intolerance are probably multiple, but they can be related to severity of injury and increased ICP (Box 29-3).[59,60] It has been reported that nasogastric feeding increases gastric residuals and promotes abdominal distention.[38] Weekes and Elia reported a twofold delay in gastric emptying and significant regurgitation of feedings into the mouth with nasogastric feeding.[39] In some cases, delayed gastric emptying is not resolved until the third week after injury.[62] Proponents of the gastric route advocate using other techniques such as elevating the head of the bed and using promotilant agents.[55,58] Because of the aforementioned factors associated with gastric feeding, several studies advocate the use of jejunal feedings via gastrojejunostomy to avoid gastric intolerances and to decrease aspiration risk. Recent studies suggest that using the jejunal route is better tolerated and overall more successful.[9,46,59] However, at this time, no definitive feeding route has been established to improve outcome.[46]

Currently controlling gastric reflux and ensuring optimal tube placement have enabled successful enteral feeding of TBI patients in the acute phase of illness. It has been reported that delayed gastric emptying may be avoided by postpyloric tube placement.[31,63] Within 36 hours of injury, TBI patients who have a clinically silent abdomen may nevertheless tolerate jejunal feeding.[31] Early jejunal enteral feedings, as compared with those delayed until bowel sounds return, increase the patient's calorie and nitrogen intake and markedly reduce the number of infections and patient days in the intensive care unit.[31,63] Blind placement of nasal feeding tubes in patients with open skull fractures should be avoided.[31] If patients have facial fractures and long-term tube feeding is anticipated, endoscopic or radiographic gastrojejunostomy tubes may be inserted into the distal duodenum or jejunum, providing a gastric port for decompression and delivery of medication during feeding into the small bowel.

In the acute phase, free water may be limited and more concentrated formula used to avoid fluid overload and increased ICP. To maintain hydration status, free water may have to be added every 8 hours. A minimum of 30 to 60 ml every 4 to 6 hours helps maintain feeding tube patency. Modular nutrition additives may be needed to achieve adequate calorie density.[31] Some clinicians have used special enteral products with glutamine, arginine, and ω-3 fatty acids to increase nutritional status and wound healing in critical care patients.[31] More controlled studies of specialized formulas in brain-injured patients are needed before conclusions can be drawn.

Parenteral Support

If enteral nutrition is not feasible because of a nonfunctioning gastrointestinal tract, PN should be initiated. PN can and should be started within 24 hours of head injury.[64] The composition of PN formula does not affect serum osmolality, ICP level, or medical therapy for TBI.[50,65,66] Total fluid intake may, however, be limited to control SIADH. In this case, the parenteral formula must maximize the concentrations of dextrose, amino acids, and fats in minimal fluid.[4] Hyperglycemia should be managed to keep the glucose level below 180 mg/dl.[10] Sodium content may need to be altered, depending on hydration status and sodium level. Phosphorus and magnesium may require replacement because of intracellular shifts after PN initiation.[31] Selenium is absent from some PN solutions and must be added to prevent deficiency with long-term PN use.[67] In conclusion, if a patient requires PN, it is important to monitor gastrointestinal function frequently so that enteral nutrition support can commence as soon as it is medically feasible.[64]

Monitoring Nutrition Support

Regardless of feeding method, serial monitoring is essential to optimize nutrition support. After the initial assessment, head-injured patients should be monitored continuously (Box 29-4). Biochemical indicators—blood glucose, electrolytes, urea nitrogen, creatinine, hematocrit, platelets and white blood cells[31]—and chart review establish the clinical picture. Nutritional status is established by monitoring prealbumin, nitrogen balance, serial weights, and indirect calorimetry.[31] Tolerance for nutrition therapy and fluid balance should be assessed daily and adjusted as necessary. Indirect calorimetry should be repeated if there is a major change in condition such as infection with fever, seizures, or drug-induced coma.[31,32]

Making the Transition to Oral Feeding

Patients who are lethargic or whose GCS is less than 12 are not suitable for transition to oral intake.[31] Head-injured patients may have a decreased gag reflex and should be assessed for dysphagia before a diet is prescribed.[64] If diet modification or

physical techniques (e.g., chin tuck, head turn) do not eliminate symptoms of aspiration, a modified barium swallow procedure is recommended. To stimulate appetite, consideration should be given to providing 50% of enteral support at night or as between-meal boluses. An initial calorie count can be done for 3 days, followed by appropriate adjustments in tube feeding. Reevaluating oral intake every 3 days ensures that the patient's needs are met while he or she is weaned from enteral support.[31]

Head-injured patients may have difficulty with oral feeding (see Box 29-4).[31,62] Fortified nutrient-dense meals; use of commercial supplements; and small, frequent feedings help meet nutrition goals. The patient should be allowed the least restrictive diet and liquid thickness that promote safe swallowing.[31]

Multiple Sclerosis

Multiple sclerosis (MS) is a demyelinating disorder of the nervous system characterized by vision difficulties, paraparesis or quadriparesis, ataxia, tremor, increasing spasticity, emotional lability, fatigue, dysarthria, and pain. Although the cause is not known, both genetics and environmental factors have been implicated.[72] Progression of disease varies, and predicting the outcome is difficult.[72,73]

Although many "therapeutic diets" have been attempted and epidemiologic studies suggest a link with the nature of dietary lipids,[74-77] no substantial data from controlled trials are available to support these assertions. The dietary guidelines of the American Heart Association are appropriate for reducing fat and cholesterol because many MS patients live into middle age.[72] Energy requirements can be estimated from the Harris-Benedict equation with activity factors of 1.2 for patients confined to bed and 1.3 for patients out of bed.[78] Suggested protein requirements for tissue integrity are approximately 1.9 g/kg for sedentary patients aged 50 years and older.[78] Weight control is a prominent concern. Overweight patients with MS are at greater risk for falls and fatigue from maneuvering excess weight. Other patients lose weight and require dietary management and supplementation to maintain weight. Patients can develop dysphagia, leading to aspiration pneumonia, which may require enteral nutrition support to meet needs.[9,72,79]

Amyotrophic Lateral Sclerosis

Amyotrophic lateral sclerosis (ALS) is a progressive neurologic disorder of unknown cause marked by muscle weakness, wasting, spasticity, hypertonicity, and hyperactive reflexes. Average age of onset is 50 years, and the disease exhibits rapid progression to tetraparalysis, dysarthria, dysphagia, and death, usually from respiratory compromise. Mean survival time after onset is 4 years.[2]

Energy and protein needs may be difficult to establish in ALS. As somatic protein tissue becomes depleted, energy needs may decrease; however, spasticity, hypertonicity, and muscle reflexes may require additional energy. Indirect calorimetry would be ideal to estimate energy needs but often is not available. The Harris-Benedict equation may be used with prudent assignment of activity factors because many of these patients have very limited energy. For patients with

---

BOX 29-4

Possible Problems with Oral Intake for Head-Injured Patients[31,68]

Oropharyngeal swallowing disorders	Oral preparatory problems
Oral transit disorders	Related oral sensory changes
Slow intake (+ 1 hr)	Pharyngeal neuromuscular
Memory deficits	abnormalities
Decreased attention span	Delayed triggering of pharyngeal
Agitation	swallow
Poor dentition	Poor motor planning
Upper extremity weakness	Slow mastication
Ataxia	Hearing and vision deficits
	Spasticity

undesirable weight loss, nutrient-dense foods and modular, commercial supplements given in small, frequent feedings are basic elements of a weight maintenance regimen.[80] Enteral feeding usually becomes necessary, with persistent weight loss and progressive dysphagia, and it can safely be provided via a percutaneous endoscopic gastrostomy[80-83] or by a percutaneous endoscopic gastrojejunostomy (PEG/J).[82] A recent study showed that a PEG/J compared with a traditional PEG or PEJ had significant benefits, including not requiring anesthesia and no disruption of the oropharynx with procedural devices.[82]

Protein needs may be similar to those of other sedentary patients, approximately 1.0 g/kg.[78] The use of special enteral formulas with branched-chain amino acids (BCAAs) in ALS is conflicting.[84] ALS alters the metabolism of the neurotransmitter glutamine. It has been proposed that certain BCAAs may indirectly correct the alteration.[85] In one study, ALS patients given supplemental BCAAs were able to maintain extremity muscle strength and sustain the ability to walk longer than ALS patients who did not receive the BCAAs.[86]

Patients with ALS may have difficulty managing their own oral secretions. Anticholinergic medications, amitriptyline, and suction may be used to moderate secretion of saliva. Delayed swallowing associated with ALS places some patients at greater risk for aspiration. Diet modifications (e.g., avoiding thin liquids and foods that do not form a bolus) and speech therapy techniques (e.g., supraglottic swallow) are useful to sustain oral intake. Hydration status may become an issue. Caregivers can be taught to include fluid-dense foods and offer additional fluids throughout the day.[80]

Parkinson's Disease

Parkinson's disease (PD) is a chronic, irreversible neurodegenerative disease caused by progressive deterioration of cells in the substantia nigra of the brain stem, where the neurotransmitter dopamine is produced.[87] Symptoms of PD include tremor, bradykinesia, rigidity, impaired postural reflexes, and occasionally dementia[88,89] and gastrointestinal motility disorders such as delayed gastric emptying, constipation, anorexia, sialorrhea, dysphagia, drooling, and aspiration.[68,89]

Treatment of PD includes oral administration of levodopa, which is converted to dopamine after crossing the blood-brain barrier. It is believed that large neutral amino acids—valine, leucine, isoleucine, tryptophan, tyrosine, and phenylalanine—compete with levodopa for transport through the blood-brain barrier.[90] Studies have reported improvement of PD symptoms among patients who consumed not more than 0.5 g/kg of protein during the day and liberal protein in the evening. In one study, 36% of patients found this very low-protein diet unpalatable and difficult to adhere to.[91] In more recent studies, symptoms of PD decreased when patients taking levodopa ate a balanced diet (dietary protein 0.8 g/kg) with a 7:1 carbohydrate-protein ratio in all meals.[87,89,92] This dietary modification is most effective for patients whose motor fluctuations are not controlled by altering the dose of levodopa.[87,92,93] Patients and care providers should be counseled on the use of the 7:1 carbohydrate-protein ratio. Total energy needs may be based on the Harris-Benedict equation using appropriate activity factors. Higher protein intake recommendations of 1.0 to 1.5 g/kg do not apply to patients following a protein-modified regimen (not more than 0.8 g/kg and a 7:1 carbohydrate-protein ratio).[94]

It has been reported that PD patients may have difficulty maintaining weight. In one study, PD patients were four times more likely to lose at least 20 lb and to have a smaller body mass index and percentages of ideal body weight (IBW) and body fat than control subjects.[95] Serial weights may be used to guide dietary adjustments for weight maintenance. Dietary measures for PD patients might include mechanical alteration of foods for easy chewing and swallowing, methods of simplifying food preparation, use of commercial supplements, easily prepared entrees and nutrient-dense snacks, and assistive devices for feeding patients with tremors.[96] Enteral support usually is not considered unless PD is advanced and weight loss significant.

PD patients risk aspiration before, during, and after swallowing. Many PD patients are unaware of this "silent aspiration" because they have a poor cough reflex, altered mental status and demonstrate no signs of choking or coughing.[96] PD patients who have frequent episodes of pneumonia may need a modified barium swallow assessment and appropriate therapy.

Cerebrovascular Accidents

Cerebrovascular accidents (CVAs; *strokes*) are sudden alterations in the blood supply to some area of the brain. Some 80% of CVAs are ischemic and highly correlated with coronary compromise, and 20% are hemorrhagic. Treatment modalities are different. The definitive diagnosis is often based on computed tomography (CT).[97] CVA signs include hemiparesis, aphasia, hemianopia, and altered LOC. Severity, loss of function, and prognosis depend on the site of occlusion or rupture and the extent of ischemia or hemorrhage.[11]

After onset of CVA symptoms, the medical goal is to stabilize the patient, determine the type of stroke, and screen for other causes or conditions through routine laboratory tests, complete blood count, coagulation studies, chemistry screen (including electrolytes), and urinalysis.[98] Abnormalities in the chemistry screen include hyperglycemia, which has been associated with increased activation of the coagulation system in acute ischemic CVA patients, and hypoalbuminemia, which is attributed to stress rather than malnutrition.[99]

Early assessment of adequate swallowing is imperative before feeding because dysphagia is found in 40% to 50% of CVA patients.[69,97] Of these patients, approximately 40% risk silent aspiration.[96] Dysphagia is more prevalent in patients with multiple, bilateral, brain stem, or large hemispheric CVAs and those with apraxia of the oral-buccal muscles or reduced LOC but is not limited to this group.[97,98,100] A bedside assessment to detect dysphagia and, if needed, a modified barium swallow procedure may be done to confirm the diagnosis. The speech therapist can recommend the safest consistency for oral feeding. Often these foods need to be fortified, nutrient-dense, and modified for consistency to meet nutrient needs. Food can be offered as small, frequent meals with snacks and monitored by nurses or therapists. Patients tire easily and may require 30 minutes' rest before meals,[101] which they take sitting to avoid aspiration.[98] Care providers may be instructed on modified diets and compensatory swallowing techniques to prevent medical complications associated with dysphagia.[102] Intake may be monitored by calorie counts and serial weights. If nutrient intake is inadequate or risk of aspiration high, enteral feeding into the small bowel may be considered to support the patient until adequate swallowing returns. Only 1% of CVA patients, usually those with bilateral lesions of the nucleus amibiguus or damage to cranial nerves IX and X, have permanent, absolute loss of swallow and need a percutaneous endoscopic gastrostomy.[98]

Early assessment of CVA patients is recommended to screen for symptoms of malnutrition that could delay recovery.[97] Barrocas and colleagues[78] noted that the RDA for moderately active persons older than 50 years is 1.5 times the resting energy expenditure (REE), or 30 kcal per kilogram of body weight. For chronically ill, sedentary, elderly persons 20 to 25 kcal/kg may be more realistic. These researchers suggest that greater accuracy can be achieved by estimating energy needs by the Harris-Benedict equation using the 1.2 activity factor for bedridden persons and 1.3 for those who are out of bed.[78] Injury and stress factors are added, if applicable. Positive nitrogen balance was not achieved in the elderly with 0.8 g/kg of protein.[94] Therefore, 1 g/kg for chronically ill persons at rest and 1.5 g/kg for moderately active elder persons are suggested. Additional protein may be needed to achieve positive nitrogen balance for patients who have pressure ulcers or are immobilized, restrained, or wheelchair or bed bound.[78]

Myasthenia Gravis

Myasthenia gravis (MG) is caused by an antibody-mediated autoimmune attack of acetylcholine receptors at the neuromuscular junction that disrupts the normal transmission of nerve impulses across those junctions.[103] Symptoms include poor muscle contraction, fatigue, weakness, and paralysis that affects principally the eyes, face, and throat. Symptoms worsen as the day progresses.[104] Occasionally, patients develop severe dysphagia that requires tube feeding before a definitive diagnosis is made.[105] Current therapy is very effective and includes anticholinesterase agents, immunosuppressant treatment,[104] and plasmapheresis for crises.[104,106] It is strongly recommended that patients between puberty and age 60 years have their thymus surgically removed. This procedure produces remission in 35% of patients and improvement in another 50%.[104]

Nutrition intervention is needed for long-term care and during respiratory crises. Energy needs for these chronically ill patients may be determined by the Harris-Benedict equation using appropriate stress and injury factors. Protein needs are expected to be similar to those of the debilitated, chronically ill patients—1.0 to 1.5 g/kg.[94] Patients with MG tend to gain weight and develop hyperglycemia from their medications.[104] Because physical exercise exacerbates symptoms, diet counseling is the mainstay of weight control management.[2] Some patients lose weight because of muscle fatigue and severe dysphagia. Strategies designed to reach calorie goals may include small, frequent, calorie-dense meals modified for appropriate consistency; commercial nutrition supplements; finger foods; easily prepared foods; and resting before meals. Patients in respiratory crisis may need mechanical ventilation for long periods.[107] Those who are too weak to meet their nutrient needs by eating may require enteral nutrition support.

Guillain-Barré Syndrome

Guillain-Barré syndrome (GB) (acute idiopathic polyradiculoneuritis) presents as demyelinating polyneuropathy manifested in acute, ascending or descending progression of symmetric motor weakness with cranial nerve involvement and dysautonomia.[2,108] Approximately 60% to 70% of patients report having had a viral illness not long before onset of GB symptoms. The patient's course deteriorates until a plateau is reached at which pathologic processes cease and reinnervation of muscle occurs.[2] GB is usually reversible, but 10% of patients develop relapse or quadriparesis.[2] The main cause of death from GB is pneumonia or adult respiratory distress syndrome.[109] Usual treatment is supportive care and plasmapheresis.[106,110]

Nutrition becomes a priority for preserving lean body mass, especially muscles of respiration. Roubenoff and coworkers found GB patients to be hypermetabolic and catabolic because of endocrine, infectious, and inflammatory components of the disease. These researchers utilized high-energy (40 to 45 nonprotein kilocalories per kilogram) and high-protein (2.0 to 2.5 g/kg) nutrition support to produce a favorable effect on visceral protein repletion, nitrogen balance, and resistance to pulmonary infection.[108] Indirect calorimetry is the preferred method of measuring energy expenditure. Protein needs may be estimated by nitrogen balance studies. In 10% of GB patients, liver function values may be abnormally high, but they resolve with recovery.[111] Enteral and parenteral nutrition support are often required because facial and oropharyngeal weakness, and possibly respirator dependency, can jeopardize adequate oral intake. One case of GB-like syndrome developed from hypophosphatemia due to inadequate phosphorus in PN solution.[112] Careful monitoring of nutrition parameters is an essential part of parenteral support.

Dementia and Alzheimer's Disease

Approximately 70% of dementia patients suffer from Alzheimer's disease—atrophy of the cerebral cortex, loss of neurons, and formation of neurofibrillary tangles and neuritic plaques.[109,113] The cause of these morphologic changes is not known.[114] Disease progression can be tracked by magnetic resonance imaging (MRI).[115] Characteristics of the disease include apathy, decreased attention span, poor judgment, sensory loss, distortions of vision, hearing, taste, smell, and tactile capabilities, marked agnosia (inability to recognize objects and sounds), and motor loss with apraxia (inability to execute purposeful movements).[116,117] Average interval between onset and death is 6 to 10 years.[114]

As the disease progresses increasing nutrition intervention is needed. At initial diagnosis, baseline weight and serum albumin measurements may be obtained. Weight can be recorded monthly thereafter.[116] Energy needs may be based on the Harris-Benedict equation with activity and stress factors.[78] Protein needs are estimated to be 1.0 to 1.25 g/kg.[118] The second phase of Alzheimer's disease is characterized by increasing agnosia and wandering, with erratic, nonpurposeful movements and weight loss. The patient may not recognize food, thirst, or satiety. Calorie expenditure can increase by as much as 1600 kcal per day.[119] It is important to offer care providers assistance in planning meals that are calorie dense, which should be taken in a quiet setting free of distractions (e.g., television, radio) that could divert the patient's attention from eating. For Alzheimer's patients, mimicking the behaviors of the care provider seated with them at the table is key to appropriate behavior and to enhancing intake. To maintain hydration, a cup of water may be handed to the patient every 2 hours. Patients who wander can carry a container of food cut in small pieces. Large pieces of food must be avoided if the patient has a tendency to bolt food.[116] As weight loss progresses, nutritional supplements can be added to the regimen.[120] Patients in the final phase who are bedridden and unable to feed themselves may require nutrition support.[121,122] However, several recent studies suggest that the placement of gastrostomy tubes provides no benefit to patients with dementia.[41,123-126] The authors argue that there is no evidence to support the belief that feeding tubes prevent aspiration or prolong life. A recent review could not find any randomized clinical trials comparing oral feeding to tube feedings in patients with dementia up until 1999,[124] while many observational studies suggest that tube feeding in this population may in fact do more harm than good.[41,123-126] Ethical questions arise regarding withdrawal of nutrition and hydration, although both are considered forms of medical therapy. Focus on quantity of life versus quality of life is often the issue.[9,123] It is clear that further study is warranted.

Spinal Cord Injury

Spinal cord injury (SCI) disrupts transmission of nerve impulses from brain to peripheral nerves. The degree of dysfunction depends on the cause, degree of transection, and level of cord injury.[11,127] The initial response to SCI is spinal shock, which may induce severe hypotension secondary to loss of sympathetic tone. Hemorrhage and other injuries complicate the clinical picture. The extent of damage and preservation of cord function may not be known until spinal shock subsides, which can take weeks. As the body seeks to repair damage and preserve function, abnormal muscle hyperactivity or spastic reflexes can occur.[128]

Nutrition Intervention in the Acute Phase

Generally the higher the level of SCI, the greater the nutrition risk.[129] Nutrition interventions focus on preserving body reserves and preventing secondary malnutrition. Anthropometrics are of little value because atrophic muscle is replaced by fat, water, and connective tissue.[129,130] Body weight may appear stable even though tissue wasting is severe.[131] Weight loss is commonly attributed to decreased lean body mass.[132,133] In one study, weight loss averaged 5.3 kg for paraplegics and 9.1 kg for quadriplegics by 18 days after injury.[132] IBW is adjusted for SCI to reflect decreased lean body mass by subtracting 5% to 10% for paraplegia and 10% to 15% for quadriplegia.[134]

A wide range of energy needs for SCI have been reported.[131,135-141] Kolpek found energy utilization among SCI patients to be 94% of predicted BEE using the Harris-Benedict equation, probably because of decreased metabolic activity of denervated muscle.[137] The validity of the Harris-Benedict equation in this patient population has been challenged.[135] In general,

the higher the cord lesion is, the more muscle is denervated and the lower the metabolic rate.[138] Indirect calorimetry is the most accurate measure of energy expenditure in SCI.[131,139,140] If indirect calorimetry is not available, Cox and colleagues reported that stable quadriplegics require 22.7 kcal/kg daily and paraplegics 27.9 kcal/kg.[139]

The metabolic response to SCI causes markedly excessive nitrogen excretion within 1 week of injury,[142] peaking at approximately 3 weeks.[143,144] During this phase, negative nitrogen balance has been noted (−14 to −21 g/day) and is improved only slightly in response to high protein intake (−11 g/day).[143] Rodriguez and coworkers suggest that positive nitrogen balance is not attainable within the first 7 weeks of SCI.[144]

Metabolic alterations from SCI also affect micronutrients. Hypercalcemia can be induced by immobilization, especially in young adolescent males. Symptoms associated with hypercalcemia are anorexia, abdominal cramps, nausea, vomiting, constipation, polydipsia, polyuria, and dehydration.[145] Treatment for hypercalcemia may include medications, hydration, and mobilization.[131,145] A calcium-restricted diet has not been shown to help,[142] and limiting calcium-rich foods can make the diet unpalatable.[131] Calciuria exceeds normal values at 4 weeks, peaks at 16 weeks, and can persist longer.[146] Excess potassium excretion and abnormal hyponatremia have been reported.[130] Chin and coworkers observed hyperphosphatemia in SCI patients but found it to be clinically insignificant.[131]

SCI patients may experience anorexia,[147] early satiety, dysgeusia, dysosmia, immobility, and depression.[131] Patients may be unable to take adequate sustenance and require enteral or parenteral support. Anemia[148] and gastrointestinal complications,[149] including stress ulcers, pancreatitis, and decreased motility, have been reported with SCI.[150] Early intravenous feeding has been shown to prevent stress ulcers, but enteral feeding should be initiated as soon as it is medically feasible.[151] Neurogenic bowel is common and incorporating 25 to 35 g of fiber and 2 to 3 L of fluid daily in the nutrition regimen promotes elimination.[152]

Nutrition and Permanent Cord Injuries

In SCI, the Harris-Benedict equation has not been found to be reliable for estimating long-term energy needs.[135] A range of energy expenditure has been reported: 19.3 to 35.8 kcal/kg, depending on the level of cord injury and physical activity.[135,139] To estimate needs, approximately 23 kcal/kg may be used for quadriplegics and 28 kcal/kg for paraplegics, adjusting as needed with monitored weight changes. Excessive weight gain must be avoided because obesity contributes to other medical problems and makes self-care and care providers' tasks more burdensome.[131] Cox and others reported that paraplegics given an unrestricted diet during rehabilitation gained 1.28 kg weekly and quadriplegics gained 1.84 kg.[139] Activity can contribute significantly to weight management for paraplegics. Olle and associates found that sedentary paraplegics had 23% body fat, whereas wheelchair athletes had 15.6% body fat.[153]

Hypercalciuria has been noted to last beyond the first year of SCI. It may contribute to osteoporosis,[154] lower extremity fractures,[155] and nephrolithiasis. High-protein diets may promote urinary calcium excretion and may indirectly contribute to osteoporosis.[131] Such a diet should be prescribed judiciously.

SCI patients are at high risk for pressure sores.[156] For them, decubitus ulcers and poor healing are closely correlated with weight loss, anemia, and hypoproteinemia.[157] Nutrition counseling, high-protein, high-calorie supplements, and diet fortification with calorie-dense modular components may be needed to attain sufficient intake.

Dysphagia with Neurologic Compromise

Dysphagia is defined as swallowing with difficulty. Neurologic diseases can compromise swallowing by altering nerve transmission to key muscle groups. Some 40% to 50% of stroke patients may have some aspect of dysphagia.[69] TBI patients can have a multitude of swallowing impairments (see Box 29-4).[31] Patients with GB syndrome, MG, ALS, MS, or CVA may have some symptoms of dysphagia during crises or as their conditions deteriorate.[70,158-160] More insidious is silent aspiration, which gives no outward indication to patients or care providers of swallowing impairments that lead to food or liquid passing into the airway beyond the true vocal folds.[71] The keys to treating dysphagia are early detection and timely follow-up to reduce the incidence of malnutrition and aspiration pneumonia, which lengthen the hospital stay.[70] Detecting dysphagia requires close collaboration with the physician, dietitian, therapists, and nursing staff.

Swallowing is a complex, well-coordinated motor activity that involves 25 facial and oral muscles and six cranial nerves and is divided into four complex phases.[69,70] Any neurologic compromise to cranial nerves V, VII, and IX to XII may result in some type of dysphagia (Table 29-3). Nerve impairment can alter saliva secretion and affect digestion. Saliva contains amylase for degradation of starch molecules; acid neutralizing capacity; and mucin, which acts as a lubricant and a selective permeability barrier. In the esophagus, saliva serves to neutralize the remaining refluxed acid and restore normal esophageal pH.[71] Other symptoms of possible dysphagia include frequent admissions to the hospital for pneumonia, history of aspiration pneumonia, complaints of pain on swallowing or swallowing difficulties, frequent heartburn, mouth odor, vomiting, and weight loss.[71]

Dietary manipulation is part of the treatment for dysphagia.[161] Diet modifications and progression of foods in dysphagia diets vary from facility to facility. The American Dietetic Association includes a dysphagia diet in its diet manual. The National Dysphagia Diet is currently under development and will be of great benefit in communicating patient tolerances as patients transfer from one facility to another.

Even with therapy, dysphagia can take a long time to resolve. Therefore patients who are unable safely to meet needs orally require nutrition support. Dysphagia patients usually have functional gastrointestinal tracts and tolerate enteral feedings. Enteral support via percutaneous endoscopic gastrostomy[81] or feeding distal to the pylorus reduces the risk of aspiration as compared with nasoenteric or gastrostomy feeding.[89] It should be noted that the aspiration risk associated with percutaneous gastrostomy is not less than that with nasogastric tubes.[162,163]

Conclusion

With severe traumatic brain and spinal cord injuries nutrition support is critical to moderate the hypermetabolic and hypercatabolic effects that waste tissues at extraordinary rates. Oral, enteral, and parenteral nutrition may be employed to preserve lean body mass and neurologic functions. In TBI, parenteral support has been the usual route because of altered gastrointestinal function and enteral intolerance; however, new data suggest that enteral feeding below the pylorus and before bowel sounds are heard is tolerated and may afford an advantage in preserving intestinal mucosa. Early support is known to increase survival with TBI, but its effect on neurologic outcome is not known. Less is known about what may be the best enteral or parenteral solution for SCI or TBI; that is, which ones provide maximum effect in (perhaps) limited volume. Future research will cast light on these unknowns.

The majority of neurologic diseases are chronic degenerative conditions or autoimmune disorders. The cause of some is unknown, and regimens to bring about complete reversal, perhaps with special therapy, remain to be developed. In the interim, nutrition plays a vital role in sustaining the patient through the course of disease. More research is needed on energy, protein, and micronutrient requirements in these conditions to establish baseline data that can be adjusted as the clinical course progresses. Perhaps nutrition components can help to slow the progression of Alzheimer's or MS or form a basis for rapid cure of GB syndrome. For PD, careful structuring of dietary intake around a 7:1 carbohydrate-protein ratio offers hope to some patients who now take levodopa to ameliorate symptoms. Perhaps as more of these new therapies and treatments are developed, the role of nutrition will become an even greater part of the solution.

TABLE 29-3

Effects of Dysphagia in Phases of Swallow[69-71]

Oral and Oral Preparatory Phases		Pharyngeal Phase	Esophageal Phase
Facial drooping	Difficulty in controlling saliva	Food stuck in throat	Food collects in the esophagus and enters the reopened airway after swallow Cycle is completed
Drooling	Thick, excessive saliva	Nasal regurgitation	
Piecemeal deglutition	Insufficient saliva	Coughing or choking with swallow	
Spilling of food or fluid from mouth	Inability to move food around in mouth	Weak cough	
Inability to form bolus	Avoidance of food or fluids	Voice sounds "wet" or hoarse	
Unchewed/inadequately chewed food	Mumbled speech	Frequent throat clearing	
Multiple swallows with each bite			

REFERENCES

1. Walleck CA: Preventing secondary brain injury, *AACN Clin Issues* 3: 19-28, 1992.
2. Cammermeyer M, Appledorn C (eds): *Core curriculum for neuroscience nursing,* ed 3, Chicago, 1990, American Association of Neuroscience Nurses, pp Ie1-3, Ii1-I5, Ij1-2, Is1-3, IIId1-3, IVf1-2.
3. Jennett B: Diagnosis and management of head trauma, *J Neurotrauma* 8:(suppl 1)15-S19, 1991.
4. Ott L, Young B: Nutrition in the neurologically injured patient, *Nutr Clin Pract* 6(6):223-229, 1991.
5. Friedman AH: Craniocerebral injuries. In Sabiston D (ed): *Textbook of surgery,* ed 14, Philadelphia, 1991, WB Saunders, pp 323-326.
6. Miller JD: Barbiturates and raised intracranial pressure, *Ann Neurol* 6(3):189-193, 1979.
7. Varella L: Barbiturate therapy and nutritional support in head-injured patients, *Nutr Clin Pract* 6(6):239-244, 1991.
8. Sundberg S: The use of steroids in severe head trauma, *Clin Trends Hosp Pharm* 1(1):9-12, 1987.
9. Evans NJ, Compher CW: Nutrition and the neurologically impaired patient. In Torosian MH (ed): *Nutrition for the hospitalized patient,* New York, 1995, Marcel Dekker, pp 567-590.
10. Suchner U, Senftleben U, Eckart T, et al: Enteral versus parenteral nutrition: effects on gastrointestinal function and metabolism, *Nutrition* 12(1):13-22, 1996.
11. Samuels MA (ed): *Manuel of neurologic therapeutics with essentials of diagnosis,* ed 3, Boston, 1986, Little, Brown, pp 243-257.
12. Brain Trauma Foundation: Nutritional support of brain injured patients, *J Neurotrauma* 13(11):721-729, 1996.
13. Deutschman CS, Konstantinides FN, Raup S, Cerra FB: Physiological and metabolic response to isolated closed-head injury, *J Neurosurg* 66(3):388-395, 1987.
14. Fried RC, Dickerson RN, Guenter PA, et al: Barbiturate therapy reduces nitrogen excretion in acute head injury, *J Trauma* 29(11):1558-1563, 1989.
15. Dempsey DT, Guenter P, Mullen JL, et al: Energy expenditure in acute trauma to the head with and without barbiturate therapy, *Surg Gynecol Obstet* 160(2):128-134, 1985.
16. Fried R, Dempsey D, Guenter D, et al: Barbiturates improve nitrogen balance in patients with severe head trauma, *J Parenter Enteral Nutr* 8(1):86, 1984 (abstract).
17. Magnuson B, Hatton J, Zweng T, Young B: Pentobarbital coma in neurosurgical patients: nutrition considerations, *Nutr Clin Pract* 9(4):146-150, 1994.
18. Shapiro BA, Warren J, Egol AB, et al: Practice parameters for intravenous analgesia and sedation for adult patients in the intensive care unit: an executive summary, *Crit Care Med* 23(9):1596-1600, 1995.
19. Mirenda J, Broyles G: Propofol as used for sedation in the ICU, *Chest* 108(2):539-548, 1995.
20. Lowrey TS, Dunlap AW, Brown RO, et al: Pharmacologic influence on nutrition support therapy: use of propofol in a patient receiving combined enteral and parenteral nutrition support, *Nutr Clin Pract* 11(4):147-149, 1996.
21. Clifton GL, Robertson CS, Grossman RG, et al: The metabolic response to severe head injury, *J Neurosurg* 60(4):687-696, 1984.
22. Long CL, Schaffel N, Geiger JW, et al: Metabolic response to injury and illness: estimation of energy and protein needs from indirect calorimetry and nitrogen balance, *J Parenter Enteral Nutr* 3(6):452-456, 1979.
23. Ott L, Young B, McClain C: The metabolic response to brain injury, *J Parenter Enteral Nutr* 11(5):488-493, 1987.
24. Borzotta AP, Pennings J, Papasadero B, et al: Enteral versus parenteral nutrition after severe closed head injury, *J Trauma* 37(3):459-468, 1994.
25. Robertson CB, Clifton GL, Grossman RG: Oxygen utilization and cardiovascular function in head injured patients, *Neurosurgery* 15(3):307-314, 1984.
26. Boulanger BR, Nayman R, McLean RF, et al: What are the clinical determinations of early energy expenditures in critically injured adults? *J Trauma* 37(6):969-974, 1994.
27. Young B, Ott L, Norton J, et al: Metabolic and nutritional sequelae in the non-steroid treated head injury patient, *Neurosurgery* 17(5):784-791, 1985.
28. Bruder N, Dumont JC, Francois G: Evolution of energy expenditure and nitrogen excretion in severe head-injured patients, *Crit Care Med* 19(1):43-48, 1991.
29. Chiolero R, Schutz Y, Lemarchard T, et al: Hormonal and metabolic changes following severe head injury or non-cranial injury, *J Parenter Enteral Nutr* 13(1):5-12, 1989.

30. Raurich JM, Ibanez J: Metabolic rate in severe head trauma, *J Parenter Enteral Nutr* 18:521-524, 1994.
31. Harper RA, Magnuson B, Loan T: Nutrition support for traumatic brain injury, *Support* 17(4):12-17, 1995.
32. Annis K, Ott L, Kearney PA: Nutritional support of the severe head-injured patient, *Nutr Clin Pract* 6(6):245-250, 1991.
33. Young B, Ott L, Dempsey R, et al: Relationship between admission hyperglycemia and neurological outcome of severe brain-injured patients, *Ann Surg* 210(4):466-473, 1989.
34. Teasdale G, Jennett B: Assessment of coma and impaired consciousness: a practical scale, *Lancet* 2(7872):81-84, 1974.
35. Mamelak AN, Pitts LH, Damron S: Predicting survival from head trauma 24 hours after injury: a practical method with therapeutic implications, *J Trauma Injury Infect Crit Care* 41(1):91-99, 1996.
36. Kueffner C, Braunschweig C: Metabolic alterations in head injured patients, *J Am Diet Assoc* 95(S)9:A-87, 1995 (abstract).
37. Godbole KB, Berbiglia VA, Goddard L: A head-injured patient: caloric needs, clinical progress and nursing care priorities, *J Neurosci Nurs* 23(5):290-294, 1991.
38. Young B, Ott L, Twyman D, et al: The effect of nutritional support on outcome from severe head injury, *J Neurosurg* 67(5):668-676, 1987.
39. Weekes E, Elia M: Observations on the patterns of 24-hour energy expenditure changes in body composition and gastric emptying in head-injured patients receiving nasogastric feeding, *J Parenter Enteral Nutr* 20(1):31-37, 1996.
40. Rapp RP, Young B, Twyman D, et al: The favorable effect of early parenteral feeding on survival in head-injured patients, *J Neurosurg* 58(6):906-912, 1983.
41. Kearnes P: Nutrition in neurolgical injury, *Nutr Clin Pract* 6(6):211-212, 1991.
42. American Association of Neurological Surgeons and the Congress of Neurological Surgeons, Joint Section on Neurotrauma and Critical Care: *Guidelines for the management of severe head injury. Nutritional support of brain-injured patients,* New York, 1995, Brain Trauma Foundation, pp 14-1 to 14-15.
43. Hester DD: Suggested guidelines for use by dietitians for the interpretation of indirect calorimetry data, *J Am Diet Assoc* 89(1):100-101, 1989.
44. Harris JA, Benedict FG: *Biometric studies of basal metabolism in man,* Carnegie Institute of Washington, Pub. No. 279, 1919.
45. Hadley MN: Nutrition support of head-injured patients. Nutrition, *Int J Appl Basic Nutr Sci* 12:126-127, 1996.
46. The Brain Trauma Foundation, The American Association of Neurological Surgeons, The Joint Section on Neurotrauma and Critical Care: Nutrition, *J Neurotrauma* 17(6-7):539-547, 2000.
47. Twyman D, Young AB, Ott L, et al: High protein enteral feedings. A means of achieving positive nitrogen balance in head injured patients, *J Parenter Enteral Nutr* 9(6):679-684, 1985.
48. Ford EG, Jennings LM, Andrassy RJ: Steroid administration potentiates urinary nitrogen losses in head-injured children, *J Trauma* 27(9):1074-1077, 1987.
49. Hadley MN, Grahm TW, Harrington T, et al: Nutritional support and neurotrauma: a critical review of early nutrition in forty-five acute head injury patients, *Neurosurgery* 19(3):367-373, 1986.
50. Shapira Y, Artru AA, Cotev S, et al: Brain edema and neurologic status following head trauma in rat: no effect from large volumes of isotonic or hypertonic intravenous fluids with or without glucose, *Anesthesiology* 77(1):79-85, 1992.
51. McClain CJ, Twyman DL, Ott LG, et al: Serum and urine zinc response in head injured patients, *J Neurosurg* 64(2):224-230, 1986.
52. McClain CJ, Henning B, Ott LG, et al: Mechanisms and implications of hypoalbuminemia in head-injured patients, *J Neurosurg* 69(3):386-392, 1988.
53. Varella L, Jastremski CA: Neurological impairment. In Gottschlich, MM (ed): *The science and practice of nutrition support: a case-based core curriculum,* Dubuque, 2001, American Society for Parenteral and Enteral Nutrition, pp 421-444.
54. Kirby DF: As the gut churns: feeding challenges in the head-injured patient, *J Parenter Enteral Nutr* 20(1):1-2, 1996.
55. Klodell CT et al: Routine Intragastric feeding following traumatic brain injury is safe and well tolerated, *Am J Surg* 179(3):168-171, 2000.
56. Moore RA, Moore EE, Jones TN, et al: TEN versus TPN following major abdominal trauma-reduced septic morbidity, *J Trauma* 29(7):916-923, 1989.
57. Akkersdijk JA, Roukema JA, Werken C: Percutaneous endoscopic gastrostomy for patients with severe cerebral injury, *Injury* 29(1):11-14, 1998.

58. Pepe JL, Barba CA: The metabolic response to acute traumatic brain injury and implications for nutritional support, *J Head Trauma Rehabil* 14(5):462-474, 1999.

59. Ott L, et al: Postpyloric enteral feeding costs for patients with severe head injury: blind placement, endoscopy, and PEG/J versus TPN, *J Neurotrauma* 16(3):233-242, 1999.

60. Norton JA, Ott LA, McClain C, et al: Intolerance to enteral feeding in the brain injured patient, *J Neurosurg* 68:62-66, 1988.

61. Breen JP, MacCracken K (eds): *Nutrition support manual,* Eugene OR, 1992, Sacred Heart Medical Center, pp 2-40.

62. Ott L, Young B, Phillips R, et al: Altered gastric emptying in the head-injured patient: relationship to feeding intolerance, *J Neurosurg* 74(5):738-742, 1991.

63. Kirby DF, Clifton GL, Turner H, et al: Early enteral nutrition after brain injury by percutaneous endoscopic gastrojejunostomy, *J Parenter Enteral Nutr* 15:298-302, 1991.

64. Konvolinka CW, Morell VO: Nutrition in head trauma, *Nutr Clin Pract* 6:251-255, 1991.

65. Shenkin HA, Bezier HS, Bouzarth WF: Restricted fluids intake: rational management of the neurosurgical patient, *J Neurosurg* 45(4):432-436, 1976.

66. Young B, Ott L, Haack D, et al: Effect of total parenteral nutrition upon intracranial pressure in severe head injury, *J Neurosurg* 67(1):76-80, 1987.

67. Abrams CK, Siram SM, Galsim C, et al: Selenium deficiency in long-term total parenteral nutrition, *Nutr Clin Pract* 7(4):175-178, 1992.

68. Choy C: The head-injured patient: nutritional care considerations, *Network* 12(1):7, 1993.

69. Gauwitz DF: How to protect the dysphagic stroke patient, *Am J Nurs* 95(8):34-38, 1995.

70. Kintzer T, Wood P: Dysphagia, *Network* 12:10-11, 1993.

71. Tripp F, Cordero O: Dysphagia and nutrition in the acute care geriatric patient, *Topics Clin Nutr* 6(2):60-69, 1991.

72. Lynch SG, Rose JW: Multiple sclerosis, *Disease a Month* (1):1-33, 1996.

73. Weinshenker BG, Issa M, Baskerville J: Long-term and short-term outcome of multiple sclerosis; a 3-year follow-up study, *Arch Neurol* 53(4):353-358, 1996.

74. Esparza ML, Sasaki S, Kesteloot H: Nutrition, latitude and multiple sclerosis mortality: an ecologic study, *Am J Epidemiol* 142(7):733-737, 1995.

75. Harbige LS, Jones R, Jenkins R, et al: Nutritional management in multiple sclerosis with reference to experimental models, *Ups J Med Sci Suppl* 48:189-207, 1990.

76. Bates D: Dietary lipids and multiple sclerosis, *Ups J Med Sci Suppl* 48:173-187, 1990.

77. Marshall BH: Lipids and neurological diseases, *Med Hypotheses* 34(3):272-274, 1991.

78. Barrocas A, Craig LD, Foltz MB: Nutrition support, supplementation and replacement, *Primary Care* 21(1):149-173, 1994.

79. Henderson CT: Safe and effective tube feeding of bedridden elderly, *Geriatrics* 46(8):56-66, 1991.

80. Kintzer T, Wood P: Amyotrophic lateral sclerosis (ALS), *Network* 12(1):12-13, 1993.

81. Mathus-Vliegen LMH, Louwerse LS, Merkus MP, et al: Percutaneous endoscopic gastrostomy in patients with amyotrophic lateral sclerosis and impaired pulmonary function, *Gastrointest Endosc* 40(4):463-469, 1994.

82. Strong MJ, Rowe A, Rankin RN: Percutaneous gastrojejunostomy in amyotrophic lateral sclerosis, *J Neurol Sci* 169(1-2):128-132, 1999.

83. Silani V, Kasarskis EJ, Yanagisawa N: Nutritional management in amyotrophic lateral sclerosis: a worldwide perspective, *J Neurol* 245:S13-S19, 1998.

84. Testa D, Caraceni T, Fetoni V: Branched-chain amino acids in the treatment of amyotrophic lateral sclerosis, *J Neurol* 236(8):445-447, 1989.

85. Rothstein JD, Tsai G, Kuncl RW, et al: Abnormal excitatory amino acids metabolism in amyotrophic lateral sclerosis, *Ann Neurol* 28(1):18-25, 1990.

86. Plaitakis A, Smith J, Mandeli J, Yahr MD: Pilot trial of branch-chained amino acids in amyotrophic lateral sclerosis, *Lancet* 1(8593):1015-1018, 1988.

87. Burk-Shull KA: Protein distribution to improve quality of life for those with Parkinson's disease, *Topics Clin Nutr* 10(1):65-70, 1994.

88. Atienza-Mantero E, Maitland T, Beach RS, et al: Nutritional considerations of Parkinson's disease. Proceedings of meeting, National Parkinson's Foundation, Los Angeles, CA, May 1990.

89. Lieberman A: Roundtable discussion, Saturday, Oct 16, 1993, Boston, MA, Protein distribution diets in the management of fluctuations in levodopa response. Session I. Metabolic determinants of fluctuations in levodopa response. Session II. Development of dietary alternatives to improve levodopa response. *Drugs & nutrients in neurology, special report,* Cedar Knolls, NJ, Feb 1994, National Med Info Network, pp 3-47.

90. Fernstrom JD: Dietary amino acids and brain function, *J Am Diet Assoc* 94(1):71-77, 1994.

91. Riley D, Lang AE: Practical application of a low protein diet for Parkinson's disease, *Neurology* 38(7):1026-1031, 1988.

92. Feldman RG: A pilot study of EL-422. Roundtable discussion, Saturday, Oct 16, 1993, *Drugs & nutrients in neurology. Special report,* Boston MA, Feb 1994, National Med Info Network, pp 36-42.

93. O'Brien CF: A multicenter trial of EL-422. Roundtable discussion, Saturday, Oct 16, 1993, *Drugs & nutrients in neurology. Special report,* Boston MA, Feb 1994, National Med Info Network, pp. 43-47.

94. Gersovitz M, Motil K, Munro HH, et al: Human protein requirements: assessment of the adequacy of the current recommended dietary allowance for dietary protein in the elderly men and women, *Am J Clin Nutr* 35(1):6-14, 1982.

95. Beyer PL, Palarino MY, Michalek D, et al: Weight change and body composition in patients with Parkinson's disease, *J Am Diet Assoc* 95(9):979-983, 1995.

96. Kintzer T, Wood P: Dysphagia in Parkinson's disease, *Network* 12(1):15-16, 1993.

97. Adams HP, Brott TG, Crowell RM, et al: Guidelines for the management of patients with acute ischemic stroke; a statement for healthcare professionals from a special writing group of the Stroke Council, American Heart Association, *Stroke* 25(9):1901-1913, 1994.

98. Futrell N, Milliken CH: Stroke is an emergency, *Disease a Month* XLII(4):197-264, 1996.

99. Feinburg WM, Ozturk S, Bruck D: Diabetes, hyperglycemia and hemostatic markers in acute stroke, *Stroke* 26(1):171, 1995 (abstract).

100. Wreford K. Aging. In Gines DJ (ed): *Management in rehabilitation,* Rockville, MD, 1990, Aspen Publishers, pp 209-216.

101. Kintzer T, Wood P: Dysphagia management for post CVA patients with right hemisphere brain injury, *Network* 12(1):14-15, 1993.

102. DePippo KL, Holas MA, Reding MJ, et al: Dysphagia therapy following stroke: a controlled trial, *Neurology* 44(9):1655-1660, 1994.

103. Novorian EL: Myasthenia gravis: a nursing prospective, *J Neurol Sci Nurs* 18:74-80, 1986.

104. Drachman DB: Myasthenia gravis, *N Engl J Med* 330(25):1797-1810, 1994.

105. Khan OS, Campbell WW: Myasthenia gravis presenting as dysphagia: Clinical considerations, *Am J Gastroenterol* 89(7):1083-1085, 1994.

106. Consensus Conference on Therapeutic Plasmapheresis: The utility of therapeutic plasmapheresis for neurological disorders, *JAMA* 256(10):1333-1337, 1986.

107. Mayer SA, Thomas CE, Swarup R, et al: Risk factors for prolonged intubation in myasthenic crisis, *Neurology* 27:A383-A384, 1996 (abstract).

108. Roubenoff RA, Borel CO, Hanley DF: Hypermetabolism and hypercatabolism in Guillain-Barré syndrome, *J Parenter Enteral Nutr* 16(5):464-472, 1992.

109. Geldmacher DS, Whitehouse PJ: Evaluation of dementia, *N Engl J Med* 1996:333(5):330-336.

110. Bril V, Ilse WK, Pearce R, et al: Pilot trial of immunoglobin versus plasma exchange in patients with Guillain-Barré syndrome, *Am Acad Neurol* 46:100-103, 1996.

111. Oomes PG, Van Der Meche FGA, Kleyweg RP and the Dutch Guillain-Barré Study Group: Liver function disturbances in Guillain-Barré syndrome: a prospective longitudinal study in 100 patients, *Am Acad Neurol* 46:96-100, 1996.

112. Hoff SD, Rowlands BJ: Guillain-Barré syndrome due to hypophosphatemia following intravenous hyperalimentation, *J Parenter Enteral Nutr* 12(4):414-416, 1988.

113. Gray GE: Nutrition and dementia, *J Am Diet Assoc* 89(12):1795-1802, 1989.

114. Litchford MD, Wakefield LM: Nutrient intakes and energy expenditures of residents with senile dementia of the Alzheimer's type, *J Am Diet Assoc* 87(2):211-213, 1987.

115. Fox NC, Freeborough PA, Rosser MN: Visualization and quantification of rates of atrophy in Alzheimer's disease, *Lancet* 348(9020):94-97, 1996.

116. Finely B: Nutritional needs of the person with Alzheimer's disease: practical approaches to quality care, *Network* 16(2):1-3, 8-10, 1996.

117. Mega MS, Cummings JL, Fiorello T, Gornbein J: The spectrum of behavioral changes in Alzheimer's disease, *Neurology* 46(1):130-135, 1996.

118. Campbell WW, Crim MC, Dallal GE, et al: Increased protein requirements in elderly people: new data and retrospective reassessments, *Am J Clin Nutr* 60(4):501-509, 1994.

119. Rheaume Y, Riley ME, Volicer L: Meeting nutritional needs of Alzheimer's patients who pace constantly, *J Nutr Elderly* 7:43-52, 1987.

120. Riley ME, Volicer L: Evaluation of a new nutritional supplement for patients with Alzheimer's disease, *J Am Diet Assoc* 90(3):433-435, 1990.

121. Bucht G, Sandman P: Nutritional aspects of dementia, especially Alzheimer's disease, *Age Ageing* 19(4):S32-S36, 1990.

122. Barrett JJ, Whaley WE, Powers RE: Alzheimer's disease, patients and their caregivers: medical care issues for the primary care physician, *South Med J* 89(1):1-9, 1996.

123. Gillick MR: Sounding Board: Rethinking the role of tube feeding in patients with advanced dementia, *N Engl J Med* 342(3):206-210, 2000.

124. Finucane TE, Christmas C, Travis K: Tube feeding in patients with advanced dementia: a review of the evidence, *JAMA* 282(14):1365-1370, 1999.

125. Meier DE, et al: High short-term mortality in hospitalized patients with advanced dementia: lack of benefit of tube feeding, *Arch Intern Med* 161(4):594-599, 2001.

126. Sanders DS, et al: Survival analysis in percutaneous endoscopic gastrostomy feeding: a worse outcome in patients with dementia, *Am J Gastroenterol* 95(6):1472-1475, 2000.

127. Oreskovich MR, Carrico JC: Trauma: management of the acutely injured patient. In Sabiston DC (ed): *Textbook of surgery,* ed 14, Philadelphia, 1991, WB Saunders, pp 323-326.

128. Atkinson PP, Atkinson JLD: Spinal shock, *Mayo Clinic Proc* 71:384-389, 1996.

129. Pfeiffer SC, Blust P, Leyson JFJ: Nutritional assessment of the spinal cord injured patient, *J Am Diet Assoc* 78(5):501-505, 1981.

130. Cardus D, McTaggart WG: Body sodium and potassium in men with spinal cord injury, *Arch Phys Med Rehabil* 66(3):156-159, 1985.

131. Chin DE, Kearns P: Nutrition in the spinal-injured patient, *Nutr Clin Pract* 6(6):213-222, 1991.

132. Kearns PJ, Thompson JD, Werner PC, et al: Nutritional and metabolic response to acute spinal cord injury, *J Parenter Enteral Nutr* 16(1):11-15, 1992.

133. Claus-Walker J, Halstead LS: Metabolic and endocrine changes in spinal cord injury: IV. Compounded neurologic dysfunctions, *Arch Phys Med Rehabil* 63(12):632-638, 1982.

134. O'Brien RY. Spinal cord injury. In Gines DJ (ed): *Nutrition management in rehabilitation,* Rockville, MD, 1990, Aspen, pp159-173.

135. Lee BY, Agarwal N, Corcoran L, et al: Assessment of nutritional and metabolic status of paraplegics, *J Rehab Res Dev* 22:11-17, 1985.

136. Kearns PJ Jr, Pipp TL, Quirk M, Campolo M: Nutritional requirements in quadriplegics, *J Parenter Enteral Nutr* 6:577, 1982 (abstract).

137. Kolpeck JH, Ott LG, Record KE, et al: Comparison of urinary urea nitrogen excretion and measured energy expenditure in spinal cord injury and nonsteroid-treated severe head trauma patients, *J Parenter Enteral Nutr* 13:277-280, 1989.

138. Mollinger LA, Spurr GB, El Ghatit AZ, et al: Daily energy expenditure and basal metabolic rates of patients with spinal cord injury, *Arch Phys Med Rehabil* 66(7):420-426, 1985.

139. Cox, SAR, Weiss, SM, Posuniak EA, et al: Energy expenditure after spinal cord injury: an evaluation of stable rehabilitating patients, *J Trauma* 25(5):419-423, 1985.

140. Shizgal HM, Roza A, Leduc B, et al: Body composition in quadriplegic patients, *J Parenter Enteral Nutr* 10:364-368, 1986.

141. Dietz JM, Bertschy M, Gschaedler R, Dollfus P: Reflections on the intensive care of 106 acute cervical spinal cord injury patients in the resuscitation unit of a general traumatology center, *Paraplegia* 24(6):343-349, 1986.

142. Schneider AB, Sherwood LM: Calcium homeostasis and pathogenesis and management of hypercalcemic disorders, *Metabolism* 23(10):975-1007, 1974.

143. Kaufman HH, Rowlands BJ, Stein DK, et al: General metabolism in patients with acute paraplegia and quadriplegia, *Neurology* 16:309-313, 1985.

144. Rodriquez DJ, Clevenger FW, Osler TM, et al: Obligatory negative nitrogen balance following spinal cord, *J Parenter Enteral Nutr* 15:319-322, 1991.

145. Maynard FM, Imai K: Immobilization hypercalcemia in spinal cord injury, *Arch Phys Med Rehabil* 58(1):16-24, 1977.

146. Claus-Walker J, Halstead LS, Rodriquez GP, Henry YK: Spinal cord injury hypercalcemia: therapeutic profile, *Arch Phys Med Rehabil* 63(3):108-115, 1982.

147. Dunn D, Ridout J: Increased incidence of anorexia in spinal cord injured adults, *Arch Phys Med Rehabil* 75:718, 1994 (abstract).

148. Huang CT, DeVivo MJ, Stover SL: Anemia in acute phase of spinal cord injury, *Arch Phys Med Rehabil* 71(1):3-7, 1990.

149. Carey ME, Nance FC, Kirgis HD, et al: Pancreatitis following spinal cord injury, *J Neurosurg* 47(6):917-922, 1977.

150. Weingarden SI: The gastrointestinal system and spinal cord injury, *Phys Med Rehabil Clin North Am* 3(4):765-781, 1992.

151. Kuric J, Lucas CE, Ledgerwood AM, et al: Nutrition support: a prophylaxis against stress bleeding after spinal cord injury, *Paraplegia* 27(2):140-145, 1989.

152. Blisset PA: Nutrition in acute spinal cord injury, *Crit Care Nurs Clin North Am* 2:375-384, 1990.

153. Olle MM, Pivarnik JM, Klish WJ, Morrow JR Jr: Body composition of sedentary and physically active spinal cord injured individuals estimated from total body electrical conductivity, *Arch Phys Med Rehabil* 74(7):706-710, 1993.

154. Leslie WD, Nance PW: Dissociated hip and spine demineralization: a specific finding in spinal cord injury, *Arch Phys Med Rehabil* 74(9):960-964, 1993.

155. Ragnarsson KT, Sell GH: Lower extremity fractures after spinal cord injury: a retrospective study, *Arch Phys Med Rehabil* 62(9):418-423, 1981.

156. Yarkony GM: Pressure ulcers: a review, *Arch Phys Med Rehabil* 75(8):908-917, 1994.

157. Moolten SE: Bedsores in the chronically ill patient, *Arch Phys Med Rehabil* 53(9):430-438, 1972.

158. Spofford B: History and physical examination. In Cummings CW, Fredrickson JM, Harker LA, et al. (eds): *Otolaryngology: head and neck surgery,* St Louis, 1993, CV Mosby.

159. Horner J, Bouyer FG, Alberts MJ, Helms MJ: Dysphagia following brainstem stroke: clinical correlates and outcome, *Arch Neurol* 48:1170-1173, 1991.

160. Scott A, Heughan A: A review of dysphagia in four cases of motor neuron disease, *Palliative Med* 7:41-47, 1993.

161. Curran J, Gropher ME: Development and dissemination of an aspiration risk, reduction diet, *Dysphagia* 5(1):6-12, 1990.

162. Ciocon JO, Silverstone FA, Graver LM, Foley CJ: Tube feedings in elderly patients: Indications, benefits, and complications, *Arch Intern Med* 148(2):429-433, 1988.

163. Raha SK, Woodhouse K: The use of percutaneous endoscopic gastrostomy (PEG) in 161 consecutive elderly patients, *Age Ageing* 23(22):162-163, 1994.

Pulmonary and Cardiac Failure

30

Denise Baird Schwartz, MS, RD, FADA, CNSD

NUTRITION is intricately linked to pulmonary function because underfeeding and overfeeding affect outcomes. Malnutrition is common in persons with respiratory disease and, if prolonged, can result in decreased respiratory muscle mass and decreased ventilatory drive. Malnutrition can cause pulmonary failure, and, conversely, pulmonary failure can lead to malnutrition. The effects of nutritional status on metabolism and pulmonary physiology are evident in all patients with ventilatory impairment. Refeeding improves functional capacities and can be critical for weaning patients from mechanical ventilation. Overfeeding can increase ventilatory demand, rendering the patient "unweanable" from mechanical ventilation. The goals of nutrition support in pulmonary failure are to improve the patient's overall nutritional status, enhance the immune system and promote respiratory muscle function. Early assessment of nutritional status in patients with pulmonary failure is essential, and early enteral feeding may be beneficial.[1-3]

Nutrition support in cardiac failure focuses on preventing exacerbation of clinical symptoms with reducing fluid and limiting sodium intake in the alimentation. Adequate nutrition support in patients undergoing cardiac surgery who have postoperative complications is prime. This chapter provides an overview of the respiratory system and the role of nutrition in optimizing organ function for patients with pulmonary failure, aspects of heart failure, and those undergoing cardiac surgery.

Overview of the Respiratory System and Function

Structure and Function

The respiratory system can be divided into three basic functional components. The drive mechanism attempts to maintain homeostasis via various feedback controls. Carbon dioxide, oxygen, and hydrogen ion concentrations determine the rate of respiration by acting directly on the respiratory center in the brain and by acting on chemoreceptors in the carotid arteries and aorta. The muscles of respiration are several paired muscles or muscle groups in the neck, around the rib cage, and in the abdomen, plus the diaphragm, which separates the chest from the abdomen. The diaphragm is the principal muscle of respiration. The lungs provide the surface over which oxygen can move from the external environment into the body and carbon dioxide produced in the tissues can pass to the outside. Removal of carbon dioxide and provision of oxygen for metabolic needs are dependent on an adequate quantity of ventila-

tion reaching the gas-exchange surface in the lung. Through the process of gas exchange, the respiratory system provides oxygen for transport to the tissues. Alveoli are the functional units of the lungs responsible for the exchange of gases between the air and the blood. Thus the prime function of the respiratory system is to allow oxygen to move from the air into the venous blood and carbon dioxide to move out.[4-6]

Blood Gas Analysis

Analysis of blood gas values includes evaluation of both acid-base balance and oxygenation in comparison with normal values (Table 30-1). Three components of arterial blood gases are analyzed to determine the acid-base balance: $Paco_2$, HCO_3, and pH.[7] $Paco_2$ is a direct indicator of the effectiveness of ventilation. HCO_3 is a reflection of renal participation in maintenance of acid-base balance. pH is a measurement of free hydrogen ion concentration in the blood.

Types of Pulmonary Failure

Pulmonary failure is the inability of the respiratory system to provide adequate oxygenation of the arterial blood, with or without adequate elimination of carbon dioxide. Acute respiratory failure occurs when arterial carbon dioxide rises above 50 torr (mm Hg) and arterial oxygen drops below 60 torr. It should be noted that normal values for these parameters can be altered by the age of the individual. Pulmonary failure can result from various primary or secondary disorders of the airways, lung parenchyma, chest wall, and neural processes involved in breathing. Respiratory muscle fatigue secondary to an imbalance in respiratory muscle energetics has been suggested as a

---

TABLE 30-1

Blood Gas Glossary[4,7,8]

Term	Definition
pH	Negative logarithm of the hydrogen ion concentration expressed as a positive number
$Paco_2$	Partial pressure of carbon dioxide in arterial blood
Pao_2	Partial pressure of oxygen in arterial blood
O_2 saturation	Oxygen content carried in arterial blood in combination with hemoglobin
Base excess (BE)	Provides an additional method of quantifying the metabolic contribution to acid/base changes, determination of BE includes accounting of pH, $Paco_2$ and the total hemoglobin
1 torr	Pressure of 1 mm of mercury under standard conditions of temperature and atmospheric pressure

Acknowledgment: A special thank you is extended to Deborah W. Silverman, MS, RD, LD, FADA, who contributed to the first edition chapter.

cause of pulmonary failure in patients with pulmonary disease.[7,9,10]

Among the many causes of pulmonary failure are altered function of the brain, spinal cord, neuromuscular structures, thorax, upper and lower airways, and cardiovascular system. Chronic obstructive pulmonary disease (COPD), a disorder characterized by persistent obstruction of bronchial airflow, affects the lower airways. The three disorders that most often cause COPD are bronchial asthma, chronic bronchitis, and pulmonary emphysema.[5,11]

Pulmonary Component of Multisystem Organ Failure

Acute Respiratory Distress Syndrome

Acute respiratory distress syndrome (ARDS, also known as *adult respiratory distress syndrome*) is a multisystem syndrome that can be triggered by both traumatic and nontraumatic events. All patients who develop ARDS initially have an acute lung injury, but not all patients with acute lung injury develop ARDS. ARDS describes the onset of acute respiratory failure characterized by pulmonary edema secondary to increased microvascular permeability. The most significant risk factor for development of ARDS appears to be sepsis. ARDS probably develops from varied insults at the cellular level: initially, a direct or indirect injury to the lungs, followed by a systemic response including release of chemical mediators such as complement fragments, endotoxins, and tumor necrosis factors.[12,13]

ARDS can occur in isolation, but more frequently it is associated with multisystem organ failure (MSOF). ARDS can incite the development of MSOF, or it can develop secondary to pathophysiologic derangements accompanying the MSOF.[14] Treatment goals for ARDS are to identify and treat the underlying condition while supporting physiologic function. Generally, this can be accomplished by maintaining optimal tissue oxygen delivery, minimizing pulmonary edema, providing nutrition support, and preventing or managing infection, along with emotional support. Managing ARDS is never easy. Maintaining oxygenation and ventilation, tissue perfusion, and organ function requires coordination of ventilator and oxygen therapy changes, pharmacologic intervention, and nutrition support, all while trying to resolve the underlying pathology.[12] Meduri and colleagues[15] studied 27 consecutive patients with severe medical ARDS and found that unfavorable outcome in acute lung injury is related to the degree of inflammatory response at the onset and during the course of ARDS. Inflammatory cytokines have been related to the development of ARDS, shock, and MSOF.

Mangialardi and associates[16] found hypoproteinemia to predict ARDS development, weight gain and death in patients with sepsis. Low or borderline serum total protein levels (< 6 g/dl) was found in 92% of the 178 patients that developed ARDS. Patients with low serum total protein levels may be more prone to develop pulmonary edema even when elevated hydrostatic pressures are not present. It appears that the degree of hypoproteinemia and the change in the protein levels over time are the most significant predictors of weight change, ventilator dependence, and survival in sepsis-induced ARDS.

Vasilyev and coworkers[17] analyzed the results of an international, multicenter, prospective survey conducted to determine the hospital survival rates of patients with potentially reversible acute respiratory failure. The most important predictors of in-hospital survival for patients in acute respiratory failure supported by mechanical ventilation were found to be (1) severity of lung dysfunction, (2) actual cause of the acute failure, (3) high degree of mechanical ventilation required to achieve acceptable arterial blood gas values, (4) existence and severity of hypoxemia when the patient is receiving maximum safe ventilator support, (5) length of time on mechanical ventilation before the patient shows significant improvement in natural lung function, and (6) MSOF.

McIntyre and associates[18] systematically reviewed clinical trials in ARDS to determine the effect of various therapies on outcome. Studies were graded for scientific evidence. Based on the analysis, lung protective ventilator strategy was the first therapy found to improve outcome in ARDS and was supported by improved outcome in a single large, prospective trial and a second smaller trial. However, other therapies for ARDS, such as noninvasive positive pressure ventilation, inverse ratio ventilation, fluid restriction, inhaled nitric oxide, almitrine, prostacyclin, liquid ventilation, surfactant, and immune-modulating therapies were not recommended at this time. One of the major concerns in analyzing ARDS studies is the need to identify patient subgroups with similar pathophysiologic and biochemical mechanisms of disease that react differently to various therapies. Future strategies in this population may include one or a combination of the following interventions such as high-frequency ventilation, lung recruitment maneuvers, β_2-adrenergic stimulation, protein kinase inhibition, phosphatidic acid generation inhibition, antagonism of neutrophil endothelium adhesion, complement inhibition, IL-10, and elastase inhibition.

Multisystem Organ Failure

MSOF generally has a predictable course beginning with the lungs and followed by hepatic, intestinal, and renal failure, in that order. Pulmonary criteria for dysfunction include hypoxia requiring respirator-assisted ventilation for at least 3 to 5 days, with progressive ARDS requiring positive end-expiratory pressure (PEEP) greater than 10 cm H_2O and F_{IO_2} greater than 50% oxygen concentration. Hemodynamic and heart failure are usually later manifestations of MSOF, whereas onset of central nervous system alterations can occur either early or late. Physiologically, these patients are hypermetabolic and have increased cardiac output with decreased systemic vascular resistance. The actual sequence pattern of organ failure may be modified by the presence of chronic disease or by the nature of the precipitating clinical event.[19]

The patient with MSOF has a very characteristic reduction in peripheral oxygen extraction. It is now apparent that the reduction is associated with a switch from normal supply-independent oxygen consumption to pathologic supply-dependent oxygen consumption. It is this change in physiology that is associated with the high cardiac output observed in these patients. The question remains, what level of oxygen transport is high enough to ensure that residual pockets of ischemic tissue are not present?[20]

This imbalance between oxygen supply and demand occurs when the body cannot supply organs with the oxygen they need to meet the demands of a higher metabolic rate, tissue damage, and fever. Oxygen supply is limited by hypotension and poor control of blood flow in the microcirculation. This oxygen supply is also compromised by lung abnormalities. Because the pulmonary capillaries are leaky, too much fluid moves into the lung tissue and alveoli. Collapsed alveoli, pulmonary edema, and thick secretions hinder gas exchange.[21]

The most essential point in MSOF is that the cause of the continued leukocyte system activation is probably major wounds and marginally viable tissue. This can include inadequately resuscitated gut mucosa on a hidden gut wound that may be atrogenic. Early enteral feeding can play a major role in maintaining adequate gut function and preventing MSOF.[20] To give the patient the best chance at recovery from MSOF, the entire health care team must optimize and coordinate all aspects of patient care.[21]

Mechanical Ventilation and Weaning

Mechanical Ventilation

Mechanical ventilation is a method of managing the gas exchange ($Paco_2$ and Pao_2) in the lungs with a machine (Table 30-2). It is used to overcome a patient's inability to breathe or oxygenate adequately. Therapy must be individualized to the needs of the patient. Several aspects of ventilator therapy must be considered when tailoring the mechanical ventilation therapy to the patient.[7,22] Routine management of a mechanically ventilated patient includes monitoring breath sounds, chest wall movement, vital signs, and comfort; suctioning the endotracheal tube and oropharynx; monitoring ventilator settings and function; and assessing changes in pulse oximetry and arterial blood gas values.[12]

The management of patients who require mechanical ventilation is obviously geared toward ensuring adequate gas exchange as a priority while optimizing efforts to improve lung function. Regardless of the cause, whether acute respiratory failure is due to primary pulmonary disease or to lung injury as a consequence of systemic disease, the principal goal of mechanical ventilation is to restore normal gas exchange until the primary disease process is controlled.[23]

Once the acute illness is controlled, the patient must make the transition from mechanical ventilation to full spontaneous breathing; this is *weaning*. The duration of weaning from mechanical ventilation is a function of the patient's general condition, the severity of acute respiratory failure, and the length of time on mechanical ventilation.[23] Despite many investigators' attempts to identify weaning predictors and weaning modes for long-term (more than 3 days) mechanically ventilated patients, none has emerged as superior. Therefore, guidelines for care of these patients have yet to be developed.[24] Because successful weaning depends on multiple physiologic systems—pulmonary, cardiovascular, skeletal, muscle, neurologic, and metabolic—it is likely that no single parameter can accurately represent homeostasis in all of these systems.[25]

Burns and associates[26] focused on identifying the four stages of weaning: acute, prewean, wean, and outcome. They attempted to define these distinct stages by using clinical

instruments designed to quantify severity of illness, patient stability, or weaning readiness. Data from 97 adult patients requiring more than 3 days mechanical ventilation were collected prospectively. The goal was to be able to better determine appropriate interventions for the four stages, as well as predict weaning outcomes. Nutrition intervention, including oral, tube feeding, and parenteral nutrition (PN), was addressed in each of the four phases. Respiratory factors alone were found to be insufficient to facilitate, identify, and optimize decision making about the four stages; physiologic and respiratory factors were both required (Table 30-3).

TABLE 30-2

Mechanical Ventilation Glossary

Term	Definition
Controlled mechanical ventilation (CMV)	Patient's alveolar ventilation is determined solely by the settings on the ventilator. CMV abolishes the respiratory drive. The patient is often sedated to allow the ventilator to control the respirations.
Intermittent mandatory ventilation (IMV)	During IMV the patient remains connected to the ventilator and breathes spontaneously between controlled breaths (called *mandatory breaths*). During IMV the spontaneous breath and the mandatory breath are not necessarily synchronized, and a mandatory breath may be delivered anywhere in the patient's respiratory cycle. A large tidal volume is given at relatively infrequent intervals. It is often combined with PEEP or CPAP. This pattern may be useful in weaning a patient from a ventilator.
Synchronized intermittent mandatory ventilation (SIMV)	Ventilator breaths are synchronized with the patient's spontaneous breaths. The ventilator is informed of the patient's respiratory cycle and stacking of breaths is eliminated.
Positive end-expiratory pressure (PEEP)	Maintenance of greater than atmospheric pressure at the airway opening at the end of expiration during positive-pressure ventilation. Its primary purpose is to prevent collapse of airways and alveoli. It increases the functional residual capacity to allow more surface area across which O_2 can diffuse.
Continuous positive airway pressure (CPAP)	Low positive-pressure applied continuously to the airway while a ventilated patient breathes spontaneously. The airway pressure is held constant above atmospheric pressure throughout the entire respiratory cycle.
Pressure-support ventilation (PSV)	Patient's spontaneous breaths are assisted by having the pressure at the airway opening held relatively constant during inspiration.
High-frequency ventilation (HFV)	Mode of ventilation that delivers small tidal volumes at very rapid respiratory rates (60-100 breaths per minute).
Fractional inspired oxygen concentration (FIO_2)	Fraction of inspired oxygen or oxygen concentration; delivery of a concentration of oxygen of 21% to 100% to satisfy patient's oxygen demands.
Tidal volume (VT)	Volume of air inspired or expired with a normal breath.
Dead-space ventilation	Portion of ventilation in the tracheobronchial tree that is not involved in gas exchange.
Vital capacity (VC)	Maximal volume of air that can be expired following a maximal inspiration.
Minute ventilation (VE)	Measurement of total amount of air inspired and expired in a minute.

Reasons for Ventilator Dependence

Ventilator dependence exists for several reasons. Extra-respiratory factors include cardiovascular dysfunction, psychologic dysfunction, malnutrition, and multiple organ failure.[27] Most authors would agree that adequate nutrition is a necessary prerequisite for successful weaning and that markers such as serum albumin, which is also linked to total body fluid less than 3.0 g/dl, correlate with inability to be weaned and death; yet few indices incorporate this marker.[24] Both overfeeding and underfeeding have been linked with the inability to wean patients from mechanical ventilation. Increased carbon dioxide production as a result of excessive carbohydrate intake and especially with excessive total kilocalories has been identified as a factor in preventing successful weaning from mechanical ventilation. The clinical presentation is excessive ventilatory demand with a high minute ventilation requirement to keep the $Paco_2$ normal;[28] however, pulmonary failure, rather than overfeeding, is probably the most important reason for ventilator dependency.

Goals for Weaning from Mechanical Ventilation

In deciding whether to extubate the ventilated patient recovering from pulmonary failure, the clinician must consider two factors: the patient's ability to provide adequate gas exchange during spontaneous ventilation and the patient's ability to provide and protect a patent upper airway. Weaning and extubation should be approached as two separate decision processes, both of which must be independently assessed before extubation is attempted.[25] Goals for weaning from long-term mechanical ventilation include reducing the amount of support, decreasing the invasiveness of support, increasing independence from mechanical devices, preservation of function, and maintaining medical stability.[29]

Collaborative Care of Mechanically Ventilated Patients

Coordinated and collaborative care has been linked to improved outcome and mortality rates in critical care units. The use of a collaborative, multidisciplinary team to effect timely communication and promote comprehensive care planning for long-term mechanical ventilation patients has been reported. Another way to manage patients with complicated problems who also require long-term mechanical ventilation is to assign them to special care units. Such units often use protocols, standardized weaning plans, or critical pathways to expedite weaning. Regardless of which option is selected, care delivery systems that provide efficient, systematic, coordinated, and comprehensive planning are attractive to consumers and health care providers.[24]

Respiratory System Pharmacology
Pulmonary Failure Medications

Three specific drug groups are commonly used for COPD (Table 30-4). Various drug therapies, conventional and unconventional, have been used in attempts to reverse ARDS. Corticosteroids were once used to try to blunt the inflammatory response during the acute injury phase by decreasing complement activation and neutrophil aggregation, but research has shown that, in most patients corticosteroids do not prevent ARDS and high-dose steroids may even be harmful for patients with septic ARDS. Vasodilators may be ordered to manage pulmonary hypertension, but they dilate systemic vessels, too, causing hypotension. To prevent hemodynamic instability, they are typically given with inotropic drugs such as dopamine and dobutamine. In preliminary studies of patients with sepsis-induced ARDS, use of aerosolized artificial surfactant has been associated with decreased shunting, increased lung compliance, and improved survival rates. This is given to patients on ventilators and is dispensed during inspiration.[12]

Pharmacologic Role in Preventing Postoperative Pulmonary Complications

A variety of pharmaceutical interventions have been tried for postoperative prevention and treatment of pulmonary complications. These include respiratory stimulants, mucolytics, and surfactant stimulants. Drugs such as aminophylline, caffeine, and β_2-agonists have been shown to enhance diaphragm activity and

TABLE 30-3

Clinical Pathway: Mechanical Ventilation Nutrition Components[26]

	Outcomes: Phase 1 Intubation/acute	Outcomes: Phase 2 Prewean	Outcomes: Phase 3 Wean	Outcomes: Phase 4 Rehabilitation
Problem: Nutrition	Tolerating tube or PN Receiving adequate nutrition as evidenced by increasing albumin or normal prealbumin	→	→	Taking PO diet →
Interdisciplinary Communication: Consults	Nutrition Support Services		Speech therapy for swallow	
Dressing tubes/drains	Insert NGT or small bore feeding tube	→	D/C NGT; assess for gastrostomy	
Nutrition	Initiate tube feed by day 3 Initiate PN if unable to tolerate TF by day 7	→	→	Maintain tube feed at night until cleared for adequacy of nutrition; begin soft or mechanical soft diet if not a risk for aspiration; as tolerated.

D/C, Discontinue; *NGT,* nasogastric tube, *PO,* per os (by mouth); *TF,* tube feeding; *PN,* parenteral nutrition.

TABLE 30-4

Most Common Types of Medications Used in COPD[11]

Medications	Mode of Action
Bronchodilators	Open airways by relaxing muscle walls and loosening mucus by increasing airflow
Steroids	Open breathing tubes by decreasing swelling
Antibiotics	Fight infections by killing bacteria (sometimes used prophylactically)

prevent respiratory muscle fatigue. Despite these effects, no data support their routine use in reducing postoperative pulmonary complications. At this time few data support specific pharmaceutical interventions to prevent or minimize postoperative pulmonary complications.[30]

Pharmacotherapy Considerations for Preventing Stress Ulcers and Nosocomial Pneumonia

Patients with acute respiratory failure have several risk factors that result in microbial colonization of the lower respiratory and gastrointestinal tracts. Endotracheal tubes or tracheostomy sites can easily become colonized with microbes, introducing bacteria into the lower respiratory tract. Nasogastric tubes placed for decompression of the stomach may allow microbes to migrate into the gastrointestinal tract. Also, use of histamine H_2-receptor antagonists or antacids to prevent stress ulcers can increase gastric pH and allow microbes to proliferate. This may contribute to the development of nosocomial pneumonia; the organisms are thought to move from the stomach to the respiratory tract. Sucralfate is an alternative therapy for stress-ulcer prophylaxis that does not alter gastric pH and may be beneficial in preventing this type of infection.[2]

A second pathway for microbial overgrowth is across the gut lumen, causing hematogenous or lymphatic spread, which can contribute to bacteremia or sepsis. Several studies have evaluated the effect of selective gut decontamination with two to three drugs applied topically to the oropharynx or the stomach. Although selective gut decontamination may reduce the incidence of nosocomial infection, further research is needed to define optimal regimens and duration of therapy.[2]

Enteral feeding may be effective in preventing stress ulceration. Even feedings into the small bowel appears to assist in maintaining an intragastric pH greater than 4 and may decrease the incidence of stress-related mucosal damage, possibly through a humoral mechanism.[2]

Patients who are on ventilator therapy with PEEP may be at increased aspiration risk. Many medications such as theophylline, anticholinergics, calcium channel blockers, β-agonists, and α-antagonists cause reduction in lower esophageal sphincter pressure. All of these factors can increase the risk of life-threatening pulmonary aspiration.[31]

Pharmacologic Approaches to Promote Weaning

A long list of pharmacologic agents commonly used in the intensive care unit (ICU) can interfere with weaning. Those most often encountered are sedatives, narcotics, tranquilizers, and hypnotics, and all are capable of depressing central ventilatory drive. Neuromuscular blocking agents such as pancuronium, vecuronium, and atracurium render patients incapable of somatic muscle activity and thus cause ventilatory muscle weakness or paralysis. In the presence of even mild renal insufficiency, clearance can be delayed, sometimes for days, resulting in persistent ventilatory muscle weakness. Prolonged muscle weakness following use of these agents during mechanical ventilation is a recently appreciated syndrome that can substantially increase a patient's requirement for ICU care.[28] Medications such as vecuronium may paralyze the gut and decrease tube feeding tolerance, in addition to reducing energy requirements.

Anxiolytic, neuroleptic, and antidepressant medications all have a role in treating anxiety, agitation, and depression in the ICU; however because they have the potential for respiratory depression and for some psychological dysfunctions such as sleep disturbances, they should be used with caution during weaning. Opiates are particularly good at blocking dyspnea, especially dyspnea associated with lung edema and irritant dysfunction, and have been used to make patients with chronic dyspnea more comfortable. Yet, because of associated neurologic depression and decreased respiratory drive, their role in the weaning process may be limited. Aerosolized opiates may be an attractive alternative; however, more research is needed in this area.[32]

Use of recombinant human growth hormone is being investigated in severely malnourished patients with COPD. In initial studies it appears that malnourished patients with COPD respond to growth hormone therapy with improved nitrogen balance and a significant increase in maximum inspiratory pressure. Further long-term placebo-controlled trials are necessary to confirm these results.[2]

The use of aminophylline and β-agonists for enhancing respiratory muscle contractility and preventing fatigue has been the focus of several early studies. The usefulness of these agents in weaning patients to prevent or offset fatigue has yet to be determined. A wide variety of drugs such as anxiolytics and bronchodilators are used to promote weaning, but few studies have associated specific categories of pharmacologic agents with weaning ability or outcomes.[24]

Role of Malnutrition in Pulmonary Failure
Muscle Compromise

Decreased strength, greater fatigability, and reduced endurance of the respiratory muscles are associated with severe malnutrition.[33] It now appears that the respiratory muscles (diaphragm, intercostals, accessory muscles of respiration) are subject to the same catabolic effects as other skeletal muscles during starvation or stress. Diaphragmatic mass decreases with body weight, diminished inspiratory and expiratory muscle strength, and reduction in vital capacity and endurance. It is not clear whether inadequate fuel availability or increased utilization is responsible for the respiratory muscle changes associated with malnutrition.[34] Murciano and colleagues[35] studied 15 patients with anorexia nervosa and found diaphragmatic function to be markedly impaired in severely malnourished patients free of any disease, particularly respiratory disease.

Malnutrition has several adverse effects on the entire pulmonary system, affecting respiratory muscle function. The nutrition-mediated respiratory muscle dysfunction begins to occur within days of deprivation. One is the loss of muscle mass secondary to the negative nitrogen balance of semistarvation. A second effect of malnutrition is to deplete energy reserves such as energy-rich phosphates and glycogen, which limits metabolic efficiency and endurance. Impaired function of the respiratory muscles because of malnutrition can result in a reduction of alveolar ventilation, which can be evident clinically as hypercarbia. Under normal circumstances, the respiratory muscles serve as bellows, which move atmospheric gas in and out of the lungs at a rate that allows the lungs to effect the appropriate gas exchange necessary to support cellular metabolism. Respiratory insufficiency develops as parenchymal lung disease and associated ventilation-perfusion mismatch increase respiratory muscle work to compensate for the reduced efficiency of gas exchange. If the ventilation-perfusion mismatch is severe, the respiratory muscles become fatigued, causing a vicious cycle with worsening gas exchange; increasing work of breathing; and, eventually, pulmonary failure.[23]

Micronutrient status must also be evaluated because severe hypophosphatemia results in neuromuscular dysfunction and may exacerbate pulmonary failure. Hypophosphatemia can result in decreased delivery of oxygen to the tissues and decreased contractility of the respiratory muscles. In addition, magnesium deficiency is associated with abnormalities of respiratory muscle strength.[23]

Severe Hypoalbuminemia-Altering Function

When combined with critical illness, nutritional depletion is associated with expansion of extracellular fluid and reductions in the intracellular fluid space. Sodium balance is positive and total body sodium is increased in this setting. These pathophysiologic changes result in anasarca and increased interstitial lung water. Low serum albumin levels lead to decreased colloid osmotic pressure and possible pulmonary edema. This increased extravascular lung water reduces functional residual capacity and pulmonary reserve.[23,36]

Impaired Immunocompetence

The principal immune functions impaired in protein-calorie malnutrition are cell-mediated immunity, secretory immunoglobulin A (IgA) antibody response, the complement system, and bactericidal capacity of neutrophils.[37] Dysfunctions of both T and B cells are well documented. The integrity of the respiratory epithelium and its ciliary function are compromised during starvation, with consequential impairment of the pulmonary defense system.[38]

Death from starvation is often due to pneumonia. Malnutrition associated with critical illness impairs the immune response. Anergy is commonly manifested in impaired T-lymphocyte response to mitogens. These effects have a detrimental impact on alveolar defenses. The respiratory epithelium of malnourished patients has increased bacterial adherence and decreased IgA secretion. The predisposition to lung infection has further consequences for patients with malnutrition because of alterations in the sequence of injury and repair. Damaged fibers of the lung matrix are removed by enzymes such as proteinases and collagenases, which are activated in the immune response process. Malnutrition or critical illness can deplete circulating antiproteinases, resulting in unopposed proteinase activity. Each pulmonary infection is then met with an exaggerated amount of lung fiber destruction, leading to a weakened and structurally abnormal matrix.[1] Deficiencies of individual nutrients, such as vitamin A, pyridoxine, zinc, and others, can also impair immunocompetence and increase vulnerability to lung infection.[37]

Surfactant Deficit

Biochemical measurements in progressive malnutrition demonstrated a reduction in desaturated lecithin, which is a major component of surfactant.[3] Even during short-term starvation, capacity to both synthesize and secrete surfactant seems to be decreased.[38]

The function of pulmonary surfactant is emphasized because of its role in maintaining alveolar stability; reducing the work of breathing; and, perhaps, protecting against fluid transudations. The importance of surfactant is underscored by the fact that, with experimental malnutrition there is a marked initial reduction in surfactant phospholipid production within the type II cells of the lung, which eventually return to normal.[37]

Additional effects of work on breathing are due to changes in lung surface recoil and pressure-volume curves. This also apparently relates to a decrease in surfactant production. Surfactant is stored in the lamellar bodies of the granular alveolar pneumocyte. Decreased volume and quantity of these organelles have been found when malnutrition is present.[34]

Altered Antioxidant Defense System

The damage effect by oxygen, at least as it relates to free radical mechanisms, occurs directly through reactions with cellular lipids, proteins, and nucleic acids. Indirectly, this damage can occur through inflammatory cells that are attracted to the area of injury and have the capacity to either form additional free radicals or release proteolytic enzymes into surrounding tissue. Free radicals are produced in the body as byproducts of normal metabolism; however, because they are highly reactive, they can damage cellular components and are implicated in a variety of diseases.[39] It is clear that antioxidant protective mechanisms can be compromised by nutritional deficiencies of sulfur-containing amino acids, copper, selenium, iron, vitamin E, carotenes, and ascorbic acid, fatty acid saturation in lipids, and calories. Decreased concentrations of serum vitamin E associated with increased lipid peroxidation have been reported in patients with sepsis-induced ARDS. Patients with processes such as ARDS may need more antioxidants to meet demands of excessive free radical production and the effects of acute-phase alterations in vitamin uptake and mobilization.[37,40] Goode and colleagues[41] studied 16 consecutive patients with septic shock and found decreased antioxidant status in the face of enhanced free radical activity.

Assessment of Nutritional Status in Pulmonary Compromise

Indicators of Malnutrition in Respiratory Disease

Hospitalized patients who have COPD have a high prevalence of nutritional depletion. Patients with COPD who develop pulmonary failure are more likely to be protein-calorie malnourished. Studies show that patients with COPD, and particularly emphysema, are frequently malnourished. Patients with emphysema are found to be somatically protein depleted, and the degree of nutritional depletion is significantly correlated with the degree of lung dysfunction. Iatrogenic perpetuation of malnutrition occurs with surprising frequency in the critical care setting, particularly among patients who are mechanically ventilated.[33,42,43]

In patients with COPD, after the airflow limitation is accounted for, body weight is significantly correlated with many functional variables. Specifically, greater body weight is associated with greater exercise capacity, better diffusing capacity, and less hyperinflation of the lungs; less body weight is associated with more hyperinflation, lower diffusing capacity, poor exercise performance, and increased mortality.[44]

Nutritional status was assessed prospectively on hospital admission in 59 consecutive COPD patients who presented with acute respiratory failure, 27 of whom required mechanical ventilation.[45] Malnutrition, defined on a multiparameter nutritional index, was observed in 60% of all patients and in 39% of those whose body weight was equal to at least 90% ideal body weight. The multiparameter nutritional index included the following assessment tools: percentage of ideal body weight, triceps skinfold, midarm muscle circumference, creatinine height index, albumin, prealbumin, and retinol-binding protein. Malnutrition was more common in those who required mechanical ventilation than in those who did not require ventilatory support. Subcutaneous fat stores decreased, and indices of lean body mass such as midarm muscle circumference and creatinine height index were decreased as well. Patients were also found to be depleted in prealbumin, retinol-binding protein, and albumin, the more profound deficits being in prealbumin and retinol-binding protein. Patients with cor pulmonale may increase or maintain body weight despite severe protein depletion.[42]

Mannix and associates[46] demonstrated relative hypermetabolism of malnourished COPD patients. Ten patients were divided into two groups based on nutritional status as determined by body mass index (BMI). Significant correlations were observed that implicated the increased oxygen cost of ventilation as a cause of tissue wasting. The authors concluded that the increased oxygen cost of ventilation was linked with poor lung function, a state of hypermetabolism, and that the hypermetabolism state was linked with the reduction in BMI.

Pulmonary evaluation of patients with malnutrition and chronic lung disease must focus on both problems. In addition to routine pulmonary function testing, maximal voluntary ventilation and maximal inspiratory and expiratory pressure measurements could be done. Other studies more appropriate to a research setting include assessment of the oxygen consumption of the ventilatory muscles and measurements of the transdiaphragmatic pressure difference and diaphragm electromyography.[42]

Mechanisms for Weight Loss

Several theories have been advanced to explain weight loss in patients with COPD, yet the actual cause has not been established. Dyspnea, as quantified by a dyspnea index, is significantly correlated with calorie intake, but others have found that the underweight patients with COPD consume enough calories to meet their average energy expenditure during periods of clinical stability. A substantial portion of the increase in energy expenditure can be attributed to the work and cost of breathing. Another hypothesis for the weight loss is that patients with COPD lose weight when they are acutely ill and do not regain it later. It seems unlikely that episodic weight loss is the only explanation because patients with emphysema are most apt to lose weight, yet they generally do not experience episodes of acute infection or heart failure. It has been postulated that intestinal malabsorption is responsible for weight loss in COPD, but this hypothesis has not been substantiated. Additional abnormalities such as inability to appropriately increase food intake or inability to utilize nutrients, perhaps because of a lack of tissue oxygen supply, may also be involved.[37,44,47]

The possible contribution to weight loss of increased, diet-induced thermogenesis in patients with COPD has been studied. Diet-induced thermogenesis can be defined as the net increase in energy expenditure after a meal because of the processing of the ingested nutrients through various biochemical pathways. It has been hypothesized that the extra energy expenditure was due to the increased work of breathing induced by the postprandial rise in carbon dioxide production and in minute ventilation. Hugli and colleagues studied 11 patients with COPD in a stable clinical state and 11 healthy control subjects and found that the COPD patients did not show increased diet-induced thermogenesis.[48] Although the diet-induced thermogenesis in response to a single balanced meal may be slightly higher than in control subjects, data suggest that its contribution to the malnutrition and weight loss in this disease is unlikely.

It is evident from several studies that the patient with COPD has an increased oxygen consumption of the respiratory muscles. The work of breathing is elevated in patients recovering from pulmonary failure, also, and is well-documented. Compromised pulmonary function, particularly reduced efficiency of gas exchange, may exert stress on homeostasis similar to that experienced by healthy persons during vigorous exercise. Both the increased resistive load and the reduced respiratory muscle efficiency contribute to increased cost of breathing.[42,49]

Clinical and Laboratory Data

Nutrition assessment should be designed to identify patients who exhibit clinical consequences of the malnutrition and who might reasonably stand to benefit from nutrition support. In pulmonary failure, malnutrition has major clinical consequences, and nutrition support certainly improves nutritional status.[38]

Important information to be obtained includes usual stable weight for comparison with current and ideal weight. In patients with chronic diseases such as COPD, baseline anthropometric measurements are useful in serial assessment of nutritional status. It is important to determine the amount of weight gain or loss and the period of time during which the weight change occurred. Restrictions on the usual home diet and use of food supplements can be useful to optimize the current food selection and enhance appetite. In addition, specific questions about teeth, dentures, chewing, swallowing, smell, taste, and bowel function are important. Increased dyspnea while eating may be a sign of arterial oxygen desaturation during meals and could explain poor appetite. Psychosocial factors surrounding preparation of meals and eating arrangements are also important.[42,44]

Clinicians have long had a qualitative awareness of the significance of increased respiratory work. The usual sequelae to sustained increases in respiratory work are progressive respiratory muscle fatigue and deteriorating gas exchange. Often, the clinical signs of increased work of breathing develop long before exhaustion and deterioration of arterial blood gases values. For this reason, many feel that clinically apparent increased respiratory work is an indication for institution or continuation of mechanical ventilation. Because increased work of breathing is clinically important, many investigators have attempted to quantify respiratory work.[49]

Indirect Calorimetry

Indirect calorimetry is a valuable tool for assessing energy expenditure, evaluating how the body uses nutrient fuel, and designing nutrition regimens that best fit the clinical condition of patients with pulmonary failure. The best metabolic studies are achieved by controlling the testing environment, accounting for the many clinical factors that can affect measurements, and eliminating potential sources of error. For example, a percentage of the resting energy expenditure (REE) is attributable to the work of breathing. Normally, this accounts for only 2% to 3% of the REE, but with impending pulmonary failure, as much as 25% of REE can be related to the work of breathing. Once patients are mechanically ventilated and the work of breathing is being done for them, REE may be expected to decrease by an equal amount.[50] Prolonged 24-hour metabolic rate studies in critically ill intensive care patients on mechanical ventilation have shown that true basal energy expenditure occurs only during deep sleep.[51]

Indirect calorimetry is a relatively simple, reliable bedside technique for determining the oxygen cost of breathing. In one study, the oxygen cost of breathing was found to be a reliable predictor of weaning and extubation in patients recovering from pulmonary failure. The measurement may be clinically useful in identifying who will not be able to sustain spontaneous ventilation because of excessive respiratory work.[49]

Indirect calorimetry can guide nutrition management in patients in acute respiratory failure. An indirect calorimeter analyzes the energy expenditure by measuring the concentration of inhaled oxygen and exhaled carbon dioxide gas. Through multiplying these concentrations by the exhaled minute ventilation, the metabolic cart can determine the rates of oxygen utilization and carbon dioxide production.[33]

Wilson and colleagues[52] compared REE in stable, adequately nourished COPD patients and undernourished ones. The researchers identified a hypermetabolic state in stable,

malnourished COPD patients that is not present in adequately nourished ones, and their finding was confirmed by indirect calorimetry. Results of indirect calorimetry in malnourished COPD patients have suggested that their REE is significantly higher than values predicted by the Harris-Benedict equation.[53] Malnourished COPD patients appear to have an REE approximately 20% above predicted values. The calorie requirements of stable, malnourished COPD patients are best determined by indirect calorimetry or, when indirect calorimetry is unavailable, estimated by the Harris-Benedict equation with a 20% stress factor.

In critically ill patients, the inaccuracy of predictive formulas for nutrition assessment often leads to inappropriate and potentially detrimental feeding regimens. Use of the metabolic cart determines precisely the metabolic state, identifies problems with substrate utilization, and enables the design of the most efficacious nutrition regimen[51] by a collaborative health care team.

Nutrient Requirements and Substrate Impact on Pulmonary Function

Protein and Amino Acids

The protein requirement of patients with pulmonary disease is not significantly different from that of other patients. Optimal nutrition support would be to establish homeostasis or positive nitrogen balance, depending on the need for repletion. A reasonable initial protein goal would be 1.2 to 1.5 g/kg body weight (actual or ideal body weight, whichever is lower) per day. Actual determination of a positive nitrogen balance, approximately +2 g for repletion, is desirable.

Because patients with COPD are hypermetabolic but not hypercatabolic, one can assume that they would respond readily to a repletion regimen with a moderate amount of protein intake. Data suggest that, in severely malnourished patients with COPD, the weight loss does not depend on increased rates of skeletal muscle protein degradation; nevertheless, degradation rates attenuate with positive nitrogen balance during nutrition repletion.[54]

In addition to serving as substrate for protein synthesis, amino acids were reported to increase minute ventilation, oxygen consumption, and ventilatory response to hypoxia and hypercarbia. It has been demonstrated that branched-chain amino acids have specific stimulation of ventilatory drive. This stimulation of respiratory function might well improve ventilatory efficiency, but it could also induce muscle fatigue and create difficulty weaning the patient from the ventilator. Thus, the amount of protein supplied should be advanced slowly and respiration monitored for possible deterioration.[40]

Fats

Maintenance and repletion regimens for ambulatory patients with COPD can contain 35% to 50% of total calories from fat. For patients whose ventilatory reserve is marginal, it may be useful to provide a regimen in which half the calories are supplied by fat. The high-fat regimen is most likely to benefit patients who are having difficulty with weaning from mechanical ventilation and ambulatory COPD patients whose $PaCO_2$ is greater than 50 torr.[44]

If pulmonary failure is caused by intercostal and diaphragmatic muscle depletion or by dysfunction of chemoreceptors, there is no reason to substitute fat for glucose beyond approximately 20% to 30% of calories, just to reduce carbon dioxide production. Mechanical ventilator settings should instead be adjusted to compensate for any increase in carbon dioxide production. If pulmonary failure is caused by acute parenchymal disease, overfeeding should be avoided, but the primary goal is maintenance of normal nutritional status while pulmonary membrane function is restored. If pulmonary failure is caused by COPD in a limited number of patients, overfeeding, especially excessive glucose infusion, can increase carbon dioxide production enough to affect ventilatory status. If careful adjustment of calorie support is not sufficient, the nutrient formula should be modified to provide as much as approximately 50% of calories in the form of lipid. To avoid lipid-induced injury to the reticuloendothelial system from the currently available long-chain fatty acids solutions, the lipid emulsion should not be given faster than 2 kcal per minute. If carbon dioxide production is not a concern, as in a patient who is ventilator dependent for other reasons, standard nutrition formulas should be given that do not contain excessive lipid.[3]

In one animal study, chemically defined structured lipids improved function of the reticuloendothelial system and a lesser bacterial sequestration in the lungs than nonstructured lipids.[55] These structured lipids consisted of different fatty-acid groups bound to the same glycerol backbone. The increase in lung sequestration of bacteria after a decrease in liver sequestration observed has already been demonstrated. It has been shown that lungs trap bacteria very efficiently; however, their ability to kill sequestrated bacteria is relatively poor as compared with the liver. The advantage of structured lipids over a physical mixture seems to be the absence of pure long-chain triglycerides. This avoids the problems caused from the mixture's high rate of triglyceride-free fatty acid cycling, its tendency to be stored, and its poor availability as a metabolic fuel. Nonoxidized polyunsaturated fatty acids, linoleic acid in particular, may serve as precursors for prostaglandin synthesis. The prostaglandins can lead to neutrophil activation and margination into the pulmonary circulation. Activation of pulmonary neutrophils can lead to increased sequestration of bacteria in the lungs. The activation of the nonspecific immune function in the lungs may therefore be a result of, or may result in, a more extensive bacterial sequestration in the lungs. Bacteria trapped by the lungs, or the remains of killed bacteria, can induce the cascade of inflammation and so alter the morphology and function of the lungs.

Indirect evidence indicates that in acutely ill patients intravenous fat infusion can aggravate existing gas exchange abnormalities. Hwang and colleagues[56] studied 48 patients with several types of respiratory failure who were on mechanical ventilation while also receiving intravenous fat infusion. Fat infusion in patients with disrupted alveolar capillary membrane resulted in decreased oxygenation, increased intrapulmonary shunting, and increased mean pulmonary artery pressure. The decreased diffusion capacity has been attributed to changes in alveolar capillary membrane secondary to deposition of fat particles in the reticuloendothelial system and alterations in red blood cell membranes.

Carbohydrates

Administration of glucose to cover REE increased (1) minute ventilation in proportion to the increase in carbon dioxide production and (2) the ventilatory response to hypoxia. This increase in respiratory work is one of the major reasons for the current practice of feeding mixed glucose-fat formula to critically ill patients, particularly mechanically ventilated ones. Excessive carbohydrate given to mechanically ventilated patients has been reported to cause accumulation of carbon dioxide and difficulty weaning them from mechanical ventilation, but this is probably true for only a minority of patients, particularly those whose previous pulmonary dysfunction rendered respiratory function and reserve marginal.[40] Maintenance and repletion regimens for ambulatory patients with COPD can be 35% to 50% of the total calories from carbohydrate.[44] It has been recommended to limit glucose intake to a maximum of 4 to 5 mg/kg per minute, although even this amount and rate might prove excessive in patients with limited respiratory reserve.[40]

Kilocalories

Patients with COPD who are stable and whose nutritional status is normal require calorie intake about 1.3 times their REE to maintain body weight. This factor takes into account the energy expenditure during periods of increased activity. Even patients on mechanical ventilation expend 5% more energy over 24 hours than their REE. To achieve nutritional repletion it may be necessary to provide at least 50% more calories than the REE.[44] However, providing the actual REE with close monitoring of the effect on the $PaCO_2$ and respiratory quotient (RQ) is useful during the weaning phase from mechanical ventilation. Additional calories beyond the REE for repletional therapy would be more appropriately used before the weaning phase begins or after extubation, when the patient's respiratory status is stable.

To make weaning easier for patients with marginal respiratory function, it has been recommended (although it has not been proven in a clinical study) that calorie intake be about 50% of needed calories. This reduction in protein and caloric intake fits well with the need for gradual return of the sodium pump function deranged by malnutrition. With excessive refeeding of malnourished patients, shift of large amounts of sodium from the intracellular to the extracellular compartment contributes to the development of edema and makes weaning more difficult. Thus, it is important at this stage to limit protein, calories, fluids, and sodium.[40]

Vitamins and Minerals

Of particular interest with pulmonary failure is hypophosphatemia, which can affect respiration of patients receiving nutrition support. Cellular phosphate uptake is enhanced with exogenous substrate administration, especially carbohydrate, increasing insulin secretion and an anabolic state. Hypophosphatemia may be associated with altered red blood cell oxygen transport (increased hemoglobin-oxygen affinity and impaired release of oxygen to tissues) secondary to decreased levels of adenosine triphosphate and 2,3-diphosphoglycerate. Acute respiratory failure has been described in hypophosphatemic patients.[57]

Magnesium and calcium play dynamic roles in pulmonary structure and function. Magnesium inhibits vasoconstriction through calcium regulation. Magnesium deficiency enhances the action of calcium, whereas magnesium excess blocks it. Magnesium is a weak antagonist to entry of calcium into the vascular smooth muscle cells. Calcium bindings to sites that release acetylcholine initiate smooth muscle contractility. By competing for these sites, magnesium may regulate bronchial activity. Other actions ascribed to magnesium include an antihistamine effect on mast cells and an overall calming influence because of central nervous system depression.[58]

Fluids

Patients with pulmonary disease may need moderate to severe fluid restriction. For cor pulmonale, congestive heart failure, or ARDS, the nutrition regimen may have to be delivered in concentrated and sodium-restricted formulas.[40] Fluid management in ARDS is controversial, however. One study demonstrated that weight change and cumulative intake-output were significant predictors of survival.[59] In particular, weight gain and large cumulative intake and output were very bad prognostic indicators. Although weight gain and large positive fluid balance correlated with poor clinical outcome, one must be careful not to infer a cause-and-effect relationship. It is possible that large fluid requirements may be a sign of severity of capillary leakage. Also, positive fluid balance may be an effect of a subsequent complication such as gastrointestinal bleeding, vascular collapse, or myocardial pump function failure.

Effect of Refeeding on Pulmonary Function

Restoration of nutritional status in patients with pulmonary failure requires an understanding of effects of substrates on metabolism. These patients often appear malnourished and the desire to succumb to the "tank them up" syndrome, resulting in over feeding, must be avoided. The single most important cause of nutrition-related respiratory distress is overfeeding. Because patients with respiratory compromise may be overwhelmed by the physiologic stress induced by overzealous feeding, gradual repletion of lean body mass is better tolerated. If the patient is severely depleted, long-term nutrition support may be required.

Lung protein synthesis has been found to respond to overnight fasting but not to acute provision of nutrients as solid food or enteral or parenteral formulas. Insulin appears to modulate proteolysis rather than protein synthesis in perfused lung.[60]

The effects of malnutrition and refeeding on nutritional indices, pulmonary function, and diaphragmatic contractile properties were studied in severely malnourished patients with anorexia nervosa.[35] The diaphragmatic impairment caused by the undernutrition was completely reversed during refeeding. It appears that alterations in muscle contractile and endurance properties are not simply or solely due to changes in lean tissue. Refeeding studies after hypocaloric dieting or fasting and severe starvation (anorexia nervosa) document improved muscle performance at a time when significant changes in body composition (e.g., percent mean ideal body weight) could not be detected; however, the response of malnourished patients with COPD to nutrition support may be different from that of patients with anorexia nervosa.

When deficiencies of potassium and phosphorus are corrected, muscle function rapidly improves. In contrast, it takes several weeks for the effects of nutritional repletion to become apparent. Moreover, the benefits of nutrition repletion continue to accrue if it is maintained for several months. When patients resume their "baseline diet," they lose the benefits of nutrition repletion at about the same rate as they improved during repletion. Therefore, to maintain the repleted state, caloric intake should probably be about 1.4 times REE.[44]

Guidelines for Nutrition Support in Pulmonary Failure

Inability to Consume Sufficient Nutrients Orally

It is difficult to provide adequate oral dietary supplementation to some persons with pulmonary disease. For example, although some patients with COPD were able to increase their calorie intake to well over 1.5 times REE, others could not. Patients often felt dyspneic, satiated, or bloated, or had diarrhea. Thus, not all COPD patients are able to get enough calories from a regular diet or a regular diet with liquid supplements, to benefit from nutritional repletion.[44]

Creutzberg and associates[61] investigated prospectively the nonresponse to 8 weeks of oral nutrition therapy with respect to lung function impairment, body composition, energy balance, and systemic inflammatory response in depleted patients (5 of 24) with COPD. The supplementation consisted of 500 to 750 kcal/day extra and was part of an inpatient pulmonary rehabilitation program. Nonresponse to increased calorie intake in the patient with COPD should be considered as a multifactorial problem. Factors that may have contributed to the nonreponse included the presence of acute-phase response, elevated systemic inflammatory response, aging, relative anorexia, and shifting in body water compartments.

Goal of Nutrition Therapy

A major goal of nutrition therapy is to prevent or minimize loss of respiratory muscle mass and function so the patient can breathe without mechanical assistance. To achieve this goal for a patient with pulmonary failure these recommendations are offered:

1. Evaluate the nutritional status of all patients with COPD and other chronic respiratory system diseases, patients with acute respiratory failure, and other critically ill patients.
2. Identify and treat reversible complications that cause muscle weakness and wasting. Typical examples include metabolic disarray, infection, and circulatory and gastrointestinal dysfunction.
3. Initiate protein-calorie repletion for all severely undernourished patients. (However, optimal results occur only when the underlying disease can be controlled to the extent that patients ingest the needed calories and achieve positive nitrogen balance.)[44]

Determine Appropriate Route for Alimentation

The enteral route is preferred whenever nutrition support is indicated. The advantages of enteral feeding include not only low expense and less risk of sepsis but also better preservation of the gut mucosal barrier. Maintenance of this barrier is believed to reduce gastrointestinal bleeding from stress ulcer and to protect against translocation of luminal bacteria or their toxins through the intestinal wall into the lymphatic system or portal blood. Although the bacterial translocation hypothesis remains attractive as an explanation for septic morbidity in critically ill patients, it is nevertheless a hypothesis. The exact relationship between bacterial translocation and enteral nutrition support in humans is unclear; yet, some clinicians believe breakdown of the mucosal barrier to be an important event in development of sepsis, ARDS, and MSOF.[3,62] When the functioning area of the gastrointestinal tract of a compromised pulmonary failure patient is not accessible, parenteral alimentation should be considered. Generally, central access is preferred to peripheral alimentation because of the need for fluid restriction and maximum macronutrient concentration formulations for pulmonary failure patients.

Risks of placing central venous access include air embolus, hemothorax, arterial puncture, hydromediastinum, brachial plexus injury, hydrothorax, catheter embolus, pneumothorax, hemomediastinum, and thoracic duct injury. It might be expected that a patient with pulmonary failure would be at higher risk for complications because of the associated patient agitation, commonly present coagulopathy, and hyperinflation of the lung with emphysema or positive inspiratory pressures; however, when the access device is placed by an experienced physician, the risks are no greater for patients with pulmonary failure than for other patients.[3]

Enteral Alimentation Considerations

With a nasogastric tube, there is always the possibility of aspiration into the trachea. Cuffed endotracheal tubes may reduce the volume of aspirate, but they certainly do not prevent the complication. The extent of the aspiration problem depends much on the gastric residual, maintaining proper tube placement and the head of the patient's bed greater than 30 degress during feeding infusion. Transpyloric feedings have been suggested to prevent aspiration, but the patient could still aspirate oral secretions. Diarrhea, decreased bowel sounds, and abdominal distention were observed in about half of all acute respiratory failure patients. Antacid therapy was identified as the major contributing cause of diarrhea in one study, and it was recommended that antacids not be given to such patients.[44] Medications containing sorbitol, such as theophylline elixirs, have been found to increase diarrhea occurrence.[63]

Monitoring of these patients to determine that the ordered amount of enteral feeding is actually infused is essential. Although gastrointestinal intolerance may limit infusion in the intensive care unit (ICU) patient, in a study done by Jonghe and associates,[64] two thirds of the causes of inadequate nutrition were related to extra intestinal reasons. The reasons included diagnostic procedures, airway management, and mechanical problems.

Specific enteral formulas have been designed for patients with pulmonary compromise, but they may not be appropriate for all patients with pulmonary compromise (see Chapter 20.) The original concept for the care of these patients—a low-carbohydrate, high-fat enteral formula—originated from the early use of parenteral alimentation with a primary calorie source of a dextrose-rich component. During this period patients were

also grossly overfed in total calories. Now, it is more accepted to feed a more modest amount of total calories.[65] As patients with acute lung injury are weaned from mechanical ventilators, some 2% benefit from an alimentation regimen containing approximately 50% to 60% fat because of its effect on carbon dioxide production and the increased work of breathing.[66]

Parenteral Alimentation Factors

Increased concentrations of the macronutrients (protein, fat, carbohydrate) with central line administration are preferred. Supplementation beyond standard components may be warranted for electrolyte depletion. Once the patient has been weaned from mechanical ventilation, calories and protein should be increased gradually to the full support regimen while attempting to achieve positive nitrogen balance and repletion of nutrition deficits. After the patient's overall condition and disease improve, enteral feeding of a commercial formula should be initiated. A transition period of combined enteral and PN follows, and, with return of appetite, complete enteral or oral nutrition[40] (see Chapter 22).

Practice Parameters, Guidelines, and Outcome Measures

Practice parameters, based on published standards and guidelines, and outcome measurements are two tools for quality and utilization management. Practice parameters are management strategies that help clinicians make clinical decisions. Such parameters were conceived as a solution to provision of unnecessary care. The idea is to consolidate all medical knowledge about a particular illness or injury and to draft a statement about the best approach to management. Outcome measures evaluate the delivery of care.[67] Critical pathways have been developed at many institutions to link provision of care to outcomes for specific patient populations. These critical pathways are a sequence of important key events in the treatment process that must be accomplished to achieve the desired outcomes. If a particular treatment modality is not linked to an optimal care outcome, it is considered nonessential and, in the future, probably will not be used in that patient population.

The American Society for Parenteral and Enteral Nutrition (ASPEN) published practice guidelines for respiratory failure.[68] Five clinical guidelines were developed to provide practical advice to clinicians who administer oral, enteral (tube), or PN support to patients in respiratory failure. The guidelines represent the authors' best effort to summarize the state of the art of parenteral and enteral nutrition support for such patients. Strength of evidence was identified for each practice guideline. The type of evidence supporting each recommendation was identified as (1) *good research-based,* (2) *fair research-based,* or (3) *expert opinion and panel consensus* (Box 30-1).

Dietitians in Nutrition Support (DNS), a dietetic practice group of The American Dietetic Association, suggested a clinical indicator for the nutrition management of patients with compromised pulmonary function: increase in $Paco_2$ over baseline value during enteral or PN support. In field testing, no patients on PN support had increased $Paco_2$. In the data available for 73% of those receiving enteral nutrition no changes in $Paco_2$ were noted. On a scale of 1 (least important) to 5 (most important), field test-site participants

---

BOX 30-1

ASPEN Practice Guidelines for Respiratory Failure[68]

Good research-based evidence supports the following recommendation:
- Meet protein and energy requirements in acute ventilatory stress to limit wasting of respiratory muscles.

Fair research-based evidence supports the following recommendation:
- Selected patients with chronic stable ventilatory stress due to COPD or cystic fibrosis should receive nutrition support, which has been associated with measurable improvements in muscle strength and endurance.

Expert opinion and panel consensus support the following recommendations:
- Monitor nutrient intake in patients with borderline ventilatory status to prevent excessive CO_2 production. The significance of modifying formula respiratory quotient through changes in the proportion of total calories as fat and carbohydrate is undetermined in controlled trials; however, it may reduce CO_2 production in some patients.
- Essential nutrients such as potassium, calcium, phosphate, and magnesium should be provided in adequate amounts to meet muscle requirements and thereby maintain optimal respiratory muscle force.
- Parenteral lipid formulations should be administered cautiously to patients with severe oxygenation defects.

BOX 30-2

Objectives of Metabolic Measurements by Indirect Calorimetry[70]

1. To accurately determine the REE of mechanically ventilated patients to guide appropriate nutritional support
2. To accurately determine RQ to allow nutrition regimens to be tailored to patient needs
3. To accurately determine REE and RQ to monitor adequacy and appropriateness of current nutritional support
4. To allow determination of substrate utilization when urinary nitrogen values are measured concurrently
5. To determine the oxygen cost of breathing as a guide to the selection of ventilator mode, settings, and weaning strategies
6. To monitor the oxygen consumption as a guide to targeting adequate oxygen delivery

---

ranked this indicator 3.8 for monitoring and improving patient care and 2.8 for patient outcome. The field test participants felt that this indicator would be most useful in patients who were having difficulty being weaned from mechanical ventilation.[69]

The American Association for Respiratory Care developed clinical practice guidelines and objectives for metabolic measurement using indirect calorimetry during mechanical ventilation (Box 30-2).[70] A physician or nutritionist may evaluate assessment of outcome by interpretation and confirmation or manipulation of the patient's nutrition support regimen based on the measurement results. Additionally, the outcome can be assessed by successful manipulation of the mechanical ventilator settings or hemodynamic management based on the measurement of the oxygen consumption.

The Task Force on Guidelines of the Society of Critical Care Medicine developed standards of care for critically ill patients with acute respiratory failure receiving mechanical ventilation in a critical care unit. Because these are minimum standards, all of these guidelines must be met, and many critical care units exceed most or all of them. The following aspects of the standards relate directly to nutrition support:[71]

1. Having the capacity to monitor, on an intermittent basis, weight of bedridden and ambulating patients
2. Utilization of nutrition support, enteral and parenteral, at intervals to be determined by individual clinical circumstances
3. Utilization of objective measurements of nutritional status at intervals to be determined by individual clinical circumstances

Simplified Guidelines for Patient Instruction

The patient must be alerted to the following aspects of pulmonary disease that could decrease appetite, limit food intake, and result in weight loss:

1. Shortness of breath with exertion (limiting shopping for food, meal preparation, and eating)

2. Easy fatigue and reduced endurance of respiratory muscles
3. Early satiety caused by a flattened diaphragm or air swallowing
4. Alteration of taste by medications
5. Abdominal discomfort caused by bronchodilator or corticosteroid medications
6. Feeling of fullness after eating only a few bites

Guidelines for appropriate meal scheduling and food selections are discussed with patients:[68]

1. Consume five or six small meals per day.
2. Rest before and after meals, to avoid fatigue.
3. Use oxygen during meals at home or in the hospital if ordered by the physician.
4. Separate liquids and solid foods at meals to avoid distention.
5. Use soft, easy-to-chew foods to avoid exertion while eating.
6. Use nutrient-dense convenience foods as necessary if meal preparation is exhausting.
7. Restrict salt only if the physician orders.

Patient must be educated in the role of nutrition in maintaining optimal lung function, along with the other aspects of health care prescribed by the patient's physician:

1. Focus on the relationship between nutrition and pulmonary function.
2. COPD patients need to consume more calories, and if they do not, they will lose weight.
3. Work with the patient and family members to provide support for reinforcement of adequate oral intake.

Heart Failure Description

Heart failure results when cardiac function is impaired resulting in the heart's inability to pump blood at a rate sufficient to meet the requirements of tissue at rest or during exercise. It is a complex syndrome, resulting in shortness of breath, fatigue, and abnormal heart function.[72] For many years, heart failure was known as congestive heart failure. Pulmonary congestion is not always present with this condition. The more common terms used now are acute heart failure and chronic heart failure.[73] There are different types of heart failure, and the failure is

---

BOX 30-3

Heart Failure Classifications[72,73]

Backward failure	Failure of ventricle to empty
Forward failure	Inadequate delivery of blood into the arterial system
Acute heart failure	Decrease in left ventricular function due to acute myocardial infarction or acute valvular dysfunction
Chronic heart failure	Inability of heart to compensate over time, caused by valvular disease, high blood pressure, or chronic obstructive pulmonary disease
Low-output syndrome	Response to high blood pressure, evidenced by impaired peripheral circulation and peripheral vasoconstriction
High-output syndrome	Conditions that require heart to work harder to supply blood, such as hyperthyroidism, fever, pregnancy, arteriovenous fistula, anemia, and beriberi
Shock	Tissue perfusion is inadequate to meet needs of cells, extreme end of forward failure
Systolic dysfunction	Impaired pump function, due to coronary heart disease, dilated cardiomyopathy, and hypertension
Diastolic dysfunction	Increased resistance to filling, mainly due to long-standing hypertension; increased age appears to be a factor

---

BOX 30-4

Clinical Manifestations of Heart Failure[72,73]

Dysfunction	Signs and Symptoms
Failure of left ventricle as a pump	Dyspnea, weakness, fatigue, dizziness, confusion, pulmonary congestion, hypotension, orthopnea nocturia
Failure of right ventricle as a pump	Weakness, anorexia, indigestion, weight gain, mental changes, hepatomegaly, dependent peripheral edema, ascites
Pulmonary venous congestion	Interstitial edema, progressing to alveolar edema, engorged pulmonary vessels, elevated pulmonary artery pressure, reduced lung compliance causing increased exertional dyspnea
Systemic venous congestion	Jugular venous distention, volume in distensible organs, hepatomegaly, splenomegaly, serous effusion, peripheral edema

---

classified based on specific dysfunctions and factors that contribute to the failure (Box 30-3). Clinical manifestations of the heart failure result in different signs and symptoms (Box 30-4).

Medical Management of Heart Disease

Determining the type and severity of the underlying condition causing the heart failure and extent of the damage is the initial goal in assessing a patient with heart failure.[72] Focus is placed on relieving the heart failure symptoms, enhancing cardiac performance, and correcting the precipitating causes of acute heart failure. Symptom management involves controlling fluid overload and improvement of cardiac output by decreasing systemic vascular resistance and increasing contractility. Medications, fluid reduction, and even an intraaortic balloon pump may be required.[73] Various diagnostic procedures and

---

BOX 30-5

Diagnostic and Laboratory Tests[72,73]

Electrocardiogram	Measures the heart's activity as wave forms; can be used to identify myocardial ischemia and infarction, rhythm and conduction disturbances, chamber enlargement, electrolyte imbalances, and drug toxicity
Echocardiogram	Assesses dysrhythmias, diagnoses cardiac valvular changes, pericardial effusion, chamber enlargement, and ventricular hypertrophy
Cardiac catheterization	Used in patients with angina or large areas of ischemic or hibernating myocardium
Electrolytes	Increase in total body water results in decreased serum sodium; potassium and magnesium alterations due to medications or impaired kidney function
Complete blood count	Anemia resulting in decreased oxygen carrying capacity
Urinalysis	Proteinuria, red blood cells, and high specific gravity indicate kidney involvement
Liver panel	Elevated levels result from hepatic congestion
Thyroid stimulating hormone	Heart failure may be due to hypothyroidism or hyperthyroidism

---

laboratory test provide insight into the factors contributing to the heart failure and assist in management of the disease process (Box 30-5).

Hemodynamic Monitoring

Hemodynamic monitoring involves direct determination of intraarterial pressure with an arterial line. It uses invasive techniques to measure pressure, flow, and resistance within the cardiovascular system. The variables measured with this catheter are cardiac output by thermodilution; right atrial pressure; and pulmonary artery systolic, diastolic and wedge pressures.[72,74]

Cardiac output is the amount of blood ejected by the heart. This measurement helps evaluate cardiac function. Pulmonary artery pressures provide important information about left ventricular function and preload. This measurement is especially useful for hemodynamically unstable patients, for fluid and cardiac drug management. Direct arterial blood monitoring is desired when highly accurate or frequent blood pressure measurements are needed, such as in patients with low cardiac output and high systemic vascular resistance.[74]

Hemodynamic monitoring systems consist of four components: (1) an invasive catheter in the patient and high pressure tubing connection to the transducer, (2) a transducer that receives the physiologic signal from the catheter and converts it into electrical energy, (3) the flush system for maintaining catheter patency, and (4) the beside monitor.[75]

Cardiac Surgery Complications—Nutrition Implications

Preadmission nutrition screening of this population is desirable to identify patients scheduled for elective surgery who could benefit from intervention before admission for nutrition deficits. Most patients undergoing cardiac surgery have short, uncomplicated hospital stays and then discharge home. Nutrition goals at this time are to consume an adequate oral intake for surgery wound healing with sodium and fluid restrictions. Future adherence to a prudent diet with sodium restriction and fat and cholesterol limitations is necessary when adequate oral intake has been achieved over the next several weeks.

Doering and associates[76] found that a significant portion of the variance in the ICU length of stay after coronary artery bypass graft (CABG) surgery was attributable to preoperative mortality risk, intubation hours, presence of arrhythmias, early hemodynamic instability, and 12-hour fluid balance. Increasing age and the presence of comorbidities such as hypertension, poor ejection fraction, and COPD have been found to contribute to the ICU length of stay in patients following CABG surgery. Preoperative factors associated with prolonged ICU stay in CABG surgery patients include: recent MI, smoking, number of diseased arteries, and preoperative left-ventricular end diastolic pressure. Low cardiac output syndrome, postoperative use of inotropes, atrial arrhythmias, respiratory complications, and renal insufficiency are postoperative factors that contribute to prolonged ICU stay.

Sternal wound infection following coronary artery bypass surgery usually occurs 4 to 14 days after surgery and is manifested by fever, leukocytosis, and inflammatory wound with purulent drainage.[77] Glucose control may be a factor in preventing deep wound infections in diabetic patients undergoing cardiac surgery. In a study of nearly 9000 cardiac surgery patients there was a higher incidence of deep sternal wound infections in diabetic patients (1.7%) versus nondiabetics (0.4%). Infected diabetic patients had a higher mean blood glucose level through the first 2 postoperative days than noninfected diabetic patients. Incidence of deep wound infections in diabetic patients was reduced by implementation of a protocol to maintain the blood glucose level less than 200 mg/dl in the immediate postoperative period.[78]

Postoperative bleeding from media sternal chest tubes can be caused by inadequate hemostasis, suture line disruption, or coagulopathy dysfunction. Depending on the quantity of blood loss and despite normalization of clotting studies, reexploration of the surgical site may be required.[72]

Adequacy of gastrointestinal tract function after cardiac surgery is a concern for patients requiring enteral nutrition, especially for those individuals exhibiting altered hemodynamic status. Gastrointestinal function appears to be altered after cardiac surgery. In a group of 39 cardiac patients, pyloric closure was the main clinical finding and adsorptive capacity of the intestinal mucosa was not abolished by hemodynamic failure. The initial altered pyloric function was attributed to opiates. Mechanisms required for enteral absorption may be maintained despite hemodynamic compromise in the cardiac surgery.[79]

Long-term survival and functional health status was evaluated in adult patients who required more than 7 days of mechanical ventilation after cardiac surgery. Nineteen out of 124 patients died in the hospital. Survival was 59% at 5 years. Patients who died after discharge were more likely to have had preoperative renal dysfunction or stroke, remained on the ventilator longer, and had more postoperative complications such as stroke or renal dysfunction. These individuals had more difficulty with walking and eating because of debilitation.

Interestingly, patients with chronic obstructive pulmonary disease (COPD) were less likely to die in the hospital. It was speculated that the patients without COPD who required more than 7 days mechanical ventilation had problems such as renal failure, stroke, or sepsis that were more likely to have fatal outcomes. This study has implications for nutrient adequacy during the hospitalization and after discharge.[80]

Nutrition Support Interventions in Heart Failure

Individuals with heart failure are at increased risk for nutrition deficits if shortness of breath or dyspnea has been present, resulting in decreased nutrient intake. Weight maintenance and weight gain may occur more readily in this population because of fluid retention, despite inadequate intake, loss of muscle mass, and fat stores. If the individual is unable to consume an adequate low sodium diet, with small frequent feedings and nutrient dense supplements, initiation of enteral tube feeding should be considered. Nutrient density and decreased sodium content are desirable characteristics of an enteral formula for this population. PN would be provided only if the gastrointestinal tract was impaired or access was not available. Fluid restriction would be achieved with using concentrated macronutrient substrates for the amino acids, lipids, and dextrose. Electrolyte modification, especially focusing on sufficient levels of potassium and magnesium, would be used. Vitamins and minerals, with an emphasis on thiamine if depletion was anticipated, would be added, especially if the patient had a history of alcohol abuse.

Conclusion

Incorporation of nutrition therapy into the total management of persons with pulmonary and cardiac failure is essential to improve outcomes in all health care settings. Ideally, educating patients about the role of nutrition in maintaining optimal lung function before acute illness and hospitalization would be beneficial. During the acute hospital phase of the illness, possible intubation, and subsequent weaning period, clinicians need to be aware of the intricate relationship between undernutrition and overnutrition effects of various substrates. The role of nutrition support regimens in individuals with heart failure requires reducing fluid and sodium content of alimentation solutions. Patients undergoing CABG surgery who develop postoperative complications with prolonged intubation require timely nutrition support therapy.

REFERENCES

1. Stacy KM: Pulmonary disorders. In Urden LD, Stacy KM (eds): *Priorities in critical care nursing,* ed 3, St Louis, 2000, Mosby, pp 224-246.
2. Mowatt-Larssen CA, Brown RO: Specialized nutritional support in respiratory disease, *Clin Pharm* 12:276-292, 1993.
3. Grant JP: Nutrition care of patients with acute and chronic respiratory failure, *Nutr Clin Pract* 9(1):11-17, 1994.
4. West JB: Structure and function—how the architecture of the lung serves its function. In *Respiratory physiology: the essentials,* Philadelphia, 2000, Lippincott Williams & Wilkins, pp 1-9.
5. Schwartz DB: Pulmonary failure. In Gottschlich MM, Matarese LE, Shronts EP (eds): *Nutrition support dietetics core curriculum,* ed 2, Silver Spring, MD, 1993, ASPEN, pp 251-260.

6. Klocke RA: Ventilation, pulmonary blood flow, and gas exchange. In Fishman AP: *Pulmonary diseases and disorders,* ed 2, vol I, New York, 1988, McGraw-Hill, pp 185-198.

7. Stacy KM, Maiden JM: Pulmonary assessment and diagnostic procedures. In Urden LD, Stacy KM (eds): *Priorities in critical care nursing,* ed 3, St Louis, 2000, Mosby, pp 211-223.

8. In Madama VC: *Pulmonary function testing and cardiopulmonary stress testing,* Albany, NY, 1993, Delmar Publishers, pp 531-554.

9. Ingram RH, Fanta CH: VII Respiratory failure, *Sci Am* 4:1-9, 1988.

10. Ferguson GT, Irvin CG, Cherniack RM: Relationship of diaphragm glycogen, lactate, and function to respiratory failure, *Am Rev Respir Dis* 141:926-932, 1990.

11. Hahn K: Slow-teaching the COPD patient, *Nursing* 17(4):34-42, 1987.

12. Jones MA, Hoffman LA, Delgado E: ARDS revisited: new ways to fight an old enemy, *Nursing* 24(12):34-43, 1994.

13. Atkins PJ, Egloff ME, Willms DC: Respiratory consequences of multisystem crisis: the adult respiratory distress syndrome, *Crit Care Nurs Q* 16(4):27-38, 1994.

14. Morris MT: Adult respiratory distress syndrome. In Huddleston VB: *Multisystem organ failure pathophysiology and clinical implications,* St Louis, 1992, Mosby-Year Book, pp 204-221.

15. Meduri GU, Headley S, Kohler G, et al: Persistent elevation of inflammatory cytokines predicts a poor outcome in ARDS, *Chest* 107(4):1062-1073, 1995.

16. Mangialardi RJ, Martin GS, Bernard GR, et al: Hypoproteinemia predicts acute respiratory distress syndrome development, weight gain, and death in patients with sepsis, *Crit Care Med* 28(9):3137-3145, 2000.

17. Vasilyev S, Schaap RN, Mortensen JD: Hospital survival rates of patients with acute respiratory failure in modern respiratory intensive care units, *Chest* 107(4):1083-1088, 1995.

18. McIntyre Jr RC, Pulido E, Bensard DO, et al: Thirty years of clinical trials in acute respiratory distress syndrome, *Crit Care Med* 28(9):3314-3331, 2000.

19. Deitch EA: Multiple organ failure. Pathophysiology and potential future therapy, *Ann Surg* 216(2):117-134, 1992.

20. Border JR: Multiple systems organ failure, *Ann Surg* 216(2):111-116, 1992.

21. Huddleston VB: Multisystem organ failure. What you need to know, *Nursing* 21(9):34-42, 1991.

22. Tesauro J: Mechanical ventilation and blood gas analysis, *Dietitians Nutr Support* Feb:4, 12, 1988.

23. Benotti PN, Bistrian B: Metabolic and nutritional aspects of weaning from mechanical ventilation, *Crit Care Med* 17(2):181-185, 1989.

24. Burns SM, Clochesy JM, Hanneman SKG, et al: Weaning from long-term mechanical ventilation, *Am J Crit Care* 4(1):4-26, 1995.

25. Sharar SR: Weaning and extubation are not the same thing, *Respir Care* 40(3):239-243, 1995.

26. Burns SM, Ryan B, Burns JE: The weaning continuum use of Acute Physiology and Chronic Health Evaluation III, Burn Wean Assessment Program, Therapeutic Intervention Scoring System, and Wean Index scores to establish stages of weaning, *Crit Care Med* 28(7):2259-2267, 2000.

27. MacIntyre NR: Respiratory factors in weaning from mechanical ventilatory support, *Respir Care* 40(3):244-248, 1995.

28. Pierson DJ: Nonrespiratory aspects of weaning from mechanical ventilation, *Respir Care* 40(3):263-270, 1995.

29. Pierson DJ: Long-term mechanical ventilation and weaning, *Respir Care* 40(3):289-295, 1995.

30. Brooks-Brunn JA: Postoperative atelectasis and pneumonia, *Heart Lung* 24(2):94-115, 1995.

31. Berry SM, Lacy JA, Nussbaum MS: Basic concepts of enteral and parenteral nutrition. In Torosian MH (ed): *Nutrition for the hospitalized patient,* New York, 1995, Marcel Dekker, pp 255-269.

32. MacIntyre NR: Psychological factors in weaning from mechanical ventilatory support, *Respir Care* 40(3):277-281, 1995.

33. Hagaman M, Christman JW: Nutrition support in acute respiratory failure, *Cont Intern Med* 6(7):29-41, 1994.

34. Rochester DF, Esau SA: The respiratory muscles. In Baum GL, Wolinsky E (eds): *Textbook of pulmonary disease,* vol I, Boston, 1989, Little, Brown, pp 73-103.

35. Murciano D, Rigaud D, Pingleton S, et al: Diaphragmatic function in severely malnourished patients with anorexia nervosa. Effects of renutrition, *Am J Respir Crit Care Med* 150(6):1569-1574, 1994.

36. Schwartz DB: Respiratory disease and mechanical ventilation. In Skipper A (ed): *Dietitian's handbook of enteral and parenteral nutrition,* Rockville, MD, 1989, Aspen Publishers, pp 137-150.

37. Edelman NH, Rucker RB, Peavy HH: Nutrition and the respiratory system, *Am Rev Respir Dis* 134:347-352, 1986.

38. Askanazi J, Mullen JL: Nutrition and acute respiratory failure. In Fishman AP: *Pulmonary disease and disorders,* ed 2, vol III, New York, 1988, McGraw-Hill, pp 2387-2396.

39. Sardesai VM: Role of antioxidants in health maintenance, *Nutr Clin Pract* 10(1):19-25, 1995.

40. Freund HR: Nutritional support in cardiac and pulmonary disease. In Fischer JE (ed): *Total parenteral nutrition,* ed 2, Boston, 1991, Little, Brown, pp 203-216.

41. Goode HF, Cowley HC, Walker BE, et al: Decreased antioxidant status and increased lipid peroxidation in patients with septic shock and secondary organ dysfunction, *Crit Care Med* 23(4):646-651, 1995..

42. Wilson DO, Rogers RM, Hoffman RM: Nutrition and chronic lung disease, *Am Rev Respir Dis* 132(6):1347-1365, 1985.

43. Askanazi J, Goldstein S, Kvetan V, et al: Respiratory disease. In Kinney JM, Jeejeebhoy KN, Hill GL: *Nutrition and metabolism in patient care,* Philadelphia, 1988, WB Saunders, pp 522-530.

44. Rochester DF: Nutritional repletion, *Semin Respir Med* 13(1):44-52, 1992.

45. Laaban JP, Kouchakji B, Dore MF, et al: Nutritional status of patients with chronic obstructive pulmonary disease and acute respiratory failure, *Chest* 103(5):1362-1368, 1993.

46. Mannix ET, Manfredi F, Barber MO: Elevated O_2 cost of ventilation contribute to tissue wasting in COPD, *Chest* 115(3):708-713, 1999.

47. Congletion J: The pulmonary cachexia syndrome: aspects of energy balance, *Proc Nutr Soc* 58: 321-328, 1999.

48. Hugli O, Frascarolo P, Schutz Y, et al: Diet-induced thermogenesis in chronic obstructive pulmonary disease, *Am Rev Respir Dis* 148(6):1479-1483, 1993.

49. Lewis WD, Chwals W, Benotti PN, et al: Bedside assessment of the work of breathing, *Crit Care Med* 16(2):117-122, 1988.

50. McClave SA, Snider HL: Use of indirect calorimetry in clinical nutrition, *Nutr Clin Pract* 7(5):207-221, 1992.

51. Makk LJK, McClave SA, Creech PW, et al: Clinical application of the metabolic cart to the delivery of total parenteral nutrition, *Crit Care Med* 18(12):1320-1327, 1990.

52. Wilson DO, Donahoe M, Rogers RM, Pennock BE: Metabolic rate and weight loss in chronic obstructive lung disease, *J Parenter Enteral Nutr* 14(1):7-11, 1990.

53. Donahoe M, Rogers RM: Laboratory evaluation of the patients with chronic obstructive pulmonary disease. In Cherniack NS: *Chronic obstructive pulmonary disease,* Philadelphia, 1991, WB Saunders, pp 373-386.

54. Aguilaniu B, Goldstein-Shapses S, Pajon A, et al: Muscle protein degradation in severely malnourished patients with chronic obstructive pulmonary disease subject to short-term total parenteral nutrition, *J Parenter Enteral Nutr* 16(3):248-254, 1992.

55. Pscheidl E, Med PDD, Hedwig-Geissing M, et al: Effects of chemically defined structured lipid emulsions on reticuloendothelial system function and morphology of liver and lung in a continuous low-dose endotoxin rat model, *J Parenter Enteral Nutr* 19(1):33-40, 1995.

56. Hwang TL, Huang SL, Chen MF: Effects of intravenous fat emulsion on respiratory failure, *Chest* 97(4):934-938, 1990.

57. Whitmore SF: Fluid and electrolytes. In Gottschlich MM (ed): *The science and practice of nutrition support,* Dubuque, 2001, Kendall/Hunt Publishing, Co. pp 53-83.

58. Landon RA, Young EA: Role of magnesium in regulation of lung function, *J Am Diet Assoc* 93(6):674-677, 1993.

59. Simmons RS, Berdine GG, Seidenfeld JJ, et al: Fluid balance and the adult respiratory distress syndrome, *Am Rev Respir Dis* 135(4):924-929, 1987.

60. Preedy VR, Garlick PJ: Ventricular muscle and lung protein synthesis in vivo in response to fasting, refeeding, and nutrient supply by oral and parenteral routes, *J Parenter Enteral Nutr* 19(2):107-113, 1995.

61. Creutzberg EC, Schols AMWJ, Weling-Scheepers CAPM, et al: Characterization of nonresponse to high calorie oral nutritional therapy in depleted patients with chronic obstructive pulmonary disease, *Am J Respir Crit Care Med* 161(3):745-752, 2000.

62. Lipman TO: Bacterial translocation and enteral nutrition in humans: an outsider looks in, *J Parenter Enteral Nutr* 19(2):156-165, 1995.

63. Hill DB, Henderson LM, McClain CJ: Osmotic diarrhea induced by sugar-free theophylline solution in critically ill patients, *J Parenter Enteral Nutr* 15(3):332-336, 1991.

64. Jonghe BD, Appere-De-Vechi C, Fournier M, et al: A prospective survey of nutritional support practices in intensive care unit patients: What is prescribed? What is delivered? *Crit Care Med* 29(1):8-12, 2001.

65. Bell SJ, Apour CH, Burke PA, et al: Enteral formulas: an update. In Torosian MH (ed): *Nutrition for the hospitalized patient,* New York, 1995, Marcel Dekker pp 293-306.

66. Murray MJ, Kumar M: Omega-3 fatty acids and pulmonary disease, *Nutr MD* 21(8):1-3, 1995.

67. Hirshfeld EB: Practice parameters versus outcome measurements how will prospective and retrospective approaches to quality management fit together? *Nutr Clin Pract* 9(6):207-215, 1994.

68. ASPEN Board of Directors: Guidelines for the use of parenteral and enteral nutrition in adult and pediatric patients, *J Parenter Enteral Nutr* 17(suppl 4):1SA-52SA, 1993.

69. Colaizzo-Anas T: Assessment and nutrition management of the patient with compromised pulmonary function. In Winkler MF, Lysen MK (eds): *Suggested guidelines for nutrition and metabolic management of adult patients receiving nutrition support,* ed 2, Chicago, 1993, American Dietetic Association, pp 80-90.

70. American Association for Respiratory Care: Clinical practice guidelines: metabolic measurement using indirect calorimetry during mechanical ventilation, *Respir Care* 39(12):1170-1175, 1994.

71. Task Force on Guidelines Society of Critical Care Medicine: Guidelines for standards of care for patients with acute respiratory failure on mechanical ventilatory support, *Crit Care Med* 19(2):275-278, 1991.

72. Laurent-Bopp D: Heart failure. In Wood SL, Froelicher ESSA, Motzer SA (eds): *Cardiac nursing*, ed 4, Philadelphia, 2000, Lippincott, pp 560-577.

73. O'Donnell M, Dirks J: Cardiovascular disorders. In Urden LD, Stacy KM (eds): *Priorities in critical care nursing,* ed 3, St Louis, 2000, Mosby, pp 146-179.

74. Milford C, Purvis G: Cardiovascular care. In *Nursing procedures,* ed 3, Springhouse, 2000, Springhouse Corporation, pp 343-417.

75. Bloomquist J, Love MM: Cardiovascular assessment and diagnostic procedures. In Urden LD, Stacy KM (eds): *Priorities in critical care nursing,* ed 3, St Louis, 2000, Mosby, pp 99-144.

76. Doering LV, Esmailian F, Imperial-Perez, et al: Determinants of intensive care unit stay after coronary artery bypass graft surgery, *Heart Lung* 30(1):9-17, 2001.

77. Ledoux D, Luikart H: Cardiac surgery. In Wood SL, Froelicher ESSA, Motzer SA (eds): *Cardiac nursing,* ed 4, Philadelphia, 2000, Lippincott, pp 580-595.

78. Zerr KJ, Furnary AP, Grunkemeier, et al: Glucose control lowers the risk of wound infection in diabetics after open heart operations, *Ann Thorac Surg* 63(3):356-361, 1997.

79. Berger MM, Berger-Gryllaki M, Wiesel PH, et al: Intestinal absorption in patients after cardiac surgery, *Crit Care Med* 28(7):2217-2223, 2000.

80. Engoren M, Buderer NF, Zacharias: Long-term survival and health status after prolonged mechanical ventilation after cardiac surgery, *Crit Care Med* 28(8):2472-2749, 2000.

Gastrointestinal and Pancreatic Disease 31

Elizabeth Wall-Alonso, MS, RD, CNSD
Mary M. Sullivan, MPH, RD
Theresa A. Byrne, DSc, RD, CNSD

IN healthy humans, nutrients are absorbed from ingested foods by the gastrointestinal (GI) tract through a series of mechanical, enzymatic, hormonal, and neural mechanisms. Persons with a healthy, functioning GI tract who consume a well-balanced diet can maintain adequate nutritional stores without supplements or alternative alimentation. Because normal digestion and absorption depend on fine integration of GI function and accessory organs plus the nervous, endocrine, and circulatory systems, many diseases and surgical procedures can cause malnutrition. This chapter provides general information and nutrition support recommendations for the many diseases, treatments, and surgeries that can cause GI or pancreatic dysfunction.

Normal Gastrointestinal Function

The GI tract starts at the mouth, ends at the anus, and includes the salivary glands, the liver, the pancreas, and the gallbladder. Digestion begins in the mouth, where the salivary glands secrete amylase, which initiates digestion of carbohydrates. Once food is chewed and moistened, the bolus is moved past the pharynx into the esophagus by a swallow. The food bolus is then propulsed through the esophagus by peristalsis, which is regulated by cholinergic nerves. When the food reaches the end of the esophagus, the lower esophageal sphincter muscle relaxes and allows the food to pass into the stomach.

The stomach is an expandable reservoir. The empty stomach's capacity is about 50 ml, but it can normally accommodate 1.0 to 1.5 L after a meal. The gastric mucosa contains cells that secrete mucus and bicarbonate to protect the epithelium from acidic gastric juices. The gastric mucosa contains various glands that secrete gastric acid, intrinsic factor, digestive enzymes, hormones, and mucus (Tables 31-1 and 31-2). The stomach has three sections: fundus, body, and antrum. The fundus and the body are reservoirs for ingested food and the site of initial mixing of food and enzymes. The lower portion of the stomach, the antrum, is where the food and digestive enzymes are churned together by powerful gastric contractions to form chyme. Approximately every 30 seconds the chyme and small food particles are emptied through the pyloric sphincter into the duodenum in 1 to 5 ml boluses. Gastric emptying is mainly controlled by neural reflexes and GI hormones (see Table 31-2).

The adult small intestine measures approximately 20 to 22 feet. The first and shortest portion, the duodenum, measures only 8 to 10 inches. Of the remaining small intestine, approximately 8 feet is jejunum and 12 feet is ileum. The epithelial

surface area of the small intestine is approximately 300 m². Large mucosal folds, fingerlike projections throughout the mucosa (villi), and microscopic projections covering the villi (microvilli) impart to the small intestine its massive absorptive surface. The microvilli (or "brush border") produce intestinal enzymes that achieve final digestion before nutrients are absorbed. Blood capillaries and lymphatic ducts run the length of the villi and are the means of nutrient transport after absorption. When the acid chyme enters the duodenum, glands in the mucosa secrete an alkaline substance, thus neutralizing the chyme and protecting the epithelial surface of the intestine. As the chyme progresses through the duodenum, cholecystokinin (CCK) and secretin (see Table 31-2) are released, which trigger secretion of pancreatic enzymes and bile. Segmental contractions of the circular muscles in the intestine and peristalsis facilitate mixing of the chyme and digestive enzymes while moving the chyme through the intestine. Absorption occurs at nutrient-specific sites throughout the intestine (Fig. 31-1), although the majority of nutrients are absorbed in the proximal portion of the small intestine.

Chyme moves through the ileocecal valve into the first portion of the colon (cecum). The chyme is still fluid when it enters the cecum, but as it moves sequentially through the colon, by way of muscle contractions, the colonocytes absorb water, sodium, and potassium (see Fig. 31-1).Some 90% to 95% of the fluid that enters the colon is absorbed by the time the fecal matter enters the rectum.[1] Feces are stored in the rectum until defecation.

The Esophagus

Various diseases and injuries can affect swallowing. Some of the more common medical problems that compromise esophageal function are corrosive injuries and perforation, achalasia, gastroesophageal reflux disease (GERD), and partial or full obstruction.

Corrosive Injuries

Corrosive injuries to the esophagus are caused by swallowing caustic chemicals and are most often associated with suicide attempts. Swallowed caustics can damage the oropharynx, esophagus, and stomach, and when large amounts of chemicals are consumed, the damage can extend into the small intestine and surrounding organs and tissues.[2] Extensive damage is often fatal because of imbalances of fluids, electrolytes, and acid-base status.[2] Treating caustic chemical ingestion by giving water or gastric lavage to dilute it or by inducing vomiting is

Digestive Enzymes and Their Actions

Enzymes or Secretory Product	Site of Secretion	Action	
Salivary amylase (plyalin)	Mouth (salivary glands, three pairs)	Cooked starch Glycogen Dextrin	→ Branched oligosaccharides: some maltose
Lingual lipase (important only in neonates)	Mouth (lingual serous glands)	Fats*	→ Fatty acids, monoglycerides, glycerol
Hydrochloric acid	Stomach, (oxyntic glands o-parietal cells)	Pepsinogen Fe^{+3} Swelling of proteins Antibacterial effects	→ Pepsin → Fe^{+2}
Pepsinogen	Stomach (oxyntic glands, chief cells)	Hydrolyzes peptide bonds between aromatic and dicarboxylic acids	→ Large polypeptides and amino acids
Trypsinogen (activated to trypsin by enterokinase and free trypsin)	Pancreas	Protein and polypeptides	→ Small polypeptides
Chymotrypsinogen (activated to chymotrypsin by trypsin)	Pancreas	Protein and polypeptides	→ Small polypeptides
Procarboxypeptidase (activated to carboxypeptidase A and B by trypsin)	Pancreas	(A) Polypeptides with free carboxyl group (B) Polypeptides with free carboxyl	→ Smaller peptides and aromatic amino acids → Smaller peptides and dibasic amino acids
Elastase	Pancreas	Hydrolyzes fibrous proteins	
Collagenase	Pancreas	Hydrolyzes collagen	
Ribonuclease	Pancreas	Ribonucleic acid	→ Nucleotides
Deoxyribonuclease	Pancreas	Deoxyribonucleic acids	→ Nucleotides
Alpha-amylase	Pancreas	Starch	→ Maltose and dextrins
Lipase and colipase	Pancreas	Fats	→ Monoglycerides, fatty acids, and glycerol
Phospholipase A and B (require bile salts)	Pancreas	Removal of fatty acids from lecithin	
Cholesterol esterase† (requires bile salts)	Pancreas	Free cholesterol	↔ Cholesterol esters (fatty acids)
Retinyl ester hydrolase	Pancreas	Hydrolyzes retinyl esters	
Aminopeptidases	Small intestine (localized in brush border and cytoplasm of absorptive cells)	Polypeptides with free amino group	→ Smaller peptides and free amino acids
Dipeptidases	Small intestine (primarily in cytoplasm of absorptive cells)	Dipeptides	→ Amino acids
Nucleotidase	Small intestine (localized for most part in brush border of villi)	Nucleotides	→ Nucleosides + H_3PO_4
Nucleosidase		Nucleosides	→ Purines, pyrimidines, pentose
Alkaline phosphatase		Organic phosphates	→ Free phosphates
Monoglyceride lipase		Monoglycerides	→ Fatty acid and glycerol
Lechithinase		Lecithin	→ Fatty acids, glycerol, phosphoric acid, choline
Disaccharidases	Small intestine (brush border of villi)	Sucrose	→ Glucose + fructose
Sucrase alpha-dextrinase‡		Maltose and maltotriose	→ Glucose
Lactase		Branched dextrin	→ Maltotriose + glucose
		Lactose	→ Galactose + glucose
Bile	Liver (gallbladder is storage site from which bile moves into small intestine)	Emulsifies fats Stabilizes emulsions Coordinates action of lipase and colipase	

From Hunt SM, Groff JL: *Advanced nutrition and human metabolism*, ed 1, © 1990. Reprinted with permission of Wadsworth an imprint of the Wadsworth Group, a division of Thomson Learning. Fax 800-730-2215.
* Site of action is stomach and small intestine rather than secretion site.
† Enzyme can hydrolyze esters of vitamins A and D, as well as hydrofyzing all three ester linkages of triglycerides.
‡ Enzyme necessary for breaking one to six glucose linkages in dextrins.

controversial. Most of the tissue damage occurs upon contact, and forced emesis can cause complications such as aspiration of the chemical.[2] Surgical resection of the affected tissue is often necessary; however, mild injuries can be managed conservatively with antibiotics and esophageal rest.[3]

Nutrition support recommendations for patients who have suffered a corrosive injury to the esophagus depend on its extent. Indirect calorimetry, when available, should be used to measure energy expenditure, which can vary greatly depending on the extent of the injury. Protein requirements are high because of catabolism and healing (1.5 g protein per kilogram body weight).[3] Patients with mild to moderate injuries that do not require surgery can usually start sipping a liquid diet within 7 to 10 days of injury and can progress to soft foods.[4] Patients

TABLE 31-2

Actions of Gastrointestinal Hormones

Hormone	Site of Secretion	Stimulus	Action
Gastrin	Antrum, duodenum	Peptides, proteoses	Gastric acid secretion
Cholecystokinin (CCK)	Proximal small intestine	Fat, amino acids	Pancreatic enzyme secretion and gallbladder contraction
Secretin	Proximal small intestine	Duodenal acidification	Pancreatic bicarbonate secretion
Gastric inhibitory polypeptide (GIP)	Proximal small intestine	Carbohydrate and fat	Decreases gastric motility, insulin secretion
Motilin	Proximal small intestine	Duodenal alkalinity	Stimulates gastrointestinal motility
Vasoactive intestinal polypeptide (VIP)	Small intestine	Unknown	Vasodilation and smooth muscle relaxation
Glucagon	Pancreas	Plasma insulin and glucose concentrations	Inhibition of motility and stimulation of hepatic glycogenolysis
Enteroglucagon	Small intestine	Carbohydrate and fat	Inhibition of motility
Pancreatic polypeptide	Pancreas	Unknown	Inhibition of gallbladder contraction and pancreatic secretion
Bombesin	Small intestine	Unknown	Gastrin release
Somatostatin	Stomach, small intestine, pancreas	Unknown	Inhibition of other hormone release

Adapted from Klein S, et al; The alimentary tract in nutrition. A tutorial. In Shils M, et al (eds): *Modern nutrition in health and disease*, ed 9, Baltimore, 1999, Williams & Wilkins, p. 613; and Rowlands B, Miller T: The physiology of eating. In Rombeau J, Caldwell M (eds): *Enteral and tube feeding*, Philadelphia, 1984, WB Saunders, p. 16.

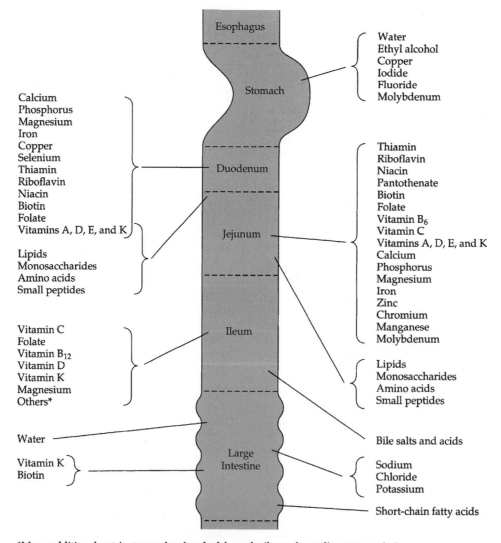

*Many additional nutrients may be absorbed from the ileum depending on transit time.

FIGURE 31-1 Sites of nutrient absorption in the gastrointestinal tract. (From Groff JL, Gropper S: *Advanced nutrition and human metabolism,* ed 3, copyright © 2000. Reprinted with permission of Wadsworth, an imprint of the Wadsworth Group, a division of Thomson Learning. Fax 800-730-2215.

who require surgical resection of the injured tissue often must be hospitalized for long periods and require enteral, if not parenteral, nutrition support.

Feeding via jejunostomy tube is often recommended for those who require long-term esophageal rest.[3,4] Nasoenteric tube feeding is not recommended because the tube can irritate or erode the conduit and cause reflux of gastric contents. Endoscopically placed feeding tubes are not ideal because passing the scope through the esophagus can further damage already injured tissue. Most patients tolerate standard polymeric enteral formulas well. It is best to initiate feedings with an isotonic solution at a slow infusion rate (20 to 30 ml per hour). Feeding volume and concentration can be advanced gradually over 48 to 72 hours to meet the patient's nutrient requirements. When esophageal rest will be short lived or for patients who cannot tolerate enteral feedings, nutrition can be sustained with mixed-nutrient parenteral nutrition (PN).

Esophageal Perforation

Esophageal perforation can be life threatening and difficult to treat. Its causes are varied: esophageal instrumentation (43%); trauma (19%); spontaneous perforation (16%); intraoperative injury (8%); ingestion of foreign bodies (7%); esophageal carcinomas (4%); and other less common causes, such as infection (3%).[5] The treatment plan often depends on the cause of the perforation, the interval between perforation and diagnosis, and the overall condition of the esophagus and surrounding tissues.[5] Both conservative, nonsurgical treatment and definitive surgical repair require esophageal rest. Nutrition support therapy for esophageal perforations is the same as that previously discussed for corrosive injuries. Jejunal feeding is preferable if esophageal rest is required for more than 7 to 10 days.[3,4] PN can be used if enteral access is not available. Radiographic documentation of no leakage in the area of repair is usually required before oral feeding can be initiated.[4]

Achalasia

Achalasia is a disease that affects the lower esophageal sphincter (LES) and peristalsis in the middle and distal esophagus. The sphincter muscles do not relax during swallowing, and the sphincter does not open. Patients with achalasia often suffer from dysphagia, frequent vomiting, feelings of chest fullness or pain, and weight loss. In severe cases, some patients develop protein-calorie malnutrition and pulmonary infections secondary to reduced oral intake and aspiration of food and saliva. The medical treatment includes endoscopic dilation of the LES, surgical release of the muscle, or botulinum toxin injection of the LES.[6]

Nutrition support of patients with achalasia varies with the severity of disease and the mode of treatment. In general, nutrient-dense liquids and semisolid foods, taken at moderate temperatures, in small quantities, and at frequent intervals are usually tolerated by patients with achalasia.[7] Foods that can irritate the esophagus, very spicy or very coarse-textured ones, should be avoided. In some cases, more aggressive treatment may be indicated. Such therapies can include enteral nutrition (EN) or PN support until esophageal emptying improves and nutrient stores are repleted.

Gastroesophageal Reflux Disease

Gastroesophageal reflux is a very common disease that affects at least 21% to 59% of the general population.[8] GERD describes the symptoms that result from reflux of gastric juices, and sometimes duodenal contents, into the esophagus. Reflux occurs with reduced LES pressure and a hiatal hernia or with frequent transient LES relaxations.[9] The symptoms of GERD include substernal burning (heartburn), epigastric pressure sensation, and severe epigastric pain. Prolonged and severe GERD can lead to esophageal bleeding, perforation, strictures, Barrett's epithelium, adenocarcinoma, and pulmonary fibrosis (from aspiration).[9,10] Patients with GERD experience these symptoms at least twice a week. First line therapy for GERD is the use of a proton pump inhibitor (PPI).[11] Severe complications associated to the GERD or persistent symptoms may warrant more invasive evaluation or treatment procedures.

Dietary and lifestyle modifications may provide symptomatic relief of GERD when used in conjunction with PPI therapy. Traditional advise to patients with GERD were to reduce weight if obese and restrict carbonated beverages, caffeine, fatty foods, peppermint, chocolate, and ethanol to promote symptomatic relief of increasing LES pressure. However, more recent analysis of evidence-based medicine supports more limited dietary modifications, which include avoidance of carbonated beverages, alcoholic drinks, and large meals.[9,11] Other lifestyle changes that may benefit some people with GERD are smoking cessation, weight loss if obese, and elevation of the head of the bed for people with nocturnal symptoms.[9,11] Nevertheless, clinicians should treat patients as an individual and advise other dietary or lifestyle modifications if they are identified as triggers of GERD symptoms.

In patients whose GERD symptoms persist or recur after optimal medical therapy or whose LES is documented to be mechanically defective, an antireflux operation may be considered.[11] The purpose of antireflux surgery is to provide permanent relief of all symptoms and complications of GERD secondary to LES incompetence. The Nissen fundoplication, the Belsey Mark IV repair, and the Hill posterior gastropexy are the most widely used antireflux repairs, each associated with 80% to 90% success in providing relief of reflux.[11]

Esophageal Obstruction

Esophageal obstruction can be caused by tumors in or near the esophagus, strictures or scarring of the esophagus, and congenital anomalies. Partial and total obstructions of the esophagus can lead to dysphagia, severe malnutrition, and aspiration pneumonia. Surgical resection of the esophagus with reconstruction provides palliation by permitting normal passage of food and saliva. Various techniques are used to replace the esophagus. The stomach, colon, and jejunum have been successfully used as conduits after total thoracic esophagectomy.[12] When the stomach is mobilized, pyloroplasty or pyloromyotomy is usually done to prevent gastric stasis induced by vagotomy.[12] Reflux may occur through the gastric conduit because it is drained solely by gravity. Once the stomach is pulled into the thoracic cavity, the capacity for gastric expansion decreases. This condition exacerbates gastric reflux and limits the capacity for ingested food.

Colonic interposition, utilization of the colon as a conduit following removal of the esophagus, is performed when the stomach is not suitable for use as a conduit, as when it has been resected or contains tumor.[12] Operative mortality is greater for a colonic interposition than for a gastric conduit, likely because two more anastomoses (colojejunostomy and colocolostomy) must be created during the colonic interposition surgery. Long-term function of colonic interpositions performed for benign obstructions has been excellent.[12] Jejunal interposition is utilized infrequently if neither the stomach nor the colon is appropriate for use. Anastomotic leaks, a complication of esophagectomy, are associated with increased morbidity and mortality.[12,13] Long-term complications of bowel interposition surgery include swallowing difficulty (because of the difference in bowel and esophageal musculature and enervation) and, frequently, stricture formation.[3]

Resurgence of interest in EN has led to the common use of feeding jejunostomy tubes for nutrition support following esophagectomy. Postoperative feedings have been initiated successfully with full-strength isotonic polymeric enteral formulas infused at a slow, continuous rate of 20 to 30 ml per hour. The feeding can be advanced as tolerated over 2 to 3 days to meet the patient's fluid and nutrient requirements. With respect to energy and protein requirements, esophagectomy is major surgery. Indirect calorimetry should be used to measure energy expenditure. Protein requirements can range from 1.0 to 1.5 g/kg body weight.[14]

Ultimately, most esophagectomy patients can take oral liquids and soft solid foods. Small, frequent meals are best tolerated in the perioperative period. Hypertonic oral supplements may not be tolerated well because patients often exhibit dumping syndrome after surgery. Total esophagectomy patients are at risk of reflux through the conduit because the LES is removed during surgery. These patients should be instructed to avoid reclining for 1 hour after a meal and to elevate the head of the bed 30 to 45 degress.[12] Patients able to consume part of their nutrient requirements orally can be managed with cyclic, nocturnal tube feedings until oral intake is sufficient. Those who are able to eat enough orally to fulfill their calorie requirements can discontinue enteral feedings; however, if the patient is to have adjunctive treatments such as chemotherapy, it may be useful to leave the jejunostomy in place in case the treatment impedes oral intake.

The Stomach

The stomach, where food and gastric secretions are mixed and churned together, has secretory functions, which include secretion of intrinsic factor for the absorption of vitamin B_{12} and of hydrochloric acid. Hydrochloric acid is important for several digestive processes, including transformation of ferric iron to ferrous iron and activation of pepsinogen to pepsin (see Table 31-1). Hydrochloric acid also has an immunoprotective role: it kills bacteria and parasites,[15] thus reducing microbial penetration into the intestinal tract.

Gastric Emptying

For the purpose of defining gastric emptying, the stomach can be divided into two compartments: the proximal stomach, consisting of the fundus and upper body of the stomach, and the distal stomach, which includes the lower body and antrum. The proximal stomach accepts and stores ingested food and delivers it to the distal stomach, at a controlled rate, for digestion. Neural reflexes in the proximal stomach allow for receptive relaxation and accommodation, which allow the stomach to relax and accept a food bolus and to accommodate large changes in volume without major fluctuations in intragastric pressure.[15,16] These reflexes are mediated by the vagus nerve and, so, are affected by vagotomy. Intragastric pressure generated by slow, sustained contractions in the proximal stomach is thought to be responsible for emptying of liquids from the stomach. Increased intragastric pressure causes rapid emptying of liquids, whereas decreased intragastric pressure delays emptying of liquids.[16] The hormone motilin stimulates proximal gastric contractions while various other hormones—gastrin, secretin, gastric inhibitory peptide (GIP), vasoactive intestinal peptide, glucagon, and somatostatin—suppress the same contractions (see Table 31-2).[3,16]

Contractions of the distal stomach represent peristalsis. Besides transport functions, peristaltic contractions have an important mixing and grinding effect on solid foods. It is in the distal stomach that solids are reduced to a particle size of 1 to 7 mm.[1,17] The peristaltic waves propel chyme against the antrum wall and down toward the pylorus, where emptying into the duodenum is controlled. Solids that cannot be reduced to smaller than 3 mm are emptied from the stomach between meals by the migrating motor complex (MMC), which produces strong, interdigestive contractions that slowly move from the LES to the ileocecal valve, sweeping intestinal contents through the system.[16,18]

Several factors determine the rate of gastric emptying. Liquids are usually emptied more rapidly than solids, isotonic solutions more quickly than hypotonic or hypertonic ones, and neutral solutions more rapidly than acidic ones.[16,17] With respect to macronutrients, carbohydrates are generally emptied more rapidly than proteins, which are emptied more rapidly than fats.[4,19] Postprandial gastric emptying is normally complete within 4 hours of feeding,[19] although larger, indigestible solids take longer to empty.[16,17]

Many physiologic, pharmacologic, and dietary factors can affect the rate of gastric emptying. Table 31-3 lists some factors commonly associated with increased or decreased gastric emptying. Symptoms of delayed gastric emptying include anorexia, nausea, vomiting, weight loss, and abdominal pain. Several conditions are associated with delayed gastric emptying. Pyloric obstruction like that associated with gastric carcinoma, pyloric stenosis, or bezoar formation can result in gastric retention. Other clinical conditions associated with delayed gastric emptying include diabetic gastroparesis, anorexia nervosa, GERD, ulcer disease, scleroderma, and vagotomy.[18] Medications such as narcotics, somatostatin, and anticholinergic agents can delay gastric emptying.[18] Abnormal serum glucose or electrolytes can transiently delay gastric emptying as well.

Metoclopramide is a cholinergic agent that has been used successfully to treat delayed gastric emptying. It affords symptomatic relief and accelerates gastric emptying in patients with diabetic or postsurgical gastroparesis. In the event of gastro-

TABLE 31-3

Factors Determining the Rate of Gastric Emptying

Decrease Emptying	Increase Emptying
FOODS	
Fat > protein > carbohydrate	In stomach
Thicker consistency (solids > liquids)	Liquids
High osmolality > 800 mOsm/L	Change in temperature
	In duodenum
	High osmolality
	High volume
	Low pH
	Irritant
DRUGS	
Anticholinergics	Cholinergics
Ganglion blockers	Metoclopramide
GASTROINTESTINAL HORMONES	
Secretin	Gastrin
Cholecystokinin	Motilin
Glucagon	
DISEASES OR SURGERY	
Vagotomy	"Irritable colon"
Pseudoobstruction	Pyloroplasty
Diabetic neuropathy	Partial gastrectomy
Autonomic neuropathy	
Scleroderma	
MECHANICAL	
Peptic ulcer	Gravity
Extrinsic pressure	Gastric distention

From Greene HL, Moran JR: The gastrointestinal tract: regulator of nutrient absorption. In Shils ME, Olson JA, Shike M (eds): *Modern nutrition in health and disease*, ed 8, Malvern, PA, 1994, Lea & Febiger, p 556.

paresis refractory to pharmacologic therapy, enteral feeding via jejunostomy tube may be used to provide adequate nutrition to the patient.

Rapid gastric emptying is associated with duodenal ulcers, Zollinger-Ellison syndrome, and gastric surgery.[18,19] The term *dumping syndrome* describes a constellation of postprandial symptoms that result from rapid emptying of hyperosmolar gastric contents into the duodenum.[15,20] The hypertonic load in the small intestine promotes reflux of vascular fluid into the bowel lumen, which rapidly creates symptoms of abdominal cramping, nausea, vomiting, palpitations, sweating, weakness, and osmotic diarrhea.[16,20] Symptoms of early dumping syndrome begin 10 to 30 minutes after eating; late dumping syndrome occurs 1 to 4 hours after a meal.[16,21] Late dumping syndrome is a result of insulin hypersecretion in response to the carbohydrate load dumped into the small intestine. Once the carbohydrate is absorbed, the hyperinsulinemia causes hypoglycemia, which results in vasomotor symptoms such as diaphoresis, weakness, flushing, and palpitations.[15,16]

Dietary manipulation can be useful in preventing dumping syndrome. The following dietary modifications are recommended to prevent rapid emptying of hypertonic solutions into the intestine: (1) eat five or six small meals per day; (2) take liquids 45 to 60 minutes after a meal; (3) avoid simple sugars

TABLE 31-4

Drugs for Peptic Ulcer Disease

Drug	Action
Antibiotics	Bactericidal for *Helicobacter pylori*
Metronidazole	
Amoxicillin	
Tetracycline	
Clarithromycin	
H₂-receptor antagonists	Competitive inhibition of histamine-controlled hydrochloric acid and pepsin production in parietal cells
Cimetidine	
Famotidine	
Nizatidine	
Ranitidine	
Proton pump inhibitors	Blocks H^+-K^+ exchange at parietal cell membrane, thus reducing production of hydrochloric acid
Omeprazole	
Lansoprazole	
Mucosal protectors	Coats stomach to protect healthy and ulcerated mucosa against gastric acid and pepsin
Sucralfate	
Antacids	Neutralizes gastric acids
Magnesium–aluminum hydroxide	
Aluminum hydroxide	

and hypertonic fluids; (4) plan meals that combine complex carbohydrates, protein, or fat; (5) avoid lactose; and (6) recline and rest for 15 to 20 minutes after a meal.[20,22] Recently, octreotide, a long-acting somatostatin analog, has been cited as effective for preventing dumping syndrome.[21] It is thought that somatostatin inhibits secretion of hormones associated with the rapid gastric emptying of dumping syndrome.

Peptic Ulcer Disease

Peptic ulcer disease (PUD) is a common disorder characterized by erosion of the mucosal tissue in the distal esophagus, stomach, and proximal duodenum. *Helicobacter pylori (H. pylori)* infection has been identified as the major cause of PUD. Hypersecretion of hydrochloric acid and pepsin and prolonged or excessive use of nonsteroidal anti-inflammatory drugs may play a role in the development of PUD. Traditionally, PUD was treated with a bland, milk-based diet or surgery; however, research has shown that milk actually causes rebound hyperacidity that can exacerbate the ulcer.[23] Management of PUD includes antibiotics to irradicate *H. pylori* and medications to control the physiologic causes and symptoms (Table 31-4). People with PUD should consume a balanced diet that eliminates only the foods that cause individual symptoms.[7,24]

Gastric Surgery

With the advent of medications to suppress gastric acid secretion, surgeries for benign gastric disease have declined.[24] Currently, gastric surgery is performed for refractory PUD, malignancy, perforation, Zollinger-Ellison syndrome, gastric polyposis, and Mentrier's disease.[3] The common operations are subtotal and total gastrectomy, vagotomy, and pyloroplasty. Each has particular effects on normal function of the stomach and can affect the patient's nutritional status.[1,15]

Most partial gastrectomy procedures remove the distal portion of the stomach and the pylorus and are followed by

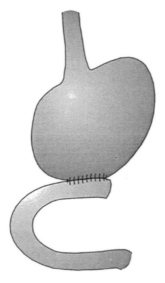

FIGURE 31-2 Billroth I reconstruction after distal gastrectomy.

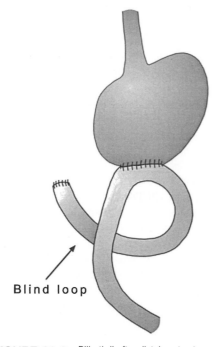

Blind loop

FIGURE 31-3 Billroth II after distal gastrectomy.

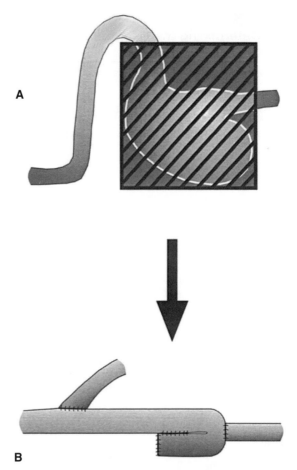

FIGURE 31-4 *A,* Total gastrectomy removes the entire stomach, the distal esophagus, and the proximal duodenum. *B,* Jejunostomy pouch formation and Roux-en-Y reconstruction after total gastrectomy.

Billroth I or Billroth II reconstruction. In the Billroth I reconstruction (gastroduodenostomy), the distal end of the remaining stomach is anastomosed to the duodenum (Fig. 31-2); the Billroth II operation (gastrojejunostomy) forms an anastomosis between the distal stomach and the side of the jejunum, which creates a blind loop (Fig. 31-3). The type of procedure that is performed depends on the primary disease, the condition of the remaining stomach and intestine, and the surgeon's expertise. Both procedures can be associated with early satiety, dumping syndrome, maldigestion, malabsorption, anemia, and metabolic bone disease.[20] Blind loop syndrome is a complication of the Billroth II procedure secondary to stasis in the afferent loop of bowel. The stagnant environment of the blind loop of bowel

permits bacterial overgrowth and infection.[20] Common symptoms of this complication are abdominal pain and bloating, diarrhea, and weight loss. Primary treatment of blind loop syndrome is antibiotic treatment for the bacterial overgrowth or in severe cases surgical repair of the loop of bowel.[20]

NUTRITIONAL CONSEQUENCES AND SUPPORT AFTER GASTRIC SURGERY. Proximal gastrectomy can be performed for distal esophageal cancers or strictures and proximal gastric tumors or anomalies. The resection diminishes the stomach's capacity to receive and store food. This causes increased postprandial intragastric pressure, which ultimately leads to rapid emptying of liquids.[16] Depending on the extent of the resection, gastric peristalsis can be affected, which could impair digestion and emptying of solid foods. Another complication of proximal gastric resection is loss of the LES, which can lead to gastroesophageal reflux.

Total gastrectomy, resection of the entire stomach from the distal esophagus to the duodenum, can cause significant protein-calorie malnutrition.[20] Maldigestion, malabsorption, dumping syndrome, anemia, and metabolic bone disease are reported complications of total gastrectomy.[20] In a randomized, prospective clinical trial, Jivonen and associates[25] studied postgastrectomy patients who had one of two types of reconstructive surgery (simple Roux-en-Y or Roux-en-Y with jejunal pouch formation). Results of this study indicate that the jejunal pouch formation and Roux-en-Y reconstruction (Fig. 31-4) allowed for fewer postoperative symptoms and increased eating capacity compared with the simple Roux-en-Y group. In Jivonen's study, patients who received the jejunal pouch formation and Roux-en-Y reconstruction had delayed emptying that reduced dumping syndrome symptoms, early satiety, and dysphagia. These results are likely due to the fact that the jejunal pouch acts as a reservoir for food and liquids, and the Roux-en-Y facilitates biliary drainage. Interestingly, despite the increased eating capacity, the Roux-en-Y and pouch group did not have significantly different postoperative weight gain or serum albumin concentrations as compared with the simple Roux-en-Y group.[25] However, contrary to these findings, Liedman and colleagues found similar weight loss in the first year after total gastrectomy for both simple Roux-en-Y and Roux-en-Y with a pouch, but over a 5-year postoperative period, individuals in the pouch group were found to regain weight with greater ease.[26,27]

The vagus nerve is a major modulator of the enteric nervous system. Vagotomy is often performed to eliminate gastric acid secretion. Vagotomy at certain levels can alter the normal physiologic function of the stomach, small intestine, pancreas, and biliary system.[16] The three operations commonly performed to block nerve function at various sites of the intestinal tract are proximal gastric, total gastric, and truncal vagotomy.[16] The proximal gastric vagotomy eliminates the stomach's receptive relaxation and accommodation reflexes and thus reduces its capacity to regulate intragastric pressure and store food in the proximal part.[16] Increased intragastric pressure leads to rapid emptying of hypertonic liquids but does not alter emptying of solids.[16] The total gastric and truncal vagotomy procedures impair proximal and distal motor function of the stomach. Thus, digestion and emptying of solids is retarded, while emptying of liquids is accelerated.[19] Total gastric and truncal vagotomy procedures are generally accompanied by a drainage procedure (antrectomy or pyloroplasty) that helps the stomach empty. Nutritional complications associated with vagotomy and pyloroplasty include dumping syndrome and bacterial overgrowth (from total gastric or truncal only).[20]

Postoperative nutrition support is important for gastric surgery patients, regardless of the underlying disease. The potential for maldigestion and malabsorption may necessitate energy intake levels as high as 40 kcal/kg body weight.[28] Measurement of energy expenditure utilizing indirect calorimetry may more precisely estimate energy requirements. Protein requirements range from 1.0 to 1.5 g/kg of body weight.[14]

Patients who have undergone partial or total gastrectomy may require PN or EN support. PN support may be indicated when small bowel resection accompanies gastric surgery or when severe diarrhea develops from EN support. A feeding jejunostomy tube may be placed during gastric surgery. Continuous EN support has been found to be effective after gastric surgery.[29,30] Isotonic, polymeric enteral formulas are usually well tolerated. Feedings should be initiated with full strength isotonic formula at a continuous infusion rate of 20 to 30 ml per hour. The feeding rate can be advanced as tolerated over 2 or 3 days to meet nutrient requirements. Once oral intake is initiated, partial enteral support can be given by cycling the

tube feedings at night. At this time, calorie counts should be taken to quantitate and document oral intake. EN therapy may be required for months after discharge, until adequate oral intake can be maintained. The standard oral diet for gastric surgery patients is one that includes multiple, small, nutrient-dense meals.[3] This recommendation is based on the fact that gastric surgery often reduces the stomach's capacity to accommodate large volumes of food. Additional dietary modifications should be based on individual complications such as dumping syndrome, which is observed in approximately half of all gastric surgery patients.[3,6]

All gastric surgeries carry potential for development of malnutrition. Common consequences of gastric surgery include weight loss, dumping syndrome, maldigestion, malabsorption, anemia, and metabolic bone disease.[3,16,20] Dumping syndrome, epigastric fullness, nausea, and vomiting often occur in the early postoperative period. These symptoms are managed with dietary modifications as previously described for dumping syndrome and with antiemetic medications.

Persons who have had a gastrectomy generally weigh less than normal healthy people.[28,31] Loss of as much as 25% to 30% of premorbid weight is not uncommon after total gastrectomy.[3] The weight loss is the result of reduced dietary intake secondary to epigastric discomfort, early satiety, anorexia, and malabsorption.[3,31] Diet therapy often is not sufficient to produce significant weight gain, and hypertonic oral supplements can cause dumping syndrome and diarrhea. Some patients may require long-term supplemental support via enteral feedings.

Malabsorption after gastric surgery has many causes. Dumping syndrome plays a key role because foods that empty rapidly into the small intestine are not digested well (mechanically or chemically).[26,31] This renders many nutrients unavailable for absorption. Also, the dumping decreases transit time of nutrients, so they are not in contact with the bowel lumen long enough to maximize absorption. Metabolic balance studies suggest that protein, fat, and carbohydrates are incompletely absorbed after gastric surgery.[20,31] Maldigestion is likely the cause. Inadequate pancreatic and biliary stimulation from fast emptying of chyme into the intestine can result in poor mixing of bile and pancreatic enzymes, which may contribute to malabsorption after Billroth II or total gastrectomy[20,31] Finally, bacterial overgrowth from blind loop syndrome can result in fat malabsorption because the bacteria may alter bile salts structurally.[32]

Anemia is a common consequence of gastric surgery. As many as 30% of partial gastrectomy patients develop anemia that can be attributed to a deficiency or malabsorption of one or more nutrients, including iron, vitamin B_{12}, and folate.[20] Hypochromic, microcytic anemia is a consequence of iron deficiency. Gastric surgery patients tend to have reduced intake of foods containing iron as their total dietary intake decreases.[20] After vagotomy, because of decreased gastric acidity, less ferric iron is reduced to ferrous iron and less iron complexed with proteins is liberated. Iron is absorbed in the duodenum (see Fig. 31-1), so either reconstruction that bypasses the duodenum or the dumping syndrome could prevent iron absorption.

Macrocytic anemia can result from vitamin B_{12} malabsorption and folate depletion. Assimilation of vitamin B_{12} requires liberation of the vitamin from protein and binding of the vitamin to intrinsic factor, both of which occur in the stomach. Failure of either of these reactions to occur results in vitamin B_{12} malabsorption, which with time produces anemia. Total gastrectomy patients require periodic intramuscular vitamin B_{12} injections.[15] The efficiency of folate absorption is decreased after some stomach operations because the process requires an acidic environment, and folate intake is often reduced as patients generally eat less.[31] Oral folate supplementation can help increase total absorption and prevent deficiency.

Metabolic bone disease can be a late complication for some 1% to 25% of gastric surgery patients.[3,31] Osteomalacia, osteoporosis, or the combination can result from gastric resection.[33] The cause of metabolic bone disease varies with the surgical procedure. The Billroth II procedure is associated with more complications than is Billroth I because it bypasses the duodenum and upper jejunum (the site of calcium absorption). Procedures that destroy the pylorus can result in rapid gastric emptying that may contribute to development of metabolic bone disease. Rapid gastric emptying not only reduces absorption time but also, when fats are malabsorbed, can lead to formation of insoluble calcium soaps.[20] Fat malabsorption can also result in vitamin D malabsorption, which leads to impaired metabolism of calcium and phosphorus.[33] Finally, prolonged reduced calcium intake, which can lead to metabolic bone disease, is common in gastrectomy patients. Plasma alkaline phosphatase levels have been found to be useful in identifying patients at risk for metabolic bone disease.[33] For patients with elevated alkaline phosphatase values, a diagnostic trial of calcium and vitamin D can be useful to confirm bone disease. If osteomalacia is present, the plasma alkaline phosphatase level drops to normal, after which maintenance levels of calcium and vitamin D should be continued.[33] For those patients at risk, screening and routine monitoring using dual energy x-ray absorptiometry (DEXA) should be advised.

The Small and Large Intestines.

In making nutritional recommendations for the patient with intestinal disease, knowledge of how intestinal pathology impacts digestion, absorption, and metabolism is required. Fig. 31-1 provides information about specific nutrient absorption throughout the GI tract that is helpful in understanding the nutritional sequelae of intestinal disease.

Inflammatory Bowel Disease

The term *inflammatory bowel disease* (IBD) encompasses at least two forms of chronic intestinal inflammation: Crohn's disease (CD) and ulcerative colitis (UC). Although related, these diseases are clinically and pathologically distinct.[34] In the United States, the shared prevalence of CD and UC is approximately 50 per 100,000 population.[35,36] There are approximately 15,000 to 30,000 new cases of IBD in the United States every year.[37] Both diseases occur in all age groups but have a peak incidence in the second and third decades of life.[35] The exact etiologies of both CD and UC unclear. Both CD and UC are believed to result from altered immune responses in the body. A current hypothesis for the etiology of IBD holds that the disease process is a dysregulated immune response to common intraluminal antigens.[38] Given that immune factors are felt to contribute to the pathology of CD and UC, many nutritional and pharmacologic therapies are directed at altering host immunity.

CROHN'S DISEASE. Crohn's disease (CD) is characterized by transmural inflammation—often granulomatous—of the GI tract.[34] CD can attack any region of the GI tract, but it most frequently involves the terminal ileum and proximal colon.[39,40] The chronic inflammatory nature of CD frequently leads to scarring or strictures of the bowel with occasional fistula formation.[34] Symptoms of CD include diarrhea, fever, abdominal pain, growth failure (in children), joint pain, and skin lesions. Some 65% to 75% of Crohn's patients are undernourished, with undernutrition being related to disease severity.[41,42] Many patients with CD require at least one intestinal resection during the course of the disease;[34] however, because of the relapsing nature of the disease, resection is rarely curative and may put the patient at risk of developing short-bowel syndrome (SBS).[34,43]

ULCERATIVE COLITIS. Symptoms of UC include anorexia, nausea, abdominal pain, vomiting, and bloody diarrhea with mucus and purulence.[40] Unlike CD, the inflammation of UC is superficial and limited to the mucosal layer of the large intestine.[34,39] Children with UC may exhibit growth failure as a complication of the disease or of corticosteroid therapy.[44] Weight loss, occurring in approximately 18% to 62% of patients with UC, is less common than is seen with CD.[45] Serious complications of UC include toxic megacolon, severe bleeding, and colonic perforation. Unlike CD, in which intestinal resection is not curative, total colectomy is curative for UC.[34,43]

DRUG THERAPY OF INFLAMMATORY BOWEL DISEASE. Aside from antibiotics, almost all conventional drug treatments for IBD involve direct suppression or modification of the host immune or immunoinflammatory response.[46] Because so many of the drugs used to treat IBD are associated with nutrition-related side effects, a review of medications should be included in the nutrition assessment of patients. Table 31-5 provides an overview of medications commonly used to treat IBD.

NUTRITION ASSESSMENT IN INFLAMMATORY BOWEL DISEASE. Malnutrition is often associated with IBD. The reasons for malnutrition may be related to disease process or may be iatrogenic (Box 31-1). Nutrition therapy of IBD is aimed at providing adequate macronutrients and micronutrients, establishing normal growth in children, and relieving intestinal symptoms. Traditionally, diet therapy of IBD consisted of dietary fiber and lactose restrictions. In reality, controlled studies have not supported the use of low-fiber diets, and the most prudent approach is for IBD patients to exclude only those foods to which they have had a negative clinical response.[38] Similarly, lactose should not be excluded unless evidence of lactose intolerance exists as the incidence of lactose intolerance is no greater in persons with IBD than in the general population.[54]

Individual dietary counseling is key to the dietary management of IBD. A diet history should be taken from each patient to determine which foods are associated with aggravation of GI symptoms. In providing nutritional counseling, the dietitian should be cognizant of which areas of the patient's bowel are affected by disease. For example, presence of ileal disease may predict problems with bile salt or vitamin B_{12} absorption,

TABLE 31-5

Drugs for Inflammatory Bowel Disease[39,47-53]

Drug	Indications	Potential Nutrition-Related Side Effects
Corticosteroids (antiinflammatory)		
Prednisone	Short-term use for induction of remission of	Fluid, salt retention
Prednisolone	Crohn's disease, ulcerative colitis	Increased K, Ca excretion, decreased CHO tolerance, increased
Hydrocortisone		protein catabolism, electrolyte disturbance
Budesonide		Weight gain, dry mouth, vomiting, taste alteration
Aminosalicylate		
Sulfasalazine	Mild to moderate ulcerative colitis, colonic	Decreased absorption of folic acid, nausea, appetite loss, dyspepsia
Mesalamine	Crohn's disease	
Mesalazine		
Immunosuppressants		
Mercaptopurine	Ulcerative colitis, Crohn's disease	Anorexia, diarrhea, nausea, thrombocytopenia, leukopenia
Azathioprine		
Cyclosporine A	Acute, severe ulcerative colitis refractory to steroids	Nausea, vomiting, leukopenia
Methotrexate		Liver damage, megaloblastic anemia, IDDM, hypertension,
Tacrolimus		hyperkalemia, hypomagnesemia, nausea, diarrhea
Antibiotics		
Metronidazole	Ulcerative colitis, perianal Crohn's disease	Nausea, painful oral mucosa, GI upset
Ciprolloxacin		
Resin, bile acid sequestrant		
Cholestyramine	Cholerheic diarrhea (secondary to small bowel	Decreased absorption of vitamins A, D, E, and K
Colestid	resection)	
Biological therapies	Crohn's disease	Abdominal pain, diarrhea, nausea, dehydration, weight loss,
Infliximab		anemia
Antidiarrheals		
Loperamide		Constipation, nausea, vomiting, anorexia
Diphenoxylate HCL		

BOX 31-1

Factors in the Malnutrition of Inflammatory Bowel Diseases[36,43,72]

Decreased nutrient intake
  Restricted oral intake to reduce GI symptoms
  Prescribed dietary restrictions
Increased losses
  Loss of absorptive surface because of active disease or resection
  Small bowel bacterial overgrowth
  Drug-induced losses
  Protein-losing enteropathy
  Bile salt loss secondary to ileal disease or resection
Increased nutrient requirements
  Fever
  Infection
  Postsurgical stress

which may necessitate dietary modifications or additional supplementation. If intestinal stenosis or stricture is present, restriction of high-fiber foods may be indicated to prevent obstructive symptoms.[34,37,55]

Body composition appears to be altered in IBD, particularly CD, in which patients have been shown to have a lower fat mass compared with disease-free controls of the same weight.[56] This finding indicates that patients typically have a higher proportion of lean body mass (LBM) to fat than the general disease-free population. Therefore, when interpreting energy metabolism studies, it is important to compare metabolic rates between patients and controls on a basis of LBM rather than total body weight. Generally, metabolic studies have failed to show significant hypermetabolism in patients with quiescent IBD compared with controls when LBM is controlled for.[57-59] In their study of stable outpatients with CD, Kushner and Schoeller found total energy expenditure (TEE) to be 1.78 times the metabolic rate predicted by the Harris-Benedict equation. This compared with a TEE for healthy controls of 1.70 times the predicted value.[57] The TEEs of both groups included energy expenditure for physical activity. In a more recent trial, measured resting energy expenditure (REE) in patients with stable CD was similar to that of controls; however, higher rates of diet-induced thermogenesis and lipid oxidation were noted in the those with CD.[56] It is hypothesized that these alterations in substrate metabolism provide an explanation for the decreased fat mass associated with the disease and general difficulty CD patients have in maintaining nutritional status.[56] Although energy metabolism in UC has not been studied as extensively as CD, significant hypermetabolism has not been observed in UC either. An REE 19% greater than predicted by the Harris-Benedict equation was observed in patients with active UC.[60] In either CD or UC the presence of sepsis, concurrent infection, or surgical stress increases energy requirements. However, in the absence of those conditions, energy intakes of 30 to 35 kcal per kilogram of body weight has been shown to be sufficient to meet the calorie needs of patients with stable IBD.[45,58,60]

Protein requirements for patients with IBD may be elevated, even in the presence of normal or nearly normal energy requirements. Factors that increase the protein requirements of persons with CD or UC include blood loss, protein-losing enteropathy, fever, infections, and corticosteroid therapy. Protein requirements for most patients with CD or UC typically range from 1.0 to 1.5 g/kg body weight per day. Septic or malnourished patients may require protein intakes up to 2.0 g/kg body weight per day.[60]

Physiologic derangements of IBD predispose patients to electrolyte loss, vitamin D malabsorption, impaired folic acid absorption, niacin deficiency, hypocalcemia, hypomagnesemia, vitamin B_{12} deficiency, or selenium deficiency, among others.[54,61] Before performing a nutrition assessment and counseling IBD patients, the clinician should have a full understanding of the diseased area of bowel, previous resections, and any dietary restrictions, so that appropriate vitamin and mineral supplements can be suggested. A high-potency multivitamin with minerals is recommended for most persons with active IBD. Additional supplementation of other micronutrients is frequently necessary. Decreased bone mineral density and metabolic bone disease is a common complication of both CD and UC and is particularly prevalent in pediatric patients. Reasons for decreased bone mineral density include undernutrition, prolonged corticosteroid use, hypogonadism, malabsorption of calcium and vitamin D, and the effects of inflammatory cytokines.[62-64] Upon diagnosis of IBD, it is recommended that a measurement of bone density be performed to establish a baseline value.[65] Patients receiving corticosteroids should be supplemented with 1 to 2 g calcium daily.[55] As previously stated, calcium-rich milk-based foods should not be excluded from the diet unless lactose intolerance is documented. If there is a risk of fat-soluble vitamin malabsorption either because of small bowel disease or resection, serum 25-hydroxyvitamin D should be measured every 2 to 3 years. If it is below normal or in the low-normal range and parathyroid hormone level is elevated, replacement with 25,000 to 50,000 units of vitamin D orally once daily to once weekly should be instituted.[55] Anemia is commonly seen in IBD and may be due to iron deficiency from blood loss, folate deficiency or vitamin B_{12} malabsorption from ileal disease.[62] Anemia should be assessed with a complete blood count (CBC) and serum ferritin. Iron, vitamin B_{12}, or folate supplements should be prescribed as appropriate. Sulfasalazine, commonly used in UC, decreases folate absorption and so patients receiving this medication should receive at least 1 mg folate daily. A baseline height and weight should be recorded on every patient with a new diagnosis of IBD. Weight should be recorded at frequent intervals. For children, height, weight, sexual maturation, and bone age should be documented on a routine basis as well. The following laboratory studies should be performed to identify nutritional deficiencies: CBC; ferritin; calcium; magnesium; zinc; total protein; albumin; prothrombin time, and levels of vitamin B_{12}, folate, vitamins A, D, and E, and zinc.[62] Consultation with a dietitian is indicated for the person with newly diagnosed IBD. Reconsultation should occur with any change in clinical course such as surgery, unexplained weight loss, or failure to thrive in children.

NUTRITION AS PRIMARY THERAPY FOR INFLAMMATORY BOWEL DISEASE. Because a theoretic cause of IBD, particularly CD, is that of a "dietary antigen" thought to provoke immune-mediated damage to gut mucosa,[66,67] therapies that manipulate dietary protein have been investigated. In the late 1970s and

early 1980s, parenteral nutrition (PN) was considered an important advance in the treatment of refractory CD. Although PN with "bowel rest" was considered primary therapy, most patients so treated also took corticosteroids, confounding the benefits of PN and "bowel rest."[34,68] In trials using PN to induce remission of CD, initial remission rates averaged 60% and body weight and serum albumin were improved.[69] However, in addition to being expensive and associated with complications, the use of PN for CD was associated with a fairly high relapse rate.[34,68] Enteral nutrition (EN) as primary therapy (in place of corticosteroids) has been shown to be an effective means of inducing remission in CD and may provide more nutritional benefits than PN with bowel rest. Compared with PN, EN has been shown to better improve total body nitrogen and replenish body reserves of protein in malnourished persons with CD, suggesting that the gut may be the preferred route for nutrient administration to malnourished patients.[68] The nutritional benefits of EN, combined with greater safety and lower costs as compared with PN, make it the preferred nutrition therapy for IBD for most patients. Early clinical trials of EN as primary therapy for CD centered around chemically defined ("elemental") diets, under the premise that a hydrolyzed protein source of peptides or amino acids lessened or eliminated protein antigenicity. O'Morain and coworkers have demonstrated a chemically defined diet to be as effective as prednisolone in inducing remission of acute CD.[70] Other investigators using "elemental" or "semi-elemental" diets have shown similar results.[71-75] Teahon and colleagues reported 15 years' experience with chemically defined diets in the treatment of CD. In more than 150 patients, remission rates with chemically defined diets averaged 80%.[76]

Despite the apparent effectiveness of chemically defined diets in promoting remission of CD, certain practical considerations make it undesirable for some patients and clinicians. Chemically defined diets are generally expensive and relatively unpalatable, making them unacceptable for many patients. For these reasons, many studies that have addressed the effectiveness of these diets for IBD have been plagued by high dropout rates and poor compliance.[45,66,67] Polymeric diets have been used as an alternative to chemically defined diets in the treatment of CD because they are generally less expensive and more palatable. Meta-analysis applied to multiple clinical trials enabled a comparison of chemically defined and polymeric diets. In two separate meta-analyses, there was no statistically significant difference between the two types of diets in achieving remission of CD or in subsequent relapse rates.[77,78] Both types of diets were inferior to standard drug treatment (corticosteroids) in inducing clinical remission of Crohn's.[77] The suggested reasons that EN is effective as a primary treatment modality in CD include reversal of malnutrition, modification of gut flora, decreased gut permeability, and the provision of trophic nutrients.[78,79] In practice, a short course of corticosteroids is likely to be more effective in inducing remission of CD than is EN therapy. Although this may be acceptable to adults, corticosteroid therapy has more devastating sequelae such as growth failure in pediatric patients. For pediatric patients, especially, EN with a liquid formula in lieu of corticosteroids may be preferable as a primary therapeutic modality in active Crohn's disease.

Nutrition as primary therapy for UC has been disappointing. Studies investigating the use of PN for UC have generally shown it to be ineffective in reversing the course of the disease.[80-82] Similarly, EN using chemically defined diets has not been demonstrated to be effective in the treatment of colitis, as it has in CD.[44,82] Current research indicates that the theory of "bowel rest" or dietary restriction may in fact exacerbate colitis by starving colonocytes of their primary energy source, short-chain fatty acids (SCFAs), which are an end product of bacterial fermentation of unabsorbed carbohydrate.[44] It has been postulated that UC may be a manifestation of enterocyte fuel deficiency.[83] This theory would support feeding the colon, rather than resting it, during treatment of UC. There is much interest in the provision of SCFAs in UC; however, no nutritional formulations currently available provide this substrate to the colon.

THERAPY WITH SPECIFIC NUTRIENTS IN INFLAMMATORY BOWEL DISEASE. Provision of specific nutrients that exert trophic effects on the bowel or modulate immunity have been investigated in the treatment of both CD and UC.

Short-chain fatty acids. Short-chain fatty acids (SCFAs) appear to play a significant role in normal colon function and in the treatment of bowel inflammation. SCFAs are produced by bacterial fermentation of dietary fiber and resistant starches that escape absorption in the intestine.[84,85] SCFAs are the preferred fuel for human colonocytes, providing about 4.4 kcal/g.[86] The primary SCFAs—acetate, propionate, and butyrate—compose about 90% to 95% of total SCFAs.[84] SCFAs appear to have several roles that affect the nutritional state and general health of humans.

By enhancing sodium and water absorption, SCFAs counteract diarrhea.[84,85] The addition of pectin, a soluble fiber metabolized to SCFA, to isotonic tube feedings of 13 normal adults significantly reduced the incidence of liquid stools and promoted normalization of colonic fluid composition.[87]

Animal and human studies have demonstrated enhanced bowel motility when SCFAs are introduced into the small bowel or colon. In healthy volunteers, a mixture of SCFAs infused into the ileum produced more motor events than infusion of air or water. The amount of SCFAs used in this study was similar to the concentration normally found in the colon.[84]

There is evidence that SCFAs have a trophic effect on normal colon mucosa. In animal studies, bacterial carbohydrate fermentation has been shown to be necessary for raising cell turnover.[84] Pectin supplementation of elemental diets has been shown in rat studies to enhance intestinal adaptation after bowel resection by increasing mucosal weight and deoxyribonucleic acid (DNA), ribonucleic acid (RNA), and protein content of the mucosa.[88] Bursting pressures of colonic anastomoses in rats have been shown to increase when pectin is added to the diet.[89] Additionally, SCFAs appear to prevent or improve inflammatory changes of the large bowel. In patients with UC, twice-daily rectal instillation of a mixture of SCFAs promoted clinical and histologic improvement of disease.[83] Harig and colleagues reported clinical and histologic improvement of diversion colitis in four patients after SCFAs irrigation for 2 to 3 weeks.[90]

In summary, preliminary evidence exists to support the benefits of providing substrate (fermentable carbohydrate) for

bacterial fermentation to SCFAs in some patients with colonic disease. Although successful use of pectin in tube feedings has been reported,[87,91] routine commercial use of it or other soluble fiber is limited by its viscosity. Parenteral infusion of SCFAs has been used experimentally, but formulas are not yet commercially available.[86] Until practical forms of fermentable fibers or SCFAs become available, clinicians must be wary of unnecessarily restricting dietary fiber in patients with colonic disease and thus depriving the colon of its preferred fuel.

Fish oils (ω-3 fatty acids). Omega-3 (ω-3) fatty acids (Chapter 9) have been found to have a number of anti-inflammatory effects and have therefore been of interest as a nutritional therapy in inflammatory disorders such as IBD.[92] Two main types of ω-3 fatty acids are found in fish oil, eicosapentanoic acid and docosahexaenoic acid, which are important inhibitors of proinflammatory leukotriene B4 and thromboxane A2. Modification of leukotriene production results in downregulation of the intestinal immunoinflammatory response.[58,92,93] Because of its ω-3 fatty acid content, the use of fish oil has been investigated in CD and UC. One study compared patients with CD who took fish oil capsules (2.7 g per day) with patients taking placebo capsules. Relapse of disease was significantly lower in the fish oil group than in the placebo group. Furthermore, significantly more patients taking the fish oil remained in remission after 1 year as compared with those taking placebo.[94] When studied in patients with UC, fish oil was associated with improvement in clinical and sigmoidoscopic score compared with placebo. Moreover, patients taking fish oil required less steroid medication than those treated with placebo.[65] A study looking at the prophylactic use of fish oil in quiescent UC was less encouraging and did not show significant benefits.[60] Although it appears that use of fish oil supplements may confer some benefit in reducing the inflammation of IBD, problems have been cited with its use. Unpleasant side effects such as halitosis, flatulence, and diarrhea have been reported, resulting in poor patient compliance.[93] Although the trials to date have shown promise that fish oil supplementation may be an effective adjunct in IBD therapy, more controlled trials are necessary before its use is routinely recommended in IBD.

Glutamine. Glutamine is the primary energy substrate for the small intestine and has been shown to prevent gut permeability and protect against intestinal mucosal atrophy, and it may improve gut immune function.[95-97] In catabolic states, enteral or parenteral glutamine supplementation has been shown to improve immune function of the gut.[60] Although it would seem reasonable that glutamine might exert benefits in IBD, controlled trials have yet to demonstrate this. Akobeng and colleagues[96] randomized 18 children with active CD to receive a 4-week course of either a standard polymeric diet with a low-glutamine content or an isocaloric isonitrogenous glutamine-enriched polymeric diet. The proportion of patients achieving remission was no different between groups. Improvement in mean pediatric CD activity index was actually greater in the group receiving the low-glutamine diet. Although more studies are indicated, it would appear at present that the beneficial effects demonstrated with glutamine in the catabolic patient may not apply in IBD.[96]

Growth hormone and dietary protein. Recently, the use of growth hormone (somatropin) has been shown to benefit persons with active CD. Thirty-seven adults with moderate to severe active CD were randomized to receive self-administered injections of growth hormone or a placebo. Both groups were instructed to increase protein intake to at least 2 g/kg body weight per day. Patients received treatment for 4 months. Patients in the growth hormone group had significant improvement in disease activity (as indicated by the Crohn's Disease Activity Index tool) within the end of the first month. Improvement continued during the subsequent 3 months. Additionally, clinical improvement enabled a reduction in the amount of medications required by the patients in the growth hormone group.[97] It is not clear specifically how growth hormone improves symptoms of CD, but in general growth hormone enhances uptake of amino acids by the intestine, decreases intestinal permeability, and increases intestinal protein synthesis. Because all subjects consumed a high-protein diet, the beneficial effect of dietary protein was presumed to be enhanced by the administration of growth hormone.[97] This preliminary study shows great promise, but additional research is needed to confirm the results.

Probiotics. There is evidence that the contents of the intestinal luminal microenvironment is responsible for the initiation and perpetuation of IBD, particularly CD.[46] Therefore, novel therapies for IBD such as probiotics are being investigated that attempt to alter the microenvironment of the intestine. Probiotics are defined as nonpathogenic microorganisms that, when ingested, exert a positive influence on the health or physiology of the host.[98] They can influence intestinal physiology either directly or indirectly through modulation of the endogenous ecosystem or immune system. Different strains of probiotics have been identified that are associated with a variety of clinical benefits. Intracolonic administration of the probiotics *L. reuteri* and *L. plantarum* into rats with methotrexate-induced enterocolitis was associated with lower intestinal permeability, bacterial translocation, and plasma endotoxin concentrations compared with rats with enterocolitis that did not receive the probiotic infusions.[98] Human probiotic studies in patients with IBD have been conducted as well. In a 20-patient study, patients with active, moderate CD were randomized to receive either oral *S. boulardii* or placebo for 7 weeks in addition to their routine medical therapy. Patients receiving the probiotic had a significant reduction in disease activity, which was not observed in the patients receiving placebo.[99] In UC, an oral nonpathogenic *E.coli* preparation was found to be as effective as mesalazine in inducing remission and preventing relapse of disease.[100] Several studies are currently being conducted to further investigate the effects of probiotics on IBD.[98]

CONSEQUENCES OF SURGERY FOR INFLAMMATORY BOWEL DISEASE

Ileal pouch–anal anastomosis. Total proctocolectomy is necessary for some medical conditions. In recent years, abdominal colectomy together with ileal pouch–anal anastomosis (IPAA) has become routine surgery for uncontrolled UC or familial adenomatous polyposis.[101,102] During IPAA, the diseased colon and rectum are removed and a pelvic reservoir (pouch) is constructed from the healthy ileum and anastomosed to the anal sphincter.[57] With this procedure, permanent ileostomy is avoided and normal bowel function may

be retained. Normally, the colon is the principal site of sodium, potassium, and water absorption and the formation and absorption of bacteria-produced vitamin K;[101] however, after removal of the colon, the constructed ileal reservoir apparently adapts to the absorptive capacity of the colon.[101] No dietary restrictions are necessary after the procedure, with the possible exception of concentrated carbohydrates and large volumes of fluids with meals. These measures may help avoid osmotic diarrhea after surgery.[101] Minor iron-deficiency anemia has been reported after IPAA. Oral iron supplementation is usually corrective. Serum vitamin B_{12} levels may also be low, possibly because of changes in the terminal ileum from pouch reconstruction.[103] A finding of low serum vitamin B_{12} warrants further workup of B_{12} absorption, with appropriate therapy.

"Pouchitis." Approximately 20% of patients with an IPAA develop pouchitis, a mucosal inflammation of the pouch characterized clinically by diarrhea, bloody stools, malaise, fecal urgency, and fever.[83,102,104] Drug therapy of pouchitis typically consists of antibiotics.[83,104]

Reduced levels of SCFAs in acute pouchitis led to the theory that it may be a manifestation of enterocyte fuel deficiency. Reduced levels of fecal SCFAs have been demonstrated in acute pouchitis, as well as UC, and correlate closely with mucosal villus atrophy.[83] In one study, three of nine patients with pouchitis showed good clinical response to treatment with SCFAs (butyrate) suppositories.[83] Preliminary data, along with recent research in UC, support enteral feeding rather than "bowel rest" as preferred therapy for large bowel IBD.

Malabsorption

Malabsorption is a syndrome in which normal products of digestion do not traverse the intestinal mucosa and enter the lymphatic or portal venous branches.[24] *Maldigestion,* which may be clinically similar to malabsorption, describes defects in the intraluminal phase of the digestive process caused by inadequate exposure of chyme to bile salts and pancreatic enzymes. The term *malabsorption* generally includes maldigestive processes. The following discussion provides general information about the clinical presentation and nutrition support of malabsorption and detailed descriptions of three malabsorption disorders: SBS, radiation enteritis, and celiac sprue. Box 31-2 describes conditions associated with malabsorption and the mechanisms by which nutrient loss occurs.

Clinical symptoms of malabsorption typically include diarrhea, steatorrhea, and weight loss.[24,105,106] Laboratory signs of malabsorption may include depressed serum fat-soluble vitamin levels, accelerated prothrombin time, hypomagnesemia, and hypocholesterolemia. Patients with symptoms of malabsorption should have a laboratory workup to determine presence and degree of nutrient loss. Details of a "malabsorption workup" (Table 31-6) include tests of fat absorption, small bowel and pancreatic function, and disaccharidase activity.

STEATORRHEA. Steatorrhea—excessive fat in the feces—may be the most common sign of malabsorption. Normally, approximately 94% of fat consumed is absorbed. Fecal fat output greater than 7 to 8 g/day (with a 100-g fat per day diet) is associated with disease.[107] When steatorrhea is greater than 25 g/day, it is usually associated with pancreatic rather than intestinal

Pathophysiology of Malabsorption

Pathologic Condition	Mechanism of Malabsorption
Gastric surgery	No feedback control of chyme release
Billroth I	Improper mixing of chyme with digestive enzymes
Billroth II	Duodenal bypass
Roux-en-Y	Duodenal bypass
Zollinger-Ellison syndrome	Pancreatic enzymes inactive due to low pH
Bacterial overgrowth	Bile acid deconjugation, mucosal damage
Chronic pancreatitis	Insufficient digestive enzymes or bile
Pancreatic carcinoma	Insufficient digestive enzymes or bile
Chronic cholestasis	Insufficient digestive enzymes or bile
Biliary tract disease	Insufficient digestive enzymes or bile
Endocrine disorders	Rapid transit, decreased contact time
Hormonally active tumors	Rapid transit, decreased contact time
Jejunoileal bypass	Bypass of absorbing sites
Ileal resection	Loss of absorbing sites
Short bowel syndrome	Loss of surface area
Infectious enteritis	Mucosal damage
Crohn's disease	Transmural inflammation and mucosal atrophy
Celiac sprue	Transmural inflammation and mucosal atrophy
Giardiasis	Unknown
Whipple's disease	Infiltration of lamina propria by bacteria
Eosinophilic enteritis	Inflammation
Small bowel lymphoma	Loss of brush border enzymes
Radiation enteritis	Submucosal fibrosis
Lymphangiectasia	Blocked lymphatic drainage
Abetalipoproteinemia	Blocked transport from bowel target tissue

From Cerda J: Diet and gastrointestinal disease, *Med Clin North Am* 77:881, 1993.

disease.[107] Steatorrhea rarely exists independently of malabsorption of other nutrients, so persons with steatorrhea are at risk of developing protein-calorie malnutrition and other micronutrient deficiencies.[107] Steatorrhea may cause other physical and metabolic problems unrelated to the underlying disease process, such as hyperoxaluria. When fatty acids are absorbed, as during normal bowel function, intraluminal oxalate forms complexes with calcium to make an insoluble compound that is then excreted in the feces. During fat malabsorption, however, unabsorbed fatty acids bind with calcium, to form soaps in a process called *saponification.* Free oxalate then binds with sodium, forming a salt that is absorbed in the colon.[105,107,108] Persons with hyperoxaluria are at risk of developing calcium oxalate kidney stones. Steatorrhea can also contribute to increased loss of the divalent cations calcium, magnesium, and zinc. Divalent cations saponify with fatty acids, resulting in excessive loss of the divalent cations through stool. Steatorrhea aggravates diarrhea in patients whose colon is intact to the small bowel. Unabsorbed fatty acids enter the large bowel and undergo hydroxylation by colonic bacteria, which increase water and electrolyte secretion.[109]

CARBOHYDRATE MALABSORPTION. Malabsorption of carbohydrate by the intestinal mucosa is fairly uncommon. Maldigestion of carbohydrate (or carbohydrate "intolerance"), however, is much more common and can cause bloating, flatulence, and diarrhea. Usually, carbohydrate intolerance is due to disaccharidase deficiency, most often lactase. Lactase deficiency, or lactose intolerance, can be primary or secondary to medications, radiation therapy, or abdominal surgery.[110]

Lactose intolerance is easily diagnosed by serum or breath tests. The lactose breath test is a simple, noninvasive method of determining tolerance to lactose. After a dose of lactose is consumed, breath hydrogen is measured. If lactose remains unabsorbed, hydrogen is released by lactose fermentation by colonic bacteria. A high level of hydrogen (usually more than 20 ppm) indicates lactose intolerance.[111]

PROTEIN MALABSORPTION. Maldigestion of protein may occur during pancreatic insufficiency secondary to inadequate breakdown of dietary protein by protease; however, intestinal malabsorption of protein is less common. Like carbohydrate, protein is absorbed very efficiently in the proximal small bowel without bile salts. When protein malabsorption does occur, it is usually secondary to postoperative inflammatory conditions such as gastritis or jejunitis that disrupt mucosal integrity.[106]

FLUID AND ELECTROLYTE MALABSORPTION. Extensive fluid and electrolyte losses can occur during malabsorption. Approximately 7 to 9 L of fluid is presented to the small bowel daily. Of this volume, all but 100 to 200 ml is absorbed, which is then excreted in stool.[108,112] When intestinal absorptive capacity is diminished, increased GI losses can frequently cause dehydration, hyponatremia, hypokalemia, hypomagnesemia, hypocalcemia, and metabolic acidosis.[108]

NUTRITION MANAGEMENT OF MALABSORPTION. If possible, the disease underlying the malabsorption syndrome should be treated. Nutrition support is aimed at decreasing fecal losses while correcting nutrient deficiencies. Steatorrhea has traditionally been treated with a low-fat diet (25 to 40 g/day), frequently with the addition of medium-chain triglycerides (MCTs) as the calorie source. Besides being unpalatable and difficult to comply with, an extremely fat-restricted diet is frequently hypocaloric. A less radical approach to nutrition management of steatorrhea should first be attempted. Patients with steatorrhea should be counseled on modest fat restriction (30% of total caloric intake). If symptoms continue, fat can be further restricted.

MCT oil traditionally has been an adjunct to the low-fat diet used to treat malabsorption. MCTs have the theoretic advantage of increasing the palatability and energy intake of the diet without promoting steatorrhea and the mineral loss associated with consumption of long-chain fatty acids (LCFAs). MCTs are fatty acids that range in length from 6 to 12 carbon molecules and do not require bile salt micelle formation for absorption.[107] They are absorbed directly into the portal vein instead of through the lymphatic system.[107] Disadvantages of MCT oil include its cost, lack of essential fatty acids, and cathartic effect in some persons.[107,108] Reasons for the poor tolerance to MCTs have not been well understood. A recent study compared intestinal transit times of medium-chain and long-chain triglycerides (LCTs) in normal, healthy volunteers. Both lipids were infused intraduodenally to eliminate differences caused by varying rates of gastric emptying. Transit time for MCTs was significantly shorter than that of long-chain fats, which may explain the symptoms of borborygmi, abdominal pain, and diarrhea associated with its use.[113] It is possible that MCTs induce a secretory response in the bowel or that hydrolysis of MCTs creates osmotically active fatty acids, resulting in osmotic diarrhea.[113] The current

TABLE 31-6

Tests for Malabsorption: Typical Findings

Test	Normal Values	Malabsorption (Nontropical Sprue)	Maldigestion (Pancreatic Insufficiency)	Comments
Stool examination				
Qualitative				
Neutral fat	1+	Normal	↑ ↑	Reliable screening test if properly performed; not sensitive enough to detect minimal steatorrhea
Fatty acid	1+	↑ ↑	↑	
Undigested muscle fibers	<5	<5	>5	
Quantitative				
Determination of stool fat	≤6 g/24 hr; 95% coefficient of fat absorption	>6 g/24 hr	>6 g/24 hr	Most reliable test for documenting steatorrhea
Carbohydrate absorption				
D-Xylose absorption test (25-g dose)	Urinary excretion ≥4.5 g/5 hr; blood level ≥30 mg/dL	↓	Normal	Good screening test for carbohydrate absorption; spurious low values may be obtained with incomplete urine collections, renal failure, ascites, bacterial overgrowth in small bowel, and certain drugs (e.g. indomethacin)
Oral glucose tolerance test (GTT)	USPHS criteria; O'Sullivan criteria	Frequently flat	Frequently diabetic	Approximately 10% of normal subjects have a flat GTT
Gastrointestinal roentgenograms of stomach and small bowel		Malabsorption pattern	May see malabsorption pattern or pancreatic calcification	Malabsorption pattern is nonspecific; may be present in several disorders
Peroral jejunal mucosal biopsy		Abnormal	Normal	
Pancreatic function tests				
Secretin test	Volume ≥1.8 mL/kg/hr [HCO$_3$] ≥80 mEq/L	Normal	Abnormal	A sensitive test for demonstration of exocrine pancreatic insufficiency
Duodenal perfusion with essential amino acids	Trypsin and lipase output	Frequently normal	↓	Abnormal volumes found when ≤10% of the exocrine pancreas is functioning
Schilling test for vitamin B$_{12}$ absorption	>10% urinary excretion ^{60}Co in 48 hr	Frequently ↑	Frequently ↑	Useful in screening for gastric disorders (pernicious anemia) bacterial overgrowth, and ileal diseases (regional ileitis)
Blood tests				
Serum iron	80-150 µg/dL	Frequently ↓	Normal	Blood tests are fairly satisfactory screening tests for malabsorption; abnormalities should raise the question of malabsorption; however, such tests provide little help with differential diagnosis
Serum folate	5-21 ng/ml	Frequently ↓	Frequently ↓	
Serum calcium	9-11 mg/dL	Frequently ↓	Usually normal	
Serum cholesterol	150-250 mg/dL	Frequently ↓	Frequently ↓	
Serum albumin	3.5-5.5 g/dL	Frequently ↓	Occasionally ↓	
Prothrombin time	12-15 sec	Frequently prolonged	Occasionally prolonged	
Serum carotenes	100 IU/dL	↓	Frequently ↓	
Serum vitamin A	100 IU/dL	↓	Occasionally ↓	
Urine test				
Urine 5-hydroxyindoleacetic acid (5-HIAA)	2-9 mg/24 hr	Frequently ↑	Normal	Greatly increased values characteristic of carcinoid syndrome; slightly increased levels (12-18 mg/24 hr) frequently found in sprue
Specialized tests				
Culture of jejunal contents	≤10^3 organisms per ml	Negative cultures	Negative cultures	Abnormal cultures (≥10^7 microorganisms per mL) characteristically found in bacterial overgrowth syndromes
Duodenal or jejunal fluid analysis				
Conjugated bile salts	≥2 mm/ml	Usually normal	Normal	May be decreased in sprue due to sequestration in gallbladder; characteristically decreased in ileal inflammatory disease and ileal resection
Unconjugated bile salts	Not present	Not present	Normal	Increased with bacterial overgrowth
Micellar lipid	≥50% dietary lipid ingested in micellar phase	Usually normal	Decreased	Decreased with a deficiancy of steapsin or bile salts
^{14}C-glycolic acid breath test	<1% of dose excreted as ^{14}CO$_2$ in 4 hr	Normal	Normal	Increased ^{14}CO$_2$ excretion with bacterial overgrowth syndromes or bile acid malabsorption; determination of fecal bile acids aid in identifying the latter
Breath hydrogen test (after 50 g of lactose)	Minimal breath hydrogen	May be ↑	Normal	Secondary to lactase deficiency

From Stralovich A: Gastrointestinal and pancreatic disease. In Gottschlich M, Matarese L, Shronts E (Eds): *Nutrition Support Dietetics Core Curriculum*, ed 2, Silver Spring, MD: ASPEN, 1993, pp 275-310.

availability of low-fat commercial products, such as bakery items and snack foods, which can increase the caloric density of a fat-restricted diet, minimizes the value of MCTs in the diets of patients with malabsorption.

Symptoms of carbohydrate intolerance will disappear if the offending carbohydrates are avoided. In the case of lactase deficiency, however, restriction of foods containing lactose can reduce calcium consumption if dairy foods are eliminated from the diet. Most persons with diagnosed lactose intolerance can tolerate small amounts of lactose without developing symptoms. A recent study found that lactose maldigesters could tolerate as much as 6 g of lactose (equivalent to 1/2 cup of milk) without symptoms of intolerance.[114] Larger doses of lactose may be tolerated as well if they are consumed with other foods, which serve to delay gastric emptying and delivery of lactose to the colon. Lactase tablets are available commercially that, when taken with foods containing lactose, decrease symptoms of lactose intolerance. Patients may have to titrate dosing to food, depending on the severity of their symptoms.

Patients with malabsorption require fairly high levels of calories and protein to maintain nutritional status. The requirements of macronutrients and micronutrients increase with the magnitude of malabsorption. A reasonable goal for a person who initially presents with malabsorption is an energy intake of approximately 40 to 45 kcal/kg body weight per day and a protein level of at least 1.5 g/kg per day. Alternatively, 500 kcal per day may be added to the total Harris-Benedict equation (BEE × activity factor × stress factor) as an "allowance" for malabsorptive losses. Close follow-up is required, and modifications must be made in prescribed energy and protein recommendations, as anthropometry, laboratory parameters, and clinical status dictate.

Micronutrient deficiencies are common with malabsorption. Patients with steatorrhea are at risk for deficiencies of fat-soluble vitamins, folic acid, and divalent cations.[107] Vitamin B_{12} deficiency may occur if the terminal ileum is diseased or has been resected. Calcium status may be adversely affected by fatty acid saponification and vitamin D deficiency. All patients with malabsorption should have full laboratory assessment of nutrition parameters. Recommendations for vitamin and mineral supplementation should be individualized based on laboratory parameters (Table 31-7).

In general, most patients with malabsorption benefit from small, frequent feedings during the day. Oral calorie supplements may be useful in some patients, although hypertonic formulas can cause osmotic diarrhea in patients with rapid gastric emptying and intestinal transit. Theoretically, chemically defined or peptide-based nutritional supplements may benefit patients with significant malabsorption secondary to mucosal damage like that associated with radiation enteritis or celiac sprue; however, the increased osmolarity of many of these formulas can contribute to increased diarrhea.

With malabsorption, maintenance of fluid balance is especially important. Patients with malabsorption and diarrhea are frequently treated with antimotility medications, including opiates, synthetic opiates, hydrophilic colloids, and octreotide (a somatostatin analog). In some cases, stool output is related to increased gastric secretion, which can be controlled by the administration of PPI or H_2 receptor blocker therapy. Hydration

TABLE 31-7

Suggested Vitamin and Mineral Supplements for Malabsorption

Nutrient	Dosage
Calcium	Normal replacement is 1-2 g/d
Magnesium	Magnesium gluconate, 500 mg q.i.d. Each tablet contains 29 mg magnesium
Iron	Ferrous sulfate, one 320 mg tablet q.i.d. for repletion OR Polysaccharide iron, 150 mg b.i.d./t.i.d.
Vitamin A*	25,000-U tablets; for severe deficiency, 25,000-100,000 U/day maintenance dose is 3,000-5,000 U/d
Vitamin D*	Initial dose is 50,000 U 2-3 times/wk for repletion Dosage varies based on patient response as determined by serum and urinary calcium.
Vitamin K*	Vitamin K_1, 10 mg/d PO or SC or vitamin K_3, 10 mg/PO
Folate	1-5 mg/d PO for 4-5 wk for repletion; maintenance dose is 1 mg/d
Vitamin B_{12}	100-100 µg/d IM for 2 wk as a loading dose; maintenance dose is 100-1000 µg/day IM each month
Vitamin B complex	Any multivitamin preparation that contains daily requirements should be administered twice daily

*Available in water-miscible form.
Adapted from Willis J: Gastrointestinal diseases. In Carey CF, Lee HH, Woeitje KF (eds). The Washington manual of medical therapeutics, Philadelphia, ed 29, Lippincott Williams & Wilkins, 1998.

status should be monitored routinely in patients with malabsorption, particularly those with significant diarrhea. Patients unable to maintain hydration despite optimal diet and pharmacologic treatment require PN or parenteral administration of fluid and electrolytes.

Short-Bowel Syndrome

SBS is a constellation of symptoms resulting from a functional or absolute loss of intestinal absorptive surface. It is characterized by severe diarrhea, malabsorption, dehydration, electrolyte abnormalities, and progressive weight loss. In adults, the most common causes of SBS are intestinal resection after vascular infarct to the small intestine and multiple bowel resections for CD.[115] The clinical outcome of SBS depends as much on what site is resected as on how much bowel is resected, making precise definition of *short bowel* difficult. In practice, residual small bowel shorter than 200 cm can lead to nutritional complications and can be considered "short bowel."[116,117] Several factors can influence the severity of SBS, and therefore, its impact on nutritional status and metabolism.[115]

THE SITE AND EXTENT OF RESECTED BOWEL. In general, the more bowel that is lost, the greater is the loss of surface for absorption of nutrients and fluid; however, what region of bowel is resected may be more significant for nutrient absorption than the extent of resection alone. The loss of jejunum is usually tolerated well if the remainder of the bowel is healthy.[112] Transit time is slower in the ileum, and the ileum can adapt morphologically much better to the loss of jejunum than jejunum can to loss of ileum.[117] Loss of ileum has more nutritional and metabolic consequences than loss of jejunum because it is the only site of absorption of conjugated bile salts and vitamin B_{12}.[107,115] With ileal resection of less than 100 cm, bile salt or "cholerrheic" diarrhea can occur.[107,112] Unabsorbed bile salts reaching the colon impair water and ion absorption and can produce secretory diarrhea.[112] With ileal resection of greater than 100 cm, loss of bile salts exceeds the capability of the liver to synthesize them, resulting in steatorrhea.[107,112]

PRESENCE OF THE ILEOCECAL VALVE. The ileocecal valve is a specialized muscle that increases the pressure gradient between ileum and colon.[112] Loss of the ileocecal valve appears to have important metabolic consequences. Decreased transit time of luminal contents in its absence may result in malabsorption by decreasing the time that nutrients are in contact with mucosal surface.[112,115] Furthermore, loss of the valve may result in bacterial overgrowth in the small intestine, causing deconjugation of bile salts and reduced absorption of fat and fat-soluble vitamins. Vitamin B_{12} can also be metabolized by increased bacteria in the small intestine, resulting in deceased absorption.[112,115]

PRESENCE OF THE COLON. The presence or absence of the colon can have a significant effect on the patient's ability to maintain fluid and electrolyte balance after massive bowel resection. Removal of part or all of the colon, in addition to part of the small intestine, can increase the risk of developing sodium and potassium depletion and dehydration.[115] This can occur in two ways: from the loss of colonic absorptive surface and from the effect of the colon on gastric emptying. Patients with distal ileal and colonic resections have significantly faster gastric emptying of liquid than short-bowel patients with colon in situ.[118] This rapid rate of early gastric emptying further decreases intestinal transit time and increases intestinal output. The terms *colonic brake* and *ileal brake* have been used to describe the delaying effect on GI transit that these bowel segments have in normal anatomy.

CONDITION OF THE REMAINING BOWEL AND OTHER DIGESTIVE ORGANS. After loss of small intestine, it is important that the remaining bowel be functional. In patients with SBS due to resection for CD or radiation injury, presence of disease in the remaining bowel further impedes absorption of nutrients and water. Any impairment in pancreatic, gastric, or hepatic function, for example, would also worsen the sequelae of SBS.[115]

DEGREE OF ADAPTATION OF THE REMAINING BOWEL. The severity of SBS is also influenced by the degree to which the bowel adapts following resection. The adaptive response is characterized by elongation and dilation of the remnant bowel and an increase in villus height, crypt depth, cell proliferation, and enzyme activity. These alterations in mucosal hyperplasia, bowel morphology, and bowel function, are achieved by the interaction of various factors (e.g., hormones, enteric nutrients, pancreaticobiliary secretions), which together allow the small bowel to compensate for the loss of absorptive surface area.[119]

Clinically, the patient typically progresses through three postoperative phases. Phase I begins during the immediate postoperative period and typically lasts for approximately 3 months. This phase is characterized by massive diarrhea and severe fluid and electrolyte abnormalities, necessitating that all fluid and nutrient needs be met parenterally. Luminal nutrients are provided to enhance the process of bowel adaptation. The second phase is one of decreasing diarrhea and malabsorption. The enteral and/or oral diet is typically advanced and PN is gradually reduced, but often still required to maintain the patient's nutritional and hydration status. This phase can last

for 3 to 24 months following resection. The third phase is one of complete adaptation, where the patient is able to maintain adequate nutritional and hydration status via an enteral and/or an oral diet. Some patients are never able to maintain themselves via an oral/enteral diet, and thus become dependent on long-term parenteral support.[120-123]

NUTRITION ASSESSMENT. A complete nutrition assessment should be done on all patients with SBS: weight history; standard laboratory assessments; an evaluation of vitamin, trace element, and essential fatty acid levels; and in some cases, a detailed workup of the malabsorption (see Table 31-7). To make appropriate dietary management decisions (Table 31-8), the dietitian should be familiar with the surgical history, including the time (months/years) from resection, length and section of remaining bowel, presence or absence of ileocecal valve and colon, and any residual disease. All medications should be recorded and checked for potential drug-nutrient interactions. Because oral/enteral medications may not be properly absorbed in patients with short bowel, serum levels of drugs should be monitored, if possible.

ENTERAL NUTRITION SUPPORT. Absorption of food energy may vary widely in persons with SBS. Messing and colleagues reported energy absorption equal to 67% of energy intake in SBS patients.[124] Woolf reported total energy absorption of 62% of intake in SBS patients, absorption of protein, carbohydrate, and fat, being 81%, 61%, and 54%, respectively.[125] Some patients may require as much as 60 kcal/kg per day to maintain their weight. In one study, 10 ambulatory patients with SBS required calorie intakes equivalent to 2.5 times BEE to maintain energy balance.[124] It has been recommended that protein intake for SBS patients be 1.5 to 2.0 g/kg per day.[116,125]

For a patient with SBS whose colon is intact, a high-carbohydrate diet may be of great benefit for the production of SCFAs. Nordgarrd and coworkers compared the effects of a high-fat and low-carbohydrate diet with those of a high-carbohydrate and low-fat diet in 16 patients with SBS. In patients whose colon was intact, the high-carbohydrate diet improved energy absorption from 49% to 69% (of ingested calories) as compared with the low-carbohydrate diet. This finding was attributed to the fermentation of carbohydrate in the colon and resulting production of SCFAs.[126,127]

In patients with rapid transit or disturbed gastric emptying, simple sugars can cause osmotic diarrhea. Restriction of hypertonic fluids and lactose can reduce osmotic diarrhea or stomal output.[116] Lactose malabsorption is prevalent in SBS secondary to loss of brush border disaccharidase, so lactose restriction may help decrease output.

The subject of fat restriction in SBS is rather controversial. Historically, a low-fat diet (40 g per day) was recommended routinely to minimize steatorrhea.[108] For patients with documented fat malabsorption, dietary recommendations depend on whether the patient has colon in continuity with small bowel. When the colon is in continuity with the small intestine, fat restriction can help reduce diarrhea by decreasing the volume of bile salts and hydroxylated fatty acids that enter the colon. Fat restriction also helps decrease oxalate absorption in the colon and minimizes loss of divalent cations.[116] As with diet therapy for malabsorption (above), modest fat restriction (30% of calories) should be attempted initially. This level can be

TABLE 31-8

Dietary Management of Malabsorption

	Short-Bowel Syndrome		Pancreatic Insufficiency	Celiac Sprue
	Colon Intact	**Ileostomy Jejunostomy**		
Meal Pattern	5-6 small feedings/day	5-6 small feedings/day	5-6 small meals/day Pancreatic enzyme replacement with meals and snacks	Small, frequent meals initially. As malabsorption improves, meal pattern may be as desired.
Dietary Fat	Moderate restriction necessary. Start with 30% of calories from fat, and modify if necessary based on clinical response.	Restriction not necessary for most stable patients.	Restriction necessary. Titrate enzyme replacement to fat intake.	Initial restriction may be necessary to decrease stool output. As malabsorption improves, fat restriction can be relaxed or eliminated.
Carbohydrate	Fiber intake may be beneficial, as it increases production of SCFA. Lactose restriction if lactase deficient.	Restrict concentrated sweets and hypertonic liquids in cases of rapid intestinal transit and high output.	Lactose restriction if lactase deficient. Carbohydrate modified if DM present. Excessive fiber content of diet may decrease activity of pancreatic enzymes and bile salts, worsening steatorrhea.	Gluten-free diet. Patients are frequently lactose intolerant initially but may become lactose tolerant as intestinal lesion improves.
Vitamins/minerals	1 g/d calcium to bind oxalate. Avoid excess Vitamin C. May need Vitamin B_{12} shots if >50% illeum resected. Supplement other vitamins and minerals per matabsorption workup.	Vitamin B_{12} shots necessary. Supplement vitamins and minerals as per malabsorption workup. Carefully monitor serum, calcium, magnesium, and zinc; supplement as necessary.	High-potency multivitamin mineral. Take with meals and enzymes.	Initial supplementation per malabsorption workup. After deficiencies corrected and sprue symptoms controlled, change to standard multivitamins and mineral daily. Check gluten content of vitamins.
Other	Restrict dietary oxalate.		Avoid alcohol.	Lifelong adherence to gluten/gliadin-free diet necessary.

DM, diabetes mellitus, *SCFA*, short-chain fatty acids.

adjusted as necessary, depending on the clinical response to the diet.

Patients with a jejunostomies or SBS and no colon typically do not benefit from a significant resriction of fat in the diet. For these patients, percentage of fat absorption appears to be the same with either a low-fat or a high-fat diet. Simko and colleagues studied the effects of different dietary fat levels on short-bowel patients. On a low-fat diet (64 g per day), fat absorption was 44 g per day. On a high-fat diet (200 g per day) fat absorption was 133 g per day. Not only did the high-fat diet result in greater energy absorption, it also *decreased* ostomy fluid output. Additionally, there was a 2.5-fold *decrease* of bile acids in the ostomy effluent on the high-fat diet.[128] Other researchers have reported good tolerance to a high-fat diet in short-bowel patients whose colon was not in continuity with the small bowel.[124,125,129] What is less clear is the impact of a high-fat diet on divalent cation balance in SBS. Woolf found that a high-fat diet did not decrease divalent cation absorption in SBS, whereas Cosnes reported a significant incidence of hypocalcemia and hypomagnesemia in SBS patients who ate an unrestricted diet.[129,130] On balance, research suggests that a high-fat diet can be beneficial in maintaining energy and fluid balance in stable SBS patients with a high output jejunostomy; however, the gain of energy may be associated with risk for divalent cation loss. Appropriate calcium, magnesium, and zinc supplements should be given and the serum levels monitored (Table 31-7).

Maintaining adequate hydration can be the most challenging problems for some patients with SBS, particularly for those

with end jejunostomies. Often the fluid losses of these patients exceed their oral/enteral fluid intake, making them dependent on intravenous support. However, in an effort to limit their stomal output, high sodium, glucose-containing, isotonic oral rehydration solutions are recommended. If colon is present, sodium absorption may be adequate, provided enough sodium is included in the diet. For these individuals, the composition of the oral fluid intake is typically not as critical; however, it is often recommended that these patients avoid hyperosmolar beverages.[131,132]

Depending on the site and extent of bowel resection, patients with SBS may be at risk for vitamin deficiency. Ileal resections more extensive than 60 to 100 cm lead to inadequate absorption of vitamin B_{12}. Failure to provide parenteral vitamin B_{12} in this situation can lead to megaloblastic anemia, peripheral neuropathy, and spinal cord degeneration.[115] Patients with limited ileal resections should be assessed for vitamin B_{12} absorption with Schilling's test. Fat-soluble vitamins are malabsorbed when steatorrhea is present. Vitamin D deficiency affects calcium bioavailability. Deficiencies and/or prolonged inadequate intake place patients with SBS at increased risk of developing metabolic bone disease. Serum levels of vitamins A, D, and E, or tocopherol, should be routinely monitored in patients with SBS and malabsorption. Prothrombin time may be used as an indirect indication of vitamin K status.[108] Table 31-7 provides guidelines for vitamin and mineral supplementation. Serum levels should be monitored in patients with SBS.

The site and extent of bowel resection govern absorption of minerals. The divalent cations calcium, zinc, and magnesium are malabsorbed in the presence of steatorrhea. Supplements of these minerals can be taken orally, but because oral magnesium supplementation is associated with increased diarrhea, parenteral magnesium may be preferable for some patients. Calcium supplementation is desirable to correct calcium balance and bind luminal oxalate, preventing its absorption in the colon. SBS patients should take at least 1 g of elemental calcium per day and should be counseled on selection of the supplement. Of the available calcium preparations, calcium carbonate contains the greatest percentage of elemental calcium (by weight); however, it is relatively insoluble, especially at neutral pH.[133] Patients who are achlorhydric or taking H_2 blockers should take a more soluble form of calcium, such as calcium citrate. Patients with SBS, particularly after proximal resection, are frequently anemic and require iron supplementation. Unfortunately, oral iron sulfate supplements are often associated with GI symptoms. Iron polysaccharide is a more easily absorbed form of iron and may eliminate the unpleasant side effects of iron sulfate supplements.

Patients who have all or part of their colon and who exhibit fat malabsorption are at increased risk of hyperoxaluria and nephrolithiasis. Restriction of dietary oxalate decreases oxalate absorption and should be recommended in concert with fat restriction for those at risk of hyperoxaluria. Calcium supplementation further decreases available oxalate through luminal binding (see previous discussion). Ascorbic acid supplements should be avoided because ascorbic acid is a precursor of oxalate. Adequate fluid intake should be maintained.

Tube feeding may be used for nutrition support for some SBS patients. There is no consensus about whether a polymeric or hydrolyzed formula is preferable. Patients must be assessed individually, and tube feeding formula recommendations must be based on extent of resection, presence of colon, presence and degree of steatorrhea, condition of remaining bowel, and length of time from resection. The provision of continuous enteral feedings during the early adaptive phase of SBS appears to encourage enteral autonomy. Levy and coworkers[120] suggested that elemental formulas offered no advantage over polymeric formulas. However, patients with rapid intestinal transit may benefit from a more hydrolyzed formula that is more readily absorbed, although the tonicity of these formulas may in some cases further exacerbate the diarrhea.[108] Hydrolyzed formulas generally provide protein in the form of free amino acids or peptides. It has been suggested that peptide-based diets utilize different protein carrier systems for absorption that make the protein more readily bioavailable than free amino acid diets; however, when selecting an enteral product, the clinician must look at features other than the protein source, such as fat, MCTs, fiber content, and osmolality, all of which can affect a patient's tolerance to feeding. SBS patients receiving enteral tube feedings may have increased intestinal output despite appropriate selection of formula. In these cases, antidiarrheal medications can be administered by mouth or by tube (Table 31-9). Continuous, rather than intermittent, feeding is preferable in the early phases of SBS. Continuous feedings are tolerated better and may enhance intestinal adaptation.[134]

STANDARD MEDICAL TREATMENT OF SHORT BOWEL SYNDROME. Like the oral/enteral diet, standard drug therapy of SBS is aimed at reducing intestinal nutrient and fluid losses.

TABLE 31-9

Antidiarrheal Medications for Adults

Medication (Generic/Trade Names)	Usual Adult Dose	Administration
Bismuth subsalicylate (Pepto-Bismol)	*Original Strength*: Liquid, 30 ml; caplets, 2 caplets *Maximum Strength*: Liquid, 30 ml	Original strength: One dose up to 8 times/day Maximum: (maximum strength) One dose up to 4 times/day
Attapulgite (Kaopectate)	30 ml	Take one dose after first diarrheal stool and one dose after subsequent stool, not to exceed 6 doses/day
Loperamide HCl (Imodium, Pepto Diarrhea Control)	Liquid, 10 ml; caplet, 1 caplet	Two doses after first loose stool, one dose after each subsequent stool, not to exceed 4 caplets/day
Camphorated opium tincture (Paregoric)	Liquid, 5-10 ml	One dose 1-4 times/day
Tincture of opium (Laudanum)	Liquid, 0.3-1.0 ml (usually 0.6 ml)	One dose up to 4 times/day
Diphenoxylate-atropine (Lomotil)	Liquid, 10 ml; tablets, 2 tablets	One dose

Adapted from American Dietetic Association: Handbook of clinical dietetics, ed 2, New Haven, 1992, Yale University Press, p 140.
Note: Compalibility of these medications with enteral tube feeding formulations has not been established.
Sources: 1996 Physicians Desk Reference for Nonprescription Drugs. Medical Economics. 1996; *1996 Physicians Desk Reference for Prescription Drugs*, Medical Economics, 1996; *Drug Information for the Health Care Professional*, United States Pharmacopeial Convention, Inc., Rockville, MD, 1997.

Antidiarrheal medications, such as loperamide and codeine phosphate, reduce intestinal motility.[135] After bowel resection, gastric acid hypersecretion often occurs at least transiently, although in some patients a hypersecretory state persists. Gastric hypersecretion adds to increased intestinal volume and may deactivate pancreatic enzymes by decreasing duodenal pH. Administration of intravenous or oral H2 receptor blockers can help decrease fluid and electrolyte losses by decreasing gastric output.[112,115,136] For patients with cholerrheic diarrhea, cholestyramine, a bile salt sequestrant, can be effective in controlling diarrhea; however, in patients with steatorrhea, cholestyramine can worsen diarrhea by further depleting the bile salt pool.[108,112] Somatostatin and octreotide (a somatostatin analog) have been used with some success in SBS. Octreotide reduces intestinal fluid and electrolyte losses and therefore, has primarily been recommended for patients with end-jejunostomies.[137]

Bowel Rehabilitation

In addition to the standard medical management of patients with SBS, there has been, over the past decade, much interest in developing noninvasive treatment modalities (which utilize growth factors, specific nutrients and/or diets) to "rehabilitate" (improve the function) the diseased and/or shortened bowel. Because specific hormones (e.g., growth hormone, glucagon-like peptide-2, insulin-like growth factor-I [IGF-1], keratinocyte), and luminal nutrients (e.g., glutamine, soluble fibers, and SCFAs) appear to influence the growth, adaptation, and repair of the intestinal mucosa,[135] much of the original research in the area of bowel rehabilitation has focused on determining the potential role that these agents might play in the management of patients with SBS.

Two prospective, randomized clinical trials evaluating the effect of growth hormone and glutamine failed to demonstrate a significant improvement in small bowel morphology[138] or nutrient absorption;[138,139] however, both studies were conducted in a very small (n = 8), heterogenous group of patients (some with colon and some without). In addition, the prescribed diet was either unrestricted[132] or did not control for the presence or absence of colon,[138] making it difficult to interpret the results, particularly the studies of nutrient absorption.

However, in an open-label evaluation, others demonstrated that the use of growth hormone and glutamine, when combined with a modified oral diet resulted in significant improvement in nutrient and fluid absorption in a group of 8 patients with severe short bowel (mean jejunal-ileal length = 37 cm), all with colon.[140] These patients were prescribed a diet high in carbohydrate, which has been shown to be advantageous to patients with remnant colon (but to have an adverse effect on fluid absorption and stool/ostomy volume for those without).[126]

In a larger study (n = 45), with an average follow-up period of approximately 2 years, Wilmore and associates demonstrated that the use of growth hormone and glutamine, when administered with an appropriate oral diet, allowed 40% of the patients with severe short bowel to remain independent of PN and another 40% of the patients to experience a reduction in the parenteral requirements.[141] To better differentiate the individual effects of this treatment approach, prospective randomized, placebo-controlled trials, which control for the influence of diet, are underway. In addition to the potential role of growth hormone and glutamine, the application of other growth factors and luminal nutrients are also being studied.

Despite the limitations in our current understanding of the role that a given growth factor or luminal nutrient might have on bowel morphology, transit time, and/or nutrient absorption, the positive clinical outcomes of some of these early studies in the area of bowel rehabilitation have encouraged the application of these noninvasive treatment modalities, particularly in patients at risk of significant complications related to their long-term PN and/or before pursuing intestinal transplantation. The in-house treatment of nearly 400 patients at a single center has allowed investigators not only to evaluate the role of various growth factors and/or a specific nutrient, but also to observe the influence of various diet prescriptions (and perhaps more importantly, specific foods and fluids and meal patterns) on nutrient absorption and stool output.[132] In addition to identifying the optimal food and fluid regimen via careful 24-hour monitoring of all intake and output, these authors have recognized the importance of providing patients with education and programs aimed at behavior modification to encourage long-term compliance.

Thus, today, the concept of bowel rehabilitation has moved beyond the administration of a given growth factor and/or nutrient, and embraces a concept of patient care in which the primary problems that define the SBS (diarrhea, malabsorption, dehydration, electrolyte abnormalities, vitamin and trace element deficiencies, weight loss), as well as the secondary medical problems that confront this patient population (bacterial overgrowth, D-lactic metabolic acidosis, kidney stones, bone disease, and the myriad complications associated with long-term PN—liver dysfunction, catheter-related events, and so on), are managed by a team of specialized clinicians. The optimal treatment plan for these patients is often achieved with repeated 24-hour measurements of all intake and output and then adjustment and readjustments in medications and the diet. Patient education and behavior modification, particularly related to the oral diet, has become an integral part of bowel rehabilitation. This noninvasive approach appears to lessen or eliminate the need for long-term PN in some patients with severe short bowel. Ongoing and future research will help clarify the role that specific growth factors and/or nutrients play in further advancing the care of patients with this debilitating problem.

Radiation Enteritis

Radiation is an important treatment modality for many cancers: about half of all patients diagnosed with cancer undergo radiation therapy.[142] Irradiation to abdominal or pelvic areas can cause radiation injury, which is associated with considerable morbidity. Radiation to the intestine can be classified as acute or chronic. Acute injury is evident either during or immediately following radiotherapy. Cell turnover in the healthy intestine is normally rapid: reepithelialization of the villus occurs every 2 to 5 days.[142,143] When the intestine is exposed to radiation, cell replacement is delayed, the intestinal villi are shortened, and the total epithelial surface is reduced, resulting in symptoms of radiation enteritis. Symptoms of acute radiation enteritis, which commonly include abdominal pain, diarrhea, and tenesmus, usually resolve within 2 to 6 weeks after completion of treatment. Complete histologic recovery of acute radiation injury usually occurs within 6 months.[142]

Late or chronic effects of radiation therapy have a different mechanism of injury. In addition to acute cellular injury, radiation causes progressive arteritis and submucosal fibrosis that may lead to thrombosis of the intestinal arteries, resulting in ischemia or necrosis of the bowel wall.[142] The chronic effects of radiation may not be seen until several months to several years after completion of radiation therapy. Chronic radiation changes can include dense adhesions or perforation. Symptoms of chronic radiation enteritis include diarrhea, weight loss, and malabsorption. Bacterial overgrowth of the small intestine can follow radiation injury, which contributes to malabsorption and malnutrition.

NUTRITION THERAPY OF RADIATION ENTERITIS. Evidence of malabsorption should be sought whenever a patient with radiation enteritis presents with diarrhea and weight loss (see Table 31-7). Levels of mucosal lactase have been shown to be reduced in patients with radiation enteritis despite a radiographically normal jejunum.[144] Therefore, a lactose tolerance test is a useful diagnostic tool when patients have diarrhea. A fecal fat determination and serum assay of fat-soluble vitamins can detect fat malabsorption. Hematologic studies are recommended because radiation injury can cause chronic blood loss.[144] Dietary modifications of fat and lactose and the addition of vitamin and mineral supplements should be based on the results of the malabsorption workup. If steatorrhea is present and the colon is intact, fat restriction helps reduce fecal losses. Bile salt malabsorption may be present, which can increase fluid loss in the colon; however, bile salt sequestrant, a resin, should be used only with extreme caution if there is narrowing or stricture of the bowel as this treatment could rsult in obstruction. Similarly, when the irradiated bowel is involved by stenosis or stricture, fiber restriction may be necessary to prevent obstructive symptoms.

Research interest in radiation enteritis has involved the use of chemically defined diets and glutamine for prophylaxis against radiation changes in the bowel. McArdle and colleagues[144] studied the effects of a peptide-based diet in 20 patients receiving presurgical radiation therapy. The patients were fed the peptide-based diet for 3 days before and 4 days during a short course of high-dose radiation therapy for invasive bladder cancer. Additionally, the diets were resumed by jejunostomy tube 24 hours after patients underwent radical cystectomy and ileal conduit procedures. Various histologic examinations were conducted in the peptide diet fed patients following radiation and compared with a retrospective control group of patients. The patients fed the peptide-based diet had maintenance of normal ileal mucosa with normal enzyme activity in the intestinal brush border, as demonstrated by biopsy. Bloody or severe diarrhea was absent in the peptide-diet group, but not in the control group. Other parameters, such as nitrogen balance and return of bowel sounds postoperatively were positively impacted by alimentation with the peptide-based diet. This study indicated that not only was enteral feeding with a peptide-based diet feasible in this patient group, both preoperatively and postoperatively, but also that it provided a prophylaxis against acute radiation enteritis during high-dose, short-course radiation therapy.[145]

Glutamine also shows promise in the nutrition support of radiation therapy patients. In an animal study, rats were randomized to receive diets containing either 3% glutamine or 3% glycine before they were irradiated. The experimental diets were isocaloric and isonitrogenous. Following radiation, survival in the glutamine-treated animals was 100%, but in the glycine group only 45%. Other signs of radiation injury, such as bloody diarrhea and bowel perforation, were present in the glycine-treated group but not in the glutamine group. Favorable histologic changes in the bowel, including greater villus height and number, were markedly improved in the glutamine group.[146] More recent animal studies have confirmed the beneficial effect of glutamine in radiation enteritis, and demonstrated a therapeutic effect of dietary arginine as well.[147,148] Although peptide-based and arginine- and glutamine-enriched diets have shown promise in the treatment of radiation enteritis, more human studies are needed before they become accepted as standard treatment.

Celiac Disease

Celiac disease (celiac sprue or gluten-sensitive enteropathy) is an autoimmune enteropathy that is initiated by ingestion of gluten, the protein in flour and grains (particularly wheat, rye, and barley–possibly oats), which consists of four peptides: gliadins, glutenins, albumins, and globulins.[107,149,150] People with celiac disease have an inappropriate T cell–mediated

immune response to gluten.[150, 151] The disease is characterized by mucosal lesions of the small intestine.[149,152] The classical histology of these lesions show villous atrophy and hyperplastic crypt cells.[152] Measurement of circulating antiendomysial antibodies is used to screen patients for celiac disease, but given the reports of both false-positive and false-negative results, these tests should not replace small bowel mucosal biopsy for a definitive diagnosis.[152] Clinical symptoms of celiac disease include diarrhea, abdominal pain, fatigue, and steatorrhea.[152] Secondary nutrition disorders may include anemia, osteoporosis, and osteopenia. Common laboratory abnormalities in sprue include low serum levels of cholesterol, folate, iron, carotene, calcium, potassium, and albumin.[152]

The cornerstone of treatment is lifelong avoidance of gluten ingestion.[150] Details of the diet have been published elsewhere.[153] Because of the complexities of the diet, all newly diagnosed celiac disease patients should have thorough diet counseling by a registered dietitian. Initially many patients presenting with celiac disease have steatorrhea and lactase deficiency secondary to untreated disease. Restriction of fat and lactose, in addition to gluten, helps control diarrhea. After clinical response to the diet is observed, lactose and fat restrictions can be relaxed and ultimately eliminated. GI symptoms usually improve within 1 to 2 weeks of gluten withdrawal from the diet.[154] Patients who fail to respond clinically after 4 to 6 weeks on the diet should be evaluated by a dietitian for diet compliance. A small group of patients with celiac disease exhibit clinical and histologic persistence of disease despite strict adherence to the diet. It has been reported that up to 30% of adult patients have refractory sprue (RS).[155] A common cause of RS is voluntary or inadvertent gluten ingestion for which a reconsultation with a clinical dietitian is indicated. For true refractory cases, anti-inflammatory or immunosuppressive agents such as corticosteroids, azathioprine, and cyclosporine have been used.[154] Celiac disease is associated with increased risk of intestinal malignancies, although early diagnosis and strict dietary compliance may decrease the risk.[156]

Because malabsorption is such a prevalent feature of celiac disease, full laboratory assessment of nutritional status should be performed at diagnosis. Patients who require vitamin and mineral supplementation to correct deficiencies should be cautioned about "hidden" gluten in vitamins and other pharmaceutical preparations, and instructed to contact manufactueres for more detailed information about "inert" ingredients as needed.

The Pancreas

The pancreas synthesizes and secretes enzymes and hormones necessary for the digestion of nutrients, maintenance of carbohydrate homeostasis, and regulation of intraluminal bowel transit.[157] To appreciate the rationale for nutrition support in pancreatic disorders, it is important to have a basic understanding of exocrine pancreatic function.

Control of the exocrine pancreas is both hormonal and neural.[157,158] Exocrine pancreatic secretion occurs in four related phases: basal, cephalic, gastric, and intestinal.[159] Basal pancreatic secretion occurs in the fasted state at a low rate.[159] The cephalic phase, which is initiated by the sight and smell of food, is mediated through cholinergic stimulation of the pancreatic acinar cells by the vagus nerve.[160] The gastric phase of pancreatic secretion begins when distention of the gastric antrum by food triggers the release of gastrin and hydrochloric acid. Following the gastric phase, the intestinal phase starts when the acidified stomach contents enter the duodenum, stimulating the release of secretin and cholesystokinin (CCK). CCK is the primary stimulus for pancreatic enzyme secretion.[159] Maximum CCK release occurs with response to amino acids, intact protein, triglycerides, and LCFAs; MCTs minimally stimulate pancreatic secretions.[161,162]

Secretion of pancreatic enzymes diminishes the farther distal that food is introduced into the small bowel. This has implications in the enteral feeding of persons with pancreatitis or pancreatic insufficiency.

Acute Pancreatitis

Acute pancreatitis (AP) is an acute inflammatory process of the pancreas that may involve peripancreatic tissues and/or remote organs.[163] The pathophysiology of pancreatitis is not completely understood, but it appears that intrapancreatic activation of enzymes results in release of enzymes into the interstitium, leading to "autodigestion" of the organ and peripancreatic tissues.[164,165] The most common causes of pancreatitis are gallstones and alcohol abuse. Drugs are another common cause of pancreatitis; more than 85 medications are associated with pancreatitis.[164] Metabolic derangements including hyperlipidemia and hypercalcemia may contribute to the development of pancreatitis.[164]

AP is characterized by abdominal pain, vomiting, and anorexia, and may be associated with prolonged ileus.[157,160] AP is characterized as mild or severe and can range from mild inflammation of the gland to a necrotizing hemorrhagic process.[157] Mild pancreatitis occurs in approximately 80% of patients hospitalized for AP with the remainder being considered as having severe disease. A combination of clinical and laboratory data, known as Ranson's criteria, are commonly used to indicate the severity of pancreatitis within the first 48 hours following hospital admission (Box 31-3).[166] Patients with fewer than three of these risk factors have a very low mortality. As the number of risk factors increases, mortality rises.[164] Other tools such as Glasgow Score and APACHE II (Acute Physiology and Chronic Health Evaluation) are also used in assessing severity of disease in AP.[167,168] In general, mortality in severe AP is estimated to be 10% to 20% and is associated with sepsis and systemic inflammatory response syndrome (SIRS).[169,170]

BOX 31-3
Ranson's Criteria

On admission:
 Age >55 yr
 White cell count >16,000/mm³
 Glucose >200 mg/dL
 Lactic dehydrogenase >350 µg/L
 Aspartate aminotransferase >250 µ/L

Within 48 hr of hospitalization:
 Decrease in hematocrit >10 points
 Increase in BUN >5 mg/dl
 Calcium <8 mg/dL
 Po_2 <60 mm Hg
 Base deficit >4 mmol/L
 Fluid deficit >6 L

From Ranson JHC, Rilkind KM, Roses DF, et al.: Prognostic signs and the role of operative management in acute pancreatitis, *Surg Gynecol Obstet* 139:69-81, 1974.

NUTRITION SUPPORT FOR ACUTE PANCREATITIS. Nutrition support for patients with AP has been a subject of much interest and debate in the medical literature. Following the concern that pancreatic stimulation by oral intake would exacerbate the disease by increasing the synthesis of proteolytic enzymes and promoting pancreatic autodigestion, the cornerstone of therapy in AP has been "pancreatic rest"—avoidance of exocrine stimulation from oral or gastric intake and blockade of exocrine secretion by nasogastric suction and use of antacids.[159,169] Pancreatic rest has been further supported by clinical experience that exocrine stimulation by oral intake exacerbates symptoms of pancreatitis, such as abdominal pain. Additionally, the prevalence of delayed gastric emptying and adynamic ileus in AP makes oral and gastric feeding undesirable or unattainable during the acute phase of the disease.[157,160,171] The practice of pancreatic rest has traditionally been facilitated by bypassing the cephalic, gastric, and intestinal phases of pancreatic secretion through fasting with intravenous hydration alone or with the provision of parenteral nutrition (PN). Several clinical trials have studied the safety and efficacy of the use of PN for AP. Improved outcomes have been demonstrated with the use of PN when compared with fasting.[172-174] PN appears not to stimulate pancreatic secretions and promotes positive nitrogen balance in patients with AP.[169,175] While some studies support use of PN, others have identified a prevalence of complications such as hyperglycemia, hyperlipidemia, and catheter-related sepsis and other septic complications when PN is administered during pancreatitis.[176] The use of PN and its association with bacterial translocation and sepsis have been reported and are discussed in detail in Chapter 21. The relationship between PN, the lack of enteral nutrients, and the development of bacterial and endotoxin translocation may be especially significant in patients with AP. AP drives release of proinflammatory cytokines, possibly from the mucosa or the immune cells within the gut. This gut-derived release of cytokines and the response of the liver to AP amplifies the systemic inflammatory response, which further serves to suppress gut immune surveillance and exacerbate bacterial translocation.[169] Therefore, maintaining integrity of the gut mucosa appears to be especially important in the treatment of patients with AP for whom sepsis is the primary cause for morbidity. Preliminary experience suggests that the institution of enteral nutrition (EN) administered beyond the ligament of Treitz within 48 hours of the onset of severe AP attenuates endotoxin exposure and the cytokine and systemic inflammatory responses.[177]

Clinical studies have shown improved outcomes when enteral feeding is administered during AP. Given that pancreatitis is associated with high gastric output and delayed gastric emptying, enteral feeding with a jejunally placed feeding tube, bypassing the stomach, is preferred over gastric enteral feeding. An additional benefit of feeding jejunally is the presumed diminution of pancreatic secretions compared with feeding proximally. A recent study assessed the feasibility and effectiveness of jejunal feedings in patients with severe pancreatitis who required laparotomy for peritonitis or for failed conservative treatment for pancreatitis.[167] Thirty patients were randomized to receive a jejunostomy tube (JT) during laparotomy with initiation of full-strength, whole protein formula feedings within 12 hours of surgery. An additional thirty patients served as a control group, receiving only intravenous hydration until resumption of oral intake. Caloric intake was higher in patients receiving the JT feedings; 1294.6 kcal/day compared with 472.8 kcal/day in the control group. Recovery of bowel transit postoperatively was more rapid in the JT group. Incidence of systemic inflammatory response syndrome (SIRS) was not different between groups, but outcomes differed significantly. Mortality was 3.3% in those patients receiving early jejunostomy feedings while the control group had a mortality rate of 23%. Interestingly, early JT feedings appeared to have a beneficial impact on renal function. All four patients with acute renal failure in the JT group experienced improved renal function during the postoperative period. Conversely, three control patients who suffered from acute renal failure later developed multiple organ dysfunction syndrome.[167] Tolerance to JT feeding was enhanced by ensuring proper tube placement before feeding and initiating feedings at a low rate. This study demonstrated that when managed carefully, jejunostomy tube feeding can be safely done in patients with severe pancreatitis. Furthermore, the provision of enteral nutrients in the early postoperative period may have conferred immunomodulatory benefits that improved outcome. A limitation of this study is that control patients were fasted initially, making it difficult to separate the benefits of provision of enteral nutrients specifically with the provision of calories and nitrogen.

Another recent controlled study compared outcomes of jejunally fed AP patients to outcomes of AP patients given PN.[168] Sixteen patients were randomized to receive polymeric enteral feeding administered through nasojejunal feeding tube. Eighteen patients were randomized to receive PN. Groups were comparable with regard to age, gender, and disease severity. In the enterally fed patients, SIRS was present in 11 patients before nutrition support, but in only two patients at the end of nutrition support ($p < .05$). C-reactive protein, a marker of the acute-phase response, was significantly reduced, as was the APACHE II injury score, following 7 days of enteral feeding ($p<.005$, $p<.001$, respectively). There was no significant change in SIRS incidence, C-reactive protein, or APACHE II score in the parenterally fed group following 7 days of nutrition support. Three patients in the PN group developed intraabdominal sepsis. Five parenterally fed patients also developed organ failure; two of whom died. No septic complications were noted in the enteral group. In general, enteral feeding with the polymeric diet was successful. Five patients in the enterally fed group who developed ileus had transient episodes of nausea and fullness for which the feeding rate was temporarily reduced with subsequent resumption to previous rate. No enterally fed patient had diarrhea. As with the aforementioned clinical study, these results demonstrated that enteral feeding with a jejunally placed feeding tube can be accomplished safely and effectively in the setting of AP. Furthermore, compared with PN or fasting, outcomes were improved when jejunal feedings were administered; ostensibly because of maintenance of the gut barrier, reduction in the risk of bacterial translocation, and attenuation of the inflammatory response.

The selection of formula for jejunal feeds during AP is subject to debate. There is no clear consensus as to which type of formula is preferable for the patient with pancreatitis. Early studies used low-fat, hydrolyzed protein ("chemically defined," "elemental" or "semielemental") diets.[178,179] The use of these formulas was supported by the observation that pancreatic output is decreased with their administration when compared with higher fat or polymeric feedings.[180,181] The previously discussed studies demonstrated that polymeric diets can safely be administered through jejunal tubes in patients with AP.[167,168] In a published case report, jejunal pancreatic exocrine secretion with a jejunally fed polymeric "immune-enhancing" diet was not different from that observed with PN.[182] Given the lack of studies comparing the use of chemically defined and polymeric diets, recommendations for the use of a hydrolyzed protein versus intact protein formula cannot be made at the current time. However, given the abundance of data implicating the use of ω-6 fatty acids in the inflammatory response (see Chapter 35), it may be prudent to avoid formulas containing a high level of ω-6 fatty acids in this patient group with a high risk of SIRS and sepsis.

Despite the evidence for the benefits of enteral feeding during AP, it is not feasible for every patient. PN may be necessary for nutrition support for some individuals. Preclusions to enteral feeding may include high nasogastric aspirates and superseding complications such as fistulation and ileus.[167,183] For those patients for whom enteral feeding cannot be initiated, the risk of providing PN must be weighed against the risk of fasting. Most patients with mild severity of the disease typically recover and are able to resume oral diet within several days of conventional supportive therapy of analgesia and hydration.[159,170] Early initiation of PN is beneficial for malnourished patients whose pancreatitis is so severe that enteral feeding is likely to be delayed longer than a week.

Provision of intravenous lipid emulsions with PN has been controversial because of the temporal association between lipid emulsions and hypertriglyceridemia, a potential etiology of pancreatitis. Generally, data indicate that lipid emulsions are a safe means of providing energy to patients with nonhyperlipidemic AP.[158,169,175,184] Serum triglyceride levels should be checked at baseline and after lipid infusion, to ensure proper triglyceride clearance (less than 400 mg/dl).[185] Hypertriglyceride-induced pancreatitis is usually seen only with serum triglyceride levels greater than 1000 mg/dl.[163] Should hypertriglyceridemia (>400 mg/dl) occur following lipid emulsion, lipid infusion should be discontinued. If serum triglyceride levels remain elevated for more than 2 weeks, approximately 1 g/kg of lipid emulsion should be provided twice each week to prevent essential fatty acid deficiency.[163] Prolonging the length of infusion time for lipid emulsion helps promote triglyceride clearance.

ENERGY EXPENDITURE AND PROTEIN REQUIREMENTS IN ACUTE PANCREATITIS. AP is a catabolic, hypermetabolic disease process during which risk of deterioration of nutritional status is high. AP is associated with a metabolic picture similar to that of gram-negative sepsis.[157,165,170,186] The characteristics of this response include increased cardiac output, increased oxygen consumption, and generalized hypermetabolism characterized by changes in carbohydrate, protein, fat, and energy metabolism.[165] Deterioration of nutritional status adversely effects host defenses, immunocompetence, and resistance to infection, which may lead to complications in the clinical course of the disease.[170]

Dickerson and colleagues assessed the resting energy expenditure (REE) of 48 hospitalized patients with AP. The patients tended to be hypermetabolic with REE 20% greater than predicted by the Harris-Benedict equation.[186] A smaller study of six patients with AP demonstrated greater increases in energy expenditure. Patients with AP complicated by sepsis had REEs 58% greater than expected, whereas those without sepsis had REEs 39% greater than predicted by the Harris-Benedict equation.[187]

In calculating energy requirements for patients with AP, calories and nitrogen should be increased according to degree of stress and sepsis. Therefore, consideration should be given to body temperature and other indicators of sepsis such as leukocytosis, peritonitis, and positive blood cultures. The Harris-Benedict equation alone underestimates basal energy expenditure (BEE) in AP.[186] In addition to an appropriate activity factor, a stress factor of 30% to 50% generally must be added to the calculated BEE to ensure that metabolic demands will be met.[163]

Protein requirements are elevated in AP because increased protein catabolism has been reported as a concomitant of the disease.[186,187] In the absence of renal or hepatic insufficiency, a protein level of 1.4 to 2 g/kg of body weight is suggested.[163]

Chronic Pancreatitis

Chronic pancreatitis is a destructive inflammatory disorder that may lead to loss of pancreatic exocrine and endocrine functions.[188] Symptoms of chronic pancreatitis include persistent abdominal and back pain, anorexia, nausea, vomiting, and diarrhea. Malnutrition is frequently present in chronic pancreatitis and is generally related to nutrient loss or decreased intake. Patients with chronic pancreatitis may have pancreatic insufficiency from diminished production or release of pancreatic enzymes, resulting in maldigestion. Steatorrhea, and to a lesser degree, azotorrhea, may be present.[160,189] Steatorrhea usually does not occur until lipase output is below 10% of normal.[157,188,189] Aside from the deficiencies expected in the face of steatorrhea (e.g., dietary fat and fat-soluble vitamins), vitamin B_{12} malabsorption may also be present secondary to deficiency of pancreatic protease.[188] Diabetes mellitus may be associated with chronic pancreatitis, and the overall incidence of impaired glucose tolerance with chronic pancreatitis is 40% to 90%.[157]

NUTRITION SUPPORT OF CHRONIC PANCREATITIS. The malnutrition frequently associated with chronic pancreatitis is multifactorial. Maldigestion of fat and protein with secondary malabsorption of micronutrients may be present. Persons with pancreatitis frequently limit oral intake because eating is associated with pain.[157,189] Chronic pancreatitis is not generally associated with hypermetabolism unless sepsis or other concurrent illness is present.[186] Goals of therapy for chronic pancreatitis include pain management, nutrition support, and treatment of complications.[161]

Pancreatic enzyme supplementation and balanced nutrition are the basics of therapy for the pain and malnutrition of pancreatic insufficiency. Adequate doses of oral pancreatic enzymes can relieve pain and enhance fat digestion and absorption.[160,190,191] Pancreatic enzyme supplements may take the form of enteric-coated microspheres designed to withstand the acidity of the stomach and be released at duodenal pH.[188] Conventional enzyme preparations are destroyed by the acidity of the stomach and for maximum effectiveness are usually administered with antacids, H_2-receptor blockade, or a prokinetic agent. It is recommended that adults take approximately 30,000 USP units of lipase with each meal, assuming no inactivation of enzymes in the stomach or small bowel.[160,190,191] Enzymes should also be taken with snacks. Table 31-10 lists currently available enzyme preparations.

If symptoms of steatorrhea fail to improve on enzyme therapy, patients should be interviewed to discern compliance to enzyme therapy. If noncompliance is ruled out, other causes for malabsorption, such as bacterial overgrowth should be investigated. If steatorrhea persists, a "last resort" is to further reduce dietary fat.[190]

TABLE 31-10
Pancreatic Enzyme (Pancrelipase) Supplements

Manufacturer	Product Name	Dosage Form	Enzyme Content (USP Units)		
			Lipase	Protease	Amylase
Ortho-McNeil	Pancrease	Capsule	4,500	25,000	20,000
	Pancrease MT-4	Enteric-coated microspheres	4,000	12,000	12,000
	Pancrease MT-10	Enteric-coated microspheres	10,000	30,000	30,000
	Pancrease MT-16	Enteric-coated microspheres	16,000	48,000	48,000
	Pancrease MT-20	Enteric-coated microspheres	20,000	44,000	56,000
Solvay	Creon-5	Enteric-coated microspheres	5,000	18,750	16,600
	Creon-10	Enteric-coated microspheres	10,000	37,500	33,200
	Creon-20	Enteric-coated microspheres	20,000	75,000	66,400
Axcan Scandipharm	Viokase 8	Tablet	8,000	30,000	30,000
	Viokase 16	Tablet	16,000	60,000	60,000
	Viokase	Powder (.7 g)	16,800	70,000	70,000
	Ultrase MT 12	Capsule	12,000	39,000	39,000
	Ultrase MT 18	Capsule	18,000	58,500	58,500
	Ultrase MT 20	Capsule	20,000	65,000	65,000
A.H. Robins	Donnazyme	Tablet	1,000	12,500	12,500

Physician's desk reference, ed 56, Montrale, NJ, 2002, *Medical Economics*, 835-839, 2580-2581, 2931, 3521.

Diabetes mellitus calls for attention to balanced carbohydrate intake and insulin administration to prevent ketoacidosis and other complications.[188] Patients with chronic pancreatitis who take insulin may be at risk for hypoglycemia secondary to inadequate glucagon release.[157] Nutrition counseling should be individualized to address symptoms and any complications, but typically the prescription is frequent small meals consisting of a moderate amount of fat (30% of calories), reduced carbohydrate, and high protein.[157,188,190] Patients should abstain from drinking alcohol.[157,190] For patients with chronic pancreatitis, a multivitamin-mineral supplement is generally prescribed to compensate for dietary deficits and increased losses caused by malabsorption. More aggressive vitamin and mineral supplementation may be required if malabsorption is significant despite pancreatic enzyme therapy (see Table 31-7).

Pancreatic Resection
Pancreatic resection may be performed for treatment of or palliation of pancreatic cancer or chronic pancreatitis. Major pancreatic resection can cause pancreatic enzyme insufficiency with fat malabsorption resulting in symptoms of abdominal pain, steatorrhea, and weight loss that may be extremely debilitating.[192] Nutritional status is usually negatively impacted by pancreatic resection.

WHIPPLE'S PROCEDURE. Whipple's procedure, pancreaticoduodenectomy, is a standard pancreatic resection procedure. Whipple's procedure consists of gastric resection, vagotomy, extrahepatic bile duct resection, and total duodenectomy plus partial pancreatic resection. For this reason, it is associated with multiple postoperative GI complications, including dumping syndrome, diarrhea, peptic ulceration, disturbed GI hormone regulation, and diabetes mellitus.[193]

PYLORUS-SPARING PANCREATICODUODENECTOMY. In pylorus-sparing pancreaticoduodenectomy (PPD), the stomach and the first portion of the duodenum are preserved, and pancreatic enzyme patterns and gastric emptying are normal. A recent review of 26 patients compared nutritional status of those who underwent PPD with those who underwent traditional pancreaticoduodenectomy.[194] After the PPD, patients had significantly greater nutrient absorption than those who had the alternative procedure. Furthermore, long-term maintenance of nutritional status was better in the pylorus-sparing group.

TOTAL PANCREATECTOMY. Brittle diabetes mellitus and maldigestion are two unavoidable consequences of total pancreatectomy.[195] The metabolic sequelae of total pancreatectomy are associated with increased morbidity and mortality, so the procedure is done rarely and only as a last resort.[193]

NUTRITION SUPPORT AFTER PANCREATIC RESECTION. A patient undergoing pancreatic surgery is likely to be malnourished as a result of the underlying condition. Following surgery, patients may become further malnourished as a result of decreased intake or maldigestion, or both. Nutrition recommendations for patients with pancreatic resections should be driven by the type of resection and the presence and degree of malabsorption or maldigestion symptoms. After Whipple's procedure, multiple small feedings, avoidance of concentrated sweets, and avoidance of fluids with meals help prevent the dumping symptoms associated with gastric and duodenal resections. Patients who have undergone total pancreatectomy have very brittle diabetes

because the body produces neither insulin nor glucagon, a counter-regulatory hormone. These patients also benefit from taking small, frequent meals, and they must be counseled on the symptoms and treatment of hypoglycemia. Diarrhea following pancreatic resection should raise suspicion of steatorrhea, and if confirmed by fecal fat analysis, pancreatic enzyme therapy should be initiated.

Jejunostomy tube feedings have been used successfully to maintain or restore nutritional status in the postoperative period. Placing a jejunostomy tube during surgery permits early institution of enteral feeding and more rapid advancement to calorie goals than oral feeding generally can. For patients with maldigestion, enzyme therapy must be titrated to the tube feeding. Alternatively, a low-fat, chemically defined diet may be used, which in many cases obviates enzyme therapy during the feeding.

Most patients who have undergone pancreatic resection are at risk for vitamin and mineral deficiencies, and a multivitamin-mineral supplement should be prescribed routinely. Routine laboratory monitoring of nutritional parameters should be performed and deficiencies treated as necessary (see Table 31-7). Because persons with pancreatic disorders are at risk for malnutrition, medical nutrition therapy should be an ongoing and routine part of their medical care.

Cystic Fibrosis
Cystic fibrosis (CF) is a hereditary, autosomal-recessive disorder of exocrine gland secretion.[196-199] CF is characterized clinically by recurrent respiratory tract infections, pancreatic insufficiency, and excessive losses of electrolytes in sweat.[198,200] Long-term survival with CF is associated with nutritional status, thus frequent and ongoing nutritional assessment is an important part of treatment to prevent malnutrition and compromise of pulmonary function.

Nutritional Status in Cystic Fibrosis
Poor nutritional status in CF may be multifactorial. Energy deficits can be attributed to three basic causes: increased losses, decreased intake, and increased requirements.[198]

INCREASED LOSSES. Pancreatic insufficiency is present in approximately 80% to 85% of persons with CF.[199] Thus pancreatic enzyme replacement therapy (PERT) is an important part of the nutritional management of most CF patients. The clinical aim of PERT is to correct symptoms of steatorrhea and associated abdominal pain and to reduce volume and frequency of stools. Despite maximum PERT, 10% to 20% of ingested calories can still be malabsorbed.[196] PERT should be individualized and modifications based on clinical response with respect to stool pattern and growth velocity in children.[196,201] Initial dosing of pancreatic enzyme supplements should begin with 500 lipase u/kg per meal, using enteric-coated microsphere products. The recommended maximum dose of enzyme is 2500 lipase u/kg per meal or 10,000 lipase u/kg per day.[202] Lipase doses exceeding these limits have been associated with fibrosing colonopathy (colonic strictures). Patients whose lipase intake exceeds 2500 u/kg per meal should be evaluated and the enzyme dose adjusted.[203] Table 31-10 lists commercially available pancreatic enzymes.

Diabetes mellitus (DM) can be a complication of CF. Many studies have illustrated an association between diabetes and increased morbidity and mortality in CF.[204] Glucose intolerance in CF increases with age and may occur in as many as 75% of adult CF patients.[205,206] Therefore, screening for DM should be a part of the routine management of CF patients. The 1998 Consensus Conference participants developed guidelines for DM screening in CF patients that has been described elsewhere.[204] Poor control of diabetes results in increased weight loss secondary to glycosuria, deteriorating pulmonary function, and overall decline in clinical status. Patients with CF-related DM should be treated with insulin and a calorie-dense diet to maintain body composition or growth velocity as well as euglycemia. Carbohydrate counting or the exchange system can be used effectively so that insulin dosing is based on actual carbohydrate intake, thus allowing more flexibility of dietary intake.

DECREASED INTAKE. Anorexia is frequently a feature of CF. Several factors can decrease oral intake with CF. Recurrent vomiting, gastroesophageal reflux, chronic infections, and psychic stress have all been identified as possible reasons.[207]

INCREASED REQUIREMENTS. Generally, energy requirements of patients with CF are believed to be approximately 120% to 150% of recommended daily allowances.[208-211] In one study, REEs and TEEs of 25 children with CF were measured and compared to those for 25 healthy controls. TEE was 12% higher for the entire CF group as compared with controls. In CF patients of the homozygous delta 508 genotype (the most common genotype), TEE was 23% higher than for controls.[211] Naon and colleagues studied REE and nutritional parameters in 13 patients hospitalized for exacerbation of CF. All patients received intravenous antibiotics during hospitalization, which were administered based on sputum culture findings. At hospital discharge, REEs were significantly lower than they had been on admission, suggesting that REE is correlated with clinical status and presence of infection.[212] Kane and coworkers measured BEE in 10 hospitalized CF patients. BEEs averaged 120% of predicted values and increased with severity of clinical status.[213] Increased diet-induced thermogenesis may contribute to increased energy expenditure in CF. A recent study of seven children with CF demonstrated increases in energy expenditures between 20% and 34% associated with feeding.[214]

Nutrition Support in Cystic Fibrosis

Whenever possible, an unrestricted diet with at least 35% to 40% of total calories from fat is recommended.[215] "Grazing" food behavior makes PERT difficult for patients who require enzyme replacement. They should aim for three meals per day and two or three snacks. High-fat, low-carbohydrate feedings may benefit patients with CF complicated by diabetes or significant lung disease. Kane and colleagues compared the effect of three commercial enteral formulas on respiratory parameters in young adults with CF.[213] The formulas represented high-fat, standard, and low-fat compositions and were administered nocturnally by tube. The high-fat formula increased V_{CO_2} by 29%, the standard formula by 49%, and the low-fat formula by 53%. The rate of increase in V_{CO_2} was directly related to the carbohydrate-fat ratio in the formula.[213]

In a separate study, 10 hospitalized CF patients taking oral nutrition supplements had milder increases in V_{CO_2}, respiratory quotient, and minute ventilation following ingestion of a high-fat, low-carbohydrate "pulmonary" commercial formula as compared with a higher-carbohydrate, lower-fat feeding.[216] These studies indicate that high-fat, reduced-carbohydrate feedings may be preferable for CF patients with respiratory compromise. Milla and coworkers compared high-fat, low-carbohydrate oral supplements with standard oral supplements in five adult CF patients with diabetes.[217] The high-fat supplements were associated with a lower glucose excursion rate and lower serum insulin levels than the higher-carbohydrate supplements. The authors suggest that glucose-intolerant CF patients be fed a high-fat formula with a carbohydrate-fat ratio of not more than 0.5.[217]

It is important that adequate energy intake be provided in CF, particularly for pediatric CF patients. The Cystic Fibrosis Consensus has established the following guidelines for determining energy requirements of patients with growth failure or poor weight gain (Box 31-4).

In the event that oral diet is insufficient to maintain weight, oral nutrition supplements should be tried to increase calorie

---

BOX 31-4

Calculating Energy Requirements for Cystic Fibrosis[203,207]

Age Range (yr)	Females	Males
PART A: BASAL ENERGY EXPENDITURE (KCAL)		
0-3	61 (wt) − 51	60.9 (wt) − 54
3-10	22.5 (wt) + 499	22.7 (wt) + 495
10-18	12.2 (wt) + 746	17.5 (wt) + 651
18-30	14.7 (wt) + 496	15.3 (wt) + 679
30-60	8.7 (wt) + 829	11.6 (wt) + 879

PART B: ACTIVITY COEFFICIENTS (AC)

Level of Activity	Activity Coefficient
Confined to bed	1.3
Sedentary	1.5
Active	1.7

PART C: DISEASE COEFFICIENTS (DC)

Lung Function*	Disease Coefficient
Essentially normal (FEV >80% predicted)†	0
Moderate lung disease (FEV 40-79% predicted)	0.2
Severe lung disease (FEV 40% predicted)	0.3

* Pulmonary function tests not available, assess severity of lung disease clinically.
† FEV, Forced expiratory volume.

TO CALCULATE TOTAL ENERGY REQUIREMENTS (TEE)
1. Calculate the BEE (Part A above).
2. Calculate TEE by multiplying BEE by the activity coefficient (AC) plus disease coefficient (DC):

$$TEE = BEE \times (AC + DC)$$

For example, the TEE for a patient who is active, with moderate lung disease, would be:

$$TEE = BEE \times (1.7 + 0.2), \text{ or } BEE \times 1.9$$

content of the diet. If oral intake continues to be poor with supplementation, enteral tube feedings are recommended. A 1992 Cystic Fibrosis Foundation registry revealed that 6.4% of patients received home supplemental feedings. In this group, approximately 72% received gastrostomy tube feedings, and 9% received PN.[218] Although there has been no controlled trial of nutrition support by enterostomal methods, improved body composition, increased strength, and improved body image are among the benefits observed.[217] For the patient with pancreatic insufficiency who is receiving EN support, PERT must be titrated to the feeding to control steatorrhea. Steinkamp and colleagues followed 14 CF patients who underwent long-term nocturnal tube feedings via percutaneous endoscopic gastrostomy tube. Each night, patients received 800 to 1500 calories of polymeric formula containing 35% of total calories from fat. Enteric-coated pancreatic microsphere capsules were given orally just before bedtime (and initiation of feeding). Feedings were tolerated and body weight increased by an average of 6 kg after 1 year of nocturnal feedings.[219] Oral PERT may be taken just before and during the feeding cycle. The addition of pancreatic enzyme preparations to tube feeding generally is not recommended because of the potential for tube occlusion. PN is associated with weight gain in CF patients but also with increased risk of sepsis.[220] In a retrospective review of medical records, pulmonary function, antibiotic use, and weight gain were assessed in 25 CF patients receiving PN. PN promoted weight gain, but the weight was lost when the feedings were discontinued. Antibiotic use and sepsis rates were clearly increased with PN.[220] As in other patient groups, PN should be limited to CF patients who are unable to tolerate EN.

Micronutrient deficiencies are common in CF patients with poorly controlled fat malabsorption. The Cystic Fibrosis Foundation has recommended the vitamin supplementation regimen outlined in Tables 31-11 through 31-13.

Because much salt is lost in the sweat of CF patients it should be replaced in the diet. Breast-fed infants should be supplemented with 1/4 to 1/2 teaspoon salt per day. The salt may be added to expressed breast milk, which is then given in small volumes throughout the day. Children and adults should be advised to use salt liberally. In hot weather or periods of increased physical activity, an additional 1 to 2 teaspoons of salt should be added to the usual diet of children and adults.[221]

Monitoring of nutritional status should be routine in children and adults with CF. Anthropometry, including midarm circumference, triceps skinfold, head circumference (in infants), and weight and height should be monitored at least every 3 months. Laboratory studies, including complete blood count, serum retinol, and serum alpha-tocopherol, should be performed at diagnosis and annually in stable patients. Serum levels of albumin, electrolytes, and acid-base balance and fecal fat studies are indicated if weight loss, growth failure, or clinical deterioration occurs.[221]

Advances in medical treatment have enabled persons with CF to live into adulthood. Improvement of nutritional status through thorough assessment and intervention has allowed people with CF to achieve stature and body composition indices within a desirable range,[200] thus contributing to an increased life expectancy of CF patients.

TABLE 31-11

Multivitamin Supplementation for Cystic Fibrosis*[203,207]

Age (yr)	Recommended Dosage
<2	Standard pediatric liquid multivitamin 1 mL/d
2-8	Standard multivitamin containing 5000 IU vitamin A and 400 IU vitamin D
Older children	Standard adult multivitamin 1-2 times daily
Adolescents	Standard adult multivitamin 1-2 times daily
Adults	Standard adult multivitamin 1-2 times daily

* For patients who cannot maintain serum vitamin A levels with a standard multivitamin preparation, water-miscible vitamin A preparations are available.

TABLE 31-12

Vitamin E Supplementation* for Cystic Fibrosis[203,207]

Age	Dose† (IU/day)
0-6 mo	25
6-12 mo	50
1-4 yr	100
4-10 yr	100-200
Children >10 yr	200-400
Adults	200-400

* Excessive doses of vitamin E can exacerbate coagulopathy associated with vitamin K deficiency.
† Water-miscible form.

TABLE 31-13

Vitamin K Supplementation for Cystic Fibrosis

Age (yr)	Patients on Antibiotic Therapy*	Patients Not on Antibiotic Therapy
0-12 m	2-5 mg twice a wk	2-5 mg once a wk
>12 m	5.0 mg twice a wk	–

Data from Cystic Fibrosis Foundation: Consensus Conference: Concepts in Care, vol VI, Session I, March 23-24, 1995.
* Or if cholestatic liver disease is present.

Other Related Diseases

Enteric Fistulas

Enteric fistulas (EF) are abnormal communications between a portion of the intestinal tract and another organ (internal) or between the intestinal tract and the surface of the body (external or enterocutaneous). EFs can originate anywhere along the intestinal tract, although the small and large intestines and the pancreas are the most common sites of origin.[222,223] Most EFs are a result of surgical wound dehiscence or unintentional enterotomies.[224] IBD, cancer, trauma, and radiation to the abdomen can also lead to development of EFs. Major complications associated with EFs are fluid and electrolyte losses, malnutrition, and sepsis.[225] The fluid and electrolyte losses vary, depending on the volume of digestive secretions lost. Fistulas can be classified as high-output, moderate-output, or low-output, based on the amount of intestinal effluent lost each day (high-output is more than 500 ml per day, moderate-output is considered 500 to 200 ml per day, and low-output less than 200 ml per day).[224] These losses usually are most severe when the fistula first develops, and they decrease with time. GI and pancreatic secretions can be exacerbated by oral nutrition or EN, so complete bowel rest may be necessary to facilitate fluid and electrolyte corrections and fistula closure. Despite optimal medical therapy, elderly patients and those with high-output fistulas in the distal small bowel or colon stemming from malignancy or IBD are unlikely to exhibit spontaneous closure and are likely to require corrective surgery.[223]

Malnutrition can be both a cause and a consequence of EFs. Surgical wound dehiscence and fistula formation have been observed in malnourished patients after surgery.[226] Malnutrition can rapidly develop after fistula formation as a result of inadequate nutrient intake, hypermetabolism, and nutrient losses through the fistula. The typical signs of malnutrition—weight loss and hypoproteinemia—are due to inadequate intake, increased GI losses, and increased energy expenditure for healing and sepsis.[225] Clinical outcomes in patients with fistulas and malnutrition were first observed by Edmunds and colleagues,[227] who cited a 42% mortality rate in all fistula patients, but this rate increased to 64% in the malnourished subpopulation. Randomized, prospective clinical studies to investigate the true effects of nutrition support on malnutrition in fistula patients are not available because of ethical impediments, although it makes sense that optimal nutrition support may enhance the healing process and prevent additional complications related to malnutrition.

Nutrient requirements for patients with fistulas vary with body size, presence of hypermetabolism, and degree of activity. Indirect calorimetry provides information on actual energy expenditure and should be used when available. If indirect calorimetry measurement is not possible, a multifactorial calculation of BEE multiplied by factors of 1.5 to 2.0 should provide adequate calories.[225] Protein requirements are elevated because of enteric losses and hypermetabolism. Nitrogen balance studies, which account for enteric effluent losses, can help determine protein requirements. Daily protein requirements as high as 2.0 g/kg ideal body weight have been recommended.[225,228]

The preferred method of alimentation depends on the site of the fistula. Because the goal is to avoid or limit GI stimulation, enteral feedings may be limited to patients with colocutaneous or low-output fistulas.[3,223,229] The type of enteral formula fed depends on the site of the fistula. Polymeric formulas have been well tolerated by patients with colocutaneous and proximal intestinal fistulas. For patients with distal small bowel EFs, in whom at least 4 feet of functioning bowel are proximal to the fistula, a trial of enteral feeding with a chemically defined formula may be appropriate.[225] If fistula output increases after initiation of enteral feedings, the feedings should be discontinued and PN instituted, with bowel rest. A trial of partial enteral feedings or oral intake may be warranted when the fistula output is minimal or closure has been documented.[224] PN support is indicated for patients with high-output, small bowel fistulas; patients with esophageal, gastric, or pancreatic fistulas who do not have enteral access; and patients who cannot tolerate enteral feedings.[223,224] A mixed-fuel parenteral formula is generally appropriate for these patients. Some fistulas take

more than 4 weeks to close, so home nutrition support may be necessary.

Pharmacologic therapy with H_2 blockers and somatostatin can help decrease secretion of intestinal and pancreatic juices.[3,229-231] As previously discussed, H_2 blockers reduce the gastric secretion of hydrochloric acid (see Table 31-4). Somatostatin (see Table 31-2) works by inhibiting GI endocrine and exocrine secretions and reducing GI motility. These actions decrease the volume of GI secretions and, thus, fistula output. Reduction of output facilitates fluid, electrolyte, and trace mineral management and reduces nitrogen losses.[228] However, a recent review of seven clinical trials designed to test the usefulness of octreotide, a somatostatin analog, in EF closure rates demonstrated octreotide's utility in reducing fistula output, but its role in shortening the time for closure remains to be proven.[232] In a recent randomized, controlled study by Alvarez and colleagues,[233] 13 patients with complicated EF were treated with octreotide and matched to 13 similar patients with EFs who were not treated with octreotide. The results of this study show an acute reduction in fistula output from octreotide use, but no benefit of octreotide in fistula closure. In fact, the octreotide group had a significantly higher rate of mortality as compared with the control group. Somatostatin has few adverse effects, although patients receiving it should be monitored for hypoglycemia.

In summary, the goals of therapy for patients with EFs are to correct fluid and electrolyte disturbances, control fistula drainage with pharmacologic agents, minimize stimulation of GI secretions, and provide adequate nutrients. Enteral feedings can be attempted in patients with low-output and colocutaneous fistulas, and possibly proximal fistulas if enteral access is available below the fistula site. PN may be necessary for high-output fistulas and those that drain more after initiation of enteral feedings, or when appropriate enteral access is not available. The ultimate goal of nutrition therapy is to provide adequate nutrients to support wound healing and prevent deterioration of the patient's nutritional status.

Chylous Ascites and Chylothorax

Chylous leaks into the peritoneal and thoracic cavities can follow surgical injury or trauma to the lymphatic ducts and as a result of obstruction caused by cancer or congenital anomalies. The lymph vessels collect excess tissue fluid, extravasated protein, and fat chylomicrons. The chylomicrons are formed in the intestinal villi from absorbed LCTs and very low-density lipoproteins, and they flow into the thoracic duct as a cloudy, white liquid called *chyle*. The thoracic duct ultimately empties into the venous system at the internal jugular or subclavian vein.[234] Leakage of chyle into the abdominal or thoracic cavity can cause ascites, pleural effusions, abdominal pain, anorexia, hypoalbuminemia, hyponatremia, hypocalcemia, hypocholesterolemia, and elevated alkaline phosphatase.[235] Chylous leaks may resolve with conservative management alone, although surgical repair can be required to ligate the duct.

Conservative management involves reducing the chyle flow, which is normally 1500 to 5500 ml per day. Dietary fluid and fat intake, blood pressure, and portal blood flow contribute to the production of chyle; thus, dietary modification is a primary means of conservatively managing chyle flow.[234] Because nutrient requirements vary, indirect calorimetry should be performed when available. Calorie requirements may be elevated as much as 1.7 to 1.8 times BEE.[3] Protein requirements are normally elevated for wound healing, but they vary depending on how much chyle is secreted. Nitrogen balance studies, which account for excessive protein losses, can help determine requirements.

The goal of nutrition support for patients with chylous leaks is to provide adequate nutrients without stimulating chyle flow. Because chyle production is directly related to oral intake, conservative practice dictates feeding nothing by mouth and support from PN. If oral intake is permitted, strict reduction of LCT intake to less than 20 g per day is recommended.[3,235] This level of dietary fat is very restrictive and compliance may be difficult for patients discharged from the hospital with chyle leakage. Enteral feeding practices are controversial because some formulas can stimulate chyle production. If enteral support is to be instituted, an elemental low-fat formula is recommended.[234-236] MCTs are absorbed directly into the portal vein circulation (thus bypassing the lymphatic system) and can therefore be added to oral diets or enteral formulas for calorie supplementation. Because chyle production is sensitive to fluids, tolerance to volumes of enteral formula may be limited. If prolonged low-fat feedings are required, parenteral supplementation of essential fatty acids and fat-soluble vitamins may be required.[235] PN can allow for bowel rest and facilitate lymphatic vessel closure (conservative or surgical). A mixed nutrient source (including lipid emulsions) is recommended. Intravenous lipids are tolerated well because infusion is via central or peripheral vein, which bypasses the lymphatic system. Resolution of lymphatic leaks can take 6 weeks or more. Thus, home nutrition support may be an option to improve quality of life and reduce health care costs.

Conclusion

The nutrition assessment, support, and counseling of patients with GI disease provides a unique challenge to dietitians. In some conditions—celiac sprue or SBS—nutrition support may be primary therapy. Even when it is only supportive therapy, as in CF, it can dramatically improve quality of life. The role of nutrition in GI disease has evolved rapidly in the last 20 years. Many theories about nutrition therapy that have been posed require further research and clarification; however, virtually all the research of the last several years has one common theme: the benefit of feeding the patient *and* feeding the bowel whenever possible. It is now apparent that unnecessarily restricting the diet or resting the bowel may be deleterious to GI disease. Previously accepted approaches, such as restricting dietary fat for CF and ileostomy patients and treating IBD with PN, are outdated. In combining knowledge of current nutrition research with knowledge of the functions of the GI tract, the dietitian is in a position to positively impact patients' health and well-being.

REFERENCES

1. Groff J, Gropper S: The digestive system: mechanism for nourishing the body. *Advanced nutrition and human metabolism*, ed 3, Belmont, CA, 2000, Wadsworth/Thomson Learning, pp 24-52.
2. Wu M, Lai W: Surgical management of extensive corrosive injuries of the alimentary tract, *Surg Gynecol Obstet* 177(1):12-16, 1993.
3. Stralovich A: Gastrointestinal and pancreatic disease. In Gottschlich M, Matarese L, Shronts E (eds): *Nutrition support dietetics core curriculum*, ed 2, Silver Spring, MD, 1993, ASPEN, pp 275-310.
4. Gerndt S, Orringer M: Tube jejunostomy as an adjunct to esophagectomy, *Surgery* 115(2):164-169, 1994.
5. Jones W, Ginsberg R: Esophageal perforation: a continuing challenge, *Ann Thorac Surg* 53(3):534-543, 1992.
6. Imperiale TF, et al: A cost minimization analysis of alternative treatment strategies for achalasia, *Am J Gastroenterol* 95(10):2737-2745, 2000.
7. Williams S: Gastrointestinal diseases. In Smith J (ed): *Diet therapy*, St Louis, 1995, CV Mosby, pp 96-118.
8. Heading R: Prevalence of upper gastrointestinal symptoms in the general population: a systematic review, *Scand J Gastroenterol* 34(Suppl 231): 3-8, 1999.
9. Meining A, Classen M: The role of diet and lifestyle measures in the pathogenesis and treatment of gastroesophageal reflux disease, *Am J Gastroenterol* 95(10):2692-2697, 2000.
10. Flynn C: The evaluation and treatment of adults with gastroesophageal reflux disease, *J Fam Pract* 50(1):57-58, 61-63, 2001.
11. Dent J, Brun J, Fendrick A, et al: An evidence-based appraisal of reflux disease management the Genval Workshop Report, *Gut* 44(suppl 1):1-32, 1999.
12. Roth J, Putnam J: Surgery for cancer of the esophagus, *Semin Oncol* 21(4):453-461, 1994.
13. Vigneswaran W, Trastek V, Pairolero P, et al: Transhiatal esophagectomy for carcinoma of the esophagus, *Ann Thorac Surg* 56(4):838-846, 1993.
14. Nutrition assessment of adults. In Hornich B, et al: (eds): *Manual of clinical dietetics*, ed 6, Chicago, 2000, The American Dietetic Association, pp 3-38.
15. Stenson W: The esophagus and stomach. In Shils M, et al: (eds): *Modern nutrition in health and disease*, ed 9, Baltimore, 1999, Williams & Wilkins, pp 1125-1133.
16. Cullen J, Kelly K: Gastric motor physiology and pathophysiology, *Surg Clin North Am* 73(6):1145-1160, 1993.
17. Klein S, Cohn S, Alpers D: The alimentary tract in nutrition: a tutorial. In Shils M, et al: (eds): *Modern nutrition in health and disease*, ed 9, Baltimore, 1999, Williams & Wilkins, pp 605-629.
18. Minami H, McCallum R: The physiology and pathophysiology of gastric emptying in humans, *Gastroenterology* 86(6):1592-1610, 1984.
19. Summers G, Hocking M: Preoperative and postoperative motility disorders of the stomach, *Surg Clin North Am* 72(2):467-486, 1992.
20. Grant J, Chapman G, Russel M: Malabsorption associated with surgical procedures and it treatment, *Nutr Clin Pract* 11(2):43-52, 1996.
21. Greer R, Richards W, O'Dorisio T, et al: Efficacy of octreotide acetate in treatment of severe postgastrectomy dumping syndrome, *Ann Surg* 212(6):678-687, 1990.
22. Gastric Surgery. In Hornich B, et al: (eds): *Manual of clinical dietetics*, ed 6, Chicago, 2000, The American Dietetic Association, pp 395-400.
23. Ippoliti A, Maxwell V, Isenberg J: The effect of various forms of milk on gastric acid secretion, *Ann Intern Med* 84(3):286-289, 1976.
24. Cerda J: Diet and gastrointestinal disease, *Med Clin North Am* 77(4): 881-887, 1993.
25. Jivonen M, Koskinen M, Ikonen T, et al: Emptying of jejunal pouch and Roux-en-Y limb after total gastrectomy—a randomized, prospective study, *Eur J Surg* 165(8):742-747, 1999.
26. Liedman B: Symptoms after total gastrectomy on food intake, body composition, bone metabolism, and quality of life in gastric cancer patients— Is reconstruction with a reservoir worthwhile? *Nutrition* 15(9):677-682, 1999.
27. Liedman B, Bosaeus I, Hugosson I, et al: Long-term beneficial effects of a gastric reservoir on weight control after total gastrectomy. A study on potential mechanisms, *Br J Surg* 85(4):542-547, 1998.
28. Wechsler J: Dietary treatment following gastrectomy, *Nutrition* 4:324, 1989.
29. Daly J, Weintraub F, Shou J, et al: Enteral nutrition during multimodality therapy in upper gastrointestinal cancer patients, *Ann Surg* 221(4): 327-338, 1995.
30. Kornowski A, Cosnes J, Genore J, et al: Enteral nutrition in malnutrition following gastric resection and cephalic pancreaticoduodenectomy, *Hepato-Gastroenterol* 39(1):9-13, 1992.
31. Meyer J: Nutritional outcome of gastric operations, *Gastroenterol Clin North Am* 23(2):227-260, 1994.

32. Kim Y, Spritz N, Blum M, et al: The role of altered bile acid metabolism in the steatorrhea of experimental blind loop, *J Clin Invest* 45(6): 956-962, 1966.

33. Tovey F, Hall M, Ell P, et al: A review of postgastrectomy bone disease, *J Gastroenterol Hepatol* 7(6):639-645, 1992.

34. Sitrin MD: Nutrition support in inflammatory bowel disease, *Nutr Clin Pract* 7(2):53-60, 1992.

35. Hanauer SB: Inflammatory bowel disease. In Bennet JC, Plum F (eds): *Cecil textbook of medicine,* ed 20, Philadelphia, 1996, WB Saunders.

36. Glickman R: Inflammatory bowel disease (ulcerative colitis and Crohn's disease). In Isselbacher K, Braunwald E, Wilson JD (eds): *Harrison's principles of internal medicine,* ed 13, New York, 1994, McGraw Hill, pp 1403-1407.

37. Goldner F, Kraft SC: Idiopathic inflammatory bowel disease. In Stein JH (ed): *Internal medicine,* ed 2, Toronto, 1987, Little, Brown, p 141.

38. Griffiths AM: Inflammatory bowel disease, *Nutrition* 14(10):788-791, 1998.

39. Hanauer SB, Peppercorn MA, Present DH: Current concepts, new therapies in IBD, *Patient Care* 15:79-103, 1992.

40. Dudrick SJ, Latifi R, Schrager R: Nutritional management of inflammatory bowel disease, *Surg Clin North Am* 71(3):609-623, 1991.

41. Fleming RC: Nutrition in patients with Crohn's disease: another piece of the puzzle, *J Parenter Enteral Nutr* 19:93-94, 1995.

42. Royall D, Greenberg GR, Allard JP, et al: Total enteral nutrition support improves body composition of patients with active Crohn's disease, *J Parenter Enteral Nutr* 19(2):95-99, 1995.

43. Kahng KU, Roslyn JJ: Surgical treatment of inflammatory bowel disease, *Med Clin North Am* 78(6):1427-1441, 1994.

44. Hanauer SB: Medical therapy of ulcerative colitis, *Lancet* 342(8868): 412-417, 1993.

45. Lewis JD, Fisher RL: Nutrition support in inflammatory bowel disease, *Med Clin North Am* 78(6):1443-1456, 1994.

46. Rigaud D, Angel LA, Cerf M, et al: Mechanisms of decreased food intake during weight loss in adult Crohn's disease patients without obvious malabsorption, *Am J Clin Nutr* 60(5):775-781, 1994.

47. Shanahan F: Probiotics and inflammatory bowel disease: is there a scientific rationale? *Inflamm Bowel Dis* 6(2):107-115, 2000.

48. Hanauer SB: Inflammatory bowel disease revisited: newer drugs, *Scand J Gastroenterol* 25(suppl 175):97-106, 1990.

49. Lennard-Jones JE: Inflammatory bowel disease: medical therapy revisited, *Scand J Gastroenterol* 27(suppl 192):110-116, 1992.

50. Hanauer SB, Baert F: Medical therapy of inflammatory bowel disease, *Med Clin North Am* 78(6):1413-1426, 1994.

51. Hanauer SB: Inflammatory bowel disease, *N Engl J Med* 334(13): 841-848, 1996.

52. *Physician's Desk Reference,* ed 56, Montvale, NJ, 2002, Medical Economics.

53. Bonner GF: Current medical therapy for inflammatory bowel disease, *South Med J* 89(6):556-566, 1996.

54. Meyers S: Inflammatory bowel disease: complications and their management. In Haubrich WS, Schaffner F, Berk JE (eds): *Bockus gastroenterology,* ed 5, vol 2, Philadelphia, 1991, WB Saunders, p 1499.

55. Dieleman LA, Heizer WD: Nutritional issues in inflammatory bowel disease, *Gastro Clin North Am* 27(2):435-451, 1998.

56. Mingrone G, Caprista E, Greco AV, et al: Elevated diet-induced thermogenesis and lipid oxidation rate in Crohn's disease, *Am J Clin Nutr* 69(2):325-330, 1999.

57. Kushner RF, Schoeller DA: Resting and total energy expenditure in patients with inflammatory bowel disease, *Am J Clin Nutr* 53(1): 161-165, 1991.

58. Stokes MA, Hill GL: Total energy expenditure in patients with Crohn's disease: measurement by the combined body scan technique, *J Parenter Enteral Nutr* 17(1):3-7, 1993.

59. Schneeweiss B, Lochs H, Zauner C, et al: Energy and substrate metabolism in patients with active Crohn's disease, *J Nutr* 129(4):844-848, 1999.

60. Han PD, Burke A, Baldassano RN, et al: Nutrition and inflammatory bowel disease, *Gastroenterol Clin North Am* 28(2):423-433, 1999.

61. Geerling BJ, Badart-Smook A, Stockbrugger RW, Brummer R-JM: Comprehensive nutritional status in recently diagnosed patients with inflammatory bowel disease compared with population controls, *Eur J Clin Nutr* 54(6):514-521, 2000.

62. Kelly DG. Nutrition in inflammatory bowel disease, *Curr Gastroenterol Rep* 1(4):324-330, 1999.

63. Gokhale R, Favus MJ, Karrison T, et al: Bone mineral density assessment in children with inflammatory bowel disease, *Gastroenterology* 114(5): 902-911, 1998.

64. Schoon EJ, Muller MC, Vermeer C, et al: Low serum and bone vitamin K status in patients with longstanding Crohn's disease: another pathogenic factor of osteoporosis in Crohn's disease? *Gut* 48(4):473-477, 2001.

65. Stein RB, Lichtenstein GR, Rombeau JL: Nutrition in inflammatory bowel disease, *Curr Opin Clin Nutr Metab Care* 2(5):367-371, 1999.

66. Gorard DA, Hunt JB, Payne-James JJ, et al: Initial response and subsequent course of Crohn's disease treated with elemental diet or prednisolone, *Gut* 34(9):1198-1202, 1993.

67. Fernandez-Banares F, Cabre E, Gonzalez-Huix F, Gassull MA: Enteral nutrition as primary therapy in Crohn's disease, *Gut* 35(1 suppl): S55-S59, 1994.

68. Greenberg GR: Nutritional support in inflammatory bowel disease: current status and future directions, *Scand J Gastroenterol* 27(suppl 192):117-122, 1992.

69. Bengoa J, Rosenberg IH: Parenteral nutrition therapy in gastrointestinal disease, *Adv Intern Med* 28:363-385, 1983.

70. O'Morain C, Segal AW, Levi AJ: Elemental diet as primary treatment of acute Crohn's disease: a controlled trial, *Br Med J Clin Res* 288: June (Pt 2):1859-1862, 1984.

71. Saverymuttu S, Hodgson HJF, Chadwick VS: Controlled trial comparing prednisolone with an elemental diet plus non-absorbable antibiotics in active Crohn's disease, *Gut* 26(10):994-998, 1985.

72. Seidman EG: Nutritional management of inflammatory bowel disease, *Gastroenterol Clin North Am* 18(1):129-155, 1989.

73. Sanderson IR, Udeen S, Davies PSW, et al: Remission induced by an elemental diet in small bowel Crohn's disease, *Arch Dis Child* 62(2): 123-127, 1987.

74. Alun Jones V: Comparison of total parenteral nutrition and elemental diet in induction of remission of Crohn's disease, *Dig Dis Sci* 32(12 suppl):100S-107S, 1987.

75. Hunt JB, Payne-James JJ, Palmer KR, et al: A randomized controlled trial of elemental diet and prednisone as primary therapy in acute exacerbations of Crohn's disease, *Gastroenterology* 96(No. 5, Pt. 2):A 224, 1989.

76. Teahon K, Pearson M, Levi AJ, Bjarnson I: Practical aspects of enteral nutrition in the management of Crohn's disease, *J Parenter Enteral Nutr* 19(5):365-368, 1995.

77. Raouf AH, Hildrey V, Daniel J, et al: Enteral feeding as sole treatment for Crohn's disease: controlled trial of whole protein versus amino acid based feed and a case study of dietary challenge, *Gut* 32:702-707, 1991.

78. Griffiths AM, Ohlsson A, Sherman PM, Sutherland LR: Meta-analysis of enteral nutrition as a primary treatment of active Crohn's disease, *Gastroenterology* 108(4):1056-1067, 1995.

79. O'Sullivan MA, O'Morain CA: Nutritional therapy in Crohn's disease, *Inflamm Bowel Dis* 4(1):45-53, 1998.

80. Sitzmann JV, Converse RL, Bayless TM: Favorable response to parenteral nutrition as the sole therapy in Crohn's colitis, *Gastroenterology* 99(6):1647-1652, 1990.

81. McIntyre PB, Powell-Tuck J, Wood SR, et al: Controlled trial of bowel rest in the treatment of severe acute colitis, *Gut* 27(5):481-485, 1986.

82. Meyers S: Inflammatory bowel disease: medical management. In Haubrich WS, Schaffner F, Berk JE (eds): *Bockus gastroenterology,* ed 5, vol 2, Philadelphia, 1995, WB Saunders, pp 1479-1513.

83. Sagar P, Macfie J: Pouchitis, colitis and deficiencies of fuel, *Clin Nutr* 14:13-16, 1995.

84. Scheppach W: Effects of short-chain fatty acids on gut morphology and function, *Gut* 37 (suppl 1):S35-S38, 1994.

85. Nordgaard-Andersen I, Clausen MR, Mortense PB: Short-chain fatty acids, lactate, and ammonia in ileorectal and ileal pouch contents: a model of cecal fermentation, *J Parenter Enteral Nutr* 34(4):324-331, 1993.

86. Evans MA, Shronts EP: Intestinal fuels: Glutamine, short chain fatty acids, and dietary fiber, *J Am Diet Assoc* 92(10):1239-1249, 1992.

87. Zimmaro DM, Rolandelli RH, Koruda MJ, et al: Isotonic tube feeding formula induces liquid stool in normal subjects: reversal by pectin, *J Parenter Enteral Nutr* 13(2):117-123, 1989.

88. Koruda MJ, Rolandelli RH, Settle RG, et al: The effect of a pectin-supplemental elemental diet on intestinal adaptation to massive small bowel resection, *J Parenter Enteral Nutr* 10(4):343-350, 1986.

89. Rolandelli RH, Koruda MJ, Settle G, Rombeau JL: The effect of enteral feedings supplemented with pectin on the healing of colonic anastomoses in the rat, *Surgery* 99(6):703-707, 1986.

90. Harig JM, Soergel KH, Komorowski RA, Wood CM: Treatment of diversion colitis with short-chain fatty acid irrigation, *N Engl J Med* 320(1):23-28, 1989.

91. Finkel Y, Brown G, Smith HL, et al: The effects of a pectin-supplemented elemental diet in a boy with short gut syndrome, *Acta Pediatr Scand* 79:983-986, 1990.

92. Ling SC, Griffiths AM: Nutrition in inflammatory bowel disease, *Curr Opin Clin Nutr Met Care* 3:339-344, 2000.

93. Kim Y-I: Can fish oil maintain Crohn's disease in remission? *Nutr Rev* 54(8):248-257, 1996.

94. Belluzzi A, Brignola C, Campieri M, et al: Effect of an enteric coated fish-oil preparation on relapses in Crohn's disease, *N Engl J Med* 334(24):1557-1560, 1996.

95. Bernstein CN, Shanahan F: Critical appraisal of enteral nutrition as primary therapy in adults with Crohn's disease, *Am J Gastroenterol* 91(10):2075-2079, 1996.

96. Akobeng A, Miller V, Stanton J, et al: Double-blind randomized controlled trial of glutamine-enriched polymeric diet in the treatment of active Crohn's disease, *J Pediatr Gastroenterol Nutr* 30(1):78-84, 2000.

97. Slonim AE, Bulone L, Damore MB, et al: A preliminary study of growth hormone therapy for Crohn's disease, *N Engl J Med* 342(22):1633-1637, 2000.

98. Marteau PR, deVrese M, Cellier C, et al: Protection from gastrointestinal diseases with the use of probiotics, *Am J Clin Nutr* 73 (suppl): 430S-436S, 2001.

99. Plein K, Hotz J: Therapeutic effects of *Saccharomyces boulardii* on mild residual symptoms in a stable phase of Crohn's disease with special respect to chronic diarrhea-a pilot study, *Z Gastroenterol* 31:129-134, 1993.

100. Rembacken BJ, Snelling AM, Hawkey PM, et al: Non-pathogenic *Escherichia coli* versus mesalazine for the treatment of ulcerative colitis: a randomized trial, *Lancet* 354(9179):635-639, 1999.

101. Faller MC, Welling RE, Lambert CE: Nutritional implications and dietary management postproctocolectomy and ileal reservoir construction, *J Am Diet Assoc* 86(9):1235-1236, 1986.

102. Sandborn WJ, Tremaine WJ, Batts KP, et al: Pouchitis after ileal pouch–anal anastomosis: a pouchitis disease activity index, *Mayo Clin Proc* 69(5):409-415, 1994.

103. Setti-Carraro P, Ritchie JK, Wilkinson KH, et al: The first 10 years' experience of restorative proctocolectomy for ulcerative colitis, *Gut* 35(8):1070-1075, 1994.

104. Luukkonen P, Jarvinen H, Tanskanen M, Kahri A: Pouchitis—recurrence of the inflammatory bowel disease? *Gut* 35(2):243-246, 1994.

105. Hermann-Zaidins MG: Malabsorption in adults: etiology, evaluation and management, *J Am Diet Assoc* 86(9):1171-1178, 1181, 1986.

106. Shikora SA, Blackburn GL: Nutritional consequences of major gastrointestinal surgery. Patient outcome and starvation, *Surg Clin North Am* 71(3):509-521, 1991.

107. Marotta R, Floch MH: Dietary therapy of steatorrhea, *Gastroenterol Clin North Am* 18(3):485-512, 1989.

108. Bernard DK, Shaw MJ: Principles of nutrition therapy for short bowel syndrome, *Nutr Clin Pract* 8(4):153-162, 1993.

109. Zeman F: Conditions common to many gastrointestinal disorders. In Zeman FJ (ed): *Clinical nutrition in dietetics,* ed 2, New York, MacMillan, 1991, pp 230-243.

110. Tamm A: Management of lactose intolerance, *Scand J Gastroenterol* 202:55-63, 1994.

111. Strocchi A, Levitt MD: Digestion and absorption of lipid, protein and carbohydrate, *Support Line* 13(1):2-6, 1991.

112. Purdum PP, Kirby DF: Short-bowel syndrome: A review of the role of nutrition support. *J Parenter Enteral Nutr* 15(1):93-100, 1991.

113. Ledeboer M, Masclee AM, Jansen BM, Lamers CBHW: Effect of equimolar amounts of long-chain triglycerides and medium-chain triglycerides on small-bowel transit time in humans, *J Parenter Enteral Nutr* 19(1):5-8, 1995.

114. Hertzler SR, Huynh BC, Savaiano D: How much lactose is low lactose? *J Am Diet Assoc* 96(3):243-246, 1996.

115. Brasitus TA, Sitrin MD: Short-bowel syndrome. In Yamada T (ed): *Textbook of gastroenterology,* Philadelphia, 1990, JB Lippincott, pp 1541-1554.

116. Lennard-Jones JE: Review article: practical management of the short bowel, *Aliment Pharmacol Ther* 8:563-577, 1994.

117. Nightingale JM, Lennard-Jones JE: The short bowel syndrome: what's new and old? *Dig Dis* 11(1):12-31, 1993.

118. Nightingale JM, Kamm MA, van der Sijp JR, et al: Disturbed gastric emptying in the short bowel syndrome. Evidence for a "colonic brake," *Gut* 34(9):1171-1176, 1993.

119. Lentze MJ: Intestinal adaptation in short bowel syndrome, *Eur J Pediatr* 148(4):294-299, 1989.

120. Levy E, Frileux P, Sandrucci S, et al: Continuous enteral nutrition during the early adaptive stage of the short bowel syndrome, *Br J Surg* 75(6):549-553, 1988.

121. Dudrick SJ, Latifi R, Fosnocht DE: Management of short bowel syndrome. *Current Strategies in Surgical Nutrition* 71:625-643, 1991.

122. Gouttebel MC, Saint Aubert B, Colette C, et al: Intestinal adaptation in patients with short bowel syndrome, *Dig Dis Sci* 34(5):709-715, 1989.

123. Gouttebel MC, Saint Aubert B, Astre C, et al: Total parenteral nutrition needs in different types of short bowel syndrome, *Dig Dis Sci* 31(7): 718-723, 1986.

124. Messing B, Pigot F, Rongier M, et al: Intestinal absorption of free oral hyperalimentation in the very short bowel syndrome, *Gastroenterology* 100(6):1502-1508, 1991.

125. Woolf GM, Miller C, Kurian R, et al: Nutrition absorption in short bowel syndrome. Evaluation of fluid, calorie and divalent cation requirements, *Dig Dis Sci* 32(1):8-15, 1987.

126. Nordgaard I, Hansen BS, Mortensen PB: Colon as a digestive organ in patients with short bowel, *Lancet* 343(8894):373-376, 1994.

127. Nordgard I, Hansen BS, Mortinsen. Importance of colonic support for energy absorption as small-bowel failure proceeds, *Am J Clin Nutr* 64(8):222-231, 1996.

128. Simko V, McCarroll AM, Goodman S, et al: High-fat diet in a short bowel syndrome, *Dig Dis Sci* 25(5):333-339, 1980.

129. Cosnes J, Gendre JP, Evard D, LeQuintrec YL: Compensatory enteral hyperalimentation for management of patients with severe short bowel syndrome, *Am J Clin Nutr* 41(5):1002-1009, 1985.

130. Woolf GM, Miller C, Kurian R, et al: Diet for patients with short bowel syndrome: high fat or high carbohydrate? *Gastroenterology* 84(4): 823-828, 1983.

131. Lennard-Jones JE. Oral rehydration solutions in short bowel syndrome, *Clin Ther* 12(suppl A):129-138, 1990.

132. Byrne T, Veglia L, Camelio M, et al: Beyond the prescription: optimizing the diet of patients with short bowel syndrome, *Nutr Clin Pract* 15(6):306-311, 2000.

133. Levenson DI, Bockman RS: A review of calcium preparations, *Nutr Rev* 52(7):221-232, 1994.

134. Rodriguez DJ, Clevenger FW: Successful enteral refeeding after massive small bowel resection, *West J Med* 159(2):192-194, 1993.

135. Zeigler TR, Estivariz CF, Jonas CR, et al: Interactions between nutrients and growth factors in intestinal growth, repair and function, *J Parenter Enteral Nutr* 23(6):S174-S183, 1999.

136. Jeejeebhoy KN: Intestinal disorders: short bowel syndrome. In Shils ME, Olson JA, Shike M (eds): *Modern nutrition in health and disease,* ed 8, vol 2, Philadelphia, 1994, Lea & Febiger, 1994, pp 1036-1042.

137. O'Keefe S, Peterson ME, Fleming CR: Octreotide as an adjunct to home parenteral nutrition in the management of permanent end-jejunostomy syndrome, *J Parenter Enteral Nutr* 18(1):26-34, 1994.

138. Scolapio JS, Camilleri M, Fleming CR et al: Effect of growth hormone, glutamine and diet on adaptation in short-bowel syndrome: a randomized, controlled study, *Gastroenterology* 113(4):1074-1081, 1997.

139. Szkudlarek J, Jeppesen PB, Mortensen PB: Effect of high dose growth hormone with glutamine and no change in diet on intestinal absorption in short bowel patients, a double blind, crossover, placebo-controlled study, *Gut* 47(2):199-205, 2000.

140. Byrne TA, Morrissey TB, Nattakom TV, et al: Growth hormone, glutamine and a modified oral diet enhance nutrient absorption in patients with severe short bowel syndrome, *J Parenter Enteral Nutr* 19(4):296-302, 1995.

141. Wilmore DW, Lacey JM, Soultanakis RP, et al: Factors predicting a successful outcome after pharmacological bowel compensation, *Ann Surg* 226(3):288-293, 1997.

142. Nusbaum M, Campana T, Weese J: Radiation induced intestinal injury, *Clin Plast Surg* 20(3):573-580, 1993.

143. Jackson WD, Grand RJ: The human response to enteral nutrients: a review, *J Am Coll Nutr* 10(5):500-509, 1991.

144. McArdle AH, Reid EC, Laplante MD, Freeman CR: Prophylaxis against radiation injury. The use of elemental diet prior to and during radiotherapy for invasive bladder cancer and in early postoperative feeding following radical cystectomy and ideal conduit, *Arch Surg* 121(8):879-885, 1986.

145. Beer W, Fan A, Halsted C: Clinical and nutritional implications of radiation enteritis, *Am J Clin Nutr* 41(1):85-91, 1985.

146. Klimberg VS, Salloum RM, Kasper M, et al: Oral glutamine accelerates healing of the small intestine and improves outcome after whole abdominal radiation, *Arch Surg* 125(8):1040-1045, 1990.

147. Gurbuz AT, Kunzelman J, Ratzer EE: Supplemental dietary arginie accelerates intestinal mucosal regeneration and enhances bacterial clearance following radiation enteritis in rats, *J Surg Res* 74(2):149-154, 1998.

148. Ersin S, Tuncyurek P, Esassolak M, et al: The prophylactic and therapeutic effects of glutamine- and arginine-enriched diets on radiation-induced enteritis in rats, *J Surg Res* 899(2):121-125, 2000.

149. Trier, JS: Diagnosis of celiac sprue, *Gastroenterology* 115(1):211-216, 1998.

150. Fasano A, Catassi C: Current approaches to diagnosis and treatment of celiac disease: an evolving spectrum, *Gastroenterology* 120(3):636-651, 2001.

151. Shuppan D: Current concepts of celiac disease pathogenesis, *Gastroenterology* 119(1):234-242, 2000.

152. Godkin A, Jewell D: The pathogenesis of celiac disease, *Gastroenterology* 115(1):206-210, 1998.

153. Celiac disease. In Hornick B, et al: (eds): *Manual of clinical dietetics,* ed 6, Chicago, 2000, The American Dietetic Association, pp 182-191.

154. Trier JS: Celiac sprue, *N Engl J Med* 325(24):1709-1719, 1991.

155. Ryan B, Kelleher D: Refractory celiac disease, *Gastroenterology* 119(1):243-251, 2000.

156. Green, PHR, Stavropoulos, SN, Panagi SG, et al: Characteristics of adult celiac disease in the USA: results of a national study, *Am J Gastroenterol* 96(1):126-131, 2001.

157. Latifi R, McIntosh JK, Dudrick SJ: Nutritional management of acute and chronic pancreatitis, *Surg Clin North Am* 71(3):579-595, 1991.

158. Corcoy R, Sanchez JM, Domingo P, Net A: Nutrition in the patient with severe acute pancreatitis, *Nutrition* 4:269-275, 1988.

159. Abou-Assi S, O'Keefe SJ: Nutrition in acute pancreatitis, *J Clin Gastroenterol* 32(3):203-209, 2001.

160. Marulendra S, Kirby DF: Nutrition support in pancreatitis, *Nutr Clin Pract* 10(2):45-53, 1995.

161. Shea JC, Hopper IK, Blanco PG, Freedman SD: Advances in nutritional management of pancreatitis, *Curr Gastroent Rep* 2: 323-326, 2000.

162. Fried M, Mayer EA, Jansen JBM, et al: Temporal relationships of cholecystokinin release, pancreatobiliary secretion, and gastric emptying of a mixed meal, *Gastroenterology* 95(5):1344-1350, 1988.

163. Seidner DL, Fish JA: Nutritional management of patients with feeding-induced pain: acute pancreatitis, *Semin Gastrointest Dis* 9:200-209, 1998.

164. Steinberg W, Tenner S: Acute pancreatitis, *N Engl J Med* 330(17): 1198-1210, 1994.

165. Pisters PWT, Ranson JHL: Nutritional support for acute pancreatitis, *Surg Gynecol Obstet* 175(3):275-284, 1992.

166. Ranson JHC, Rifkind KM, Roses DF, et al: Prognostic signs and the role of operative management in acute pancreatitis, *Surg Gynecol Obstet* 139(1):69-81, 1974.

167. Pupelis G, Selga G, Austrums E, Kaminski A: Jejunal feeding, even when instituted late, improves outcomes in patients with severe pancreatitis and peritonitis, *Nutrition* 17(2):91-94, 2001.

168. Windsor ACJ, Kanwar A, Li AGK, et al: Compared with parenteral nutrition, enteral feeding attenuates the acute phase response and improves disease severity in acute pancreatitis, *Gut* 42(3):431-435, 1998.

169. Lehocky P, Sarr MG: Early enteral feeding in severe acute pancreatitis: can it prevent secondary pancreatic (super) infection? *Dig Surg* 17(6):571-577, 2000.

170. McClave SA, Ritchie CS: Artificial nutrition in pancreatic disease: what lessons have we learned from the literature? *Clin Nutr* 19(1):1-6, 2000.

171. Kudsk KA, Campbell SM, O'Brien TO, Fuller R: Postoperative jejunostomy feedings following complicated pancreatitis, *Nutr Clin Pract* 5(1):14-17, 1990.

172. Feller JH, Brown RA, MacLaren-Toussant GP, et al: Changing methods in the treatment of severe pancreatitis, *Am J Surg* 127(2):196-201, 1974.

173. Blackburn GL, Williams LF, Bistrian BR, et al: New approaches to the management of severe acute pancreatitis, *Am J Surg* 131(1):114-124, 1976.

174. Grant JP, James S, Grabowski V, et al: Total parenteral nutrition in pancreatic disease, *Ann Surg* 200(5): 627-631, 1984.

175. Sitzmann JV, Steinborn PA, Zinner MJ, et al: Total parenteral nutrition and alternate energy substrates in treatment of severe acute pancreatitis, *Surg Gynecol Obstet* 168(4):311-317, 1989.

176. Sax HC, Warner BW, Talamini MA, et al: Early total parenteral nutrition in acute pancreatitis: lack of beneficial effects, *Am J Surg* 153(1): 117-124, 1987.

177. Guillou PJ: Enteral versus parenteral nutrition in acute pancreatitis, *Baillieres Best Pract Res Clin Gastroenterol* 13(2):345-355, 1999.

178. McClave SA, Snider H, Owens N, Sexton LK: Clinical nutrition in pancreatitis, *Dig Dis Sci* 42(10):2035-2044, 1997.

179. Kalfarentzos F, Kehagias J, Mead N, et al: Enteral nutrition is superior to parenteral nutrition in severe acute pancreatitis. Results of a randomized prospective trial, *Br J Surg* 84(12):1665-1669, 1997**.**

180. Keith RG: Effect of a low fat elemental diet on pancreatic secretion during pancreatitis, *Surg Gynecol Obstet* 151(3):337-343, 1980.

181. Grant JP, Davey-McCrae J, Snyder PJ: Effect of enteral nutrition on human pancreatic secretions, *J Parenter Enteral Nutr* 11(3): 302-304, 1987.

182. Duerksen DR, Bector S, Yaffe C, Parry DM: Does jejunal feeding with a polymeric immune-enhancing formula increase pancreatic exocrine output as compared with TPN? A case report, *Nutrition* 16(1):47-49, 2000.

183. Schneider H, Boyle N, McCluckie A, Beal R, Atkinson S: Acute severe pancreatitis and multiple organ failure: total parenteral nutrition is still required in a proportion of patients, *Br J Surg* 87(3):362-373, 2000.

184. Burns GP, Stein TA: Pancreatic enzyme secretion during intravenous fat infusion, *J Parenter Enteral Nutr* 11(1):60-62, 1987.

185. Practice Guidelines: Pancreatitis. Guidelines for the use of parenteral and enteral nutrition in adult and pediatric patients, *J Parenter Enteral Nutr* 17(4 suppl):16SA, 1993.

186. Dickerson RD, Vehe KL, Mullen JL, Feurer ID: Resting energy expenditure in patients with pancreatitis, *Crit Care Med* 19(4):484-490, 1991.

187. Bouffard YH, Delafosse BX, Amant GJ, et al: Energy expenditure in severe acute pancreatitis, *J Parenter Enteral Nutr* 13(1):26-29, 1989.

188. Holt S: Chronic pancreatitis, *South Med J* 86(2):201-207, 1993.

189. Toskes PP: Medical management of chronic pancreatitis, *Scand J Gastroenterol* 208(suppl): 74-80, 1995.

190. Lankesh PG: Chronic pancreatitis. In Haubrich WS, Schaffner F, Berk J (eds): *Bockus gastroenterology,* ed 5, vol 4, Philadelphia, 1995, WB Saunders, pp 2930-2958.

191. *Physician's desk reference,* ed 56, Montvale, NJ, 2002, Medical Economics, 835-839; 2580-2581, 2931, 3521.

192. Ghaneh P, Neoptolemos JP: Pancreatic exocrine insufficiency following pancreatic resection, *Digest* 60(suppl 1):104-110, 1999.

193. Berger HG, Buchler MW: Surgical management of chronic pancreatitis. In Haubrich WS, Schaffner F, Berk J (eds): *Bockus gastroenterology,* ed 5, vol 4, Philadelphia, 1995, WB Saunders, 2959-2968.

194. Crucitti F, Doglietto G, Bellantone R, et al: Digestive and nutritional consequences of pancreatic resections, *Int J Pancreatol* 17(1):37-45, 1995.

195. Braga M, Cristallo M, De Franchis R, et al: Correction of malnutrition and maldigestion with enzyme supplementation in patients with surgical suppression of exocrine pancreatic function, *Surg Gynecol Obstet* 167(6):485-492, 1988.

196. Dowsett J: Nutrition in the management of cystic fibrosis, *Nutr Rev* 54(1):31-33, 1996.

197. Winklhofer-Roob B, Tuchschmid PE, Molinari L, Shmerling DH: Response to a single oral dose of all-rac-α-tocopheryl acetate in patients with cystic fibrosis and in healthy individuals, *Am J Clin Nutr* 63(5): 717-721, 1996.

198. Dowsett J: An overview of nutritional issues for the adult with cystic fibrosis, *Nutrition* 16(7-8):566-570, 2000.

199. Stutts J: Gastrointestinal considerations in the patient with cystic fibrosis, *Support Line* 21(1):3-5, 1999.

200. Richardson I, Nyulasi I, Cameron K, et al: Nutritional status of an adult cystic fibrosis population, *Nutrition* 16(4):255-259, 2000.

201. Kalivianakis M, Minich D, Bijleveld C, et al: Fat malabsorption in cystic fibrosis patients receiving enzyme replacement therapy is due to impaired intestinal uptake of long-chain fatty acids, *Am J Clin Nutr* 69(1):127-134, 1999.

202. Cystic Fibrosis Foundation: Consensus conference on pancreatic enzyme supplementation, vol VI, sect. I, March 23-24, 1995.

203. Cystic Fibrosis Foundation: Consensus conference: Concepts in care, vol VI, sect I, March 23-24, 1995.

204. Hardin DS, Moran A: Diabetes mellitus in cystic fibrosis. *Endocrinol Metab North Am* 28(4):787-799, 1999.

205. Webb AK, David TJ: Clinical management of children and adults with cystic fibrosis, *BMJ* 308(6925):459-462, 1994.

206. The Consensus Committee: Consensus conference on cystic fibrosis related diabetes mellitus. Concepts in care, Cystic Fibrosis Foundation, vol I, sect IV, Jan 11-12, 1990.

207. Ramsey BW, Farrell PM, Pencharz P, and the Consensus Committee: Nutritional assessment and management in cystic fibrosis, *Am J Clin Nutr* 55(1):108-116, 1992.

208. Smith J: Nutrition management of cystic fibrosis, *Support Line* 21:6-10, 1999.

209. Hogg J, Klapholz A, Reid-Hector J: Pulmonary disease. In Shils M, et al: (eds): *Modern nutrition in health and disease,* ed 9, Baltimore, 1999, Williams & Wilkins, pp 491-516.

210. Shepherd RW, Greer, RM, McNaughton SA, et al: Energy expenditure and body cell mass in cystic fibrosis, *Nutrition* 17(1):22-25, 2001.

211. Tomezsko JL, Stallings VA, Kawchak DA, et al: Energy expenditures and genotype of children with cystic fibrosis, *Pediatr Res* 35(4):451-460, 1994.

212. Naon H, Hack S, Shelton MT, et al: Resting energy expenditure. Evolution during antibiotic treatment for pulmonary exacerbation in cystic fibrosis, *Chest* 103(6):1819-1825, 1993.

213. Kane RE, Hobbs PJ, Black PG: Comparison of low, medium and high carbohydrate formulas for night time enteral feeding in cystic fibrosis patients, *J Parenter Enteral Nutr* 14(1):47-52, 1990.

214. Horswill CA, Kien L, Zipf WB, McCoy KS: Feeding-induced changes in energy expenditure in children with cystic fibrosis, *J Parenter Enteral Nutr* 18(6):497-502, 1994.

215. Cystic Fibrosis Foundation Consensus Conference: Nutritional assessment and management in cystic fibrosis, *Clinical Practice Guidelines for Cystic Fibrosis* 1:1-15, 1997.

216. Kane RE, Hobbs PJ: Energy and respiratory metabolism in cystic fibrosis: the influence of carbohydrate content of nutritional supplements, *J Pediatr Gastro Nutr* 12(2):217-223, 1991.

217. Milla C, Doherty L, Raatz S, et al: Glycemic response to dietary supplements in cystic fibrosis is dependent on the carbohydrate content of the formula, *J Parenter Enteral Nutr* 20(3):182-186, 1996.

218. Rettammel AL, Marcus MS, Farrell PM, et al: Oral supplementation with a high fat, high energy product improves nutritional status and alters serum lipids in patients with cystic fibrosis, *J Am Diet Assoc* 95(4):454-459, 1995.

219. Steinkamp G, von der Hardt H: Improvement of nutritional status and lung function after long term nocturnal gastrostomy feedings in cystic fibrosis, *J Pediatr* 124(2):244-249, 1994.

220. Allen ED, Mick AB, Nicol J, McCoy KS: Prolonged parenteral nutrition for cystic fibrosis patients, *Nutr Clin Pract* 10(2):73-79, 1995.

221. Cystic Fibrosis Foundation: *CF consensus conference. Concepts in care,* vol I, sect V, Bethesda, MD, Jan 11-12, 1990, Cystic Fibrosis Foundation, pp 11-14.

222. Fukushi S, Seeburger J, Parquet G, et al: Nutrition support of patients with enterocutaneous fistulas, *Nutr Clin Pract* 13(2):59-65, 1998.

223. Rombeau J, Rolandelli R: Enteral and parenteral nutrition in patients with enteric fistulas and short bowel syndrome, *Surg Clin North Am* 67:551, 1987.

224. Tulsyan N, Abkin AD, Storch KJ: Enterocutaneous fistulas, *Nutr Clin Pract* 16(2):74-77, 2001.

225. Dudrick SJ, Maharaj AR, McKelvey AA: Artificial nutrition support in patients with gastrointestinal fistulas, *World J Surg* 23(6):570-576, 1999.

226. Torres-Garcia A, Landa I, Moreno-Azcoita I, et al: Somatostatin in the management of gastrointestinal fistulas, *Arch Surg* 127(1):97-100, 1992.

227. Edmunds L, Williams G, Welch C: External fistulas arising from gastrointestinal tract, *Ann Surg, Sept* 152(3):445-471, 1960.

228. Cresci GA, Martindale RG: Metabolic and nutritional management of patients with multiple enterocutaneous fistulas, *Nutrition* 13(5):446-449, 1997.

229. Charney P, Martindale R: Nutrition support in patients with enterocutaneous fistulas, *Support Line* 15:1, 1993.

230. Ottery F: Nutritional consequences of reoperative surgery in recurrent malignancy, *Semin Oncol* 20(5):528-537, 1993.

231. Ysebaert D, Van Hee R, Hubens G, et al: Management of digestive fistulas, *Scand J Gastroenterol* 29(suppl 207):42-44, 1994.

232. Martineau P, Shwed JA: Is octreotide a new hope for enterocutaneous and external pancreatic fistulas closure? *Am J Surg* 172(4):386-395, 1996.

233. Alvarez C, McFadden DW, Reber HA: Complicated enterocutaneous fistulas: failure of octreotide to improve healing, *World J Surg* 24(5):533-538, 2000.

234. DeHart M, Lauerman W, Conely A, et al: Management of retroperitoneal chylous leakage, *Spine* 19(6):716-718, 1994.

235. Spain D, McClave S: Chylothorax and chylous ascites. In Gottschlich, et al (eds): *The science and practice of nutrition support,* Silver Spring, MD, 2001, ASPEN, pp 479- 490.

236. Marts B, Naunheim K, Fiore A, et al: Conservative versus surgical management of chylothorax, *Am J Surg* 164(5):532-534, 1992.

Sandra M. Raup, RD, CNSD
Peggy Kaproth, MS, MBA, RPh, RD

THE liver is responsible for multiple functions that impact other organ systems. It regulates substrate availability, synthesizes proteins, and maintains an intimate relationship with the gastrointestinal (GI) tract. Hepatic dysfunction can affect any of these activities. It can be acute or chronic and has various causes.

Nutrition assessment is important in this patient population because the resulting information can be used to develop nutrition intervention strategies that may improve medical outcomes. In a review by McCullough and Bugianesi, malnutrition was identified as an independent predictor of survival and operative mortality in several studies of patients with chronic liver disease, ascites, and hepatic transplants.[1] Improved nutritional status has been shown to correlate with improved survival.[2] However, expected outcomes and appropriate nutrition interventions may vary with the type and degree of liver failure. Evaluation of the progress toward goals should take into account the pathophysiology and metabolic alterations typical of the extent and type of liver damage. The following steps describe an effective intervention strategy for persons with liver disease:

1. Recognize the type and severity of liver dysfunction.
2. Assess nutritional status and identify potential effects of hepatic dysfunction on substrate utilization and tolerance.
3. Formulate a nutrition intervention plan to accommodate metabolic abnormalities, minimize nutritional depletion, and improve nutritional status, when possible.
4. Evaluate the response to intervention and adjust the care plan if necessary.

Hepatic Failure

Hepatic failure can be classified in various ways because of the complexity of the liver's multiple functions and the number of possible causes of failure. Early liver failure from hepatocellular damage results in loss of control of portal and systemic hormone mechanisms.[3] In later phases of failure, the liver loses its capacity to perform basic functions such as glucose homeostasis (hypoglycemia or hyperglycemia may occur). Vascular effects of a fibrotic liver, such as increased portal resistance, have major effects on the ability of the liver to function in chronic failure.[4]

Hepatocellular Injury

Hepatocellular injury results from various insults including microbes, toxins, and ischemia. Acute hepatic failure (AHF) is defined as severe liver dysfunction (coagulation factor V < 50%) without encephalopathy. AHF may progress to fulminant hepatic failure (FHF) or subfulminant hepatic failure (SFHF). If coagulation factor V remains greater than 50% encephalopathy is rare and prognosis is better. Prognosis is also improved when the course of the illness lasts less than 2 weeks.[5] In AHF, both systemic protein catabolism and synthesis of acute phase proteins are increased. Cytokines, especially interleukin-1 (IL-1), interleukin-6 (IL-6), and tumor necrosis factor-α (TNF-α) are released in response to tissue necrosis and are responsible for the initial inflammatory response. These cytokines may have a prolonged effect because of delayed clearance by the liver. Normally, sinusoidal stroma are quickly repopulated with hepatocytes after hepatocellular necrosis. If regeneration is delayed, the stroma become fibrotic and cannot support hepatocellular regeneration. Cytokines play a role by inhibiting hepatic regeneration. Synthetic function is not seriously compromised until considerable damage has occurred.[6]

Acute viral hepatitis usually presents with GI symptoms such as anorexia, nausea, and weight loss. Jaundice can occur as symptoms improve, although malaise may persist. Acute hepatitis can progress to FHF (discussed later). If the virus persists, chronic hepatitis develops. It is defined as liver inflammation persisting without improvement for 6 months or more. This is especially likely if humoral or cell-mediated immunity is compromised, as seen in patients with leukemia, organ transplantation, AIDS, or immunosuppressive therapy. Chronic hepatitis may also be related to drug reactions.[7]

Ischemic hepatitis can occur in association with acute heart failure or shock related to trauma, hemorrhage, or sepsis. Although injury mainly results from lack of oxygen, insufficient substrates and accumulating metabolites may also contribute to the damage. Additional damage can occur during reperfusion. Duration of ischemia is significant in terms of outcome. If the ischemia is present for less than 10 hours, damage is uncommon. After 24 hours, damage is almost always present. Jaundice occurs in up to 15% of cardiac surgery patients, although it is usually not related to ischemia alone. It is most often associated with multiple valve replacement, higher blood transfusion requirements, and a longer time on cardiac bypass support.[8,9]

Ethanol is hepatotoxic independent of nutrition deficits. Long-term ethanol consumption causes liver injury whether the diet is inadequate or enriched. Ethanol is oxidized by the alcohol dehydrogenase pathway, producing the reduced form of nicotinamide adenine dinucleotide, and by liver microsomes by an ethanol-inducible cytochrome P_{450} (P-450IIE1). Ethanol intake equal to or greater than 80 g/day may induce liver damage. This is equivalent to 240 ml of whiskey or 2000 ml of beer. Liver damage is also more likely to occur with daily ethanol ingestion. Abstaining for at least 2 days/week greatly reduces the risk of liver damage. Liver damage begins with fatty liver (steatosis), progresses to hepatitis, and may eventually lead to cirrhosis, usually micronodular.[10] Also, the increase in hepatic microsomal enzyme activity resulting from chronic ethanol consumption increases the toxicity of other potentially toxic agents, including medications such as acetaminophen and vitamins such as vitamin A.[11] Total abstinence from ethanol is essential to stop the progression of disease and to possibly reverse damage that has already occurred.

Liver damage progresses differently among individuals. Females are more susceptible to ethanol-induced liver damage than males. Some studies have shown that a diet higher in fat and lower in carbohydrate and protein may increase the risk of developing cirrhosis in those individuals with high ethanol intake and a history of chronic hepatitis C infection.[12] Those with an intake of pork and beer were more likely to develop cirrhosis than those who consumed either beef with beer or pork with wine when all groups had high intakes of ethanol.[13] This may be due to the fat content of the meat. Studies in rats have shown that rats fed ethanol and fat from pork suffered significant liver injury, but those fed ethanol and fat from beef did not.[13]

NUTRITION INTERVENTIONS. Because acute hepatic injury usually is self-limiting, nutrition care is supportive. Time is required to resolve the inflammatory process, and nutrition support may improve protein synthesis. Micronutrients should be assessed for depletion and supplemented as necessary, especially when ethanol intake has been significant or if dietary intake has been inadequate for some time. Nutrition intervention during the progression of hepatic failure to FHF, cirrhosis, or cholestasis is addressed later.

Ethanol's high caloric contribution to the diet may result in diminished food intake, thus reducing vitamin and mineral intake. It may interfere with absorption of fat-soluble vitamins (i.e., A, D, E, K), minerals (e.g., calcium, phosphorus, magnesium, selenium, zinc), and water-soluble vitamins (e.g., folate, thiamine, vitamin C). Hormonal effects of ethanol favor increased calcium urinary excretion. In fact, magnitude of hypercalciuria indicates the severity of ethanol dependence.[14] Osteoporosis and osteomalacia are possible under these circumstances. Intake and serum concentrations of the bone minerals calcium, phosphorus, and magnesium should be kept at optimal levels. Intake of vitamin D should also be optimized, in addition to exposure to sunlight, if possible, to facilitate endogenous vitamin D synthesis. Activity and adequate protein intake will help maintain adequate muscle mass, which is important for maintenance of bone mass and optimal nutritional status.[15] Normally, absorption of nutrients increases as ethanol intake decreases. Social and familial aspects may also affect the nutritional status of patients. Santolaria and colleagues reported that the presence of irregular meals and cirrhosis with ascites independently predicted malnutrition. The level of ethanol intake and disruption in family and social situation predicted irregularity in feeding habits.[16]

Fulminant Hepatic Failure

FHF complicates AHF when encephalopathy occurs within 2 weeks of the onset of acute hepatic failure. SFHF occurs if encephalopathy occurs 2 to 12 weeks after the onset of acute hepatic failure. If encephalopathy progresses only to grade 2, prognosis for recovery is excellent (see Hepatic Encephalopathy in the section on complications). Acute-onset, fulminant failure is a devastating condition with systemic effects. Increased intracranial pressure is the most dangerous complication and it is the most common cause of death in patients with FHF. Other complications include metabolic problems (e.g., hypoglycemia and metabolic acidosis), hemodynamic changes, hypoxemia, coagulopathy, immunosuppression, and oliguric renal failure. Renal failure may be caused by prerenal azotemia, acute tubular necrosis, or hepatorenal syndrome.[17] Sepsis is a risk for immunosuppressed patients, especially during the recovery period.[18]

NUTRITION INTERVENTIONS. Medical and nutrition intervention involves stabilization and metabolic management of the patient until the liver recovers or transplantation occurs. Fluid status is a concern because both dehydration and overhydration can cause complications. Dehydration may lead to inadequate perfusion of other organs, which may contribute to multiorgan failure. On the other hand, overhydration may contribute to cerebral edema and intracranial hypertension. Changes in fluid distribution are difficult to predict. Central pressure monitoring is usually required. Rapid fluid administration is to be avoided whenever possible. Serum calcium, phosphorus, and magnesium concentrations may fluctuate, exacerbated by GI and renal losses as well as multiple blood product transfusions. Generally, electrolytes require monitoring and replacement, as necessary. Sodium replacement should be avoided if possible because it may only serve to increase total body sodium. Serum potassium concentrations may require frequent monitoring because potassium shifts can occur quickly. Necrosis may lead to hyperkalemia and lactic acidosis. Factors that contribute to hypokalemia include GI losses (via nasogastric tube and/or diarrhea) and renal losses of potassium, bicarbonate, and acid. In the presence of hypoglycemia, a glucose infusion of 4 mg/kg per minute usually provides adequate support without causing hyperglycemia. Serum glucose levels should be checked every hour if the patient is comatose, and every 4 hours if he or she is conscious. Protein (amino acid) support should not be considered until the third day after onset of acute FHF, and it may be avoided until the seventh day of nutritional deprivation.[19]

Cirrhosis

Cirrhosis is a chronic disease characterized by disruption of hepatic architecture and systemic effects. Cirrhosis can be compensated or decompensated. Compensated cirrhosis exhibits minimal signs and symptoms of disease and is usually identified incidentally or not at all. Patients with decompensated cirrhosis present with weakness, muscle wasting, and weight loss. Patients often seek medical attention after experiencing symptoms of ascites or jaundice. Cirrhosis of unknown etiology is "cryptogenic" with an incidence reported as 5% to 30%. In a recent study, obesity and type 2 diabetes were identified as the most prevalent risk factors for cryptogenic cirrhosis.[20]

Cirrhosis is characterized by diffuse destruction and regeneration of hepatic parenchymal cells, as well as increased connective tissue and disorganization of the lobular and vascular architecture. Liver cells are regenerated in nodules that are responsible for the disruption of hepatic architecture.[4] Systemic effects may occur as a result of decreased hepatocyte function, altered circulation, and altered immune status. Hepatocytes are regenerated after necrosis, but their level of function may not be optimal.

Glucose homeostasis is compromised by a greatly decreased ability to store glycogen. There is also decreased insulin clearance by the liver, peripheral insulin resistance that is compensated by increased insulin secretion, and decreased insulin sensitivity in fat and muscle tissue. Body composition is changed because fat stores are increased in relation to lean body mass in those with hyperinsulinemia.[21] Serum growth hormone (GH) concentrations, both basal and stimulated, are increased as the liver and kidneys are responsible for its degradation and insulin-like growth factor (IGF-1) levels are decreased.[22] The net effect is insulin resistance, glucose intolerance, and hyperglycemia. Patients with hepatitis C–related cirrhosis have been found to have a tenfold greater chance of having overt diabetes mellitus than those with cirrhosis from other causes. Patients who develop diabetes have a higher mortality rate from hepatocellular failure.[23]

Fatty acid metabolism is regulated by the liver. Serum fatty acid concentrations are increased in patients with cirrhosis because of alterations in carbohydrate metabolism and increased cytokine levels. Continued ethanol ingestion increases fatty acid and triglyceride values. Fatty acid transport is also influenced by the liver because it is responsible for synthesis of apolipoproteins, including cell surface receptors, triglycerides, phospholipids, cholesterol and its esters, and lecithins. Lipoprotein, triglyceride, and total cholesterol concentrations are altered in cirrhosis.[24]

Hepatic protein synthesis is altered as well. Albumin synthesis is normally 10 g/day, but can fall to 4 g/day in patients with cirrhosis.[25] Serum values are depressed not only because of decreased synthesis, but also because of a shift of albumin to the extravascular compartment (including ascites), increased total body water, and increased renal and GI losses. Acute phase protein synthesis is increased because of chronic inflammation mediated by cytokines. Globulin synthesis and serum concentrations are increased because of the liver's decreased ability to clear intestinal antigens. Albumin synthesis is partially regulated by oncotic pressure, so increased serum globulins, which contribute to oncotic pressure, will also decrease albumin synthesis.[7] Increased serum concentration of methionine and decreased clearance of it have been observed in patients with cirrhosis. This may be explained by an inactivation of methionine adenosyltransferase resulting in decreased synthesis of S-adenosylmethionine, which, in turn, may lead to depletion of hepatic glutathione.[26] Some studies have shown that administering various antioxidants and S-adenosylmethionine can slow the progression of disease and allow patients to delay the time to transplantation.[27]

Circulatory changes are responsible for multiple systemic changes. As the fibrotic liver remodels, portal vein resistance increases dramatically, resulting in portal hypertension. Portal veins normally supply 70% of blood to the liver, almost all from the digestive tract between the proximal stomach and the upper rectum. Portal hypertension causes dilated collateral veins, which may result in esophageal varices, gastric varices, portal hypertensive gastropathy, and enterocolopathy, all possible sources of bleeding. The liver usually takes up nutrients from the portal veins and metabolizes or modifies them for storage in the liver or peripheral tissues. In the fasting state, the liver normally will maintain metabolic requirements by releasing stored fuel or synthesizing substrates. In patients with cirrhosis, the liver becomes almost totally dependent on blood from the hepatic arteries as portal vein perfusion is lost. Portal-systemic shunting occurs when portal venous pressure exceeds systemic venous pressure. Peripheral tissues receive nutrients first, before they can be modified in the liver. The process of substrate management is greatly altered, thus affecting nutrient needs and optimal nutritional support. In approximately 10% of patients, portal venous blood enters hepatic arterial blood flow. These patients have the highest risk for impaired hepatic function and encephalopathy.[28]

Portal hypertension also results in hyperdynamic circulation, resulting in increased cardiac output, decreased arterial blood pressure, and increased total body water and sodium. Two theories are used to explain this phenomenon. The "underfill" theory states that arterial vasodilation contributes to decreased central volume and is the primary cause leading to increased sodium, blood volume, and cardiac output. The "overflow" theory states that retention of sodium and water is directly caused by portal hypertension, and leads to an increase in cardiac output. Studies indicate that both theories are partially correct.[29] These hyperdynamic changes may progress to multisystem organ dysfunction (kidney, brain, and lungs).[30]

NUTRITION INTERVENTIONS. Goals of nutrition care in cirrhosis include arresting nutrient depletion, repleting lost stores, and minimizing the effects of portal-systemic shunting. Liver failure itself causes nutritional depletion in virtually all patients because of its effect on substrate metabolism and the involvement of inflammatory mediators.[31] Therapies and medications may interfere with optimal nutritional status as well.[32]

In fasting patients with cirrhosis, carbohydrate accounts for 2% of energy expended (compared with 38% without cirrhosis), and fat accounts for 86% of energy expended (compared with 45% without cirrhosis) because of the limited amount of glycogen available.[20] High carbohydrate intake and frequent high carbohydrate feedings limit time spent in the fasting state, potentially limiting gluconeogenesis and maintaining muscle mass. Adding a late evening meal to the nutrition regimen improves nitrogen balance. The European Society of Parenteral and Enteral Nutrition (ESPEN) guidelines suggest no more than 6 hours of fasting for patients with cirrhosis.[33-35]

Strategies to control blood glucose levels may include oral hypoglycemic agents. These drugs are metabolized by the liver, so adjustment in the timing and dosing of these agents may be required. Shorter-acting agents are preferred. Biguanides should be avoided to avoid the risk of lactic acidosis.[2,20] Insulin may be required to control blood glucose levels, but it will act differently than in those without cirrhosis.[22] Although rigorous control of blood glucose concentration may not be a priority compared with maintaining nutritional status, blood glucose concentration that is high enough to affect fluid and electrolyte status should be avoided.

Sodium restriction is usually encouraged for patients with cirrhosis to manage sodium and water retention manifested by edema and ascites. In one study, patients with preascitic cirrhosis had less water and sodium excretion and weight loss than normal subjects, after initiation of a very low sodium diet (20 mEq/day).[36] These patients tolerated a very low sodium diet better than normal controls.[36] However, a low sodium diet alone is not adequate to mobilize fluid in patients with cirrhosis.[37] Diets with less than 90 mEq of sodium per day are not recommended because of their effect on nutrient intake. These very low sodium diets are likely to be associated with inadequate energy and protein intake leading to body cell mass (BCM) depletion.[29]

Adequate protein is important because protein requirements for maintenance are usually greater than normal for patients with cirrhosis. A study of malnourished patients with alcoholic cirrhosis, without encephalopathy, was conducted to assess the benefits and adverse effects of aggressive refeeding of energy and protein. The refeeding occurred over a mean of 38 days. Energy intake increased from 123 to 190 kJ/kg per day (29 to 45 kcal/kg per day), and protein increased from 0.98 to 1.78 g/kg per day. Protein kinetics indicated that the protein requirement for maintenance is higher than normal, but there is no change in the ability to use protein for new protein synthesis. Overall, there was 84% retention of protein consumed, and protein retention was as efficient with increasing intake. Only one patient was protein intolerant, demonstrating encephalopathy at the increase from 80 to 95 g/day of protein.[38] Another study showed that patients with mild cirrhosis had significant protein-calorie malnutrition (PCM), even though they had near normal intake. When the protein intake of these patients was increased, both nitrogen retention and protein synthesis were improved.[39]

Patients with cirrhosis are likely to be energy and protein depleted. It is important to maintain nutrient intake to maintain or replete tissue stores, if possible, especially if patients are candidates for transplantation. Outcomes of liver transplantation were studied to assess whether pretransplant nutritional and metabolic status, in addition to edema, ascites, and Child-Pugh scores, could predict survival. Only patients who exhibited hypermetabolism (measured resting energy expenditure [REE] greater than 120% of predicted) together with a low BCM of less than 35% of body weight (BW) (BCM%BW) demonstrated reduced survival at 1 and 5 years. BCM%BM did not correlate with degree of hypermetabolism. With hypermetabolism and low BCM%BW, 63% survived at 1 year and 46% at 5 years. Without hypermetabolism and low BCM%BW, 86% survived at 1 year and 83% at 5 years. The group of patients with hypermetabolism and low BCM%BW experienced more postsurgical and septic complications. The difference, however, was not statistically significant. This study identified those most likely to do well after transplantation versus those who should receive intensive nutritional intervention while waiting for transplantation.[40] Attention to lean body tissue and bone mass is especially important because these are the most depleted posttransplant. Another study assessing optimal support for patients who received transplants found that negative nitrogen balance persisted at least 28 days posttransplant. Nitrogen loss was determined to be primarily from skeletal muscle catabolism, while corticosteroid therapy was probably responsible for the severity and persistence of the nitrogen losses.[41] Because it is virtually impossible to replace these losses, attention to preservation of lean body tissue is imperative to limit the risk of complications and optimize the chances of survival.[42,43]

Cholestasis

Cholestasis is defined as decreased flow of bile from the gallbladder and larger bile ducts or an accumulation of bile in liver tissue. It can be due to extrahepatic biliary obstruction such as a tumor, intrahepatic mechanical obstruction (e.g., a common bile duct stone or primary biliary cirrhosis), or intrahepatic cholestasis without obstruction (e.g., sepsis-related cholestasis or complications related to parenteral nutrition [PN]).[44] If severe, retained bile acids cause hepatocyte death.[45]

Cholestasis related to infections may be mediated by cytokines. Interleukin-6 inhibits hepatocellular bile acid transport. In sepsis, however, many factors may be involved in worsening liver function, such as ischemia, multiple blood transfusions, and drug therapy. Jaundice associated with increased bilirubin production is not caused by liver dysfunction, but is related to the load of unconjugated bilirubin (indirect) that overwhelms the ability of hepatocytes to conjugate it. The liver will function normally and jaundice will clear spontaneously if complicating factors that increase bilirubin production (e.g., hemolysis, multiple blood transfusions, resolving hematoma) are not present.[9]

The eventual effect of cholestasis is liver damage, leading to biliary cirrhosis over months or years. In primary biliary cirrhosis (PBC), the intrahepatic bile ducts are progressively destroyed. It is associated with a profound immunologic disturbance, mediated by cytokines from activated T lymphocytes.[44]

Sclerosing cholangitis is characterized by diffuse inflammation of the biliary system, and it is distinguished from PBC by a negative mitochondrial antibody test. Primary sclerosing cholangitis (PSC) has an unknown cause, and it may or may not be associated with ulcerative colitis, Crohn's disease, an autoimmune process, transplant rejection, or graft-versus-host disease associated with blood and marrow transplantation. PSC is most often identified in late stages when symptoms appear. Fibrosis of intrahepatic and/or extrahepatic ducts is progressive and may cause ducts to disappear. PSC can lead to cholangiocarcinoma, so surveillance for this is recommended.[46]

Cholestasis interferes with enterohepatic circulation of bile acids. Bile acids are retained in the liver, are increased in plasma, and deficient in the small bowel. Inadequate bile acids in the small bowel may result in fat malabsorption. Fat malabsorption may subsequently lead to inadequate energy absorption at a time when energy intake is already compromised. Fat malabsorption may also lead to diarrhea and reduced calcium absorption, as a result of soap formation (calcium and unabsorbed fatty acids in the small bowel). Oxalate absorption increases when calcium is unavailable to form the insoluble salt. The patient's risk for developing kidney stones increases under these conditions. Absorption of fat-soluble vitamins is impaired and deficiencies are likely to develop over time.

Osteopenia becomes a risk because both calcium and vitamin D absorption are impaired, resulting in a net loss of bone. Chronic cholestasis leads to marked hyperlipidemia, although atherosclerotic disease is not common.[15,45]

NUTRITION INTERVENTIONS. Cholestasis associated with a self-limiting condition requires no intervention because it will resolve with the primary cause. Nutrition effects become substantial if cholestasis is chronic. Significant fat malabsorption and steatorrhea can be debilitating, leading to fluid and electrolyte depletion, as well as decreased oral intake. Fat intake should be limited while providing adequate energy and protein. Tolerance for fat consumption will improve if fats are taken in small amounts throughout the day. Medium-chain triglycerides can be used to provide additional energy, either by adding them directly to the diet or incorporating them into oral supplements or enteral support.[32] Oxalates and excessive oral ascorbic acid should also be restricted because of the increased risk for developing kidney stones. Supplementing oral calcium to a total of 1500 mg/day will allow adequate amounts for absorption and oxalate binding, as well as for that which is saponified with fatty acids. Calcium taken between meals is more likely to be absorbed. If a fat-restricted diet does not decrease the patient's stool volume or improve its consistency, the restricted diet should be discontinued.[15]

The fat-soluble vitamins A, D, E, and K may be depleted because of decreased absorption and intake. Serum values should be monitored routinely and supplemented when necessary.[15] An increased prothrombin time (PT) may be the result of vitamin K deficiency. If PT is not normalized after treatment with intravenous vitamin K, it indicates that hepatocellular dysfunction is compromised enough to limit coagulation factor synthesis.[9] Thus, underlying liver disease is the cause of increased PT rather than vitamin K deficiency. Please see Chapters 11 and 12 for more information about vitamins and minerals.

Bile acid therapy may be used in the treatment of chronic cholestatic disease. Ursodeoxycholic acid is most often used to alter the balance of circulating bile acids. It decreases the cytotoxicity of bile acids in the circulation.[45]

Hyperlipidemia is usually present in chronic cholestatic disease, and it becomes more pronounced as the disease progresses. Because hyperlipidemia is not accompanied by an increase in atherosclerotic disease, an attempt to lower serum lipid concentrations with diets that are low in fat and cholesterol is not necessary.[15]

Steatosis/Steatohepatitis

When the liver is composed of greater than 5% of its weight as triglyceride, steatosis is present. It occurs when excess fat is delivered to or synthesized by the liver, or when lipid transport out of the liver is impaired.[47] In obese individuals, excess caloric intake is believed to be responsible for this condition; in fact, steatosis is present in 40% of morbidly obese individuals undergoing surgery for weight reduction.[48] Nonalcoholic steatohepatitis develops when inflammation is present in addition to steatosis, which leads to fibrosis resembling alcohol-induced hepatitis. It is found more frequently in those with type 2 diabetes, in those with hypertriglyceridemia, and in females.[49]

On autopsy, 12% of those with cirrhosis had only obesity as a risk factor for the development of liver disease.[48] Steatosis alone does not necessarily lead to disease. It appears that one or more episodes of steatohepatitis are required to develop cirrhosis. Steatosis may progress to more severe liver damage in some obese individuals, yet not in others. Matteoni and associates suggest that both excessive fat accumulation and oxidative stress are required to stimulate collagen production, fibrosis, and cirrhosis.[50] Studies indicate that inflammation may have more toxic effects in genetically obese mice and rats than in nonobese animals. This abnormal response may be due to sensitization of hepatocytes to TNF-α, dysfunction of Kupffer cells, and/or leptin deficiency. It is likely that the interaction of cytokines (including TNF-α, IL-1, IL-10, IL-12) from Kupffer cells and hepatocytes are involved, and they exert effects on insulin production, substrate utilization, and immune function.[51]

NUTRITION INTERVENTIONS. Prevention is the most effective treatment for steatosis/steatohepatitis. Avoiding obesity and related conditions (e.g., diabetes, hypertriglyceridemia) significantly reduces the risk of developing fatty liver. For those with fatty liver alone, restricted diet and exercise to reduce weight have demonstrated statistically significant improvement in blood chemistries (e.g., glucose, triglycerides, aspartate aminotransferase, alanine aminotransferase) and the degree of steatosis after 3 months of treatment. However, no evidence at this time indicates that weight loss will reverse steatohepatitis.[52]

Complications of Hepatic Failure

Hepatic Encephalopathy

Hepatic encephalopathy is one of the earliest identified complications of liver failure and has been recognized for its protein intolerance for centuries. Grades of encephalopathy vary from mild impairment (1+) to coma (4+) and are based on level of consciousness, intellectual function, personality or behavior, and neuromuscular abnormalities. With grade 1 encephalopathy, sleep disturbances, slight personality changes, and tremor may be present. In grade 2, an overt personality change develops, with slurred speech, hypoactive reflexes, ataxia, and lethargy. Somnolence, confusion, bizarre behavior, hyperactive reflexes, and rigidity may occur in grade 3, and coma in grade 4. Encephalopathy is a process, so individuals may not manifest all components at once. Signs may vary slightly, depending on the underlying pathology.[53]

The causes of encephalopathy have not been definitively established. Encephalopathy is most commonly precipitated by electrolyte imbalance or by, among other things, GI bleeding, infections, procedures such as surgery, and drugs (including ethanol).[54] The relationship between nitrogenous products in the GI tract and effects on the brain is complicated, possibly involving several factors. Ingestion of increased amounts of dietary protein has been identified as the factor that precipitated encephalopathy in 7% to 9% of patients. GI bleeding was associated with encephalopathy in another 18% to 34% of patients.[55]

Because ammonia accumulation is involved in encephalopathy, lowering serum ammonia levels is of primary concern. The ability of the liver to convert ammonia to urea is not the primary defect. With portosystemic shunting, ammonia is delivered to peripheral tissues before it can be cleared and converted to urea by the liver. Most ammonia is generated in the small and large intestines. In descending order, it is generated in the greatest amounts from blood, meat, milk products, and finally vegetable sources of protein. Uremia increases diffusion of urea into the colon. It is then converted to ammonia by colonic bacteria. Serum pH and colonic pH affect ammonia levels as well. Hypokalemia and alkalosis favor cellular uptake of ammonia.[56] Lower pH in the colon favors ammonium ion formation, which is not as readily absorbed as ammonia.[19] The amount of muscle mass itself affects ammonia levels because muscle is an important source of ammonia clearance. As muscle mass decreases, less ammonia is cleared by muscle and uptake of ammonia by the brain is subsequently increased.[56] Serum ammonia values are lowered by minimizing ammonia and ammonia precursors in the GI tract, and by reducing ammonia absorption. Lactulose, lactitol, and lactose (in lactase-deficient individuals) produce an acidic environment in the colon, which favors ammonium formation. In addition, bacterial proliferation is enhanced. Ammonia substrate is incorporated into nitrogen by bacteria, and they are subsequently excreted via the GI tract.[19] Water-soluble fiber may be used in the same manner, so increasing this fiber in the diet also increases nitrogen excretion.[32] It is important to remember that bacteria in the gut are required to produce the nitrogen-lowering effect of these agents. Therefore, antibiotics may eliminate the intended therapeutic effect.

Because hepatic encephalopathy has been associated with high nitrogen ingestion, limiting protein has traditionally been a component of therapy for this condition. However, this practice may exacerbate malnutrition. The association between higher protein intake and hepatic encephalopathy has been studied with patients who had moderate or severe alcoholic hepatitis. Patients were enrolled in the study and encouraged to increase both protein and energy intake. The lowest protein intake was 0.338 g protein/kg dry body weight, and the highest protein intake was 1.067 g protein/kg dry body weight. Sixty-three percent of these patients had encephalopathy upon entry into the study. Low protein intake, elevated blood urea nitrogen, and elevated creatinine were independently associated with worsening encephalopathy. Higher protein intake was actually associated with an improvement in hepatic encephalopathy; however, it is important to note that these patients did not have cirrhosis.[57] Some patients with end-stage liver disease are protein sensitive, but protein restriction is not necessary if protein sensitivity is not demonstrated.[15]

Under conditions of hepatic encephalopathy, amino acid levels are also abnormal: serum branched-chain amino acid (leucine, isoleucine, valine) values are decreased and aromatic amino acid (phenylalanine, tyrosine, tryptophan) values are increased. A molar ratio of branched-chain amino acids (BCAAs) to aromatic amino acids (AAAs) of 1.4 to 2.0 is usually present with significant liver dysfunction, and a ratio of 1.0 or less is associated with presence of hepatic encephalopathy.[58] Kawamura-Yasui and associates[59] used branched-chain amino acid/tyrosine ratio (BTR) to assess severity of hepatic injury in chronic hepatitis and cirrhosis. They found that BTR

was significantly decreased in both groups compared with normal controls and significantly correlated with Child-Pugh score. BTR increased after administration of an oral BCAA-enriched supplement; however, the presence of encephalopathy was not addressed in this study. It is still unclear whether normalizing serum amino acid levels has clinical benefits for patients with encephalopathy beyond improvement in nutritional status. Many of the studies done in this area, especially with parenteral support, did not provide nutrition support to those in the control groups.

A double-blind placebo-controlled crossover study used an oral BCAA supplement for latent portosystemic encephalopathy. Psychometric testing was used to assess changes in mental status, with improvement in those receiving BCAA treatment. The study period, however, was too short to extrapolate results to long-term benefit.[60] Another trial of BCAA-enriched enteral support versus oral diet was undertaken with the goal of assessing effects of BCAAs on nutritional status and rate of complications and survival. Those in the treatment group tolerated the formula well and had a significantly higher survival rate and better nutritional status, although the rate of complications was not different. Only severely malnourished cirrhotics were included in this trial.[2] The use of specialized nutrition support formulas is discussed in detail in Chapter 20.

Ascites

Cirrhosis is the most common cause of ascites, although it may occur as a result of various conditions. Rapid onset of ascites is associated with a better outcome than slow onset because the cause is more likely to be a reversible. Ascites with cirrhosis is related to portal pressure, which correlates closely to the serum-ascites albumin gradient (may be calculated from albumin levels in ascites fluid and serum). Portal pressure treatment strategies begin with fluid and sodium management. Sodium restriction is an important first-line treatment, aiming for sodium intake levels as low as possible without compromising calorie and protein intake. A sodium restriction less than 2000 mg or 90 mEq/day is usually not recommended. Negative sodium balance is the goal, although it is nearly impossible to attain because sodium excretion is close to nil. Diuretic therapy is almost always needed. The degree of peripheral edema is used as a measure of the effectiveness of diuresis, which should be slow. Diuresis of greater than 900 ml/day (or weight loss >1 lb per day) may lead to intravascular dehydration, which could precipitate encephalopathy. The magnitude of sodium excretion required guides the selection of a diuretic. Aldosterone antagonists such as spironolactone are the most effective in facilitating sodium excretion, however, hyperkalemia and mild hyperchloremic metabolic acidosis are possible in the presence of renal insufficiency. Paracentesis can be used to treat ascites if sodium restriction and diuretic therapy fail. Different protocols including plasma expansion are used, depending on cost concerns, physician preference, and proximity to a center where the procedure can be performed.[29] Spontaneous bacterial peritonitis is not uncommon in patients who have cirrhosis-related ascites, and it has been identified in 10% to 20% of routine paracentesis for cirrhotic ascites.[61]

If sodium and fluid management fail to decrease portal pressure, strategies to mechanically decrease pressure are used.

Shunts, including peritoneovenous (LeVeen) shunt, portosystemic shunt, and, most recently, transjugular intrahepatic portosystemic shunt, help relieve ascites but they are unlikely to provide a long-term solution.[61] All protocols have risks, including protein depletion, so liver transplantation may be the only good option for long-term survival.

Gastrointestinal Tract Bleeding

Portal hypertension leads to increased collateral circulation, which in turn, may result in engorged veins (varices) along the GI tract. The most common varices are esophageal, gastroesophageal, and anorectal. Esophageal varices are most likely to be the source of GI tract bleeding. Patients with decompensated liver disease are more likely to bleed, and they have a worse prognosis if bleeding occurs. Variceal bleeding is the most serious complication of portal hypertension, accounting for approximately 20% to 35% of all deaths in patients with cirrhosis. Treatment includes resuscitation, endoscopic sclerotherapy or endoscopic variceal ligation, and pharmacologic therapy. To prevent rebleeding that is most likely within the first 5 days, early management is important. Shunts may be used to control variceal bleeding, although long-term success is unlikely. Patients with esophageal varices are advised to avoid aspirin and nonsteroidal anti-inflammatory drugs.[21,62]

Hepatorenal and Hepatopulmonary Syndromes

Hepatorenal syndrome is functional renal failure in the setting of portal hypertension and ascites. It may be difficult to differentiate from prerenal azotemia. Intractable ascites may indicate that hepatorenal syndrome is imminent.[63] Patients do better after transplantation if hepatorenal syndrome is not present, so transplantation is more likely to be successful if it is done before hepatorenal syndrome develops.

Hepatopulmonary syndrome involves pulmonary vasodilation associated with a hyperdynamic state, which leads to arterial hypoxemia. It is usually associated with ascites. Large ascites can also affect lung mechanics. Hepatopulmonary syndrome may be the primary indication for liver transplantation, although transplantation may not be possible if hypoxemia is severe.[56]

Clinical and Laboratory Assessment of Liver Disease

Overview

Assessment of liver disease is complex. A number of clinical and laboratory findings are often required before a diagnosis is made. In addition to the condition itself, the stage in the disease process is also critical for determining the optimal treatment plan, including nutrition interventions.

Jaundice is often the first sign of liver or biliary tract disease. It is a yellow discoloration of skin, sclerae, and mucous membranes, which occurs as a result of increased serum bilirubin. Bilirubin is the product of heme degradation, and it is eventually secreted into bile for disposal via the GI tract. Unconjugated bilirubin is conjugated with glucuronate in hepatocytes to make it water-soluble. Conjugated bilirubin can then be excreted via bile. In serum, unconjugated bilirubin is tightly bound to albumin. Measurement of direct bilirubin estimates the conjugate, while indirect bilirubin estimates the unconjugated form. In patients with liver disease, total bilirubin may be elevated in conjunction with global hepatocellular dysfunction or when cholestasis is the primary problem.[9]

Child's classification was developed to assess hepatocellular function and predict complications and other outcomes. It includes serum bilirubin, serum albumin, ascites, neurologic disorder, and nutritional status.[64] The Child-Pugh classification was developed for similar uses. It includes bilirubin, albumin, PT, ascites, and encephalopathy.[65] Both are used to grade the severity of cirrhosis. Clinical signs and laboratory values are used to assign a grade or classification. They have been shown to predict outcomes such as complications and mortality better than any other method of assessment.

Laboratory Tests

Several biochemical tests are used to determine the type and extent of liver dysfunction, and they may provide useful information in the process of determining the cause(s) of dysfunction (Table 32-1). They provide information about the extent of cell damage, but not the degree of dysfunction. Biochemical tests are of little use in determining the presence or severity of complications.[66]

Serum aminotransferases are the primary markers of hepatocellular necrosis. Aspartate aminotransferase (AST) is found in tissues other than the liver, while alanine aminotransferase (ALT) is specific to the liver. Three times the upper limits of normal (ULN) for either aminotransferase is considered to be a mild elevation. A moderate elevation is 10 times ULN, and a severe elevation is more than 10 times ULN. The degree of elevation, however, correlates poorly with the extent of hepatocyte necrosis. In most incidences of acute liver injury, the AST:ALT ratio is less than or equal to 1, but will usually be greater than 2 in patients with alcoholic hepatitis.[66] Of those with AST levels greater than 100 times ULN, 90% have been shown to be due to liver disease. Of this group, hypotension due to myocardial infarction or cardiac surgery was the most common cause, with hypotension due to sepsis being the second most common.[67]

Serum alkaline phosphatase (AP) is the primary marker of cholestasis, although it will not be elevated in the first few days after obstruction and remains elevated for up to a week after. Very high elevations are usually present with an infiltrative hepatic disorder, such as a tumor, or biliary obstruction. γ-Glutamyl transpeptidase is usually elevated under the same conditions as AP; however, it is usually even more pronounced in alcoholic liver disease. Bilirubin levels are elevated in cholestasis and in various hepatic or nonhepatic conditions as discussed previously.[66]

PT, albumin, and prealbumin all have been used in evaluations of hepatic synthetic capacity. In addition, vitamin K deficiency, warfarin, and consumptive coagulopathy should be evaluated because they may be the cause of increased PT. Serum albumin is not a good indicator of synthetic function because it can be influenced by many other factors.[66]

TABLE 32-1

Clinical Significance of Common Liver Tests

Test (Normal Range)	Basis of Abnormality	Associated Liver Diseases	Extrahepatic Sources
Aminotransferases (0-35 IU/L, 0-0.58 μkat/L for both ALT and AST	Leakage from damaged tissue	Modest elevations—many types of liver disease Marked elevations—hepatitis (viral, autoimmune, toxic, and ischemic) AST/ALT > 2 and each < 300 U suggests alcoholic liver disease or cirrhosis of any cause	ALT—relatively specific for hepatocyte necrosis AST—muscle (skeletal and cardiac), kidney, brain, pancreas, red blood cells
Alkaline phosphatase (AP) (30-120 IU/L, 0.5-2.0 μkat/L)	Overproduction and leakage into serum	Modest elevations—many types of liver disease Marked elevations — extrahepatic and intrahepatic cholestasis, diffuse infiltrating disease (e.g., tumor, MAI), occasionally alcoholic hepatitis	Bone growth or disease (e.g., tumor, fracture, Paget's disease), placenta, intestine, tumors
γ-Glutamyl transpeptidase (GGT) (0-30 IU/L, 0-0.50 μkat/L)	?Overproduction and leakage into serum	Same as for alkaline phosphatase; induced by ethanol, drugs, GGT/AP > 2.5 suggests alcoholic liver disease	Kidney, spleen, pancreas, heart, lung, brain
5'-Nucleotidase (0-17 IU/L, 0-0.28 μkat/L)	?Overproduction and leakage into serum	Same as for alkaline phosphatase	Found in many tissues but serum elevation relatively specific for liver disease
Bilirubin (0.1-1.0 mg/dL, 2-18 μmol/L)	Decreased hepatic clearance	Modest elevations—many types of liver disease Marked elevations—extra and intrahepatic bile duct obstruction, alcoholic, drug-induced or viral hepatitis, inherited hyperbilirubinemia	Increased breakdown of hemoglobin (due to hemolysis, ineffective erythropoiesis, resorption of hematoma) or myoglobin (due to muscle injury)
Prothrombin time (10.9-12.5 sec)	Decreased synthesis	Acute or chronic liver failure (unresponsive to vitamin K) Biliary obstruction (usually responsive to vitamin K administration)	Vitamin K deficiency (secondary to malabsorption, malnutrition, antibiotics), consumptive coagulopathy
Albumin (4.0-6.0 g/dl, 40-60 g/L)	Decreased synthesis ?Increased catabolism	Chronic liver failure Liver failure of at least several weeks' duration	Decreased in nephrotic syndrome, protein-losing enteropathy, vascular leak malnutrition, malignancy, and inflammatory states

From Davern II TJ, Scharschmidt BF: Biochemical liver tests. In Feldman M, Scharschmidt BF, Sleisenger MH (eds): *Sleisenger & Fordtran's gastrointestinal and liver disease,* ed 6, vol 2, Philadelphia, 1998, WB Saunders, pp 1112-1122.
ALT, Alanine aminotransaminase; *AST,* aspartate aminotransaminase; *MAI, mycobacterium avium-intracellulare; AP,* alkaline phosphatase; *GGT,* gamma-glutamyltransferase

Nutrition Assessment

A wide range in the prevalence of malnutrition (10% to 100%)[68-77] has been reported for patients with chronic liver disease of various etiologies, which may be a reflection of the different patient populations and methods of nutrition assessment that were used.[69,73-76,78] An accurate, quantitative nutrition assessment is difficult to achieve because conventional markers of nutritional status, such as weight and serum albumin concentration, are often influenced by nonnutritive factors (e.g., ascites, extent of liver damage, renal insufficiency, metabolic abnormalities).[15,68,79,80] Therefore, a composite analysis based on clinical criteria and anthropometric standards such as midarm muscle circumference, may more accurately determine nutritional status than individual biochemical parameters.[77,81]

Assumptions about nutrition interventions based on patient type or by extrapolating results from one study to different patient populations may not be useful in developing nutrition care plans for individual patients. Although categorization may serve as a gross identifier of potential nutritional deficits, each patient should be assessed using tools that have demonstrated utility in identifying such deficits. Parameters that are selected for monitoring should be appropriate for the outcomes being evaluated. Various tools, ranging from those found in research facilities to those that can be utilized in most clinical settings, are available.

Subjective Global Assessment and Anthropometric Indices

Subjective global assessment (SGA) is a clinical evaluation of PCM that has demonstrated benefit in evaluating patients before liver transplantation.[77] Information comprising the SGA is obtained primarily by interviewing patients and their families, and it covers four broad categories. These include nutrition history, physical appearance, existing conditions, and additional information such as history of diabetes mellitus, dietary supplement use, and current diet and medications. In a study of 20 adult liver transplant candidates, this tool was determined to be reliable by the Cronbach coefficient α-test (0.707). Muscle wasting and fat depletion were determined to be the strongest predictors of the final SGA rating ($p < .0001$).[77] Using SGA, investigators identified 15% of the patients as being well nourished, 70% were moderately malnourished, and 15% were severely malnourished.[77]

Other work using SGA methodology to assess 1402 patients with cirrhosis of various origins and severity produced inaccurate results in 37% of patients (with midarm muscle area and/or fat area below the 5th percentile.)[72] In addition, 29% of females and 18% of males appeared to be overnourished, yet one third of these patients demonstrated a significant reduction in fat stores when midarm fat area and/or muscle mass was estimated using midarm muscle area. Overall, clinical judgment parameters differed from anthropometric assessment in 23% of patients. The authors concluded that anthropometric measurements in addition to SGA might improve accuracy in the identification of malnutrition among patients with cirrhosis.[72]

It is beyond the scope of this review to provide a detailed discussion of SGA or anthropometric technique. Please see Chapter 2 for an overview of potential SGA components, such as health history and nutritional deficiencies that may be revealed by physical examination. A study by Hasse and coworkers describes the reliability of an SGA tool for liver transplant candidates and the discussion includes SGA criteria used in the study.[77] Chapter 3 provides a discussion of anthropometry and body composition analysis.

Body Compartment Approach

There has been renewed interest in body composition analysis for patients with liver disease because it may provide a reliable quantitative measure of nutritional status.[75] The two most important metabolic and nutritional body compartments are the BCM and body fat stores.[75]

BODY FAT STORES. One of the functions of body fat is to provide a reservoir of energy. Body fat provides more than 75% of calories that are used after the first few days of food deprivation.[82] Therefore, measurement of body fat stores indicates current energy reserves, and subsequent monitoring may be used to evaluate progress toward nutrition therapy goals.[83] Global assessment of fat stores is possible using various techniques including anthropometric evaluation (e.g., body mass index, triceps skinfold thickness) and body composition methodology.[72,74,75,77,78,83]

BODY CELL MASS. The BCM represents oxygen-exchanging, glucose-oxidizing, and work-performing tissue. It serves as a reference for expressing rates of metabolic processes.[84] Because BCM is composed primarily of muscle and viscera, which are affected by periods of nutritional deprivation, it is useful as a marker in initial and subsequent assessments of progress toward nutrition therapy goals.[85] Evidence indicates that reliable measurements of BCM can be made in patients with cirrhosis by using total body potassium counting. Apparently, the intracellular potassium content of red blood cells, muscle, and leukocytes is not decreased because of cirrhosis, even in the presence of edema or following diuretic use.[84,86,87]

Many studies of body composition in patients with cirrhosis have used the fat-free mass (FFM) (e.g. arm muscle area) as a surrogate marker for BCM.[75] However, cirrhosis is often characterized by an increase in extracellular water, which disrupts the fixed relationship between total body water, total body potassium, and the FFM in normal subjects.[75] Consequently, in cirrhotic patients for whom this situation exists, it has been suggested that the BCM compartment itself must be measured, rather than extrapolated from single anthropometric and body water measurements to a value for FFM.[75]

SELECTED STUDIES OF BODY COMPOSITION AND ENERGY EXPENDITURE IN PATIENTS WITH LIVER DISEASE. In a study of 123 patients with biopsy-proven cirrhosis, Muller and others evaluated hypermetabolism, REE, and FFM in relation to the cause of cirrhosis, duration of disease, liver function, and clinical staging of the disease.[74] Although the focus of the study was REE, body composition was also evaluated using four different methods. Anthropometry, 24-hour urinary creatinine

excretion, bioelectrical impedance, and FFM were determined in 20 patients using total body potassium (TBK) in a whole body counter, with a precision in the order of 2%. A close correlation was found between bioelectrical impedance analysis (BIA) and TBK-determined FFM.[74] However, BIA results exceeded TBK-determined FFM at low FFM values.[74] Chapters 3 and 4 provide additional information about these assessment tools.

The REE varied between 1090 and 2300 kcal/day, and it was closely related to FFM.[74] REE differed from the Harris and Benedict predicted values in 70% of patients.[88] Different amounts of ascites did not affect REE. Other studies have demonstrated normal estimated energy requirements among patients with chronic and stable cirrhosis, hypermetabolism or hypometabolism, and an inverse relationship between the severity of liver disease and energy expenditure in other patient populations of cirrhosis.[74,89,90] As reported by Muller and associates, 18% of patients with cirrhosis were hypermetabolic and 31% were hypometabolic. Hypermetabolism did not show a strict association with the cause of cirrhosis, the duration of disease, liver function, cholestasis, cell damage, clinical staging (Child's classes), blood hemoglobin, plasma thyroid hormone levels, or human leukocyte antigens. An increased REE was associated with significant losses of muscle, BCM, and extracellular mass, in the presence of unchanged body fat. Fat and FFM were increased in hypometabolic patients when compared with normometabolic patients.[74]

In the previously described study, malnutrition was characterized by predominant losses in muscle tissue and BCM, whereas fat mass was conserved in most patients with chronic liver disease.[74] Patients with alcoholic liver cirrhosis frequently had increased subcutaneous and intra-abdominal fat mass, whereas those with biliary cirrhosis had decreased subcutaneous and intra-abdominal fat mass, as well as reduced body weight. Patients with significant losses in BCM frequently had normal body weight. Biochemical parameter values used to evaluate liver function were independent of the nutritional state of patients.[74] Parameter values varied between different subgroups of patients, and they worsened with advanced stages of disease (Child class B and C versus Child class A).[74] Differences in mean BCM or body fat stores were not observed between groups of patients with class A, B, or C disease. However, these results have been criticized by other investigators who have demonstrated such differences between lower class C patients and the other classes when corrections are made for sex, age, height, and weight.[75]

In summary, the work described indicates that properly conducted BIA may be used in a clinical practice setting to assess FFM because results appear to be closely correlated with those from bench-mark methodology (TBK-determined FFM). Furthermore, REE has demonstrated a close relationship to FFM. REE may provide a more accurate assessment of energy expenditure for individual patients than Harris and Benedict predicted values. As assessed by REE, hypermetabolism does not appear to be strictly associated with various markers used to assess the progression or severity of liver disease. Therefore, a particular metabolic state may not be presumed for individuals with liver disease.

Vitamin and Mineral Status

As described earlier in this chapter, malabsorption combined with suboptimal dietary intake places some patients with liver disease at risk for nutritional deficiencies. Patients with cirrhosis may have exocrine pancreatic insufficiency with reduced lipase production, which impairs digestion and absorption of nutrients. Steatorrhea predisposes patients with cholestatic liver disease to losses of fat-soluble vitamins and minerals (e.g., calcium, iron, zinc).[91,92]

In an evaluation of serum vitamin concentrations, Jorgenson and colleagues reported that certain vitamin deficiencies were prevalent among patients with primary sclerosing cholangitis.[91] Vitamins A, D, and E were deficient in 82%, 57%, and 58% of the patients, respectively.[91] Cholestyramine, when used as a bile-sequestrant in cholestatic diseases, can also contribute to fat-soluble vitamin and calcium malabsorption.[92] Although zinc, calcium, and magnesium status may be difficult to assess because they bind to albumin (which may be low), it is reasonable to provide supplementation if serum levels are low and there is a history of poor dietary intake or malabsorption. Conversely, subclinical malabsorption may be a consideration if dietary intake appears to be adequate but serum fat-soluble vitamin and mineral values are less than normal. Patients with advanced liver disease should be screened for fat-soluble vitamin deficiencies and supplemented with water-miscible forms when deficiencies are identified.[15] Serum vitamin concentrations should be monitored routinely to evaluate whether supplementation is adequate.[15] Of note, several specialized enteral formulas that may be used for patients with hepatic disease are lacking in vitamin content. Please see Chapter 20 for more information about specialized formulas and Chapter 2 for a review of nutritional deficiencies that may be revealed by physical examination.

Other Considerations in Nutrition Assessment

INTERPRETATION OF CREATINE-DERIVED VALUES OF MUSCLE MASS.

In clinical practice, the 24-hour urinary creatinine approach and the anthropometric estimation of whole body skeletal muscle mass are the most common methods of assessing muscle mass in patients with cirrhosis.[93] Validity of the creatinine approach has not been demonstrated for use in patients with cirrhosis. It has been suggested that reduced liver function rather than reduced muscle mass may explain the low levels of urinary creatinine excretion that is frequently observed in these patients.[84] However, because a rate-limiting biosynthetic step of the creatine precursor is predominantly located in the kidney,[93] its function rather than reduced liver function may affect the validity of the creatinine approach in patients with cirrhosis.

In an evaluation of cirrhotic patients ($n = 102$) under standard clinical conditions including many degrees of liver and renal function, possible systematic errors associated with the creatinine method were studied.[93] Muscle mass was assessed by 24-hour urinary creatinine excretion as compared with anthropometry (arm muscle area), and with BCM that was estimated by BIA and TBK. Whole body muscle mass, as estimated from urinary creatinine excretion, was found to be significantly correlated with anthropometric estimates of muscle mass and with BCM obtained by TBK. Arm muscle

area and 24-hour urinary creatinine excretion in this study population was lower (19% and 10.4%, respectively) than expected according to predicted values. Differences between results did not show any correlation with parameters of liver function or the severity of liver disease (i.e., Child-Pugh score). In contrast, renal function was strongly correlated with the differences between creatinine and anthropometric muscle mass ($r = .64$, $p < .001$). Sixty-two percent of the study population had normal renal function. This population had significantly higher creatinine and muscle mass (estimated by anthropometric measurement) as compared with 38% of the patients who had reduced renal function. In addition, significantly higher differences between measured and predicted values of urinary creatinine excretion and arm muscle area were found in the subgroup with impaired renal function. Investigators concluded that renal dysfunction, but not reduced liver function, systematically affected the urinary creatinine method for estimating skeletal muscle mass in patients with cirrhosis.[91] In view of the high prevalence of renal dysfunction in patients with cirrhosis, judicious interpretation of creatinine-derived values of muscle mass is required.

PROGNOSIS VERSUS RESPONSIVENESS TO NUTRITION THERAPY.

When reviewing literature that reports methodology for nutrition assessment, it is important to consider whether study parameters used are known to be responsive to nutrition therapy or if they are primarily prognostic indicators. This concept is illustrated in the work of Mendenhall and associates, who reported findings regarding the use of nutrition-related parameters in patients with severe alcoholic hepatitis.[70] The authors concluded that nutrition therapy improved both outcome (prognosis) and overall nutritional status. Prognosis was best addressed using information from the initial creatinine height index, total peripheral blood lymphocyte count, handgrip strength, and serum prealbumin. Parameters most responsive to effective treatment were parameters related to muscle and body mass (i.e., midarm muscle area, creatinine height index, and percent of ideal body weight).[70] Appropriate measures must be selected to provide meaningful information about the adequacy of nutritional support.

INSULIN-LIKE GROWTH FACTOR AND GROWTH HORMONE.

For patients without liver failure, serum IGF-1 has been identified as a sensitive marker of malnutrition.[94] Serum IGF-1 levels normalize within 8 days after nutritional repletion. In patients with hepatic failure, serum IGF-1 levels continue to be depressed after long-term refeeding. Depressed serum IGF-1 levels, along with insulin-like growth factor binding protein (IGFBP-3), appear to be more related to hepatocyte function than malnutrition in those with cirrhosis. IGF-1 levels correlate closely with visceral proteins, such as transferrin and albumin, but IGF-1 is depleted more rapidly than other proteins synthesized by the liver.[94] In alcohol abusers who do not have liver disease, IGF-1 values are depressed, even though other visceral proteins are not. In the presence of decreased IGF-1, fasting basal GH levels increase, and they further increase after oral glucose tolerance testing. Normally, GH levels would decrease. Both decreased serum IGF-1 and raised urinary GH levels are associated with hepatic insufficiency and poor prognosis in patients with cirrhosis.[21]

Summary

Studies that have been described demonstrate the importance of making individualized assessments to determine the nutritional needs of patients with liver disease because requirements may vary considerably even among seemingly homogeneous patient populations. Despite heterogeneity among patients, certain generalizations may be made about the utility of nutrition assessment tools. Reports from studies of nutritional status with patients who had alcoholic hepatitis,[70] or alcoholic[16,78] or virus-related cirrhosis,[78] indicate that various nutritional assessment tools are useful in these populations. Parameters that have been shown to independently predict malnutrition include irregular feeding habits and liver cirrhosis with ascites;[17] anthropometry (e.g., triceps skinfold, midarm muscle area);[70,78] and TBK,[74,75] creatinine excretion, and BIA, which have been used in determinations of BCM.[69,74,93] As previously discussed, SGA has also shown utility in the nutrition assessment of liver transplant candidates.[42,77] After initial assessment, these parameters may also be used to monitor progress toward nutrition-related objectives.

Nutrition Support in the Medical Management of Liver Disease

Although studies have shown that a significant proportion of patients with advanced liver disease have PCM, relatively few studies have been designed to evaluate the effect of nutrition on outcome in advanced liver disease or after transplantation. Although some studies have demonstrated improved outcomes, particularly in patients with moderate or severe malnutrition,[2,42,57,95,96] some have not.[97] However, nutrition therapy should not be thought of as an isolated part of a patient's care plan. It is important to consider the benefit of nutrition support as an adjunct to the overall medical management of patients. The following discussion is not intended to be a comprehensive description of this concept, but rather as thought-provoking examples from which other opportunities may be explored to enhance medical outcomes for patients.

Refeeding Syndrome

Refeeding syndrome refers to the unique metabolic and functional aberrations that occur when chronically malnourished patients are refed.[98] The syndrome is not unique to patients with liver disease; however, given the prevalence of malnutrition in this population it should be considered whenever carbohydrate substrate such as dextrose is a part of the nutritional regimen or the medical plan for hydration. Refeeding syndrome is precipitated by an acute increase in insulin, which stimulates the uptake of cellular potassium into skeletal and hepatic tissue for the synthesis of glycogen and lean body tissue (3 mEq potassium and 0.5 mg of magnesium per gram of nitrogen and 1 mEq of potassium per 3 g of glycogen).[99] Acute repletion of these patients with carbohydrate substrate may be fatal (cardiac arrest) because serum concentrations of potassium, magnesium, and phosphorus decline precipitously.[98,100-102] Other nutrients such as thiamine may be depleted and are also required for carbohydrate metabolism.[55,103]

When refeeding begins, protein can be initiated at 1.5 g/kg of normal weight when hepatic and renal function are normal.[100] Caloric intake should be increased slowly, usually starting at 20 kcal/kg of ideal body weight. Carbohydrate intake, including that from intravenous solutions, should be approximately 150 to 200 g/day or 2 mg/kg per minute. Fat intake provides additional calories and essential fatty acids, but it is not necessary to increase fat intake beyond customary provision at this time. Carbohydrate substrate may be gradually increased over several days to meet estimated caloric needs of the patient, while monitoring and adjusting the regimen regularly in response to electrolyte shifts and repletion needs (see Box 32-1 and Chapter 10). If weight gain in the refed patient is greater than 1 kg/week, it is usually a result of fluid retention. Fluid and sodium are often restricted initially to 800 to 1000 ml/day and 20 mEq of sodium/day, respectively.[100,101]

Oxandrolone and Adequate Caloric Intake

In a study of malnourished male patients with alcoholic hepatitis, the efficacy of oxandrolone in combination with an enteral food supplement was evaluated.[96] At the end of 6 months treatment, 79.7% of the patients who had initially been categorized as moderately malnourished were still alive, as compared with 62.7% of the placebo-treated patients ($p = .037$). Improvements in both the severity of liver injury ($p = .03$) and malnutrition ($p = .05$) also occurred. No significant improvement occurred in severely malnourished patients.[96]

The previously described group was compared with a nearly identical patient population, in which subjects received oxandrolone but not the food supplement. After 6 months of treatment with oxandrolone, mortality was 4% in the moderately malnourished patient group that had adequate caloric intake versus 28% in the placebo group ($p = .002$).[96] Oxandrolone had no effect on mortality among patients who had inadequate caloric intake. In cases of oxandrolone treatment and severe malnutrition, mortality was 51% among those with inadequate intake and 19% among those with adequate caloric intake ($p = .0001$).[96]

Osteopenia

Metabolic bone disease occurs in a broad spectrum of digestive disorders affecting the biliary system, liver, intestine, and pancreas.[103] With the advent of liver transplantation, there is a new clinical syndrome of metabolic bone disease in the postliver transplant population.[15,103] Because patients with chronic liver disease are living longer and surviving liver transplantation, osteopenia has become a significant management and morbidity issue.[15] This is predominantly true for patients with cholestatic liver disease, but it also applies to those with corticosteroid-treated autoimmune hepatitis, alcoholic hepatitis, and hemochromatosis.[15] Patients may be at risk for osteoporosis for multiple reasons (e.g., malabsorption due to steatorrhea, concomitant drug therapy, inadequate dietary intake of calcium and vitamin D, alcohol consumption, smoking, lack of exercise, and age or hormonal status).[15,104] In many cases, neither pharmacologic management alone nor behavioral modification alone is adequate to effectively manage such assaults on bone density and microarchitecture. Generally, several approaches are required.[15,104] It is beyond the scope of this discussion to provide an exhaustive review of bone pathology and therapy for osteoporosis; however, the reader may refer to other publications on the subject if additional information is desired.[105]

BOX 32-1

Preventing Refeeding Syndrome[98-101]

Carbohydrate	Potassium*	Phosphorus*	Magnesium*
• Limit carbohydrate to ≈150-200 g/day or 2 mg/kg/min	• Intravenous supplementation may be necessary with severe hypokalemia	• Intravenous supplementation may be necessary with severe hypophosphatemia	• Intravenous supplementation may be necessary with severe hypomagnesemia
• Increase carbohydrate provision to the desired goal over several days, as tolerance dictates	• 160 mEq/day of potassium may be required for the first 2-3 days of feeding	• 0.5 mmol/kg (15 mg/kg) of phosphorus may be required	• 2-4 mEq/kg of magnesium may be required
	• Subsequent provision may stabilize at 40-90 mEq/day	• Approximately 20.4 mmol/1000 kcal of carbohydrate	

*Recommendations assume that patients have normal renal function and that laboratory monitoring occurs at regular intervals until caloric goals are achieved and serum electrolytes are within normal limits. Oral intake with supplemental amounts of these minerals may result in diarrhea. Consider providing them orally in divided daily doses as serum values stabilize and supplemental requirements diminish.

BOX 32-2

An Approach to Nutrition Intervention for Patients with Liver Disease

Question or Concern	How to Address
What is the type and severity of liver dysfunction? Is it self-limiting? Is the goal survival until transplant?	Consult with the medical team to appraise the significance of liver dysfunction. Develop an appropriate plan for nutrition care. Consider the risks and benefits of interventions.
ACUTE LIVER FAILURE	
What are the primary concerns?	Fluid and electrolytes are primary concerns. Watch for hypoglycemia or hyperglycemia. Assess whether the patient is in a catabolic or anabolic stage. Consider the protein and electrolyte load of GI tract blood, if present. Assess whether the patient is a candidate for enteral, parenteral, or no support.
What is the patient's pre-illness status?	Ethanol abuse—Increased risk of micronutrient deficiencies. Electrolyte abnormalities may require more frequent monitoring.
	Malnutrition—Difficult to assess because of acute changes. History and physical examination are the most useful. Acute weight changes and serum proteins are not helpful.
	History of chronic diseases—Consider the presence of diabetes, kidney, lung, or heart failure.
What should be monitored?	Monitor progress and watch for intervention-induced complications (e.g., fluid, electrolytes, blood glucose levels, GI tract function).
CHRONIC LIVER FAILURE	
Is there malnutrition?	Assess protein/energy status, metabolic status, micronutrient status. Consider the history (including micronutrient intake) and physical examination.
Is there malabsorption?	Adjust the diet to improve tolerance if diarrhea or steatorrhea are present. Supplement nutrients (including fat-soluble vitamins, Ca^{++}) if needed.
Are there metabolic alterations?	Manage blood glucose to within normal limits, as possible.
	Minimize fasting to < 6 hr.
	Maintain adequate protein (if possible) and energy intake (especially carbohydrate).
Are there complications?	Encephalopathy—Maintain adequate protein as much as possible. Watch for protein sensitivity. Use oral BCAA-enriched supplements if they are better tolerated by those who are protein-sensitive.
	Ascites/Edema—Sodium restriction to 2000 mg or 90 mEq/day. Avoid rapid diuresis. Fluid restriction is rarely required.
What should be monitored?	Nutritional status should be monitored with the goal of maintenance or repletion, if possible (especially protein and bone mass).
	Serial measurements are important to evaluate progress.
	Maintain status through episodes of acute complications as much as possible.
	Watch for fluctuations and trends in blood glucose levels, fluids, and electrolytes as needed.
	Monitor response to changes in diet (such as fat or sodium restriction) and adjust if needed.

Relatively recent studies of pharmacologic osteoporosis preventive agents invariably include calcium and vitamin D supplementation in study protocols, in recognition that many people do not consume adequate calcium and vitamin D.[106-109] Efficacy of pharmacologic therapy is enhanced by the provision of adequate substrate. In the case of patients with liver disease, 1500 mg/day of calcium (diet and supplements) and enough water-miscible 25-hydroxyvitamin D to keep serum values within the normal range have been recommended (~50,000 ergocalciferol IU 3 times per week).[15] Postmenopausal women are at increased risk for osteoporosis because of their hormonal status alone; therefore, estrogen replacement therapy is indicated, unless individual risk factors constitute a contraindication to therapy (e.g., smoking, clotting disorder). Newer agents, such as bisphosphonates, offer unique attributes for this patient population. Bisphosphonates have proven efficacy in reducing the risk of fractures and increasing bone mineral density in both men and women.[106,107] At this time, two bisphosphonates have FDA approved indications for the prevention of glucocorticoid-induced osteoporosis.[106,107] Bisphosphonates do not appear to be metabolized by the liver, dosage adjustment is unnecessary for patients with mild to moderate renal insufficiency, and they have not been shown to affect clotting mechanisms.[106,107]

Conclusion

Managing nutrition intervention in liver failure is complex. In acute failure, etiology may not be known when the initial intervention is being planned. In chronic failure, progression of the disease and complications will cause plans to change. Social situations such as finances, family dynamics, and/or chemical use often affect your ability to make optimal plans for discharge. Box 32-2 presents a checklist of factors and suggestions to consider when planning nutrition interventions for patients with liver disease.

REFERENCES

1. McCullough AJ, Bugianesi E: Protein-calorie malnutrition and the etiology of cirrhosis, *Am J Gastroenterol* 92(5):734-738, 1997.
2. Cabre E, Gonzales- Huix F, Abad-Lacruz A: Effect of total enteral nutrition on the short-term outcome of severely malnourished cirrhotics, *Gastroenterology* 98:715-720, 1990.
3. Farrell GC: Liver disease caused by drugs, anesthetics, and toxins. In Feldman M, Scharschmidt BF, Sleisenger MH (eds): *Sleisenger & Fordtran's gastrointestinal and liver disease,* ed 6, vol 2, Philadelphia, 1998, WB Saunders, pp 1221-1253.
4. Friedman SL: Hepatic fibrosis. In Schiff ER, Sorrell MF, Maddrey WC (eds): *Schiff's diseases of the liver,* ed 8, vol 1, Philadelphia, 1999, Lippincott-Raven, pp 371-385.
5. Latifi R, Killam RW, Dudrick SJ: Nutrition support in liver failure, *Surg Clin North Am* 71(3):567-578, 1991.
6. Sherlock S, Dooley J: Hepatic cirrhosis. In Sherlock S, Dooley J (eds): *Diseases of the liver and biliary system,* ed 10, Oxford, 1997, Blackwell Science Ltd, pp 371-384.
7. Sherlock S, Dooley J: Chronic hepatitis. In Sherlock S, Dooley J (eds): *Diseases of the liver and biliary system,* ed 10, Oxford, 1997, Blackwell Science Ltd, pp 303-335.
8. Nyberg LM, Pockros PJ: Postoperative jaundice. In Schiff ER, Sorrell MF, Maddrey WC (eds): *Schiff's diseases of the liver,* ed 8, vol 1, Philadelphia, 1999, Lippincott-Raven, pp 599-605.
9. Lidofsky S, Scharschmidt BF: Jaundice. In Feldman M, Scharschmidt BF, Sleisenger MH (eds): *Sleisenger & Fordtran's gastrointestinal and liver disease,* ed 6, vol 2, Philadelphia, 1998, WB Saunders, pp 220-232.
10. Sherlock S, Dooley J: Alcohol and the liver. In Sherlock S, Dooley J (eds): *Diseases of the liver and biliary system,* ed 10, Oxford, 1997, Blackwell Science Ltd, pp 385-403.
11. Jorquera F, Culebras JM, Gonzalez-Gallego J: Influence of nutrition on liver oxidative metabolism, *Nutrition* 12(6):442-447, 1996.
12. Corrao G, Ferrari PA, Galatola G: Exploring the role of diet in modifying the effect of known disease determinants: application to risk factors of liver cirrhosis, *Am J Epidemiol* 142:1136-1146, 1995.
13. Bode C, Bode JC, Erhardt JG, et al: Effect of the type of beverage and meat consumed by alcoholics with alcoholic liver disease, *Alcohol Clin Exp Res* 22(8):1803-1805, 1998.
14. Schapira D: Alcohol abuse and osteoporosis, *Semin Arthritis Rheum* 19(4):371-376, 1990.
15. Haase J, Weseman B, Fuhrman P, et al: Nutrition therapy for end-stage liver disease: a practical approach, *Support Line* 19(4):8-15, 1997.
16. Santolaria F, Perez-Manzano JL, Milena A, et al: Nutritional assessment in alcoholic patients. Its relationship with alcoholic intake, feeding habits, organic complications and social problems, *Drug Alcohol Depend* 59:295-304, 2000.
17. Detry O, Margulies JE, Arkadopoulos N, et al: Acute hepatic encephalopathy: treatment. In Demetriou A, Watanabe FD (eds): *Support of the acutely failing liver,* ed 2, Georgetown, 2000, Eurekah.com, pp 35-44.
18. Kramer DJ, Aggarwal S, Martin M, et al: Management options in fulminant hepatic failure, *Transplant Proc* 23(3):1895-1898, 1991.
19. Watanabe FD, Kahaku E, Demetriou A: Medical management of acute liver failure. In Demetriou A, Watanabe FD (eds): *Support of the acutely failing liver,* ed 2, Georgetown, 2000, Eurekah.com, pp 45-54.
20. Sherlock S, Dooley J: Nutritional and metabolic liver diseases. In Sherlock S, Dooley J (eds): *Diseases of the liver and biliary system,* ed 10, Oxford, 1997, Blackwell Science Ltd, pp 427-454.
21. Campillo B, Bories PN, Leluan M, et al: Short-term changes in energy metabolism after 1 month of a regular oral diet in severely malnourished cirrhotic patients, *Metabolism* 44(6):765-770, 1995.
22. Santolaria F, Gonzalez-Gonzalez G, Gonzales-Reimers E, et al: Effects of alcohol and liver cirrhosis on the GH-IGF-1 axis, *Alcohol Alcohol* 30(6):703-708, 1995.
23. Marks JB, Skyler JS: The liver and the endocrine system. In Schiff ER, Sorrell MF, Maddrey WC (eds): *Schiff's diseases of the liver,* ed 8, vol 1, Philadelphia, 1999, Lippincott-Raven, pp 477-488.
24. Stoltz A: Liver physiology and metabolic function. In Feldman M, Scharschmidt BF, Sleisenger MH (eds): *Sleisenger & Fordtran's gastrointestinal and liver disease,* ed 6, vol 2, Philadelphia, 1998, WB Saunders, pp 1061-1082.
25. Sherlock S, Dooley J: Assessment of liver function. In Sherlock S, Dooley J (eds): *Diseases of the liver and biliary system,* ed 10, Oxford, 1997, Blackwell Science Ltd, pp 17-32.
26. Lauterburg BH, Velez ME: Glutathione deficiency in alcoholics: risk factor for paracetamol hepatotoxicity, *Gut* 29:1153-1157, 1988.
27. Mato JM, Camara J, de Paz JF, et al: S-Adenosylmethionine in alcoholic liver cirrhosis: a randomized, placebo-controlled, double-blind, multicenter clinical trial, *J Hepatol* 30:1081-1089, 1999.
28. Wanless IR: Anatomy and developmental anomalies of the liver. In Feldman M, Scharschmidt BF, Sleisenger MH (eds): *Sleisenger & Fordtran's gastrointestinal and liver disease,* ed 6, vol 2, Philadelphia, 1998, WB Saunders, pp 1055-1060.
29. Aiza I, Perez GO, Schiff ER: Management of ascites in patients with chronic liver disease, *Am J Gastroenterol* 89(11):1949-1956, 1994.
30. Bass NM, Somberg KA: Portal hypertension and gastrointestinal bleeding. In Feldman M, Scharschmidt BF, Sleisenger MH (eds): *Sleisenger & Fordtran's gastrointestinal and liver disease,* ed 6, vol 2, Philadelphia, 1998, WB Saunders, pp 1284-1309.
31. Silk DBA, OKeefe SJD, Wicks C: Nutritional support in liver disease, *Gut Suppl* S29-S33, 1991.
32. Munoz SJ: Nutritional therapies in liver disease, *Semin Liver Dis* 11(4):278-291, 1991.
33. Madden AM, Morgan MY: Patterns of energy intake in patients with cirrhosis and healthy volunteers, *Br J Nutr* 82:41-48, 1999.
34. McCullough AJ, Tavill AS: Disordered energy and protein metabolism in liver disease, *Semin Liver Dis* 11(4):265-277, 1991.
35. Verboeket-van de Venne WPHG, Westerterp KR, van Hoek B: Energy expenditure and substrate metabolism in patients with cirrhosis of the liver: effects of the pattern of food intake, *Gut* 36:110-116, 1995.
36. Wong F, Liu P, Allidina Y, et al: The effect of posture on central blood volume in patients with preascitic cirrhosis on a sodium-restricted diet, *Hepatology* 23(5):1141-1147, 1996.
37. Garcia-Pagan JC, Salmeron JM, Feu F, et al: Effects of low-sodium diet and spironolactone on portal pressure in patients with compensated cirrhosis, *Hepatology* 19(5):1095-1099, 1994.
38. Kondrup J, Nielsen K, Juul A: Effect of long-term refeeding on protein metabolism in patients with cirrhosis of the liver, *Br J Nutr* 77:197-212, 1997.
39. Dichi I, Dichi JB, Papini-Berto SJ, et al: Protein-energy status and ^{15}N-glycine kinetic study of child a cirrhotic patients fed low- to high-protein energy diets, *Nutrition* 12:519-523, 1996.
40. Selberg OS, Bottcher J, Tusch G, et al: Identification of high- and low-risk patients before liver transplantation: a prospective cohort study of nutritional and metabolic parameters in 150 patients, *Hepatology* 25(3):652-657, 1997.
41. Plevak DJ, DiCecco SR, Wiesner RH, et al: Nutritional support for liver transplantation: identifying caloric and protein requirements, *Mayo Clin Proc* 69:225-230, 1994.
42. Harrison J, McKiernan J, Neuberger JM: A prospective study on the effect of recipient nutritional status on outcome in liver transplantation, *Transpl Int* 10:369-374, 1997.
43. Driscoll DF, Palombo JD, Bistrian BR: Nutritional and metabolic considerations of the adult liver transplant candidate and organ donor, *Nutrition* 11(3):255-263, 1995.
44. Sherlock S, Dooley J: Cholestasis. In Sherlock S, Dooley J (eds): *Diseases of the liver and biliary system,* ed 10, Oxford, 1997, Blackwell Science Ltd, pp 217-237.

45. Lehman GA, Sherman S: Motility and dysmotility of the biliary tract and sphincter of Oddi. In Feldman M, Scharschmidt BF, Sleisenger MH (eds): *Sleisenger & Fordtran's gastrointestinal and liver disease,* ed 6, vol 2, Philadelphia, 1998, WB Saunders, pp 929-936.

46. Bass NM: Sclerosing cholangitis and recurrent pyogenic cholangitis. In Feldman M, Scharschmidt BF, Sleisenger MH (eds): *Sleisenger & Fordtran's gastrointestinal and liver disease,* ed 6, vol 2, Philadelphia, 1998, WB Saunders, pp 1006-1025.

47. Ueno T, Sugawara H, Sujaku K, et al: Therapeutic effects of restricted diet and exercise in obese patients with fatty liver, *J Hepatology* 27:103-107, 1997.

48. Yang SQ, Lin HZ, Lane MD, et al: Obesity increases sensitivity to endotoxin liver injury: Implications for pathogenesis of steatohepatitis, *Proc Natl Acad Sci USA* 94:2557-2562, 1997.

49. Angulo P, Keach JC, Batts KP, et al: Independent predictors of liver fibrosis in patients with nonalcoholic steatohepatitis, *Hepatology* 30(6):1356-1362, 1999.

50. Matteoni CA, Younossi ZM, Gramlich T, et al: Nonalcoholic fatty liver disease: a spectrum of clinical and pathological severity, *Gastroenterology* 116:1413-1419, 1999.

51. Loffreda S, Yang SQ, Lin HZ, et al: Leptin regulates proinflammatory immune responses, *FASEB J* 12:57-65, 1998.

52. Okolo III P, Diehl AM: Nonalcoholic steatohepatitis and focal fatty liver. In Feldman M, Scharschmidt BF, Sleisenger MH (eds): *Sleisenger & Fordtran's gastrointestinal and liver disease,* ed 6, vol 2, Philadelphia, 1998, WB Saunders, pp 1215-1220.

53. Mullen KD, Dasarathy S: Hepatic encephalopathy. In Schiff ER, Sorrell MF, Maddrey WC (eds): *Schiff's diseases of the liver,* ed 8, vol 1, Philadelphia, 1999, Lippincott-Raven, pp 545-581.

54. Sherlock S, Dooley J: Hepatic encephalopathy. In Sherlock S, Dooley J (eds): *Diseases of the liver and biliary system,* ed 10, Oxford, 1997, Blackwell Science Ltd, pp 87-102.

55. Mullen MB, Weber FL: Role of nutrition in hepatic encephalopathy, *Semin Liver Dis* 11(4):292-304, 1991.

56. Fitz G: Systemic complications of liver disease. In Feldman M, Scharschmidt BF, Sleisenger MH (eds): *Sleisenger & Fordtran's gastrointestinal and liver disease,* ed 6, vol 2, Philadelphia, 1998, WB Saunders, pp 1334-1354.

57. Morgan TR, Moritz TE, Mendenhall CL, et al: Protein consumption and hepatic encephalopathy in alcoholic hepatitis, *J Am College Nutr* 14(2):152-158, 1995.

58. Guidelines for the use of parenteral and enteral nutrition in adult and pediatric patients, *J Parenter Enteral Nutr* 17(4):14SA, 1993.

59. Kawamura-Yasui N, Kaito M, Nakagawa N, et al: Evaluating response to nutritional therapy using the branched-chain amino acid/tyrosine ratio in patients with chronic liver disease, *J Clin Lab Anal* 13:31-34, 1999.

60. Egberts EH, Schomerus H, Hamster W, et al: Branched chain amino acids in the treatment of latent portosystemic encephalopathy: a double-blind placebo-controlled crossover study, *Gastroenterology* 88:887-895, 1985.

61. Olafsson S, Blei AT: Diagnosis and management of ascites in the age of TIPS, *Am J Roentgenol* 165:9-15, 1995.

62. Groszmann RJ, de Franchis R: Portal hypertension. In Schiff ER, Sorrell MF, Maddrey WC (eds): *Schiff's diseases of the liver,* ed 8, vol 1, Philadelphia, 1999, Lippincott-Raven, pp 387-442.

63. Sherlock S, Dooley J: Ascites. In Sherlock S, Dooley J (eds): *Diseases of the liver and biliary system,* ed 10, Oxford, 1997, Blackwell Science Ltd, pp 119-134.

64. Sherlock S, Dooley J: The portal venous system and portal hypertension. In Sherlock S, Dooley J (eds): *Diseases of the liver and biliary system,* ed 10, Oxford, 1997, Blackwell Science Ltd, pp 135-180.

65. Sabesin SM: Hepatic metabolism. In Stein JH (ed): *Internal medicine,* ed 5, St Louis, 1998, Mosby, p 2143.

66. Davern II TJ, Scharschmidt BF: Biochemical liver tests. In Feldman M, Scharschmidt BF, Sleisenger MH (eds): *Sleisenger & Fordtran's gastrointestinal and liver disease,* ed 6, vol 2, Philadelphia, 1998, WB Saunders, pp 1112-1122.

67. Schafer DF, Sorrell MF: Vascular diseases of the liver. In Feldman M, Scharschmidt BF, Sleisenger MH (eds): *Sleisenger & Fordtran's gastrointestinal and liver disease,* ed 6, vol 2, Philadelphia, 1998, WB Saunders, pp 1188-1198.

68. McCullough AJ, Mullen KD, Smanik EJ, et al: Nutritional therapy and liver disease, *Gastroenterol Clin North Am* 18(3):619-643, 1989.

69. Mendenhall LL, Anderson S, Weesner RE, et al: Protein-calorie malnutrition associated with alcoholic hepatitis. Veterans Administration Cooperative Study Group on alcoholic hepatitis, *Am J Med* 76:211-222, 1984.

70. Mendenhall CL, Moritz TE, Toselle GA, et al: Protein energy malnutrition in severe alcoholic hepatitis: diagnosis and response to treatment, *J Parenter Enteral Nutr* 19(4):558-265, 1995.

71. Simko V, Connell AM, Banks B: Nutritional status in alcoholics with and without liver disease, *Am J Clin Nutr* 35:197-203, 1982.

72. Nutritional status in cirrhosis: Italian multicentre cooperative project on nutrition in liver cirrhosis, *J Hepatol* 21:317-325, 1994.

73. Sarin SK, Khingra N, Bansai A, et al: Dietary and nutritional abnormalities in alcoholic liver disease: a comparison with chronic alcoholics without liver disease, *Am J Gastroenterol* 92(5):777-783, 1997.

74. Muller MJ, Lautz HU, Plogmann B, et al: Energy expenditure and substrate oxidation in patients with cirrhosis: the impact of cause, clinical staging and nutritional state, *Hepatology* 15(5):782-794, 1992.

75. Crawford DH, Shepherd RW, Halliday JW, et al: Body composition in nonalcoholic cirrhosis: the effect of disease etiology and severity on nutritional compartments, *Gastroenterology* 106(6):1611-1617, 1994.

76. Muller MJ: Malnutrition in cirrhosis, *J Hepatol* 23(1):31-35, 1995.

77. Hasse J, Strong S, Gorman MA, et al: Subjective global assessment: alternative nutrition-assessment technique for liver-transplant candidates, *Nutrition* 9(4):339-343, 1993.

78. Caregaro L, Alberino F, Amodio P, et al: Malnutrition in alcoholic and virus-related cirrhosis, *Am J Clin Nutr* 63:602-609, 1996.

79. Crawford DHG, Cuneo RC, Shepherd RW: Pathogenesis and assessment of malnutrition in liver disease, *J Gastroenterol Hepatol* 8:89-94, 1993.

80. Campillo Bernard, Sommer F, Bories PN, et al: Nutritional and metabolic consequences of basal hyperinsulinemia in alcoholic liver cirrhosis: relationship with postprandial changes in erythrocyte insulin-receptor affinity, *Nutrition* 10(6):532-537, 1994.

81. Baker JP, Detsky AS, Wesson DE, et al: Nutritional assessment: a comparison of clinical judgment and objective measurements, *N Engl J Med* 306:969-972, 1982.

82. Cahill GF: Starvation in man, *N Engl J Med* 282:668-675, 1976.

83. Detsky AS, McLaughlin JR, Baker JP, et al: What is subjective global assessment of nutritional status? *J Parenter Enteral Nutr* 11(1):8-13, 1987.

84. Heymsfield SB, Waki M, Reinus J: Are patients with chronic liver disease hypermetabolic? *Hepatology* 11:502-505, 1990.

85. Shizgal HM: Nutritional assessment with body composition measurements, *J Parenter Enteral Nutr* 11:42S-47S, 1987.

86. Mas A, Bosch J, Piera C, et al: Intracellular and exchangable potassium in cirrhosis, *Dig Dis Sci* 26:723-727, 1981.

87. Vitale GC, Neill GD, Fenwick MK, et al: Body composition in the cirrhotic patient with ascites, *Am J Surg* 51:675-681, 1985.

88. Harris JA, Benedict FG: *Biometric study of basal metabolism in man,* Washington, DC, 1919, The Carnegie Institute, pp 1-266.

89. Schneeweiss B, Graninger W, Ferenci P, et al: Energy metabolism in patients with acute and chronic liver disease, *Hepatology* 11:387-393, 1990.

90. Merli M, Riggio O, Romiti A, et al: Basal energy production rate and substrate use in stable cirrhotic patients, *Hepatology* 12:106-112, 1990.

91. Jorgenson R, Lindor KD, Sartin J, et al: Serum lipid and fat-soluble vitamin levels in primary sclerosing cholangitis, *J Clin Gastroenterol* 20(3):215-219, 1995.

92. Hay JE: Bone disease in cholestatic liver disease, *Gastroenterology* 108:276-283, 1995.

93. Pirlich M, Selberg O, Boker K, et al: The creatinine approach to estimate skeletal muscle mass in patients with cirrhosis, *Hepatology* 24(6):1422-1427, 1996.

94. Caregaro L, Alberino F, Amodio P, et al: Nutritional and prognostic significance of insulin-like growth factor 1 in patients with liver cirrhosis, *Nutrition* 13:185-190, 1997.

95. Pikul J, Sharpe M, Lowndes R, et al: Degree of perioperative malnutrition is predictive of post-operative morbidity and mortality in liver transplant recipients, *Transplantation* 57:469-472, 1994.

96. Mendenhall CL, Moritz TE, Roselle GA, et al: A study of oral nutritional support with oxandrolone in malnourished patients with alcoholic hepatitis: results of a Department of Veteran's Affairs Cooperative Study, *Hepatology* 17(4):564-576, 1993.

97. Cerra FB, McMillen M, Angelico R, et al: Cirrhosis, encephalopathy, and improved results with metabolic support, *Surgery* 94:612-618, 1983.

98. Brooks MJ, Melnik G: The refeeding syndrome: an approach to understanding its complications and preventing its occurrence, *Pharmacotherapy* 15(6):713-726, 1995.

99. Rudman D, Millikan WJ, Richardson TJ, et al: Elemental balances during intravenous hyperalimentation of underweight adult subjects, *J Clin Invest* 55:94-104, 1975.

100. Apovian CM, McMahon MM, Bistrian BR: Guidelines for refeeding the marasmic patient, *Crit Care Med* 18:1030-1033, 1990.

101. Havala T, Shronts E: Managing the complications associated with refeeding, *Nutr Pract* 5:23-29, 1990.

102. Weinsier RL, Krumdieck CL: Death resulting from overzealous total parenteral nutrition: the refeeding syndrome revisited, *Am J Clin Nutr* 34:393-399, 1980.

103. Lipkin EW: Metabolic bone disease in gut diseases, *Gastroenterol Clin North Am* 27(2):513-523, 1998.

104. National Osteoporosis Foundation: *Physician's guide to prevention and treatment of osteoporosis,* Belle Med, NJ, 1998, Excerpta Medica, Inc.

105. Rao DS, Honasoge M: Metabolic bone disease in gastrointestinal, hepatobiliary, and pancreatic disorders. In Favus MJ (ed): *Primer on metabolic bone diseases and disorders of mineral metabolism,* New York, 1996, Lippincott-Raven, p 306.

106. Actonel product information. Procter & Gamble Pharmaceuticals, Aug 2000.

107. Fosamax product information. Merck & Co., Oct 2000.

108. Evista product information. Eli Lilly & Co., Dec 1998.

109. Nieves JW, Komar L, Cosman F, et al: Calcium potentiates the effect of estrogen and calcitonin on bone mass: a review and analysis, *Am J Clin Nutr* 67:18-24, 1998.

Renal Failure 33

D. Jordi Goldstein-Fuchs, DSc, RD

Beth McQuiston, MS, RD, LD

THE objective of this chapter is to review how aberrations in kidney function affect nutritional status and clinical management. Clinical management is emphasized. To accomplish this objective the chapter is divided into four main sections. The first section briefly reviews normal renal anatomy and physiology. The second section reviews principles of nutrition care for the patient with acute renal failure. The third section discusses altered nutrient requirements in chronic renal failure. This is followed by a discussion of nutrition assessment techniques and guidelines for nutrition management of both the predialysis and dialysis adult patient populations.

The relationship between renal pathology, nutritional status, and requirements is complex and continually challenges nutrition clinicians and researchers to identify new therapies and tools for intervention. This chapter identifies the challenges, presents current practices of nutrition care, and highlights areas where additional research is needed for the renal patient population.

The Kidney

The kidneys, two retroperitoneal organs the size of a fist, each consist of approximately 1.25 million nephrons (the functioning units of the kidney). Each nephron has a glomerulus attached to the filtering unit of tiny blood vessels, the tubules (Fig. 33-1). The glomerulus is a tuft of capillaries, which forms an ultrafiltrate. The composition of this filtrate is regulated by the tubules.[1] These complex functions are vital for survival and can be replaced only by a successful kidney transplant.

The kidney has three types of functions: excretory, metabolic, and endocrine. Compromise of these functions by renal disease requires special nutrition and medical management. Advanced impairment of kidney function may cause edema, uremia, metabolic acidosis, hypertension, anemia, bone disease, hyperphosphatemia, hyperkalemia, and muscle wasting.[2-5]

Excretion and regulation of body water, minerals, and organic compounds are the most important functions of the kidney. Without excretory function, a patient rarely survives longer than 4 or 5 weeks, especially if the patient is hypercatabolic.[6] Intermittent dialysis therapy, such as hemodialysis (HD) or peritoneal dialysis (PD), can maintain life once end-stage renal disease (ESRD) sets in, even though endocrine and meta-

bolic functions of the kidney are not totally replaced. The kidneys remove nonessential solutes from the blood and conserve those essential to the body. Solutes that are freely filtered from the blood by the glomeruli are either reabsorbed by the tubules or excreted in the urine to maintain fluid and electrolyte balance.[1]

Metabolic Functions

In addition to maintaining electrolyte and fluid balance, the kidney produces important hormones, including 1,25-dihydroxycholecalciferol and erythropoietin. Patients with renal disease are therefore likely to develop anemia and vitamin D deficiency if they are not treated.

The active form of vitamin D (1,25-dihydroxycholecalciferol, $1,25(OH)_2D_3$) is synthesized in the kidney after the inactive direct precursor (25-hydroxycholecalciferol, $25(OH)D_3$) is

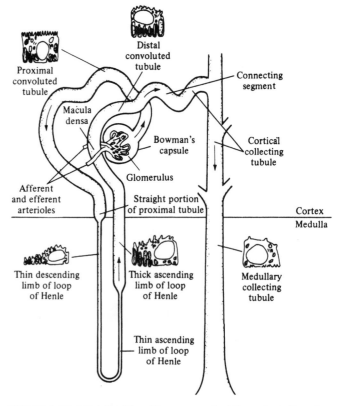

FIGURE 33-1 Relationships of the components of the nephron. (From Rose B: Clinical assessment of renal function. In Rose B [ed]: *Pathophysiology of renal disease,* New York, 1987, McGraw-Hill, pp 1-39.) Reprinted with permission.

Acknowledgment: A special thank you is extended to Christine Abrahamian-Gebeshian, MS, RD, who contributed to the first edition chapter.

hydroxylated in the liver. Deficiency of the active form of vitamin D is associated with impaired intestinal calcium absorption and secondary hyperparathyroidism, both of which contribute to the development of renal osteodystrophy.[2,6,7]

Erythropoietin is a glycoprotein synthesized in the kidneys that stimulates erythropoiesis in the bone marrow. In renal failure erythropoietin is not synthesized; the result is the anemia of chronic renal failure (CRF). Recombinant DNA human erythropoietin is commonly administered to patients to sustain the hemoglobin at normal levels.[8-11]

Regulation of Fluid Balance, Volume, and Tonicity

Extracellular fluid volume is affected by the amount of sodium and other cations in the extracellular space.[12] Confined to extracellular fluid, sodium is the osmotic determinant of how much water will be contained in the extracellular fluid space.[12] When sodium is added to or lost from the body, the resulting change in osmolarity in the extracellular space dictates, in the former case, activation of the thirst mechanism and, in both cases, a specific renal response involving several hormones, which is described subsequently.

Changes in extracellular volume are accompanied by alterations in intravascular volume, cardiac output, and organ perfusion.[12] For example, a decrease in intravascular volume sends sympathetic neural signals to the kidneys. Baroreceptors in the afferent glomerular arterioles sense reduced perfusion pressure. Juxtaglomerular cells from the same area secrete a very important proteolytic enzyme called *renin*.[12,13] An additional stimulus for renin release is increased sympathetic neural tone in the kidneys and decreased sodium delivery to the distal convoluted tubule secondary to a reduction in the glomerular filtration rate (GFR).[12]

Renin, a proteolytic enzyme, cleaves a decapeptide, angiotensin I, from a circulating renin substrate produced by the liver, angiotensinogen. Angiotensin-converting enzyme, a converting enzyme in the lungs, plasma, kidneys, and other tissues, converts angiotensin I to an octapeptide, angiotensin II. Angiotensin II mediates renal sodium and water retention by stimulating the secretion of aldosterone from the adrenal cortex. Aldosterone stimulates renal sodium retention.[12]

Atrial natriuretic factor may be released from the cardiac atria in response to volume expansion. This hormone increases sodium excretion by raising GFR and by reducing tubular reabsorption of sodium. It also opposes renin and aldosterone secretion and the sodium-retaining action of aldosterone.[12]

The kidney is important in maintaining osmolality of all body fluids by virtue of its ability to excrete urine with an osmolality different from that of plasma. In response to increased osmolality, osmoreceptors in the hypothalamus promote secretion of antidiuretic hormone (ADH) by the neurohypophysis.[5,13] Once released, ADH binds to specific receptors in the collecting duct. The net effect is increased water permeability, which results in net water reabsorption into the interstitium.[5,12]

Renal failure secondary to kidney disease is grouped into two categories: acute renal failure (ARF) and CRF. Patients with ARF are more likely to regain kidney function, although recovery and survival do depend on the nature of the original

insult.[6,14] Patients with CRF who develop ESRD require maintenance dialysis treatment or kidney transplantation to survive.

Acute Renal Failure
Clinical Characteristics and Morbidity

ARF is characterized by abrupt cessation or reduction in GFR and accumulation of nitrogenous wastes. ARF is dominant in the clinical setting. Its reported prevalence is 1% of hospitalized patients; 3% to 5% in general medical-surgical patients; 5% to 25% in intensive care units; 5% to 20% in open heart surgery; 10% to 30% with aminoglycoside therapy; 20% to 60% in severe burns; 20% to 30% in rhabdomyolysis; and 15% to 25% for those treated with cisplatinum, bleomycin, and vinblastine.[15-17]

Statistics indicate that the mortality rate from ARF has remained around 50% for the past 25 years.[14,18] This is attributed to the fact that many patients who present with ARF are older and have a difficult medical or surgical course. In addition, patients with ARF who do not survive often die from extrarenal disease rather than from ARF itself. It has been estimated that death occurs in 40% of nonsurgical patients with severe ARF, in as many as 80% of surgical patients, and in 20% of those with noncatabolic conditions. The high morbidity is associated with the degree of hypercatabolism and infection.[14,19] No method has yet proved to reduce the catabolism observed in this patient population. Interventions that have been tried include special nutrition formulations such as ketoacids and parenteral nutrition (PN) formulations that contained a large percentage of branch-chain amino acids or were supplemented with glutamine.[19] Still under study is the use of hormones to decrease protein breakdown (e.g., growth hormone) and therapies directed at reducing metabolism of inflammatory mediators such as thromboxane antagonists, anti–tumor necrosis factor antibodies, and cyclooxygenase inhibitors.[19]

Correct dialysis technique may reduce the mortality rate. Leblanc and colleagues[18] reviewed data suggesting that the dialysis dose has a strong impact on outcome. Of 58 consecutive patients admitted to an intensive care unit with ARF, only 34 survived. The survivors received a dialysis dose or KT/V of 1.09; the nonsurvivors a KT/V of 0.89. Other areas being studied for impact on outcome include type of dialysis (chronic renal replacement therapy [CRRT] or intermittent) and membranes (biocompatible or not).[18]

Consequences of Hypercatabolism

ARF rapidly causes severe nutritional imbalances, regardless of cause.[14] Within a short time the patient's nutritional status declines because of nitrogen losses (up to 30 g per day), leading to loss of lean body mass, toxicity-related symptoms (anorexia, nausea, vomiting, bleeding), loss of essential and nonessential amino acids and plasma proteins during intervention dialysis therapy, and intermediary metabolic disturbances (impaired glucose utilization and protein synthesis) from uremia toxins. Energy and protein malnutrition often result, although one may predominate.

The increase in nutrient requirements characteristic of hypercatabolic patients with ARF results from a combination of increased nutrient demands and reduced supply.[14,20-22] Box 33-1 lists factors related in part to alterations in metabolism. In the hypercatabolic state, normal metabolic functions are altered. The metabolic priorities become maintenance of energy status through gluconeogenesis, synthesis of enzymes and structural and secretory proteins (at the expense of preserving lean body mass), and maintenance of physiologic homeostasis through hormone-substrate interactions. Energy expenditure is often increased, so it could be difficult to maintain and improve the nutritional status of these patients by enteral nutrition (EN) or PN.[6]

Treatment options and nutrition support should be based on the underlying cause of renal failure, the specific metabolic changes of each patient, and other complications associated with the illness.[14,15,19] It is imperative to be aware of the medical intervention planned for each patient, particularly to the type of dialysis therapy to be used, if any. The nutrition requirements of patients with ARF are directly affected by whether the patient receives HD, PD, or CRRT.

ARF patients are likely to develop fluid and electrolyte disorders, uremic toxicity (azotemia), and wasting, particularly if they are both oliguric and hypercatabolic (common complications of ARF). Normal urine output is 1 to 1.5 L per day. With oliguria, urine output is less than 400 ml per day; with anuria, less than 100 ml per day; and with polyuria, more than 3 L per day.[22,23]

The catabolic ARF patient, most frequently encountered in the intensive care setting, presents a management challenge to the entire team of physicians, nurses, dietitians, respiratory therapists, dialysis staff, pharmacists, and other technicians. These patients are in negative nitrogen balance and generate much urea resulting from the catabolic process. Infection is a major threat, and it aggravates the existing malnutrition.[21,22]

Because available data on nutrition therapy for ARF are both limited and conflicting, no treatment plan can be enthusiastically advocated for such patients. Depending on whether the dialysis is initiated or not, general recommendations for protein are 0.6 to 1.4 g/kg per day.[24] Adequate kilocalories should also be provided (126 to 147 kg/kg per day).[15] The percentage of increases in protein and calorie needs in catabolic ARF patients is generally related to the precipitating event. Not only must protein and calorie requirements be estimated, but also altering intake of vitamins and electrolytes should be considered in view of the degree of renal dysfunction. Strategies for fluid and electrolyte management include CRRTs such as continuous arteriovenous hemodialysis (CAVHD). These treatment modalities can allow for sufficient nutrition while avoiding fluid and electrolyte complications. Dialysis interventions require close monitoring and assessment to allow ongoing adjustment of the total treatment regimen.[14,15]

Patients who are metabolically stable may not require dialysis therapy if normal fluid and electrolyte balance can be maintained and the blood urea nitrogen (BUN) level does not exceed 80 mg/dl.[19] Noncatabolic ARF generally results from ingestion of nephrotoxic drugs or exposure to contrast dyes used for diagnostic imaging.[14] These patients are not normally nutritionally depleted and have lower urea generation rates. Oral and enteral feedings are preferred as long as the gastrointestinal (GI) tract is functioning normally. However, catabolic ARF patients are most frequently encountered in the intensive care setting.

Assessment of Nutritional Status

Assessment of the nutritional status of patients with ARF is individualized. The best ways of identifying which patients would benefit from early and aggressive nutrition support have not yet been identified. Monitoring the appropriate laboratory data over time is useful so that each patient serves as his or her own control for comparison.

It is important to classify patients according to their nutrition diagnosis. Clinically available nutrition assessment tools allow for an initial determination of nutritional status and provide baseline data that can be used to follow the effects of therapy.

ANTHROPOMETRY. Anthropometry in the setting of ARF includes body weight, triceps skinfold, midarm circumference, and midarm muscle circumference. Fluid overload and fluid shifts in patients with anuric or oliguric ARF compromise these measurements, so anthropometric data should be interpreted with caution. Serial measurements can be useful for determining changes in euvolemic patients.

PHYSICAL AND CLINICAL EVALUATION. Patients with ARF who were adequately nourished before trauma or injury frequently develop kwashiorkor-like malnutrition. These patients need to be evaluated and monitored for signs of muscle wasting, depleted adipose tissue stores, macronutrient and micronutrient deficiencies (hair loss; dry, flaky skin), and fluid imbalances

---

BOX 33-1

Sources of Increased Nutrient Demands and Decreased Nutrient Availability That Characterize Hypercatabolic Patients with Acute Renal Failure[18,21,22]

INADEQUATE USE OF NUTRIENTS SECONDARY TO:
Insulin resistance
Increased glucose production (glycogenolysis)
Decreased insulin-mediated amino acid uptake/protein synthesis
Reduced clearance of long-and medium-chain triglycerides

CATABOLIC FACTORS:
Associated medical illness or surgical procedure
Sepsis, hypotension, ischemia
Circulating hormones: glucagon, cortisol, epinephrine, parathyroid hormone
Metabolic acidosis
Proteases
Cytokines

DRUG THERAPY:
Steroids
Tetracyclines

DIALYSIS MEMBRANE:
Amino acid losses (hemodialysis, peritoneal dialysis, continuous dialysis)
Protein losses (peritoneal)
Cytokine induction with use of bioincompatible membranes

DECREASED SUPPLY:
Preexisting nutritional deficiencies
Inaccurate assessment of nutritional requirements
Withholding nutrition based on presumption of rapid resolution of ARF
Withholding nutrition to limit or delay dialysis therapy

(poor skin turgor, peripheral edema, hypertension, shortness of breath, increased thirst).

DIET HISTORY. Information might be obtained from the patient or a caretaker on the adequacy of food intake before the morbid event. Such information does not typically become clinically useful until the patient is stabilized and able to eat. At that time, usual intake data might help the patient identify foods he or she can tolerate and eat regularly to reach pre-discharge nutrition goals.

BIOCHEMICAL PARAMETERS. Although there are obvious pitfalls in applying the parameters for nutrition assessment of CRF patients to the ARF patients, evidence indicates that the use of biochemical indicators is appropriate. These include albumin, fasting glucose, lipid profile, serum electrolytes, and measures of cellular immunity. These parameters should be used in conjunction with anthropometry, diet history, and data obtained from clinical and physical evaluation.

SERUM PROTEINS. Serum albumin and transferrin are routinely used to assess visceral protein. The limitation of these and other serum proteins is that they all decrease in response to stress, inflammation, injury, and infection. In addition, serum albumin has a long half-life (about 20 days) and is affected by hydration status. Another serum protein available to assess visceral stores of ARF patients is prealbumin. The elevated levels observed in dialysis patients with ESRD have not been reported in ARF patients. One advantage of prealbumin is that it has a short half-life (2 to 3 days) and has been observed to respond more rapidly than serum transferrin in response to nutrition support.[20]

Patients with ARF have changes in serum proteins—low albumin, transferrin, total protein, and low plasma essential–nonessential amino acid ratio, histidine, leucine, isoleucine, valine, lysine, and threonine.[19]

Stress results in a transient fall in serum albumin caused by a shift of fluid from the intravascular to the extravascular space. Hydration status affects both albumin and transferrin. Although transferrin has a shorter half-life, it is affected by iron status. Severe iron deficiency causes the serum level to increase, whereas iron overload causes it to decrease. Despite all the factors that could invalidate the results, albumin and transferrin are useful if they are carefully evaluated in the context of the patient's overall condition.

IMMUNE SYSTEM PROFILE. Decreased total lymphocyte count and delayed cutaneous sensitivity to skin test antigens are thought to be indicators of protein-calorie malnutrition. Values of total lymphocyte counts less than 1500 per cubic millimeter have been associated with protein-calorie malnutrition and are useful for predicting risk for increased morbidity and mortality in general hospital admissions. Non-nutritional artifacts such as drug therapy, acute illness, stress, infections, and neoplastic disease also alter total lymphocyte count values.[20,21]

Delayed cutaneous hypersensitivity is assessed by intradermal injection of common antigens. Anergy to recall antigens has been correlated with body cell mass depletion and increased postoperative morbidity. Uremic toxicity, infection, and medications can independently affect the immune response and alter the sensitivity and reliability of this parameter as a reflection of nutritional status.[20,21]

Nitrogen Balance Studies

Nitrogen balance is a useful indicator of the degree of catabolism and a guide to nutrition support for critically ill patients with or without ARF.[20] Nitrogen balance studies can also be useful in stable dialysis patients to determine optimal protein intake.[25] What method is best for calculating nitrogen balance depends on whether a patient is being treated with dialysis and, if so, which type.

For critically ill patients with normal renal function, nitrogen balance can be calculated in the standard way by measuring 24-hour urinary urea nitrogen (UUN), adding a factor for insensible and nonurea urinary nitrogen losses, and subtracting nitrogen losses from nitrogen delivered.

The validity of using UUN values to calculate urea nitrogen losses is compromised when creatinine clearance drops to less than 50 ml per minute.[20] In patients with ARF, nitrogen balance can be determined by calculating the urea nitrogen appearance (UNA) or the protein catabolic rate (PCR). Both the UNA and PCR are only *estimates* of protein catabolism. The calculations do not factor into the respective equations, the 3 to 4 g/kg per day of endogenous protein turnover that occurs in catabolic adult ARF patients.

The UNA can also be used to calculate nitrogen balance for patients receiving CRRT. CRRT treatment modalities include continuous ambulatory peritoneal dialysis (CAPD), continuous arteriovenous hemofiltration (CAVH), and continuous arteriovenous hemofiltration (CAVHD). The technical details of these different therapies are described elsewhere.[23] The dialysate used in some types of CRRT contains dextrose, which is absorbed and contributes to the total calorie load. Dextrose absorption during PD and CAVHD must be accounted for to avoid metabolic consequences of overfeeding and to accurately calculate carbohydrate requirements. Although dextrose absorption depends on concentration and the dialysate flow rate, in general, administered at the rate of 1 L per hour, a 1.5% dextrose solution contributes 525 kcal per day (43% absorbance), and a 2.5% dextrose dialysate provides 920 kcal per day (45% uptake).[26] In addition to accounting for dextrose absorption, amino acid loss across the dialyzer membrane must also be factored into the calculation of nitrogen balance.

INDIRECT CALORIMETRY. Determining energy requirements using indirect calorimetry is a useful element of nutrition assessment in patients with catabolic ARF. Accurate measurements of oxygen consumption, carbon dioxide production, resting energy expenditure, and respiratory quotient guide nutrition support for these patients. In critically ill, mechanically ventilated patients, indirect calorimetry must be meticulous to ensure accuracy (Chapter 6). Factors that can invalidate the results include leaking of chest or endotracheal tubes and mechanical ventilation with high fractional inspired oxygen concentrations.[20]

If indirect calorimetry is not available, basal energy expenditure (BEE) can be calculated indirectly using the Harris-Benedict equation, adjusting for stress by multiplying by an activity factor of 1 to 2 (Box 33-2). It is unlikely that energy requirements will ever exceed 130% of the calculated BEE.

TRACE MINERALS AND VITAMINS. The optimal vitamin and mineral requirements of patients with ARF are not known.

Manual Calculation of Energy Requirements for Patients with Impaired Renal Function

1. Calculate basal energy expenditure (BEE) using the Harris-Benedict equation:
   Females: $655.1 + (9.56 \times BW) + (1.85 \times height) - (4.67 \times age)$
   Males: $66.47 + (13.75 \times BW) + (5 \times height) - (6.76 \times age)$
2. Multiply BEE by appropriate activity factor:
   a. Sleeping, reclining: 1.0
   b. Very light; sitting, standing, driving: 1.5
   c. Light; walking 2-3 mph, shopping: 2.5
   d. Moderate: walking 3-4 mph, biking: 5.0
   e. Heavy; running, climbing, swimming: 7.0
3. Multiply product of #2 above using stress factor to approximate total calorie requirements:
   Postoperative (no complications)   1.0
   Long-bone fracture   1.15-1.3
   Cancer   1.10-1.3
   Peritonitis/sepsis   1.10-1.3
   Severe infection/polytrauma   1.2-1.4
   Multiple organ failure syndrome   1.2-1.4
   Burns (approximate BEE + % surface area burned) 1.2-2.0
4. Corrected energy requirements (kcal/day) = BEE × activity factor × stress factor

Modifed from Protein and calories: requirements, intake, and assessment. In Alpers D, Stenson W, Bier D (eds): *Manual of nutritional therapeutics,* Boston, 1995, Little, Brown, p 83.
BW, Body weight.

Patients with ARF can develop trace mineral toxicity because of reduced renal clearance of these nutrients; thus, daily infusion of trace minerals is not recommended. Vitamin A levels can be increased secondary to enhanced hepatic release of retinol and retinol-binding protein, decreased renal catabolism, and decreased degradation of vitamin A transport protein by the kidneys.[19] Levels of vitamin D may be decreased with ARF because of impaired activation of 1,25-dihydroxycholecalciferol. Vitamin K deficiency has been reported in postoperative nonuremic patients receiving antibiotics and no enteral feedings; however, plasma levels are usually elevated and supplementation is rarely indicated. Water-soluble vitamin deficiencies can also develop because of dialysis losses, the exception being vitamin C, which is metabolized to oxalate. Vitamin C supplements greater than 250 mg per day may cause ARF from secondary oxalosis. The majority of multivitamin preparations for parenteral solutions contain the vitamin dietary reference intakes (DRIs) and can be used without ill effect for ARF patients.[19]

Electrolytes

Serum levels of potassium, magnesium, and phosphorus are generally elevated in patients with ARF because of decreased renal clearance and marked net protein breakdown. Decreased levels of serum potassium, magnesium, and phosphorus may occur as a result of intracellular shifts associated with carbohydrate delivery and anabolism. In addition, serum phosphorus may be decreased secondary to severe respiratory alkalosis as a result of increased clearance across the dialysis membrane with CRRT or of intracellular shifts. Hypophosphatemia also occurs in the refeeding syndrome, malnutrition, and diuretic therapy. Serum levels of potassium, magnesium, and phosphorus should therefore be monitored frequently to assess the need for addi-

tional supplementation. Delivery of potassium, magnesium, and phosphorus should be individualized according to serum levels.[23,27,28]

Blood Urea Nitrogen and Creatinine

BUN and creatinine are elevated in ARF, although the ratio of BUN to creatinine may be normal (10:1 or higher). Insufficient dietary calories and protein and altered blood levels of proteases contribute to high levels of protein catabolism. Dialysis may be required to remove metabolic wastes and excess water. When recovery of renal function is expected to take several weeks or when wasting is severe, aggressive dialysis is often recommended. Medical and nutrition management typically aim to maintain BUN in the range of 80 to 100 mg/dl.[23]

Triglycerides

The type and amount of fat delivered to catabolic ARF patients is important. Serum levels of triglycerides should be within the normal range. High doses of ω-6 fatty acids may result in hypoxemia, bacteremia, and suppression of tests of immune function in vitro. Serum triglyceride levels can be useful to monitor the efficiency of hepatic removal of long-chain and medium-chain triglycerides. Elevated serum triglyceride levels suggest reduced hepatic capacity for intravenous lipids. When this is observed, a lipid-free nutrition formula might be in order or the amount of total lipid infused might initially be reduced. Which route is selected depends on the degree of dyslipidemia and on other clinical indices such as liver enzymes (serum glutamic-oxaloacetic and pyruvic transaminases and alkaline phosphatase).[24]

NUTRITION REQUIREMENTS. The ARF patient's nutrition requirements are directly influenced by the type of renal replacement therapy (if any), nutritional and metabolic status, and the degree of hypercatabolism. The current recommendations for protein and calories for this patient population are defined below.

Protein is expressed as grams per kilogram of ideal body weight per day. Protein sources containing both essential and nonessential amino acids should be provided. For patients whose ARF is expected to resolve in a few days and who will not need dialysis, 0.6 to 1 g of protein is recommended.[15,29-31] The patient's nutrition and metabolic status and the renal diagnosis determine the exact dose. For patients receiving acute HD, the recommendation is 1.2 to 1.4 g of protein, for those on acute intermittent or continuous cycling peritoneal dialysis (CCPD), 1.2 to 1.5 g, and for those on CRRT, 1.5 to 2.0 g.[30]

When energy requirements cannot be measured directly, calorie requirements can usually be met by providing 35 to 50 kcal/kg ideal body weight,[29,30] reserving the upper limit of the range for patients who are severely catabolic and whose nitrogen balance does not improve at lower intakes. In general, 60% of calories should be provided as carbohydrate and 20% to 35% as fat.[29,30] Any patient receiving PN for more than 5 to 7 days should receive 50 to 100 g of lipids as an emulsion to avoid essential fatty acid deficiency.[29]

The total fluid intake for any patient depends on the amount of residual renal function (i.e., is the patient oliguric? anuric?) and fluid and sodium status. In general, fluid intake can be calculated by adding to the 24-hour urine output 500 ml for insensible losses.[30]

Supplementation of minerals, electrolytes, and trace elements is determined by monitoring serum and urine levels, when appropriate, to prevent excess or deficiency states from arising. While the specific vitamin requirements of ARF patients are not known, the following guidelines are available:[29]

1. Supplementation of vitamin A is not recommended for at least 2 weeks because levels are elevated with chronic renal failure.
2. Vitamin K supplements should be given, particularly to patients who are taking antibiotics that suppress intestinal growth of bacteria that usually synthesize it.
3. To avoid vitamin B_6 deficiency, 10 mg per day of pyridoxine hydrochloride (8.2 mg per day of pyridoxine) is recommended.
4. Limiting ascorbic acid to 60 to 100 mg per day prevents increased oxalate production and serum oxalate levels.[29]

ROUTE OF NUTRITION SUPPORT. The criteria for deciding which route of nutrition support to use (enteral or parenteral) for critically ill patients has become increasingly complex. In addition to the increased costs associated with the parenteral route, some studies report an increased incidence of infectious complications with parenteral, as compared with enteral, nutrition. PN has also been associated with atrophy of gut mucosa, reduced levels of secretory immunoglobulin A, enhanced bacterial and endotoxin translocation, and exaggerated hormonal and metabolic responses to septic challenge.[20] Therefore, patients with catabolic ARF should be evaluated for route of nutrient delivery; EN should be used unless contraindicated.

Because uremia is a potent catabolic signal, metabolic studies in patients with ARF and CRF have traditionally limited the intake of nonessential amino acids in an attempt to reduce urea production. Proteins of high biologic value, but in quantities much smaller than are usually given (< 0.5 g/kg per day), were administered along with adequate calories, usually in the form of glucose. The same approach was used with PN. A central venous infusion of an essential amino acid solution and a hypertonic dextrose solution was frequently administered to provide calories and a small quantity of essential nitrogen. It was thought that this approach would prevent malnutrition and at the same time reduce protein catabolism and minimize the rise in BUN.[19]

This clinical approach to nutrition therapy has not reduced mortality rates. In the mid-1990s aggressive use of dialysis (early intervention and large doses) and parenteral solutions containing mixed amino acids, dextrose, and lipids was becoming standard practice. Dialysis therapy can be adjusted to the patient in terms of clearing catabolic products and allowing for increased administration of protein and calories. CRRT therapy has made possible aggressive nutrition support for hypercatabolic patients who have failing kidney function.[23]

Debate goes on about the optimal amino acid composition of PN solutions. Despite some question about the relative nephrotoxicity of certain amino acids, current recommendations call for formulations containing mixed amino acids, essential and nonessential. Currently, no conclusive evidence indicates that specialized formulations such as those addition-

---

BOX 33-3

Sample Parenteral Formulations for Renal Failure

ARF OR PREDIALYSIS CRF:

- 500 ml, 70% dextrose, 250 ml EAA,
  97% carbohydrate, 3% protein
  (provides 1640 kcal/L, 13.3 g protein/L)
- *For patients with glucose intolerance:*
  500 ml 50% dextrose, 250 ml EAA
  96% carbohydrates, 4% protein
  (provides 1187 kcal/L, 13.3 g protein/L)
  (Use no longer than 6 days.)
- As BUN stabilizes or decreases, mixed AA solution:
  500 ml 70% dextrose, 250 ml EAA, 250 ml 8.5% MAA
  90% carbohydrate, 10% protein
  (provides 1315 kcal/L, 31.3 g protein/L)
- *For patients with glucose intolerance:*
  500 ml 50% dextrose, 250 ml EAA, 250 ml 8.5% MAA
  87% carbohydrate, 13% protein
  (provides 975 kcal/L, 31.3 g protein/L)

DIALYSIS INITIATED, FLUID RESTRICTION REQUIRED:

- 500 ml 70% dextrose, 500 ml 8.5% MAA
  87% carbohydrate, 13% protein
  (provides 1360 kcal/L, 42.2 g protein/L)

  500 ml 70% dextrose, 10.0% MAA
  85% carbohydrate, 14% protein
  (provides 1390 kcal/L, 50 g protein/L)
- *For patients with glucose intolerance:*
  250 ml 70% dextrose, 500 ml 8.5% MAA
  240 ml 20% fat emulsion
  47% carbohydrate, 13% protein, 40% fat
  (provides 1265 kcal/L, 42.5 g protein/L)

DIALYSIS INITIATED, NO FLUID RESTRICTION REQUIRED:

- 500 ml 50% dextrose, 500 ml 8.5% MAA
  83% carbohydrate, 17% protein
  (provides 1020 kcal/L, 42.5 g protein/L)

  500 ml 50% dextrose, 500 ml 10% MAA
  81% carbohydrate, 14% protein
  (provides 1050 kcal/L, 50 g protein/L)
- *For patients with glucose intolerance:*
  250 ml 50% dextrose, 500 ml 10% MAA
  250 ml 20% fat emulsion
  38% carbohydrate, 18% protein, 44% fat
  (provides 1125 kcal/L, 50 g protein/L)

Data from Liftman C, Hood S: Parenteral nutrition for the patient with renal failure. In Stover J (ed), *Nutrition care in end-stage renal disease*, ed 2, Chicago, 1994, American Dietetic Association, pp 111-121.
EAA, essential amino acids; *MAA*, mixed amino acids (essential + nonessential).

---

ally enriched with branched-chain amino acids have a beneficial effect on outcome.[32-34] Box 33-3 lists parenteral solutions commonly used for patients with ARF.

Principles of Nutrition Management

ARF patients on nutrition support therapy must be monitored closely. The monitoring schedule depends on the nutrition regimen being used. In addition to considerations of nutrient content of oral or tube feedings or parenteral intake, particular attention to the subsequently described indices is in order.

DETERMINING NUTRITION INTERVENTION GOALS. Energy and protein intake should meet the patient's nutrition requirements, which are likely to be greater than normal. The amount of nutrition administered depends on the patient's nutritional status, catabolic rate, residual GFR, and medical and/or surgical interventions (i.e., dialysis therapy and type). Patients with ARF (particularly those with underlying catabolic illness) frequently have metabolic derangements that promote degradation of protein and amino acids and consumption of fuel substrates. Protein, amino acids, and energy substrates may not be utilized efficiently, so it may be difficult to maintain or improve the nutritional status of these patients by enteral or parenteral support. When feasible, patients with ARF should receive oral nutrition. If a patient cannot eat enough, a liquid formula diet, elemental diet, and tube or enterostomy feeding should be considered. Nutrient recommendations for ARF, based on the degree of catabolism, are reviewed in Table 33-1.

MANAGING FLUID AND MINERAL REPLACEMENT. Fluid and mineral balance need to be carefully monitored in ARF to prevent overhydration and electrolyte disorders. Total fluid input is recommended to equal output from urine and all other measured sources (e.g., nasogastric aspirate or fistula drainage) plus 400 to 500 ml per day. This regimen takes into consideration the contributions of endogenous water production from metabolism and insensible water losses in breath and perspiration. If the patient is catabolic, weight can be allowed to drop by 0.2 to 0.5 kg per day to avoid excessive accumulation of fluid.[20,37] Records of daily intake and output, weight changes, serum electrolyte levels, and blood pressure are useful for assessment of fluid tolerance and requirements.

SERUM PARAMETERS. Indices that reflect renal function must be checked daily: BUN, creatinine, creatinine clearance, electrolytes, bicarbonate, calcium, phosphorus, and magnesium. Serum iron, leukocyte count, occult blood, triglycerides, and glucose values are needed to evaluate response to the infusion. Because of the hormone and metabolic changes that often accompany institution of PN, serum levels of potassium, magnesium, and other electrolytes may decline despite impaired

renal function and may require supplementation via GI or intravenous therapy. As part of the anabolic response, hypophosphatemia may result as metabolism shifts to deriving energy from glucose. As potassium is deposited into newly synthesized cells, the serum potassium level may drop if it is not supplemented.[38] Insulin therapy is initiated if hyperglycemia develops.

Feeding formulations can be changed or manipulated to achieve the desired physiologic result. This type of intervention, referred to as *nutritional pharmacology,*[39] continues to be explored for the treatment of critically ill patients.

Weekly liver function tests and other parameters that would alert to multisystem organ failure are important because the results might indicate modification of the nutrition intervention.

NUTRITIONAL STATUS. Weekly serum albumin and prealbumin (if available) values are recommended. Thrice weekly nitrogen balance calculations are useful to verify that the nutrition plan is in fact meeting the patient's needs and to determine whether nutritional needs have changed. Once positive nitrogen balance is achieved, a weekly calculation is sufficient to monitor the patient's progress.

Special monitoring is required for patients receiving CRRT and intermittent dialysis intervention. With many types of CRRT, standard nutrition support solutions may overfeed carbohydrate because of significant dextrose absorption from the dialysate. Modification of PN and EN formulas is necessary to prevent potentially deleterious consequences. PN solutions with low dextrose concentrations may be used. When nutrition is delivered via the enteral route, formulas with a low calorie-nitrogen ratio provide more protein without excessive carbohydrate. Modular protein supplements may need to be added to protein-dense enteral formulas to meet the catabolic needs of dialysis patients.[23,30]

With CRRT, adequate fluid, solute, and electrolyte removal generally obviates parenteral or enteral formulas with reduced

---

TABLE 33-1

Nutrient Recommendations for Patients with Acute Renal Failure[3,35,36]

	Degree of Catabolism			
	None/Mild	**Moderate**	**Severe**	**Burn/Sepsis**
GFR	5-10 ml/min			
UNA	4-5 g/day		5 g N/day+	10 g N/day+
Dialysis	None	As needed	Hemodialysis/PD	CRRT
Protein g/kg/day	0.6-0.8	1.0-1.2	1.2-1.5	1.5-2.0
Carbohydrates (% of kcal)	60 or for all conditions, calculate 5-7 mg/kg/min/day			
		60	60	60
Fat (% of kcal)	35	20-30	20-30	20
kcal/kg/IBW	30	35	40-50	40-50
or BEE x stress factor calculated or measured via indirect calorimetry (energy requirements unlikely to exceed 130% of the calculated BEE)				
Sodium (1.1-3.3 g/day)	Individualized; in the absence of edema, sodium should match urinary losses			
Potassium (780-2000 mg/day)	Individualized			
Fluids	24-hour urine output + 500 ml (insensible losses) (depends on urinary sodium; total fluid output, including urine; and modality of dialysis treatment, if any)			
Vitamin and minerals	Fat-soluble vitamins A, D, K, and trace minerals if ARF patients receive nutrition support ≥2 weeks. Vitamins similar to CRF. Electrolytes and minerals supplemented as indicated by laboratory values; extra needed with CRRT			

ARF, Acute renal failure; *BEE,* basal energy expenditure; *CRF,* chronic renal failure; *CRRT,* continuous renal replacement therapy; *GFR,* glomerular filtration rate; *g N/day +,* the minimum plus grams of nitrogen per day expected for the degree of catabolism indicated; *IBW,* ideal body weight; *PD,* peritoneal dialysis; *UNA,* urea nitrogen appearance.

quantities of fluid, protein, and electrolytes; however, with intermittent HD, enteral and parenteral solution volumes must be limited. Likewise, the electrolyte composition of enteral formulas must be evaluated and electrolytes must be added carefully and judiciously to parenteral solutions. Both fluid and electrolyte control are essential to maintain acceptable levels of serum electrolytes and to avoid fluid overload.[20,30]

Future Trends

Use of exogenous recombinant human growth hormone for critically ill or malnourished HD patients is currently being explored.[40-44] Growth hormone is a potent anabolic agent that accelerates growth in uremic children and increases nitrogen balance in nonuremic patients.[29,44] Exogenous administration of this hormone has also been found to benefit dietary protein utilization and reduce urea generation when administered to stable HD patients.[41-43]

The anabolic properties of growth hormone are thought to be mediated by insulin-like growth factor 1 (IGF-1). IGF-1 exerts its somatogenic effect on target tissues via endocrine, paracrine, and autocrine mechanisms.[44] Growth hormone has been found to improve the biologic activity and circulating levels of IGF-1 in uremic children. Some evidence suggests that the biologic activity of IGF-1 is reduced in HD patients. Therefore, the anabolic effects observed after growth hormone administration to dialysis patients might be mediated through normalization of IGF-1 properties. Research in this area appears promising and could lead to a new type of treatment for malnutrition in dialysis patients.[45,46] Clinical studies of the effects of growth hormone on outcome in critically ill ARF patients have not yet been reported.

Chronic Renal Failure

CRF is a syndrome of progressive and irreversible loss of the excretory, endocrine, and metabolic functions secondary to kidney damage. Renal function is measured by the GFR, which is reflected in clearance tests that measure the rate at which substances are cleared from the plasma by the glomeruli. Clearance, defined as the volume of plasma cleared of a particular solute in a given time, is expressed in moles, or weight of the substance per volume per time.[4,47] The mean GFR, expressed in milliliters per minute per 1.73 m^2, can be calculated.[1,47,48]

GFR = 122.49 − 0.37 (age) for adults younger than 45 years

GFR = 153.9 − 1.07 (age) for those 45 and older

In the clinical setting, endogenous creatinine clearance is measured to approximate the actual GFR. The formula most often used to calculate creatinine clearance is:[4]

$$(140 - age) \times (weight)/72 \times PCr,$$

where age is stated in years, body weight is in kilograms, and PCr is plasma creatinine concentration in milligrams per deciliter.[4,49] This formula applies to white males. For women and black males, the result should be multiplied by 0.85 and 1.12, respectively. The formula overestimates GFR for persons who have edema or are obese.[49,50]

Plasma creatinine concentration varies inversely with GFR. The normal range of serum creatinine is 0.8 to 1.2 mg/dl for males and 0.6 to 1.0 for females. Many different laboratory techniques are available for measuring serum creatinine, and the upper limit of normal varies significantly. Although the serum creatinine value cannot be used as a measure of GFR, levels start to increase as kidney function decreases. The clinical definition of CRF includes a long-term reduction in GFR, decreased creatinine clearance, and a corresponding increase in serum creatinine concentration.[2]

CRF progresses slowly over time, and there may be intervals during which kidney functions remain stable. The onset of renal failure is not usually apparent until 50% to 70% of renal function is lost. Once the disease progresses to end stage, maintenance dialysis or kidney transplantation is indicated. Dialysis only partially replaces the excretory and regulatory functions of the kidney. Absence of other functions requires medications and a special diet to maintain homeostasis.[2]

Blachley and Knochel[51] described four stages through which the average patient with chronic, progressive renal failure passes. The first stage is characterized by decreased renal reserve. The excretory and regulatory functions of the kidney remain stable, and the only observed change may be decreased creatinine clearance. Normal values for creatinine clearance are 115 ± 20 ml per minute. In the second stage, renal insufficiency, creatinine clearance falls to less than 50 ml per minute and azotemia (elevation of urea and other products of protein in the blood without uremic symptoms), inability to concentrate the urine, nocturia, and mild anemia occur. In the third stage of renal failure, creatinine clearance ranges from 10 to 15 ml per minute or less and corresponds to a serum creatinine of 5.5 to 11.0 mg/dl. In this stage symptoms of uremic toxicity begin to appear: fatigue, nausea, vomiting, loss of appetite, hypocalcemia, hyperphosphatemia, metabolic acidosis, and polyuria. The fourth (and last) stage is uremia, when all the consequences of uremic toxicity overtly affect the patient. Creatinine clearance is usually less than 10 ml per minute. Multisystemic symptoms occur, such as pericarditis, neuropathy, digestive disorders, glucose intolerance, hyperlipidemia, soft tissue calcification, and bleeding disorders.

The decision to initiate dialysis depends on the severity of symptoms. Unnecessary delay should be avoided to prevent medical complications of advanced uremia and subsequent patient debilitation and deterioration. Many patients require dialysis once the serum creatinine reaches 6 mg/dl or creatinine clearance is less than 15 ml per minute for nondiabetics and diabetics, respectively.[4] Symptoms considered to be definite indications for dialysis therapy include pericarditis, uncontrollable fluid overload, pulmonary edema, uncontrollable and repeated hyperkalemia, coma, and lethargy. Less severe symptoms such as azotemia, nausea, and vomiting require a subjective determination that takes into consideration the patient's quality of life.

Uremia

Uremia is a form of systemic intoxication caused by retention in the blood of substances that are normally excreted in urine. Uremia describes the phase of CRF when overt symptoms of toxicity such as those described earlier begin to appear. The remarkable regulatory function of the kidney is well-demonstrated by the fact that the uremic syndrome is not usually manifested until 90% of kidney function has been lost.[51]

Uremic disorders and symptoms are not due to kidney failure per se. Uremic serum has toxic effects on biologic systems in vitro and in vivo. Observations that uremic symptoms improve following dialysis treatment suggest a role of toxic molecule retention. Dialysis therapy was derived from the concept that uremia is a function of concentration of retained solutes.[52]

Which molecules are actually uremia toxins? Chemical identification of these molecules has been going on for more than 60 years and is still incomplete. However, the number of substances known to play a part in the uremia syndrome has increased, and many of them have been found to be products of nitrogen catabolism. Examples of metabolites suspected to be toxins include urea, guanidines, uric acid, aliphatic amines, purine derivatives, and middle molecules (substances with a molecular weight between 300 and 5000 daltons). Despite this identification of retained compounds, a cause-and-effect relationship between molecules and specific uremic symptoms has not been conclusively demonstrated.[53]

The major end-product of protein metabolism in humans is urea. Although urea may not be toxic in the levels found in dialysis patients, its presence implies the existence of other, more toxic, protein metabolites. Symptoms of uremia appear to increase with a high-protein diet, and they resolve when protein intake is restricted. This clinical observation supports indications that many uremia toxins are nitrogen compounds or their derivatives. Symptoms of excessive protein intake include high BUN levels, anorexia, nausea, vomiting, weakness, taste change, confusion, lethargy, and generalized itching.[52]

Controlling the amounts of end products of protein and nutrient metabolism (e.g., phosphorus and hydrogen ion) that accumulate in CRF patients is critical for treatment. Diet therapy is a major component of medical management intended to return the patient to a homeostatic condition. Patients requiring renal replacement therapy for acute or chronic renal failure have altered nutrient requirements and require special nutrition management. The nutrient recommendations for the predialysis and dialysis patient populations are summarized in Table 33-2.

Renal Replacement Therapies

Simply stated, dialysis is a procedure that removes excessive and toxic by-products of metabolism from the blood, thus replacing the filtering function of healthy kidneys. During the

TABLE 33-2

Daily Nutrient Recommendations for CRF Based on Treatment Modality[54, 55, 56]

Nutrient	Predialysis	Hemodialysis	Peritoneal Dialysis
Protein (g/kg)	Prescribed according to GFR: GFR: 25-55 ml/min/m²: >0.8 g/kg/day GFR: <25 ml/min/m²: 0.6 g/kg/day If unable to maintain an adequate energy intake: 0.75 g/kg Nephrotic syndrome: 0.8-1.0 g/kg	1.2; at least 50% high biologic value	1.2-1.3; at least 50% high biologic value
Energy (kcal/kg) If patient <90% or greater than 115% of median standard weight, use aBW$_{ef}$*	35-40 kcal/kg, depending on nutritional status and stress factors GFR<25 ml/min, 35 kcal/kg for those younger than 60 years of age and 30-35 kcal/kg for those 60 years and older	30-35 (125-145) if ≥ 60 yr and 35 (145) if < 60 yr	30-35 (125-145) if ≥ 60 yr and 35 (145) if < 60 yr For continuous ambulatory peritoneal dialysis (CAPD) and automated or "cycler" peritoneal dialysis (APD) include dialysate calories
Phosphorus	10-20 mg/g protein	800-1200 mg/day or <17 mg/kg	1200 mg/day or <17 mg/kg
Sodium	Varies with cause; usual is NAS 2-4 g/day	2000-3000 mg/day (88-130 mmol/day)	Individualized based on blood pressure and weight; CAPD and APD, 3000-4000 mg/day (130-175 mmol/day)
Potassium	Usually not restricted until GFR is <10 ml/min	40 mg/kg or approximately 2000-3000 mg/day (50-80 mmol/day)	Generally unrestricted with CAPD and APD (approximately 3000-4000 mg/day [80-102 mmol/day]) unless serum level is increased or decreased
Fluid	As indicated by medical status	500-1000 ml/day plus daily urine output	CAPD and APD approximately 2000-3000 ml/day based on daily weight fluctuations, urine output, ultrafiltration, and blood pressure; Unrestricted if weight and blood pressure are controlled and residual renal function is 2-3 L/day
Calcium	1-1.5 g/day	Approximately 1000-1800 mg/day; supplement as needed to maintain normal serum level	Same as for hemodialysis
Vitamins and minerals	RDA for B complex, C, D, and iron; individualize zinc, calcium, and vitamin D	Vitamin C, 60-100 mg; B$_6$, 5-10 mg; folic acid; 0.8-1 mg; RDA for others; individualize zinc, calcium, and vitamin D	Same as for hemodialysis

HBV, High biologic value; *NAS,* no added salt.

*aBW$_{ef}$= adjusted edema-free body weight

removal of unwanted solutes, fluid and electrolyte balance must be maintained. This is accomplished by passing blood across a selective membrane that is exposed to some rinsing fluid (dialysate). Dialysates have varying ion and mineral compositions.[56] The dialysate does not come into direct contact with the blood.

Currently two major types of dialysis replacement therapy are used for outpatients with ESRD: HD and PD.[4] Of the latter, there are two main types: continuous ambulatory peritoneal dialysis (CAPD) and continuous cycling peritoneal dialysis (CCPD).[57,58]

Regardless of the dialysis technique, all methods require a selective, permeable membrane that allows passage of water and small-molecular weight molecules and ions but excludes large-molecular weight molecules such as proteins. In HD, this membrane is a man-made dialyzer sometimes referred to as *an artificial kidney*. The most common types are the hollow fiber and parallel-plate dialyzers.[46] In PD, the lining of the patient's peritoneal wall serves as the selective membrane.[57-58]

Dialysis replacement therapy requires access to the patient's circulatory system. For HD, the preferred permanent access site is an arteriovenous (AV) fistula, created surgically by fashioning in the forearm a subcutaneous anastomosis of the radial artery and the cephalic vein.[56,59] If the patient's veins are not adequate for this procedure, an arteriovenous graft can be created with polytetrafluoroethylene (Teflon).[59]

The grafts can be punctured repeatedly by the arterial and venous needlesticks required for each dialysis treatment (typically 3 times per week for 3 to 4 hours). Blood travels through a needle placed into the arterial side of the graft. The needle is attached to tubing that leads to the hollow fibers of the dialyzer, or between the sheets of membranes in the parallel plate design.[60] While blood passes through the dialyzer, dialysate simultaneously passes around the artificial membrane. Pressure gradients applied to the dialysate affect fluid and solute removal.[61] The blood then returns to the patient through the venous side (Fig. 33-2).

In PD, access to the patient's blood supply is gained via a catheter of silicone rubber or polyurethane, placed surgically into the peritoneal cavity.[57-58] The Tenckhoff catheter is one of the most widely used peritoneal access devices. In this procedure, dialysate is introduced into the peritoneum through the peritoneal catheter. Solutes from the plasma circulating in the vessels and capillaries perfusing the peritoneal wall pass across the peritoneal membrane into the dialysate, which is subsequently removed and discarded (Fig. 33-3).[57-58]

The dialysate for PD is available with a range of dextrose concentrations, which alter the osmolality of the dialysate and assist in fluid removal.[57-58] In addition, the dwell time (i.e., how long the dialysate remains in the peritoneum) and the number of exchanges (i.e., how many bags of dialysate and the total volume of each) used in 24 hours also affect the amount of fluid and solute removal.

A wide variety of renal replacement therapies are available for use with ARF, including intermittent hemodialysis (IHD), intermittent peritoneal dialysis (IPD), intermittent hemofiltration (IHF), and CRRT.[62-64] Currently nine different CRRT methods are available to treat ARF. They differ in route of access to the circulatory system (arteriovenous versus venovenous) and method of solute clearance.[23] The effects of these dialysis procedures on nutrient requirements and nutrition management are reviewed in the sections that follow.

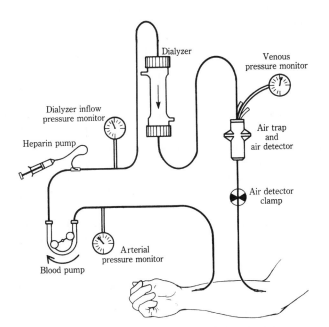

FIGURE 33-2 The blood circuit, showing the usual location of the pressure monitors. The alternative location of the "arterial" pressure monitor between the blood pump and the dialyzer is also shown. (From Daugirdas J, Van Stone J, Boag J: Hemodialysis apparatus. In Daugirdas JT, Blake PG, Ing TS [eds]: *Handbook of dialysis,* ed 3, Philadelphia, 2001, Lippincott Williams & Wilkins, pp 61.)

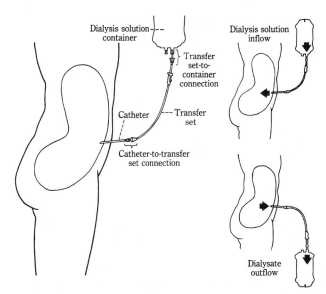

FIGURE 33-3 Basic continuous ambulatory peritoneal dialysis system with catheter, a "straight" transfer set, and dialysis solution container. On the right, inflow and outflow are depicted. Adapted from Cogan MG, Garovoy MR [eds]: *Introduction to dialysis,* New York, 1985, Churchill Livingstone.

Altered Nutrient Requirements in Chronic Renal Failure

SODIUM AND WATER. Healthy kidneys normally maintain sodium balance by adjusting sodium excretion in relation to dietary intake. When dietary salt intake increases, urinary sodium excretion increases proportionally over a 3-day period, as does fluid intake, resulting in weight gain. When salt intake is reduced, sodium excretion decreases and body water and body weight are lost.[65]

As kidney function declines (as evidenced by decreased GFR), the ability of the nephrons to maintain sodium balance through sodium excretion falls. However, until late stages of CRF, an adaptive mechanism permits continued sodium excretion. The undamaged nephrons excrete a higher percentage of filtered sodium, with the effect being decreased fractional reabsorption of sodium by the renal tubules and increased fractional excretion. It is when the GFR falls to less than 4 to 10 ml per minute that dietary sodium restriction is usually necessary to maintain sodium balance. At this level of kidney function, adequate sodium excretion cannot usually occur if the patient's sodium intake is a typical 160 mEq (4 g) per day.[65,66] However, the decision to implement dietary sodium restriction depends on the patient's fluid status, urinary sodium excretion, and the presence or absence of hypertension.

During renal replacement therapy urine output usually continues to decline in proportion to the decline in the GFR. Many patients become anuric. Fluid intake must be controlled and prescribed individually. Balance of both sodium and water is maintained by dietary intake equaling removal by dialysis plus any losses incurred via residual renal function.[67-69]

Sodium and water intake that exceeds the failing kidney's regulatory and excretory capacity can have detrimental effects. Symptoms that reflect this include shortness of breath, hypertension, congestive heart failure, and edema. These symptoms are due in part to the expansion of intravascular and interstitial fluid volume. A high sodium intake may cause thirst, which prompts the person to drink and, subsequently, to develop hypervolemia. Fluid intake is best controlled by restricting salt intake.[67-69]

The average dialysis patient without extra losses has insensible water losses (via respiration, sweat, and stool) of 400 to 500 ml per day. Daily fluid intake for dialysis patients should equal urinary output plus 500 to 1000 ml to cover insensible losses, or the amount needed to avoid more than a 2.5-kg weight gain between dialysis treatments.[12,67] Recommended sodium intake is 86.9 to 130 mEq (2.0 to 3.0 g) per day for HD patients and 130.4 to 173.9 mEq (3 to 4 g) for those receiving PD.[70] Predialysis patients typically do not require fluid restriction. Salt restriction is determined individually and might be indicated for blood pressure control or medical management of conditions associated with fluid retention.[12,70]

POTASSIUM. The kidneys regulate potassium balance by excreting potassium in an amount equal to that absorbed in the GI tract. Normally, potassium absorption is 90% to 95% complete, the remainder being excreted in the stool. Potassium balance depends on kidney tubule potassium secretion, unlike sodium regulation, which is dependent upon the excretory functional ability.[1,12,67]

As kidney failure progresses, the ability of the tubules to secrete potassium decreases. Nephron adaptation occurs to maintain potassium balance by increasing the amount secreted by the tubules and by increasing the amount excreted into the stool. As much as 20% to 50% of ingested potassium can appear in the stool when the GFR drops to less than 5 ml per minute. These two adaptations are sufficient to maintain potassium balance with normal potassium intake (100 mEq per day, 3900 mg) when the GFR is greater than 10 ml per minute, and the patient has a urine output of at least 1000 ml per day. Once the patient becomes oliguric or GFR drops to less than 10 ml per minute, dietary potassium restriction is necessary to maintain serum levels in the normal range of 3.5 to 5.0 mEq/L.[67,71]

Dietary potassium restriction for HD patients is required to avoid the consequences of hyperkalemia. Potassium accumulates in the body between dialysis treatments unless the patient has GI losses or a urine output greater than 500 ml/day. Hyperkalemia can be caused by eating potassium-dense foods or potassium supplements or can be secondary to catabolism, hemolysis, acidemia, or oliguria.[67,71]

The recommended potassium intake for HD patients is 51.2 to 75 mEq (2000 to 3000 mg) per day.[70] Consuming too much potassium induces hyperkalemia, which can be life threatening. Symptoms include cardiac arrhythmias and neurologic disturbances such as muscle weakness and flaccid quadriplegia. Patients must be monitored for hypokalemia and treated appropriately. Because of the number of exchanges and dwell times, PD results in a more continuous potassium clearance than does IHD. Therefore, patients receiving PD therapy can have a more liberal diet intake of potassium, 76.9 to 102.5 mEq (3000 to 4000 mg) per day, or in some cases, an unrestricted intake.[70]

PHOSPHORUS, CALCIUM, AND VITAMIN D. The metabolic derangements of calcium, phosphorus, and vitamin D associated with CRF result in bone disease referred to as *renal osteodystrophy*. The disease affects the skeletal system in a combination of four potential forms in varying proportions: osteitis fibrosa cystica secondary to classic hyperparathyroidism; osteomalacia, which results from excessive and unclarified bone matrix; osteopenia, or decreased bone mass; and osteosclerosis, increased bone density.[72-76] A brief overview of the events believed to precipitate renal osteodystrophy follows.

The kidney filters approximately 7 g of phosphorus daily, of which 80% to 90% is reabsorbed by the renal tubules and the remainder is excreted in the urine. In early renal failure, hyperphosphatemia is prevented by an adaptive increase in kidney phosphate excretion and decreased tubular phosphate resorption. Not until the GFR falls to less than 20 ml per minute does hyperphosphatemia usually become evident.[67]

There is an important relationship between serum phosphate and calcium levels. As phosphate is retained and the serum level rises, serum calcium decreases as a result of calcium-phosphate salt precipitation and deposition in bone and soft tissue. The low serum calcium level stimulates secretion of parathyroid hormone (PTH), which reduces tubular phosphate reabsorption by the kidney tubules and enhances bone resorption of calcium. A new steady state of calcium and phosphorus is then achieved at the expense of elevated circulating levels of PTH, which are needed to maintain calcium and phosphorus homeostasis as renal failure progresses. This sequence of events occurs early in the course of renal failure and may be a major factor in the development of renal osteodystrophy and ultimately mortality.[72,77,78]

As renal failure progresses, the damaged kidney does not respond to PTH for increased excretion. Phosphorus continues to accumulate as less is being filtered by the kidney. Serum phosphorus levels rise and dietary restriction becomes necessary. Dietary phosphorus restriction of 800 to 1200 mg/day or less than 17 mg/kg of body weight per day is commonly recommended.[70] Diet restriction alone is not sufficient to maintain normal serum levels. Phosphate-binding medications (e.g. calcium-containing agents or noncalcemic agents such as sevelamer hydrochloride), which prevent GI absorption of dietary phosphorus, are also frequently prescribed. Elevated phosphorus, calcium X phosphorus product (the calcium phosphorus product is the product of the serum calcium level multiplied by the serum phosphorus level), and PTH levels have been demonstrated to be independently associated with increased morbidity and mortality.[75,79]

Problems related to bone resorption and impaired mineralization of newly formed bone are exacerbated by the decreased availability or absence of the active form of vitamin D (1,25-dihydroxycholecalciferol). The kidney is the major site of conversion of the biologically inactive form of vitamin D (25-hydroxycholecalciferol) to the biologically active one. A deficiency of this metabolite is responsible for the development of osteomalacia and disorders of calcium, phosphorus, magnesium, and muscle metabolism.[72,77,78]

Vitamin D is available for pharmaceutical administration in the form of vitamin D_2 (ergocalciferol), vitamin D_3 (cholecalciferol), dihydrotachysterol, and the active form 1,25-dihydroxycholecalciferol (calcitriol). They all increase intestinal calcium and phosphorus absorption. Recently, vitamin D analogs have become available for use including paracalcitol and doxercalciferol. Both the oral and intravenous forms of calcitriol and vitamin D analogs suppress PTH and can normalize elevated levels. The latter have minimal impact on calcium and phosphorus. A usual starting dose of any of these products is dependent on the severity of the disease.[78,80-85] Of interest, new calcimimetic agents that act directly on the parathyroid calcium receptors to decrease PTH production are currently under investigation and may prove beneficial in this area.[86]

Careful monitoring of calcium, phosphorus, and PTH levels and subsequent titration of vitamin D or vitamin D analogs is essential in managing secondary hyperparathyroidism. The specific clinical indices are currently under reexamination, with recommendations forthcoming from the National Kidney Foundation's Kidney Disease Outcomes Quality Initiative (K/DOQI).

PROTEIN AND CALORIES. Malnutrition is a long-standing problem in kidney disease patients. Recent surveys report the prevalence of mild to moderate malnutrition at 18% to 59% for the CAPD patient population and 33% for the HD patient.[87] Approximately 8% to 37% of patients are severely malnourished.[87] Factors that contribute to this problem include anorexia of unknown cause, the use of bioincompatible membranes, metabolic acidosis, protein and amino acid losses into dialysate, intercurrent illness, and endocrine disorders.[54,87,88]

Inadequate dietary intake is a major cause of wasting. Anorexia associated with chronic disease, uremia, and psychologic depression as well as alterations in GI function and taste can lead to inadequate oral intake. In addition, malnutrition and wasting may increase morbidity including loss of vigor; poor rehabilitation; poor quality of life; and ultimately, mortality.[87-91]

Protein requirements for adults receiving maintenance dialysis are affected by several factors related to the process itself, such as the type of dialyzer membrane (biocompatible or incompatible) and the method of dialyzer reuse.[54,92,93] HD induces loss of amino acids, the degree depending on the type of dialyzer membrane, blood flow rate, and dialyzer reuse procedure. Mean losses of 7.2 g of dialysate amino acid losses per dialysis using a traditional cellulosic membrane, 6.1 g per dialysis using low-flux polymethylmethacrylate membrane, and 8.0 g per dialysis using a high-flux polysulfone membrane have been reported. The difference in amino acid loss between the cellulosic membranes and the high-flux dialyzer was statistically significant. Patients receiving CAPD lose approximately 5 to 12 g of total protein including 2 to 4 g of free amino acids per day.[94]

Additional factors in protein requirements include alterations in amino acid metabolism and gut resorption. For example, loss of amino acids during HD is believed to alter intracellular amino acid pools and to affect protein metabolism. Metabolic acidosis, common in dialysis patients, has been shown to induce muscle catabolism.[94,95] The recommended dietary protein intake for dialysis patients is 1.2 to 1.3 g of protein per kilogram of body weight per day.[54,70]

The dietary protein recommendations for predialysis patients are somewhat controversial. Results from the Modification of Diet in Renal Disease (MDRD) study indicate that patients whose GFR is 25 to 55 ml per minute per 1.73 m^2 should eat at least 0.8 g of protein per kilogram per day, and for those whose GFR is less than 25 ml per minute per 1.73 m^2 and not receiving dialysis, 0.6 g of protein per kilogram per day is recommended.[54,96-98] A study group of the National Kidney Foundation's Kidney Disease Outcomes Quality Initiative (K/DOQI) has recently reviewed the medical literature and published a dietary protein recommendation for predialysis patients by 2002. (See Table 33-2).

Fifty percent of protein ingested by renal patients is recommended to be of high biologic quality. The biologic value of a protein expresses the percentage of absorbed nitrogen that is retained by the body for growth and maintenance. If an adequate amount of high-biologic value protein is not consumed, negative nitrogen balance may result, which causes an increase in BUN secondary to tissue catabolism.

A similar situation results when calorie intake is inadequate. Once protein requirements are met, carbohydrates and fats are needed to provide the remainder of calories. Inadequate dietary intake of carbohydrates and fats leads to protein catabolism for energy and accumulation of nitrogenous wastes in the blood stream.

Energy expenditure of predialysis patients is comparable to that of normal healthy persons. Nitrogen balance becomes more positive as energy intake is increased. Predialysis patients tend to have inadequate intakes and may become malnourished by the time dialysis is started; the daily calorie intake recommended is 35 kcal/kg of ideal body weight for individuals less than 60 years old and 30 to 35 kcal/kg for those 60 years old or older.[54] The exceptions are obese persons (more than 120% of ideal body weight) and malnourished ones. The latter group may require more calories for repletion.[6]

It is well accepted that adequate energy intake is imperative to maintaining energy stores and optimizing protein metabolism.[54,99,100] The measured energy expenditure of dialysis patients is the same as that of healthy persons.[99] Based on available research, current caloric recommendations for dialysis patients are 35 kcal/kg per day for patients less than 60 years of age and 30 kcal/kg per day for those 60 years of age or older.[54] Dialysis patients, however, typically consume 23 to 27 kcal/kg per day.[101] Depending on the results of ongoing research, the current caloric recommendations may be modified.

Because nitrogen balance depends so much on adequate calorie intake, proper calorie and protein intake are extremely important for predialysis and dialysis patients. This is true regardless of the route of nutrient administration (oral, enteral, or parenteral). Table 33-2 summarizes nutrient recommendations for stable adult patients with kidney disease based on treatment modality. The ideal diet prescription takes into account the patient's age, sex, weight, ethnic origin, dialysis protocol, disease, nutritional and metabolic status, and activity level.

WATER AND FAT-SOLUBLE VITAMINS. Adult dialysis patients usually have low blood levels of the water-soluble vitamins unless they take a vitamin supplement. The causes include losses induced by dialysis; dietary restrictions of protein, potassium, and phosphorus; anorexia and reduced food intake; and alterations in metabolism. Supplementation is in order at levels of the National Academy of Sciences/National Research Council Recommended Dietary Allowances (RDA) for water-soluble vitamins. Additional amounts are needed for pyridoxine (B_6), folate, and ascorbic acid.[101,102] The recommended amounts for each of these for dialysis patients are 10 mg for vitamin B_6, 0.8 to 1 mg for folate, and 60 mg for ascorbic acid.[102,103] The same amounts are recommend for patients with chronic disease, except that 5 mg of pyridoxine is recommended.[6]

Increased requirement for vitamin B_6 by dialysis patients is evidenced by low plasma and red blood cell pyridoxine levels and low plasma levels of the vitamin's coenzyme, pyridoxine phosphate. Abnormal lymphocyte function, depressed immune response, and abnormal plasma leucine and valine levels in this patient population have been ameliorated by pyridoxine supplementation.[104]

Reduced plasma and leukocyte ascorbic acid levels have been reported in dialysis patients and are most likely due to restriction of fruits and vegetables necessary for control of potassium intake and to dialysis losses. Dietary supplementation in excess of 60 mg per day of ascorbic acid is not recommended, however, to avoid hyperoxalosis.[103]

Inadequate dietary intake, dialysis-induced losses of approximately 37% per session, and altered metabolism are possible causes of folate deficiency. Low plasma and serum folate levels and inhibition in membrane transport of this vitamin by anions such as phosphate have been observed in dialysis patients.[103,105]

Vitamin A and retinol-binding protein are normally cleared by the kidneys and therefore become elevated as renal function

deteriorates. Vitamin A supplementation should be avoided to prevent vitamin A toxicity.[102,106,107] Vitamin K replacement is not indicated unless intestinal flora are suppressed by antibiotic therapy. Although vitamin E supplementation has not been shown to be required, it may prove to be of some benefit.[108-110] Special vitamin supplements for dialysis patients that meet these requirements are available, depending on the formulation, either over the counter or by prescription.

Minerals and Trace Elements

The dietary requirements for trace elements are not known, and, with the exception of iron, supplementation is not usually recommended. Adequacy of diet and the nutritional and medical status of the predialysis patient determine the need for supplementation of vitamins and minerals.[101,102]

Hypermagnesemia may be present because magnesium normally is excreted mainly by the kidneys. Although the "renal diet" tends to contain less magnesium than a typical American diet, active restriction of dietary magnesium usually is not necessary to maintain normal serum levels. Hypermagnesemia has been induced by ingestion of magnesium-containing antacids, enemas, and laxatives.

The requirement for iron is affected by intake, dialysis-induced blood losses, frequent laboratory testing, decreased production of erythropoietin, shortened erythrocyte life span, hemolysis, impaired intestinal iron absorption, and occult GI bleeding. All of these factors are likely to cause iron-deficiency anemia.[11]

Replacement therapy with recombinant human erythropoietin (rHuEPO) has been shown to reverse the anemia associated with CRF. As the hemoglobin mass increases, more iron is needed.[8,111-113] Certain laboratory parameters must be evaluated regularly to determine whether patients need supplemental iron and how much. Percentage of transferrin saturation (iron/total iron-binding capacity × 100), indicating bone marrow iron stores (or "available" iron) and serum ferritin levels (indicating tissue iron stores), must be closely monitored.[11] If the serum ferritin level declines, intravenous iron supplementation may be necessary.

Low plasma zinc levels observed in dialysis patients may be due to the diet restriction of protein, impaired zinc absorption, redistribution of the body pool zinc, or a change in zinc binding to plasma protein. Uremic symptoms of hypogeusia, sexual impotence, and anorexia have been reported to improve when subjects were given zinc supplementation in clinical trials. Routine zinc replacement is not generally prescribed.[104]

The effects of aluminum retention are a concern for dialysis patients. Accumulation of aluminum in cerebral gray matter may be responsible for the dialysis encephalopathy syndrome. Aluminum has also been noted to accumulate in bone and may play a role in renal osteodystrophy. Medications containing aluminum should not be prescribed to these patients.[114]

CARNITINE. L-Carnitine (1-3-hydroxy-4-N-trimethylaminobutyrate) is an amino acid whose main function is to transfer long-chain fatty acids from the cytoplasm through the inner membrane of the mitochondria for oxidation.[22,54,115] A carnitine deficiency can result in inefficient energy production, impaired oxidation of long-chain fatty acids, and abnormal lipid metabolism.[56] The high incidences of cardiomyopathy, skeletal myopathy, and dyslipidemia that characterize the dialysis patient population have prompted investigators to question whether carnitine deficiency contributes to these problems.

Predialysis patients do, indeed, have elevated plasma levels of free carnitine. Elevated levels of acyl carnitine have been observed in predialysis, HD, and PD patients.[56] HD has been found to decrease plasma carnitine; however, the losses do not exceed those that would occur with normal urinary excretion.[56] Total skeletal muscle carnitine content can be low or normal in HD patients. It appears that a small subpopulation of HD patients has severe carnitine deficiency.[54] The prevalence in predialysis and PD patients is less clear.

The National Kidney Foundation's K/DOQI Nutrition Work Group evaluated the literature on carnitine. The expert panel concluded that evidence is insufficient to recommend the routine use of carnitine for any clinical disorders, including elevated triglycerides, cardiovascular disease, or anemia.[54] A trial of L-carnitine may be considered in specific individuals who are symptomatic of a carnitine deficiency and have not responded to standard therapies.[54] The most promising area of carnitine use is its use in erythropoietin resistant anemia.[54,116] Several outcomes-based studies have been proposed regarding carnitine use and may suggest an expanded role for L-carnitine therapy in the future.

Nutrition Assessment and Management of Predialysis and Dialysis Patients

The following principles are applicable to patients who can maintain oral intake of the prescribed diet or who require nutrition support with enteral or parenteral intervention. Current nutrition assessment and management of adult dialysis patients routinely rely on analysis of biochemical parameters reflected by blood indices. These values are usually reported monthly for stable patients. Ideally, the blood sample should be obtained before the dialysis treatment (i.e., predialysis), after the longest interdialytic interval. It is following this period of time that peak nutrient accumulation will occur and nutrition assessment and management will be based on these values.

Serum values commonly reviewed for nutrition evaluation are BUN, creatinine, serum proteins, potassium, phosphorus, calcium, sodium, cholesterol, triglycerides, glucose, and alkaline phosphatase. Other important elements in nutrition assessment include anthropometrics, physical and clinical evaluation, and food intake information. These values are incorporated with the patient's dry weight (i.e., weight at which the patient is free of detectable peripheral edema and has normal blood pressure without postural hypotension), interdialysis weight gains, blood pressure, and food intake information to evaluate nutrition and fluid status. These values, together and alone, are reviewed in the context of the patient's previous ranges and current clinical status. The same values are collected for patients with CRF. Use of these values is discussed in the following sections. The National Kidney Foundation's K/DOQI project recently published nutrition assessment and monitoring guidelines (Table 33-3).

BLOOD UREA NITROGEN. A significant correlation between dietary protein intake and the predialysis BUN concentration has been observed when patients are clinically stable.[32,117] This value can be used to indirectly monitor the patient's protein intake. Normal BUN values for adult dialysis patients are in the range of 60 to 80 mg/dl. A BUN value higher than 100 mg/dl suggests excessive dietary protein intake, an inadequate dialysis prescription, catabolism, or gastrointestinal bleeding. A BUN value less than 60 mg/dl suggests inadequate protein intake, anabolism, residual renal function not accounted for in the dialysis prescription, or an inappropriate dialysis prescription. For CRF patients, previously normal BUN values begin to rise as kidney function deteriorates. For these patients, creatinine clearance is regularly calculated to monitor renal function.

The predialysis BUN value, which correlates with dietary protein intake, is relied on to assess and manage dialysis patients. A major drawback is that, by itself or with other assessment parameters, the BUN value cannot quantify the deviation in protein intake, nor does it describe the cause for its variance. It is the dietitian's responsibility to integrate BUN

TABLE 33-3

K/DOQI Recommended Measures for Monitoring Nutritional Status of Maintenance Dialysis Patients

Category	Measure	Minimum Frequency of Measurement
I. Measurements that should be performed routinely in all patients	● Predialysis or stabilized serum albumin	● Monthly
	● % of usual postdialysis (MHD) or postdrain (CPD) body weight	● Monthly
	● % of standard (NHANES II) body weight	● Every 4 months
	● Subjective global assessment (SGA)	● Every 6 months
	● Dietary interview and/or diary	● Every 6 months
	● nPNA	● Monthly MHD; every 3-4 months CPD
II. Measures that can be useful to confirm or extend the data obtained from the measures in Category I	● Predialysis or stabilized serum prealbumin	● As needed
	● Skinfold thickness	● As needed
	● Mid-arm muscle area, circumference, or diameter	● As needed
	● Dual energy x-ray absorptiometry	● As needed
III. Clinically useful measures, which, if low, might suggest the need for a more rigorous examination of protein-energy nutritional status	● Predialysis or stabilized serum —Creatinine —Urea nitrogen —Cholesterol	● As needed
	● Creatinine index	● As needed

MHD, maintenance hemodialysis, *CPD*, chronic peritoneal dialysis, *NHANES II* = National Health and Nutrition Examination Survey, *nPNa*, normalized protein nitrogen appearance.
From Recommended measures for monitoring nutritional status of maintenance dialysis patients, Adult Guidelines, *Am J Kidney Diseases*, 35(6), s19, 2000.

with other laboratory and clinical parameters, develop the clinical picture, and counsel the patient in nutrition management.[118]

Even when the BUN value is integrated with the serum albumin and dry body weight, early detection of compromised protein intake may not be accomplished. The BUN may be low for the patient but still within normal range. The albumin concentration may not decrease that particular month in response to the decreased protein intake, nor might a change in the patient's dry weight be noticed. It could be a few months before the clinical parameters reflect a compromised protein intake, preventing the dietitian from functioning in a preventive fashion. Calculation of the normalized protein catabolic rate (nPCR) can assist in identifying patients with compromised protein intake, before the onset of malnutrition becomes apparent. The nPCR should be incorporated into the nutrition assessment procedure for both the predialysis and dialysis patient whenever it can be made available.

CREATININE/CREATININE INDEX. The serum level of creatinine, a by-product of normal muscle metabolism, can be used to evaluate the nutritional status of stable, noncatabolic dialysis patients. Creatinine is formed at a fairly constant rate and may be used to assess muscle mass.[54] Creatinine index is the creatinine synthesis rate and is also related to muscle mass.[54] Low values may reflect inadequate somatic protein stores. Of note, if a patient is catabolic or anabolic over time, these values may decrease or increase accordingly and should be interpreted with caution.

SERUM PROTEINS. Total protein, transferrin, albumin, and prealbumin levels are all commonly used for nutrition assessment of visceral stores. In patients with renal disease, the specificity and reliability of these parameters for nutritional status is questionable because of the metabolic derangements associated with the uremic state. For example, transferrin, albumin, and prealbumin levels are all affected by hydration status. Serum transferrin levels are altered by iron status. With iron deficiency, transferrin is falsely elevated, whereas it becomes falsely depressed in the presence of iron overload. Serum albumin has a long half-life (18 to 20 days) and often is a late marker of malnutrition. However, low serum albumin levels are often accompanied by abnormal levels of other indices that reflect malnutrition (e.g., anthropometrics, total lymphocyte count, serum transferrin) and are usually interpreted to indicate a state of poor nutrition. The sensitivity of serum albumin in this regard continues to be challenged.

Nonnutritional factors affecting serum albumin metabolism of renal patients and the implications of these factors on the utility of serum albumin as a marker of malnutrition have recently been identified. These factors include responses to inflammation (i.e., synthesis of acute-phase reactant proteins such as C-reactive protein and cytokine release), acute metabolic acidosis, and the hormonal milieu.[38]

Serum prealbumin has a shorter half-life (2 days) than albumin and for this reason has been considered to be a more sensitive nutritional measure. It may be falsely elevated in euvolemic patients with CRF because the serum level is associated with the level of kidney function.[7,26] Nonetheless, prealbumin levels less than 30 mg/dl in dialysis patients are associated with increased mortality.[54] In addition, because prealbumin has been directly correlated to changes in nutritional status, it can be useful to serially monitor a patient with stable renal function over time.[7]

Of these three serum proteins, serum albumin is currently the parameter most frequently used to assess visceral stores in both predialysis patients and ESRD patients receiving renal replacement therapy. This is most likely because of its wide availability and association with outcome. Serum albumin levels have been extensively correlated with mortality in HD patients.[54,119,120] Lowrie and Lew[119] reported a twofold increase in the relative risk of death for patients with serum albumin levels in the normal range of 3.5 to 4.0 g/dl, as compared with the upper range of normal, 4.0 to 4.5 g/dl. For patients whose serum albumin is in the range of 2.5 g/dl, the risk of death was nearly 20 times that for patients whose albumin levels were 4.0 to 4.5 g/dl. These and other studies that document a direct relation between malnutrition and outcome in kidney patients have heightened awareness of the magnitude of the problem and of the need to identify interventions for malnutrition.

IGF-1, a serum protein with mitogenic properties and insulin-like activities, may be a sensitive biochemical indicator of nitrogen balance. A serum IGF-1 concentration less than 200 ng/ml has been reported to indicate poor nutritional status.[26] Moreover, current research suggests treatment with recombinant human IGF-1 may induce an anabolic response in malnourished dialysis patients.[40,45,46] However, serum IGF-1 and recombinant IGF-1 injections are not readily available in the majority of clinics. Additional research is needed before definitive recommendations can be offered.

SODIUM, POTASSIUM, PHOSPHORUS, AND CALCIUM. Sodium, potassium, phosphorus, and calcium values, along with the patient's dry weight, blood pressure, intradialytic weight gain, and BUN, are typically monitored monthly for stable patients. The nonserum parameters can be monitored more frequently because of their greater availability; dry weight, interdialytic weight gain, and predialysis and postdialysis blood pressure are all recorded at each treatment. Causes of fluctuations in these values must be determined and discussed with the patient. The causes of abnormal values dictate nutrition management. For example, if the values for BUN, potassium, and phosphorus are all elevated, this might be due to tissue catabolism; inadequate dialysis; and/or excessive oral, enteral, or parenteral protein intake. The different combinations of altered serum values and their implications are described elsewhere.[7]

LIPIDS. The most prevalent abnormal lipid profile observed in the renal patient population is increased serum triglyceride, low-density lipoprotein (LDL), very low-density lipoprotein (VLDL), and a low serum high-density lipoprotein (HDL) cholesterol.[121] Patients receiving CAPD treatment may also have high total cholesterol and VLDL levels.[6] The alterations in lipid metabolism observed in uremia patients that are thought to contribute to the development of dyslipidemia in renal disease include enhanced hepatic production of triglyceride-rich lipoproteins (VLDL, LDL), impaired catabolism of lipoproteins, decreased activity of lipoprotein lipase in plasma and adipose tissue, and decreased levels of hepatic lipase and lecithin-cholesterol acyltransferase.[121,122]

Low cholesterol levels are associated with malnutrition, morbidity, and mortality.[119,123,124] Hypocholesterolemia is common in CRF patients, especially those undergoing HD.

Lowrie and Lew[119] reported doubling of the risk for death in this population when serum cholesterol levels were less than 150 mg/dl. Normal cholesterol and triglyceride values are difficult to maintain but that is the goal for these patients.

GLUCOSE. Abnormal carbohydrate metabolism is frequently observed in renal disease, especially for patients approaching ESRD because of uremia, infection, or peripheral insulin resistance. Patients with insulin-dependent diabetes may require a smaller insulin dose or discontinuation of insulin because of decreased insulin clearance by the kidneys. On the other hand, glucose levels may be higher in nondiabetic patients approaching ESRD because of altered glucose metabolism secondary to altered insulin response and secretion. Therefore, close monitoring of insulin and diet is necessary. Both may have to be adjusted during progression of renal disease. Ideally, normal glucose levels should be maintained in kidney patients with and without diabetes to prevent the complications of hypoglycemia or hyperglycemia.[5]

Patients undergoing peritoneal dialysis may develop glucose intolerance and gain weight because they absorb glucose from the dialysate. Thus, calculation of energy requirements for PD patients must take into consideration the amount of glucose absorbed during the procedure.[70]

Glucose adsorption varies among patients on the same dialysis regimen because of variability in the permeability characteristics of an individual peritoneal membrane. However, various methods are available to approximate glucose absorption and, thus, the contribution of calories from the dialysis procedure. An example of this calculation in shown in Box 33-4.

ALKALINE PHOSPHATASE. Alkaline phosphatase is an enzyme produced mainly in the liver, bones, and kidneys. Renal failure can disrupt normal skeletal metabolism, resulting in renal osteodystrophy. When this occurs, increased quantities of alkaline phosphatase are secreted. This elevation can be used as an indicator of bone disease in kidney patients. Liver abnormalities may need to be investigated when serum alkaline phosphatase levels are increased, especially if other indices indicate liver dysfunction.[72]

BOX 33-4

Sample Calculation of Calories Contributed from the Dextrose Exchanges Used in Peritoneal Dialysis[125]

---

1. Calculate the total grams of dextrose in each exchange used by the patient over the course of 24 hours.
2. Multiply the total number of grams of dextrose by 3.4 kcal (monohydrous dextrose; for anhydrous dextrose, the conversion factor is 3.7 kcal/g dextrose).
3. Multiply the total kilocalories by the estimated absorption rate of 70%. The product is the estimated number of calories gained from the dialysate (referred to as *exchanges*.)

EXAMPLE: If a patient dialyzed with two 1-L exchanges of 1.5%, one 2-L exchange of 4.25%, and one 2-L exchange of 2.5%, the total amount of dextrose would be

Two 1-L exchanges of 1.5% = 30 g dextrose (15 g/L × 2)
One 2-L exchange of 4.25% = 85 g dextrose (42.5 g/L × 2)
One 2-L exchange of 2.5% = 50 g dextrose (25 g/L × 2)
  Thus, 30 + 85 + 50 g dextrose = 165 g dextrose × 3.4 kcal/g = 561 kcal dextrose × 0.70 (estimated absorption rate, 70%) = 392.7 kcal
This patient took in approximately 393 kcal during the dialysis procedure.

ANTHROPOMETRY. Anthropometry includes body weight (dry weight for dialysis patients), height, triceps skinfold, abdominal circumference, calf circumference, midarm muscle circumference, elbow breadth, and subscapular skinfold and provides information about the distribution of body fat and skeletal muscle mass.[36,54,126,127] Over time, these measurements identify nutrition deficiencies or excesses in calorie and protein reserves compared with standardized percentiles.

One of the problems with using anthropometrics to assess the nutritional status of kidney disease patients is that the reference values used are from measurements obtained on healthy individuals. It is less than ideal to assess the nutritional status of a renal patient by comparing the measurements to those of age- or sex-matched healthy persons because of the known alterations in body composition associated with uremia and the presence of edema.

A special procedure is recommended for taking anthropometric measures of patients receiving maintenance HD. In other patients, anthropometry is performed on the nondominant arm, whereas in HD patients the dominant arm is often used because the contralateral one is used for venous access. Experts recommend that to minimize the problem of edema, measurements be made during the last hour of dialysis.[118] For all of these reasons, the best use of anthropometrics for CRF patients who do not yet require or are receiving renal replacement therapy is to monitor for changes in body composition over time. For routine care, measurements are recommended every 3 to 6 months.[118]

Other methods of assessing body composition include dual-energy x-ray absorptiometry and bioelectrical impedance.[54,128,129] These techniques are accurate, but they are not without limitations that prevent widescale use. Limitations include cost, safety, radiation dose, patient acceptance, equipment availability, and facilities.[7] As a result, these techniques are used principally in research and their routine use is not recommended.[54]

PHYSICAL AND CLINICAL EVALUATION. Wasting syndrome, a protein-calorie malnutrition prevalent in the dialysis population, is sometimes seen in predialysis patients. It is characterized by decreased relative body weight (patient's body weight divided by "normal of weight" for the same age range, height, gender, and skeletal frame size), skinfold thickness, arm muscle mass, and total body nitrogen.[6]

Clinical evaluation of muscle wasting, depleted adipose stores, signs of macronutrient and micronutrient deficiencies (hair loss; dry, flaky skin), and fluid status (as reflected by skin turgor, peripheral edema, hypertension, shortness of breath, and increased thirst) are all important components of the physical examination.[7]

Another method of assessment used to assess protein-energy status is *subjective global assessment* (SGA).[7,54,129,130] SGA requires evaluating subjective and objective patient information, including the medical history and physical examination. On completion of the evaluation, the patient is classified into various nutritional status categories from well-nourished to severely malnourished. This technique was originally devised for nutrition assessment of general surgery patients but has been validated for use in peritoneal dialysis patients. The National Kidney Foundation's K/DOQI recommends the SGA as part of routine nutrition monitoring.

PATIENT-REPORTED FOOD INTAKE. Obtaining patient-reported food intake is an important component of the nutrition care of the patient with CRF.[7] In addition to providing the opportunity to quantitate food intake, food records reveal sources of problems related to food intake and tolerance, food habits, patterns, and allergies. The interactive nature of reported food intake provides the dietitian with an opportunity to establish a rapport with each individual patient. All of this information can be used to formulate an individual meal plan to help the patient meet his or her nutritional needs. Reported food intake can be obtained in the form of a 24-hour recall, a multiple-day food record, diet history, or food frequency. Which tool provides the most reliable and valid data is not known because the use of these different methods has not been widely studied in the renal patient population. Recently however, a Food Frequency Questionnaire was found useful in evaluating the diet intake in a cohort of HD patients.[131] More studies in this area are needed.

Regardless of the reporting method, the data should include current nutrient intake, factors that affect intake (e.g., difficulty chewing or swallowing, physical impediments to adequate intake, nausea, vomiting, diarrhea, allergies), current resources and other support systems, current medications, food preferences, cultural influences on food intake, meal patterns, meals eaten away from home, and portion sizes. Fluid intake should be reported in the same detail. Whenever possible, diet information is collected directly from the patient. Otherwise family members or caregivers are interviewed.

UREA KINETIC MODELING. The rationale for dialysis therapy is the idea that uremia is due to the accumulation of toxic substances, a function of solute concentration. How much dialysis is needed to remove which toxins, and what dialysis prescription is optimal are not known.[118]

Historically, individual patient control and adjustment of dialysis therapy were not possible. The patient had to adjust to the dialysis therapy because treatment could not be adjusted to meet the needs of the patient. In addition, evaluation for determining the adequacy of dialysis therapy and the relative importance of the various monitored outcome measurements lacked universal medical criteria. The need to develop a quantitative way to prescribe dialysis therapy on an individual basis was recognized.[60,118]

Urea kinetic modeling (UKM) was developed largely by Gotch and Sargent in the 1970s. It is a mathematical model that determines urea generation rate and uses urea nitrogen as a marker and control substance to guide dialysis treatments. It permits individualized dialysis prescription and adjustment, based on the solute kinetics of urea.[118]

The main premise underlying the model is based on the facts that urea is the major product of protein metabolism and that excessive protein intake is associated with uremic symptoms. The basic assumption of the urea kinetic model is that the requirement of dialysis is proportional to the patient's normalized protein catabolic rate (nPCR) or urea nitrogen appearance (UNA) relative to lean body mass. Being a measurable product of protein catabolism, urea can be used to monitor and define the patient's metabolic status.[60,132]

UKM provides valuable nutrition information because it measures a patient's urea generation rate, which has direct linear correlation to the nPCR. UKM has been used in a number of studies to monitor, adjust, and improve nutrition intervention and patients' nitrogen balance.[118]

The original premise was that because urea is the primary product of protein catabolism and there is a correlation between urea generation rate and nPCR, nPCR can be used to estimate nitrogen balance. When the patient is in zero nitrogen balance, nPCR equals dietary protein intake. The desired range is 1.2 to 1.3 g of protein per kilogram of dry body weight per day. In general, a stable patient's nPCR is equal to his dietary protein intake, a catabolic patient's (evidenced by weight loss, decreased serum albumin, onset of medical illness) nPCR is greater than dietary protein, and an anabolic patient's nPCR is less than protein intake. Protein balance can be calculated from the difference between dietary protein intake and nPCR. This method is best used to monitor nitrogen balance of noncatabolic patients because catabolized protein can be either endogenous or exogenous.[37,53]

Nutrition Support

In the past, particularly for predialysis and ARF patients, the principal goal of nutrition intervention was to prevent development or exacerbation of uremia symptoms, sometimes at the expense of adequate nutritional status. The rationale for this approach stemmed from the observation that limiting dietary protein might minimize generation of uremia toxins and nonessential nitrogen, delaying the start of dialysis, and perhaps even preventing progression of renal failure.

As a result, it was common to give predialysis and dialysis patients with ARF nutrition solutions that contained only essential amino acids, and dextrose if indicated. These hypocaloric, low-protein formulas did not accomplish either of the original goals. Hypercatabolism was not diminished by feeding formulas that were restricted in protein and calories, despite their being rich in essential amino acids.

In clinical practice today, the tendency is to treat patients aggressively with dialysis and to liberalize diet to meet the increased nutrient needs of the hypercatabolic state, without inducing metabolic, fluid, and electrolyte imbalances. PN formulas containing mixed amino acids (rather than essential ones only) are now used more often than those high in essential amino acids. The same is true for enteral products. However, research still continues in this area to try to identify the optimal nutrition intervention for these patients, and many issues, both new and old, continue to be topics of debate.

The key to successful nutrition support for the CRF and ARF patient populations requires:

1. Completion of a comprehensive nutrition assessment
2. Keeping current with medical and surgical care plans by participating in daily (or at least weekly) patient care rounds with medical staff and by communicating with other members of the health care team as often as needed
3. Accurate calculation of each patient's individual nutritional needs
4. Careful identification of necessary restrictions of fluid, vitamin, mineral, and electrolyte tolerance
5. Astute identification of the formulation that best meets the patient's needs without exacerbating uremia symptoms

The laboratory values required to monitor patient progress and response to nutrition intervention are the same as those outlined in the preceding section on the nutrition assessment and management of adult renal failure patients.

The monitoring protocols for patients receiving routine care and for those receiving nutrition support differ mainly in the frequency of laboratory value monitoring. When a new intervention is initiated and a patient is first demonstrating medical stability, the patient who is in the hospital should be monitored every 24 to 48 hours for weight, serum sodium, potassium, calcium, phosphorus, glucose, bicarbonate, BUN, and creatinine. Upon demonstration of proven tolerance and medical stability, thrice weekly monitoring is acceptable, except that the patient should be weighed daily. Other laboratory values, including serum albumin, lipids, and alkaline phosphatase should also be checked. Upon discharge, once or twice monthly laboratory monitoring is appropriate as long as the patient's status remains stable. Body weight should be checked once a week. Dialysis patients should be weighed before and after each treatment.

Guidelines for Enteral Nutrition Support

The enteral route for nutrient delivery should be used whenever possible.[19] Diet restrictions should be minimized to improve the overall appeal of food. In addition to enteral formulations for oral feeding, modular supplements of protein, carbohydrate, or fat can be useful to increase nutrient density.

If the patient is unable to maintain adequate oral diet intake, tube feedings should be initiated, provided that the GI tract is functioning. The feeding tube (nasoenteric or enterostomy) and administration method (continuous drip, intermittent, cyclic method) should be selected according to standard medical criteria (see Principles of Nutrition Management).

Selection of the formula depends largely on the patient's fluid allowance. If a HD patient is restricted to 1000 ml per day, a 2-kcal/ml formula of moderate protein content and low in electrolytes such as Nepro (Ross Laboratories, Columbus, Ohio) might be considered. In contrast, if fluid restriction is not an issue (e.g., for a predialysis patient) but controlling potassium and protein intake is important, Osmolite HN (Ross Laboratories) might be a good choice. Other factors that affect formula selection include protein and energy requirements; electrolyte, vitamin, and mineral status; and planned medical interventions (e.g., surgery, dialysis). Table 33-4 includes a list of enteral and modular products appropriate for ARF and CRF patients. Table 33-5 lists the supplements most often prescribed for malnourished patients receiving maintenance dialysis.

Metabolic Complications of Enteral Nutrition Support for Kidney Disease

Patients with renal failure may have delayed gastric emptying, particularly those who have diabetes and are particularly susceptible to GI disorders. Dialysis procedures, high BUN levels, and hyperglycemia have been shown to contribute to impaired gastric emptying.[62] Medications such as metoclopramide (Reglan) may be prescribed to promote gastric motility. Tube feeding must stop if decreased gastric motility does not respond to medication or if vomiting or other indications of gastric obstruction occur.[63]

Hemodynamic instability is common during HD. This is one reason why eating is not permitted during treatment in many dialysis units across the country. To avoid the potential for hypotension, tube feedings should stop 1 hour before the scheduled treatment. From the practical and the medical standpoint, patients receiving PD, which is frequently continuous or takes longer than 8 hours, do not have to discontinue tube feedings during treatment. Hypotension is uncommon during PD.[63]

Despite the fact that kidney disease patients typically exhibit abnormal retention of many substances, hypomagnesemia, hyponatremia, hypocalcemia, and hypophosphatemia can occur during EN. This would not be unexpected, for example, in a malnourished predialysis (or even dialysis) patient being given nutrients to support repletion. Adding supplements of these elements directly to the enteral solution should correct the abnormality. Thus it is very important to monitor patients' serum values regularly.

The majority of enteral products available for nutrition support provide 100% of the RDAs for most vitamins and minerals in 1 L of formula. As for dialysis patients, the recommendations of folic acid and pyridoxine are higher than the RDAs, thus supplementation of these nutrients is recommended.

Parenteral Nutrition Support

PN is indicated for CRF patients when EN fails to achieve or to maintain adequate nutritional status. Specific nutrition requirements vary, depending on the metabolic status of the patient (nonstressed or hypercatabolic) and on whether or not the patient is to receive dialysis therapy and of which type (HD, PD, CAVDH). CRF patients who are stressed have requirements similar to those of hypercatabolic patients with ARF. Recommended nutrient intake, nutrition solutions, and monitoring are described in detail in the section on PN support of ARF patients.

Nonstressed predialysis patients receiving PN should get 0.6 to 0.8 g of protein per kilogram of body weight per day and HD patients receiving PN require 1.2 to 1.4 g/kg per day. Patients on PD should receive protein in the range of 1.2 to 1.5 g/kg per day. As previously discussed, depending on age, all patients, whether they receive dialysis or not, should receive 30 to 35 kcal/kg per day. One exception is the obese patient who weighs more than 120% of relative body weight, for whom 25 to 28 kcal/kg per day may be more appropriate.[64]

The specific formulation selected to achieve the above goals is determined by whether the patient is receiving renal replacement therapy, the daily fluid allowance, glucose tolerance, metabolic status, and specific nutrient goals. Box 33-3 includes sample parenteral formulations for predialysis and dialysis patients.

Regular clinical monitoring of laboratory values and fluid status is essential for all patients receiving nutrition support. Any change in a patient's medical care or clinical status can dramatically affect serum parameters. The monitoring protocol described in this chapter for kidney disease patients receiving EN support is also appropriate for predialysis and dialysis patients receiving PN. One exception is tolerance to intravenous lipid emulsions. Many patients are hyperlipidemic at baseline. Any elevation in serum triglycerides or hepatic

TABLE 33-4

A Sampling of Enteral Products for Acute and Chronic Renal Failure

Product	Kcal (ml)	Protein (g/L)	Na (mg/L)	K (mg/L)	(Ca) (mg/L)	PO (mg/L)
Amino-acid (100% essential amino acids)	2.0	19.4	None	None	None	None
Travasorb Renal (67% essential, 33% nonessential amino acids)	1.1	22.8	None	None	None	None
Vivonex T.E.N.	1.0	38	460	780	500	500
Vivonex Plus (100% free amino acids)	1.0	45	610	1100	560	560
SandoSource-Peptide (26% free amino acids, 34% peptide chains of 2-4, 40% peptide chains of more than 4)	1.0	50	1100	1490	570	570
Alitraq (elemental, fortified with glutamine and arginine)	1.0	52.5	1000	1200	733	733
Vital High Nitrogen	1.0	41.7	566	1400	667	667
Criticare High Nitrogen	1.06	38	630	1320	530	530
Tolerex (free amino acids)	1.0	21	470	1200	560	560
Impact (contains arginine, fish oil, and dietary nucleotides for ventilator-dependent patients)	1.0	56	1100	1400	800	800
Pulmocare	1.5	62.6	1310	1730	1056	1056
Respalore	1.52	76	1270	1480	710	710
Traumacal	1.5	82	1180	1390	750	750
Deliver 2.0	2.0	75	800	700	1000	1000
*Nepro	2.0	70	845	1060	1370	685
Nutrirenal	2.0	70	740	1256	1400	700
TwoCal High Nitrogen	2.0	83.7	1310	2456	1052	1052
*Ensure	1.06	37.2	846	1564	530	530
*Ensure Plus	1.5	54.9	1050	1940	705	705
*Ensure High Nitrogen	1.06	44.4	802	1564	758	758
*Ensure Plus High Nitrogen	1.5	62.6	1188	1850	1056	1056
Ensure High Protein	0.94	50	1208	2833	1042	1042
*Isocal	1.06	34	530	1320	630	530
*Isocal High Nitrogen	1.06	44	930	1610	850	850
*Osmolite	1.06	37	640	1020	530	530
*Osmolite High Nitrogen	1.06	44.3	930	1570	758	758
Renalcal	2.0	34.4	–	–	–	–
Sustacal liquid	1.01	61	930	2100	1010	930
*Sustacal Basic	1.06	37	850	1610	530	530
Sustacal Plus	1.52	61	850	1480	850	850
*Resource	1.1	37	890	1600	530	530
Resource Plus	1.5	55	1300	2100	700	700
MODULAR PRODUCTS						
Protein						
*ProMod (per 6.6 g, or 1 scoop)	28	5	6	15	44	44
Casec (per 100 g of powder)	370	88	120	10	1600	1600
Fat						
Lipisorb powder	2.0	16.8	360	600	330	330
			(per 60 ml reconstituted with water)			
*MCT oil	116/tbsp	None	None	None	None	None
Carbohydrate						
*Moducal	30/tbsp	None	184	13.2	None	None
*Polycose (powder 263 g/1000 kcal)	2.0	None	289	10	78.9	13
(liquid 500/ml/1000 Kcal)	None	None	350	30	100	15

Data from Novartis Enteral Product Reference Guide, 2001, Novartis Nutrition Corp., Minneapolis, MN, 55440-0370.
*Appropriate for use with predialysis and dialysis patients. Ultimate selection of formula depends on patient's fluid and electrolyte status and protein and calorie requirements.

enzymes upon introduction or during administration of PN containing lipids suggests impaired hepatic clearance of the lipid load. Thus, upon initiation of PN containing a lipid emulsion, the serum triglycerides, serum glutamic oxaloacetic transaminase (SGOT), serum glutamic-pyruvic transaminase (SGPT), and alkaline phosphatase should initially be monitored at 24-hour intervals for 72 hours. After tolerance is demonstrated, once weekly monitoring of the indices should prove sufficient.[133]

Peripheral Parenteral Nutrition

Peripheral parenteral nutrition (PPN) is normally indicated for short-term feeding for renal disease patients who are unable to maintain adequate dietary intake and are not eligible for central access placement. The use and efficiency of PPN for CRF patients have not been adequately documented, but if PPN is elected, the laboratory values previously described should be monitored according to the same schedule.

TABLE 33-5

Composition of Enteral Products Commonly Prescribed as an Oral Supplement for Poorly Nourished Dialysis Patients*

Product	Energy (Kcal/ml)	CHO (g)	Protein (g)	Fat (g)	Na+ (mg)	K+ (mg)	PO4+ (mg)
Alterna	0.363	11.2	2.35	3.7	96	260	<120
Ensure	1.06	34.3	8.8	8.8	200	370	125
Ensure HN	1.06	33.4	10.5	8.4	190	370	179
Ensure Plus	1.5	47.3	13.0	12.6	250	460	167
Ensure Plus HN	1.5	47.3	14.8	11.8	280	430	250
Isocal	1.06	31.9	8.16	10.56	127	317	127
Isocal HN	1.06	29.76	10.56	10.8	223	382	204
Magnacal Renal	2.0	48	18	24.2	192	305	192
Replete(250 ml)	1.0	28.2	15.6	8.3	125	388	180
Resource	1.06	34.3	8.8	8.8	163	275	130
Suplena	2.0	61.2	7.2	22.9	190	269	175
Sustacal	1.0	33.0	14.5	5.5	220	490	220
Sustacal HC	1.5	45.0	14.4	13.6	200	350	200

Data from Novartis Enteral Product Reference Guide, 2001, Novartis Nutrition Corp., Minneapolis, MN, 55440-0370
*Composition is per 240 ml, except for Replete, 250 ml.

Solutions for PPN usually consist of 10% dextrose with as much as 8.5% amino acids or 20% dextrose with a maximum of 5.5% amino acids. Concentrations of amino acids and dextrose must be low because of the hypertonic nature of solution constituents. The risk of vein thrombosis is significant. Lipids are useful to add to PPN formulations to help boost the energy content. Intravenous lipids are hypotonic and thus reduce the osmolality of the infusion. The specific solution composition and volume must be calculated for each patient.[64]

Intradialysis Nutrition Support

In addition to being a means of nutrition support for patients with CRF and ARF, intravenous nutrition is sometimes used as an intervention for malnutrition in patients receiving maintenance HD or PD.[133] For the former group, intravenous amino acids, carbohydrate, and fat are infused directly into the venous drip chamber of the HD machine during treatment. This therapy is referred to as *intradialytic parenteral nutrition* (IDPN). In peritoneal dialysis, amino acids are used as a dialysis solution in rotation with dextrose-enriched dialysate exchanges. This approach is referred to as *intraperitoneal nutrition.*

HISTORY. The forerunner of intravenous nutrition supplementation for uremia patients was high-calorie, low-protein oral regimens including rice, sugar, and potatoes. These did not alleviate malnutrition, in large part because they were unpalatable. Emphasis was later directed toward supplementing renal patients with essential amino acids and ketoacids. When added to a low-protein diet, these substances were found to reduce production of urea and other metabolites while maintaining nitrogen balance.

One of the first applications of intravenous nutrition was done by Borst and colleagues in 1948.[33] This group administered glucose parenterally to protein-depleted patients with CRF. A high incidence of thrombophlebitis prevented wide use of this therapy. In 1949, Bull and Joekes[34] gave anuric patients glucose and peanut oil via the enteral route for up to 3 weeks. This was reported to reduce protein catabolism. In 1969, Josephson and colleagues[134] administered essential amino acids

intravenously to uremia patients. No compliance problems were reported, and nitrogen balance was more positive than with the oral route. Lacking a consistent success rate, none of these therapies became standard practice.

With the availability of dialysis therapy it was soon recognized that some problems related to nutritional status resulted directly from the therapy: protein and blood loss as part of dialysis and routine laboratory monitoring, abnormal amino acid metabolism specific to uremia, and observations that 1 g/kg per day protein intake by HD patients did not prevent development of malnutrition. Therefore, there was interest in developing nutritional therapies that would be effective for this problem.

During the 1980s clinical efforts to treat the malnutrition seen in dialysis patients included administering intravenous nutrition solutions directly into the venous drip chamber of the HD machine throughout the dialysis treatment, which became known as IDPN. Studies that were completed to determine whether IDPN resolves malnutrition were inconclusive.[135-137] This is due in part to the fact that the majority of studies were not prospective, randomized, or controlled. Other problems of study design included small sample size and short observation time. Efforts to complete statistical analyses of large numbers of patients receiving IDPN suggest it does indeed affect morbidity and mortality.[138,139] The prospective, randomized, and controlled clinical studies that are needed to clarify the potential of this therapy need to be completed. In 1996, new IDPN reimbursement regulations were devised that are so stringent and impractical that the use of IDPN therapy is rare.[140] This is an unfortunate situation because IDPN therapy should be available for study in clinical trials so that the potential and proper use of this therapy for malnutrition can be defined. Reviews of IDPN patient selection criteria, protocols for IDPN administration, and sample IDPN solutions that have been used are available.[133,141]

Intraperitoneal Parenteral Nutrition

The past 10 years have seen few studies on the use of amino acid-enriched dialysate to resolve malnutrition in peritoneal dialysis patients. Kopple and colleagues[88] completed a study that tested whether a dialysate that contained amino acids would improve the protein nutrition of 19 malnourished chronic peritoneal dialysis patients. The study was completed in a metabolic ward. Each day for 20 days subjects received one or two dialysate exchanges that contained 1.1% amino acids and no glucose. While using the amino acid-enriched dialysate, patients experienced a significant increase in nitrogen balance, plasma amino acid levels became more normal, and serum total protein and transferrin concentrations increased. Some patients developed mild azotemia.

The positive findings reported in this study suggest that this type of intervention may have a positive effect on the nutritional status of malnourished peritoneal dialysis patients. Recently, a dipeptide-based intraperitoneal PN solution has been suggested.[142] The authors of this study concluded that dipeptide based solutions may provide more amino acids to the patient while having fewer side effects than amino acid based solutions.[142] It is likely that additional studies will be published in the near future that expand upon this body of work.

Conclusion

Many areas of renal nutrition require further study to devise successful clinical interventions. Good examples include malnutrition and inflammation.[143-146] Clarification of the components contributing to hypoalbuminemia that does not resolve with nutrition intervention is currently one area receiving research attention and continuing to challenge the nutrition professional. Perhaps this patient is not malnourished, but is manifesting clinical symptoms of inflammation that are affecting nutritional status, and perhaps contributing to cardiovascular status. What intervention is indicated? Additional studies are needed to properly address this question.

The National Kidney Foundation's K/DOQI project is having an impact on clinical nephrology and renal dietetics by completing expert literature review and analysis and devising clinical recommendations that can be used worldwide for the care of the renal patient. Recommendations for the nutritional management of the patient with kidney disease will continue to be a major component of the future work groups. The new approach to the assessment and treatment of nutritional status in the chronic kidney failure patient will be moving in a new direction.

REFERENCES

1. Chatoth D: Elements of renal structure and function. In Carpenter G, Griggs R, Loscalzo J (eds): *Cecil essentials of medicine,* Philadelphia, 2001, WB Saunders, pp 223-231.
2. Shaver MJ: Chronic renal failure. In Carpenter G, Griggs R, Loscalzo J (eds): *Cecil essentials of medicine,* Philadelphia, 2001, WB Saunders, pp 291-300.
3. Yousri M, Barri H, Sudhir S: Approach to the patient with renal disease. In Carpenter G, Griggs R, Loscalzo J (eds): *Cecil essentials of medicine,* Philadelphia, 2001, WB Saunders, pp 232-237.
4. Zawada E: Initiation of dialysis. In Daugirdas J, Blake P, Ing T (eds): *Handbook of dialysis,* Philadelphia, 2001, Lippincott Williams & Wilkins, pp 3-11.
5. Saulo Klahr: Effects of renal insufficiency on nutrient metabolism and endocrine function. In Mitch WE, Klahr S (eds): *Handbook of nutrition and the kidney,* 1998, Lippincott-Raven, pp 25-44.
6. Kopple J: Nutrition, diet, and the kidney. In Shils M, Olson J, Shike M (eds): *Modern nutrition in health and disease,* Philadelphia, 1994, Lea & Febiger, pp 1102-1146.
7. Goldstein DJ: Assessment of nutritional status in renal disease. In Mitch W, Klahr S (eds): *Handbook of nutrition and the kidney,* ed 4, Philadelphia, 2002, Little, Brown, pp 42-92.
8. Frankenfield, D, Johnson C, Wish J, Rocco M, Madore F, Owen W: Anemia management of adult hemodialysis patients in the U.S.: results from the 1997 ESRD core indicators project, *Kidney Int* 57:578-589, 2000.
9. Ma J, Ebben J, Hong X, Collins A: Hematocrit level and associated mortality in hemodialysis patients, *J Am Soc Nephrol* 10:610-619, 1999.
10. Tarng DC, Huang TP, Doong TI: Improvement of nutritional status in patients receiving maintenance hemodialysis after correction of renal anemia with recombinant human erythropoietin, *Nephron* 78:253-259, 1998.
11. National Kidney Foundation: Kidney disease outcomes quality initiative clinical practice guidelines for the treatment of anemia of chronic renal failure, *Am J Kidney Dis* 37 (suppl 1):S182-S235, 2001.
12. Falkenhain M, Hartman J, Hebert L: Nutritional management of water, sodium, potassium, chloride and magnesium in renal disease and renal failure. In Kopple J, Massry S (eds): *Nutritional management of renal disease,* Baltimore, 1997, Williams & Wilkins, pp 371-394.
13. Robertson GL, Berl T: Pathophysiology of water metabolism. In Brenner BM, Rector FC (eds): *The kidney,* ed 5, Philadelphia, 1996, WB Saunders, pp 873-928.
14. Shah S: Acute renal failure. In Carpenter G, Griggs R, Loscalzo J (eds): *Cecil essentials of medicine,* Philadelphia, 2001, WB Saunders, pp 283-290.
15. Albright RC: Acute renal failure: a practical update, *Mayo Clin Proc* 76:67-74, 2001.
16. Thadhani R, Pascual M, Bonventre J: Acute renal failure, *N Engl J Med* 334:1448-1460, 1996.
17. Anderson R, Schrier R: Acute tubular necrosis. In Schrier R, Gottschalk CW (eds): *Diseases of the kidney,* Boston, 1993, Little, Brown, pp 1287-1318.
18. Leblanc M, Tapolyai M, Paganini E: What dialysis dose should be provided in acute renal failure? *Adv Ren Replace Ther* 3(2):255-264, 1995.
19. Druml W: Nutritional management of acute renal failure. In Jacobson H, Striker G, Skahr S (eds): *The principles and practice of nephrology,* St Louis, 1995, CV Mosby, pp 745-753.
20. Monson P, Mehta, R: Nutrition in acute renal failure: a reappraisal for the 1990s, *J Renal Nutr* 2(4):5-77, 1994.
21. Butler B: Nutritional management of catabolic renal failure requiring renal replacement therapy, *Am Nephrol Nurses Assoc* 3(18):247-259, 1991.
22. Wolk R, Swartz R: Nutritional support of patients with acute renal failure, *Nutr Support Serv* 2(6):38-46, 1986.
23. Mehta R: Therapeutic alternatives to renal replacement for critically ill patients in acute renal failure, *Semin Nephrol* 14(1):64-82, 1994.
24. Ladefoged S, Pedersen S, Skielboe M, et al: Renal functional reserve after an acute intravenous lipid load, *J Renal Nutr* 4(3):186-190, 1993.
25. Rao M, Sharma M, Juneja R, Jacob S, Jacob C: Calculated nitrogen balance in hemodialysis patients: influence of protein intake, *Kidney Int* 58(1):336-345, 2000.
26. Ikizler TA, Hakim RM: Nutrition in end-stage renal disease, *Kidney Int* 50(2):343-357, 1996.
27. Weiner Feldman R: Nutrition in acute renal failure, *J Renal Nutr* (4)2:97-99, 1994.
28. Burge J: Parenteral micronutrient requirements in renal disease, *Support Line* (13)2:1-3, 1991.
29. Giuliano B, Leiserowitz M, Shamir E, et al: Nutritional and metabolic implications of acute renal failure. In *Renal nutrition. Report of Eleventh Ross Roundtable on medical issues,* Columbus, OH, 1991, Ross Laboratories, pp 58-64.
30. Weiner Feldman R: Nutrition in acute renal failure, *J Renal Nutr* 4(2)97-99, 1994.
31. Maroni BJ, Hirschberg R: The importance of nutritional status on outcomes from acute renal failure, *Contemp Dialysis Nephrol* 17(7):22-25, 1996.
32. Kopple J: Nitrogen metabolism. In Massry S, Sellers A (eds): *Clinical aspects of uremia and dialysis,* Springfield, IL, 1976, Charles C Thomas, pp 241-272.
33. Borst J: Protein katabolism in uraemia, *Lancet* 1:824-828, 1948.
34. Bull G, Joekes A: Conservative treatment of anuric uraemia, *Lancet* 2:229-234, 1949.
35. Iseki K, Miyasato F, Tokuyama K, Nishime K, Uehara H, Shiohira Y, Sunagawa H, Yoshihara K, Yoshi S, Toma S, Kowatari T, Wake T, Oura T, Fukiyama K: Low diastolic blood pressure, hypoalbuminemia and risk

of death in a cohort of chronic hemodialysis patients, *Kidney Int* 51:1212-1217, 1997.

36. Chumlea WC: Anthropometric assessment of nutritional status in renal disease, *J Renal Nutr* 7:176-181, 1997.

37. National Kidney Foundation: Kidney disease outcomes quality initiative. *Clinical practice guidelines for hemodialysis adequacy, Am J Kidney Dis* 37(suppl 1):S7-S46, 2001.

38. Kaysen G, Dubin J, Müller H Rosales, L, Levin N, and The HEMO Study Group. The acute-phase response varies with time and predicts serum albumin levels in hemodialysis. patients, *Kidney Int* 58:346-352, 200032.

39. Sax H, Souba W: Enteral and parenteral feeding guidelines and recommendations, *Med Clin North Am* 4(77):863-879, 1993.

40. Chen Yu, Fervenza F, and Rabkin R. Growth factors in the treatment of wasting in kidney failure, *J Renal Nutr* 11:62-66, 2001.

41. Iglesias P, Diez J, Fernandez-Reyes M, Aguilera A, Burgues S, Martinez-Ara J, Miguel J, Gomez-Pan A, Selgas R: Recombinant human growth hormone therapy in malnourished dialysis patients: a randomized prospective study, *Am J Kidney Dis* 32:454-468, 1998.

42. Fine R: Growth hormone treatment of children with chronic renal insufficiency, end-stage renal disease and following renal transplantation, *J Pediatr Endocrinol Metab* 10:361-370, 1997.

43. Ikizler T, Wingard R, Flakoll P, Schulman G, Parker R, Hakim R: Effects of recombinant human growth hormone on plasma and dialysate amino acid profiles in CAPD patients, *Kidney Int* 50:229-234, 1996.

44. Ziegler T, Lazarus J, Young L, et al: Effects of recombinant growth hormone in adults receiving maintenance hemodialysis, *J Am Soc Nephrol* 2:1130-1135, 1991.

45. Fouque D, Peng S, Shamir E, Kopple J: Recombinant human IGF-1 induces an anabolic response in malnourished CAPD patients, *Kidney Int* 57:646-654, 2000.

46. Laville M, Fouque D: Nutritional aspects in hemodialysis, *Kidney Int* 58(76)S133-S139, 2000.

47. Barri Y: Vascular disorders of the kidney. In Carpenter G, Griggs R, Loscalzo J (eds): *Cecil essentials of medicine,* Philadelphia, 2001, WB Saunders, pp 278-282.

48. Mitch WE, Walser M: Nutritional therapy for the uremic patient. In Brenner BM, Rector FC (eds): *The kidney,* ed 5, Philadelphia, 1996, WB Saunders, pp 2382-2423.

49. Kasiske BL, Keane WF: Laboratory assessment of renal disease: clearance, urinalysis, and renal biopsy. In Brenner BM, Rector FC (eds): *The kidney,* ed 5, Philadelphia, 1996, WB Saunders, pp 1137-1174.

50. Goldwasser P, Aboul-Magd A, Maru M: Race and creatinine excretion in chronic renal insufficiency, *Am J Kidney Dis* 30(1):16-22, 1997.

51. Blachley J, Knochel J: The biochemistry of uremia. In Brenner B, Stein J (eds): *Chronic renal failure, contemporary issues in nephrology,* New York, 1981, Churchhill Livingstone, pp 28-45.

52. May R, Kelly R, Mitch W: Pathophysiology of uremia. In Brenner B, Rector F Jr (eds): *The kidney,* ed 4, Philadelphia, 1991, WB Saunders, pp 1997-2018.

53. Santoro Antonio: Confounding factors in the assessment of delivered hemodialysis dose, *Kidney Int* 58(S76):S19-S27, 2000.

54. National Kidney Foundation: Kidney disease outcomes quality initiative clinical practice guidelines for nutrition in chronic renal failure. Adult guidelines, *Am J Kidney Dis* 35(suppl 2):S17-S104, 2000.

55. Goldstein DJ, McQuiston B: Nutrition and renal disease. In Coulston A, Rock C, Monsen E (eds): *Nutrition in the prevention and treatment of disease,* San Diego, 2001, Academic Press, pp 617-636.56.

56. National Kidney Foundation: K/DOQI Clinical practice guidelines for chronic kidney disease: evaluation, classification and stratification, *Am J Kidney Dis* 39:S128-S130, 2002.

57. Sorkin M, Blake P: Apparatus for peritoneal dialysis. In Daugirdas J, Blake P, Ing T (eds): *Handbook of dialysis,* ed 3, Philadelphia, 2001, Lippincott Williams & Wilkins, pp 297-308.

58. Blake P, Daugirdas J: Physiology of peritoneal dialysis: In Daugirdas J, Blake P, Ing T (eds): *Handbook of dialysis,* ed 3, Philadelphia, 2001, Lippincott Williams & Wilkins, pp 281-296.

59. National Kidney Foundation: Kidney disease outcomes quality initiative clinical practice guidelines for vascular access, *Am J Kidney Dis* 37(suppl 1):S137-S173, 2001.

60. Daugirdas J, Van Stone J, Boag J: Hemodialysis apparatus. In Daugirdas J, Blake P, Ing T, (eds): *Handbook of dialysis,* ed 3, Philadelphia, 2001, Lippincott Williams & Wilkins, pp 46-66.

61. Kinsey E, Smith M: Technical tricks. In Brain EA (ed): *Renal disease: a conceptual approach,* New York, 1987, Churchill Livingstone, pp 127-140.

62. Tzamaloukas A, Friedman E: Diabetes. In Daugirdas J, Blake P, Ing T (eds), *Handbook of dialysis,* ed 3, Philadelphia, 2001, Lippincott Williams & Wilkins, pp 453-465.

63. Levine Lewis S: Enteral nutrition in end-stage renal disease. In Stover J (ed), *Nutrition care in end-stage renal disease,* ed 2, Chicago, 1994, American Dietetic Association, pp 99-109.

64. Liftman C, Hood S: Parenteral nutrition for the patient with renal failure. In Stover J (ed), *Nutrition care in end-stage renal disease,* ed 2, Chicago, 1994, American Dietetic Association, pp 111-121.

65. Bello-Reuse E: Pathophysiology of volume regulation and sodium metabolism. In Klahr S (ed): *The kidney and body fluids in health and disease,* New York, Plenum, 1983, pp 93-118.

66. Grunfeld J: Analytical study of renal excretion of water and electrolytes. In Hamburger J, Crosnier J, Grunfeld J (eds): *Nephrology,* New York, 1979, John Wiley, pp 289-298.

67. Kopple J: Nutrition and the kidney. In Hodges RE: *Human nutrition: a comprehensive treatise: metabolic and clinical applications,* New York, 1979, Plenum, pp 409-457.

68. Hunt S, Groft J, Holbrook J: The kidney. In *Nutrition: principles and clinical practice,* New York, 1980, John Wiley, pp 358-398.

69. Delmez J: Pathophysiological principles in the treatment of patients with renal failure. In Klahr S (ed): *The kidney and body fluids in health and disease,* New York, 1983, Plenum, pp 491-520.

70. Karalis M (ed): Renal disease. In *Manual of clinical dietetics,* ed 6, Chicago, 2000, American Dietetic Association, Status project developed by the Chicago Dietetic Association and North Suburban Chicago Dietetic Association, pp 449-499.

71. Giebisch G, Malnic G, Berliner R: Renal transport and control of potassium excretion. In Brenner B, Rector FC Jr (eds): *The kidney,* ed 4, Philadelphia, 1991, WB Saunders, pp 283-317.

72. Delmez J, Kaye M: Bone disease. In Daugirdas J, Blake P, Ing T (eds): *Handbook of dialysis,* Philadelphia, 2001, Lippincott Williams & Wilkins, pp 530-547.

73. Atsumi K, Kushida K, Yamazaki K, Shimizu S, Ohmura A, Inoue T: Risk factors for vertebral factures in renal osteodystrophy, *Am J Kidney Dis* 33:287-293, 1999.

74. Slatopolsky E, Dusso A, Brown A: The role of phosphorus in the development of secondary hyperparathyroidism and parathyroid cell proliferation in chronic renal failure, *Am J Med Sci* 317:370-376, 1999.

75. Block GA, Hulbert-Shearon T, Levin N, Port F: Association of serum phosphorus and calcium X phosphate product with mortality risk in chronic hemodialysis patients: a national study, *Am J Kidney Dis* 31(4):607-617, 1998.

76. Levin N, Hulbert-Shearon T, Strawderman R, Port F: Which causes of death are related to hyperphosphatemia in hemodialysis (HD) patients? *J Am Soc Nephrol* 9:217A, 1998.

77. Gonzalez E, Martin K: Calcium, phosphorus, and Vitamin D. In Mitch W, Klahr S (eds): *Handbook of nutrition and the kidney,* Philadelphia, 1997, Lippincott-Raven, pp 87-106.

78. Brookhyser J, Pahre S: Dietary and pharmacotherapeutic considerations in the management of renal osteodystrophy, *Adv Renal Replacement Ther* 2(1):5-13, 1995.

79. Chertow G, Lazarus M, Lew N, Lowrie E: Intact parathyroid hormone (PTH) is directly related to mortality in hemodialysis, *J Am Soc Nephrol* A3025, 2000.

80. McCann L: Protocol for the administration of intravenous calcitriol, *J Renal Nutr* 4(3):143-148, 1994.

81. DeTar S, Patel C, Valdin J: A practical approach to administration of intravenous calcitriol in an outpatient dialysis setting, *J Renal Nutr* 1(4):182-186, 1991.

82. Ritz E, Mehls O: Vitamin D therapy in patients receiving dialysis, *Adv Renal Replacement Ther* 2(1):14-19, 1995.

83. Lerma E, McCormick D, Ghanekar H, Abraham M, Sprague S, Batlle D: A comparative study between 19-Nor-1 Alpha, 25-Dihydroxyvitamin D2 and intravenous calcitriol on PTH suppression in hemodialysis patients, *J Am Soc Nephrol* A3050, 2000.

84. Suki WN, Leder AJ, Khan K, Achkar GM, Nassar JM, Gonzalez TS: Suppression of secondary hyperparathyroidism by paracalcitol despite hyperphosphatemia, *J Am Soc Nephrol* A3078, 2000.

85. Martin K, Charney D, Lindberg J, Soltanek C, Llach F: Zemplar (Paracalcitol injection) dosing based on initial levels of iPTH: a safe and effective method of treating secondary hyperparathyroidism, *J Am Soc Nephrol* A3056, 2000.

86. Goodman W: A calcimimetic agent lowers plasma parathyroid hormone levels in patients with secondary hyperparathyroidism, *Kidney Int* 58:436-445, 2000.

87. Kopple J: Effect of nutrition on morbidity and mortality in maintenance dialysis patients, *Am J Kidney Dis* 24(6):1002-1009, 1994.

88. Kopple J, Bernard D, Messana J, et al: Treatment of malnourished CAPD patients with an amino acid based dialysate, *Kidney Int* 47:1148-1157, 1995.

89. Ohri-Vachaspati P, Sehgal A: Quality of life implications of inadequate protein nutrition among hemodialysis patients, *J Renal Nutr* 9:9-13, 1999.

90. Ikizler T, Wingard R, Harvell J, Shyr Y, Hakim R: Association of morbidity with markers of nutrition and inflammation in chronic hemodialysis patients: a prospective study, *Kidney Int* 55:1945-1951, 1999.

91. Herselman M, Moosa M, Kotze T, Kritzinger M, Wuister S, Mostert D: Protein-energy malnutrition as a risk factor for increased morbidity in long term hemodialysis patients, *J Renal Nutr* 10:7-15, 2000.

92. Ikizler T, Flakoll P, Parker R, Hakim R: Amino acid and albumin losses during hemodialysis, *Kidney Int* 46:830-837, 1994.

93. Kaplan A, Halley S, Lapkin R, Graeber C: Dialysate protein losses with bleach processed polysulphone dialyzers, *Kidney Int* 47:573-578, 1995.

94. Gokal R, Harty J: Nutrition and peritoneal dialysis. In Mitch W, Klahr S (eds): *Nutrition and the kidney,* Philadelphia, 1997, Lippincott-Raven, pp 269-293.

95. Alvestrand A: Nutritional requirements of dialysis patients. In Jacobson H, Striker G, Skahr S (eds): *The principles and practice of nephrology,* St Louis, 1995, CV Mosby, pp 761-766.

96. Striker G: Report on a workshop to develop management recommendations for the prevention of progression in chronic renal disease, *J Am Soc Nephrol* 5(7):1537-1540, 1995.

97. Kopple J, Levey A, Greene T, Chumlea C, Gassmann J, Hollinger D, Maroni B, Merrill D, Scherch L, Schulman G, Wang S, Zimmer G for the Modification of Diet in Renal Disease Study Group: Effect of dietary protein restriction on nutritional status in the modification of diet in renal disease study, *Kidney Int* 52:778-791, 1997.

98. Mitch W: Dietary therapy in uremia: the impact on nutrition and progressive renal failure, *Kidney Int* 57(75):S38-S43, 2000.

99. Bergstrom J: Anorexia in dialysis patients, *Semin Nephrol* 16(3):222-229, 1996.

100. Ikizler T, Hakim R: Nutritional requirements of hemodialysis patients. In Mitch WE, Klahr S (eds): *Nutrition and the kidney,* ed 3, Philadelphia, 1997, Lippincott-Raven, pp 253-268.

101. Rocco M, Blumenkrantz M: In Daugirdas J, Blake P, Ing T (eds): *Handbook of dialysis,* ed 3, Philadelphia, 2001, Lippincott Williams & Wilkins, pp 420-445.

102. Rocco M, Makoff R: Appropriate vitamin therapy for dialysis patients, *Semin Dial* 10:272-277, 1997.

103. Makoff R: Water-soluble vitamin status in patients with renal disease treated with hemodialysis or peritoneal dialysis, *J Renal Nutr* 1(2):56-73, 1991.

104. Holliday M, Mettenry-Richardson K, Portate A: Nutritional management of chronic renal disease, *Med Clin North Am* 63:954-963, 1979.

105. Fowler B: Hyperhomocysteinemia in uremia: the folate cycle and disease in humans, *Kidney Int* 59(78):S221-S229, 2001.

106. Fishbane S, Frei G, Finger M, et al: Hypervitaminosis A in two hemodialysis patients, *Am J Kidney Dis* 25(2):346-349, 1995.

107. Moth I: Implications of hypervitaminosis A in chronic renal failure, *J Renal Nutr* 1(1):2-8, 1991.

108. Roob J: Vitamin E attenuates oxidative stress induced by intravenous iron in patients on hemodialysis, *J Am Soc Nephrol* 11:539-549, 2000.

109. Yeun J, Kaysen G: C-reactive protein, oxidative stress, homocysteine, and troponin as inflammatory and metabolic predictors of atherosclerosis in ESRD, *Curr Opin Nephrol Hypertens* 9(6):621-630, 2000.

110. Trachtman H, Schwab N, Maesaka J, Valderrama E: Dietary vitamin E supplementation ameliorates renal injury in chronic puromycin aminonucleoside nephropathy, *J Am Soc Nephrol* 5(10):1811-1819, 1995.

111. Tarng D, Huang T, Chen T, Yang W: Erythropoietin hyporesponsiveness: from iron deficiency to iron overload, *Kidney Int* 55:S107-S118, 1999.

112. Fishbane S, Mittal S, Maesaka J: Beneficial effects of iron therapy in renal failure patients on hemodialysis, *Kidney Int* 55:S67-S70, 1999.

113. Vychytil A, Haag-Weber M: Iron status and iron supplementation in peritoneal dialysis patients, *Kidney Int* 55(69):S71-S78, 1999.

114. Wolfson M: Nutrition in hemo and peritoneal dialysis. In Nissenson A, Fine R, Gentile D (eds): *Clinical dialysis,* Norwalk, CT, 1984, Appleton-Century-Crofts, pp 335-350.

115. Kay J, Hano J: Musculoskeletal and rheumatologic disease. In Daugirdas J, Blake P, Ing T (eds): *Handbook of dialysis,* ed 3, Philadelphia, 2001, Lippincott Williams & Wilkins, pp 637-651.

116. Labonia W: L-carnitine effects on anemia in hemodialyzed patients treated with erythropoietin, *Am J Kidney Dis* 26:757-764, 1995.

117. Guarnieri G, Faccini L, Lipartiti T, et al: Simple methods for nutritional assessment in hemodialyzed patients, *Am J Clin Nutr* 33:1598-1607, 1980.

118. Goldstein DJ, Frederico C: The effect of urea kinetic modeling on the nutritional management of chronic hemodialysis patients, *J Am Diet Assoc* 4(87):474-479, 1987.

119. Lowrie E, Lew N: Death risk in hemodialysis patients: the predictive value of commonly measured variables and an evaluation of death rate differences between facilities, *Am J Kidney Dis* 15(5):458-482, 1990.

120. Prichard S: Comorbidities and their impact on outcome in patients with end stage renal disease, *Kidney Int* 57:S100-104, 2000.

121. Nicholls A: Heart and circulation. In Daugirdas J, Blake LP, Ing T (eds): *Handbook of dialysis,* ed 3, Philadelphia, 2001, Lippincott Williams & Wilkins, pp 583-600.

122. Mittman N, Avram MM: Dyslipidemia in renal disease, *Semin Nephrol* 16(3):202-213, 1996.

123. Avram M, Mittman N, Bonomini L, Chattopadhyay J, Fein P: Markers for survival in dialysis: a seven year prospective study, *Am J Kidney Dis* 26:209-219, 1995.

124. Fleischmann E, Bower J, Salahudeen A: Risk factor paradox in HD: better nutrition as a partial explanation, *ASAIO J* 47(1):74-81, 2001.

125. McCann L: Nutrition management of the adult peritoneal dialysis patient. In Stover J (ed), *Nutrition care in end-stage renal disease,* ed 2, Chicago, 1994, American Dietetic Association, pp 37-55.

126. Yates L: Anthropometric worksheet for use with hemodialysis patients, *J Renal Nutr* 6:162-164, 1996.

127. Feehrer C: Initial nutrition assessment, *J Renal Nutr* 9:38-42, 1999.

128. Dumler F, Kilates C: Use of bioelectrical impedance techniques for monitoring nutritional status in patients on maintenance dialysis, *J Renal Nutr* 10:116-124, 2000.

129. Stall SH, Ginsberg NS, DeVita MV, et al: Comparison of five body-composition methods in peritoneal dialysis patients, *Am J Clin Nutr* 64:125-130, 1996.

130. McCann L: Subjective global assessment as it pertains to the nutritional status of dialysis patients, *Dialysis and Transplantation* 25(4):190-202, 1996.

131. Kalantar-Zadeh, K, Kopple J, Deepak S, Block D, Block G: Food intake characteristics of hemodialysis patients as obtained by food frequency questionnaire, *J Renal Nutr* 12:17-28, 2002.

132. National Kidney Foundation: Kidney disease outcomes quality initiative, *Clinical Practice Guidelines for Peritoneal Dialysis Adequacy. Am J Kidney Dis* 37 (suppl 1):S55-S108, 2001.

133. Goldstein DJ, Strom J: Intradialytic parenteral nutrition: evolution and current concepts, *J Renal Nutr* 1(1):9-22, 1991.

134. Josephson B, Bergstrom J, Bucht H, et al: Intravenous amino acid treatment in uremia. *Proceedings of the 4th International Congress of Nephrology,* vol 2, Stockholm, Basel, Sweden, 1970, S, Karger, pp 203-211.

135. Piraino AJ, Firpo J, Power D: Prolonged hyperalimentation in catabolic chronic dialysis therapy patients, *J Parenter Enteral Nutr* 5:463-477, 1981.

136. Cherow G: Modality-specific nutrition support in ESRD: weighing the evidence, *Am J Kidney Dis* (33):193-197, 1999.

137. Berneis K, Iseli-Schaub J, Garbani E, et al: Effects of intradialytic parenteral nutrition in chronic haemodialysis patients with malnutrition: a pilot study, *Wien Klin Wochenschr* (21):876-881, 1999.

138. Capelli J, Kushner K, Camiscioli T, et al: Effect of intradialytic parenteral nutrition on mortality rates in end-stage renal disease care, *Am J Kidney Dis* (23)6:808-816, 1994.

139. Chertow G, Ling J, Lew N, et al: The association of intradialytic parenteral nutrition administration with survival in hemodialysis patients, *Am J Kidney Dis* (24)6:912-920, 1994.

140. *Regional medical policy on parenteral nutrition,* Columbia, SC, 1996, Palmetto Government Benefits Administrators.

141. Goldstein DJ, Abrahamian-Gebeshian: Nutrition support in renal failure. In Matarese L, Gottschlich M (eds): *Contemporary nutrition support practice,* Philadelphia, 1998, WB Saunders, pp 447-471.

142. Werynski A, Waniewski J, Wang T, Anderstam B, Lindholm B, Bergstrom J: Kinetic studies of dipeptide-based and amino acid-based peritoneal dialysis solutions, *Kidney Int* 59:363-371, 2001.

143. Chertow G: Renal nutrition in the new millennium, *J Renal Nutr* 10(1):1, 2000.
144. Kaysen GA, Dubin JA, Muller HG, Mitch WE, Levin NW: Levels of alpha1 acid glycoprotein and ceruloplasmin predict future albumin levels in hemodialysis patients, *Kidney Int* 60(6):2360-2366, 2001.
145. Kaysen GA: The microinflammatory state in uremia: causes and potential consequences, *J Am Soc Nephrol* 12(7):1549-1557, 2001.
146. Kaysen GA, Chertow GM, Adhikarla R, Young B, Ronco C, Levin NW: Inflammation and dietary protein intake exert competing effects on serum albumin and creatinine in hemodialysis patients, *Kidney Int* 60(1):333-40, 2001.

Cancer

34

Abby S. Bloch, PhD, RD, FADA

SCIENTIFIC evidence suggests that at least one third of the half million or more cancer deaths expected to occur in 2001 are related to nutrition, physical activity, and other lifestyle factors and could be prevented. The Harvard Health Professionals Follow-up Study estimated that a third to a half of the colon cancer risk occurring in Western countries could be decreased by lowering energy intake and increasing energy expenditure and modifying specific dietary patterns along with lifestyle changes.[1] Recently, during an international conference on nutrition and cancer, Dr. Elio Riboli estimated that 10% to 50% of digestive tract cancers could be prevented with increased consumption of fruits and vegetables, based on recent meta-analyses.[2] In this country, one in every four deaths is from cancer.[3] Cancer is the second leading cause of death in the United States, exceeded only by heart disease. If one third or more of all cancers are initiated or promoted by dietary factors, incidence and mortality rates could decrease dramatically with appropriate dietary changes.

Statistics on cancer are reported using two measures: *incidence,* or the number of new cases diagnosed, and *mortality,* the number of deaths attributable to cancer. Doll and Peto[4] suggested that as many as 70% of all cancer death may be diet induced. As long ago as 1989, the National Research Council Committee on Diet and Health reported that one third of cancer deaths may be diet related.[5] During a presentation in 1992, Doll stated that reducing the risk of cancer deaths by an average of 35% using dietary modifications remained a reasonable assumption based on available current evidence.[6] Dr. Doll went on to state, "Nothing that has happened in the last 10 years leads us to think that diet is less important than we thought 10 years ago. On the contrary, the evidence of its importance as a cause of cancer or as a defense against it has been strengthened."[6] This premise continues to be true today.

The significant roles of diet and nutrition throughout the clinical course of cancer must also be recognized. During the past 15 years, several articles have supported what many who work with this population already know, that some 40% to 80% of all cancer patients develop some degree of clinical malnutrition.[7-9] Cancer anorexia-cachexia syndrome may be present at the time of death in 80% of cancer patients.[10] The clinical effects of poor nutrition are manifested in poor wound healing and poor skin turgor, leading to skin breakdown and decubiti. Anastomotic leaks, wound dehiscence, electrolyte and fluid imbalances, and endocrine abnormalities are common in this population, as is compromised immune function.[9] The risk of malnutrition and its degree are affected by tumor type, stage of disease, and antineoplastic therapy.

The primary focus of this chapter is nutrition evaluation of cancer patients, causes of inadequate nutrition, the effects of cancer treatment, cancer-associated metabolic derangements, management concerns, and modalities available to reverse compromised nutrition of cancer patients. The role of diet in prevention by decreasing the risk of developing cancer through components found in foods is reviewed in a section at the end of this chapter. Very little has changed over the past 30 or so years in the practical management of cancer patients. More technologic methods of feeding have developed and more therapeutic options are available. However, the basic recommendations of managing the nutritional needs of the patient have altered very little. Likewise, studies on nutrition and metabolic effects of cancer that were done 15 to 20 years ago are still regarded as definitive in many areas of nutrition and cancer metabolism. For this reason, those studies are cited in the following sections in addition to any recent work available.

Nutrition Evaluation of Cancer Patients

Factors in Nutritional Status

NUTRITION SCREENING AND ASSESSMENT. Developing and implementing a screening and assessment tool is key to effective nutrition intervention and management of cancer patients. The screening and assessment tools used must be able to determine nutritional status expediently. Several tools have been developed specifically for the cancer population. The Subjective Global Assessment (SGA) developed by Detsky and his colleagues at Toronto General Hospital,[11] the modified Patient Generated–Subjective Global Assessment developed by Ottery and her team at Fox Chase Cancer Center,[12] and the Oncology Screening Tool created at Memorial Sloan-Kettering Cancer Center (MSKCC)[13] are some forms being used throughout the continuum of care (inpatient, outpatient clinics, ambulatory, or home care). The initial evaluation should seek only data to identify the patient's nutritional risk category. The SGA uses five features of history and three aspects of the physical examination.[14-16] The history consists of current weight and weight history, current and usual dietary intake, gastrointestinal (GI) symptoms that have been present for at least 2 weeks, performance status, and metabolic requirements. The three parts of the physical examination are muscle, fat, and fluid status. With these eight components the patient is categorized as (1) well-nourished, (2) moderately or possibly malnourished, or (3) severely malnourished.

For the scored Patient Generated–Subjective Global Assessment (PG-SGA), the patient or caregiver completes sections on weight history, food intake, symptoms, and activities/functions. A member of the clinical staff evaluates disease stage, metabolic demands, and physical findings, scoring the individual components and placing the individual into a global assessment category. Nutritional triage recommendations are also provided. It is hoped that a simple, easily administered form will help diagnose nutritional deficits and problems at baseline or soon after initial presentation to the clinician. This screening tool asks for weight changes over time (1 year, 6 months, and within the past 2 weeks), food intake within the past month, symptoms that would affect eating, and functional capacity. A staff member completes the form, including the diagnosis and staging, if known, metabolic stress levels, and physical findings of fat and muscle wasting, edema, and ascites. A three-level rating similar to the SGA is then determined.[12,17]

In the Oncology Screening Tool, the initial screening, performed by a nurse, dietetic professional, or other qualified person, is based on weight loss and a 2-week or longer history of decreased food intake from normal, nausea and vomiting, diarrhea, mouth sores, and chewing or swallowing difficulty. Based on these factors a patient's risk is classified as (1) low or (2) moderate to high risk. The dietetic professional's evaluation further classifies the individual into one of the two categories based on diagnosis, complications, treatment, and weight status (Table 34-1). Only the moderate- to high-risk patients are seen by a dietetic professional within 24 hours, at which time a comprehensive nutrition assessment is performed. This assessment includes general appearance, fluid status, height and weight (preillness, usual, current considering hydration status), medical history, diet history, medications, laboratory values, mechanical and physical limitations affecting intake, mental status, malabsorption status, cancer treatment plans, cultural influences to dietary practices, and ability to self-feed. From this assessment, a nutrition care plan is developed. Moderate-risk patients are reassessed by the clinical dietetic professional within 5 days; high-risk patients, within 3 days. Nutrition care plans are adjusted according to the findings. Low-risk patients are rescreened by the clinical dietetic professional on the sixth day to verify their initial risk level or recategorize them if their status has changed in the interim. By having a simple first tier screening to identify patients needing nutrition intervention versus those who are currently stable, dietetic professionals can prioritize those cases requiring their expertise and time immediately and those who can be seen at a later date or by other dietary personnel.

For comprehensive general screening and assessment information specifically for cancer patients, see references 18 and 19.

In a given clinical situation, one or more of the following categories may be most important:
- Dietary patterns, habits, current practices
- Food aversions, changes in selection, preferences
- Taste changes; impairment or distortion (dysgeusia)
- Side effects experienced with special attention to those affecting the GI tract
- The ability to consume a nutritionally adequate diet
- Actual food consumption as distinguished from the amount of food prepared or placed on the plate

- Planned anticancer modalities (surgery, chemotherapy, radiation, etc.)
- Intent of cancer care therapy—palliative versus curative

Relevant questions could be incorporated into the self-report part of the form. Any nonessential information could be obtained during follow-up monitoring. The category most likely to require personal attention by the dietetic professional is the food intake documentation. For this reason a diet history should be taken only from patients identified in the screening tool as being at high risk. This more detailed assessment is labor intensive and should be reserved for patients who will benefit most from the nutrition analysis. Food frequency questionnaires are available, but they usually encompass global intake over the past year and are more useful for deriving group averages and population-based data. A more current intake history or some form of calorie count might be more meaningful. A general diet history that records present consumption gives the dietetic professional a more accurate picture of the patient's current nutrition status.

AGE AS A FACTOR. Age is an important variable in nutritional status. Elderly persons' body composition, weight, and metabolic rate are different from those of children or young adults. Aging is associated with decreases in total body water, lean tissue, and skeletal muscle mass.[20,21] As one ages, physiologic anorexia of aging occurs, altering satiety mechanisms from elevated leptin levels and central nervous system neurotransmitters.[22] Body fat, which tends to redistribute around the waist with age can mask undernutrition in older persons. Sarcopenia (decreased muscle mass) along with loss of adipose tissue are seen after the age of 70. Elderly patients may have impaired digestive and absorptive functions such as esophageal dysmotility, atrophic gastritis, achlorhydria, or gastric dysmotility.[23] The elderly may have reduced inadequate caloric intake, a depressed sensory-specific satiety while also being functionally limited, socially isolated, or emotionally depressed.[24,25] For these reasons, age-specific variations must be taken into account when determining nutrition needs.

Physical limitations such as mobility, dexterity, visual acuity, and range of motion could limit the ability to procure or prepare food or to eat. Shopping access, financial limitations, psychologic state, and attitude all affect eating patterns. Solitary mealtimes diminish people's interest in food, especially if appetite is already poor.

MEDICAL STATUS. Another point to keep in mind during screening and initial evaluation of cancer patients' nutritional status is their overall clinical status. Cancer patients may have diabetes; hypertension; or cardiovascular, renal, or respiratory problems that predispose to nutrition deficits. Changes in food preferences, eating patterns, or food selection and pain or anxiety or depression are common with chronic, debilitating, or potentially life-threatening illnesses. Evaluating each of these areas provides a more accurate picture of the patient than does isolating the cancer diagnosis from the individual's overall medical, clinical condition.

DIET PATTERNS AND HABITS. Cancer itself can compromise nutritional status. Food aversions need to be included because they indicate a specific problem. Food intolerances, alterations in taste (dysgeusia) and decreased appetite, early satiety, and mouth, throat, or GI lesions may lead to severe

TABLE 34-1
MSKCC Nutrition Care Process

Process	Clinical Evaluation of Patient's Nutritional Risk		
MSKCC PATIENT ASSESSMENT SUMMARY NURSING REVIEW OF PATIENT HISTORY AND DATA BASE	*Low risk* Patient without weight loss/nutritional complications.	*Moderate/high nutritional risk* Nurse referral to dietitian: 1. Weight status: Patient has a weight loss of 10 or more pounds in the last 3 months, and/or 2. A 2 or more week history of food intake decreased from normal, nausea/vomiting, diarrhea, mouth sores, difficulty chewing or swallowing	
		Adult Oncology Screening Tool	
DIETITIAN'S EVALUATION OF NUTRITION RISK/	*Low risk criteria* (patient does not meet nutritional risk criteria above; without weight loss/ nutritional complications):	*Moderate nutritional risk criteria* Nutritional assessment completed within 24 hr of referral Reassessment within 5 days	*High nutritional risk criteria* Nutritional assessment completed within 24 hr of referral Reassessment within 3 days
INTERVENTION PLAN DIAGNOSIS/ COMPLICATIONS	Rescreen on 6th day Nadir fever Comfort care Cancer of the: Prostate Bladder Ovary Renal cell Lung Liver	AIDS/HIV Ascites Emesis > 3 days Diarrhea > 3 days Diabetes Decubiti stage II Edema Esophageal stricture GBM (Glioblastoma) Odynophagia Renal insufficiency Mucositis	Acute weight loss during hospitalization Chylous ascites/chylous leak Dysphagia GI (fistula, ileus, upper GI bleed, malabsorption, obstruction, short gut/dumping syndromes) Graft-versus-host disease Liver failure/hepatic encephalopathy New-onset diabetes Pancreatitis Poor wound healing documented/decubiti stage III and IV Renal failure/dialysis
TREATMENT/SURGERY	Biopsy Bronchoscopy One-day chemotherapy Head neck surgery (without complications) including: partial thyroidectomy, neck dissection, parotidectomy, craniofacial, small cheek, oral lesions, nasal polyps, sinus surgery, biopsy, tonsillectomy	Autologous BMT Head and neck surgery: Craniotomy Total thyroidectomy Free flap, skin grafts, bone grafts, palate surgeries Base of tongue, floor of mouth, partial glossectomy	Allogenic BMT Surgery for: Esophageal cancer Pancreatic cancer Head and neck surgery: Commando procedures, mandibulectomy, laryngectomy, laryngopharyngoeso- phogastrectomy/gastric pull-up After loading catheters Head and neck brachytherapy
WEIGHT STATUS	(% UBW) > 90% usual body weight (UBW)	(Loss) (1) 1%-2% UBW (over 1 wk) (2) <5% UBW (over 1 mo) (3) <10% UBW (over 6 mo)	(Loss) (1) >2% UBW (over 1 wk) (2) >5% UBW (over 1 mo) (3) >10% UBW (over 6 mo)
DIET ORDERS	Patient does not require diet instruction	Patient requires diet instruction for diet modification or drug/nutrient interaction	Enteral nutrition PN/PPN Dysphagia diet Renal diet NPO/clear liquids ≥ 5 days (without nutrition support) (*Exceptions: nephrectomy, cystectomies, hemicolectomies)

MSKCC Adult Oncology Screening Tool, Clinical Dietitian Staff 1994–1995. Courtesy Memorial Sloan-Kettering Cancer Center, Food Service Department.
BMT, Bone marrow transplant, *GI,* gastrointestinal; *IV,* intravenous; *NPO,* nil per os OIC (nothing by mouth); *PN,* parenteral nutrition; *PPN,* peripheral parenteral nutrition; *UBW,* usual body weight.

weight loss, cachexia (extreme weight loss, loss of lean body mass and adipose tissue, anorexia, anemia, and emaciation), and malnutrition.

Bowel habits, symptoms of GI distress, and previous or planned antineoplastic therapy must be factored into a comprehensive evaluation. Most of these items could easily be incorporated into the screening-assessment form with minimal cost of staff time. With cost containment playing an important role in use and support of resources and staff, every effort should be made to streamline staff involvement where possible.

Nutrition Concerns

WEIGHT CHANGES. Weight is still the most meaningful parameter in nutritional status. Weight loss greater than 10% may be present in 45% or more of hospitalized adult cancer patients.[26] The consequences of significant weight loss predisposing the patient to malnutrition are well-documented.[9,27-29] In patients with a tumor burden, weight loss independently affects morbidity and mortality.[30] In a study of 3047 adults participating in chemotherapy protocols for advanced cancer, baseline weights provided the following insights into weight loss experienced before diagnosis in several subpopulations:[30]

Lowest frequency weight loss (31% to 40%): breast, acute nonlymphocytic leukemia, sarcoma, non-Hodgkin's lymphoma

Intermediate frequency weight loss (48% to 61%): colon, prostate, lung

Highest frequency weight loss (83% to 87%): pancreas, stomach

In more recent studies looking at resting energy expenditure (REE) on specific tumor sites, variations in weight also were seen. One study assessed 21 patients with unresectable pancreatic cancer using 16 controls. The patients had an elevated REE compared with the controls. REEs were even greater in patients with an acute-phase response (C-reative protein >10 mg/L) compared with patients without a response. The investigators concluded that patients with pancreatic cancer tended to have elevated REEs contributing to their weight loss. Patients who had an acute-phase response were markedly hypermetabolic.[31]

Another study investigated the influence of malignant tumor burden in 104 patients with gastric and colorectal (GCR) cancer, 47 patients with non–small-cell lung cancer, and 40 healthy controls on REE. REE was elevated in patients with lung cancer and was similar in GCR patients compared with controls. After tumor resection, 47 patients with GCR cancer and 14 lung cancer patients had their REE measured postoperatively at 18 months and 12 months, respectively. The GCR cancer patients showed a small but significant increase in REE with or without recurrence. Lung cancer patients with no recurrence after 1 year decreased their REE, while those with lung recurrence either had no change or increased their REE. After surgery, REE again returned to normal.[32]

Seventy-five colorectal cancer patients undergoing oncologic surgery were evaluated for basal energy expenditure (BEE) postoperatively.

17 patients expended 40% to 60% estimated BEE during hospitalization

33 patients expended 60% to 80%

22 patients expended 80% to 100%

3 patients expended 100% to 125%

Sixty-seven of the 75 patients lost weight during their hospitalization. The researchers concluded that the caloric intake was insufficient to meet the BEE of these patients. They suggest that individualized nutrition care plans consistent with each patient's energy needs should be part of standard of care.[33]

Involuntary weight loss of 5% to 10% or more over 1 to 6 months places a person at nutritional risk, and such risk should be identified as early as possible. Although weight should be a straightforward measure, any health care professional who has clinical experience can appreciate the problems that can confound determining the patient's weight, but every effort should be made to record weight accurately.

Using the same scale for repeat weighing eliminates one variable. Having the patient wear the same type of clothes, with pockets empty and slippers or shoes consistently on or off, also helps. Routine policies for weighing should be established. The dietetic professional must grasp how the clinical setting "operates" and then determine how to implement a routine for weighing. Does the nutrition committee of the medical center need to draft a policy? Should a multidisciplinary team be approached on each floor? Should the nursing staff or nursing administration be consulted?

Weight is also affected by edema, ascites, pleural effusions, and hydration status. Every effort should be made to determine hydration status in conjunction with weight. A third of U.S. adults are now classified as overweight, so it is good to know how to identify undernutrition or malnutrition in overweight persons.[21] The patient must also be questioned about drugs or medications that affect weight or hydration status (and, in turn, weight).

Weight changes, the strongest correlate of nutritional status, need to be considered in a time frame. Recent unplanned weight loss of several percent alerts to a developing nutrition problem that should be addressed before it becomes severe. Involuntary weight loss of 5% within the past 3 months or a 10% weight change in the previous 6 months also places the patient in a high-risk category. Medications such as steroids that cause edema or fluid retention may create a false clinical impression of weight status.

Premorbid weight is important. In someone who has always been a thin adult, leanness can be normal or nearly normal. If a person was always heavy, that fact should be factored into the evaluation of current weight status. All possibilities should be explored before declaring the patient at risk.

In a study looking at 254 cancer patients to determine what symptoms affected weight loss, abdominal fullness, altered taste, vomiting, and dry mouth were the ones identified most frequently and were independent of whether patients had had chemotherapy.[34] The investigators concluded that oral and GI symptoms affect weight loss early in the course of disease, regardless of nutritional status, calorie intake, and prior treatment.

Breast cancer appears to be associated with little or no weight loss, even when bone involvement is present.[30] Patients who lost weight before breast cancer was diagnosed had poorer performance status and survival than those who lost little or no weight. In a study of 923 women with nonmetastatic breast cancer, only 13% were underweight, 42.2% were at their desirable weight, 22.1% were overweight, and 22.4% were obese.[35] Because of duration, type, intensity of treatment regimens, or other confounding variables such as menopausal status and nodal status, many breast cancer patients gain up to 50 pounds.[36] Overweight is associated with increased risk for recurrence and mortality. In a study of 53 premenopausal women with operable breast cancer, 36 had adjuvant chemotherapy and 17 had localized treatment. No differences were found in REE or energy intake in either group. The chemotherapy group gained twice the weight, with more accumulation of body fat and fat mass 1 year after diagnosis. The conclusion of the study was that excess intake was not attributable to the weight gain. Women undergoing chemotherapeutic regimens are at increased risk for developing sarcopenic obesity and should be counseled appropriately regarding nutrition and increasing physical activity, which was decreased.[37]

Another study of 20 premenopausal women with stage I or II breast cancer receiving adjuvant chemotherapy looked at resting metabolic rate (RMR) and energy intake. Of the original patients, the 18 completing the study showed significantly decreased RMR midway through therapy with a rebounding to baseline levels by completion of treatment. Physical activity and caloric intake were lower than baseline levels as a result of chemotherapy.[38]

An area of recent interest with postmenopausal breast cancer patients is the role of increased body mass index (BMI) and its effect on insulin and insulin-like growth factors (IGFs) modulating the cell cycle and apoptosis.[39] The incidence of breast cancer is consistent with hyperinsulinism, dyslipidemia, hypertension, and atherosclerosis—components of insulin resistance syndrome. Research indicates that hyperinsulinism can promote mammary carcinogenesis most likely by the bioactivity of IGFs.[40] The avoidance of obesity and a regular exercise regimen should be strongly encouraged for this patient population.

Women who have breast cancer may gain weight during or after treatment, which places them at higher risk for recurrence and death. A study of 535 newly diagnosed women with operable breast cancer, 147 receiving adjuvant chemotherapy only, 151 tamoxifen only, 46 both, and 168 neither, was conducted for 49.6 months. High fasting insulin was negatively correlated with BMI, tumor stage and grade, and nodal stage. Fasting insulin predicted distant disease free survival and overall survival. When adjusted for adjuvant chemotherapy or tamoxifen, the relative risk of death in upper versus lower quartiles of insulin were 7.99 and 8.46, respectively. The conclusion of this study was that fasting insulin is a strong prognostic factor and increases the risk of both recurrence and death.[41] Diet may be able to play a significant role in modulating insulin levels in this population. Other sites have also been identified as negatively responding to high insulin levels.[42] Dietetic professionals should be sensitive to dietary components that may elevate cancer patients' insulin levels.

The dietetic professional should select an appropriate method of assessing weight status and tracking weight changes in the cancer patient. Strategies should be developed for:

- Documenting weights and weight changes accurately
- Encouraging and advising patients to maintain an appropriate weight for height
- Achieving and maintaining weight for individuals who experience weight loss

BODY COMPOSITION. In addition to weight changes, underfed cancer patients exhibit alterations in body composition—loss of subcutaneous fat stores and lean body mass. Loss of muscle tissue leads to fatigue, weakness, increased risk of thrombosis, decubiti, muscle atrophy, compromised respiratory function, and GI symptoms. Cancer patients frequently present with weight and lean body losses.

Anthropometry for muscle mass is often of little value in patients with advanced undernutrition. Visible muscle wasting and fat store depletion obviously indicate advanced undernutrition.[20] If evidence of wasting is not apparent, triceps or sacral measures are of little use because changes would not be detectable over the short course during hospitalization. If the patient is to be followed as an outpatient or in a research protocol, anthropometry may detect changes or provide useful data long-term.

Height, weight, and body composition determinations must be based on appropriate standards or guidelines. Tables or nomograms developed for a healthy population at large may be biased when used for cancer patients. Tables of desirable weight for height and sex that also account for age may be better measures for patients who are not chronically malnourished. Given the high incidence of cancer among the elderly, more realistic standards for that group would be preferable.[21]

For cancer patients with active disease, the lowest weight for height in published ranges may be more appropriate than the average or higher value because the tables reflect average Americans who tend to be overweight. By such tables, thin cancer patients appear to be even more malnourished than they actually are. BMI is more appropriate for identifying obesity. It can also be useful for breast cancer patients but not for the many cancer patients who are underweight. For a more extensive review of body composition measures, see Chapter 3 and reference 29.

LABORATORY PARAMETERS. Laboratory values should be included in any patient assessment. However, they may lead to false conclusions. Most biochemical parameters do not independently reflect nutritional deficiencies.[43,44] Shike and coworkers found total serum proteins and serum albumin values to be normal in patients with small cell lung cancer who were judged malnourished by virtue of weight loss, creatinine index, negative nitrogen balance, and low potassium and fat stores. Therefore, decreased lean body tissue did not necessarily correlate with low circulating proteins as measured in the admission screening clinical chemistry panels typically available to clinicians.[45]

In many cancer patients negative nitrogen balance appears to be a result of peripheral muscle tissue loss rather than visceral protein stores.[45-47] Cohn and associates showed that changes in body composition such as increased extracellular fluid and sodium and decreased potassium and intracellular fluid were responses to severe malnutrition and cachexia. Cohn concluded that losses in skeletal muscle compartment containing 45% total body nitrogen and 85% total body potassium were accounting for the changed body composition seen in cachectic patients. Body cell mass (BCM) usually decreases with age. In cancer patients BCM decreases with weight loss, depleting protein and fat stores. The adaptive mechanism usually associated with starvation—sparing protein and utilizing fat stores—was not observed in cancer patients.[46]

Various visceral carrier proteins such as albumin, thyroxine-binding prealbumin (transthyretin), transferrin, and retinol-binding protein have been suggested for use as clinical parameters of nutritional status. Low serum albumin may be a result of so many nonnutritional medical causes such as liver disease, infection, acute and chronic inflammation, hydration status, stress, nephrotic syndrome, cirrhosis, and chronic bronchitis that its use in nutrition assessment is limited.[20] Conditions such as liver disease, metastases, kidney dysfunction, and expanded plasma volume all affect albumin status. Albumin has a half-life of about 3 weeks. Although the half-life of prealbumin is 2 days, it can be similarly affected by medical problems. In addition, inflammatory bowel disease, salicylates, and steroid hormones can affect prealbumin levels.[43,44]

Transferrin has a half-life of a week or so. Iron depletion or exogenous hormones can affect values by increasing transferrin levels. Infection, active tumorigenesis, inflammation, and hepatic or renal disease can decrease transferrin levels. Total lymphocyte counts are also affected by the patient's clinical condition. Total lymphocyte count is an indicator of immune status, but it is not generally a good indicator of nutritional status. In addition to the myriad clinical conditions that can predispose to abnormal serum protein values or total lymphocyte counts, malnutrition also contributes to compromised clinical chemistry protein measures. The difficulty arises when one attempts to sort the medically induced causes of abnormal protein values from the nutritional ones. Therefore, parameters that are more indicative of nutritional status should be selected. For an extensive review of assessment parameters, see references 35, 48, 49, 50 and Part II Assessment of Nutritional Status.

Blood levels of electrolytes and minerals, including calcium, magnesium, and phosphorus, should be measured as part of the admission screening panel or during a patient's hospital stay. Abnormalities should be accounted for in the nutrition care plan in the context of the patient's overall medical picture. Zinc testing may have to be ordered, particularly if diarrhea, scaly dermatitis, or alcohol abuse is present. If vitamin and trace element, electrolyte, or other biochemical indices are part of the screening panel, they should be incorporated into the assessment; but testing for nutrition evaluation is done only when a deficiency or abnormality is suspected and confirmation would be useful in the overall management of the patient. Using a medical nutrition therapy protocol such as the one the Oncology Nutrition Dietetics Practice Group of the American Dietetic Association (ADA) developed may be helpful in determining which parameters to monitor and how frequently they should be assessed.[19]

In summary, although many medical conditions and current nutritional status may affect the accuracy of laboratory tests and evaluations, they are a valuable part of patient care and should be considered when monitoring patients throughout treatment and recovery.

DIMINISHED INTAKE. Diminished food intake is so common among cancer patients that the dietetic professional may overlook the importance of determining the cause, which might suggest realistic, effective solutions to the problem. More than one cause may be uncovered: emotional, physical, and metabolic factors may be combined or separate issues. If the dietetic professional fails to sort out the cause or causes, an opportunity to resolve the problem may be lost.

Unexplained weight loss due to anorexia or loss of appetite suggests the possibility of an occult neoplasm. Anorexia can result from systemic responses still unexplained in the tumor process and may develop after the diagnosis is made. This can be secondary to the anxiety of confronting a life-threatening illness or to tumor activity. Anorexia (often leading to cachexia) can be present early in the course of the disease, limiting the patient's ability to eat enough to supply nutritional requirements. Management is most effective when the cause can be determined.

Early satiety is frequently experienced by the patient at risk for or already experiencing malnutrition. Delayed gastric emptying or decreased gastric transit time may contribute to the patient's inability to eat enough. Problems of GI discomfort, nausea, and vomiting are more important to quality of life than pain for many patients.[51-54]

Nausea and vomiting, diarrhea, cramping, bloating, flatulence, and general discomfort associated with eating contribute to inadequate nutrition. Use of antiemetic, antidiarrheal, orexigenic (appetite enhancers), and pain medications should be encouraged.[55,56] Drugs are now readily available for nausea, queasiness, and appetite stimulation and every effort should be made to take advantage of their benefits (Table 34-2).

Mucositis, stomatitis, and oral pain can make eating difficult. The physical discomfort caused by the irritation of eating may discourage patients from consuming enough, as can dry mouth, poor dentition, and dysphagia. Oral analgesics, topical anesthetics, antifungal medication, and ice chips may provide symptomatic relief.[57]

Aversion to the taste and smell of food frequently develops as a result of negative food experiences during or after antineoplastic therapy. The patient associates the adverse response with the food, rejecting the item when offered it again. The dietetic professional should seek the origin of the aversion and the extent of the problem.

Determining the nature of chewing or swallowing difficulty may enable the dietetic professional to recommend appropriate solutions, such as a change in consistency, texture, or amount taken with each mouthful and during each meal. The effort to prepare or consume the food or the lack of strength to cut, chew, or manipulate the utensils or food items may deter the patient from eating. Every effort should be made to assist the patient at mealtime. Volunteers, aides, or caregivers should be assigned to open containers, cut foods, and position the patient properly and comfortably for eating. The nutrition care plan should include arrangements to assist and support the patient and prevent physical deterioration after discharge. Companions, cancer care aides, or another home-bound service agency should be contacted.

Pain, either from the disease itself or the effects of treatment, can affect the desire and ability to eat. Symptomatic pain relief can be provided at mealtime with proper dosing and scheduling of medications. If the patient is suffering from uncontrolled pain, a pain consultation should be sought, and the dietetic professional should consult the physician in charge.

Fear, anxiety, and depression often alter the behavior and attitude of the patient and loved ones. One response to a devastating illness is rejection of things that nourish and nurture. If the patient is not coping well, psychiatric, spiritual, or social work consultation should be sought. If the managing physician or another team member does not pursue this, the dietetic professional should. Multidisciplinary rounds may be a good time for the issue to be raised if the dietetic professional has difficulty ordering consults independently.

DISEASE-SPECIFIC IMPACT ON NUTRITIONAL STATUS. Tumors in the GI tract can obstruct passage of nutrients or limit the patient's capability of eating. Tumors outside the GI tract such as metastatic ovarian cancer can also compromise nutrition by pressing on the GI structures and causing obstruction with the same results: inadequate intake, early satiety, and anorexia or cachexia. Tumors can also cause anorexia and cachexia secondary to remote systemic or central nervous system effects.

Metabolic Alterations

Although metabolic changes are known to occur as part of the cancer process, the mechanisms are still not fully understood,

TABLE 34-2

Emetogenic Potential of Chemotherapy Drugs

Emesis Prevalence	Agent	Dose (mg/m^2)	Onset (hr)	Duration (hr)
V. High >90%	HD-Carboplatin (CDPCA)	≥1 g/m^2		
	Carmustine (BCNU)	>200	2-4	4-24
	Cisplatin (CDDP)	≥70	1-6	24-120
	Cyclophosphamide (CTX)	≥1000	4-12	12-24
	Cytarabine (ARA-C)	>1000	Rate related	2-4
	Dacarbazine (DTIC)	≥500	1-3	1-12
	Dactinomycin (ACT-D)			
	Ifosfamide	≥3 g/m^2		
	Lomustine (CCNU)	>60	2-6	4-6
	Melphalan (L-PAM)	>140	3-6	6-12
	Nitrogen mustard (Mechlorethamine)	6	0.5-2	8-24
	Streptozocin	>500	1-4	12-24
	HD-Thiotepa	Cont. infusion		
	Tirapazamine			
IV. Moderate-High 60%-90%	5-Azacytidine*	200	1-3	3-4
	Carboplatin (CDBCA)	500-<1000		
	Carmustine (BCNU)	≤200	2-4	4-24
	Cisplatin (CDDP)	<70	1-6	24-120
	Cyclophosphamide (CTX)	750-<1000	4-12	12-24
	Cytarabine	250-1000	6-12	3-5
	Dacarbazine (DTIC)	<500	1-3	1-12
	Daunorubicin	≥75		
	Doxorubicin (ADRIA)	≥45	4-6	6+
	HD-Edatrexate*			
	Idarubicin			
	Ifosfamide	1200-<3000		
	Loboplatin*			
	Lomustine (CCNU)	<60	2-6	4-6
	Mesna			
	Methotrexate	≥1000	4-12	3-12
	Mitomycin	10	1-4	48-72
	Mitotane			
	Procarbazine	100	24-27	Variable
III. Moderate 30%-60%	Aldesleukin			
	Asparaginase	>5000 U	1-3	—
	Bleomycin			
	Busulfan	148 (4 mg/kg)	—	—
	Carboplatin (CDBCA)	<300	6-12	24
	Carmustine (BCNU)			
	Cyclophosphamide (CTX) (PO)	<750	4-12	12-24
	Cytarabine	20-<250		
	Doxorubicin (ADRIA)	20-<45	4-6	6+
	Etoposide (VP-16)	>100 or infusion	3-8	—
	5-Fluorouracil (5-FU)	>1000	3-6	—
	Hexamethylmelamine*			
	Ifosfamide	<1200	1-2	—
	Methotrexate	250-<1000	4-12	3-12
	Mitoxantrone			
	Pentostatin	2-4		
	Teniposide (VM-26)*	60-170	3-8	—

Continued.

but as a result of the explosion of knowledge in the field of molecular and cellular biology, many of the questions surrounding the mechanisms and actions of tumor cells and their effects on host cells are being explored.[58] Much is still lacking in our understanding of the myriad processes that constitute the development and clinical progression of cancer.

ENERGY EXPENDITURE. The metabolic derangements of cancer patients are different from cancer-free persons who are

starved, febrile, malnourished, or stressed. Reasons for this response remain unexplained, although research is uncovering mechanisms to explain the effects seen in this population.[28,29,59,62]

For many types of cancer, energy expenditure remains a mystery. Because of the severe weight loss typically seen in some cancer patients, hypermetabolism seemed a reasonable explanation. In the 1970s and 1980s, results of studies of REE

TABLE 34-2

Emetogenic Potential of Chemotherapy Drugs—cont'd

Emesis Prevalence	Agent	Dose (mg/m2)	Onset (hr)	Duration (hr)
II. Mild 10%-30%	9-AC*	Cont. infusion		
	Bleomycin	10 U	3-6	—
	Camptothecan (CPT-11)*			
	Cytarabine	<20	6-12	3-5
	Docetaxel*			
	Doxorubicin (ADRIA)	<20	4-6	6+
	5-Fluorouracil (5-FU)	<1000	3-6	—
	Hydroxyurea	1000-6000	6-12	—
	Irinotecan*			
	6-Mercaptopurine	100	4-8	—
	Methotrexate	<250	4-12	3-12
	Mitomycin			
	Mitomycin-C	Intrahepatic		
	Mitoxantrone	10-14	—	—
	Paclitaxel			
I. Minimal <10%	Altetamine			
	Asparaginase			
	Busulfan	2-6	—	—
	Chlorambucil	1-3	48-72	—
	Cladribine (2-CDA)	Cont. infusion		
	Edatrexate			
	Estramustine			
	Etoposide (VP-16)			
	Floxuridine (FUDR)	Intraperitoneal		
	Fludarabine			
	Fluorouracil (5-FU)	Cont. infusion		
	Goserelin			
	Idarubicin			
	Interferon (α,β,γ)	Variable	—	—
	Leuprolide acetate			
	Megestrol acetate			
	Mitotane			
	Navelbine (Vinorelbine)			
	Pegaspergase			
	PBA			
	Plicamycin			
	Suioi*	Cont. infusion		
	Suramin*			
	Tamoxifen			
	Taxotere			
	Teniposide (YM-26)*			
	Thioguanine			
	Topotecan*			
	Vinblastine (Velban)			
	Vincristine			
	Vinorelbine	6	4-8	—

Adapted from Lindley CM, Bernard S, Fields SM: Incidence and duration of chemotherapy-induced nausea and vomiting in the outpatient oncology population, *J Clin Oncol* 7:1142–1149, 1989, modified and updated by Abby S. Bloch, PhD, R.D., and Jane Nolte, Pharm. D., Memorial Sloan-Kettering Cancer Center, 1995.
*Investigational agent.
Where dosage, onset of duration information is not provided, the health professional working with a specific agent should fill in the blanks for that agent based on clinical practice at his/her facility and personal experience of patients receiving the agent.
Courtesy Memorial Sloan-Kettering Cancer Center Antiemetic Subcommittee. Pharmacy and Therapeutics Committee.

in cancer patients did not always support that hypothesis.[63-65] In a study by Knox and coworkers, the measured REE of 200 malnourished cancer patients was studied by indirect calorimetry and compared with expected energy expenditure.[59] Their findings were as follows: 26% had increased REE, 41% had normal REE, and 33% had decreased REE.

The investigators controlled for age, height, weight, sex, nutritional status, tumor burden, and presence or absence of liver metastasis and found no correlations with any of these variables. Patients who had had cancer longest were the most hypermetabolic. This led the investigators to conclude that the duration of the malignancy might have a significant effect on energy metabolism. They also proposed that energy expenditure could not be predicted by standard formulas.

Heber's group measured REE in noncachectic lung cancer patients and concluded that they were not hypermetabolic.

Heber reported, however, that a decrease in basal metabolic rate is a normal adaptation to starvation, so that even normal REEs can reflect increased REE in a malnourished cancer patient.[66] Others have reported that changes in metabolic rate depend on the type of tumor.[67] Increased REE has been associated with sarcomas, leukemia, lymphoma, lung, head and neck, lung (small cell), and stomach cancers, and decreased REE has been associated with pancreatic tumors, whereas with colon cancers, rates are normal.[45,48,65,67,68] Increases in REE seem to be associated with advanced disease and decreased food intake. Significant decreases in REE were seen in chemotherapy patients whose disease responded to treatment; nonresponders' REEs showed no change. Similarly, elevated REEs dropped after tumor resection.[68-70]

In another study in which malnourished patients with colon and non–small-cell lung cancer were compared with malnourished noncancer patients and healthy volunteers, no differences among the three groups were seen in the REE per kilogram lean body mass (LBM).[71] No significant differences were found when weight-losing or weight-stable patients with gastric and colon cancer were compared with weight-losing patients with benign GI disease when REE, REE per kilogram body weight, or REE per kilogram of fat-free mass was measured.[72] In general, it would appear that REE does not necessarily account for the cachexia seen in many cancer patients; patients with severe weight loss tend to maintain their REE instead of adapting to the starved state, which should lower the REE to preserve LBM and fat stores.[9]

CARBOHYDRATE METABOLISM. In the normal adaptation to starvation, the body uses glycogen stored in the liver and muscles to provide energy required by the brain, leukocytes, and other tissues. Once those stores are depleted, initially muscle protein is the source of fuel; then gradually it is replaced by fat and fatty acids, which are converted to ketone bodies. Ketone bodies can provide up to 95% of the fuel needed by the brain, sparing glucose and muscle protein. If cancer patients cannot utilize this adaptive mechanism, glucose production and protein catabolism continue to provide the needed energy.

Although their circulating insulin and glucose levels may or may not be normal, cancer patients appear to have glucose intolerance caused by impaired insulin sensitivity, increased insulin resistance, or inadequate insulin release. Hyperglycemia and delayed clearance of blood glucose after a glucose load is not uncommon in this population.[66,73] The importance of Cori cycling in the weight loss and cachexia of cancer patients is still not known. The Cori cycle or "futile cycle," in which glucose is converted to lactate and resynthesized to glucose in the liver, is energy wasting because six adenosine triphosphate (ATP) molecules are required to resynthesize glucose and only two ATP molecules are produced. This is a very inefficient means of producing ATP, which cells need for energy. Many reviews of abnormal carbohydrate metabolism are available.[9,74]

LIPID METABOLISM. Many cancer patients exhibit fat mobilization and loss of fat stores because of increased lipolysis. Tumor-derived lipid mobilizing factors have been identified as possible mediators of tissue wasting in cachexia by mobilizing fatty acids from adipose tissue.[75] Loss of fat stores may also be attributable to insulin resistance and increased oxidation of fatty acids. The products of lipolysis—glycerol and fatty acids—serve as the substrates for gluconeogenesis and energy production when available energy is inadequate. Waterhouse studied utilization of fatty acid, the principal substrate in cancer patients, and observed increased clearance from plasma of endogenous and exogenous fats in both fasting and fed states. These patients did not suppress lipolysis when glucose was given but continued to oxidize fatty acids.[70,76-78]

In a study by Hansell and coworkers,[29] 70 weight-losing and weight-stable cancer patients with colorectal or gastric cancer were compared to 23 control weight-losing and weight-stable cancer-free patients. The cancer group oxidized more fat and less carbohydrate than controls, findings that were independent of weight loss. The weight-losing cancer patients (including those with liver metastases) had higher fat oxidation rates than the other three groups. These findings led the investigators to conclude that the cachexia seen in these patients must be due in large part to abnormal fat and carbohydrate metabolism rather than to energy expenditure abnormalities. Cancer patients fail to suppress lipolysis even when glucose is given. This leads to the extreme fat depletion of cachectic cancer patients. Extensive reviews of rates of fatty acid oxidation in cancer patients have been published.[7,74-79]

PROTEIN METABOLISM. Protein metabolism is altered in cancer patients. Protein kinetics of undernourished cancer patients frequently are similar to those of patients who suffer trauma or infection.[9] Most patients are in negative nitrogen balance, which worsens with the degree of malignancy.[80] Norton showed that cancer patients have increased whole body protein turnover and muscle wasting and decreased in serum protein levels.[81] Fearon and coworkers, on the other hand, found no correlation between protein turnover rate, energy expenditure, and weight loss when colon and lung cancer patients were compared with controls.[72] Cohn and coworkers found that cancer patients who had lost weight had significantly decreased lean body mass; however, the percentage of nonmuscle lean body mass (i.e., visceral protein) increased.[46,47] Over 6 months, Cohn's patients lost an average of 15 kg—48% of their average total weight as water, 41% as fat, and 11% as protein.[46]

Cancer patients exhibit increased protein synthesis in the liver and decreased synthesis in muscles, with a net increase in whole-body turnover favoring the tumor at the expense of peripheral muscle. In nitrogen studies done by Brennan and Burt, muscle protein synthesis decreased and plasma aminograms appeared abnormal.[82] For more detailed information on metabolic changes in cancer, readers are referred to references 74 and 83 to 85.

Tisdale and his colleagues have developed a mouse model to study protein catabolism in cancer cachexia. They discovered that some tumors produce a circulating proteolysis-inducing factor (PIF) found in weight-losing animals. PIF was then isolated from the urine of patients with pancreatic, breast, ovarian, lung, colon, rectal, and hepatic cancer who had lost more than 1.5 kg/month. Patients who were weight stable and normal controls had no PIF in their urine. Weight-losing patients without cancer also had no detectable PIF in their urine. PIF appears to be a biologically active compound causing lean body mass depletion leading to weight loss even without a reduction in food intake. These investigators found that ω-3 fatty acids, specifically eicosapentaenoic acid (EPA), attenuated the effects of PIF by increasing total body fat and muscle mass.[86,87] In a study of 20 weight-losing patients with unresectable pancreatic adenocarcinoma who were given 1.09 g EPA, weight increased, REE fell, and performance status and appetite improved. Using EPA may be an effective supplement for cancer cachexia.[88]

CYTOKINES. Cytokines—mediators of inflammation, injury, and repair secreted by all immune cells—regulate many immune mechanisms, including intermediary metabolism, tumor growth, and metabolic derangements. It is now believed that the production of cytokines is involved in the wasting and protein, fat, and carbohydrate abnormalities that result in a net energy deficit that ultimately results in severe malnutrition and eventual death.[89] Many cytokines have been implicated in the pathophysiology of cancer cachexia, including tumor necrosis factor, interleukin-1 (IL-1), interleukin-6 (IL-6), and interferon gamma. Recently leptin, a hormone secreted by adipose tissue, which controls both dietary intake and energy expenditure through neuropeptides of the hypothalamus, has been studied in its role in cachexia. Inui hypothesized that cytokines may play a pivotal role in long-term inhibition of feeding by mimicking the hypothalamic effect of excessive negative feedback signaling from leptin.[90]

It appears that cytokines interact by overlapping physiologic activities, supporting the hypothesis that combinations rather than individual cytokines produce the devastating effects of cancer cachexia. Cytokines modulate the utilization of dietary nutrients. By modifying cytokine action, pharmacologic drugs may be effective in improving nutrition support to starving cancer patients.[91] Cytokines found in tumor models support tumor growth and may act as tumor growth factors while contributing to tissue wasting and cachexia.[89] Gogos and his group studied the effects of dietary ω-3 fatty acids and vitamin E on immune function in well-nourished and malnourished patients with generalized solid tumors. Using 18 g ω-3 fatty acids, the investigators found an immunomodulating effect with increased tumor necrosis factor levels in the malnourished patients and prolonged survival in all subjects.[92] For more extensive reviews of this emerging area of cytokines and their impact on nutrition and cancer, the reader is directed to references 9, 74, and 93 to 95.

Nutritional Effects of Cancer Therapies

As important as nutrition is to the patient with cancer, it alone cannot cure cancer. Therapeutic modalities must be provided to eradicate, control, or minimize the neoplastic process. Concomitant with the treatment, however, are detrimental effects that place the patient at risk for malnutrition. The available therapies along with their untoward effects are reviewed here.

Chemotherapy

Cytotoxic drugs destroy cancer cells by interfering directly or indirectly with the synthesis and function of nucleic acids in the cells,[93] but healthy cells (and tissues) can also be damaged, especially those with fast replication rates. Rapidly dividing cells including those of bone marrow and most parts of the GI tract are most susceptible to damage, followed by hair follicles and gonads.[93] Nutritional compromise related to chemotherapy can be attributed to direct effects of the cytotoxic agents on the GI tract plus side effects of therapy, mainly nausea, vomiting, anorexia, diarrhea, mucositis, altered taste, and food aversions. Antineoplastic drugs are classified by mechanisms of action and effects on normal and cancerous cells.[93,96] Table 34-3 lists chemotherapeutic agents and adverse effects on nutritional status.

Side effects of chemotherapy depend on the prescribed treatment regimen—single or combination agents, planned number of cycles, dose administered, the individual's response to the therapy as well as his/her current health status, including nutritional status. It is critical that the dietetic professional and other team members monitoring the oncology patient provide timely and appropriate supportive therapies and provide the patient with appropriate pharmacologic agents in the effective management of treatment-related side effects of chemotherapy.

Alkylating agents such as cyclophosphamide, the nitrosoureas (carmustine), busulfan, dacarbazine, cisplatin, and carboplatin are cell-cycle nonspecific. During G_0 phase of the cell cycle, after nucleic acids are formed, they interfere with replication of DNA and transcription of RNA by reacting with preformed nucleic acids and attacking and damaging the cells' native DNA. They remain active throughout all phases of the cell cycle. Antimetabolites such as methotrexate, 5-fluorouracil (5-FU) and cytosine arabinoside (Ara-C) replace or compete with original metabolites for the catalytic or regulatory site of a key enzyme, or they inhibit or interfere with the normal biosynthesis of nucleic acids, interrupting normal formation or function of DNA and RNA and resulting in cell death. They are most active during the S phase of the cell cycle. Dactinomycin, bleomycin, mitomycin C, and doxorubicin are examples of antibiotics that interfere with cell division by disrupting DNA replication and interfering with transcription of RNA. Other mechanisms that interfere with cell division by antitumor antibiotics are impairment of DNA repair; generation of superoxide, a damaging free radical; and their tenacious binding capability, which disrupts the cell membrane.[93] Antibiotics are active throughout the cell cycle but are most effective in the S and G_2 phases. Vinca alkaloids, vincristine, vinblastine etoposide, (VP-16), paclitaxel, to name a few, stop cell division during mitosis and are M-phase specific.

Enzymes starve certain tumor cells by hydrolyzing asparagine to aspartic acid. Cancer cells cannot synthesize asparagine and must get it from the blood. Without asparagine the tumor cells die. Normal cells can synthesize their own L-asparagine. Enzymes work in the G_1 phase of the cell cycle.

Natural and synthetic hormones such as tamoxifen, progestins, and leuprolide (Lupron) alter hormone balance or interact directly with tumor cell surface receptors to modify growth of some cancers by accelerating or retarding growth of certain cells, tissues, and target organs. Steroid hormones stimulate or suppress transcription of mRNA sequencing, leading to alterations in cell function and growth.

Miscellaneous agents, including structural analogs of existing drugs, biologic response modifiers, immune modulators,

---

TABLE 34-3

Actions and Potential Adverse Nutritional Effects of Cytotoxic Drugs

Actions	Examples	Potential for Adverse Nutritional Effects*
I. Inhibition of a stage of DNA synthesis		
A. Single carbon transfer blocking purine synthesis		
1. Inhibits H_2 folate reductase	Methotrexate†	A^+, N^+, P, M^{2+}, U, D^{2+}
2. Blocks thymidylate and inosinic acid synthesis	Methotrexate†	A^+, N^+, P, M^{2+}, U, D^{2+}
B. Inhibits purine synthesis or interconversion	6-Mercaptopurine	A, N^{2+}, M^+, D^+
	Pentostatin	A, N^{3+}
C. Blocks interconversion of pyrimidines (thymidylate synthase inhibition)	5-Fluorouracil	A, N^+, M^{2+}, D^{2+}
D. Inhibits pyrimidine metabolism	Streptozocin	A, N^{3+}, U, CT
E. DNA polymerase inhibition; also inhibits DNA strand growth	Cytarabine†	A^+, N^{2+}, M^+
F. Incorporates into RNA and inhibits protein synthesis	Azacitidine	A^{2+}, N^{2+}, D^{3+}
	Fluorouracil	A, N^2, M^+, D^+
G. Inhibits ribonucleotide reductase	Hydroxyurea†	A, N^+, M^+
II. Inhibition of DNA replication and transcription		
A. Alkylating agents react with susceptible DNA sites	Hexamethylmelamine	A, N^{3+}
	Chlorambucil	A, N^+
	Cyclophosphamide	A, N^{3+}
	Dacarbazine	A, N^{3+}, D
	Cisplatin	A, N^{3+}, Mg
	Carmustine (BCNU)	A, N^{3+}
B. Inhibiting DNA synthesis and DNA-dependent RNA synthesis by intercalating between DNA base pairs		
1. Antibiotic anthracycline glycosides	Doxorubicin	A, N^+, M^+
	Idarubicin	A, N^+, M^+
2. *Streptomyces* antibiotic	Dactinomycin	A, N^{3+}, M, D
C. Causes scission of single- and double-stranded DNA, free radical formation, and inhibition of DNA ligase	Bleomycin‡	M^{3+}, D, N^+
D. Degrades DNA by forming hydroxy radicals and inhibits DNA, RNA, and protein synthesis	Procarbazine	A, N^{2+}
E. Causes DNA strand breakage	Etoposide‡	N^+, M, D
	Amsacrine‡	A^{2+}, M^{2+}, CT
III. Enzyme inhibiting protein synthesis and delaying DNA and RNA synthesis		
A. Hydrolysis of asparagine to aspartic acid in cells lacking asparagine synthase	Asparaginase§	A^{2+}, N^{2+}
IV. Inhibition of mitosis		
A. Binds tubulin preventing microtubule assembly	Vinblastine	C, M, N, D
	Vincristine#	C^{3+}, P
B. Interferes with microtubule network	Taxol	A, M, N, D, O
C. Causes G2 phase arrest	Etoposide‡	N^+, M, D
D. Causes metaphase arrest	Teniposide‡	N^+, M, D

From Shils ME: Nutrition and diet in cancer management. In Shils ME, Olson J, Shike M (eds): *Modern nutrition in health and disease.* ed 8, Philadelphia, 1994, Lea & Febiger.
*Key: A, anorexia; C, constipation/ileus; CT, cardiac toxicity; D, diarrhea; M, mucositis/stomatitis; Mg, renal magnesium loss: N, nausea/vomiting; O, odynophagia, P, abdominal pain; U, intestinal ulceration. Letter without +, occurs uncommonly; letter with +, low potential; letter with 2+, moderate potential; letter with 3+, high potential.
† S phase specific.
‡ causes G2 phase arrest or delay.
# M phase specific.
§ G1 phase specific.

and newly discovered novel compounds are placed in this category. Colony-stimulating factors such as hematopoietic growth factors that stimulate the proliferation and differentiation of hematopoietic precursor cells and enhance the functions of mature myeloid cells may play major roles in proliferation and differentiation of progenitor cells, enhancing end-cell functions. Interleukin-3 (IL-3), granulocyte-macrophage colony-stimulating factor, and macrophage colony-stimulating factor are among the growth factors recombinant DNA technology has made available. These agents are used to support neutrophil recovery after chemotherapy and increase neutrophil counts in patients with chronic neutropenia, bone marrow myelosuppression, acute nonlymphocytic leukemia, and aplastic anemias. Another use may be as adjuncts with antibiotics for infections. Colony-stimulating factors seem to curtail neutropenia secondary to cytotoxic drug therapy.

New treatment regimens are being developed with an eye to taking advantage of drugs' different mechanisms of action, metabolic targets, and durations of activity, in the hope of reducing toxicity and maximizing antitumor activity. Attaching chemotherapeutic agents to monoclonal antibodies directed against specific tumor-associated antigens may also increase the effectiveness of some treatment modalities. The newly emerging area related to the formation of oncogenes, arising from the normal proto-oncogenes from which they are derived and their role in the deranged activity that leads to uncontrolled growth of the cell, may provide a specific target for the oncologist.[93]

SIDE EFFECTS.[9,96-98] *Nausea and vomiting* can result in decreased calorie intake, weight loss, and development of cachexia, dehydration, electrolyte and fluid imbalances, and metabolic derangements such as hypokalemia and metabolic alkalosis. Symptoms can develop within hours of administration of the drug or days later. The queasiness may be short lived or last for days. Some drugs cause dry mouth and alter the taste of food.

Diarrhea may cause fluid and electrolyte losses, dehydration, and metabolic alkalosis. *Anorexia* (which develops after chemotherapy begins) in response to treatment must be distinguished from anorexia associated with the disease process itself (depressed appetite determined in the initial screening). Distinguishing the causes of anorexia helps the dietetic professional make decisions about appropriate management and support.

Stomatitis and mucositis, inflammations of the mucous membranes of the entire alimentary tract, are very common side effects of chemotherapy. The ulceration generally lasts only several weeks; however the degree of mucositis is dose dependent and is affected by other concurrent or subsequent treatment modalities.

Constipation may result from certain chemotherapeutic drugs such as the vinca alkaloids, which cause neurotoxicity. Obstipation (severe constipation) develops within days after drugs are given and lasts several weeks.

Odynophagia (pain on swallowing), *dysgeusia* (a change in taste), and *xerostomia* (dry mouth) can limit the oral intake of individuals receiving chemotherapeutic drugs.

Cardiac toxicity, nephrotoxicity, and *hepatoxicity* may complicate the management of patients requiring monitoring of renal and hepatic function. If biochemical indices are abnormal, nutrition support should be adjusted appropriately. See Table 34-3 for nutritional consequences of chemotherapy.

Radiation
Radiation, the use of electromagnetic energy that passes through normal tissues to treat the tumor cells, may be used as the sole treatment or in combination with other therapies such as surgery or chemotherapy for nearly half of all patients treated. As Hendrickson and Withers observed, the objective of radiation therapy is "giving the maximum dose that the normal tissues can tolerate and praying that it is sufficient to control tumor."[99] Whereas chemotherapy is a system treatment, radiation therapy affects the tumor and the surrounding tissue. It is considered a "site specific treatment." Generally, treatment consists of 5-times-weekly doses for 4 to 7 weeks. (Each treatment lasts only minutes.) Side effects vary with dose, site of administration, and individual response. Areas of rapid cell proliferation such as the GI mucosa, bone marrow, and hair follicles are most vulnerable to radiation damage. When the GI tract is part of the radiation field, nutrition-related problems should be anticipated (Table 34-4).[98,100,101] These may include nausea and vomiting, diarrhea, anorexia, stenosis, radiation enteritis and malabsorption, blunted taste and smell (anosmia), difficulty or pain on swallowing or chewing, mouth blindness (loss of taste, dry mouth if head and neck area involved), mucositis, dental decay, osteoradionecrosis, oral infections, trismus, dysphagia, dysgeusia, fatigue, and strictures and fistulas.[99,102,103]

Several new techniques are being developed that irradiate tumor cells while preserving normal tissues. One such technique is three-dimensional radiotherapy, which targets the beam on a computer-generated three-dimensional image, providing more precise targeting of the tumor. Innovations in brachytherapy allow surgical implantation into the tumor of radioactive pellets (seeds) or removable thin catheters or needles into which seeds are placed after surgery. In intraoperative radiation, healthy organs are moved away from the radiation field during a surgical procedure, to protect them from the damaging effects of large doses delivered to the tumor. Hyperthermia (i.e., heat) increases the sensitivity of tumor cells to radiation. These advances should improve the outcome for many cancer patients.[93]

Surgery
Surgery, the oldest form of treatment for cancer, is still the preferred method for 60% of cases.[102,104] For undisseminated cancers, surgery can be curative. Stage and histologic features can be determined using tissue samples procured in surgical procedures. If the tumor is disseminated, surgical resection alone will not be curative. Combined modalities of therapy will be needed to control the growth of seeded cells outside the primary tumor. Resection may be curative in only 30% of patients treated with surgery alone because most solid tumors have spread beyond the primary site by the time they are resected.

When cure is not possible, palliative surgery can relieve symptoms, forestall intolerable symptoms, or prevent obstruction. Providing access to the intestinal tract, by resecting or bypassing an obstruction or inserting a feeding enterostomy, allows the GI tract to be used for feeding.

If radiation oncology, chemotherapy, or immunotherapy is used in conjunction with surgery or preoperatively or postoperatively, their contribution to nutritional compromise must be factored into the patient's clinical picture. Surgery to any part of the GI tract—from the head and neck, where mechanical or physical limitations combine with the metabolic and psychologic aspects of the disease process, to the esophagus, where severing of the vagus nerve leads to gastric atony, fat malabsorption, and diarrhea—places the patient at nutritional risk. Patients are also at increased risk for aspiration of gastric contents and gastric reflux. Gastric resection could cause rapid transit, dumping syndrome, and hypoglycemia, and possible deficiencies of iron, calcium, vitamin B_{12}, and fat-soluble vitamins. After resection, the small bowel may develop maldigestion and malabsorption of fats, fat-soluble vitamins, calcium, magnesium, and proteins, lactose intolerance, dehydration, diarrhea, blind-loop syndrome, intestinal ileus, or obstruction. Fluid and electrolyte losses, bloating, flatulence, cramping, diarrhea, bile loss, B_{12} deficiency, or bacterial overgrowth can occur in the large intestine. Finally, pancreatic function must be considered for possible maldigestion of fats and proteins, carbohydrates, fat-soluble vitamins, and minerals. Dietetic professionals providing nutrition support for patients who have undergone surgical resection for cancer often lose sight of basic physiology. The fact that the patient has cancer does not change the effect of a gastrostomy or bowel resection on the body's ability to function.[9]

TABLE 34-4

Consequences of Cancer Treatment Predisposing to Nutrition Problems

I. Radiation treatment
   A. Radiation of oropharyngeal area
      1. Destruction of sense of taste; xerostomia and odynophagia:
         loss of teeth
   B. Radiation to lower neck and mediastinum
      1. Esophagitis with dysphagia
      2. Fibrosis with esophageal stricture
   C. Radiation of abdomen and pelvis
      1. Bowel damage, acute and chronic, with diarrhea,
         malabsorption, stenosis and obstruction,
         fistulization
II. Surgical treatment
   A. Radical resection of oropharyngeal area
      1. Chewing and swallowing difficulties
   B. Esophagectomy
      1. Gastric stasis and hypochlorhydria secondary to
         vagotomy
      2. Steatorrhea secondary to vagotomy
      3. Diarrhea secondary to vagotomy
      4. Early satiety
      5. Regurgitation
   C. Gastrectomy (high subtotal or total)
      1. Dumping syndrome
      2. Malabsorption
      3. Achlorhydria and lack of intrinsic factor and R protein
      4. Hypoglycemia
      5. Early satiety
   D. Intestinal resection
      1. Jejunum
         a. Decreased efficiency of absorption of many
            nutrients
      2. Ileum
         a. Vitamin B_{12} deficiency
         b. Bile salt losses with diarrhea or steatorrhea
         c. Hyperoxaluria and renal stone
         d. Calcium and magnesium depletion
         e. Fat and fat-soluble vitamin malabsorption

      3. Massive bowel resection
         a. Life-threatening malabsorption
         b. Malnutrition
         c. Metabolic acidosis
         d. Dehydration
      4. Ileostomy and colostomy
         a. Complications of salt and water balance
   E. Blind loop syndrome
      1. Vitamin B_{12} malabsorption
   F. Pancreatectomy
      1. Malabsorption
      2. Diabetes mellitus
III. Drug treatment
   A. Corticosteroids
      1. Fluid and electrolyte problems
      2. Nitrogen and calcium losses
      3. Hyperglycemia
   B. Sex hormone analogs
      1. Fluid retention
      2. Nausea
      3. Megestrol acetate—glucocorticoid effects
   C. Immunotherapy
      1. Tumor necrosis factor
         a. Fluid retention
         b. Hypotension
         c. Nausea, vomiting
         d. Diarrhea
      2. Interleukin 2
         a. Hypotension
         b. Fluid retention
         c. Azotemia
      3. Interferons
         a. Anorexia
         b. Nausea/vomiting
         c. Diarrhea
         d. Azotemia
   D. Cytotoxic chemotherapy

From Shils ME: Nutrition and diet in cancer management. In Shils ME, Olson J, Shils M (eds): *Modern nutrition in health and disease*, ed 8, Philadelphia, 1994, Lea & Febiger.

Immunotherapy

Cancer negatively affects T cells and/or the antibody-producing B cells of the immune system. The tumor burden also alters general immune system functioning. Tumors release immunosuppressive components.[94] Immunotherapy has the potential of benefiting the host by manipulating the immune system by destroying cancer cells.

Biologic response modifiers such as interferon, interleukin-2 (IL-2), other cytokines, and monoclonal antibodies are believed to carry cytotoxic drugs selectively to the tumor site. Some side effects include fever, chills, rash, and flulike symptoms. Some of the antibodies being tested seem to have immunoregulatory effects or the capability to kill tumor cells by interacting with antibody-dependent cellular cytotoxicity (ADCC) cells.[94] For additional descriptions see references 105 to 108.

Investigative Protocols

Many new and exciting investigational approaches are on the horizon.[93,94,109-115] The therapies discussed are not available to all patient or may not be considered the "standard of care" in

general oncologic management. Until proven by randomized clinical trials or other study conditions and adopted by the oncology community as an accepted protocol, these are still to be considered investigational.

Researchers are using the biologic response modifiers in a variety of cancer treatment protocols. Interferon-α combined with chemotherapy is being tested for colorectal cancer, multiple myeloma, and melanoma. IL-2 is used to stimulate lymphocytes to produce lymphokine-activated killer (LAK) cells that can destroy tumor cells. Lymphocytes from the patient can be isolated, stimulated with IL-2, and given back to the patient as LAK cells that stimulate the immune system to fight tumor cells. Patients with renal cell carcinomas and advanced melanomas have shown good responses to this therapy. Research is being conducted into use of IL-2 as part of therapy for colorectal, ovarian, and small cell lung cancer.

Colony-stimulating factors (hematopoietic growth factors) stimulate the bone marrow to produce more white blood cells, platelets, and red blood cells. These factors are especially effective when used in combination with chemotherapy, allowing more aggressive treatment with decreased risk of infection as a result of low white blood cell counts. Colony-stimulating factors also have a role in bone marrow transplantation: patients recover faster and are discharged sooner from the hospital.

Monoclonal antibodies specific for a given antigen are being developed to react with particular cancer cells. Individual monoclonal antibodies have also been attached to radioisotopes, biologic response modifiers, or antineoplastic agents to deliver the toxin directly into the tumor. These antibodies are being tested for colorectal and lung cancer, lymphomas, leukemias, and neuroblastomas.

Molecular genetics, inserting healthy genes to treat cellular abnormalities by metabolic engineering, is a novel approach to cancer therapy. Patients will need to be treated using an individualized profile identifying molecular genetic alterations in each patient's specific tumor. By such selective treatment, patients should respond better and preserve organ function.

Tumor vaccines are being developed that will stimulate the immune system to activate T cells and B cells to destroy tumor cells. They are being studied in melanoma, renal cell, colorectal, breast, prostate, and lymphoma models. Antiangiogenic agents, small molecules with selective toxicity to endothelial cells in the G_1 phase of the cell cycle, are being studied to inhibit vascularization of the tumor. Thalidomide is one of the antiangiogenic agents being studied in prostate cancer and recurrent high-grade gliomas. The National Cancer Institute has an 800 telephone number (800-422-6237) for information on protocols and on-going clinical trials and a website: http://www.nci.nih.gov

Cyclooxygenase (COX)-2 inhibitors are being studied for their chemopreventive effects in patients at high risk for colorectal cancer. It is hypothesized that prostaglandin production will be decreased with the COX-2 inhibitors leading to reduced colorectal adenoma formation.

Pharmacologic Considerations

Metabolic Derangements Secondary to Antineoplastic Agents

Metabolic derangements from antineoplastic therapy cause serious nutrition problems (Table 34-5). In addition to the common side effects already mentioned, the responses to cytotoxic regimens discussed here must be considered when providing a comprehensive nutrition plan.

As new agents are used, the clinician should note their metabolic and nutritional implications. When drugs are used in combination protocols, synergistic effects must also be considered. Malabsorption may result from antineoplastic agents or other drugs. Impaired digestion and absorption should not be overlooked as possible causes of compromised nutritional status.

In addition to the cytotoxic drugs, cancer patients often take pain medication, drugs for other medical conditions, antidiarrheals, antiemetics, and diuretics. It is very important to obtain a complete list of medications and consider possible side-effects and untoward reactions. Frequently, the queasiness or diarrhea patients experience originates with or is exacerbated by medications prescribed for other conditions.

TABLE 34-5

Antineoplastic Drugs and Associated Metabolic Derangements

Drug	Derangements
Asparaginase	Hyperglycemia, hemorrhagic pancreatitis
Chlorotrianisene	Hypercalcemia
Cisplatin	Hyperuricemia, hypomagnesemia
Corticosteroids	Sodium retention, potassium, calcium, magnesium and zinc excretion, hyperglycemia
Diethylstilbestrol	Hypercalcemia
Methotrexate	Folate and calcium deficiency
Mithramycin	Hypocalcemia, hypokalemia
Streptozocin	Sudden hypoglycemia
Tamoxifen	Hypercalcemia
Taxol	Nausea, vomiting, mucositis
Tretinoin (all-trans retinoic acid)	Hypertriglyceridemia, elevated liver function values
Vincristine	Inappropriate antidiuretic hormone secretion, hyponatremia, water retention, decreased serum osmolality, increased urine osmolality

Antiemetic Agents

A number of antiemetics are available to alleviate some of the debilitating effects of anticipatory or treatment-induced nausea and vomiting and chronic queasiness.[55,56] Until recently, metoclopramide (Reglan), dexamethasone (Decadron), diphenhydramine (Benadryl), chlorpropamide (Compazine), and cannabinoids (Marinol) were the drugs of choice, with partial alleviation of symptoms. Serotonin antagonists, ondansetron (Zofran) used in combination with dexamethasone and granisetron (Kytril), provide very effective control of chemotherapy-induced emesis. Table 34-6 lists the emesis management regimen used at Memorial Sloan-Kettering Cancer Center.

Orexigenic (Appetite-Enhancing) Agents

Numerous pharmacologic agents have been evaluated for the anorexia of cancer patients.[55,79,116] Among the orexigenic agents (appetite stimulants) tried, corticosteroids, cyproheptadine (Periactin), hydrazine sulfate, and tetrahydrocannabinol have not proved effective for prolonged use. Steroids have the potential of worsening muscle deterioration from increased protein requirements secondary to urinary protein losses while not improving oral intake. Cyproheptadine seems to be a mild appetite stimulant, but it has not been shown to maintain body weight or improve nutritional status. Hydrazine sulfate has been shown to minimize weight loss or induce weight gain and to increase appetite in some patients, but not consistently, and it can interact with other medications. The cannabinols have been tested in several populations and have proved to alleviate the anorexia, produce weight gain, or improve nutritional status of selected patients in a given population. One agent, megestrol acetate (Megace), has shown promise in several trials. Patients in these studies who were anorexic reported increased oral intake, weight gain, and improved sense of well-being. For individuals experiencing weight loss, anabolic agents such as oxandrolone and growth hormones may be beneficial. Recent studies, although small numbers, have shown promise in

Recommended Antiemetic Regimens* Based on the Emetic Potential of Specific Chemotherapy Programs

Grade	Emetogenic Classification	Antiemetic Regimen
V	High	Granisetron 2 mg PO + Dexamethasone 20 mg PO/IV
V–CI	High—continuous infusion	Ondansetron 8 mg IVPB loading dose 30 minutes before chemotherapy × 1 dose only followed by 1 mg/hr × 24 hr for days. Dexamethasone 20 mg IVPB
IV	Moderately high	Granisetron 2 mg PO + Dexamethasone 20 mg PO/IV
III	Moderate	Granisetron 1 mg PO + Dexamethasone 20 mg PO/IV or Ondansetron 16 mg PO + Dexamethasone 20 mg PO/IV
II	Mild	Dexamethasone 20 mg PO/IV
I	Minimally	PRN antiemetics only

BREAKTHROUGH ANTIEMETIC REGIMEN:
If a patient requests additional antiemetics or vomits >3 times, give: metoclopramide 2 mg/kg IVPB × 1 dose, and every 3–4 hr as needed + diphenhydramine 50 mg IV every 30 min PRN only for dystonic reactions

DELAYED ANTIEMETIC REGIMEN:
To begin at 6:00 AM the day following chemotherapy: dexamethasone 8 mg PO BID × 2 days taper to 4 mg PO BID × 1 day + metoclopramide 0.5 mg/kg PO × 2 days OR prochlorperazine spansule 15 mg BID × 3 days

NOTE: Patients should receive dexamethasone PO or IV concurrently with a serotonin antagonist where specified. For leukemia, lymphoma, multiple myeloma, and bone marrow transplant patients, refer to individual protocols for dexamethasone use. Patients may not tolerate metoclopramide and/or prochlorperazine in delayed emesis regimens; however, dexamethasone should be used if possible.
* Antiemetic regimens are likely to change as new and more effective agents become available. Courtesy Memorial Sloan-Kettering Cancer Center, Acute Antiemetic Regimens.

helping to promote lean body mass and warrant further consideration. When anorexia is of long standing and refractory to other nutrition support, orexigenic agents might be beneficial. As more definitive studies provide better insight into the mechanisms and doses, more effective pharmacologic agents may be developed.

Determining Nutrient Requirements

Once the patient has been screened and assessed, a nutrition care plan can be developed that is tailored to the patient's present status and treatment modalities that might impact their nutritional status, thus compromising intake leading to malnutrition.

Caloric Requirements

Providing adequate caloric needs is essential for cancer patients. The obligatory energy demands of the body should be met by carbohydrates and fats without tapping protein reserves. Some use the Harris-Benedict equation to determine calorie requirements; however, the following estimates, which are simple, quick, and cover the majority of patients, may be more efficient:

- For obese patients on maintenance, 21-25 kcal/kg
- For nonambulatory or sedentary adults, 25-30 kcal/kg
- For slightly hypermetabolic patients, for those who need to gain weight, or who are clearly anabolic, 30-35 kcal/kg
- For hypermetabolic or severely stressed patients or those who have malabsorption, 35 kcal/kg adjusted upwards as indicated[117]

Protein Needs

Most cancer patients are in negative nitrogen balance and will remain so. It is nevertheless important to provide enough protein to meet protein synthesis needs and reduce protein degradation. The following guidelines may be used or adapted for determining protein requirements for the individual patient:[117]

- Hepatic or renal compromise including BUN approaching 100 mg/dl or elevated ammonia: 0.5-0.8 g/kg
- RDA reference protein: 0.8 to 0.75 g/kg
- Normal maintenance level: 0.8 to 1.0 g/kg
- Safe intake for nonstressed cancer patients: 1.0 to 1.5 g/kg
- Bone marrow transplant patients: 1.5 g/kg
- For increased protein demands (e.g., protein-losing enteropathy, hypermetabolism, extreme wasting): 1.5 to 2.5 g/kg

Fluid Status

Hydration status affects weight, which is used to determine nutritional status. Enterally fed patients risk underhydration if fluid is inadequate, whereas overhydration can develop in patients fed intravenously or given supplemental fluids by mouth. Medically induced fluid overload secondary to congestive heart failure, pulmonary disease, renal disease, or endocrine abnormalities is common. Edema can develop from sodium contained in intravenous antibiotics such as ticarcillin, carbenicillin, oxacillin, and ampicillin, which contain 3.2 to 5.2 mEq/g of sodium.

Most undiluted enteral products contain about 80% free water. Calorie-dense products contain less free water. Patients should be given adequate fluids when concentrated formulas are selected. Intake and output should be recorded daily and precisely. If a patient's weight changes more than 1 to 2 pounds in 24 hours, the values should be verified and then the patient should be checked for fluid imbalance.

Vitamins and Minerals

Patients concerned about deficiencies and effects of treatment frequently ask about vitamin and mineral supplementation. Dietary supplements should never be a substitute for whole foods. However, therapies used by cancer patients may deplete or limit utilization of nutrients. Research concerning the use of supplements during active treatment is still controversial. In addition, optimal levels of micronutrients for cancer survivors have not been established yet. Therefore, until research findings can guide the dosage of various components, levels greater than 1 to 2 times the dietary recommended intake levels should not be recommended unless by a health care professional.[97,117] The American Cancer Society published a guide to informed choices for cancer survivors in which it states "Despite the lack of firm evidence, it may be reasonable to use nutritional supplements after the active treatment phase for cancer survivors who cannot eat enough to obtain sufficient nutrients. The effects of illness and its treatment, as well as dietary deficiencies, can weaken the body, including the immune system."[97] To date little is known about specific drug responses or competition between vitamins and drugs. Patients who express interest or concern should be told what is known about pertinent drug-nutrient interactions. As new regimens become available, the clinician will have to assess their effects on other nutrients and the nutritional status of the individual.

Nutrition Support Modalities

Oral Feeding

When possible, a nutrition plan should provide for the feeding regimen most comfortable for the patient. Oral intake is the most acceptable method of feeding, but it might have to be modified from standard meals or food choices. Most patients do best with smaller, more frequent feedings instead of three large meals. By providing small frequent feedings throughout the day and evening, the caregiver can select foods that might be easily tolerated in small mouthfuls and consumed with less effort than large imposing plates of food. If early satiety, decreased appetite, or queasiness is causing poor intake, calorie-dense food choices should be offered. Patients need to be reeducated about food choices. Priorities must be revised. Information previously given about healthy eating may no longer be appropriate. Many patients try to avoid fat and eat lots of fruits, vegetables, and fiber because public health messages promote such a diet to prevent disease and ensure wellness. Patients and family members must appreciate that the nutritional challenges of the cancer patient are different from those of healthy individuals.

Concern about cholesterol, fats, and artificial colors and flavors should not deter a person from eating whatever provides needed calories, protein, and nutrients. Favorite foods should be encouraged. Supplements and high-calorie, nutritious snacks can augment a limited food regimen. Every effort should be made to maintain adequate nutrition orally. The food preparer can use cream, butter or margarine, cheese, and other high-calorie sources to increase calories without affecting portion sizes. Suggesting high-calorie snacks such as peanut butter crackers, chocolates, cheese Danish, rice pudding with whipped cream, custards made with rich ingredients, rich ice cream, or chips with sour cream dip encourages the patient to seek out appealing foods that, even eaten in small quantities, are loaded with calories. These foods might not be eaten without the dietetic professional's suggestion because weight- or health-conscious family members might be consciously avoiding them.

Enteral Nutrition

Once a patient who has been given every opportunity to meet nutrition needs by oral means has failed to do so, enteral management should be implemented as soon as possible. Because the goal of nutrition support should be to prevent malnutrition, rather than to reverse it, early intervention is crucial.

TYPES OF ENTERAL SUPPORT. If the problem that prevents adequate intake is deemed to be an acute, short-term condition, a nasoenteric tube may be the feeding method of choice.[118] Although it is a low-risk procedure and the tube is easy to insert, the patient is usually self-conscious, uncomfortable, and resistant to it. For short-term management it can be very effective once the patient is able to relax and adjust to having the tube in the throat.

If enteral support is expected to last 4 weeks or longer, an enterostomy is suggested. With the advent of the percutaneous endoscopically placed gastrostomy (PEG) procedure, patients can be given a feeding tube in an outpatient procedure and sent home the same afternoon. PEG feeding allows patients to resume whatever lifestyle or activities they are able to perform without the stigma and limitations of the feeding tube. The procedure is relatively safe, easy for a skilled endoscopist, and a very effective means of meeting otherwise unattainable nutrition requirements.[119,120] PEG insertion can be adapted to the patient's needs with modifications that allow the GI tract to be used even if normal flow of food through the GI tract is obstructed or otherwise limited.[121] This method is very effective for patients with mechanical or physical limitations of the head, neck, or esophagus. Patients who are anorexic or unable to eat adequately also find PEGs to be the answer to their nutrition problems. Although many physicians prefer parenteral nutrition (PN) for patients who are malnourished, using the GI tract is physiologically sounder, safer, and less costly.

Surgically placed enterostomy tubes are effective when placed at the time of a surgical procedure or for patients unable to undergo endoscopic placement of a PEG. For patients whose diagnosis or treatment modalities interfere with adequate nutrition, providing a feeding tube during surgery affords the clinician the option, at any time during the early postoperative course, to institute tube feeding of all or part of the patient's nutrient needs.[122] Placing the tube during the surgical procedure spares the patient endoscopic placement. Many surgeons are reluctant to place a tube prophylactically into patients who may not use it, but many types of cancer and therapy are associated with high risk of malnutrition so the likelihood of a given patient's needing enteral support is good. Dietetic professionals need to encourage surgeons to place tubes while patients are in the operating room. By determining formula choice, rate, or other logistic considerations after tube placement, the dietetic professional provides clear, concise orders, removing the burden of management from the surgeon, who may not be as well-versed on the specific details. Studies by numerous investigators reveal growing appreciation for the benefits of early enteral feeding after a surgical procedure with respect to acute-phase response to trauma, stress, and the other manifestations of major surgery (see Chapters 21 and 35).

Most absorption normally occurs in the first third of the jejunum, so a gastric tube affords a physiologic advantage. In addition, with gastric feeding, gastric secretions, bile acid, and pancreatic enzymes have more time to mix with the bolus of food. When the stomach cannot be used, a jejunostomy feeding tube can be placed. Jejunostomies can be placed endoscopically (PEJ) either as an inpatient or outpatient procedure or surgically. Endoscopic placement is technically more difficult but can be performed by a skilled endoscopist.[123] Management of the jejunostomy requires modification of the standard gastrostomy procedure. Adjustments of rate, administration, and type of feeding and tolerance must be considered. PEJ patients usually tolerate a slow-drip, pump-assisted feeding better than controlled bolus feeds.

Once an enterostomy has been placed and the patient has successfully adapted, a skin-level, low-profile feeding device may be substituted for the original PEG or PEJ. This affords the patient more freedom and comfort while he or she resumes a somewhat normal life. The patient can easily shower, wear tight-fitting clothes, go the beach, and be very active without the encumbrance of a No. 24 to 28 French, 8- to 14-inch tube dangling from the abdomen. For more details on management of enteral feeding see Part IV Principles of Nutrition Support.

An endoscopist who is creative or is committed to using the GI tract can devise some means of access. Shike and colleagues bypassed obstructed areas of patients' intestines, bile ducts, or esophagus, placing external shunts from the area proximal to the obstruction and reattaching the shunts distal to the blockage to preserve secretions, liquids, solids, and electrolytes.[124-126]

Feeding Modalities

The typical feeding modalities—bolus, intermittent, or gravity drip, pump-assisted, continuous slow infusion—for enteral formulas are chosen by the same criteria as for any other enterally fed patient.[118,127,128] The patient should be evaluated to determine if intermittent or pump-assisted feedings would serve him or her better than a bolus. Pumps were emphasized in the 1980s to heighten the awareness of institutions that were not using continuous feeding for patients who could benefit from it. In an effort to sensitize practitioners, pump-assisted feedings were stressed; however, with the increased use of PEGs for patients with anorexia or physical or mechanical limitations, the need for pump-assisted, slow-drip feeding has diminished. For the many patients using enteral feedings in home or outpatient settings, bolus feedings are much more convenient and adaptable to their caregivers and their schedules. Bolus feeding is logistically simpler and of nominal cost. Many patients at home prefer to feed themselves while they sleep, so as to be unencumbered during the day. Pump-assisted night feedings allow these patients to go about their daily activities without the feedings' interfering.

Training the patient and the caregiver in use of the equipment, care of the tube, rate, administration, schedule, and maintenance is vital to the success of the feeding program. The patient must be able to follow instructions, if complications are to be avoided and successful, long-term administration achieved. The clinical or dietetic professional can train and educate the patient and family. As the member of the multidisciplinary team with nutrition expertise, the dietetic professional is most likely to provide training and to serve as liaison between the patient and the multidisciplinary team after discharge.

If tube feedings are being used in conjunction with oral feeding, the dietetic professional should ensure that total intake is adequate. Frequently, patients decrease their enteral volume in the belief that they are eating enough when in fact they are eating considerably less than they need. They should be encouraged to sustain the volume of enteral formula, regardless

of oral consumption. If they prove that weight gain is occurring as a result of the combined intake, they can decrease enteral intake for 7 to 10 days as a trial and be monitored for response. If the patient does well, enteral volume can be adjusted appropriately. The possibility of nutritional decline, however, must be addressed by the dietetic professional monitoring the patient before severe malnutrition occurs.

FORMULAS. The array of commercially available formulas grows at a staggering rate. A formula is available for every medical need, and the composition of general and special formulas is improving as rapidly as the science is reported. Again, the cancer patient has the same considerations as other patients when enteral management is used. In a small subpopulation of cancer patients, protein needs may be higher than average, but it is of utmost importance that patients obtain their calculated caloric levels. Too often, patients do not receive adequate volume to ensure weight maintenance or gain. If they are not evaluated in a timely manner to allow identification, they may continue to lose weight and develop malnutrition. For a more complete description of enteral management and feeding methods, see Part IV Principles of Nutrition Support or references 118, 127, 129, and 130.

Parenteral Nutrition

Once the GI tract has proved ineffective in maintaining nutritional status or cannot be used, peripheral parenteral nutrition (PPN) or PN should be considered. For short-term nutritional management, supplemental, or transitional feedings, PPN may be indicated.[128] Much controversy has developed over PN for cancer patients.[131-133] Most clinicians who work with cancer patients believe that PN or PPN is appropriate for malnourished patients who are undergoing treatment. PN can support anticancer therapy in a patient who cannot be nourished via the GI tract and whose therapy could change the course of the disease, but it is not universally beneficial. In a study of chemotherapy patients with small-cell lung cancer receiving PN, increased body weight, fat, and potassium were achieved but not increased total body nitrogen.[134] In addition, when PN was discontinued, body weight, fat, and potassium decreased. Food intake was also depressed after PN. The investigators concluded that PN in conjunction with chemotherapy not only was not beneficial for improving lean body mass but had a negative effect on appetite and oral intake.[45] Indiscriminate use of PN for cancer patients does not seem warranted. Profoundly malnourished patients may benefit from adjunctive PN during cancer therapy that further compromises nutritional status.[131,135] When selected, PN requires very diligent and constant monitoring. Potential complications include fluid overload (in patients receiving blood products, chemotherapy, and IV medications via peripheral or central venous access), hyperglycemia secondary to increased dextrose content of parenteral formulas, insulin resistance secondary to severe illness, and electrolyte imbalances.

Tumor Response to Nutrition Support

Patients with active disease should receive aggressive nutrition support. Feeding patients in treatment may enhance therapy; that is, if tumor cells are more vulnerable to the therapy during proliferation, improved nutrition may enhance the therapeutic response. The host's lean body mass and organ and tissue mass and subcutaneous fat stores are preserved. Concern about the tumor's growing out of control has not been observed in humans in the same degree as in animal models. In experimental models, tumors of up to 30% of the carcass weight of the animal have been found.[136] Human tumor burdens are smaller, however, and as a result, rather than allowing patients to die of starvation, they are nourished and treated if possible. For patients in whom treatment has failed or who are terminal or refuse therapy, nutrition support may still be offered, although usually not as aggressively. Supportive care provides comfort and peace of mind to patient and family and is cost effective because it maintains hydration and electrolyte levels and avoids rehospitalization for many terminal patients in other facilities or at home. For a more detailed review of PN, its risks and benefits, see Part IV Principles of Nutrition Support.

Patient Monitoring During Nutrition Support

Once a therapeutic regimen has been established and a nutrition care plan developed and implemented, means are needed for monitoring progress and compliance. The patient should be evaluated routinely and regularly for these findings:

- Change in medical status during the course of treatment and recovery
- Change in nutritional status due to therapy, poor compliance with the nutrition care plan, or inability to meet nutritional needs because of effects of the disease process
- Change in nutrient requirements during the course of treatment and recovery
- Change in laboratory parameters during the course of treatment and recovery
- Change in psychosocial status that affects the patient's ability to meet nutritional needs adequately

When one or more of these changes are identified, steps must be taken to alter the original nutrition care plan accordingly. This might entail altering food choices, timing of meals, adding a supplement or pursuing alternative feeding options, or changing or providing medication to better control pain, nausea, diarrhea, or side effects of therapy. The patient may need a psychiatric or social work consult. If the patient's medical status is affecting nutrition, alternative feeding modalities should be suggested to the medical staff to forestall malnutrition.

As more patients are managed outside the acute-care setting, effective follow-up monitoring will be required by health care professionals. Mechanisms for monitoring should be developed similarly to screening tools and assessment forms. Databases or computer programs for tracking outpatients are convenient. Cost-effective management in choosing feeding modalities will need to be implemented. Dietetic professionals may need to "cross-train" by developing additional clinical skills to serve a broader market. Skills such as physical assessment, taking blood pressure, giving injections, drawing blood samples, and educating patients about drug-nutrient interactions and the side effects of medications prescribed afford dietetic professionals flexibility in the home care setting, where only one health professional is called on to provide services.

Clinical Indicators for Nutrition Support of Cancer Patients

In the late 1980s the ADA formed three task forces—cardiovascular, oncology, and surgical adult acute care—to determine the most effective indicators of desired outcomes of nutrition support.[137,138] In writing clinical indicators, it is necessary to distinguish differences among the terms *indicator, standard,* and *guideline. Standards* are rules or expectations for the structure or processes necessary for delivery of patient care. *Guidelines* tell what to do if inappropriate patient care occurs. *Indicators,* on the other hand, are warning flags that a system may not be functioning as well as it should and may need adjustments. Indicators are not measures of optimal care but rather help those responsible for patient care to improve areas that are less than acceptable.

For clinical indicators to be meaningful, they must be clearly defined, discrete, measurable, relevant, valid, and comprehensible. The format and more detailed explanations can be found in the *Clinical Indicator Workbook* available from the ADA.[137] Effective clinical indicators relevant to a particular facility enable dietetic professionals to better determine the efficacy of their efforts. Too often, process criteria—measures of activities or procedures—are the sole measure. We determine how many patients received calorie counts in a given time frame. How many discharge diets were administered or what percentage of screening forms were completed is recorded. But what happens to that information? Once we know how many calorie counts were done, we need to use that information to ensure that patients are getting adequate calories and nutrients or if some action is in order. Having determined how many discharge diets were devised, we need to know if our efforts were effective or if the patient went home unable to implement the diet or elected not to follow it. What is done with screening information? Are high-risk patients who are identified followed with aggressive nutrition support? Clinical indicators that are outcome oriented focus on predetermined items measurable and observable as the end result of change.

The ADA's Oncology Task Force initially identified 11 indicators as being important to monitor. Five of those were eliminated because of complexities that prohibited measuring or clearly defining the problem. Only three of the remaining six indicators survived field testing. These are listed below, followed by the three that did not pass testing. For a thorough review of the field-testing process, see reference 137.

The approved clinical indicators are as follows:

1. The patient is NPO or on a clear liquid diet without nutrition support for 5 days.
2. All patients at moderate or high risk are identified by screening and assessed within 72 hours of hospitalization.
3. Moderate or high-risk patients/caregivers demonstrate the knowledge/skills required to implement nutrition care plan for discharge.

The clinical indicators not approved are as follows:

1. The patient with weight loss greater than 10% of usual body weight continues to lose weight during current hospitalization.

2. The patient receives PN when it is documented that the gut is or will be impaired and/or dysfunctional longer than 10 days.
3. The patient screened and assessed at moderate or high risk receives no nutrition intervention within 3 days of recommendation for intervention.

As one quickly notices, issues that everyone who manages cancer patients deems important were not included in the approved list of clinical indicators. Reasons for rejection varied from logistic problems of measuring the indicator to the complexity of the indicator (having too many elements to document), such as the weight indicator. This illustrates the difficulty of creating meaningful clinical indicators. Three or more separate measurements—weight-pre-illness, admission, and ongoing hospitalized weights—were needed to complete the weight indicator. None of the field test sites used for this project was able to complete all three elements in this indicator.

Limitations were found in implementing even the indicators that were accepted. For example, several test sites struggled with the 72-hour window for completing screening and assessment. Weekends with reduced staffing and treatments that prevented access to the patient in the first 72 hours hindered assessment in some facilities. One begins to appreciate the difficulty of writing an indicator that is meaningful yet achievable. A very important aspect of this process, however, is the potential benefit that can be derived from the information.

The initial reaction of many on staff may be to justify the unsuccessful cases identified. The staff should realize that the indicators are invaluable for effecting better patient outcomes and more efficient use of the dietetic professional's time. From this documentation, better plans can be developed. Each facility can create clinical indicators appropriate for its specific problems or weaknesses. For a known problem, a clinical indicator is a means of looking at the measurable aspects, the desired outcome, and the percentage of those who meet or do not meet the indicator. Some indicators are written in the positive, others in the negative. For example, the first indicator, monitoring patients who are NPO or on a clear liquid diet for longer than 5 days, is negative, so it would not be desirable for patients to meet this indicator. Indicators should be phrased with the expectation of positive outcome. For additional information on this topic see references see 137 and 139. The ADA also publishes a manual on medical nutrition therapy.

Can Certain Foods Decrease the Risk of Cancer?

The possibility of cancers being diet-induced has led to enormous interest in the possibility that chemopreventive agents might decrease the risk of cancer. Health professionals will need to stay abreast of the literature as more is published. A vast number of phytochemicals appear to participate in cell proliferation. When a cell is exposed to a carcinogen or other mutagenic factor such as free radicals, radiation, ultraviolet light, or viruses, it is altered and the abnormality is henceforth replicated, eventually leading to the expression of tumor cells.

Phytochemicals, or chemopreventive agents, have the potential to support DNA repair and thus reverse cell damage if the change occurs during the early initiation stage of the cell cycle. If damage has already occurred, they may be able to forestall progression toward the uncontrolled proliferation of cancer by blocking or suppressing additional changes.

The positive association shown in epidemiologic studies is compelling evidence that something in foods appears to be protective. Of the 156 studies reviewed for the protective effect of fruits and vegetables, 128 showed positive outcomes.[140] Other population-based studies support these findings. Certain dietary components, such as the phytochemicals and fiber in many foods, appear to protect against specific cancers, whereas other components, such as fats and ethanol, appear to increase the risk.[2,141-143]

In the early 1980s, the National Cancer Institute created a department that was charged with systemically and scientifically studying the thousands of compounds that may protect against cancer. A five-phase program was developed: preclinical laboratory studies; assays in vivo using animal models to evaluate efficacy; toxicologic and safety evaluations; phase I-II human clinical trials; and finally, phase III full-scale intervention studies.[144]

Numerous human intervention trials have been completed to date. The Linxian, China, study, in which approximately 30,000 adults were studied for an average of 5.25 years, was two-by-four factorial design using: (1) retinol and zinc; (2) riboflavin and niacin; (3) vitamin C and molybdenum; and (4) beta-carotene, vitamin E, and selenium.[145] The α-tocopherol, beta-carotene (ATBC) study observed approximately 30,000 Finnish adult male smokers for about 6 years. The two-by-two double-blind randomized design tested (1) vitamin E (50 mg) and/or (2) beta-carotene (20 mg).[146] Another study investigated antioxidant vitamins and colorectal cancer. This randomized two-by-two factorial design studied 864 adults with adenomatous polyps for 4 years. The four arms of the study consisted of (1) beta-carotene (25 mg); (2) vitamin C (1 g) and vitamin E (400 mg); (3)beta-carotene (25 mg), vitamin C (1 g), and vitamin E (400 mg); and (4) placebo.[147] More recently, the Polyp Prevention Trial looked at consumption of low-fat, high-fiber foods and increased fruit/vegetable consumption in individuals who had a history of adenomatous colon polyps.[148] In each case the results were disappointing. Another group evaluated dietary supplements of wheat bran fiber in patients with adenomatous polyps of the colon and found no protection against recurrence of polyps.[149]

A recent conference presented findings from epidemiologic prospective cohort studies from Europe, North America, Australia, and Japan, specifically addressing the relationship between nutrition and cancer. The European Prospective Investigation into Cancer and Nutrition (EPIC) study included 10 countries involving 500,000 volunteers. Preliminary results were presented at the 2001 conference held in Lyon, France.[2] Some of the findings included that consumption of red meat has shown a very weak and nonstatistically significant increase in colorectal cancer. Those consuming a high intake of processed meats showed a modest increase in colorectal cancer. Vegetables and fruits continue to show beneficial effects on various cancer sites. Obesity and physical activity appear to have significant influence on increasing risk factors for cancer. This places emphasis on lifestyle management and changes in lieu of more specific recommendations of lowering total fat content or omitting specific foods such as animal products. Another area of interest highlighted at the conference was the role that insulin and IGFs play in cancer causation and prevention. Dietary modification would potentially have an impact on regulating insulin levels and thus cancer initiation.

In light of recent research findings and evidence from epidemiologic studies, supplements alone cannot provide the beneficial effects of the myriad components that foods contain. Cruciferous vegetables, for example, contain indoles, isothiocyanates, dithiolthiones, and phenols, among other compounds. Thousands of indoles and thousands of varieties of phenolic acids are found in nature. Supplements of individual components cannot provide the combination of compounds in foods or mimic the synergy among the components. The American Cancer Society recently provided the information in found Table 34-7 regarding dietary factors and their efficacy on specific cancer sites.[97] The AICR also provided a summary table of food, nutrition, and the prevention of cancer: an overview (Fig. 34-1).[142]

Dietary habits of Americans have not improved significantly in the last 10 to 15 years as evidenced by the epidemic of obesity, diabetes, and their concomitant increases in chronic disease risk factors. Adequate intake of vegetables and fruits and total fiber is too small to be beneficial. Dietetic professionals, public health workers, and other health professionals face a huge challenge: persuading the American people to embrace a diet containing fruits, vegetables, grains, legumes, and beans and healthy fats while restricting refined sugars and carbohydrates and calories. To that end the ADA developed this position statement:[150]

It is the position of the ADA that functional foods, including whole foods and fortified, enriched, or enhanced foods, have a potentially beneficial effect on health when consumed as part of a varied diet on a regular basis, at effective levels.

Dietetic professionals must be prepared to advise patients and clients about chemopreventive agents. This will require constant review of the scientific literature and emerging information as more studies and trials are completed and more research is conducted. Dietetic professionals must be careful in advising patients who have active cancer on the use of antioxidants and free radical quenchers until hard data confirm their effectiveness *and* safety. Health professionals must educate patients and clients in the difference between prevention of cancer in a healthy population and management of a person who has cancer. The American Cancer Society's "Nutrition During and After Cancer Treatment: A Guide for Informed Choices by Cancer Survivors" offers health professionals suggestions for this population.[97] If the survivor is not nutritionally compromised, then following a nutrition program similar to healthy eating is advised.[143] When the individual's nutritional status is compromised, then the suggestions appropriate for the specific side effect or problem may be helpful.

Conclusion

As we enter the twenty-first century, dietetic professionals will face issues such as biotechnology and genetic engineering of foods and the use of genetic testing to develop a nutrition plan designed specifically for an individual. Regulatory and legislative issues will arise. Each of us will have to be well versed enough to voice an intelligent opinion. What will the future role of functional foods be? What does evolving science tell us about the role of foods and diet in managing wellness and disease states? Will we be ready to serve the needs of those who seek our advice and assistance? Each of us has an opportunity to provide a crucial service in the health and wellness of Americans as well as to play a key role in the support and maintenance of those who have been diagnosed and treated for cancer.

TABLE 34-7
ACS Workgroup Grades for Benefit versus Harm

Dietary Factor	Prostate Cancer	Breast Cancer	GI Cancer	Lung Cancer
Food safety	A1	A1	A1	A1
Intentional weight loss during treatment (if overweight)	E	E	E	E
Intentional weight loss after recovery (if overweight)	B	A2	A3	B
Decreased dietary fats	A3	A2	A3	B
Increased fruits and vegetables	B	A3	A2	A2
Increased physical activity	A3	A2	A2	B
Decreased alcohol	B	A3	A3	B
Fasting therapies	D	D	D	D
Juice therapies	B	A3	A3	A3
Macrobiotic therapies	C	C	C	C
Vegetarian diets	A3	A3	A2	A3
Vitamin and mineral supplements	A3	B	B	C
Flaxseed oil	B	B	B	B
Fish oils	B	B	A3	B
Ginger	B	B	B	B
Soy foods	C	C	B	B
Teas	B	B	B	B
Vitamin E supplements	A3	B	B	B
Vitamin C supplements	B	B	B	B
Beta carotene supplements	C	C	C	E
Selenium	A3	B	A3	A3

From Brown J, Byers T, Thompson K, Eldridge B, Doyle C, Williams A: Nutrition during and after cancer treatment, *CA Cancer J Clin* 2001;51:153–181, 2001.
A1, Proven benefit; *A2*, Probable benefit, but unproven; *A3*, Possible benefit, but unproven; *B*, Insufficient evidence to conclude benefit or risk; *C*, Evidence of possible harm as well as possible benefit; *D*, Evidence of lack of benefit; *E*, Evidence of harm.
Note: Information contained in this table represents studies in progress and presents the best data available at this time. This table will be updated periodically.

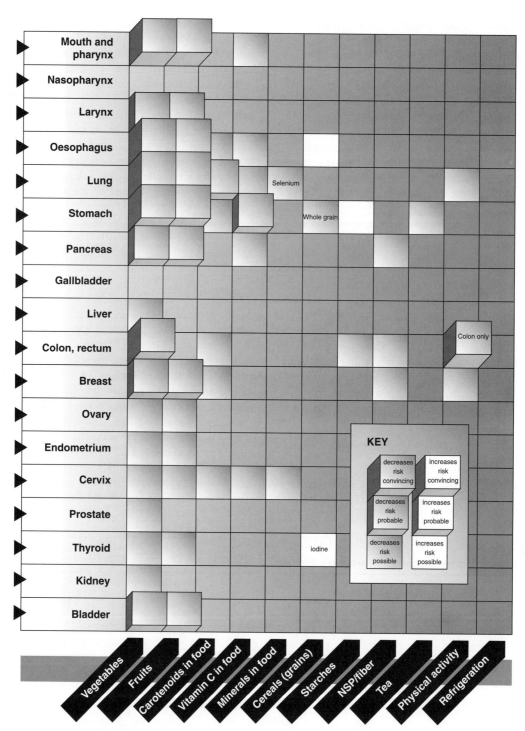

FIGURE 34-1 Food, nutrition and the prevention of cancer: an overview. (From *Food, nutrition and the prevention of cancer: a global perspective,* Washington DC, 1997, World Cancer Research Fund/American Institute for Cancer Research, pp 10-11.)

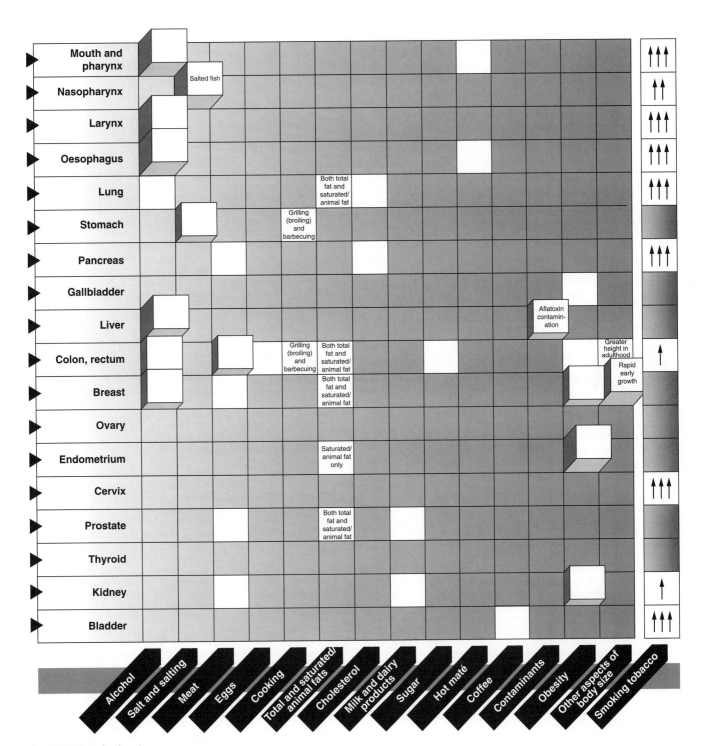

FIGURE 34-1 *Continued.*

REFERENCES

1. Platz EA, Willett WC, Colditz GA, Rimm EB, Spiegelman D, Giovannucci E: Proportion of colon cancer risk that might be preventable in a cohort of middle-aged US men, *Cancer Causes Control* 11(7):579-588, 2000.
2. Riboli E (ed): *European conference on nutrition & cancer.* Lyon, France, 2001, International Agency for Research on Cancer and Europe Against Cancer, Programme of the European Commission, pp 1-100.
3. American Cancer Society. *Cancer facts & figures 2001,* Atlanta, 2001, American Cancer Society, pp 1-42.
4. Doll R, Peto R: The causes of cancer: quantitative estimates of avoidable risks of cancer in the United States today, *J Natl Cancer Inst* 66(6):1191-1308, 1981.
5. National Research Council Committee on Diet and Health: *Implications for reducing chronic disease risk,* Washington, DC, 1989, National Academy Press, pp 1-749.
6. Doll R: The lessons of life: keynote address to the nutrition and cancer conference, *Cancer Res* 52(7suppl):2024S-2029S, 1992.
7. Kern KA, Norton JA: Cancer cachexia, *J Parenter Enteral Nutr* 12(3):286-298, 1988.
8. Ollenschlager G, Viell B, Thomas W, Konkol K, Burger B: Tumor anorexia: causes, assessment, treatment, *Recent Results Cancer Res* 121:249-259, 1991.
9. Shils ME, Shike M: Nutritional support of the cancer patient. In Shils ME, Olson J, Shike M, Ross A (eds): *Modern nutrition in health and disease,* Baltimore, MD, 1999, Williams & Wilkins, pp 1297-1325.
10. Nelson KA: The cancer anorexia-cachexia syndrome, *Semin Oncol* 27(1):64-68, 2000.
11. Detsky AS, McLaughlin JR, Baker JP, Johnston N, Whittaker S, Mendelson RA, et al: What is subjective global assessment of nutritional status? *J Parenter Enteral Nutr* 11(1):8-13, 1987.
12. Ottery FD: Cancer cachexia prevention, early diagnosis, and management, *Cancer Practice* 2(2):123-131, 1994.
13. Clinical Dietetic Professional Staff: MSKCC Adult Oncology Screening Tool, 1994.
14. Baker JP, Detsky AS, Wesson DE, Wolman SL, Stewart S, Whitewell J: Nutritional assessment: a comparison of clinical judgment and objective measurements, *New Engl J Med* 1982; 306(16):969-972.
15. Detsky AS, Baker JP, O'Rourke K, Johnston N, Whitewell J, Mendelson RA, et al: Predicting nutrition-associated complications for patients undergoing gastrointestinal surgery, *J Parenter Enteral Nutr* 11(5):440-446, 1996.
16. Hirsch S, de Obaldia N, Petermann M, Rojo P, Barrientos C, Iturriaga H, et al: Subjective global assessment of nutritional status: further validation, *Nutrition* 7(1):35-38, 1991.
17. McCallum PD: Patient-generated subjective global assessment. In McCallum PD, Polisena CG (eds): *The clinical guide to oncology nutrition,* Chicago, IL, 2000, American Dietetic Association, pp 11-23.
18. Shopbell JM, Hopkins B, Shronts EP: Nutrition screening and assessment. In Gottschlich MM, Fuhrman MP, Hammond KA HBSD (eds): *The science and practice of nutrition support: a case-based core curriculum,* Dubuque, IA, 2001, Kendall/Hunt Publishers, pp 107-140.
19. Luthringer S, Kulakowski K: Medical nutrition therapy protocols. In McCallum PD, Polisena CG (eds): *The clinical guide to oncology nutrition,* Chicago, IL, 2000, American Dietetic Association, pp 24-44.
20. Tchekmedyian NS, Halpert C, Ashley J, Heber D: Nutrition in advanced cancer: anorexia as an outcome variable and target of therapy, *J Parenter Enteral Nutr* 88S-92S, 16 (6 suppl), 1992.
21. Kuczmarski MF, Kuczmarski RJ, Najjar M: Descriptive anthropometric reference data for older Americans, *J Am Diet Assoc* 100(1):59-66, 2000.
22. Morley JE: Anorexia, body composition, and ageing, *Curr Opin Clin Nutr Metab Care* 4(1):9-13, 2001.
23. Tchekmedyian N, Zahyna D, Halpert C, Heber D: Assessment and maintenance of nutrition in older cancer patients, *Oncology* 6(suppl):105-111, 1992.
24. Roberts SB: Regulation of energy intake in older adults: recent findings and implications, *J Nutr Health Aging* 4(3):170-171, 2000.
25. Roberts SB: Regulation of energy intake in relation to metabolic state and nutritional status, *Eur J Clin Nutr* 54(S3):S64-S69, 2000.
26. Shils ME: Principles of nutritional therapy, *Cancer* 43:2093-2102, 1979.
27. Chlebowski RT: Nutritional support of the medical oncology patient, *Hematol Oncol Clin North Am* 5(1):147-160, 1991.
28. Hansell DT, Davies JW, Shenkin A, Burns HJ: The oxidation of body fuel stores in cancer patients, *Ann Surg* 204(6):637-642, 1986.
29. Hansell DT, Davies JW, Burns HJ: The relationship between resting energy expenditure and weight loss in benign and malignant disease, *Ann Surg* 203(3):240-245, 1986.
30. DeWys WD, Begg C, Lavin PT, Band PR, Bennett JM, Bertino JR, et al: Prognostic effect of weight loss prior to chemotherapy in cancer patients, *Am J Med* 69(4):491-497, 1980.
31. Falconer JS, Fearon KC, Plester CE, Ross JA, Carter DC: Cytokines, the acute-phase response, and resting energy expenditure in cachectic patients with pancreatic cancer, *Ann Surg* 219(4):325-331, 1994.
32. Fredrix EW, Soeters PB, Wouters EF, Deerenberg IM, von Meyenfeldt MF, Saris WH: Effect of different tumor types on resting energy expenditure, *Cancer Res* 51(22):6138-6141, 1991.
33. Ulander K, Jeppsson B, Grahn G: Postoperative energy intake in patients after colorectal cancer surgery, *Scand J Caring Sci* 12(3):131-138, 1998.
34. Grosvenor M, Bulcavage L, Chlebowski RT: Symptoms potentially influencing weight loss in a cancer population. Correlations with primary site, nutritional status, and chemotherapy administration, *Cancer* 63(2):330-334, 1989.
35. Senie RT, Rosen PP, Rhodes P, Lesser ML, Kinne DW: Obesity at diagnosis of breast carcinoma influences duration of disease-free survival, *Ann Intern Med* 116(1):26-32, 1992.
36. Demark-Wahnefried W, Rimer BK, Winer EP: Weight gain in women diagnosed with breast cancer, *J Am Diet Assoc* 97(5):519-26, 529, 1997.
37. Demark-Wahnefried W, Peterson BL, Winer EP, Marks L, Aziz N, Marcom PK, et al: Changes in weight, body composition, and factors influencing energy balance among premenopausal breast cancer patients receiving adjuvant chemotherapy, *J Clin Oncol* 19(9):2381-2389, 2001.
38. Demark-Wahnefried W, Hars V, Conaway MR, Havlin K, Rimer BK, McElveen G, et al: Reduced rates of metabolism and decreased physical activity in breast cancer patients receiving adjuvant chemotherapy, *Am J Clin Nutr* 65(5):1495-1501, 1997.
39. Suga K, Imai K, Eguchi H, Hayashi S, Higashi Y, Nakachi K: Molecular significance of excess body weight in postmenopausal breast cancer patients, in relation to expression of insulin-like growth factor I receptor and insulin-like growth factor II genes, *Jpn J Cancer Res* 92(2):127-134, 2001.
40. Stoll BA: Western nutrition and the insulin resistance syndrome: a link to breast cancer, *Eur J Clin Nutr* 53(2):83-87, 1999.
41. Goodwin PJ, Ennis M, Pritchard KI, Trudeau ME, Koo J, Madarnas Y, et al: Fasting insulin predicts distant disease free survival (DDFS) and overall survival (OS) in women with operable breast cancer (T1-3, N0-1, M0) who are receiving standard adjuvant therapy, American Society of Clinical Oncology, Abstract # 272, 2000, http://www.asco.org; http://www.conference-cast.com/asco/vm 2000/asco abstracts, Breast Cancer 269-314, no. 272.
42. Renehan AG, Jones J, Potten CS, Shalet SM, O'Dwyer ST: Elevated serum insulin-like growth factor (IGF)-II and IGF binding protein-2 in patients with colorectal cancer, *Br J Cancer* 83(10):1344-1350, 2000.
43. Henry JB: *Clinical chemistry. Clinical diagnosis and management, laboratory methods,* Philadelphia, 1991, WB Saunders, p 316.
44. Sacher RA, McPherson RA, Campos JM: Serum proteins of diagnostic significance in chapter 9. Widmann's clinical interpretation of laboratory tests, ed 11, 2000, FA Davis, pp 445-498.
45. Shike M, Russell DM, Detsky AS, Harrison JE, McNeill KG, Shephard F, et al: Changes in body composition in patients with small cell lung cancer: the effect of total parenteral nutrition as an adjunct for chemotherapy, *Ann Intern Med* 101(3):303-309, 1984.
46. Cohn SH, Gartenhaus W, Vartsky D, Sawitsky A, Zanzi I, Vaswani A, et al: Body composition and dietary intake in neoplastic disease, *Am J Clin Nutr* 34(10):1997-2004, 1981.
47. Cohn SH, Gartenhaus W, Sawitsky A, Rai K, Zanzi I, Vaswani A, et al: Compartmental body composition of cancer patients by measurement of total body nitrogen, potassium and water, *Metabolism* 30(3):222-229, 1981.
48. Harvey KB, Moldawer LL, Bistrian BR, Blackburn GL: Biological measures for the formation of a hospital prognostic index, *Am J Clin Nutr* 34(10):2013-2022, 1981.
49. Levy MH, Rosen SM, Ottery FD, Hermann J: Supportive care in oncology, *Curr Probl Cancer* 16(6):329-418, 1992.
50. Jeejeebhoy KN, Detsky AS, Baker JP: Assessment of nutritional status, *J Parenter Enteral Nutr* 14:193S-196S (5 suppl), 1990.
51. Tchekmedyian N, Cella DF, Heber D: Nutritional support and quality of life. In Heber D, Blackburn GL, Go VLW (eds): *Nutrition oncology,* San Diego, 1999, Academic Press, pp 587-593.

52. Brady MJ, Cella DF, Mo F, Bonomi AE, Tulsky DS, Lloyd SR, et al: Reliability and validity of the functional assessment of cancer therapy-breast quality-of-life instrument, *J Clin Oncol* 15(3):974-986, 1997.

53. Cella DF, Bonomi AE, Lloyd SR, Tulsky DS, Kaplan E, Bonomi P: Reliability and validity of the functional assessment of cancer therapy-lung (FACT-L) quality of life instrument, *Lung Cancer* 12(3):199-220, 1995.

54. List MA, D'Antonio LL, Cella DF, Siston A, Mumby P, Haraf D, et al: The performance status scale for head and neck cancer patients and the functional assessment of cancer therapy-head and neck scale. A study of utility and validity, *Cancer* 77(11):2294-2301, 1996.

55. Kennedy LD: Common supportive drug therapies used with oncology patients. In McCallum PD, Polisena CG (eds): *The clinical guide to oncology nutrition,* Chicago, IL, 2000, American Dietetic Association, pp 168-181.

56. Herrington AM, Herrington JD, Church CA: Pharmacologic options for the treatment of cachexia, *Nutr Clin Pract* 12:101-113, 1997.

57. Ottery FD: Supportive nutrition to prevent cachexia and improve quality of life, *Semin Oncol* 22:2(suppl) 3:98-111, 1995.

58. Fong Y, Moldawer LL, Lowry SF: Experimental and clinical applications of molecular cell biology in nutrition and metabolism, *J Parenter Enteral Nutr* 16(5):477-486, 1992.

59. Knox LS, Crosby LO, Feurer ID, Buzby GP, Miller CL, Mullen JL: Energy expenditure in malnourished cancer patients, *Ann Surg* 197(2):152-162, 1983.

60. Roche AF (ed): The role of nutrients in cancer treatment. *Report of the Ninth Ross Conference on Medical Research,* Columbus, Ohio, 1991, Ross Laboratories, pp 1-118.

61. Espat NJ, Moldawer LL, Copeland EM III: Cytokine-mediated alterations in host metabolism prevent nutritional repletion in cachectic cancer patients, *J Surg Oncol* 58(2):77-82, 1995.

62. Garlick PJ, McNurlan MA: Protein metabolism in the cancer patient, *Biochimie* 76(8):713-717, 1994.

63. Brennan MF: Total parenteral nutrition in the cancer patient, *N Engl J Med* 305(7):375-382, 1981.

64. Brennan MF: Uncomplicated starvation versus cancer cachexia. *Cancer Res* 37(7 Pt 2):2359-2364, 1977.

65. Young VR: Energy metabolism and requirements in the cancer patient, *Cancer Res* 37(7 Pt 2):2336-2347, 1977.

66. Heber D, Chlebowski RT, Ishibashi DE, Herrold JN, Block JB: Abnormalities in glucose and protein metabolism in noncachectic lung cancer patients, *Cancer Res* 42(11):4815-4819, 1996.

67. Shaw JM, Humberstone DM, Wolfe RR: Energy and protein metabolism in sarcoma patients, *Ann Surg* 207(3):283-289, 1988.

68. Warnold I, Lundholm K, Schersten T: Energy balance and body composition in cancer patients, *Cancer Res* 38(6):1801-1807, 1978.

69. Schersten T, Lundholm K, Eden E ES, Ekman L, Karlberg I, et al: Energy metabolism in cancer, *Acta Chir Scand* 498(suppl):130-136, 1980.

70. Arbeit JM, Lees DE, Corsey R, Brennan MF: Resting energy expenditure in controls and cancer patients with localized and diffuse disease, *Ann Surg* 199(3):292-298, 1984.

71. Nixon DW, Kutner M, Heymsfield S, Foltz AT, Carty C, Seitz S, et al: Resting energy expenditure in lung and colon cancer, *Metabolism* 37(11):1059-1064, 1988.

72. Fearon KC, Hansell DT, Preston T, Plumb JA, Davies J, Shapiro D, et al: Influence of whole body protein turnover rate on resting energy expenditure in patients with cancer, *Cancer Res* 48(9):2590-2595, 1988.

73. Tayek JA: A review of cancer cachexia and abnormal glucose metabolism in humans with cancer, *J Am College Nutr* 11(4):445-456, 1992.

74. Tayek JA: Nutritional and biochemical aspects of the cancer patient. In Heber D, Blackburn GL, Go VLW (eds): *Nutrition oncology,* San Diego, 1999, Academic Press, pp 519-536.

75. Tisdale MJ: Wasting in cancer, *J Nutr* 129(suppl 1S):243S-246S, 1999.

76. Waterhouse C: Nutritional disorders in neoplastic diseases, *Chronic Dis* 16:637-644, 1963.

77. Waterhouse C, Kemperman JH: Carbohydrate metabolism in subjects with cancer, *Cancer Res* 31(9):1273-1278, 1971.

78. Daly JM, Shinkwin M: Nutrition and the cancer patient. In Murphy GP, Lawrence W, Lenhard RE (eds): *American Cancer Society textbook of clinical oncology,* Atlanta, 1995, American Cancer Society, pp 580-596.

79. Heber D, Tchekmedyian N: Cancer cachexia and anorexia. In Heber D, Blackburn GL, Go VLW (eds): *Nutrition oncology,* San Diego, 1999, Academic Press, pp 537-546.

80. Daly JM, Redmond HP, Gallagher H: Perioperative nutrition in cancer patients, *J Parenter Enteral Nutr* 16(6 suppl):100S-105S, 1992.

81. Norton JA, Stein TP, Brennan MF: Whole body protein synthesis and turnover in normal and malnourished patients with and without known cancer, *Ann Surg* 194(2):123-128, 1981.

82. Brennan MF, Burt ME: Nitrogen metabolism in cancer patients, *Cancer Treat Rep* 65(suppl 5):67-78, 1981.

83. Pisters PW, Pearlstone DB: Protein and amino acid metabolism in cancer cachexia: investigative techniques and therapeutic interventions, *Crit Rev Clin Lab Sci* 30(3):223-272, 1993.

84. Heber D, Byerley LO, Tchekmedyian NS: Hormonal and metabolic abnormalities in the malnourished cancer patient: Effects on host-tumor interactions, *J Parenter Enteral Nutr* 16(6):60S-64S, 1992.

85. Shaw JH, Wolfe RR: Whole body protein kinetics in patients with early and advanced gastrointestinal cancer: the response to glucose infusion and total parenteral nutrition, *Surgery* 103(2):148-155, 1988.

86. Wigmore SJ, Todorov PT, Barber MD, Ross JA, Tisdale MJ, Fearon KC: Characteristics of patients with pancreatic cancer expressing a novel cancer cachectic factor, *Br J Surg* 87(1):53-58, 2000.

87. Tisdale MJ: Catabolism of skeletal muscle proteins and its reversal in cancer cachexia. In Mason JB, Nitenberg G (eds): *Cancer & nutrition: prevention and treatment,* Basel, Vevey/S. Karger AG, 135-146, 2000.

88. Barber MD, Ross JA, Voss AC, Tisdale MJ, Fearon KC: The effect of an oral nutritional supplement enriched with fish oil on weight-loss in patients with pancreatic cancer, *Br J Cancer* 81(1):80-86, 1999.

89. McNamara MJ, Alexander HR, Norton JA: Cytokines and their role in the pathophysiology of cancer cachexia, *J Parenter Enteral Nutr* 16(6 suppl):50S-55S, 1992.

90. Inui A: Cancer anorexia-cachexia syndrome: are neuropeptides the key? *Cancer Res* 59(18):4493-4501, 1999.

91. Moldawer LL, Copeland EM III: Proinflammatory cytokines, nutritional support, and the cachexia syndrome. interactions and therapeutic options, *Cancer* 79(9):1828-1839, 1997.

92. Gogos CA, Ginopoulos P, Salsa B, Apostolidou E, Zoumbos NC, Kalfarentzos F: Dietary omega-3 polyunsaturated fatty acids plus vitamin E restore immunodeficiency and prolong survival for severely ill patients with generalized malignancy: a randomized control trial, *Cancer* 82(2):395-402, 1998.

93. Cooper MR: Basis for current major cancer therapies: systemic therapy. In Lenhard RE, Osteen RT, Gansler TG (eds): *The American Cancer Society's clinical oncology,* Atlanta, 2001, The American Cancer Society, pp 175-215.

94. Herberman RB: Basis for current major cancer therapies: immunotherapy. In Lenhard RE, Osteen RT, Gansler TG (eds): *The American Cancer Society's clinical nutrition,* Atlanta, 2001, The American Cancer Society, pp 215-223.

95. Beutler B: Summary of the 5th International Congress on TNF and related cytokines: scientific advances and their medical applications, *J Leukocyte Biol* 57(1):11-12, 1995.

96. Eldridge B: Chemotherapy and nutrition implications. In McCallum PD, Polisena CG (eds): *The clinical guide to oncology nutrition,* Chicago, IL, 2001, American Dietetic Association, pp 61-69.

97. Brown J, Byers T, Thompson K, Eldridge B, Doyle C, Williams A: Nutrition during and after cancer treatment: a guide for informed choices by cancer survivors— American Cancer Society Workgroup on nutrition and physical activity for cancer survivors, *CA Cancer J Clin* 51(3):153-187, 2001.

98. Bloch AS, Charuhas PM: Cancer and cancer therapy. In Gottschlich MM, Fuhrman M, Hammond KA HBSD (eds): *The science and practice of nutrition support: a case-based core curriculum,* Dubuque, IA, Kendall/Hunt Publishers, 2001, pp 643-661.

99. Hendrickson FR, Withers HR: Principles of radiation oncology. In Holleb AI, Fink DJ, Murphy FP (eds): *American Cancer Society textbook of clinical oncology,* Atlanta, 1991, American Cancer Society, pp 35-46.

100. Polisena CG: Nutrition concerns with the radiation therapy patient. In McCallum PD, Polisena CG (eds): *The clinical guide to oncology nutrition,* Chicago, IL, 2000, American Dietetic Association, pp 70-78.

101. Darbinian JA, Coulston AM: Impact of radiation therapy on the nutrition status of the cancer patient: acute and chronic complications. In Bloch AS (ed): *Nutrition management of the cancer patient,* Gaithersburg, MD, 1990, Aspen Publishers Inc, pp 181-197.

102. Fleming ID, Brady LW, Mieszkalski GB, Cooper MR, Cooper MR: Basis for major current therapies for cancer. In Murphy GP, Lawrence W, Lenhard RE (eds): *American Cancer Society textbook of clinical oncology,* Atlanta, 1995, American Cancer Society, pp 96-134.

103. Mieszkalski GB, Brady LW, Yaeger TE: Basis for current major cancer therapies: radiotherapy. In Lenhard RE, Osteen RT, Gansler TG (eds):

The American Cancer Society's clinical oncology, Atlanta, 2001, The American Cancer Society, pp 165-174.

104. Fleming ID: Basis for current major cancer therapies: surgical therapy. In Lenhard RE, Osteen RT, Gansler TG (eds): *The American Cancer Society's clinical oncology,* Atlanta, 2001, The American Cancer Society, pp 160-165.

105. Rosenberg SA: Immunotherapy and gene therapy of cancer, *Cancer Res* 51(18 suppl):5074S-79S, 1991.

106. Rosenberg SA: The gene therapy of cancer, *Preventive Med* 23(5):624-626, 1994.

107. Hwu P, Rosenberg SA: The use of gene-modified tumor-infiltrating lymphocytes for cancer therapy, *Ann NY Acad Sci* 716:188-197, 1994.

108. Hwu P, Rosenberg SA: The genetic modification of T cells for cancer therapy: an overview of laboratory and clinical trials, *Cancer Detection & Prevention* 18(1):43-50, 1994.

109. Herberman RB: Principles of tumor immunology. In Murphy GP, Lawrence W, Lenhard RE (eds): *American Cancer Society textbook of clinical oncology,* Atlanta, 1995, American Cancer Society, pp 135-145.

110. Rosenberg SA, Blaese RM, Brenner MK, Deisseroth AB, Ledley FD, Lotze MT, et al: Human gene marker/therapy clinical protocols, *Hum Gene Ther* 11(6):919-979, 2000.

111. Cordon-Cardo C: Applications of molecular diagnostics: solid tumor genetics can determine clinical treatment protocols, *Mod Pathol* 14(3):254-257, 2001.

112. Wang F, Raab RM, Washabaugh MW, Buckland BC: Gene therapy and metabolic engineering, *Metab Eng* 2(2):126-139, 2000.

113. Fazzari M, Heller G, Scher HI: The phase II/III transition. Toward the proof of efficacy in cancer clinical trials, *Control Clin Trials* 21(4):360-368, 2000.

114. Hwu P: Current challenges in cancer gene therapy, *J Intern Med Suppl* 740:109-114, 1997.

115. Lynch PM: COX-2 inhibition in clinical cancer prevention, *Oncology (Huntington)* 15(suppl 5):21-26, 2001.

116. Murphy S, Von Roenn JH: Pharmacological management of anorexia and cachexia. In McCallum PD, Polisena CG (eds): *The clinical guide to oncology nutrition,* Chicago, IL, 2000, American Dietetic Association, pp 127-133.

117. Martin C: Calorie, protein, fluid, and micronutrient requirements. In McCallum PD, Polisena CG (eds): *The clinical guide to oncology nutrition,* Chicago, IL, 2000, American Dietetic Association, pp 45-52.

118. Piazza-Barnett R, Matarese L: Enteral nutrition in adult medical/surgical oncology. In McCallum PD, Polisena CG (eds): *The clinical guide to oncology nutrition,* Chicago, IL, 2000, American Dietetic Association, pp 106-118.

119. Levy H: Nasogastric and nasoenteric feeding tubes. In Shike M, Bloch AS (eds): *Gastrointestinal endoscopy clinics of North America,* Philadelphia, 1998, WB Saunders, pp 529-550.

120. Safadi BY, Marks JM, Ponsky JL: Percutaneous endoscopic gastrostomy. In Shike M, Bloch AS (eds): *Gastrointestinal endoscopy clinics of North America,* Philadelphia, 1998, WB Saunders, pp 551-568.

121. Kirby DF, Teran JC: Enteral feeding in critical care, gastrointestinal diseases, and cancer. In Shike M, Bloch AS (eds): *Gastrointestinal endoscopy clinics of North America,* Philadelphia, 1998, WB Saunders, pp 623-644.

122. Georgeson K, Owings E: Surgical and laparoscopic techniques for feeding tube placement. In Shike M, Bloch AS (eds): *Gastrointestinal endoscopy clinics of North America,* Philadelphia, 1998, WB Saunders, pp 581-592.

123. Shike M, Latkany L: Direct percutaneous endoscopic jejunostomy. In Shike M, Bloch AS (eds): *Gastrointestinal endoscopy clinics of North America,* Philadelphia, 1998, WB Saunders, pp 569-580.

124. Shike M: Percutaneous endoscopic stomas for enteral feeding and drainage, *Oncology* 9(1):39-45, 1995.

125. Shike M, Miodownik S, Pantason P, Schiano TD, Salk L: An active esophageal prosthesis, *Gastrointest Endosc* 41(1):64-67, 1995.

126. Bloch AS: Creative enteral access in the cancer patient, *Support Line* 16:1-5, 1994.

127. Charney P: Enteral nutrition: indications, options, and formulations. In Gottschlich MM, Fuhrman M, Hammond KA HBSD (eds): *The science and practice of nutrition support: a case-based core curriculum,* Dubuque, IA, 2001, Kendall/Hunt Publishers, pp 141-166.

128. Bloch AS, Mueller C: Enteral and parenteral nutrition support. In Mahan LK, Escott-Stump S (eds): *Krause's food, nutrition, and diet therapy,* Philadelphia, 2000, WB Saunders, pp 463-482.

129. Olree K, Vitello J, Sullivan J, Kohn-Keeth C: *Enteral formulations. The ASPEN nutrition support practice manual,* Silver Spring, MD, 1998, American Society for Parenteral and Enteral Nutrition, pp 41-49.

130. Matarese LE: Enteral feeding solutions. In Shike M, Bloch AS (eds): *Gastrointestinal endoscopy clinics of North America,* Philadelphia, 1998, WB Saunders, pp 593-610.

131. American College of Physicians: Parenteral nutrition in patients receiving cancer chemotherapy, *Ann Intern Med* 110(9):734-736, 1989.

132. Klein S, Kinney J, Jeejeebhoy KN, Alpers D, Hellerstein M, Murray M, et al: Nutrition support in clinical practice: review of published data and recommendations for future research directions, *J Parenter Enteral Nutr* 21(3):133-156, 1997.

133. Klein S, Koretz RL: Nutritional support in patients with cancer: what do the data really show? *Nutr Clin Pract* 9:91-100, 1994.

134. Russell DM, Shike M, Marliss EB, Detsky AS, Shephard FA, Feld R, et al: Effects of total parenteral nutrition and chemotherapy on the metabolic derangements in small cell lung cancer, *Cancer Res* 44(4):1706-1711, 1984.

135. National Advisory Group on Standards and Practice Guidelines for Parenteral Nutrition: Safe practices for parenteral nutrition formulations, *J Parenter Enteral Nutr* 22(2):49-66, 1998.

136. Báracos VE, LeBricon T: Animal Models for Nutrition in Cancer. In Mason JB, Nitenberg G (eds): *Cancer & nutrition: prevention and treatment,* Basel, Switzerland, 2000, Vevey/S. Karger AG, pp 167-182.

137. Hummell AC, Bloch AS, MacInnis P, Winkler MF: *Clinical indicator workbook for nutrition care systems,* Chicago, IL, 1994, American Dietetic Association, pp 1-151.

138. Queen PM, Caldwell M, Balogun L: Clinical indicators for oncology, cardiovascular, and surgical patients: report of the ADA Council on Practice Quality Assurance Committee, *J Am Diet Assoc* 93(3):338-344, 1996.

139. Kushner RF, Ayello EA, Beyer PL, Skipper A, Van Way CW III, Young EA, et al: National coordinating committee for nutrition standards clinical indicators of nutrition care, *J Am Diet Assoc* 94(10):1168-1177, 1994.

140. Block G, Patterson B, Subar A: Fruit, vegetables, and cancer prevention: a review of the epidemiological evidence, *Nutr Cancer* 18(1):1-29, 1992.

141. Steinmetz KA, Potter JD: Vegetables, fruit, and cancer prevention: a review, *J Am Diet Assoc* 96(10):1027-39, 1996.

142. Food, Nutrition and the Prevention of Cancer: a global perspective. Washington, DC, 1997, World Cancer Research Fund/ American Institute for Cancer Research, p 1-16.

143. American Cancer Society: The American Cancer Society guidelines on nutrition and physical activity for cancer prevention, California, 2002, *A Journal for Clinicians* 52(2):92-119, 2002, The American Cancer Society.

144. Malone WF: Studies evaluating antioxidants and β-carotene as chemopreventives, *Am J Clin Nutr* 53(1 suppl):305S-313S, 1991.

145. Blot WJ, Li J-Y, Taylor PR, et al: Nutrition intervention trials in Linxian, China; supplementation with specific vitamin/mineral combinations, cancer incidence, and disease-specific mortality in the general population, *J Natl Cancer Inst* 85(18):1483-1492, 1993.

146. The Alpha-Tocopherol Beta Carotene Cancer Prevention Study Group: The effect of vitamin E and beta carotene on the incidence of lung cancer and other cancers in male smokers, *N Engl J Med* 330(15):1029-1035, 1994.

147. Greenberg ER, Baron JA, Tosteson TD, Freeman DH, Beck GJ, Bond JH, et al: A clinical trial of antioxidant vitamins to prevent colorectal adenoma, *N Engl J Med* 331(3):141-147, 1994.

148. Schatzkin A, Lanza E, Corle D, Lance P, Iber F, Caan B, et al: Lack of effect of a low-fat, high-fiber diet on the recurrence of colorectal adenomas, Polyp Prevention Trial Study Group, *N Engl J Med* 342(16):1149-1155, 2000.

149. Alberts DS, Martinez ME, Roe DJ, Guillen-Rodriguez JM, Marshall JR, van Leeuwen JB, et al: Lack of effect of a high-fiber cereal supplement on the recurrence of colorectal adenomas. Phoenix Colon Cancer Prevention Physicians' Network, *N Engl J Med* 342(16):1156-1162, 2000.

150. Thomson C, Bloch AS, Hasler CM: Position of The American Dietetic Association, *J Am Diet Assoc* 99(10):1278-1285, 1999.

Inflammatory Response and Sepsis

35

Charles M. Mueller, PhD, RD, CNSD, CDN

SEPSIS has been characterized as a condition of progressive physiologic disorders that often culminate in organ dysfunction. Presumably, the cause is an infectious agent in the bloodstream. Although often blood cultures do not grow identifiable organisms, patients' systemic responses are similar to those of persons who have a confirmed septic source. Patients without detectable infection (those who have severe burns, trauma, or acute pancreatitis) display clinical, hemodynamic, and metabolic alterations like those of septic patients. The host of endogenous proteins and phospholipids that participate as mediators of these derangements provide a common link to the syndrome of symptoms despite the absence of a clearly identifiable initiating factor. Evidence suggests that these mediators mobilize substrate and initiate an immune response to ensure the host's survival.[1-5]

Modern medical technology appears to be able to sustain life beyond the point that human immunity has evolved to be of benefit to critically ill patients. Investigators have hypothesized that in the late stages of critical illness, immune and inflammatory responses to an insult, rather than microbes or injury, are most important to the development of morbid consequences. Much research has focused on interventions to interrupt or modulate production of endogenous mediators of immunity and inflammation in an effort to decrease mortality. These interventions have included the effects that parenteral and enteral nutrition and specific nutrients have on mediation of inflammation and immunity.[1-6]

Terminology

The constellation of clinical, hematologic, metabolic, and organ function abnormalities associated with gram-negative and gram-positive sepsis or sepsis of unknown origin is called *the inflammatory response,* even though it is not clear that infection is always the source of the phenomenon. In an effort to promote consistency and communication among investigators and clinicians, the American College of Chest Physicians and Society of Critical Care Medicine have defined *sepsis, organ failure,* and related terms.[1] These operational definitions are used in this chapter.

Systemic Inflammatory Response Syndrome

The responses characteristic of sepsis are not peculiar to sepsis (Fig. 35-1). Several insults can lead to the same sequelae (Box 35-1). *Systemic inflammatory response syndrome* (SIRS) has no clearly identifiable cause. When SIRS is conclusively the result of an identifiable infection, the term *sepsis* is used.

Thus, *sepsis* is defined as the systemic response to infection. *Septic shock* is a severe form of sepsis distinguished by persistent hypotension despite adequate fluid resuscitation and concurrent hypoperfusion that may precipitate abnormalities such as lactic acidosis, oliguria, and acute changes in mental status.[1]

Multiple Organ Dysfunction Syndrome

As life-support technology has developed in intensive care units, the major cause of death has become progressive failure of organ systems rather than the primary illness.[7-10] In the literature, criteria for describing organ failure often fail to distinguish between organ failure and organ dysfunction, which is an important distinction because organ failure is usually a continuous process affected both by host responses to injury and by medical intervention. The term *syndrome* has been applied to organ dysfunction because the condition is characterized by several progressive signs and symptoms that are thought to be pathologically related.[1] Multiple organ dysfunction syndrome (MODS) can be primary or secondary.[1] *Primary* MODS results from an early direct insult to an organ, as in trauma (e.g., pulmonary contusion, renal failure caused by rhabdomyolysis, or coagulopathy caused by multiple transfusions). Patients may also have underlying organ dysfunction such as cirrhosis of the liver or chronic obstructive pulmonary disease. *Secondary* MODS reflects an inflammatory response in organs remote from an original site of infection or insult. In this scenario, SIRS is viewed as part of a continuous process that results in MODS (e.g., sepsis originating from a wound abscess leading to organ dysfunction, severe trauma leading to organ dysfunction).

Causes

Gram-negative sepsis is induced by lipopolysaccharide (LPS) endotoxin on the outer membrane of the bacterium. As bacteria multiply in the host, membrane fragments and LPS release increase. The destruction of organisms associated with antibiotic treatment also causes LPS to surge. In humans, only a few micrograms of LPS per kilogram of body weight are required to cause septic shock.[3] In 1953, Bennett and Beeson[11] discovered that macrophages exposed to LPS released endogenous substances (*endogenous pyrogens*[12]) that were associated with fever in uninfected animals. This was the first evidence that endotoxin alone was not responsible for the clinical sequelae of sepsis.

Early studies correlated occult infection with MODS.[7,9,10,13] In more recent studies, MODS was demonstrated in the absence of an infectious source[14,15] and organ failure was

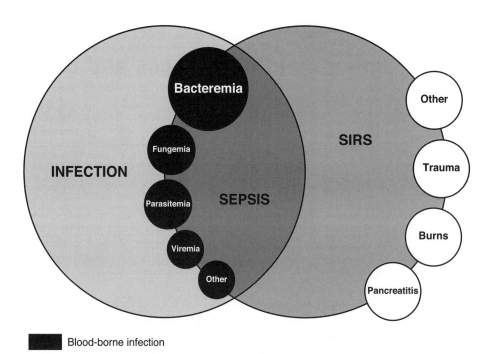

Blood-borne infection

FIGURE 35-1 Relationships among systemic inflammatory response syndrome (SIRS), sepsis, and infection. (American College of Chest Physicians/Society of Critical Care Medicine Consensus Conference: definitions for sepsis and organ failure and guidelines for the use of innovative therapies in sepsis, *Crit Care Med* 20:864-874, 1992.)

BOX 35-1

Manifestations of Sepsis and Systemic Inflammatory Response Syndrome

---

Temperature <36°C or >38°C
Heart rate >90 bpm
Respiratory rate >20 breaths/min or $Paco_2$ <30 mm Hg
Leukocyte count >12,000 cells/mm^3, <4000 cells/mm^3, or 10% immature (bands) forms

---

Adapted from American College of Chest Physicians/Society of Critical Care Medicine Consensus Conference Committee: American College of Chest Physicians/Society of Critical Care Medicine Consensus Conference: definitions for sepsis and organ failure and guidelines for the use of innovative therapies in sepsis, *Crit Care Med* 20:864-874, 1992.

reproduced by experimentally infusing endogenous mediators of the inflammatory response.[16] This supports the concept and definition of SIRS. Deitch[2] proposed three hypotheses to explain the development of MODS. *The macrophage hypothesis* attributes failure to prolonged SIRS caused by continual macrophage stimulation culminating in tissue injury at the cellular level. *The microcirculatory hypothesis* holds that organ dysfunction is caused by tissue and cellular oxygen deprivation, ischemia-reperfusion phenomenon, and endothelium-leukocyte interactions. Tissue ischemia and subsequent injury can enhance host inflammatory responses by activating neutrophils and stimulating macrophages. *The gut hypothesis* proposes that bacteria originating in the intestine initiate and sustain a SIRS state that culminates in organ dysfunction. Deitch revised this hypothesis in the late 1990s. Originally the hypothesis stated that bacteria and endogenous mediators breaching the gastrointestinal (GI) barrier entering systemic circulation via portal circulation cause and sustain SIRS. More recently Deitch and colleagues have speculated that endogenous mediators, derived from mesenteric lymph and the GI

mucosa during GI ischemia-reperfusion phenomenon, have the primary role in GI injury and SIRS. They hypothesize that ischemia-reperfusion and subsequent cytokine-mediated responses precede and indeed cause GI injury and that this injury is more significant than bacterial translocation to subsequent SIRS.[17-19]

Mediation of Systemic Inflammatory Response Syndrome

The endogenous substances that appear to mediate SIRS, and ultimately MODS, may explain the failure of antibiotic treatment for identifiable pathogens. The cascade of humoral and cellular mediators released early in the infection process is believed to be the ultimate cause of tissue injury and (septic) shock. The most extensively investigated of these mediators are cytokines, endogenous proteins or glycoproteins released in very small concentrations by a variety of host cells (e.g., macrophages, lymphocytes, endothelial cells, and Kupffer cells). They participate in the metabolic, hemodynamic, immunologic, and wound healing responses to injury and infection. Thus, cytokines are essential to the normal healing process. They have complex interrelations that appear to ensure their actions. For example, one cytokine may produce another cytokine, which in turn, stimulates production of more of the first. They function principally as paracrine (cell to cell) and autocrine (cell to self) mediators.[3,12] In one theory, cytokines are released in the local environment to promote wound repair and mediate defense against pathogens. They may also be released in small amounts into the circulation, for the purpose of recruiting macrophages and platelets. These responses are regulated by the cytokines themselves and by receptor antagonists and antibodies. On occasion, control is lost and the result is SIRS.[20]

TABLE 35-1

Biologic Effects of Cytokines During SIRS

TNF	IL-1	IL-6
Fever	Fever	Fever
Anorexia	Anorexia	↑ Acute-phase protein synthesis
Tissue injury and inflammation	Tachycardia	B and T lymphocytes activation
Tachycardia	↑ Cardiac output	
↓ Cardiac output	Shock (with TNF)	
Shock	↑ Capillary permeability	
↑ Capillary permeability	Generates eicosanoids	
Generates eicosanoids	Generates IL-2, IL-6, TNF	
Generates IL-2, IL-6, TNF	↑ Acute-phase protein synthesis	
↑ Acute-phase protein synthesis	Sequestration of Zn and Fe	
Sequestration of zinc and iron	↑ Corticotropin-releasing hormone	
↑ Corticotropin-releasing hormone	↑ Counterregulatory hormones	
↑ Counterregulatory hormones	Lactic acidosis	
Lactic acidosis	↓ Lipoprotein lipase	
↓ Lipoprotein lipase	↑ Host resistance	
Host resistance	↑ Margination and chemotaxis	
Margination and chemotaxis	↑ T lymphocytes	

Developed from Tracey KJ, Lowry SF: The role of cytokine mediators in septic shock, *Adv Surg* 23:21-56, 1990; Chrousos GP: The hypo-thalamic-pituitary-adrenal axis and immune-mediated inflammation, *N Engl J Med* 332: 1351-1362, 1995.
IL-1, Interleukin 1; *IL-6,* interleukin 6; *TNF,* tumor necrosis factor.

Tumor necrosis factor-alpha (TNF-α), or cachectin, is the cytokine studied most extensively and, thus far, appears to play the most significant role in SIRS. Many other cytokines have been associated with the inflammatory process, as have secondary mediators such as platelet-activating factor (PAF), eicosanoid metabolites, and complement components.[3,12] TNF, interleukin-1 (IL-1), and interleukin-6 (IL-6) are also the primary cytokine stimulants of the hypothalamic-pituitary-adrenal (HPA) axis, which, in conjunction with the noradrenergic system, makes up the core system for neuroendocrine stress-related responses.[21] Table 35-1 lists some of the major biologic activities mediated by the cytokines.

Tumor Necrosis Factor

TNF (cachectin) is produced by activated cells, monocytes, Kupffer cells, and macrophages stimulated by LPS (endo-toxin) or bacterial exotoxin, viruses, and fungi. TNF, in con-trast to a toxin such as LPS, initiates inflammatory responses by stimulating production of secondary cytokine mediators;[22] PAF,[23] prostaglandins[24] and leukotrienes;[25] activating neu-trophils and endothelial cells;[26,27] stimulating synthesis of acute-phase proteins;[28] and activating the coagulation cascade.[29] TNF also plays a role in decreasing skeletal muscle membrane potential,[30] increasing capillary membrane perme-ability,[3,12] and stimulating catabolism of skeletal muscle,[31] leading to accumulation of extracellular and extravascular fluid and to cachexia. The exact role of TNF in muscle catab-olism is not yet clear, but it probably involves other cytokine mediators.[32]

Secondary Cytokine Mediators

IL-1 production by endothelial cells and monocytes is induced by TNF. IL-1 and TNF work synergistically, producing many immunologically beneficial effects, such as T-lymphocyte pro-liferation, during an ineffective event, and potentially detri-mental inflammatory changes.[12] IL-1 induces fever by stimulating prostaglandin production in the anterior hypothala-mus.[33] IL-6 produces several inflammatory effects, including hepatic acute-phase protein synthesis,[34] B- and T-lymphocyte activation,[12,35,36] and stimulation of hematopoiesis.[37] IL-1, IL-6, and TNF have been investigated as predictors of morbidity[38] and mortality[39] in patients with the SIRS and septic shock. More recently IL-18 levels have been correlated with severity of illness score in sepsis, which suggests a role for this cytokine in SIRS.[40,41]

Other Secondary Mediators

PAF is produced by monocytes, macrophages, neutrophils, endothelial cells, and platelets from TNF and immune complex stimuli. PAF has been implicated in mediation of septic shock because of its contribution to hypotension,[42] bowel necrosis,[43] capillary permeability,[44] and TNF pro-duction (secondarily) during experimentally induced sepsis. Many of the effects of PAF are caused by eicosanoid produc-tion, which is also stimulated by cytokines. Prostaglandins and thromboxanes are synthesized via cyclooxygenase path-ways and leukotrienes via lipoxygenase pathways from the membranes of activated macrophages, neutrophils, platelets, and mast cells. Several of these eicosanoids have been linked to endotoxin-induced septic shock[45] because of their role in vasodilation and vasoconstriction, vascular permeability, platelet aggregation, chemotaxis, leukocyte adhesion, and edema.[46,47] Complement has been associated with exacer-bation of SIRS and has been proposed as a measure of sever-ity of sepsis.[48] The complement cascade, which includes the anaphylatoxins, stimulates production of TNF and IL-1, which in turn increases neutrophil expression of complement receptors.[49] Complement has been implicated in the develop-ment of the acute respiratory distress syndrome,[50] cardiac dysfunction, and septic shock.[51] Finally, the hormone pro-calcitonin has recently been suggested to be a secondary mediator that might enhance the septic response.[52]

Neuroendocrine Mediation

All cell types that participate in the inflammatory syndrome, both systemically (monocytes, neutrophils, basophils, eosinophils, lymphocytes) and locally (endothelial cells, mast cells, tissue fibroblasts, macrophages), produce TNF, IL-1, and IL-6. These cytokines, in conjunction with cholinergic and serotoninergic neurotransmitters, stimulate the hypothalamus to produce corticotropin-releasing hormone and arginine vasopressin. Both hormones work synergistically to produce corticotropin, which stimulates the adrenal cortex to produce cortisol. Corticotropin-releasing hormone and the noradrenergic system, which is responsible for catecholamine production, stimulate each other. Thus, cytokines play a role in catecholamine and glucocorticoid hormone secretion.[21] The glucocorticoids, including cortisol, suppress the functions of many immunoactive cells[53] and the production of cytokines.[54] The glucocorticoids therefore have antiinflammatory and immunosuppressant properties. The catecholamines, epinephrine and norepinephrine, stimulate IL-6, which inhibits TNF and IL-1, ultimately inhibiting inflammation.[53] Figure 35-2 illustrates the complexity of the interactions between cytokines, catecholamines, and glucocorticoids in SIRS.

Glucocorticoids, catecholamines, and glucagon, the counterregulatory hormones, function to mobilize energy reserves. They oppose the anabolic action of insulin, which transports glucose into cells, stimulates protein synthesis, and controls lipolysis. Cortisol mobilizes amino acids from skeletal muscle, which provides substrate for hepatic acute-phase protein and glucose synthesis. Epinephrine and norepinephrine increase metabolic rate, stimulate gluconeogenesis and glycogenolysis, and participate in lipolysis. β-Adrenergic activation increases glucagon release from pancreatic islet cells. Glucagon increases hepatic glycogenolysis and gluconeogenesis and increases hepatic mitochondrial uptake of long-chain fatty acids for oxidation.[55]

Hemodynamic and Metabolic Characteristics of Systemic Inflammatory Response Syndrome

In the manner previously described, humoral and neuronal stimulation collectively mediate the physiologic and metabolic alterations listed in Table 35-1 and Box 35-2. Patients with SIRS have elevated metabolic rates and increased tissue oxygen needs. If these oxygen demands are not met, then an ischemic condition resulting in anaerobic respiration results.[54] The altered substrate metabolism and hemodynamic irregularities described next are characteristic of hyperdynamic metabolism in SIRS and provide some of the rationale for nutrition support intervention.

In general, glucose oxidation in SIRS is decreased when compared with that of simple starvation. Pyruvate dehydrogenase activity is decreased, which increases the amount of pyruvate available for conversion to alanine and lactate. These two substrates, along with increased amino acid load from catabolized muscle, support increased gluconeogenesis. The result of decreased glucose oxidation and increased glucose production is hyperglycemia that is resistant to exogenous insulin.[56]

Amino acids are an important energy source in SIRS. They are derived from proteolysis of skeletal muscle, connective

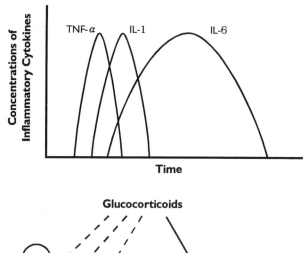

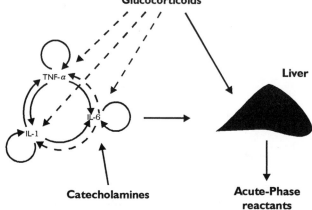

FIGURE 35-2 Interactions among the inflammatory cytokines and the effects of glucocorticoids and catecholamines. The *upper panel* shows the sequence of cytokine, TNF-α, IL-1, and IL-6 release at an inflammation site. Each of the inflammatory cytokines stimulates its own production *(lower panel)*. TNF-α and IL-1 stimulate each other, and both stimulate IL-6. IL-6 inhibits secretion of both TNF immune α and IL-1. Glucorticoids, the end-products of the hypothalamic-pituitary-adrenal axis, inhibit the production of all three inflammatory cytokines and their effects on target tissues, except for the effect of IL-6 on the production of acute-phase proteins by the liver, which is potentiated by glucocorticoids. Catecholamines, the other end-products of the stress system, have a major role in the control of inflammation through stimulation of IL-6, which inhibits the other two cytokines, stimulates glucocorticoids, and induces the acute-phase response. The *solid lines* denote stimulation and the *broken lines,* inhibition. (Chrousos GP: The hypothalamic-pituitary-adrenal axis and immune-mediated inflammation, *N Engl J Med* 20:1351-1362, 1995. Massachusetts Medical Society. All rights reserved.

tissue, and intestinal viscera, which results in significant loss of lean body mass. These losses are poorly attenuated by provision of exogenous protein or amino acids.[57] Hepatic acute-phase protein synthesis increases and lean body losses continue, even in fed patients, because protein synthesis is redistributed to the degree that inflammatory responses require acute-phase proteins.[55] The branched-chain amino acids leucine, isoleucine, and valine are oxidized peripherally, and the major gluconeogenic amino acids, alanine, glycine, and cystine, are transported to the liver. Increased glutamine release from lean body mass provides ammonia for renal excretion of metabolic acids and energy substrate for enterocytes.[56]

Lipolysis and oxidation of free fatty acids are accelerated and attendant lipogenesis is decreased. Ketosis of unstressed starvation is minimal. As SIRS progresses to severe sepsis and

Metabolic and Substrate Alterations in SIRS

↑ Metabolic rate
↑ Oxygen consumption
↓ Glucose oxidation
↑ Muscle, connective tissue, and visceral protein catabolism
↑ Hepatic (acute-phase) protein synthesis
↓ Ketogenesis
↑ Lipolysis

Developed from Beal AL, Cerra FB: Multiple organ failure syndrome in the 1990s. Systemic inflammatory response and organ dysfunction, *JAMA* 271:226-233, 1994.

MODS, plasma clearance of triglycerides decreases and hepatic lipogenesis increases. Unproductive cycling of triglycerides (lipolysis and lipogenesis without fatty acid oxidation) also occurs, which may be the result of increased catecholamines stimulating lipolysis with concomitant triglyceride synthesis caused by high levels of insulin. In the later stages of MODS, hypertriglyceridemia is common.[56,58]

When patients progress to septic shock with hypotension, depressed systemic vascular resistance, and possibly respiratory decompensation and myocardial dysfunction, oxygen utilization appears to decrease despite increased oxygen demand.[57] This may be caused by disturbances in normal cell respiration and oxidative phosphorylation[59] or disorders in microcirculatory function causing maldistribution of blood, and therefore oxygen, to tissues with variable oxygen needs.[58,59] In nonseptic (healthy) patients, red cell delivery of oxygen to all tissues is more than adequate. When severe sepsis or septic shock imposes vasoactive irregularities and increased tissue oxygen needs, available oxygen does not match cellular need, resulting in lactic acidosis and anoxic tissue damage.[60,61] Supply of exogenous substrate, particularly dextrose, may appropriate vitally required oxygen, compounding the problem.[58] Therefore, delivery of nutrients to these patients may be problematic.

Prevention and Treatment

Timely intervention is the most logical initial strategy to prevent SIRS. Depending on the patient population, accurate monitoring, maximization of ventilation-perfusion status and organ function, timely and appropriate use of antibiotics, proper surgical technique, and rapid resuscitation when necessary decrease complications in the critically ill patients highest risk for SIRS. The general strategy is to treat primary insults as quickly and effectively as possible, to avoid or limit SIRS.[2,56,62]

Several interventions—preventive, supportive, and therapeutic—have been discussed in the literature. Selective gut decontamination has been discussed as a method of preventing acquired infections and bacterial colonization.[63] Investigators have evaluated strategies for interrupting the cascade of SIRS mediation in an effort to decrease morbidity and mortality;[3,64] however, these tactics have been minimally effective.[65,66] The route of nutrition support (parenteral or enteral) figures prominently into a theorized mechanism for attenuating mediator (endocrine and paracrine) production in patients at risk for developing SIRS.[4,62] Finally, several clinical trials[5,67,68] have addressed formulation of enteral nutrition (EN) products with specific amino acid, lipid, and micronutrient components designed to affect infectious morbidity and mortality, possibly by modifying inflammatory mediators.

Gut Decontamination

Combining oral antibiotics, such as tobramycin, polymyxin, and nystatin, has been advocated as a way of selectively decontaminating the GI tract to reduce the risk of acquired infections in critically ill persons.[56] Studies of this practice report variable results in terms of length of hospitalization, mortality, and cost.[63] Rocha and coworkers[69] observed fewer nosocomial infections, more resistant microbes, and no reduction in costs for the antibiotic-treated group. Hammond and colleagues[70] found no differences in infection rates, length of stay, or mortality in a similar experiment. Thus, selective gut decontamination for critically ill populations remains controversial.[56]

Alteration of Mediators

Treatment strategies targeted directly at interrupting the cascade of SIRS mediators have formulated several hypotheses. TNF and IL-1 are the most proinflammatory of such mediators and so have been the focus of research designed to investigate regulation of their activity. Much of this research derives from what is known about endogenous inhibition of both TNF and IL-1 through mechanisms that appear to regulate cytokine activity.[71]

Glucocorticosteroids inhibit production of both TNF and IL-1. IL-6 activity in response to LPS is attenuated with exogenous provision of glucocorticosteroids.[72] Several proteins have been isolated and cloned that exhibit inhibitory functions on both TNF and IL-1. These proteins include TNF cell-surface receptors with very short half-lives that are shed from cell surfaces in response to inflammatory stimuli[73] and proteins that compete with IL-1 to bind to the receptors themselves.[74] TNF and IL-1 frequently are not detectable in septic patients, but TNF receptor, TNF-receptor complexes,[75] and IL-1 receptor antagonists[76] usually are. Lowry states the failure to detect free cytokines during sepsis is partially explained by the presence of the binding proteins, by the fact that cytokine activity frequently occurs only at the tissue level, and by the short half-lives of cytokines.[71]

In a bacteria-induced septic shock experiment,[77] recombinant IL-1 receptor blockade improved hemodynamic parameters and survival. Inhibition of phosphodiesterases, the enzymes involved in regulation of TNF production, has decreased TNF levels and improved morbidity and mortality in murine models of acute and chronic inflammation.[78] Lexipafant, a PAF antagonist, reduced the incidence of MODS and increased rates of recovery from organ failure in a randomized, double-blind trial of humans with acute pancreatitis.[79] Experts have suggested that timing of the intervention is critical.[3,56,71] For example, in animals, steroids given before, but not after, bacterial challenge abrogate TNF production.[80] Box 35-3 summarizes experimental strategies designed to interrupt the proinflammatory effects of LPS, TNF, IL-1, and PAF leading to SIRS.

The complex interactions among the various identified mediators of SIRS make it unlikely that a single treatment will successfully reduce inflammatory responses.[3] Cytokine

BOX 35-3

Experimental Treatments for SIRS

Monoclonal antibodies: TNF, LPS
Antireceptor antibodies: IL-1
Synthesis reduction: IL-1
Receptor antagonists: TNF, IL-1, PAF
Corticosteroid (synthesis block): TNF, IL-1

Developed from Giroir BP: Mediators of septic shock: new approaches for interrupting the endogenous inflammatory cascade, *Crit Care Med* 21:780-789, 1993; Beal AL, Cerra FB: Multiple organ failure syndrome in the 1990s. Systemic inflammatory response and organ dysfunction, *JAMA* 271:226-233, 1994; Lowry SF: Anticytokine therapies in sepsis, *New Horiz* 1:120-126, 1993; Dinarello CA, Gelfand JA, Wolff SM: Anticytokine strategies in the treatment of the systemic inflammatory response syndrome, *JAMA* 269:1829-1835, 1993.

blockade may also interfere with fundamental host immunity.[81] The mechanisms of cytokine function are not fully understood,[82] and blockade of one mediator may not decrease morbidity. For example, treatment of septic shock with pentoxifylline decreased TNF concentrations as compared with those of controls. But there were no significant differences between hemodynamic and oxygenation measurements or serum IL-6 and IL-8 concentrations in the treatment and control groups.[83]

In 1996, Bone expanded the definition of SIRS, in part to explain the failure thus far of cytokine blockade in the treatment of SIRS. He stated that investigators have assumed that responses to provocative events are all proinflammatory when, in fact, evidence indicates the body also produces a compensatory response to inflammation. Further, the magnitude of this response is proportionate to the magnitude of inflammation and may be great enough to suppress immunity. Bone characterized this phenomenon as the *compensatory antiinflammatory response syndrome* (CARS). Attempts at cytokine blockade have been too crude to affect the entire sequelae of SIRS, CARS, and the restoration of homeostasis.[65]

Recent research has evaluated the concept of overstimulation and subsequent compensation. Muller Kobold et al. hypothesized that poor outcome in sepsis is related to the severity of CARS. They confirmed this hypothesis by demonstrating that poor prognosis in septic patients was associated with a lower expression of activation markers on monocytes and neutrophils, i.e. CARS predominated.[84] Several cytokines have been identified that have primarily antiinflammatory functions. IL-10, synthesized by lymphocytes and monocytes, inhibits proinflammatory cytokines in several leukocytes.[85] IL-4, IL-11, and IL-13 have antiinflammatory properties as well, although they are not as well defined as IL-10, nor are all their metabolic effects understood.

Nutrition Assessment and Support

Metabolic support of patients with SIRS (and CARS) is necessary to minimize nutritional morbidity. To a certain extent, providing energy and protein is futile because of obligate hypermetabolism and proteolysis that lead to loss of lean body mass. Provision of macronutrients and micronutrients is necessary to replace losses in hyperdynamic patients and promote tissue anabolism when SIRS abates. The use of anthropometric measurements and serum transport protein levels (albumin, transferrin, and prealbumin) for assessment of nutritional status

is problematic in the critically ill. Capillary permeability, dilution of intravascular proteins, increased hepatic acute-phase protein synthesis, and decreased transport protein synthesis collectively diminish the value of weight and serum protein measurements as markers of nutritional status. Often, patients are nutritionally depleted at the onset of SIRS.[56,57,86,87]

Energy requirements for patients with SIRS are generally elevated between 20% and 50% above their basal energy requirements, and their day-to-day, indeed, hour-to-hour requirements fluctuate dramatically. The optimal amounts of macronutrients are difficult to determine because of increased proteolysis, relatively increased dependence on lipid for energy metabolism, and decreased ability to utilize glucose for energy metabolism. Recommended nonprotein kilocalorie:nitrogen ratios are 100:1 to 150:1, reflecting increased protein requirements to replace nitrogen losses. For example, 1.5 g of protein and 24 nonprotein kilocalories per kilogram of body weight or 2.0 g of protein and 32 nonprotein kcal provide a 100:1 nonprotein kilocalorie:nitrogen ratio. Carbohydrate provision should not exceed 5 mg/kg per minute, and insulin should be given to maintain serum glucose to less than 200 mg/dl. Lipid should make up 30% to 50% of nonprotein calories, depending on the patient's clinical status. Overfeeding should be avoided, lest organ dysfunction be exacerbated. Nutrition support may be futile, or even detrimental, for patients with marginal oxygen transport secondary to severe sepsis or septic shock.[2,56,88]

Enteral Versus Parenteral Nutrition Support

Providing adequate amounts of essential nutrients to appropriately identified patients is part of the process of caring for patients with SIRS or MODS. The route of nutrition support selected to provide these nutrients may have different effects on the patient.[2,4,89] Since the late 1980s, investigators have examined the metabolic and physiologic effects of EN and parenteral nutrition (PN) on laboratory animals and critically ill humans. The explanations for these differences converge on discussions of GI integrity and bacterial translocation[90,91] and alterations in paracrine and endocrine expression associated with lack of GI feeding.[4,67] The former explanation focuses on a causative link to SIRS, and the latter on mediation of SIRS. As previously mentioned, the role that the GI tract plays before and during inflammation is evolving. Recent literature implicates gastrointestinally derived inflammatory factors produced in response to ichemia/reperfusion phenomenon with inflammation rather than translocated bacteria.[92-95]

Several papers have examined outcomes associated with early posttrauma nutrition support that are relevant to prevention of SIRS. In 1986, Moore and colleagues[96] randomized patients with major abdominal trauma to receive either early enteral feeding via needle catheter jejunostomy or PN if oral intake was inadequate by posttrauma day 5. The prevalence of infectious complications, principally intraabdominal abscesses, was 9% in the early enteral group and 29% in the delayed-feeding (parenteral) group. In a follow-up study with a similar population, 75 patients were randomized to receive either EN or PN within 12 hours of celiotomy.[97] The enteral group had significantly fewer infectious complications (largely pneumonia) than the group fed parenterally. A 1992 meta-analysis published by the same group using data from eight clinical centers found that EN was associated with fewer total complications ($p < .007$) and fewer septic complications ($p < .0001$).[89] In the same year, Kudsk and coworkers[98] published similar results from an abdominal trauma population. Collectively, these results indicate that EN, as compared with PN, is associated with a lower incidence of infection and decreased risk of SIRS in trauma patients.

The gut hypothesis, previously described as a possible cause of MODS, may explain the protective benefits of EN in critically ill populations. Bacteria originating in the GI tract initiate and sustain SIRS, which can lead to MODS. Organisms or endotoxins from the GI lumen move to mesenteric lymph nodes and portal circulation. This phenomenon is called *bacterial translocation.*[2] Theoretically, EN, as opposed to PN, may reduce translocation (see Chapter 21). Many investigators have examined the protective properties of EN on the GI mucosa in animal models. In general, bacterial translocation appears to occur more frequently with PN and monomeric enteral formulas. Crude fiber and rat chow appeared to be protective, but the results have not been duplicated in human studies, so the hypothesis of bacterial translocation as a source of SIRS in humans remains to be confirmed.[93] Indeed, recent reports from Deitch's group focus on ischemia/reperfusion rather than bacterial translocation as the primary GI-tract event affecting SIRS. Cytokines derived from mesenteric lymph rather than portal circulation led to lung injury as well as increased ileal permeability in rodent models of intestinal ischemia/reperfusion.[92-94] Finally, intestinal bacterial overgrowth increased GI cytokine production in a burn injury model.[95] These conclusions, like those of bacterial translocation, were derived from animal models.

Evidence of bacterial translocation in humans is indirect. Permeability of the epithelial lining of the GI tract has been evaluated by testing the movement of compounds across the mucosal barrier under pathologic conditions and normal control conditions. Endotoxin (LPS) produced by bacteria would be equivalent to this type of compound. Benign compounds that have been used under experimental conditions include lactose, rhamnose, chromium ethylenediamine-tetraacetic acid (Cr EDTA), polyethylene glycol, and cyanocobalamin (vitamin B_{12}). O'Dwyer and colleagues[99] administered intravenous *Escherichia coli* endotoxin to healthy humans and observed increased absorption and excretion of orally administered lactulose and mannitol. Dietch[100] produced similar results in burn patients with the same two sugars. Unfortunately, the mechanisms that explain mucosal permeability and bacterial translocation are not completely understood, and the two phenomena do not necessarily occur at the same time. Therefore, these studies cannot be interpreted as confirmation of bacterial translocation in humans.[101]

In 1990, Lowry proposed a hypothesis to explain exaggerated inflammatory responses via enhanced proinflammatory mediator production associated with PN or GI rest.[4] In this hypothesis, lack of EN and intestinal stimulation disrupt the mucosal barrier, exposing mononuclear cells of the submucosa, mesenteric lymph nodes, and splanchnic tissue to antigenic stimulus. Figure 35-3 illustrates enhanced Kupffer cell produc-

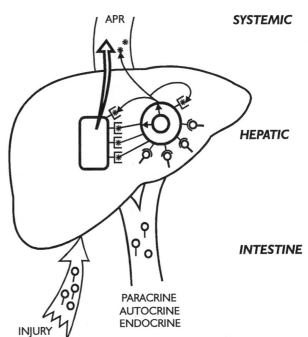

FIGURE 35-3 A proposed mechanism for enhanced hepatic cytokine responses during loss of enteral stimulation and concomitant injury. Under these conditions, the predisposition to enhance cytokine *(asterisks)* production by Kupffer cells *(large circles)* is amplified by inducing antigen *(small circles with line)* exposure from the intestine and injury sites. Demonstrable evidence of increased hepatic injury responses, such as acute-phase protein (APR) production, is evident in circulation. With this level of cytokine production, soluble mediator is detectable and systemic responses consistent with cytokine appearance are observed. (Lowry SF: The route of feeding influences injury responses, *J Trauma* 30(suppl):10S-15S, 1990.)

tion of cytokines in response to a gastrointestinally derived stimulus (i.e., translocated antigen). Low-level cytokine activity maintains metabolic homeostasis and immune regulation in normal GI function. Exaggerated antigenic exposure of immunocompetent GI and liver cells may boost local cytokine expression above normal levels and exacerbate SIRS. This hypothesis is not completely supported by Deitch's (previously discussed) investigations published subsequent to publication of Lowry's hypothesis. Deitch's work suggests that ischemia and reperfusion are the sentinal events of GI compromise and increased cytokine production. Mesenteric lymph and not portal vein plasma was cytotoxic to endothelial cells in these studies. However, prevention of bacterial overgrowth by enteral or oral feeding to minimize GI cytokine production would suggest that EN still plays a role in attenuating inflammation.

A human model of sepsis supports the use of EN, as opposed to PN, to decrease inflammation. Normal adult volunteers and stable hospitalized patients fed parenterally for a week exhibited a moderate increase in cortisol levels. There was no increase in cytokine concentrations in normal volunteers, and no significant increases in cytokine concentrations in all patients studied;[102] however, endotoxin administration produced higher peak concentrations of epinephrine, glucagon, and TNF in parenterally fed normal subjects than in a similarly treated group, fed enterally.[103] The parenteral group also displayed inflammatory symptoms such as malaise and fever. More recently, Santos and colleagues[104] tested the same hypothesis in parenterally and enterally fed normal subjects and found no significant differences in tested counterregulatory hormone and cytokine levels; however, patients were challenged with endotoxin after 2 days' feeding in the enteral group and after 10 days' feeding in the parenteral group, as compared with 7 days' feeding in both groups in the previous study.

Additional investigations that support this hypothesis can be found in two animal studies of the effects of early enteral feeding on endocrine responses to stress. Mochizuki and coworkers[105] found lower plasma cortisol and glucagon levels, and lower urinary vanillylmandelic acid (VMA) in severely burned guinea pigs fed enterally early (2 hours) after the burn rather than late (72 hours). Saito and associates[106] found lower plasma cortisol and glucagon levels and lower urinary VMA in similarly burned guinea pigs fed enterally as opposed to parenterally. The authors of both papers attributed their findings to breach of GI barrier function (rather than ischemia reperfusion phenomenon), macrophage activation, and subsequent catabolic hormone production. These studies were performed in animals, which weakens their clinical significance for critically ill humans. Nevertheless, the fact that SIRS occurs following a variety of insults, including severe burns (see Fig. 35-1), suggests that similar mechanisms are causing the syndrome.[1]

Nutrient Formulation of Enteral Products

Supplementation of enteral formulas with specific nutrients has been hypothesized to have a beneficial effect on paracrine and endocrine responses of stressed patients.[107] Several clinical trials have investigated these formulations, heretofore referred to as immune-enhanced enteral formulas (IEEFs), for their effect on systemic immune function, morbidity, and mortality. However, despite numerous investigations, the clinical utility of these formulas remains controversial. In 2000, a group of nutrition support experts convened to develop a consensus on the clinical use of these IEEF.[108] The nutrients supplemented in commercially available formulas with research-based claims for immune-enhancement are ω-3 fatty acids, arginine, ribonucleic acid, glutamine, and antioxidant vitamins.

Dietary fatty acids are a concentrated source of energy, part of cell membranes, and they provide substrate for eicosanoid (prostaglandins, thromboxane, leukotriene) synthesis. The lipids most commonly used in enteral formulas and parenteral solutions are rich in the ω-6 fatty acid linoleic acid, which is thought to be an immunosuppressant.[109] Spielmann and coworkers[110] have suggested that excessive linoleic acid inhibits δ[6]-desaturase activity (the rate-limiting enzyme in the biosynthesis of polyunsaturated fatty acids), ultimately producing eicosanoid metabolites in ratios unfavorable to optimal human immune responses.

Research, predominantly in animals, has examined whether the use of alternative lipids, such as fish oils rich in the ω-3 fatty acids eicosapentaenoic and docosahexaenoic acid, avert the immunosuppressive effects of linoleic acid. Burned guinea pigs had improved immune parameters and less weight loss when fed fish oil rather than safflower oil, which is greater than 70% linoleic acid.[111] Guinea pigs fed fish oil survived better after exposure to endotoxin challenge.[112] A rat model of chronic sepsis showed decreased mortality in animals fed menhaden oil (ω-3 fatty acid) as compared with animals fed safflower oil (ω-6 fatty acid).[113] However, no improvement in survival was observed in mice with induced peritonitis fed fish oil.[114] In an acute peritonitis guinea pig model, mixture of equal parts fish oil and safflower oil improved survival rates over those of single-oil preparations.[115] Thus far, the use of ω-3 fatty acids in human enteral formulas for the purpose of improving septic outcome remains controversial.

The amino acid arginine, essential to growth, may also play an important role in wound healing and immune responses; however, definitive evidence of a beneficial effect for sepsis or severe stress is lacking.[5] Rats with peritonitis fed an arginine-enriched enteral diet survived longer than rats fed an arginine-poor diet only when fed before cecal ligation and puncture.[116] In a peritonitis model, guinea pigs that received the most arginine had the worst survival rate.[117]

Arginine supplementation of enteral diets may not be advantageous to patients with SIRS because arginine is the nitrogen donor for nitric oxide synthesis. Nitric oxide has several functions during SIRS, among them vasorelaxation (and potential hypotension), oxygen radical binding, inhibition of cellular respiration and of platelet aggregation, and prevention of neutrophil adhesion to endothelium. Because of these functions, it is not yet known whether exogenous arginine is beneficial or detrimental to patients with SIRS.[118]

The theoretically beneficial effect of nucleotides in enteral regimens derives from their ability to enhance natural killer cell activity and T lymphocyte-mediated immunity.[119] A study using septic mice that compared nucleotide-depleted diets; nucleotide-depleted diets enriched with RNA, adenine, or uracil; and normal chow diets found mice fed nucleotide-depleted diets had the highest mortality rate. The supplemented group did not exhibit better survival than the chow (control) group.[120] Mice fed enterally with nucleic acid-free enteral formula supplemented with RNA did not have lower mortality rates than animals fed the unsupplemented formula in another murine sepsis model.[121]

Many studies have examined the use of glutamine in the maintenance of GI mucosal integrity and the prevention of bacterial translocation in animals. Prevention of continual macrophage stimulation caused by translocation of enteric bacteria and/or endotoxin provides the link between a role for glutamine and the prevention of SIRS. Experimental results are inconclusive.[5] Animal models have shown that enteral glutamine reduced translocation after radiation-induced colitis[122] and prolonged survival with methotrexate-induced enterocolitis.[123] Glutamine supplementation did not benefit rats challenged with endotoxin,[124] and a glutamine-free diet (as opposed to a glutamine-rich diet) did not produce structural damage to the GI mucosa in a tissue injury rat model.[125]

Several clinical studies examined the effects of parenterally supplemented glutamine, mostly in bone marrow transplant (BMT) patients. Scheltinga and coworkers[126] reported that

BMT patients not given supplemental glutamine in their parenteral formulas had expanded extracellular fluid volume, more positive microbial cultures ($p < .01$), and higher rates of clinical infection than patients who received supplemental glutamine. Using similar methods, Ziegler and associates[127] found improved nitrogen balance ($p = .002$), less infection ($p = .041$), and shorter hospitalization in the glutamine-supplemented BMT patients. Schloerb and Amare[128] reported increased total body water in BMT patients who received standard parenteral formula and decreased total body water in those who received glutamine-supplemented PN. The supplemented group also had shorter lengths of hospitalization after transplantation ($p < .05$). Finally, patients with short-bowel syndrome treated with glutamine, growth hormone, and a modified diet exhibited significantly increased absorption of total calories, protein, carbohydrate, and water and sodium, compared with patients treated with a modified diet alone.[129] Collectively, these studies appear to demonstrate a role for glutamine in certain patient populations.

The antioxidant vitamins retinol, tocopherol, ascorbate, and carotenoids have been added to enteral formulas to, in theory, minimize free radical damage to patients with SIRS. Briefly, free radicals are believed to contribute to reperfusion injury.[130] Antioxidant status may be compromised during SIRS because of decreased synthesis of hepatic proteins, which transport antioxidants, and by concurrent increased need for antioxidants.[131] Inhibition of lipid (membrane) peroxidation after reperfusion of heart tissue has been shown to decrease reperfusion injury on the cellular level.[132] In a population of patients with septic shock, retinol, tocopherol, and beta-carotene levels were significantly lower than in healthy controls, with evidence of increased lipid peroxidation in the septic group. The authors suggest a therapeutic role for antioxidants in critically ill patients.[133]

More than 20 published clinical trials were used to develop a consensus on the clinical utility of IEEF at the previously mentioned meeting of experts in 2000.[108] Early studies[134-137] were criticized because the nitrogen content of the control and experimental (immune-enhanced) formulas were not equal.[5] The consensus panel pointed out that mortality was actually increased among critically ill patients receiving IEEF in two studies.[137,138] A more recent study in the same population contradicts these results.[139] IEEF decreased mortality when compared with controls. However, the best results were obtained in the least sick patients. One possible explanation for these contradictory results may be timing of the administration of IEEF to critically ill patients. Some have suggested that the supplemented nutrients in IEEFs may enhance inflammation if infused during SIRS, contributing to subsequent MODS and increased mortality.[140]

Recommendations on the clinical use of IEEF were provided by the consensus panel for patients who should receive IEEF, those for whom insufficient data are insufficient but may benefit from these formulas, and those who should not receive IEEF.[141] These recommendations and more are reviewed in Box 35-4.

Subsequent to publication of the consensus panel's recommendations, a comprehensive evaluation was published on the efficacy of IEEFs in critically ill patients.[142] The relationship

---

BOX 35-4

Recommendations for the Use of Immune-Enhanced Enteral Formulas (IEEF)

SHOULD RECEIVE IEEF
Moderately or severely malnourished receiving elective gastrointestinal surgery
Blunt and penetrating abdominal trauma with injury severity score ≥18; abdominal trauma index ≥20

INSUFFICIENT DATA EXIST, BUT MIGHT BENEFIT FROM IEEF
Aortic reconstruction with known COPD and anticipated prolonged mechanical ventilation
Major head and neck surgery with preexisting malnutrition
Severe head injury; Glasgow Coma Scale <8 with abnormal head CT scan
Burns ≥ 30%
Ventilator dependent, nonseptic at risk for subsequent infectious morbidity

SHOULD NOT RECEIVE IEEF
Severe sepsis
Oral intake to resume within 5 days
Bowel obstruction distal to site of enteral access
Incomplete resuscitation or splanchnic hypoperfusion
Major upper GI hemorrhage

WHEN TO BEGIN IEEF
Before insult when possible (i.e., 5-7 days preoperatively or as early as clinically possible postoperatively)

MINIMUM DOSE OF IEEF
1200-1500 ml or 50%-60% calculated nutrient goals

Adapted from Galban C, Montejo JC, Mesejo A, et al: An immune-enhancing enteral diet reduces mortality rate and episodes of bacteremia in septic intensive care patients, *Crit Care Med* 28:643-648, 2000.
COPD, Chronic obstructive pulmonary disease; *CT*, computed tomography; *GI*, gastrointestinal;

---

between IEEFs and infectious complications and mortality was systematically reviewed in 22 randomized trials, which compared IEEFs and standard formulas in elective surgery patients, severe trauma patients, and critically ill intensive care unit (ICU) patients.

The conclusions derived from the evaluation were made for the aggregate of studies and for studies in subgroup populations. The authors emphasized that conclusions based on subgroup evaluations are appropriately viewed as hypotheses rather than definitive confirmation of efficacy in each subgroup. Aggregate results indicated that IEEFs were not associated with decreased mortality, were associated with decreased infectious complications, and were associated with decreased length of hospitalization.[142]

Subgroup analysis for high-arginine IEEFs versus low-arginine IEFFs found no difference in mortality, but *higher* mortality in IEEFs that were low in arginine. Infectious complications were lower in high-arginine IEEFS, and no difference was found in infectious complications in IEEFs low in arginine. High-arginine IEEFs decreased length of hospitalization and low-arginine IEEFs *increased* length of hospitalization.[142]

Subgroup analysis of patients in mechanically ventilated ICU patients found no relationship between IEEFs and mortality or infectious complications. However IEEFs were associated with decreased length of hospitalization. Mortality was *increased* in subjects on low-arginine IEEFs. Mortality was also *increased* in studies with high methodologic scores and decreased in studies with lower methodologic scores. *Methodologic score* refers to a score given to each study that evaluated the quality of a study's methods.[142]

The results and conclusions from the expert panel and the IEEF efficacy evaluation suggest that the appropriate use of these formulas in critical care populations remains elusive. In fact, the use of IEEFs low in arginine in critically ill ICU patients may be detrimental to outcome. The optimal use of the appropriate combination of immune-enhancing nutrients is likely to become more apparent as the understanding of inflammation increases.

Practical Application of Nutrition Support

Nutrition support recommendations for SIRS (and CARS) rely to a great extent on use of clinical judgment, in the face of less-than-conclusive research and speculation about the possible benefits of modifying the mediators of SIRS. Nutrition support may play a role in attenuation of mediators. The less controversial purpose of nutrition support is to minimize nutritional morbidity by providing appropriate metabolic support. Although sepsis is in some ways comparable to major trauma, SIRS from a septic source is not predictable, nor is severe sepsis or shock. Thus, timing of nutrition support is irrelevant (i.e., early feeding either by the enteral or parenteral route and use of immune-enhanced enteral formulas). Nevertheless, it is prudent to use the enteral route as much as possible in patients at risk for sepsis. EN does not carry the risk of catheter sepsis, may help maintain GI immunity, may decrease the risk of gut-derived sepsis, and may attenuate inflammatory mediator production in patients exposed to an inflammatory challenge.

Nutrition support should begin when oxygen transport is adequate or has been restored by maximizing cardiac function, correcting anemia, and maximizing arterial oxygen saturation. Patients with inadequate oxygen transport are also likely to be hemodynamically unstable, which refers to instability of intravascular plasma volume and flow resulting in inadequate tissue perfusion and hypotension. Such conditions are often accompanied by decreased visceral blood flow.[143] Under normal conditions, the presence of food in the intestinal lumen stimulates visceral blood flow. During conditions of sepsis and shock, EN may stimulate intestinal blood flow or cause an ischemic condition because increased oxygen demand is not met by oxygen delivery. EN has been reported to decrease intramucosal gastric pH in trauma patients requiring resuscitation, indicating tissue hypoxia.[144] Conditions of shock, inadequate oxygen transport, and (suspected) inadequate intestinal perfusion are not favorable to either PN or EN. EN should be initiated at a slow rate and advanced conservatively, and patients should be carefully monitored for pain, abdominal distention, hypermotility, and ileus.[145]

If GI function is not favorable to EN and tissue oxygenation and hemodynamics are stable, PN is necessary. Conservative carbohydrate and lipid infusion is recommended to avoid potential hepatic abnormalities.[49] A moderate amount of lipid daily in a nonprotein calorie regimen and continuous (24-hour) lipid infusion may help minimize the immunosuppressive effects associated with currently available lipid emulsions.[98]

Meticulous monitoring of patients' clinical status and appropriate modification of nutrition support are necessary to prevent potential exacerbation of organ dysfunction.

Conclusion

SIRS is a systemic response observed in patients suffering severe physiologic stress from a variety of insults, including confirmed sepsis. MODS is frequently the complication that finally causes death to patients with SIRS. To a certain extent, SIRS and MODS are the result of the capability of medical technology to effectively treat primary illnesses and sustain life in the ICU. A new body of research focusing on mediators common in several critical care diagnoses has increased understanding of the complications, and treatment strategies are being targeted toward manipulating these mediators. EN, as opposed to PN, may play a role in abrogating SIRS in its early stages. A host of nutrients believed to benefit the immune systems of critically ill patients have been investigated, principally with EN, in several clinical trials.

The challenge to nutrition support clinicians remains that of providing an appropriate amount of nutrients to minimize nitrogen loss and adverse effects on organ function. EN is the preferred route of support when the GI tract is functional. With severe sepsis and septic shock, provision of exogenous substrate may be problematic because of altered oxygen transport and utilization. Optimization of hemodynamic function and oxygen transport before initiating nutrition support may be in the best interest of these patients. The range of metabolic and physiologic abnormalities of patients with SIRS requires that the nutrition support clinician monitor patients conscientiously and adjust interventions accordingly.

REFERENCES

1. American College of Chest Physicians/Society of Critical Care Medicine Consensus Conference Committee: American College of Chest Physicians/Society of Critical Care Medicine Consensus Conference: definitions for sepsis and organ failure and guidelines for the use of innovative therapies in sepsis, *Crit Care Med* 20(6):864-874, 1992.
2. Deitch EA: Multiple organ failure. Pathophysiology and potential future therapy, *Ann Surg* 216(2):117-134, 1992.
3. Giroir BP: Mediators of septic shock: new approaches for interrupting the endogenous inflammatory cascade, *Crit Care Med* 21(5):780-789, 1993.
4. Lowry SF: The route of feeding influences injury responses, *J Trauma* 30(12 suppl):12:S10-S15, 1990.
5. Heyland DK, Cook DJ, Guyatt GH: Does the formulation of enteral feeding products influence infectious morbidity and mortality rates in the critically ill patient? A critical review of the evidence, *Crit Care Med* 22(7):1192-1202, 1994.
6. Schloerb PR: Immune-enhancing diets: products, components, and their rationales, *J Parenteral Enteral Nutr* (25 suppl):S3-S7, 2001.
7. Skillman JJ, Bushnell LS, Goldman H, Silen W: Respiratory failure, hypotension, sepsis, and jaundice. A clinical syndrome associated with lethal hemorrhage from acute stress ulceration of the stomach, *Am J Surg* 117(4):523-530, 1969.
8. Tilney NL, Batley GL, Morgan AP: Sequential system failure after rupture of abdominal aortic aneurysms. An unsolved problem in postoperative care, *Ann Surg* 178(2):117-122, 1973.
9. Fry DE, Pearlstein L, Fulton RL, Polk HC: Multiple organ system failure. The role of uncontrolled infection, *Arch Surg* 115(2):136-140, 1980.
10. Bell RC, Coalson JJ, Smith JD, Johanson WG: Multiple organ E system failure and infection in adult respiratory distress syndrome, *Ann Intern Med* 99(3):293-298, 1983.

11. Bennett IL, Beeson PB: Studies in the pathogenesis of fever, *J Exp Med* 98(11):477-492, 1953.

12. Tracey KJ, Lowry SF: The role of cytokine mediators in septic shock, *Adv Surg* 23:21-56, 1990.

13. Polk HC, Shields CL: Remote organ failure: a valid sign of occult-abdominal infection, *Surgery* 81(3):310-313, 1977.

14. Goris RJA, Boekhorst TP, Nuytinck JK, Gimbrere JS: Multiple organ failure. Generalized autodestructive inflammation? *Arch Surg* 120(10):1109-1115, 1985.

15. Norton LW: Does drainage of intraabdominal pus reverse multiple organ failure? *Am J Surg* 149(3):347-350, 1985.

16. Sculier JP, Bron D, Verboven N, Klastersky J: Multiple organ failure during interleukin-2 administration and LAK cell infusion, *Intensive Care Med* 14(6):666-667, 1988.

17. Grotz MR, Deitch EA, Ding J, Xu D, Huang Q, Regel G: Intestinal cytokine response after gut ischemia: role of gut barrier function, *Ann Surg* 229(4):478-486, 1999.

18. Xu DZ, Lu Q, Kubicka R, Deitch EA: The effect of hypoxia/reoxygenation on the cellular function of intestinal epithelial cells, *J Trauma* 46(2):280-285, 1999.

19. Maggnotti LJ, Upperman JS, Xu DZ, Lu Q, Deitch EA: Gut-derived mesenteric lymph but not portal blood increases endothelial cell permeability and promotes lung injury after hemorrhagic shock, *Ann Surg* 228(4):518-527, 1998.

20. Bone RC: Toward a theory regarding the pathogenesis of the systemic inflammatory response syndrome: what we do and do not know about cytokine regulation, *Crit Care Med* 24(1):163-172, 1996.

21. Chrousos GP: The hypothalamic-pituitary-adrenal axis and immune-mediated inflammation, *N Engl J Med* 332(20):1351-1362, 1995.

22. Waage A, Brandtzaeg P, Halstensen, et al: The complex pattern of cytokines in serum from patients with meningococcal septic shock. Association between interleukin-6, interleukin-1, and fatal outcome, *J Exp Med* 169(1):333-338, 1989.

23. Bussolino F, Camussi G, Baglioni C: Synthesis and release of platelet-activating factor by human vascular endothelial cells treated with tumor necrosis factor or interleukin-1, *J Biol Chem* 263(24):11856-11861, 1988.

24. Dayer JM, Beutler B, Cerami A: Cachectin/tumor necrosis factor stimulates collagenase and prostaglandin E$_2$ production by human synovial cells and dermal fibroblasts, *J Exp Med* 162(6):2163-2168, 1985.

25. Petersen M, Steadman R, Hallett MB, et al: Zymosan-induced leukotriene B$_4$ generation by human neutrophils is augmented by TNF-α but not chemotactic peptide, *Immunology* 70(1):75-81, 1990.

26. Gamble JR, Harlan JM, Klebanoff SJ, Vadas MA: Stimulation of the adherence of neutrophils to umbilical vein endothelium by human recombinant tumor necrosis factor, *Proc Natl Acad Sci USA* 82(24):8667-8671, 1985.

27. Dixit VM, Green S, Sarma V, et al: Tumor necrosis factor-α induction of novel gene products in human endothelial cells including a macrophage-specific chemotoxin, *J Biol Chem* 265(5):2973-2978, 1990.

28. Sheldon J, Riches P, Gooding R, et al: C-reactive protein and its cytokine mediators in intensive-care patients, *Clin Chem* 39(1):147-150, 1993.

29. Clauss M, Ryan J, Stern D: Modulation of endothelial cell hemostatic properties by TNF: insights into the role of endothelium in the host response to inflammatory stimuli. In Beutler B (ed): *Tumor necrosis factors: the molecules and their emerging role in medicine,* New York, 1992, Raven, pp 49-63.

30. Tracey KJ, Lowry SF, Beutler B, et al: Cachectin/tumor necrosis factor mediates changes of skeletal muscle plasma membrane potential, *J Exp Med* 164(4):1368-1373, 1986.

31. Warren RS, Starnes HF, Gabrilove JL, et al: The acute metabolic effects of tumor necrosis factor administration in humans, *Arch Surg* 122(12):1396-1400, 1987.

32. Moldower LL: Cytokines and the cachexia response to acute inflammation, *Support Line* 18:1-6, 1996.

33. Walter JS, Meyers P, Krueger JM: Microinjection of interleukin-1 into brain: separation of sleep and fever responses, *Physiol Behav* 45(1):169-176, 1989.

34. Marinkovic S, Jahreis GP, Wong GG, Bauman H: IL-6 modulates the synthesis of a specific set of acute phase plasma proteins in vivo, *J Immunol* 142(3):808-812, 1989.

35. Hirano T, Yasukawa K, Harada H, et al: Complementary DNA for a novel human interleukin (BSF-2) that induces B lymphocytes to produce immunoglobulin, *Nature* 324(6092):73-76, 1986.

36. Garman RD, Jacobs KA, Clark SC, Raulet DH: B-cell stimulatory (beta-2 interferon) functions as a second signal for interleukin-2 production by mature murine T cells, *Proc Natl Acad Sci USA* 84(21):7629-7633, 1987.

37. Wong GG, Witek-Gianotti JS, Temple PA, et al: Stimulation of murine hematopoietic colony formation by human IL-6, *J Immunol* 140(9):3040-3044, 1988.

38. Endo S, Inada K, Inoue Y, et al: Two types of septic shock classified by plasma levels of cytokines and endotoxin, *Circ Shock* 38(4):264-274, 1992.

39. Casey LC, Balk RA, Bone RC: Plasma cytokine and endotoxin levels correlate with survival in patients with the sepsis syndrome, *Ann Intern Med* 119(8):771-778, 1993.

40. Grobmyer SR, Lin E, Lowry SF, et al: Elevation of IL-18 in human sepsis, *J Clin Immunol* 20(3):212-15, 2000.

41. Endo S, Inada K, Yamada Y, et al: Interleukin 18 (IL-18) levels in patients with sepsis, *J Med* 3(1-2)1:15-20, 2000.

42. Chang SW, Feddersen CO, Henson PM, Voelkel NT: Platelet-activating factor mediates hemodynamic changes and lung injury in endotoxin-treated rats, *J Clin Invest* 79(5):1498-1509, 1987.

43. Sun XM, Hsueh W: Bowel necrosis induced by tumor necrosis factor in rats is mediated by platelet-activating factor, *J Clin Invest* 81(5):1328-1331, 1988.

44. Mojarad M, Hamasaki Y, Said SI: Platelet-activating factor increases pulmonary microvascular permeability and induces pulmonary edema. A preliminary report, *Bull Eur Physiopathol Respir* 19(3):253-256, 1983.

45. Klosterhalfen B, Horstmann-Jungemann K, Vogel S, et al: Time course of various inflammatory mediators during recurrent endotoxemia, *Biochem Pharmacol* 43(10):2103-2109, 1992.

46. Meyer JD, Yurt RW, Duhaney R, et al: Tumor necrosis factor-enhanced leukotriene B4 generation and chemotaxis in human neutrophils, *Arch Surg* 123(12):1454-1458, 1988.

47. Meyer J, Yurt RW, Duhaney R, et al: Differential neutrophil activation before and after endotoxin infusion in enterally versus parenterally fed volunteers, *Surg Gynecol Obstet* 167(6):501-509, 1988.

48. Nakae H, Endo S, Inada K, et al: Serum complement levels and severity of sepsis, *Res Commun Chem Pathol Pharmacol* 84(2):189-195, 1994.

49. Berger M, Wetzler EM, Wallis RS: Tumor necrosis factor is the major monocyte product that increases complement receptor expression on mature human neutrophils, *Blood* 71(1):151-158, 1988.

50. Solomkin JS, Cotta LA, Satoh PS, et al: Complement activation and clearance in acute illness and injury: evidence for C5a as a cell-directed mediator of the adult respiratory distress syndrome in man, *Surgery* 97(6):668-678, 1985.

51. Schirmer WJ, Schirmer JM, Naff GB, Fry DE: Systemic complement activation produces hemodynamic changes characteristic of sepsis, *Arch Surg* 123(3):316-321, 1988.

52. Whang KT, Vath SD, Becker KL, et al: Procalcitonin and inflammatory cytokine interaction in sepsis, *Shock* 14(1):73-78, 2000.

53. Chrousos GP: Regulation and dysregulation of the hypothalamic-pituitary-adrenal axis: the corticotropin-releasing hormone perspective, *Endocrinol Metab Clin North Am* 21(4):833-858, 1992.

54. Zitnik RJ, Whiting NL, Elias JA: Glucocorticoid inhibition of interleukin-1-induced interleukin-6 production by human lung fibroblasts: evidence for transcriptional and post-transcriptional regulatory mechanisms, *Am J Respir Cell Molec Biol* 10(6):643-650, 1994.

55. Barton RG: Nutrition support in critical illness, *Nutr Clin Pract* 9(4):127-139, 1994.

56. Beal AL, Cerra FB: Multiple organ failure syndrome in the 1990s. Systemic inflammatory response and organ dysfunction, *JAMA* 271(3):226-233, 1994.

57. Cerra FB, Siegel JH, Coleman B, et al: Septic autocannibalism; a failure of exogenous nutritional support, *Ann Surg* 192(4):570-580, 1980.

58. Schlichtig R, Ayers SM: Fuel and oxygen metabolism during health and critical illness. In Schlichtig R, Ayers SM (eds): *Nutrition support of the critically ill,* Chicago, 1988, Year Book, pp 49-74.

59. Dong YL, Sheng CY, Herndon DN, Waymack JP: Metabolic abnormalities of mitochondrial redox potential in post burn multiple system organ failure, *Burns* 18(4):283-286(4), 1992.

60. Gutierrez G, Lund N, Bryan-Brown CW: Cellular oxygen utilization during multiple organ failure, *Crit Care Clin* 5(2):271-287, 1989.

61. Nelson DP, Samsel RW, Wood LD, Schumacher PT: Pathological supply dependence of systemic and interstitial oxygen uptake during endotoxemia, *J Appl Physiol* 64:2410-2419(6), 1988.

62. Deitch EA, Goodman ER: Prevention of multiple organ failure, *Surg Clin North Am* 79(6):471-488, 1999.

63. van Saene HK, Stoutenbeek CC, Stoller JK: Selective decontamination of the digestive tract in the intensive care unit: current status and future prospects, *Crit Care Med* 20(5):691-703, 1992.
64. Faist E, Kim C: Therapeutic immunomodulatory approaches for the control of systemic inflammatory response syndrome and the prevention of sepsis, *New Horiz* 6(2 suppl):S97-S102, 1998.
65. Bone RC: Sir Isaac Newton, sepsis, SIRS, and CARS, *Crit Care Med* 24(7):1125-1128, 1996.
66. Deitch EA: Animal models of sepsis and shock: a review and lessons learned, *Shock* 9(1):1-11, 1998.
67. Lowry SF, Thompson WA: Nutrient modification of inflammatory mediator production, *New Horiz* 2(2):164-174, 1994.
68. Proceedings from summit on immune-enhancing enteral therapy, *J Parenteral Enteral Nutr* 25(2 suppl):S1-S63, 2001.
69. Rocha LA, Martin MJ, Pita S, et al: Prevention of nosocomial infection in critically ill patients by selective decontamination of the digestive tract: a randomized, double blind, placebo-controlled study, *Intensive Care Med* 18(7):398-404, 1992.
70. Hammond JMJ, Potgieter PD, Saunders GL, Forder AA: Double-blind study of selective decontamination of the digestive tract in intensive care, *Lancet* 340:5-9, 1992.
71. Lowry SF: Anticytokine therapies in sepsis, *New Horiz* 1(1):120-126, Feb 1993.
72. Barber AE, Colye SM, Fong Y, et al: Impact of hypercortisolemia on the metabolic and hormonal responses to endotoxin in humans, *Surg Forum* 41:74-77, 1990.
73. Lantz M, Malik S, Slevin ML, Olsson I: Infusion of tumor necrosis factor (TNF) causes an increase in circulating TNF-binding protein in humans, *Cytokine* 2(6):402-406, 1990.
74. Eisenberg SP, Evans RJ, Arend WP, et al: Primary structure and functional expression from complementary DNA of a human interleukin-1 receptor antagonist, *Nature* 343(6256), Jan 25, 1990.
75. Van Zee KJ, Kohno T, Fischer, et al: Tumor necrosis factor soluble receptors circulate during experimental and clinical inflammation and can protect against excessive tumor necrosis factor α in vitro and in vivo, *Proc Natl Acad Sci USA* 89(11):4845-4849, June 1, 1992.
76. Fischer E, Van Zee KJ, Marano MA, et al: Interleukin-1 receptor antagonist circulates in experimental inflammation and in human disease, *Blood* 79(9):2196-2200, 1992.
77. Fischer E, Marano MA, Van Zee KJ, et al: Interleukin-1 receptor blockade improves survival and hemodynamic performance in *Escherichia coli* septic shock, but fails to alter host responses to sublethal endotoxemia, *J Clin Invest* 89(5):1551-1557, 1992.
78. Sekut L, Yarnall D, Stimpson SA, et al: Anti-inflammatory activity of phosphodiesterase-IV inhibitors in acute and chronic murine models of inflammation, *Clin Exp Immunol* 100(1):126-132, 1995.
79. Kingsnorth AN, Galloway SW, Formela LJ: Randomized, double-blind phase II trial of Lexipafant, a platelet-activating factor antagonist, in human pancreatitis, *Br J Surg* 82(10);1414-1420, 1995.
80. Beutler B: Endotoxin, tumor necrosis factor, and related mediators: new approaches to shock, *New Horiz* 1(1):3-12, 1993.
81. Bromberg JS, Chavin KD, Kunkel SL: Anti-tumor necrosis factor antibodies suppress cell-mediated immunity in vivo, *J Immunol* 148(11):3412-3417, 1992.
82. Dinarello CA, Gelfand JA, Wolff SM: Anticytokine strategies in the treatment of the systemic inflammatory response syndrome, *JAMA* 269(14):1829-1835, 1993.
83. Zeni F, Pain P, Vindimian M, et al: Effects of pentoxifylline on circulating cytokine concentrations and hemodynamics in patients with septic shock: results from a double-blind, randomized, placebo-controlled study, *Crit Care Med* 24(2):207-214, 1996.
84. Muller Kobold AC, Tulleken JE, Kijlstra JG, et al: Leukocyte activation in sepsis: correlations with disease state and mortality, *Intensive Care Med* 26(7):883-892, 2000.
85. Opal SM, DePalo VA: Anti-inflammatory cytokines, *Chest* 117(4):1162-1172, 2000.
86. Klein S: The myth of serum albumin as a measure of nutritional status, *Gastroenterology* 99(6):1845-1846, 1990.
87. Johnson AM: Low levels of plasma proteins: malnutrition or inflammation? *Clin Chem Lab Med* 37(2):91-96, 1999.
88. Mirtallo JM: Assessing the nutritional needs of the critically ill patient, *DICP Ann Pharm* 24(11 suppl):S20-S23, 1990.
89. Moore FA, Feliciano DV, Andrassy RJ, et al: Early enteral feeding compared with parenteral reduces postoperative septic complications. The results of a meta-analysis, *Ann Surg* 216(2):172-183, 1992.
90. Fink MP: Gastrointestinal mucosal injury in experimental models of shock, trauma, and sepsis, *Crit Care Med* 19(5):627-641, 1991.
91. Lipman TO: Bacterial translocation and enteral nutrition in humans: an outsider looks, *J Parenter Enteral Nutr* 19(2):156-165, 1995.
92. Upperman JS, Deitch EA, Guo W, Lu Q, Xu D: Post-hemorrhagic shock mesenteric lymph is cytotoxic to endothelial cells and activates neutrophils (see comments), *Shock* 10(6):407-414, 1998.
93. Xu DZ, Lu Q, Kubica R, Deitch EA: The effect of hypoxia/reoxygenation on the cellular function of intestinal epithelial cells, *J Trauma* 46(2):280-285, 1999.
94. Grotz MR, Deitch EA, Ding J, et al: Intestinal cytokine response after gut ischemia: role of gut barrier failure, *Ann Surg* 229(4):478-486, 1999.
95. Magnotti LJ, Xu DZ, Deitch EA: Gut-derived mesenteric lymph; a link between burn and lung injury, *Arch Surg* 134(12):1333-1340, 1999.
96. Moore EE, Jones TN: Benefits of immediate jejunostomy feeding after major abdominal trauma: A prospective, randomized study, *J Trauma* 26(10):874-881, 1986.
97. Moore FA, Moore EE, Jones TN, et al: TEN vs. TPN following major abdominal trauma: reduced septic morbidity, *J Trauma* 29(7):916-923, 1989.
98. Kudsk KA, Croce MA, Fabian TC, et al: Enteral vs. parenteral feeding: effects on septic morbidity following blunt and penetrating trauma, *Ann Surg* 215(5):503-513, 1992.
99. O'Dwyer ST, Michie HR, Ziegler TR, et al: A single dose of endotoxin increases intestinal permeability in healthy humans, *Arch Surg* 123(12):1459-1464, 1988.
100. Deitch EA: Intestinal permeability is increased in burn patients shortly after injury, *Surgery* 107(4):411-416, 1990.
101. Fink MP: Gastrointestinal mucosal injury in experimental models of shock, trauma, and sepsis, *Crit Care Med* 19(5):627-641, 1991.
102. Coyle SM, Barber AE, Fong Y, et al: Hormone-cytokine responses to total parenteral nutrition in humans, *Abstr Clin Nutr* 9:20, 1990.
103. Fong YM, Marano MA, Barber AE, et al: Total parenteral nutrition and bowel rest modify the metabolic responses to endotoxin in humans, *Ann Surg* 210(4):449-457, 1989.
104. Santos AA, Rodrick ML, Jacobs DO, et al: Does route of feeding modify the inflammatory response? *Ann Surg* 220(2):155-163, 1994.
105. Mochizuki H, Trocki O, Dominioni L, et al: Mechanism of prevention of postburn hypermetabolism and catabolism by early enteral feeding, *Ann Surg* 200(3):297-310, 1984.
106. Saito H, Trocki O, Alexander JW, et al: The effect of route of nutrient administration on the nutritional state, catabolic hormone secretion, and gut mucosal integrity after burn injury, *J Parenter Enteral Nutr* 11(1):1-7, 1987.
107. Wilmore DW: Catabolic illness, *N Engl J Med* 325(10):695-702, 2001.
108. Kudsk, K: Introduction, *J Parenteral Enteral Nutr* 25(suppl);S1-S2.
109. Bell SJ, Mascoli EA, Bistrian BR, et al: Alternative lipid sources for enteral and parenteral nutrition: Long- and medium-chain triglycerides, structured triglycerides and fish oils, *J Am Diet Assoc* 91(1):74-78, 1991.
110. Spielmann D, Bracco U, Traitler H, et al: Alternative lipids to usual omega-6 PUFAS: gamma-linoleic acid, alpha-linoleic acid, stearidonic acid, EPA, etc, *J Parenter Enteral Nutr* 12(6 suppl):111S-23S, 1988.
111. Alexander JW, Saito H, Troki O, et al: The importance of lipid type in the diet after burn injury, *Ann Surg* 204(1):1-8, 1986.
112. Mascioli EA, Iwasa Y, Trimbo S, et al: Endotoxin challenge after menhaden oil diet: effects on survival of guinea pigs, *Am J Clin Nutr* 49(2):277-282, 1989.
113. Barton RG, Wells CL, Carlson A, et al: Dietary omega-3 fatty acids decrease mortality and Kupffer cell prostaglandin E_2 production in a rat model of chronic sepsis, *J Trauma* 31(6):768-774, 1991.
114. Clouva-Molyvdas P, Peck MD, Alexander JW: Short-term dietary lipid manipulation does not affect survival in two models of murine sepsis, *J Parenter Enteral Nutr* 16(4):343-347, 1992.
115. Peck MD, Ogle CK, Alexander JW: Composition of fat in enteral diets can influence outcome in experimental peritonitis, *Ann Surg* 214(1):74-82, 1991.
116. Madden HP, Breslin RJ, Wasserkrug HL, et al: Stimulation of T-cell immunity by arginine enhances survival in peritonitis, *J Surg Res* 44(6):658-663, 1988.
117. Gonce SJ, Peck MD, Alexander JW, Miskell PW: Arginine supplementation and its effects on established peritonitis in guinea pigs, *J Parenter Enteral Nutr* 14(3):237-244, 1990.
118. Kelly E, Morris SM, Billiar TR: Nitric oxide, sepsis, and arginine metabolism, *J Parenteral Enteral Nutr* 19(3):234-238, 1995.

119. Carver JD, Cox WI, Barness LA: Dietary nucleotide effects upon murine natural killer cell activity and macrophage activity, *J Parenter Enteral Nutr* 14(1):18-22, 1990.

120. Kulkami AD, Fanslow WC, Rudolph FB, Van Buren CT: Effect of dietary nucleotides on response to bacterial infections, *J Parenter Enteral Nutr* 10(2):169-171, 1986.

121. Adjei AA, Takamine FT, Yokoyama H, et al: The effects of oral RNA and intraperitoneal nucleoside-nucleotide administration on methicillin-resistant *Staphylococcus aureus* infection in mice, *J Parenter Enteral Nutr* 17(2):148-152, 1993.

122. Souba WW, Klimberg VA, Hautamaki RD, et al: Oral glutamine reduces bacterial translocation following abdominal radiation, *J Surg Res* 48(1):1-5, 1990.

123. Fox AD, Kripke SA, DePaula J, et al: Effect of glutamine supplemented enteral diet on methotrexate induced enterocolitis, *J Parenter Enteral Nutr* 12(4):325-331, 1988.

124. Barber AE, Jones WB, Minei JP, et al: Glutamine or fiber supplementation of a defined formula diet: impact on bacterial translocation, tissue composition, and response to endotoxin, *J Parenter Enteral Nutr* 14(4):335-343, 1990.

125. Wusteman M, Tate H, Weaver L, et al: The effect of enteral glutamine deprivation and supplementation on the structure of rat small-intestine mucosa during a systemic injury response, *J Parenter Enteral Nutr* 19(1):22-27, 1995.

126. Scheltinga MR, Young LS, Benfell K, et al: Glutamine-enriched intravenous feedings attenuate extracellular fluid expansion after standard stress, *Ann Surg* 214(4):385-395, 1991.

127. Ziegler TR, Young LS, Benfell K, et al: Clinical and metabolic efficiency of glutamine-supplemented parenteral nutrition after bone marrow transplantation, *Ann Intern Med* 116(10):821-828, 1992.

128. Schloerb PR, Amare M: Total parenteral nutrition with glutamine in bone marrow transplantation and other clinical applications (a randomized, double-blind study), *J Parenter Enteral Nutr* 17(5):407-413, 1993.

129. Byrne TA, Morrissey TB, Nattakom TV, et al: Growth hormone, glutamine, and a modified diet enhance nutrient absorption in patients with severe short bowel syndrome, *J Parenter Enteral Nutr* 19(4):296-302, 1995.

130. Manning AS: Reperfusion-induced arrhythmias: do free radicals play a role? *Free Radical Biol Med* 4(5):305-316, 1988.

131. Goode HF, Webster NR: Antioxidants in intensive care medicine, *Clin Intensive Care* 4(6):265-270, 1993.

132. Carrea FP, Lesnefsky EJ, Kaiser DG, et al: The inhibitor of lipid peroxidation attenuates myocardial injury from ischemia and reperfusion, *J Cardiovasc Pharmacol* 20(2):230-235, 1992.

133. Good HF, Cowley HC, Walker BE, et al: Decreased antioxidants status and increased lipid peroxidation in patients with septic shock and secondary organ dysfunction, *Crit Care Med* 23(4):646-651, 1995.

134. Cerra FB, Lehman S, Konstaninides N, et al: Improvement in immune function in ICU patients by enteral nutrition supplemented with arginine, RNA, and menhaden oil is independent of nitrogen balance, *Nutrition* 7(3):193-199, 1991.

135. Daly JM, Lieberman MD, Goldfine J, et al: Enteral nutrition with supplemented arginine, RNA, and omega-3 fatty acids in patients after operation: immunologic, metabolic, and clinical outcome, *Surgery* 112(1):56-67, 1992.

136. Moore FA, Moore EE, Kudsk KA, et al: Clinical benefits of an immune-enhancing diet for early postinjury enteral feeding, *J Trauma* 37(4):607-615, 1994.

137. Bower RH, Cerra FB, Bershadsky B, et al: Early enteral administration of a formula (Impact) supplemented with arginine, nucleotides, and fish oil in intensive care unit patients: results of a multicenter, prospective, randomized, clinical trial, *Crit Care Med* 23(3):436-449, 1995.

138. Atkinson S, Sieffert E, Bihari D: A prospective, randomized double-blind, controlled trial of enteral immunonutrition on the critically ill, *Crit Care Med* 26(7):1164-1172, 1998.

139. Galban C, Montejo JC, Mesejo A, et al: An immune-enhancing enteral diet reduces mortality rate and episodes of bacteremia in septic intensive care patients, *Crit Care Med* 28(3):643-648, 2000.

140. Heyland DK, Novak F: Immunonutrition in the critically ill patient: more harm than good? *J Parenteral Enteral Nutr* 25(2 suppl):S51-56, 2001.

141. Consensus recommendations from the U.S. summit on immune-enhancing enteral therapy, *J Parenteral Enteral Nutr* 25(2 suppl):S61-63, 2001.

142. Heyland DK, Novak F, Drover JW, Jain M, Su X, Suchner U: Should immunonutrition become routine in critically ill patients? A systematic review of the evidence, *JAMA* 286(8):944-953, 2001.

143. Fink MP: Adequacy of gut oxygenation in endotoxemia and sepsis, *Crit Care Med* 21(2 suppl):54-58, 1993.

144. Tappenden KA, Marvin R, Harris LL, Moore FA: Early enteral nutrition may have detrimental effects in patients with gastrointestinal hypoperfusion, American Society for Parenteral and Enteral Nutrition, 22nd Clinical Congress, *J Parenteral Enteral Nutr* 22(suppl):S9, 1998 (abstract).

145. Martindale RG: Enteral feeding during states of marginal blood flow. *Current issues in enteral nutrition support: report of the first Ross enteral device conference,* Columbus, OH, 1996, Ross Products Division, Abbott Laboratories, pp 59-61.

Human Immunodeficiency Virus Infection

36

Cade Fields-Gardner, MS, RD, LD, CD

IT is estimated that approximately 40 million people are living with human immunodeficiency virus (HIV) infection and/or advanced disease known as the acquired immuno-deficiency syndrome (AIDS) worldwide.[1] This includes the approximately 5 million new infections in the year 2001 alone. An estimated 21.8 million people have died from AIDS-related complications to date, including 3 million during the year 2001. HIV infection became an epidemic in North America during the late 1970s and early 1980s. The HIV infection prevalence rate of 0.6% suggests that nearly one million people are living with HIV disease in North America (not including the Caribbean, which accounts for an additional 420,000 HIV-infected people). The Caribbean region accounts for 60,000 new infections with HIV a year. The slight rise in HIV disease prevalence in North America has been attributed primarily to the success of antiretroviral medications in keeping HIV-infected people alive longer.

The primary mode of transmission is blood to blood through sexual contact in men who have sex with men (MSM), injection drug users (IDU), and heterosexual contact.[2] Women account for approximately 20% of those infected in North America, while accounting for nearly half of infections world-wide. The rate of perinatal infection during pregnancy and delivery has dropped from more than 20% to less than 2% with the use of anti-HIV medications.[3] Breastfeeding among HIV-infected women is considered contraindicated in developed countries where adequate nutrition support is available for adults and children.[4] In developing countries, the risk for malnutrition is too great to recommend against breastfeeding and the message of "breast is best" remains, but is being disputed.[5,6]

Antiretroviral therapy, while helping HIV-infected persons live longer, is not a cure for HIV disease. HIV disease has joined the ranks of chronic diseases with many of the same complications as other chronic or inflammatory disease states. Malnutrition and opportunistic infections are the most common manifestations of HIV disease worldwide. The contribution of malnutrition, specifically the loss of crucial lean tissues, has been more associated with the timing of death than any other complication of immune deficiency and chronic inflammation.[7] As viral load and immune destruction are better controlled with antiretroviral medications (the number of AIDS cases reported to the Centers for Disease Control [CDC] has been dramatically reduced), a person infected with HIV can survive for what is hoped to be a full lifespan. It has become clear that as people survive living with HIV disease, nutritional well-being becomes more important to the maintenance of a strong body and quality of life. At the same time, long-term survival with a chronic inflammatory disease that requires lifelong medication or chemotherapy can yield significant challenges to nutritional status maintenance.

Overview

HIV enters the bloodstream and targets many cells in the body including immune cells such as T-cells and macrophages. The primary target is the CD4 T-lymphocyte, but HIV may establish body reservoirs in lymph tissues, the gastrointestinal tract, and elsewhere in the body. As a retrovirus, HIV contains RNA, which is injected into target cells after successfully attaching and unfolding to allow the process. Once inside the cell, the ribonucleic acid (RNA) is transcribed into deoxyribonucleic acid (DNA) by "reverse transcriptase" and incorporated into the host cell's DNA using the enzyme "integrase." The cell becomes a viral breeding ground where around a billion viral particles are produced daily. The particles are cleaved for assembly by the "protease" enzyme, with typically more than 10 million viral replications achieved daily. From there, the virus must bud from the host cell, killing the host cell in the process and allowing the virus to target and infect more cells during its 6-hour life.

HIV Disease Progression

The case definition of AIDS includes immune suppression (CD4 absolute count of <200 per dl of blood), opportunistic infection or cancer (one that does not normally occur in immune competent persons), or constitutional symptoms such as wasting syndrome.[8] The CDC defines *wasting syndrome* as 10% weight loss from baseline in conjunction with diarrhea or fever for more than 30 days but without an initiating event, such as infection. It is estimated that 20% of reported AIDS cases are defined by the diagnosis of wasting syndrome, although the complication may occur in many more patients.

The continuous progression of the disease to the point of death is less common in persons adequately treated with anti-HIV therapies. The primary predictor of disease progression and risk for wasting and malnutrition is a combination of viral burden and CD4 cell destruction.[9] CD4 cell counts less than 200/dl place a patient at risk for opportunistic infection or cancers that can compromise nutritional status. Conversely, malnutrition can exacerbate immune dysfunction and increase risk of morbidity and mortality.[10-13]

Medication Management

Highly active antiretroviral therapy (HAART) plays an essential role in survival. The antiretroviral medications are used to attack the virus' life cycle at several points. Currently three classes of antiretroviral drugs are available: reverse transcriptase inhibitors (RTI), protease inhibitors (PI), and the new class of fusion inhibitors. Each class of drugs targets a specific part of the HIV lifecycle. RTIs interrupt the transcription of RNA to DNA in the host cell. Protease inhibitors prevent the cleavage of viral particles before reassembly into viable viruses. Fusion inhibitors prevent the attachment of the virus to the target cell before injection of the retrovirus contents.

At this point it appears that patients will have to remain strictly adherent to difficult multidose daily regimens of medications in order to control HIV. Many interactions affect nutritional status, and diet and nutritional status can affect the efficacy of HAART regimens. Table 36-1 shows currently available antiretroviral therapies with notes on the nutritional considerations and potential adverse effects that can impact nutritional status maintenance.

Nutrition in HIV Disease

Although it is clear that HIV infection and replication can lead to debilitating immune destruction, the overlay of malnutrition can exacerbate and cause immune suppression on its own. Viral suppression and immune reconstitution are as dependent on nutritional status as nutritional status is dependent on disease control. Malnutrition was seen as a major complication and a part of advanced disease processes in the pre-HAART era. Disease progression has been defined by the "wasting syndrome," but not by other types of malnutrition. In clinical practice, the problems associated with malnutrition may be ignored

TABLE 36-1

Selected Nutritional Concerns with Antiretroviral Medications

Generic Name (Trade name) Class of Drug (Manufacturer)	Food Interactions	Potential Nutrition-Related Side Effects
Abacavir (Ziagen) Protease inhibitor (Glaxo SmithKline)	Take with or without food; caution with alcohol.	Nausea/vomiting, loss of appetite, abdominal pain, diarrhea, anemia, pancreatitis, lactic acidosis (rare)
Amprenavir (Agenerase) Protease inhibitor (Glaxo SmithKline)	Do not take with high-fat meal; do not take vitamin E supplement when on this medication; do not take with antacids.	Diarrhea, nausea/vomiting, taste changes, stomach upset, diabetes, fatigue, high cholesterol, high triglycerides, anemia
Delavirdine (Rescriptor) NNRTI (Pharmacia & Upjohn)	Take with or without food; do not take with antacids or magnesium-containing supplements; can take with acidic beverage (such as cranberry juice); avoid alcohol.	Increased thirst, loss of appetite, dry mouth, nausea/vomiting, gastritis, diarrhea, constipation, flatulence
Didanosine (Videx) NRTI (Bristol-Myers Squibb)	Take without food on an empty stomach; do not take with acidic beverage or food, aluminum-containing antacids, or magnesium-containing supplements; avoid alcohol.	Loss of appetite, diarrhea, nausea/vomiting, constipation, dry mouth, taste changes, pancreatitis (increased risk with alcohol), lactic acidosis (rare)
Efavirenz (Sustiva) NNRTI (DuPont)	Do not take with high-fat meal; avoid alcohol.	Loss of appetite, nausea/vomiting, diarrhea, high cholesterol, high triglycerides
Emtricitabine (Coviracil) NRTI (Triangle)	None reported.	Nausea/vomiting, diarrhea
Indinavir (Crixivan) Protease inhibitor (Merck)	Take without food on an empty stomach or with very low calorie/low protein snack (Note: no food restriction when taken with ritonavir); take with plenty of fluids.	Nausea, abdominal pain, taste changes, diarrhea, kidney stones, diabetes (rare)
Lamivudine (Epivir) NRTI (Glaxo SmithKline)	Take with or without food.	Nausea/vomiting, abdominal cramps, diarrhea, pancreatitis, lactic acidosis (rare)
Lopinavir (Kaletra) Protease inhibitor (Abbott)	Take with or without food.	Abdominal pain, diarrhea, nausea, high triglycerides
Nelfinavir (Viracept) Protease inhibitor (Agouron)	Take with food; mixing powder with acidic food or beverage results in bitter taste.	Diarrhea, flatulence, nausea, abdominal pain, diabetes (rare)
Nevirapine (Viramune) NNRTI (Roxane)	Take with or without food.	Nausea/vomiting, abdominal pain, fatigue, hepatotoxicity
Ritonavir (Norvir) Protease inhibitor (Abbott)	Take with food.	Nausea/vomiting, diarrhea, taste changes, loss of appetite, upset stomach, diabetes, high triglycerides
Saquinavir (Invirase, Fortovase) Protease inhibitor (Roche)	Take with high-calorie, high-fat meal.	Nausea, diarrhea, low blood sugar
Stavudine (Zerit) NRTI (Bristol-Myers Squibb)	Take with or without food; avoid alcohol.	Nausea/vomiting, diarrhea, loss of appetite, peripheral neuropathy
Tenofovir (Viread) NRTI (Gilead)	Take with food.	Abdominal pain, lactic acidosis (rare)
Zalcitabine (Hivid) NRTI (Roche)	Take without food on an empty stomach; avoid alcohol.	Loss of appetite, oral ulcers, nausea/vomiting, diarrhea, constipation, peripheral neuropathy, lactic acidosis (rare), pancreatitis (rare), high triglycerides
Zidovudine (Retrovir) NRTI (Glaxo SmithKline)	Take with or without food, not with high-fat meal.	Loss of appetite, nausea/vomiting, upset stomach, constipation, anemias

NRTI, Nucleoside reverse transcriptase inhibitor; *NNRTI,* nonnucleoside reverse transcriptase inhibitor.

until the CDC definition of wasting is apparent. At this point in time, the case definition of AIDS serves primarily to establish the numbers of cases that have included a complication of immune deficiency and is less viable as a clinical marker for the initiation of clinical and other interventions. A diagnosis of AIDS is a criterion of eligibility for community support programs targeted to those with advanced disease.

The use of the CDC definition of "wasting syndrome" to identify nutrition-related problems does not consider the health compromise of less severe or different types of malnutrition. It has been suggested that less than 5% unintentional weight loss may increase risk of morbidity and mortality in HIV-infected persons. This level of weight loss may be a more clinically relevant landmark for treatment than other and less severe indicators of nutritional deficiency. A recent consensus publication suggests the following guidelines to redefine "wasting syndrome" in HIV-infected individuals:[14]

- >10% loss of weight over a 12-month period of time
- >7.5% loss of weight over a 6-month period of time
- >5% loss of body cell mass by bioelectrical impedance analysis (BIA) evaluation over a 6-month period of time
- body mass index <20
- body cell mass
   <35% of weight if body mass index (BMI) is <27 in males
   <23% of weight if BMI is <27 in females

The use of the CDC wasting definition is especially inadequate in the evaluation of children whose lack of growth suggests long-term malnutrition and whose drop in weight may be more detrimental to a child's health, growth, and development than a drop in weight for adults.[15-17] Nutritional status maintenance and improvement is as essential in pediatric care as medications to control disease.[18] Some clinicians have ranked nutritional status protection above antiretroviral therapy in importance, and many more rank protection of nutritional status as equivalent to disease management for children.[19]

Contrary to the currently popular perception that wasting no longer exists in treated patients, prospective data suggest that 35% to 40% of those treated with a HAART combination of drugs will newly waste body weight and crucial lean tissue stores.[20] This and other data[21,22] suggest that malnutrition and wasting should still be a concern. The two broad categories of malnutrition include starvation malnutrition and altered metabolism malnutrition.

Starvation Malnutrition

Starvation continues to exist through a number of mechanisms (Fig. 36-1). From the very first moments, HIV infection places a person at higher risk for malnutrition. Initial infection with HIV and subsequent infections or cancers result in the release of cytokines that initiate a protective immune response. At the same time these cytokines induce a loss of appetite and can lead to a reduced nutrient intake. HIV is not a dormant virus and appears to hold a "set point" level of viral particles in the blood that can result in a constant assault on nutritional well-being. Consistently higher levels of cytokines are reported in the literature and can lead to continuous suppression of appetite, hypermetabolism, and a preferential loss of lean tissues even during asymptomatic intervals of HIV disease.[23,24]

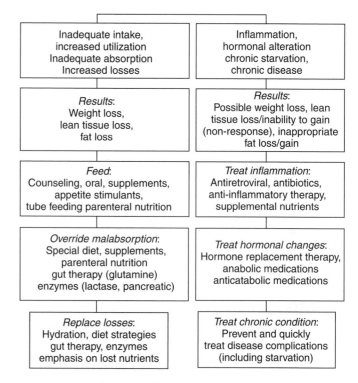

FIGURE 36-1 Examples of treatment strategies for malnutrition in HIV infection.

It would make sense that lowering viral load should reduce the level of cytokines and diminish their anorexic effects. However, with even the most effective HAART regimens, starvation continues to be a concern in patients. This could be due to inadequate intake, malabsorption, or increased losses through diarrhea or vomiting. The report on the prospective study of nutritional problems in patients on HAART regimens suggests a weight loss profile of 40% lean tissues and 60% fat, matching body composition changes seen in starvation and dieting.[25] Evidence of continued hypermetabolism with lowered viral loads was surprising, but may help explain some of the continued starvation processes.[26] There may be additional implications to managing HIV disease if the hypermetabolism is the result of unmeasured reservoirs of HIV infection within the body.

HIV is often introduced to the body through the gastrointestinal tract. It has been suggested that even before seroconversion (presence of measurable levels of HIV presence in the blood), HIV can interact with gastrointestinal immune function and ravage the gut,[27] leading to risk for malabsorptive states. Malabsorption, particularly fat malabsorption, appears to be common in HIV disease[28,29] and may contribute to the starvation process. Fat malabsorption should be suspected in patients reporting abdominal fullness and bloating or greasy, odorous, and floating stools. Additional contributors to the starvation process include depression, lack of food access, and constitutional symptoms (such as diarrhea or nausea and vomiting) related to disease and treatments.

Inadequate intake of micronutrients can also affect HIV disease management. Depletion or diminished levels of micronutrients associated with immune function and antioxidant function are associated with a poor clinical outcome.[30,31] Vitamin A, zinc, iron, and other micronutrients are essential to body functions, including immunity. Although adequacy is known to be important in supporting function and survival, the role of micronutrients in repletion or as nutraceutical treatments is unclear at this time. Minimal research has been conducted to evaluate the benefits of nutrient supplementation. Adequate micronutrient evaluation is difficult in the presence of chronic inflammatory conditions such as HIV disease.

Altered Metabolism

Even with successful ART, hypermetabolism may continue.[32] Hypermetabolism related to active infection or neoplasm can lead to a different profile of body composition changes, including a greater loss of lean tissues with the relative preservation of fat.[33] It has long been understood that continued systemic infection can reduce the effectiveness of attempts to restore nutritional status.[34,35] With long-term chronic disease, patterns of weight loss differ between men and women. Men may lose more lean tissue, while women can lose dramatic amounts of fat during the wasting process.[36] The explanation for these differences may involve baseline body composition and/or alterations in hormonal balances (including gender differences) that are seen in chronic inflammatory and infectious diseases.[37]

With any significant weight loss (10% or more), hormonal alterations may occur regardless of HIV infection or other disease states. Hypogonadism, particularly a low testosterone level, is especially detrimental to both men and women with HIV disease[38] and can occur as a consequence of weight loss or can lead to losses in lean tissues. Low testosterone levels can make it more difficult to maintain and restore crucial lean tissues, cause fatigue and depression, and lead to anemia.

Chronic inflammatory disease and high levels of cytokines can lead to the altered metabolism of nutrients.[39] Cortisol release results in resistance to endogenous anabolic hormones, including insulin, sex hormones, and growth hormone. Longer-term complications can include loss of bone density, yielding osteopenia and osteoporosis. Continued elevation in blood fats may add more nutrition-related risks of cardiovascular disease, carbohydrate intolerance, and avascular necrosis of joints and bone tissues.[40]

In addition, these and other complications may be initiated or accelerated through interactions with anti-HIV medications.[41] Patients on nucleoside analogs of reverse transcriptase inhibitors (RTIs) may experience mitochondrial toxicity, lactic acidosis, and subcutaneous fat loss.[42] Protease inhibitors have been associated with carbohydrate intolerance, diabetes, and fat accumulation in the trunk areas.[43] Alterations in body composition seem more apparent after the initiation of anti-HIV therapies, but may have occurred before the HAART era.[44] The association of these symptoms with medications is not clear. It appears that significantly lowering viral load and improving CD4 absolute count (an indicator of improved immune function) is associated with body composition changes.

Nutrition Assessment

Routine nutrition assessment should include healthy or early baselines (whenever possible) and serial measures that help evaluate the risk and impact of various factors that can adversely affect nutritional status. In addition, beneficial factors should be identified for emphasis and maintenance. Table 36-2 shows selected features of nutritional assessment categories of disease status, coexisting diagnoses, medication history, family history, physical examination, dietary history, exercise history, and psychosocial/economic factors. The complexity of malnutrition in chronic HIV disease and the appropriate integration of nutritional care may require the expertise of an HIV-specialist dietitian.

Diet Evaluation

Diet history is used to determine any deficits, excesses, potential interactions, or behavioral problems that affect diet contribution to health. Diet issues are not a primary focus if the patient is successfully treated with anti-HIV medications. However, many of the potential interactions between medications and food or medications and altered metabolism may require education, tailored diet planning, or other support for dietary adequacy while supporting medical treatments.

Medication Profile

Medications used in the treatment of HIV disease have evolved to require fewer meal restrictions. However, the health professional must be aware of food interactions to prevent the ineffective use of medications (see Table 36-1). For instance, if a patient is taking didanosine, stavudine, and indinavir, he or she will require a fairly rigid meal plan to prevent interference with medication absorption and efficacy. This combination is rarely seen because indinavir and didanosine should both be taken on an empty stomach and cannot be taken together. Indinavir must be taken every 8 hours (within a 2-hour window of time) and didanosine (taken twice daily) must not be taken within 1 hour of taking indinavir. This means that a patient on this type of HAART should refrain from eating during 11 hours of the day! It becomes difficult for a patient to maintain adequate nutrient intake with this type of regimen, and he or she is at high risk for losing weight (especially if a work schedule also restricts times when it is appropriate to eat). If meal restrictions are not adhered to, the medication may not be maintained at effective blood levels, allowing the virus to mutate and render the medication ineffective. Considering how quickly the virus runs its lifecycle, several opportunities for mutation during a missed dose exist. Lack of perfect adherence in meal and medication timing may be equivalent to a missed dose of medication and can result in failure of a medication regimen and possibly cross-resistance with other medications in the same class. Consistent lack of adherence rendering indinavir and didanosine therapies ineffective (in this example) is equivalent to providing monotherapy with stavudine alone. Monotherapy is generally considered unacceptable for long-term treatment of HIV infection. The patient may experience the adverse effects without the benefits of multidrug regimens in such cases. A meal plan to support such a difficult regimen might look like the example in Table 36-3.

Although tube feeding and parenteral nutrition (PN) have become less common in adults with HIV disease, it may be a more common consideration with small children.[45] A tube feeding regimen for children outside of the hospital setting

---

TABLE 36-2

Selected Nutrition Assessment Categories

Evaluation Category	Sample Criteria/Method	Comments
Diet history	Food recall Food diaries Food frequency Diet supplement history Use of tube feeding, PN	Compare intake to estimated needs and note special diet strategies or requirements, any intolerances or allergies, impact of cultural influences, food preferences, duration on nutrition support (tube feeding, hydration, PN).
Physical examination	Weight history Body composition and patterns Signs/symptoms of deficiency or excess nutrient intake	Compare actual to optimal or goal and note any alterations in body compartments, muscle wasting, fat patterns, dehydration or fluid shifts; note skin, hair, eyes, oral cavity, finger and toenails, and other areas sensitive to nutritional alterations.
Laboratory values	Nutritional indicators (e.g., albumin, prealbumin, hemoglobin, others) Immune function (e.g., viral load, CD4 and CD8 counts)	Both general nutrition-related laboratory values and disease-related laboratory values should be evaluated; use caution in interpreting laboratory values to determine nutritional risk to differentiate acute phase reaction from malnutrition.
Medication and medical history	Medications for HIV, complicating infections or cancers, additional medical conditions (e.g., diabetes, hyperlipidemia), and symptom management (e.g., antidiarrheals, appetite stimulants) Current and past profile of HIV disease, complicating infections or cancers, disease or medication-induced metabolic and physical changes, wasting syndrome(s)	Consider both past and present medical and medication history and note potential interactions between medications and nutritional status; allergies; past and present disease and other complications can compromise nutritional status and treatment for nutrition-related problems.
Complementary therapies	Nutraceuticals Herbal therapies Other therapies that may interact or otherwise affect nutritional status maintenance and improvement	Note all prescription, over-the-counter, and other recommended therapies and determine if there is any evidence for interaction with other prescribed or over-the-counter medications and with food and nutritional status maintenance.
Psychosocial and economic resources	Support network of friends and family Community resources used Financial limitations and support sources	Note any impact on nutritional status maintenance and any need for referral to community or other resources.

TABLE 36-3

Sample Medication Schedule

6 am	7 am	8 am	12 pm	2 pm	6 pm	8 pm	10 pm
IDV Only small nonfat, low-protein snacks should be taken with Indinavir.	ddl, d4T	Meal	Meal	IDV	Meal	ddl, d4T	IDV Snack*

ddl, Didanosine; *d4T*, stavudine; *IDV*, indinavir.*

may involve cyclic nocturnal feeding that should be paused at least 2 hours before administration of indinavir or didanosine. If the tube-feeding is administered over 24-hour cycles, the flow rate should consider interruptions that are required for 2 hours before and 1 hour after the administration of medications. Thus, the 24-hour enteral feeding regimen would have to be compressed to less than 13 hours. However, if ritonavir is added to this regimen, the meal restriction for indinavir can be lifted, although the restriction for didanosine remains. Thus, combinations of medications that *reduce* food interactions and other interruptions in daily life may be more appropriate (and, hopefully, a more common treatment strategy) for the majority of the HIV-infected population. Keeping track of

medications commonly used in HIV infection and related complications is likely to involve updates found in books published yearly or through website review. Some resources are shown in Box 36-1.

Medical History

Medical history is an important factor to determine relative risk of nutritionally challenging adverse events. Previous wasting may place a person at additional risk for wasting-related problems, such as bone density losses.[46] Hypertriglyceridemia may add risk for avascular necrosis,[47] cardiovascular disease, complications of insulin resistance or diabetes, and others. A review of family history and other risk factors for renal disease, diabetes, hypertension, and other conditions will help clinicians anticipate and monitor for such problems in the individual patient. Family history of renal disease and dialysis in a patient of African descent warrants close monitoring because the high incidence of HIV-infected African-American males on dialysis is correlated with such family histories.[48] At this point in time there are no special monitoring criteria for these complicating diseases. Persons with HIV infection should be monitored in anticipation of any conditions that may be suspected because of clinical findings, family history, or other risk factors.

The viral load and immune deficit indicators will help prioritize treatments to support immune competence and reduce

BOX 36-1
Additional Resources

Fields-Gardner C, Thomson CA, Rhodes SS: *A clinician's guide to nutrition in HIV and AIDS,* Chicago, IL, 1997, American Dietetic Association, ISBN: 0-8809-1148-4.
Joint United Nations Programme on HIV/AIDS (UNAIDS) and the World Health Organization (WHO): *AIDS epidemic update, December 2001*, ISBN: 92-9173-132-3; available at http://www.unaids.org.
McMillan L, Jarvie J, Brauer J: *Positive cooking: cooking for people living with HIV,* Garden City Park, NY, 1997, Avery Publishing Group, ISBN: 0-89529-734-5.
Pronsky ZA, Meyer SA, Fields-Gardner C: *HIV medications: food interactions,* ed 2, Birchrunville, PA, 2001, Food-Medication Interactions, Inc, ISBN: 0-9606164-9-7.
Romeyn MA: *Nutrition and HIV: a new model for treatment,* ed 2, San Francisco, CA, 1998, Jossey-Bass, ISBN 0-7879-3964-1.
Sarubin A: *The health care professional's guide to popular dietary supplements,* Chicago, IL, 2000, American Dietetic Association, ISBN: 0-88091-173-5.

General HIV-Related and Online Resources

AIDS Clinical Trials Information Service (ACTIS)
PO Box 6421
Rockville, MD 20849-6421
301-519-0459
http://www.actis.org

HIV/AIDS Bureau (HAB) of the Health Resources and Services Administration (HRSA)
5600 Fishers Lane, Room 11A-33
Rockville, MD 20857
301-443-6652 or 800-ASK-HRSA (800-275-4772)
http://hab.hrsa.gov

HIV/AIDS Treatment Information Service (ATIS)
PO Box 6303
Rockville, MD 20849-6303
301-519-0459
http://www.hivatis.org

HIV InSite
UCSF Positive Health Program
San Francisco General Hospital Medical Center
Building 80, Ward 84, 995 Potrero Avenue
San Francisco, CA 94110
415-476-4082
http://hivinsite.ucsf.edu

HIV Plus
Magazine available free of charge to organizations
Liberation Publications, Inc.
6922 Hollywood Boulevard, Suite 1000
Los Angeles, CA 90028-6148
212-242-4040 (ext 19 for subscription)
http://www.hivplusmag.com

National AIDS Fund
1030 15th Street, Suite 860
Washington, DC 20005
202-408-4848
http://www.aidsfund.org

National Association on HIV Over Fifty (NAHOF)
Chicago AIDS and Aging Project
Midwest AIDS Training and Education Center
University of Illinois at Chicago
808 South Wood Street (m/c 779)
Chicago, IL 60612
312-996-1426
http://www.hivoverfifty.org

National Pediatric and Family HIV Resource Center
University of Medicine and Dentistry of New Jersey
30 Bergen Street – ADMC #4
Newark, NJ 07103
973-972-0410
http://www.pedhivaids.org

Office of AIDS Research (OAR), National Institutes of Health (NIH)
Bethesda, MD 20892
301-496-4000
http://www.nih.gov/od/oar

Practical Nutrition Guidelines for Pediatric HIV-Infected Patients
http://www.hivpositive.com/f-Nutrition/f-3-PediatricNeut/n-Zafonte.html

nutritional risk. Support for adherence to medication regimens through meal planning is essential to successful HIV disease treatment (see Table 36-1 for food interactions with medications). Medication interactions can include direct assaults to nutritional status maintenance by decreasing available nutrients through diarrhea, vomiting, anorexia, and other symptoms. Interactions can lead to organ dysfunction, such as pancreatitis,[49] hepatic toxicity, and others, which will affect the ability to adequately and normally feed the patient.

Physical Examination

Physical examination, which includes a review of the condition of skin, hair, finger and toenails, eyes, oral mucosa, dentition, anthropometry, and body composition evaluation, provides important clues to nutritional status challenges. A general view of the patient's body weight and shape followed by specific notations on observations are part of a complete nutrition physical examination. With low CD4 count, special attention should be paid to lesions and signs of opportunistic fungal or other infections that place a patient at additional nutritional risk.

Anthropometry includes height, weight, lengths, circumferences, and fat-fold measures (Table 36-4). In addition, alterations in fat distribution should be measured and noted. Decreases in subcutaneous fat-folds and alterations in the feel or compressibility of fat-folds can help identify a patient with lipoatrophy and quantify the effect of fat losses. Hormonal (such as insulin-sensitizing agents) and calorie-based therapies to improve subcutaneous fat volume can be monitored through such measures. Examples of measures that are particularly helpful in the identification of lipoatrophy include baseline and serial measures of circumferences, lengths, and fat-folds shown in Table 36-4. Some practitioners have started to include facial fat-folds at the cheek (zygomatic) bone, next to the lips (buccal area), and along the jaw line on the mandible. From the anthropometric measures in the abdominal region, an estimate of a cross-sectional "slice" look at total abdominal circumference and area and the visceral area (under the subcutaneous fat) can help identify patients who may experience abnormal fat deposition.[50] From physical examination to identify fat deposits in the dorsocervical region along with measurements of back width and fat pad areas, identification and monitoring of the development, growth, or reduction of this type of fat pad can be accomplished. Some HIV-specialist clinicians have been using pictures and bra size in women to determine changes in breast tissues. Because a woman may not purchase additional bras to accommodate breast enlargement, it may be more appropriate to measure circumference around the torso at the nipple level of the breasts. As with other measures, monitoring trends over time may be most valuable.

Body Composition Evaluation

Lean tissue evaluation may be accomplished with anthropometry, BIA, dual energy x-ray absorptiometry (DXA), total body potassium counts (TBK+), and others. BIA has gained recognition in both the research and clinical settings and has been used to estimate either two-compartment (lean and fat tissues) or three-compartment (body cell mass, extracellular mass, and fat) volumes.[51] DXA has been used to estimate both fat-free mass

TABLE 36-4

Anthropometry to Evaluate Body Dimensions

Type of Measure	Description
Length	Height
	Back width: between acromion processes
	Dorsocervical fat pad width and height (if present)
Circumferences	Neck: at collar level
	Midupper arm
	Chest: under armpits
	Breast: across nipples
	Diaphragm: just under pectoral muscles (at bra line for women)
	Abdomen: umbilicus level
	Hip: at greater trochanter level
	Midthigh
	Calf: at largest width
Fat-folds	Infraorbital: under right eye on cheek bone (zygomatic process)
	Buccal: to right of corner of lips
	Submandible: midpoint of right jaw line
	Triceps: back of arm at midupper arm level
	Biceps: front of arm at midupper arm level
	Subscapular
	Suprailiac: at the midaxillary line
	Abdominal front: approximately 1 inch to right of umbilicus
	Abdominal sides: at abdominal circumference level on the right and left sides at the midaxillary line
	Abdominal back: approximately 1 inch to the right of the spinal column on the back
	Thigh: on top of thigh at midthigh level
	Calf: on back of calf at calf circumference level

and bone density.[52] TBK+ is rarely used outside of the research setting and is used to estimate body cell mass (BCM).

In a three-compartment model of body composition evaluation, the clinician can classify the patient into one or more of nine body composition categories (Table 36-5).[53] Three-compartment evaluations can also be used to monitor alterations and interventions over time. Identification of wasting and maintenance, restoration, and enhancement of adequate lean tissues, particularly body cell mass, is the primary justification for a body composition evaluation procedure using BIA.

At optimal weight, the proportions of each compartment should fall within a range of expected values unless the patient is in an "outlier" category. Men typically have 40% to 45% of their ideal weight as BCM, and women carry 30% to 40% of their ideal weight as BCM. Extracellular mass (ECM) comprises approximately 40% to 45% of current body weight. Fat tissues account for around 10% to 20% of a man's current weight and approximately 20% to 30% of a woman's current weight. Because there are no adequate three-compartment calculations for children, a two-compartment model may be compared with norms established for fat percentiles.[54] Serial BIA measures can help identify detrimental changes in BCM, dehydration or fluid shifts, and approximate total volume of fat. Serial measures are appropriate to identify response to treatment through the improvement and restoration of BCM and/or the return of ECM to appropriate levels. Because survival is most related to BCM stores, routine monitoring is recommended.

TABLE 36-5

Categories of Body Composition Evaluated by BIA

Body Composition Profile	Weight Change from "Normal"	BCM Change from "Normal"	ECM Change from "Normal"	Fat Change from "Normal"
Optimal	—	—	—	—
Subclinical wasting	—	Decreased	Increased	No significant changes
Athletic	—	Increased	No significant changes	Decreased
Normal obesity	Increased	Increased	Increased	Increased
Sarcopenic obesity	Increased	No significant change or decreased	—	Significantly increased
Athletic	Increased	Significantly increased	—	Slight increase to decreased
Starvation	Decreased	Decreased	Decreased	Decreased
Acute (infection, injury) weight loss	Decreased	Decreased	Significantly increased	Slow decrease
Adaptation	Decreased	Decreased	Increased	Low, normal, or high

BCM, Body cell mass; *ECM,* extracellular mass.

Clients with dehydration or a stress response (related to infection or injury) can be monitored for resolution of these health-threatening problems.

An optimal or enhanced (athletic) profile includes adequate or higher levels of BCM, the tissues most associated with survival and metabolic maintenance. Suboptimal profiles occur with starvation, stress responses due to injury or infection, and metabolic adaptation or "nonresponse" to usual and customary treatments with diet and exercise. In a patient with chronic disease, adaptive responses may be common and difficult (not to mention expensive) to overcome.[55]

Biochemistry

Laboratory values should be evaluated according to usual nutrition evaluation practices. In addition, the impact of chronic inflammatory disease should be considered when evaluating acute phase reaction indicators, such as albumin, prealbumin, zinc, and others. Laboratory evaluation of micronutrient status should consider the presence of chronic infection or other alterations and should be interpreted with caution. Laboratory evaluations that indicate the presence of common complications,[56] such as insulin resistance[57] and lactic acidosis, should be conducted when the clinician suspects these alterations. Medication interactions may alter laboratory evaluations and impact the ability to maintain and improve nutritional status (see Table 36-1).

Complementary Therapies

The use of complementary therapies by persons infected with HIV is commonplace,[58] especially in cases of unsolved problems or complications such as body pattern alterations (subcutaneous fat loss and central fat gain). Part of the nutritional evaluation should note any supplemental nutrients or other substances that have been recommended or self-prescribed. Information on potential value or adverse interactions for complementary therapies is limited, but should be investigated. The level of supplemental nutrient intake that is optimal to confer health benefit and reduce health harm of disease and its treatments remains unclear and to date no recommendations are evidence-based. It may be safe to keep recommendations below the upper limit of tolerance for nutrients.[59] Several commonly supplemented micronutrients have established upper limits of tolerance including vitamin A (3000 µg or 10,000 IU/day), copper (10 mg/day), iodine (1.1 mg/day), iron (45 mg/day), and zinc (40 mg/day).

Psychosocial and Economic Issues

As with other health and disease states, psychosocial and economic issues affecting health care and nutrition-related treatment access affect nutritional status.[60] Many community and other resources are available to assist HIV-infected persons and their families and friends in supporting access to food and other services and products. Many larger communities have home delivered meals, congregate feeding programs, and food voucher or grocery delivery services. Interfacing with the patient's case manager and/or social worker can help identify potential resources appropriate to the individual patient that will support nutritional status and health maintenance. In addition, requesting the presence of a supportive caregiver or life partner (significant other) in counseling sessions can reinforce information and help the client to better adhere to recommendations.

Nutrition Interventions

The level and type of nutrition-related interventions needed are prioritized according to the predominant problems that compromise nutritional status and the goal of the individualized health care plan. For instance, if a patient experiences insulin resistance (a fairly common finding in patients with treated HIV disease) then diet and medication therapies tailored to meet the patient's estimated nutrient requirements while diminishing the challenges of insulin resistance may be most appropriate. Estimates for fluid, calorie, protein, and micronutrient needs should be made according to patient needs for hydration, anabolism, maintenance, and tolerance. Close monitoring should allow the clinician to adjust needs according to changing priorities in care.

Nutrition Support

The goals for nutrition support depend on the goals for the individual's health care plan. If the goal is rehabilitation or enhancement of health, then aggressive nutrition interventions may be appropriate. If the goal is comfort or palliative care, then nutrition interventions should be used to support comfort rather than to rehabilitate. The use of nutrition intervention in comfort care may be confined to providing hydration, food as tolerated, or medical nutrition supplements as requested. For preventive, rehabilitative, or enhancement goals, treatments are chosen according to their efficacy in solving the problems that lead to malnutrition, wasting, and other nutrition-related complications. Guidelines for the management of nutritional status in HIV disease may be individualized according to each patient's predominant nutritional challenge.[61-63]

Once an evaluation of nutritional status and factors that challenge or compromise optimal status is completed, the role of nutrient support, exercise and activity, adjunctive medical therapies, or other resources should be defined. It is important to support the provision of adequate nutrient intake and activity whenever possible. Adherence to medication therapy is essential to controlling viral load and extending survival. Tailored nutrition strategies to optimize medication effectiveness should be implemented for each patient.

When it is determined that dietary intake is inadequate, strategies to support oral intake in the form of diet and supplements are considered to enhance fluid, calorie, protein, and/or micronutrient intake. Whenever possible, an adequate diet strategy should be used (Table 36-6 identifies selected strategies to deal with common nutrition-related symptoms). For instance, diarrhea is sometimes a long-term complication of medication therapy and an inadequate and very restrictive diet (such as the BRAT or bananas, rice, applesauce, and toast) may allow the patient to become further malnourished and further exacerbate the problem. In this case, a low-residue or similar diet can be tailored to meet the client's preferences and nutritional requirements.

Enteral nutrition (EN) is rarely used in adult patients in the United States. Enteral feeding tubes may be used to administer medications and improve adherence to prescribed medication regimens in pediatric cases. Tube placement to administer medications can also be used to improve nutrient intake.

In cases of pancreatitis, severe malabsorption, Kaposi's sarcoma of the bowel, or other conditions that make oral and EN less viable, PN may be initiated. However, it is especially important in patients with immune compromise to continue some form of oral intake to allow the gut to maintain an important function as a barrier to infection. To accomplish this process lactase, pancrelipase, or another enzyme treatment may be used with small amounts of food intake to preserve gut function and minimize the challenge to the pancreas. Potential infection with catheter placement (peripheral, peripherally inserted central, or other centrally placed catheters) in immunocompromised patients is a concern, but not a contraindication.[64]

EN and PN interventions should follow the same guidelines used in other disease states as appropriate for an HIV-infected person. Careful attention to antiseptic techniques is appropriate in patients who are immunocompromised.

Medication Support of Nutritional Status

Several medications are currently used to address some of the nutrition-related challenges in HIV disease. Symptom management may include both diet and medication strategies. Antihyperlipidemic medications have been prescribed for significant rises in blood lipids often induced by anti-HIV therapies. Antidiarrheals and antiemetics are also prescribed to

TABLE 36-6

Diet Strategies for Common Constitutional Symptoms

Symptom	Diet Strategies
Anorexia	• Eat calorie-dense foods.
	• Try small, frequent feedings.
	• Avoid food odors during food preparation and feeding times, ventilate feeding area and home.
	• Use convenience foods.
	• Eat in a pleasant atmosphere with pleasant distractions, such as television, friends, music.
	• Prepare (or have friends and family prepare) single servings of foods to store for quick use when needed.
	• Include exercise in routine.
	• Consider medical nutrition supplements, as needed.
Nausea and/or vomiting	• Eat cold or room temperature foods.
	• Avoid food odors and keep home well-ventilated.
	• Eat dry and liquid foods separately.
	• Eat small, frequent meals.
	• Try saltine crackers, dry toast, or chew on a small piece of ginger when feeling nauseated.
	• Keep still and elevate upper body after eating.
	• Try different foods to see which ones are easier to eat during nausea.
	• Minimize nausea with distractions during feeding times, such as reading, music, television, and friends/family company.
Diarrhea	• Drink plenty of fluids.
	• Replace lost nutrients (such as fluids, calories, micronutrients) with juices, gelatin, sports drinks, or other foods.
	• Avoid foods that irritate: caffeine-containing foods, citrus, some spices.
	• Reduce fat intake; choose lower-fat alternatives.
	• Reduce insoluble fiber; increase soluble fiber.
	• Avoid gassy foods (this is very individual).
	• If lactose is a problem, reduce lactose-containing foods or use reduced lactose alternatives.
	• Eat foods at room temperature.

reduce the effects of diarrhea and vomiting. Appetite stimulants have been used to promote nutrient intake. The most common appetite stimulants are megestrol acetate (Megace, Bristol-Myers Squibb, Princeton, NJ) and dronabinol (Marinol, Unimed, Deerfield, IL). Some controversy about the quality of the weight gain has prompted a look into body composition and the ability of the body to respond appropriately to refeeding. Because megestrol acetate is a progesterone-type hormone, it may favor fat accumulation, and trials have begun to attempt to hormonally balance the deposition of both fat and lean tissues through testosterone supplementation.[65]

Insulin resistance and other hormonal alterations related to disease process, host factors, and medication interactions can lead to nutrition-related problems of fat accumulation and lean tissue loss. Attempts to balance or otherwise modulate with hormonal therapies to prevent and treat nutrition-related alterations have been made. Testosterone and other hormone replacement therapies have been instituted to prevent or treat alterations caused by hormonal deficits and to encourage anabolism of lean tissues, treat anemia, and favorably affect bone density. Additionally, other anabolic agents, including testosterone analogs, growth hormone, and insulin-sensitizing agents, have

TABLE 36-7
Selected Medications to Treat Nutrition-Related Problems

Problem	Medication	Comment
Weight loss and anorexia	Appetite stimulants: megestrol acetate, dronabinol Anabolic agents: Insulin, insulin-sensitizing agents (such as metformin, rosiglitazone), testosterone and derivatives (such as testosterone cypionate, Deca-Durabolin, oxandrolone, oxymetholone, and others), growth hormone	Dosing and timing schedules for medications can be altered to increase tolerance; body composition should be monitored to ensure appropriate response to improved nutrient intake; appetite stimulants should be used with care in cases of mechanical eating difficulties; Anabolic agents should be matched to problems that lead to wasting whenever possible (e.g., hypogonadism and testosterone replacement therapy) and to the desired effect; body composition should be evaluated to monitor for effects.
Nausea and vomiting	Antiemetics: Dronabinol, timethobenzamide hydrochloride, metoclopramide, phenothiazine derivatives, ondansetron hydrochloride	Adjust timing of meals and medication to optimize medication and nutrient intake.
Diarrhea	Antidiarrheals: Antimotility agents, luminal agents, octreotide acetate Other strategies: Pancrelipase, lactase, digestive enzymes, calcium supplements	Chronic diarrhea should be evaluated whenever possible to identify the need for antidiarrheals or other medications to address the cause of the diarrhea. Other strategies should be matched to causes whenever possible; dosing and accurate instructions for taking medications can improve effect.

been used to address alterations in body composition. Table 36-7 shows some commonly used medications to address nutritional complications of HIV disease and its management.

Conclusion

HIV disease survival has been enhanced as a result of anti-retroviral medication therapies.[66] As a chronic disease, HIV infection has much in common with other chronic diseases. Complications of long-term inflammatory processes and anti-HIV treatments may include starvation-type malnutrition, altered metabolism and hormonal milieu, constitutional symptoms, and alterations in body composition and function.[67] Although there is no imminent cure, there is the need to manage the disease process and support the maintenance of a strong and functional body for survival.

Successful management of HIV disease includes viral load control, immune restoration, and support for both the body and psychosocial-economic well-being of patients. Complications of malnutrition and wasting can further compromise the ability to treat HIV infection. Prevention and treatment strategies for malnutrition, wasting, and nutrition-related risk factors are likely to involve combination therapies to address the multifactoral nature of nutritional status compromise. A multidisciplinary HIV-specialist health care team, including an HIV-specialist dietitian may be best positioned to address clinical and other issues confronting the person with HIV infection.

REFERENCES

1. United Nations Programme on HIV/AIDS and the World Health Organization: AIDS epidemic update: Dec 2001. Retrieved on May 25, 2002 from www.unaids.org/epidemic_update/report_dec01/index.html#full
2. Centers for Disease Control and Prevention: Characteristics of persons living with AIDS at the end of 1999. Retrieved on Feb 21, 2001 from http://www.cdc.gov/hiv/stats/hasrsupp71.htm
3. Ioannidis JP, Abrams EJ, Ammann A, et al: Perinatal transmission of human immunodeficiency virus type 1 by pregnant women with RNA virus loads <1000 copies/mL, J Infect Dis 183(4):539-545, 2001.
4. Mofenson LM and the Committee on Pediatric AIDS: Technical report: perinatal human immunodeficiency virus testing and prevention of transmission, Pediatrics 106(6):E88, 2000.
5. Smith MM, Kuhn L: Exclusive breast-feeding: does it have the potential to reduce breast-feeding transmission of HIV-1? Nutr Rev 58(11):333-340, 2000.
6. Dabis F, Newell ML, Fransen L, et al: Prevention of mother-to-child transmission of HIV in developing countries: recommendations for practice. The Ghent International Working Group on Mother-To-Child Transmission of HIV, Healthy Policy Plan 15(1):34-42, 2000.
7. Kotler DP, Tierney AR, Wang J, et al: Magnitude of body-cell-mass depletion and the timing of death from wasting in AIDS, Am J Clin Nutr 50(3):444-447, 1989.
8. Centers for Disease Control and Prevention: 1993 revised classification system for HIV infection and expanded surveillance case definition for AIDS among adolescents and adults, MMWR Morbid Mortal Wkly Rep 41(RR-17):961-962, 1992.
9. Perelson AS, Neumann AU, Markowitz M, et al: HIV-1 dynamics in vivo: virion clearance rate, infected cell life-span, and viral generation time, Science 271(5255):1582-1586, 1996.
10. Rivera S, Briggs W, Qian D, Sattler FR: Levels of HIV RNA are quantitatively related to prior weight loss in HIV-associated wasting, J Acquir Immune Defic Syndr Hum Retrovirol 17(5):411-418, 1998.
11. Purtilo DT, Connor DH: Fatal infections in protein-calorie malnourished children with thypolymphatic atrophy, Arch Dis Child 50(2):149-152, 1975.
12. Cunningham-Rundles S: Nutrition and the mucosal immune system, Curr Opin Gastroenterol 17(2):171-176, 2001.
13. Chandra RK: Protein-energy malnutrition and immunological responses, J Nutr 122(3 suppl):597-600, 1992.
14. Polsky B, Kotler D, Steinhart C: HIV-associated wasting in the HAART era: guidelines for assessment, diagnosis, and treatment, AIDS Patient Care STDS 15(8):411-423, 2001.
15. Henderson RA, Saavedra JM: Nutritional considerations and management of the child with human immunodeficiency virus infection, Nutrition 11(2):121-128, 1995.
16. Mintz M: Neurological and developmental problems in pediatric HIV infection, J Nutr 126(10 suppl):2663S-267S, 1996.
17. Pollack H, Glasberg H, Lee E, Nirenberg A, David R, Krasinski D, Borkowsky W, Oberfield S: Impaired early growth of infants perinatally infected with human immunodeficiency virus: correlation with viral load, J Pediatr 130(6):915-922, 1997.
18. Oleske JM, Rothpletz-Puglia PM, Winter H: Historical perspectives on the evolution in understanding the importance of nutritional care in pediatric HIV infection, J Nutr 126(10 suppl):2663S-2673S, 1996.
19. Fields-Gardner C, Romeyn MA, Bowers M: Nutrition management guidelines for pediatric HIV+ patients. Presented at the 11th Annual Conference, Association of Nurses in AIDS Care, 1998.
20. Wanke CA, Silva M, Knox TA, et al: Weight loss and wasting remain common complications in individuals infected with human immunodeficiency virus in the era of highly active antiretroviral therapy, Clin Infec Dis 31(3):803-805, 2000.
21. Schwenk A, Beisenherz A, Romer K, Kremer G, Salzberger B, Elia M: Phase angle from bioelectrical impedance analysis remains an independent

predictive marker in HIV-infected patients in the era of highly active antiretroviral treatment, *Am J Clin Nutr* 72(2):496-501, 2000.

22. Pernerstorfer-Schoen H, Schindler K, Parschalk B, Schindl A, Toeny-Lampert S, Wunderer K, Elmadfa I, Tschachler E, Jilma B: Beneficial effects of protease inhibitors on body composition and energy expenditure: a comparison between HIV-infected and AIDS patients, *AIDS* 13(17):2389-2396, 1999.

23. Ott M, Lembcke B, Fischer H, Jager R, Polat H, Geier H, Rech M, Staszeswki S, Helm EB, Caspary WF: Early changes of body composition in human immunodeficiency virus-infected patients: tetrapolar body impedance analysis indicates significant malnutrition, *Am J Clin Nutr* 57(1):15-19, 1993.

24. Beisel WR: Nutrition and infection. In Linder MC (ed): *Nutritional biochemistry and metabolism with clinical applications,* ed 2, Norwalk, CT, 1991, Appleton & Lange, pp 507-557.

25. Pritchard JE, Nowson CA, Wark JD: A worksit program for overweight middle-aged men achieves lesser weight loss with exercise than with dietary change, *J Am Diet Assoc* 97(1):37-42, 1997.

26. Pernerstorfer-Schoen H, Schindler K, Parschalk B, et al: Beneficial effects of protease inhibitors on body composition and energy expenditure: a comparison between HIV-infected and AIDS patients, *AIDS* 13(17):2389-2396, 1999.

27. Castello-Branco LR, Ortigao-de-Sampaio MB: Aspects of gastrointestinal immunology and nutrition in human immunodeficiency virust-1 infection in Brazil, *Mem Inst Oswaldo Cruz* 95(suppl 1):S171-S173, 2000.

28. Koch J, Garcia-Shelton YL, Neal EA, et al: Steatorrhea: a common manifestation in patients with HIV/AIDS, *Nutrition* 12(7-8):507-510, 1996.

29. Ribeiro Machado F, Gonzaga Vaz Coelho L, Chausson Y, et al: Fat malabsorption assessed by 14C-triolein breath test in HIV-positive patients in different stages of infection: is it an early event? *J Clin Gastroenterol* 30(4):403-408, 2000.

30. Semba RD, Tang AM: Micronutrients and the pathogenesis of human immunodeficiency virus infection, *Br J Nutr* 81(3):181-189, 1999.

31. Allard JP, Aghdassi E, Chau J, et al: Oxidative stress and plasma antioxidant micronutrients in humans with HIV infection, *Am J Clin Nutr* 67(1):143-147, 1998.

32. Garcia Luna PP, Aguayo PS, Exposito MJ, Florit AP, Garcia Lorda P, Salvado JS: Hypermetabolism and progression of HIV infection, *Am J Clin Nutr* 70(2):299-300; discussion 301, 1999.

33. Paton NI, Castello-Branco LR, Jennings G, et al: Impact of tuberculosis on the body composition of HIV-infected men in Brazil, *J Acquir Immune Defic Syndr Hum Retrovirol* 20(3):265-271, 1999.

34. Kotler DP: Cytomegalovirus colitis and wasting, *J Acquir Immune Defic Syndr* 4(suppl 1):S36-S41, 1991.

35. Kotler DP, Tierney AR, Culpepper-Morgan JA, et al: Effect of home total parenteral nutrition on body composition in patients with acquired immunodeficiency syndrome, *J Parenter Enteral Nutr* 14(5):454-458, 1990.

36. Grinspoon S, Corcoran C, Miller K, et al: Body composition and endocrine function in women with acquired immunodeficiency syndrome wasting, *J Clin Endocrinol Metab* 82(5):1332-1337, 1997.

37. Melchior JC: Metabolic aspects of HIV: associated wasting, *Biomed Pharmacother* 51(10):455-460, 1997.

38. Kopicko JJ, Momodu I, Adedokun A, et al: Characteristics of HIV-infected men with low serum testosterone levels, *Int J STD AIDS* 10(12):817-820, 1999.

39. Renard E, Fabre J, Paris F, et al: Syndrome of body fat redistribution in HIV-1-infected patients: relationships to cortisol and catecholamines, *Clin Endocrinol* 51(2):223-230, 1999.

40. Heath KV, Hogg RS, Chan KJ, et al: Lipodystrophy-associated morphological, cholesterol and triglyceride abnormalities in a population-based HIV/AIDS treatment database, *AIDS* 15(2):231-239, 2001.

41. Ridolfo AL, Gervasoni C, Bini T, et al: Body habitus alterations in HIV-infected women treated with combined antiretroviral therapy, *AIDS Patient Care STDS* 14(11):595-601, 2000.

42. Brinkman K, Smeitink JA, Romijn JA, et al: Mitochondrial toxicity induced by nucleoside-analogue reverse-transcriptase inhibitors is a key factor in the pathogenesis of antiretroviral-therapy-related lipodystrophy, *Lancet* 354(9184):1112-1115, 1999.

43. Yanovski JA, Miller KD, Kino T, et al: Endocrine and metabolic evaluation of human immunodeficiency virus-infected patients with evidence of protease inhibitor-associated lipodystrophy, *J Clin Endocrinol Metab* 84(6):1925-1931, 1999.

44. Kotler DP, Rosenbaum K, Wang J, et al: Studies of body composition and fat distribution in HIV-infected and control subjects, *J Acquir Immune Defic Syndr Hum Retrovirol* 20(3):228-237, 1999.

45. Miller TL, Awnetwant EL, Evans S, et al: Gastrostomy tube supplementation for HIV-infected children, *Pediatrics* 96(4 Pt 1):696-702, 1995.

46. Tebas P, Powderly WG, Claxton S, et al: Accelerated bone mineral loss in HIV-infected patients receiving potent antiretroviral therapy, *AIDS* 14(4):F63-F67, 2000.

47. Stovall D, Young TR: Avascular necrosis of the medial femoral condyle in HIV-infected patients, *Am J Orthop* 24(1):71-73, 1995.

48. Winston JA, Burns GC, Klotman PE: The human immunodeficiency virus (HIV) epidemic and HIV-associated nephropathy, *Semin Nephrol* 18(4):373-377, 1998.

49. Dassopoulos T, Ehrenpreis ED: Acute pancreatitis in human immunodeficiency virus-infected patients: a review, *Am J Med* 107(1):78-84, 1999.

50. Fields-Gardner C: Anthropometry. Retrieved on May 25, 2002 from http://www.Hi-R-Ed.org/sponsors.htm

51. Kotler DP, Thea DM, Heo M, et al: Relative influences of sex, race, environment, and HIV infection on body composition in adults, *Am J Clin Nutr* 69(3):432-439, 1999.

52. Visser M, Fuerst T, Lang T, et al: Validity of fan-beam dual-energy X-ray absorptiometry for measuring fat-free mass and leg muscle mass. Health, aging, and body composition study—dual-energy X-ray absorptiometry and body composition working group, *J Appl Physiol* 87(4):1513-1520, 1999.

53. Fields-Gardner C: Body composition evaluation using single-frequency tetrapolar bioelectrical impedance analysis (BIA). Retrieved on May 25, 2002 from http://www.Hi-R-Ed.org/sponsors.htm

54. Arpadi SM, Horlick MN, Wang J, et al: Body composition in prepubertal children with human immunodeficiency virus type 1 infection, *Arch Pediatr Adolesc Med* 152(7):688-693, 1998.

55. Hoh R, Pelfini A, Neese RA, et al: De novo lipogenesis predicts short-term body composition response by bioelectrical impedance analysis to oral nutrition supplements in HIV-associated wasting, *Am J Clin Nutr* 68(1):154-163, 1998.

56. Vigouroux C, Gharakhanian S, Salhi Y, et al: Diabetes, insulin resistance and dyslipidaemia and lipodystrophic HIV-infected patients on highly active antiretroviral therapy, *Diabetes Metab* 25(5):225-232, 1999.

57. Yarasheski KE, Tebas P, Sigmund C, et al: Insulin resistance in HIV protease inhibitor-associated diabetes, *J Acquir Immune Defic Syndr* 21(3):209-216, 1999.

58. Kassler WJ, Blanc P, Greenblatt R: The use of medicinal herbs by human immunodeficiency virus-infected patients, *Arch Intern Med* 151(11):2281-2288, 1991.

59. Using the tolerable upper intake level for nutrition assessment of groups. In *Dietary reference intakes: applications in dietary assessment,* 2001, National Academy Press, pp 83-92. Retrieved on May 25, 2002 from Food and Nutrition Board, Institute of Medicine, National Academies of Sciences, Washington DC, http://books.nap.edu/books/0309071836/html/83.html#pagetop.

60. Shaprio MF, Morton SC, McCaffrey DF, et al: Variations in the care of HIV-infected adults in the United States: results from the HIV Cost and Services Utilization Study, *JAMA* 281(24):2305-2315, 1999.

61. American Dietetic Association: HIV/AIDS children/adolescents medical nutrition therapy protocol. In *Medical nutrition therapy across the continuum of care,* Chicago, 1998, the American Dietetic Association and Morris Health Care, American Dietetic Association, pp 1-16.

62. American Dietetic Association: HIV/AIDS medical nutrition therapy protocol. In *Medical nutrition therapy across the continuum of care,* Chicago, IL, 1998, The American Dietetic Association.

63. Guidelines for the use of parenteral and enteral nutrition in adult and pediatric patients, *J Parenteral Enteral Nutr* 261(suppl):1SA-138A, 2002.

64. Skiest DJ, Abbott M, Keiser P: Peripherally inserted central catheters in patients with AIDS are associated with a low infection rate, *Clin Infect Dis* 30(6):949-952, 2000.

65. Murrahainen N, Mulligan K: Clinical trials update in human immunodeficiency virus wasting, *Semin Oncol* 25(2 suppl 6):104-111, 1998.

66. Kuhn L, Thomas PA, Singh T, et al: Long-term survival of children with human immunodeficiency virus infection in New York City: estimates from population-based surveillance data, *Am J Epidemiol* 147(9):846-854, 1998.

67. Behrens G, Dejam A, Schmidt H, et al: Impaired glucose tolerance, beta cell function and lipid metabolism in HIV patients under treatment with protease inhibitors, *AIDS* 13(10):F63-F70, 1999.

Pamela Charney, MS, RD, CNSD

DIABETES mellitus (DM), the most common serious metabolic disease in the world, affects more than 11 million persons in the United States alone. More than 30% of individuals with type 2 DM remain undiagnosed, leading to significant risk for development of long-term complications and blood glucose concerns during acute illness.[1] Diabetes is characterized by abnormal glucose metabolism secondary to either insulin deficiency or abnormal insulin action, which can lead to severe systemic complications, including neuropathy, nephropathy, retinopathy, and macrovascular disease. It is the most common cause of blindness in the United States. Approximately one third of new end-stage renal disease affects persons with diabetes. The costs of caring for persons with diabetes can be significant, and their life expectancy is only two thirds that of the general population.

Because of the prevalence of the disease, nutrition support teams can safely assume that they will be charged with the management of patients with diabetes. When such patients are receiving enteral nutrition (EN) or parenteral nutrition (PN) support, the challenge for clinicians is to achieve and maintain euglycemia. Acute complications of diabetes that can occur during specialized nutrition support include diabetic ketoacidosis (DKA) and hyperglycemic, hyperosmolar, nonketotic coma (HHNC) and are associated with significant morbidity and mortality. Diabetes therapy may be altered in many patients, particularly those receiving PN, so blood glucose levels must be closely monitored at all times.[2] These patients can be successfully managed with careful attention to macronutrient composition of feedings and appropriate monitoring of blood glucose levels and response to nutrition therapy.

Metabolic Control of Carbohydrate Metabolism

Postprandial

Because glucose is essential for proper function of the central nervous system, erythrocytes, and leukocytes, blood glucose levels are normally tightly regulated between 80 mg/dl after a short fast and 120 mg/dl after a meal. In normal healthy persons elevation of serum glucose after ingestion of carbohydrate (alone or as part of a mixed meal) induces increased secretion of insulin from the β-cells of the pancreas above basal levels. In the face of a small carbohydrate load, insulin release leads to suppression of hepatic glucose production, whereas a larger carbohydrate load leads to uptake of glucose by peripheral tissues, in particular, adipose tissue.[3]

After binding to target cell receptors, insulin facilitates entry of glucose into muscle and adipose tissue. Influx of glucose into the liver after a meal activates the enzyme glycogen synthetase. Hepatic glycogen synthesis and storage is one mechanism for removing excess glucose from the bloodstream. Increased insulin levels stimulate lipoprotein lipase activation and lipogenesis and fat storage in adipocytes. In addition to its role in glucose storage, insulin also inhibits proteolysis and lipolysis and stimulates further glucose storage in muscle glycogen. Amino acid uptake and intracellular protein synthesis are also stimulated in the presence of insulin.[4]

In addition to elevated serum glucose levels, other stimulators of insulin secretion include some amino acids (e.g., arginine, lysine, leucine, alanine) and certain gastrointestinal (GI) hormones (e.g., gastrin, secretin, cholecystokinin, and gastric inhibitory peptide). It appears that an oral glucose load releases more insulin than an intravenous dose, possibly because of GI stimulatory hormone release.[5] Elevated plasma unesterified fatty acid levels appeared to stimulate insulin release and acute insulin resistance in nondiabetic subjects undergoing infusion of lipid emulsion. After 24 hours, however, further increases in insulin level (which the authors felt were most likely caused by decreased clearance) led to improved peripheral glucose uptake.[6]

Insulin secretion may be inhibited by somatostatin and α-adrenergic agonists. Common medications that may inhibit insulin secretion include calcium channel blockers, diazoxide, and phenytoin.[7] Hypokalemia can also inhibit insulin secretion. Additionally, the ability of the β-cells of the pancreas to synthesize insulin can be adversely affected by prolonged exposure to hyperglycemia (glucose toxicity).

Fasting

In normal, healthy persons, blood glucose levels drop after a short (overnight) fast. Following this decrease in blood glucose, insulin levels decrease in turn, followed by slowing of peripheral glucose uptake. Glucagon is produced by the α-cells of the pancreas and released in response to falling blood glucose levels. Glucagon circulates in the bloodstream as free glucagon and has a very short half-life (5 minutes).[4] Glucagon acts as an antagonist to the activity of insulin, thus ensuring adequate energy sources for vital functions in the postabsorptive state. Lipolysis is stimulated and fatty acid levels increase (Fig. 37-1). The major activity of glucagon occurs in the liver, where it stimulates gluconeogenesis and glycogenolysis via stimulation of adenylate cyclase, which in turns activates phosphorylase. Muscle-derived alanine, lactate, and pyruvate are major sources for gluconeogenesis. Pyruvate production and acetyl coenzyme A carboxylase activity are decreased by

FASTING MAN

(24 hours, basal : — 1800 cal.)

ORIGIN OF FUEL

FUEL CONSUMPTION

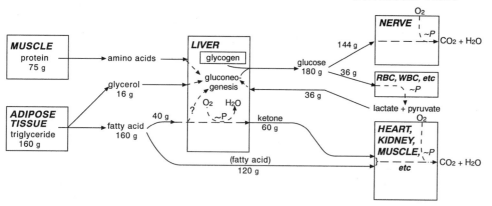

FIGURE 37-1 Approximate daily flow of fuels in a fasted man, emphasizing amino acid release from muscle as a source of glucogenic substrate for liver. (~ P) = energy. (From Cahill GF: Physiology of insulin in man, *Diabetes* 20[12]:785-799, 1971.)

glucagon, thus inhibiting fatty acid synthesis.[8] The end result of the activity of glucagon is to increase blood glucose levels. This point is important to remember because glucagon levels are elevated in persons with insulin deficiency.

Hepatic glycogen stores can provide energy needs for approximately 12 to 16 hours. Muscle glycogen is not available for systemic use because muscle lacks glucose-6 phosphatase, the enzyme necessary for glucose to leave the cell. Hepatic glucose output is equivalent to peripheral glucose uptake; this maintains euglycemia. After glycogen stores are exhausted, gluconeogenesis provides glucose for tissues that are obligate glucose users, whereas lipolysis provides fatty acids for other tissues.

A falling glucose level appears to be the most potent stimulator of glucagon secretion, but some amino acids, arginine in particular, also stimulate glucagon secretion, acetylcholine secretion, and vagal nerve stimulation.[4] Glucagon secretion is mainly inhibited by hyperglycemia, but other inhibitors are insulin, free fatty acids, somatostatin, and secretin.

In addition to glucagon, other hormones, the *counterregulatory hormones*—growth hormone, the catecholamines, and cortisol—oppose most, if not all, of the actions of insulin. The activity of glucagon was discussed previously. Growth hormone is secreted by the anterior pituitary and has anabolic functions important for protein synthesis and growth. It may also increase hepatic glucose production and turnover. Growth hormone inhibits the effects of insulin, leading to mobilization of lipid stores and catabolism. Hyperglycemia results from decreased peripheral glucose utilization and gluconeogenesis.[9] Growth hormone secretion is inhibited by somatostatin.

The catecholamines, epinephrine and norepinephrine, are secreted by the adrenal glands in response to stress, fever, or low blood glucose. Catecholamine secretion leads to hyperglycemia secondary to glycogenolysis, gluconeogenesis, and decreased utilization of glucose by peripheral tissues. Fatty acids produced by triglyceride catabolism in peripheral adipocytes help decrease tissue glucose requirements. Whereas the activity of glucagon is mainly confined to the liver, muscle is the target organ for catecholamines.

Cortisol is one of the glucocorticoid hormones, and it is released in response to stress, fever, or hypoglycemia. It increases skeletal muscle breakdown and inhibits protein syn-

thesis. Other effects are increased gluconeogenesis and glycogenolysis, leading to increased blood glucose levels.

Stress

During stress or injury, cytokines and other inflammatory mediators are released and may be responsible in part for the associated hypermetabolism, increased muscle catabolism, and hyperglycemia. These changes either abate as the patient recovers or progress to total organ failure. Levels of the counterregulatory hormones (glucagon, catecholamines, glucocorticoids, growth hormone) are also increased in response to critical illness, surgery, or trauma. Early during the stress response, blunted insulin secretion may accelerate nitrogen losses.[10] The end result of these metabolic changes is increased proteolysis, increased gluconeogenesis, and resistance to insulin's effects, leading to hyperglycemia.[11]

Classifications of Diabetes Mellitus

Box 37-1 reviews the major clinical classes of diabetes. Persons with impaired glucose tolerance may have elevated blood glucose levels that are not, however, high enough to qualify as a diagnosis of diabetes. They may be at risk for the development of diabetes and should be monitored. While the diagnosis of type 1, or insulin-dependent, diabetes is usually unequivocal, it may be difficult initially to distinguish type 2, or non–insulin-dependent diabetes, especially in older, lean patients. Diabetes may be treated by diet alone, diet plus oral hypoglycemic agents, or diet and insulin therapy. Additionally, exercise is an important component of therapy for both type 1 and type 2 DM.

Type 1 DM is characterized by a lack of insulin production by the β-cells of the pancreas, leading to lifelong reliance on exogenous insulin for survival. Type 1 DM is usually diagnosed during childhood, after the appearance of the classic symptoms triad: polydipsia, polyuria, and polyphagia. Persons with type 1 DM may be prone to develop DKA; in fact, the diagnosis is often made after an episode of DKA. Currently, it is believed type 1 DM is an autoimmune disorder caused by the development of antibodies to pancreatic β-cells and to insulin. Some trigger, possibly a viral illness, is required for the expression of the disorder.

Etiologic Classifications of Diabetes Mellitus

Type 1 diabetes mellitus*
Type 2 diabetes mellitus*
Other specific types:
Genetic defects of beta-cell function
Genetic defects in insulin action
Diseases of the exocrine pancreas
    Pancreatitis
    Trauma/pancreatectomy
    Neoplasia
    Cystic fibrosis
    Hemochromatosis
    Others
Endocrinopathies
    Acromegaly
    Cushing's syndrome
    Glucagonoma
    Pheochromocytoma
    Hyperthyroidism
    Somatostatinoma
    Aldosteronoma
    Others
Drug- or chemical-induced
    Vacor†
    Pentamidine
    Nicotinic acid
    Glucocorticoids
    Thyroid hormone
    Diazoxide
    Beta-adrenergic agonists
    Thiazides
    Phenytoin
    Alpha-interferon
    Others
Infections
    Congenital rubella
    Cytomegalovirus
    Others
Uncommon forms of immune-mediated diabetes
Other genetic syndromes sometimes associated with diabetes
    Down syndrome
    Klinefelter's syndrome
    Turner's syndrome
    Wolfram syndrome
    Friedreich's ataxia
    Huntington's chorea
    Laurence-Mood Biedl syndrome
    Myotonic dystrophy
    Porphyria
    Prader-Willi syndrome
    Others
Gestational diabetes mellitus

*Patients with any form of diabetes may require insulin treatment at some stage of the disease. Use of insulin does not, of itself, classify the patient.
†Vacor is an acute rodenticide that was released in 1975 but withdrawn as a general-use pesticide in 1979 because of severe toxicity. Exposure produces destruction of the beta cells of the pancreas, causing diabetes mellitus in survivors.
Adapted from Report of the Expert Committee on the Diagnosis and Classification of Diabetes Mellitus, *Diabetes Care* 20:1183-97 Reprinted with permission from the American Diabetes Association, 1997.

DKA is a potentially life-threatening short-term complication of diabetes that can result from insulin deficiency combined with increased activity of the counterregulatory hormones. In the presence of insulin deficiency, serum glucose, glucagon, and ketone bodies increase, leading to hyperglycemia, ketosis, and metabolic acidosis. The ketone bodies, β-hydroxybutyric acid and acetoacetic acid, are strong organic acids synthesized by the liver during ketoacidosis by β-oxidation of fatty acids.[12] Increased counterregulatory hormone levels combined with insulin deficiency permit increased entry of fatty acids into the liver, leading to pronounced ketosis. Before they are excreted, the ketone bodies are neutralized in the kidneys (with concurrent loss of bicarbonate reserves). Metabolic acidosis leads to hypocapnia and eventually to adverse effects on myocardial function.

The metabolic consequences of DKA include osmotic diuresis (leading to dehydration), hypertonicity, and electrolyte losses. In the early stages of DKA, patients with normal thirst and renal function are only mildly hyperglycemic because the kidneys are able to sustain excretion of excess glucose. If fluid intake does not match urine output, dehydration, severe hyperglycemia, and impaired renal function occur. Treatment of DKA is fluid replacement, insulin therapy, and close monitoring and replacement of electrolytes.[13]

Persons with type 1 DM require insulin therapy to survive. Several types of insulin are available in the United States (Table 37-1). Before the development of human insulin in the early 1980s, pork or beef insulin, both of which differ from human insulin by one and three amino acids, respectively, were most often used. Insulins are classified by duration of action. Regular insulin has a duration of action of 6 to 8 hours, intermediate (NPH or Lente) 18 to 26 hours, and long-acting (ultralente) 24 to 36 hours. Insulins also differ in terms of interval to onset and to peak of activity. Insulin lispro is an insulin analog that has a more rapid onset and shorter duration of action than Regular insulin.[14]

The main goal of insulin therapy for type 1 DM is to maintain adequate blood sugar control and to prevent hyperglycemia, ketoacidosis, and long-term complications. While adequate blood sugar control can be achieved with one or two injections of short- or intermediate-acting insulin, many physicians recommend intensive therapy using multiple daily injections to slow development and progression of the complications of diabetes. Selection of an insulin regimen should be individualized and tailored to optimize blood sugar levels. Over the past few years an analog of Regular insulin has been developed that has a more rapid onset and slightly shorter duration of action, which may improve mealtime management.[15] A long-acting insulin that more closely mimics basal insulin secretion is also available.[16]

Intensive therapy for type 1 DM can be initiated with three injections per day of a mixture of short- and intermediate-acting insulin in the morning, Regular insulin at dinner, and intermediate insulin at bedtime. Another option is three daily injections of Regular insulin and one of intermediate insulin. The subcutaneous continuous insulin infusion device is an alternative to multiple insulin injections.

Type 2 DM is often diagnosed in overweight persons after age 40 years, although it is becoming more common in younger populations. It is characterized by decreased insulin secretion and/or peripheral resistance to the actions of insulin.[17] Insulin resistance occurs mainly at the cellular level in both hepatic

---

TABLE 37-1

Approximate Pharmacokinetic Parameters of Currently Available Insulin Preparations Following Subcutaneous Injection of an Average Patient Dose

Type of Insulin	Onset of Action	Peak of Action	Duration of Action	Cost Per Vial for Brand Name Insulin (Generic Insulin)*	Common Pitfalls
Insulin lispro (Humalog)	5 to 15 minutes	1 to 2 hours	4 to 5 hours	$28	Hypoglycemia occurs if the lag time is too long or the patient exercises within 1 hour of administration; with high-fat meals, the dose should be adjusted downward.
Regular insulin (Humulin R)	30 to 60 minutes	2 to 4 hours	6 to 8 hours	22 (21)	Lag time is not used appropriately; the insulin should be given 20 to 30 minutes before the patient eats.
NPH insulin (Humulin N)	1 to 3 hours	5 to 7 hours	13 to 18 hours	22 (19 to 21)	In many patients, breakfast injection does not last until the evening meal; administration with the evening meal does not meet insulin needs on awakening.
Lente insulin (Humulin L)	1 to 3 hours	4 to 8 hours	13 to 20 hours	22 (18 to 21)	Zinc suspension binds with Regular insulin, which loses its effect if it is left in the syringe for more than a few minutes.
Ultralente insulin (Humulin U)	2 to 4 hours	8 to 14 hours	20 to 24 hours	22	Same as for lente insulin; in addition, peak of action is erratic in some patients.

From Hirsh IB: Type 1 diabetes mellitus and the use of flexible insulin regimens, *Am Fam Physician* 60(8):2343-2352;1999. Printed with permission from American Family Physician. All rights reserved.

*Estimated cost to the pharmacist based on average wholesale prices (rounded to the nearest dollar) in Red book, Montvale, NJ: *Medical Economics Data*, 1999. Cost to the patient will be greater, depending on prescription filling fee.

---

and muscle tissue, but a postreceptor defect can also occur. Dyslipidemia and hypertension are also often associated with type 2 DM and should be evaluated and treated accordingly.[18] Initial symptoms include polyuria and polydipsia, but asymptomatic cases are sometimes diagnosed by routine screening. Persons with type 2 DM have elevated preprandial and postprandial blood glucose levels. Elevated hepatic glucose production in the basal state leads to elevated fasting blood glucose values, whereas decreased glucose utilization and peripheral insulin resistance lead to elevated postprandial levels. Some believe that consistently elevated blood glucose levels "exhaust" the pancreas' β-cells, and that insulin reverses the effect.[19] Ketosis is rare because some endogenous insulin is present; however, severe stress can precipitate DKA in some patients with type 2 DM.

Although the majority of persons with type 2 DM do not require exogenous insulin for their immediate survival, in combination with diet, insulin and oral hypoglycemic agents are often part of therapy for type 2 DM (Table 37-2). Therapy of type 2 DM is complicated by the presence of insulin deficiency and peripheral resistance to the actions of insulin. However, it has been noted that blood glucose control can improve in overweight individuals with type 2 DM when placed on energy-restricted diets.[20,21] Therefore, caloric restriction and weight loss remain the initial treatment of choice in many individuals with type 2 DM. If dietary treatment of type 2 DM fails to achieve goals for blood glucose control and blood glucose levels are not extremely elevated, oral hypoglycemic agents are often used either singly or in combination with other medications. Until recently, sulfonylurea medications were the only oral hypoglycemic agents for treatment of type 2 DM available in the United States. Sulfonylureas increase insulin secretion and may enhance its activity.[22] There are several types of sulfonylurea medications, which differ mainly in dose, potency, and metabolism.[23] More recently another insulin secretogogue, repaglinide, has also become available.[24]

Metformin (dimethylbiguanide) acts by decreasing hepatic glucose production and increasing glucose uptake. Because metformin does not stimulate insulin production (insulin must

be present) it can be used in combination with a sulfonylurea. A beneficial effect of metformin is its potential ability to decrease triglyceride and low-density lipoprotein (LDL) levels while having no effect on high-density lipoprotein (HDL) levels, making it an appropriate line of therapy for individuals with cardiovascular disease.[25] Earlier biguanide medications had been associated with lactic acidosis in some individuals.[26] Although this is much less commonly seen now, caution should be used in patients at risk for lactic acidosis, in particular, those with renal insufficiency.

Acarbose is an oral alpha-glucosidase inhibitor used for therapy of type 2 DM. Acarbose acts by inhibiting intestinal hydrolysis of ingested carbohydrates, thus delaying absorption. Because unabsorbed carbohydrates reach the colon and are fermented there, GI side effects such as flatulence, cramps, or diarrhea may be a problem. For this reason, therapy should be initiated with a low dose and titrated up as GI symptoms allow. Acarbose was found to be effective in controlling glycemia when used alone or in conjunction with sulfonylurea medications.[27] Because absorption of disaccharides is delayed by acarbose, hypoglycemia in persons treated with acarbose must in turn be treated with glucose because absorption of oral disaccharides is affected.

Combinations of oral agents may be required to achieve optimal glucose levels in many patients with type 2 DM. Newer medications are being developed that target specific phases of insulin secretion[28] or improve insulin sensitivity.[29] Occasionally, persons with type 2 DM require insulin therapy to achieve adequate glucose control, but for them, insulin therapy can be complicated by insulin resistance and may be more effective in patients who have lost weight and have severe hyperglycemia, particularly if they are younger than 40 years of age.[30] Some patients with type 2 DM can be treated successfully with a mixture of oral agents and insulin.[31]

Persons who have type 2 DM typically are not prone to ketosis, but they may be at risk for development of hyperosmolar hyperglycemic nonketotic coma (HHNKC) (Table 37-3). HHNKC typically develops in patients with type 2 DM who have a serious illness, and it is characterized by serum glucose

TABLE 37-2

Comparison of Sulfonylureas, Repaglinide, Metformin, Troglitazone, and Acarbose When Used as Monotherapy

Effect	Sulfonylureas and Repaglinide	Metformin	Troglitazone	Acarbose
Mechanism of action	Increase in insulin secretion	Decrease in hepatic glucose production; increase in muscle insulin sensitivity	Decrease in hepatic glucose production; increase in muscle insulin sensitivity	Decrease in GI absorption
Decrease in FPG level, *mmol/L (mg/dL)*	3.3–3.9 (60–70)	3.3–3.9 (60–70)	1.9–2.2 (35–40)	1.1–1.67 (20–30)
Decrease in hemoglobin A$_{1C}$ value, *percentage points*	1.5–2.0	1.5–2.0	1.0–1.2	0.7–1.0
Triglyceride level	No effect	Decrease	Decrease	No effect
HDL cholesterol level	No effect	Slight increase	Increase	No effect
LDL cholesterol level	No effect	Decrease	Increase	No effect
Body weight	Increase	Decrease	Increase	No effect
Plasma insulin	Increase	Decrease	Decrease	No effect
Adverse events	Hypoglycemia	GI disturbances, lactic acidosis*	Anemia, hepatic toxicity†	GI disturbances

From DeFronzo R: Pharmacologic therapy for type 2 diabetes mellitus, *Ann Intern Med* 131:281–303,1999.
FPG, Fasting plasma glucose; *GI*, gastrointestinal; *HDL*, high-density lipoprotein; *LDL*, low-density lipoprotein.
*Incidence of 0.03 cases per 1000 patient-years (rare).
†Severe, idiosyncratic, sometimes irreversible hepatic failure has been reported with troglitazone, but the precise incidence is unknown. Elevated liver enzyme levels occur in about 2% of patients.

levels greater than 600 mg/dl, serum osmolality greater than 330 mOsm/kg, absence of ketosis, mild acidosis, serum bicarbonate greater than 20 mEq/L, and obtunded state.[32] Some residual insulin secretion may be responsible for the absence of ketosis in HHNKC. HHNKC should be treated promptly with volume expansion, intravenous insulin, and electrolyte replacement as needed. Treatment notwithstanding, the death rate can be as high as 50%.

Stress-induced diabetes is hyperglycemia in metabolically stressed patients who have no history of overt diabetes. Increased levels of the stress hormones blunt insulin secretion and increase hepatic gluconeogenesis and peripheral insulin resistance. The role of counterregulatory hormones in the development of stress-induced diabetes has been investigated.[33] Interaction of the counterregulatory hormones in producing hyperglycemia has been investigated in healthy volunteers. Whereas infusion of single hormones led to only mild hyperglycemia, a combined infusion caused sharply elevated blood glucose levels.[34] Additionally, stress can further impair blood glucose control for patients with known type 1 or type 2, as evidenced by an exaggerated response to glucose infusion by diabetes patients after infusion of counterregulatory hormones as compared with nondiabetic subjects.[35]

Other diseases can lead to impaired glucose tolerance. Pancreatic diseases such as cystic fibrosis and pancreatectomy are associated with variable amounts of insulin deficiency econdary to destruction of the β-cells of the pancreas. Excess counterregulatory hormone production such as that associated with pheochromocytoma, acromegaly, or Cushing's syndrome can also impair glucose tolerance. Treatment of the underlying condition usually reverses hyperglycemia in these cases. Finally, certain medications, such as corticosteroids, thiazide diuretics, and phenytoin, can induce diabetes or exacerbate blood glucose control in persons with preexisting diabetes.

Diabetes that occurs during pregnancy is called *gestational diabetes*. While blood sugar levels often return to normal after delivery, the mother is at increased risk for developing overt diabetes later in life. Adequate blood sugar control is imperative in patients with gestational diabetes to prevent complications during pregnancy. Insulin therapy is required if adequate blood glucose control cannot be achieved by diet alone. Oral hypoglycemic agents should not be used during pregnancy.

Nutrition Assessment

Appropriate nutrition assessment is vital for patients with diabetes to ensure that existing deficiencies are treated and to prevent development of nutrition-related complications during hospitalization. Nutrition assessment for patients with diabetes is in many ways similar to that for nondiabetic patients. Close attention should be given to blood glucose levels and other standard parameters because elevated blood glucose can signal smoldering infection. Glycosylated hemoglobin levels are an index of long-term blood glucose control. In addition to renal function, serum lipid levels should be evaluated because of the increased incidence of cardiovascular disease. A thorough medication history should be taken because patients frequently take multiple medications, any of which can affect nutritional status. It is important to note use of either oral hypoglycemic agents or insulin and the doses and dosing schedules of all medications. A nutrition-oriented physical assessment should focus on wound healing and skin integrity. See Table 37-4 for common nutrition assessment parameters in diabetes mellitus.

Diabetic nephropathy may affect parameters of nutrition assessment. Metabolic derangements caused by renal failure can distort serum transferrin, prealbumin, and retinol-binding protein values. Prealbumin and retinol-binding protein are both degraded in the kidneys, and levels may be increased in

TABLE 37-3

Laboratory Evaluation of DKA Versus HHNC

	DKA	HHNC
Plasma glucose	>250 mg/dl	>600 mg/dl
pH	<7.3	>7.3
Serum HCO$_3$	<15 mEq/L	>20 mEq/L
Ketonuria	≥3 +	≤1 +
Serum "ketones" (nitroprusside reaction)	Positive at 1:2 dilution	Negative at 1:2 dilution
Osmolality*	Variable	≥330 mOsm/kg
Mental obtundation	Variable	Always present

$$*\text{Calculated } 2(Na) + \frac{glucose}{18} + \frac{blood\ urea\ nitrogen}{2.8}$$

From Kitabachi AE, Murphy MB: Diabetic ketoacidosis and hyperosmolar hyperglycemic nonketotic coma, *Med Clin North Am* 72(2):1545-1564, 1988.

TABLE 37-4

Common Nutrition Assessment Parameters in Diabetes Mellitus

Parameter	Rationale
Albumin	Basic assessment parameter
Blood glucose level	Short-term glucose control
Hgb A1c	Long-term glucose control
Serum electrolyte levels	Fluid and electrolyte status
Liver function tests	Preexisting liver dysfunction may necessitate changes in feeding composition
Lipid panel	Patients with diabetes are at high risk for cardiovascular disease
BUN/creatinine	Patients with diabetes are at high risk for renal failure
UUN	Nitrogen balance; assess effectiveness of protein fed
Prealbumin (transthyrethin)	Assess changes in status or monitor therapy
Transferrin	Assess changes in status or monitor therapy

patients with end-stage renal disease. However, it is possible to monitor trends in levels of these laboratory values. Hemodialysis patients who receive exogenous albumin infusions may develop elevations in serum albumin levels that are not related to nutrition. More often, patients with nephrotic syndrome experience significant urinary protein losses (and edema) and, for them, decreased serum albumin levels do not reflect nutritional status. Patients with nephropathy may also be prone to anorexia and should be monitored closely for decreased intake and subsequent weight loss.

It may be difficult to assess the efficacy of insulin or oral hypoglycemic therapy in persons with gastroparesis because delayed gastric emptying may make it difficult to time meals and medication dosing. Acute episodes of gastroparesis can be exacerbated by increased blood glucose levels, so it is important to maintain blood glucose control. Diabetic gastroparesis or delayed gastric emptying can produce early satiety, bloating, nausea, and vomiting. Glycemic control can be difficult with gastroparesis. Patients with gastroparesis may not have severe symptoms, so gastric emptying abnormalities should be investigated in patients with unexplained poor glycemic control.[36]

Accurate estimation of energy requirements is vital to avoid the consequences of overfeeding and underfeeding. Because some patients with diabetes, particularly those with type 2 DM, may be overweight, calorie requirements are normally based on achievement and maintenance of desirable body weight. There is some controversy about the energy requirements during severe stress or illness of severely overweight persons.[37] Methods for estimating energy and protein requirements include indirect calorimetry and the Harris-Benedict equation. It would be reasonable to provide most healthy persons 25 to 30 kcal/kg for weight maintenance, with less than this amount (20 kcal/kg) if weight loss is desired.

Nutrition Management

There is no question that diet is important in the treatment of both type 1 and type 2 DM. What constitutes the appropriate diet, however, has always been controversial. Before insulin therapy was available, very low-carbohydrate diets were often recommended. With the advent of insulin and oral hypoglycemic agents, dietary recommendations for carbohydrate have varied. Current recommendations call for individualized diet prescriptions. The goal of medical nutrition therapy for individuals with DM should be to maintain blood glucose levels as near normal as possible while minimizing hypoglycemic episodes. Recommendations for DM patients are similar to those for normal healthy persons: 10% to 20% of total calories from protein, fewer than 10% of calories from saturated fats, fewer than 10% from polyunsaturated fats, and the remainder from monounsaturated fats and carbohydrate. Total fat intake should depend on blood lipid and glucose levels and on weight management goals. Patients who are obese or have elevated LDL levels may want to limit total fat intake to less than 30% of calories and saturated fat to less than 7% of calories.[38]

The carbohydrate content of the diet may vary according to energy requirements and individual glycemic response to various carbohydrates. Individuals with type 1 DM should ideally match insulin dose to the amount of carbohydrate ingested rather than the type because glycemic responses may vary.[39] It is recommended that 25 to 35 g of fiber be included.[40] Consumption of a diet consisting of 50 g total fiber (25 g soluble and 25 g insoluble) led to improved glycemic control in obese type 2 diabetic subjects.[41] Currently, the average American diet has less than 15 to 20 g of fiber. Dietary fiber is generally categorized as soluble or insoluble. Soluble fibers, such as guar gum or pectin, form a viscous gel that may assist with glucose control by slowing carbohydrate digestion and absorption. There are no recommendations on the type of fiber, although some soluble fibers may enhance blood glucose control given in large enough doses.

The use of sucrose in diets for individuals with DM has been debated. As a major source of calories (candy, soft drinks) sucrose should be avoided, but current recommendations allow modest amounts of sucrose as part of a mixed meal.[42] Other nutritive sweeteners such as fructose and sorbitol have also been used successfully in diabetes diets. Fructose is slightly sweeter than sucrose, and may cause a less rapid rise in plasma glucose than sucrose. Sorbitol is also sweeter than sucrose, but its use is limited because of GI side effects when more than 20 g are ingested.

Because patients with diabetes are at higher risk than the general population for cardiovascular disease, there is much interest in determining the appropriate level of fat in their diets. Although current diet recommendations call for a low-fat diet (not more than 30% of total calories) for most patients, there has been some research into the effects of diets high in monounsaturated fatty acids (MUFA). Such diets have been found in some studies to lower serum LDL cholesterol without changing levels of HDLs.[43,44] Garg and colleagues studied the effects of a diet high in monounsaturated fats on 10 persons with type 2 DM. Patients ate either a high-carbohydrate or high monounsaturated fat diet for 28 days. Both very low-density lipoproteins (VLDL) and triglycerides were significantly lowered on the high-MUFA diet. Additionally, the high-MUFA diet led to lower mean plasma glucose levels and insulin requirements.[45] Others have found significantly lower mean glucose levels in patients with "mild" type 2 DM who ate a diet high in MUFA for 2 weeks.[46] Long-term studies of the effects of high-MUFA diets are not currently available, although it appears that a diet high in MUFA may improve insulin sensitivity.[47]

Protein requirements of hospitalized patients with diabetes can vary with the level of stress. Normal protein requirements for individuals with diabetes are estimated to be 0.8 g/kg, or approximately 10% to 20% of calories, but the requirements may be increased to 1.2 to 2.0 g/kg per day during illness or stress.[48] Renal disease is fairly common in patients with long-standing diabetes and is in fact a leading cause of death. Some evidence indicates that mild protein restriction can slow the progression of renal disease. A recent multicenter trial of low-protein diets showed no clear-cut benefit from low-protein diets, although patients with diabetes were not analyzed separately.[49] Determining protein requirements of patients with nephropathy during stress is a challenge for the nutrition support team. Although optimal protein intake for patients with nephropathy during stress is not known, it has been recommended that no more than 1.5 g/kg per day be given to prevent excess nitrogenous waste production.[50] Protein restriction is not recommended for patients with end-stage renal disease receiving dialysis, nor should protein be restricted in critically ill patients in hopes of avoiding dialysis.[51]

Nutrition Support

Indications for nutrition support in diabetic patients are similar to those for other patients. Current recommendations are that the enteral route be utilized whenever possible, for several reasons. EN support is more "physiologic" than parenteral, leads to fewer potentially serious complications, helps maintain the gut mucosal surface, and is less expensive than parenteral feeding. There are very few absolute contraindications to enteral feeding.

Choice of Enteral Formula

Great advances have been made in the past few years in the development and marketing of enteral formulas. Until very recently, formula choices were limited to only two or three categories. As the science of nutrition support grows, the potential pharmacologic effects of individual nutrients are becoming apparent. Enteral formulas are now available for a wide variety of clinical conditions. An enteral formula for patients with diabetes should be chosen with an eye to nutrient content and the goals of nutrition therapy.

Carbohydrate sources in enteral formulas include both simple and complex carbohydrates. In general, most formulas contain 30% to 90% of total calories as carbohydrate, ranging in form from sucrose to oligosaccharides, polysaccharides, corn syrup, maltodextrins, and starches. In theory, it may be desirable initially to use more complex carbohydrates, particularly if blood glucose control has been a problem. Formulas containing a portion of carbohydrate from simple sugars can be used successfully in patients with diabetes in combination with appropriate blood glucose monitoring and judicious insulin therapy.

Protein sources in enteral formulas include complete proteins and hydrolyzed proteins, peptides of varying chain lengths, and free amino acids. There are currently no contraindications to any of these protein sources in patients with diabetes, although free L-amino acids may delay gastric emptying in some patients with gastroparesis. Intact protein sources should be used unless malabsorption is a problem. It should be remembered that formulas in which either peptides or free amino acids are the protein source often contain a large percentage of simple sugars.

Currently much controversy surrounds fat choices for enteral formulas. Most currently available standard formulas contain from 25% to 40% of total calories from fat (disease-specific formulas with more fat content are also available), often with ω-6 fatty acids as the major fat source. Corn, safflower, sunflower, and soybean oils—often used as fat sources in enteral formulas—are all rich sources of ω-6 fatty acids. Omega-6 fatty acids have many potential adverse effects on immune function and induce production of inflammatory prostanoids and leukotrienes.[52] For this reason, they may not be desirable in large quantities. Omega-3 fatty acids, found mainly in fish oils or derived from linolenic acid, most likely do not have these immunosuppressive effects and are used as a fat source in some enteral formulas.

It has been suggested that increased fat intake may enhance blood glucose control and help lower serum lipid levels in patients receiving EN support. Findings on diets high in MUFAs have been used to develop special enteral formulas for persons with diabetes and impaired glucose tolerance. Many of these products are lower in carbohydrate than most standard enteral formulas and contain MUFA as well as additional fiber. Some have found that these formulas control blood sugar better than standard enteral formulas, although response varies.[53,54] It should be remembered that they were not studied in hospitalized patients and that subjects were allowed to drink the formula. Response may be different in tube-fed patients. A more recent study using enteral feedings of a diabetic formula found no significant difference in plasma glucose or Hbg A1c when compared to a standard formula.[55] Formula composition, particularly the type of carbohydrate, may not be well-controlled in some studies. Total caloric intake may be more important than the distribution of nonprotein calories because overfeeding is likely to increase insulin requirements regardless of the distribution of nonprotein calories. Most standard enteral formulas containing 40% to 55% carbohydrate are appropriate for use in patients with DM.[56]

Increased fiber intake may improve blood sugar control, although response varies with the source of fiber. Soluble fibers such as guar and pectin have been shown to decrease postprandial blood sugar and serum insulin response in lean persons with diabetes,[57] although with varying results.[51] Most enteral formulas use soy polysaccharide, a soluble fiber that lowers blood glucose and serum lipid levels, although it appears that large amounts of soluble fiber must be ingested to produce a significant glucose response.[58] Several mechanisms have been proposed to explain the effects of soluble fiber on blood glucose control and insulin response, including delayed gastric emptying, altered intestinal transit, and increased insulin sensitivity.[59,60] More research is needed before the effects of various types of fiber are fully understood. Fiber should be given with caution to patients with gastroparesis who are receiving gastric feedings because it could further delay gastric emptying.

Initiating Enteral Feedings

It is often recommended that a feeding pump and continuous feedings be used initially, particularly in critically ill patients. Intermittent feedings may be associated with a higher risk for GI complications and with increased risk of aspiration, particularly in patients with preexisting or subclinical gastric emptying disorders, and should be used only in stable patients. If possible, the feeding tube should be placed in the small intestine to bypass potential gastric emptying abnormalities that may be exacerbated by illness. Gastric feedings are appropriate for stable patients with no evidence of gastric emptying abnormalities. Blood glucose control should be optimized before enteral feedings begin. Most enteral formulas can be started at full strength at a rate of 30 to 50 ml per hour and advanced to goal rates over 24 to 48 hours with appropriate blood glucose monitoring. There is no physiologic need to dilute enteral formulas.[61]

As enteral feedings are being initiated and advanced, blood sugar control can be achieved by modifying previous insulin dosage and using sliding-scale insulin. It is not uncommon for patients who were receiving insulin before enteral feedings to require larger insulin doses once feedings begin. Patients who previously took insulin can initially be given one fourth of the usual NPH dose every 12 hours, and sliding-scale Regular insulin can be given to maintain blood glucose levels at less than 200 mg/dl. Feedings should not be advanced until blood glucose levels are stable and less than 200 mg/dl. The NPH dose is then adjusted daily, usually by adding one fourth to one half of the previous day's Regular insulin as NPH, as a result of the previous day's Regular insulin requirements. Coverage with Regular insulin should continue as feedings are advanced to the goal rate.

Patients who did not previously take insulin can be managed with sliding-scale Regular insulin using daily adjustments based on the previous day's dose. Once blood glucose levels are stable, split doses of NPH insulin may be used. Although oral hypoglycemic agents are not recommended during continuous enteral feeding, they may be given to stable patients fed intermittently. Oral hypoglycemics should not be added to enteral formulas because compatibility may be a problem.

Certain considerations apply to all diabetic patients who receive EN. To avoid hypoglycemia, enteral feedings must not be interrupted, particularly in patients receiving insulin or oral medications. If a feeding is interrupted after insulin has been given, intravenous dextrose should be given. If oral hypoglycemic agents are used in conjunction with intermittent feedings, missing a feeding could produce dangerous hypoglycemia. For these reasons, it is imperative that careful intake and output records be kept for all diabetic patients receiving enteral feedings and that feeding tolerance be monitored carefully to avoid missed feedings or inappropriate insulin dosing. Feedings should not be advanced unless blood sugar levels are stable at an acceptable level.

Parenteral Nutrition

Adequate blood glucose control is imperative for diabetic patients who are receiving PN because they may be at increased risk for catheter infection, particularly if blood glucose levels are high. Particular attention must be given to the macronutrient composition of parenteral solutions. For nondiabetic patients, it has been suggested that the maximum glucose infusion rate be 4 to 6 mg/kg per minute. This is the rate at which hepatic glucose production is minimized and peripheral glucose uptake maximized.[62] This infusion rate may need to be decreased further to maintain glucose control in patients with diabetes. It has been recommended that dextrose in the initial PN infusion be limited to 100 to 150 g.[63] The dextrose infusion can be increased by 50 to 75 g per day once blood glucose levels are stable but less than 200 mg/dl. Other potential dextrose sources, including peripheral intravenous infusions and dextrose absorbed from peritoneal dialysis should be monitored and taken into account.

Lipid infusions, either piggybacked or as part of a three-in-one admixture, are often used to supply a portion of nonprotein energy requirements. Although infusion of more than 50% of total calories as lipid may impair reticuloendothelial system bacterial clearance,[64] it appears that infusing no more than 30% of nonprotein calories as lipid is safe and may decrease the need for exogenous insulin. Lipid emulsions currently available in the United States contain a large percentage of ω-6 fatty acids, so excessive administration should be avoided.

Insulin is often added to PN to maintain euglycemia. A certain amount of insulin can adhere to bags and tubing, but the reported percentage of insulin lost to adsorption varies. Marcuard and colleagues studied availability of insulin from a PN system consisting of an ethylene vinyl acetate (EVA) 1-L bag and polyvinyl chloride (PVC) tubing. At least 90% of insulin was recovered from the PN solutions studied.[65] Others reported smaller percentages of insulin availability, but their results may have been affected by holding PN solutions overnight in collection beakers.[66]

Insulin should be added to the initial PN infusion only for diabetic patients who required exogenous insulin before their current illness. Typically, a portion of insulin previously required is added to the PN formula as Regular insulin. Intermediate- or long-acting insulin is not added to PN. Various recommendations for determining insulin requirements are available.[67,68] One fourth to one half of the usual insulin requirement can safely be added to the initial PN solution as Regular insulin, depending on the total calorie content provided by the PN. If the PN is providing half of the patient's energy requirements, a similar proportion of insulin should be added to the formula. Blood glucose levels are then maintained with either subcutaneous injections or a separate infusion of Regular insulin. Insulin action may be delayed if given by subcutaneous injection to patients with significant edema, low albumin levels, or peripheral vascular disease.[69] The amount of additional insulin required for a 24-hour period is totaled and the insulin in the PN solution is increased by approximately one third to one half of this amount. Dextrose infusion can be increased to meet requirements once adequate blood glucose control is achieved. In this manner, wide fluctuations in blood glucose levels can be avoided.

Insulin should not be added to the initial PN solution for patients who did not require exogenous insulin before their current illness because they could have some residual insulin secretion. However the insulin response to IV dextrose is slower than if an equivalent amount of carbohydrate were taken orally because of bypassing of enteric hormonal responses to eating. Sliding-scale insulin can be given during the initial infusion of PN if blood glucose levels are greater than 200 mg/dl. On subsequent days, one third to one half of the previous day's sliding-scale insulin dose can be added to the PN solution until adequate blood sugar control is achieved. The dextrose concentration of the PN solution should not be increased until blood sugar control is achieved.

Transition Feedings

The successful transition from parenteral to enteral to oral intake (as well as from enteral to oral intake) is often overlooked. Appropriate blood glucose management is vital to ensure safe and timely transition to the feeding modality best suited to the patient. Advancement from parenteral feeding to either enteral or oral feeding requires at least minimal GI function. Trials of enteral or oral feedings can be accomplished in most patients with diabetes, using sliding-scale subcutaneous Regular insulin if insulin is needed. Once 25% to 50% of calorie requirements are met through either the enteral or the oral route, PN can be decreased accordingly. Small doses of short-acting insulin should be given because, initially, enteral or oral intake may be sporadic. Once enteral or oral intake reaches 75% to 100% of estimated requirements, PN can be discontinued after the last bag is infused.

Oral diets provided for the transitional period should be individualized and designed to encourage adequate intake meeting estimated nutrient requirements. In the past it was common to use either standard or custom "meal patterns" planned using the exchange system lists. It is probably more appropriate to use carbohydrate counting, which allows more liberal food choices. Glucose monitoring and adjusting of DM medications can optimize glycemic control during this important period. Diets using no concentrated sweets or no sugar are to be avoided.[70]

Oral hypoglycemic agents should be used only in diabetic patients who are receiving consistent oral intake or are stable on intermittent enteral feedings. Subcutaneous insulin or oral hypoglycemic agents should be used to "cover" calories given either enterally or by mouth. Insulin in TPN should be expected to cover only calories given in the PN formula.

"Tapering" PN before discontinuing it, to prevent hypoglycemia, is the subject of much controversy. In the past it was felt that abrupt discontinuation of a concentrated glucose solution would lead to rapid development of severe symptomatic hypoglycemia because of high circulating levels of endogenous insulin.[71] In nondiabetic patients, serum glucose levels returned rapidly to preinfusion levels on sudden cessation of PN. Symptomatic hypoglycemia occurred only when glucose infusion was increased significantly before it was discontinued.[72]

Serum blood glucose response to abrupt cessation of PN has been studied in patients with diabetes. Wagman and colleagues studied 48 patients who had been receiving PN for at least 7 days. Four in the study group had overt diabetes and another 11 required exogenous insulin while on PN. Plasma glucose, insulin, and serum glucagon levels were monitored for up to 8 hours after abrupt discontinuation of PN. None of the patients experienced symptoms of hypoglycemia.[73] Krzywda and colleagues studied the glucose response to abrupt discontinuation of PN in a group of 18 patients, including 6 with DM. Five patients received from 15 to 100 IU per day of insulin in the PN. For at least 1 week all had received a three-in-one solution providing 1.2 times the calculated resting energy expenditure. Blood glucose levels were measured every 5 minutes, from 10 to 120 minutes. Patients who received insulin in PN exhibited a decrease in blood glucose levels in the first 60 minutes; most of the glucose response was complete by 60 minutes. No patient became clinically hypoglycemic, which led the authors to conclude that there is no need for prolonged tapering regimens when discontinuing PN.[74] In patients with diabetes or a history of difficult glucose management on PN, it is probably wise to decrease the rate of PN for an hour or so before discontinuing it. Glucose levels should be monitored for the first 1 to 2 hours after cessation of PN because any clinically significant hypoglycemia should occur within this time. If PN is abruptly discontinued in unstable patients, it would be wise to monitor blood glucose levels closely and provide dextrose infusion to avoid hypoglycemia.

Monitoring Nutrition Support

Monitoring of nutrition support in patients with diabetes is similar to that for nondiabetic patients. Daily weight and fluid balance should be monitored carefully, especially in patients receiving PN. Mineral and electrolyte status should also be monitored. Hypokalemia and hypophosphatemia can result from entry of these elements into the cells along with glucose. The role of zinc as a cofactor for insulin underscores the need for adequate zinc in both enteral and parenteral feedings. Chromium acts as a part of the "glucose tolerance factor," and improved glucose tolerance in chromium-deficient patients receiving chromium-supplemented PN solutions has been reported.[75] However, it is difficult to determine the presence of trace element deficiency or toxicity because currently available measurement techniques often have limitations and must be interpreted in context of other signs and symptoms. Strong clinical suspicion should accompany any decision to supplement above currently recommended levels.

Blood glucose monitoring is particularly vital for DM patients because hyperglycemia can increase susceptibility to infection. A retrospective review of 235 patients with diabetes revealed a significant correlation between various infections and mean blood glucose levels checked when no infection was present. Additionally, patients with poorly controlled diabetes had higher glucose levels and diminished bactericidal activity as compared with normal controls or patients with well-controlled diabetes after challenge with endotoxin.[76] Initially, blood glucose levels should be checked every 6 hours, then, less often as blood glucose levels, insulin requirements, and clinical condition stabilize. A sudden increase in blood glucose may signify infection. Adequate blood glucose control for patients receiving PN has been defined as keeping levels between 100 and 220 mg/dl.[67] Evidence for keeping blood glucose levels as close to normal levels as possible is strong.[77-79] It has been recommended that blood glucose levels higher than 400 mg/dl be treated promptly but not overzealously, lest symptomatic hypoglycemia (requiring dextrose administration) be induced.[80] Additionally, as the stress response resolves, insulin requirement may decrease.[81]

Complications of Diabetes Mellitus with Nutritional Implications

Diabetes is associated with the development of multiple systemic complications, including neuropathy, nephropathy, retinopathy, and vascular disease. The exact mechanism of these complications is not known, but it seems that risk increases with the duration of the disease and inadequate glucose control.[82] The Diabetes Control and Complications Trial (DCCT) demonstrated that intensive therapy of patients with diabetes can delay the onset and slow the progression of complications.[83] Intensive therapy of type 2 DM, with a goal blood glucose level of less than 110 mg/dl has also been shown to decrease microvascular complications.[84,85] Nutrition support for diabetic patients becomes more complicated in the presence of neuropathy or nephropathy.

Diabetic Gastroparesis

Delayed gastric emptying, or gastroparesis, a well-recognized neurologic complication of diabetes, is most often seen in patients with long-standing type 1 DM. It has been estimated that 45% to 75% of patients with diabetes experience delayed gastric emptying.[86] Symptoms of gastroparesis include early satiety, nausea, bloating, and vomiting that may occur after every meal or in episodes lasting days to weeks that gradually resolve.[87] Using more sensitive techniques, disordered gastric emptying has been noted in the absence of overt symptoms.[87] Some believe that gastroparesis can be caused by vagal autonomic neuropathy leading to gastric motor dysfunction.[88] Preexisting delayed gastric emptying in patients receiving EN support may be aggravated by hyperosmolar feedings, solid meals, high-fat formulas, and formulas with added fiber.[89]

Treatment of gastroparesis depends on the frequency and severity of symptoms. Infrequent, mild episodes can be treated symptomatically.[90] More frequent or severe attacks may require hospitalization to replete fluid and electrolyte losses and to maintain blood glucose control. Nasogastric suction may be required in some cases. Enteral feeding may still be possible if the tip of the feeding tube can be placed in the distal duodenum. Long-term enteral feeding using a permanent jejunostomy is another alternative. If PN is required in patients with gastroparesis, it has been suggested that H_2-receptor blockers be added to the PN solution to avoid further delays in gastric emptying caused by increased gastric acid secretion.[91]

Drugs such as metoclopramide, domperidone, and erythromycin have been used, with varying degrees of success, to treat gastroparesis. Metoclopramide relieves symptoms by acting as an antiemetic and stimulating gastric emptying. It is believed that metoclopramide acts by increasing lower esophageal sphincter pressure and enhancing gastric and small bowel motility. Its effect on gastric emptying of liquids was studied in 10 patients who had type 1 DM and symptoms of gastroparesis. A single acute dose given concurrently with a liquid meal improved gastric emptying, but after 1 month of therapy this effect was lost. Most patients reported relief of symptoms after long-term administration even though gastric emptying was no longer affected. This was attributed to the drug's antiemetic effects.[92]

Domperidone is a gastrokinetic medication similar to metoclopramide but with fewer neurologic side effects. It increases the rate of emptying of both solids and liquids when given as a single 40-mg dose 1 hour before a meal. While long-term administration of domperidone did not significantly alter gastric emptying of solids, liquid emptying and subjective symptoms of gastroparesis improved.[93]

Erythromycin, an antibiotic, was found to have prokinetic effects similar to those of the GI hormone motilin. The effect of erythromycin on gastric emptying was tested in a randomized double-blind crossover trial of 10 patients with type 1 DM who had gastroparesis. Intravenous administration of erythromycin immediately after a meal significantly improved gastric emptying of solids and liquids. Long-term administration did not sustain the improvements seen early after administration, but emptying of both solids and liquids remained somewhat improved.[94]

Diarrhea

Chronic diarrhea, often occurring at night, has been reported with diabetes, and frequently no cause can be found. Usually, the diarrhea is not severe enough to warrant specialized nutrition support intervention.[95] There may be some connection between adequate blood glucose control and severity of diarrhea, as evidenced by improvement of symptoms in a patient treated with continuous subcutaneous insulin injection.[96] Antidiarrheal agents may be used in some patients, or bile salt binding agents such as cholestyramine may be used. Diarrhea in patients receiving EN support may respond to formulas containing fiber. There is no evidence that monomeric formulas are indicated for diabetic patients with diarrhea.

Renal Failure

Nephropathy develops in approximately 30% to 45% of patients with diabetes.[97] Microalbuminuria has been found as early as 5 years after onset of diabetes.[98] In many cases, end-stage renal failure eventually occurs and renal replacement therapy becomes necessary. With the development of renal failure, the insulin requirement may decrease as a result of reduced renal insulin metabolism. This may be offset by peripheral insulin resistance that can occur with uremia. Metabolism and clearance of oral hypoglycemic agents can also be altered in renal failure.[99] For these reasons, it is imperative to monitor closely the response to drugs of patients with diabetes and renal failure.

The development of renal failure in patients with diabetes leads to multiple, severe metabolic derangements. Metabolism of protein, carbohydrate, and fat is affected, as is micronutrient metabolism. Close monitoring of blood glucose levels is vital for patients with diabetic nephropathy who become critically ill because insulin resistance leading to altered glucose tolerance complicates diabetes therapy. Patients absorb some dextrose from peritoneal dialysis fluid, which should be taken into account when prescribing or monitoring diabetes therapy.

Conclusion

DM is a serious metabolic disorder that affects carbohydrate, protein, and fat metabolism. Poor blood glucose control is associated with the development of severe end-organ complications and, potentially, increased mortality. Because more than 11 million persons in the United States have DM, most nutrition support teams will be asked to manage patients with DM. Indications for nutrition support are no different in patients

with DM than for any other patient group. Long-term complications of DM may indicate the need for alterations in the nutrition care plan to optimize outcomes. It is vital that blood glucose control be optimized before EN or PN support is provided to these patients and that blood glucose levels be monitored carefully. Blood glucose should be stable before changing or advancing enteral, parenteral, or transitional feedings.

REFERENCES

1. Harris MI, Eastman RC: Early detection of undiagnosed diabetesmellitus: a US perspective, *Diab Metab Res Rev* 16(4):230-236, 2000.
2. Park RHR, Hansell DT, Davidson LE, et al: Management of diabetic patients requiring nutrition support, *Nutrition* 8(5):316-320, 1992.
3. Cahill GF: The Banting Memorial Lecture. Physiology of insulin in man, *Diabetes* 20(12):785-799, 1971.
4. Granner DK: Hormones of the pancreas and GI tract. In Murray RK, Granner DK, Mayes PA, Rodwell VW (eds): *Harper's bio-chemistry,* ed 25, Stamford, CT, 2000, Appleton & Lange, pp 610-626.
5. Tillil H, Shapiro ET, Miller MA, et al: Dose-dependent effects of oral and intravenous glucose on insulin secretion and clearance in normal humans, *Am J Physiol* 254(3 Pt 1):E349-357, 1988.
6. Boden G, Chen X, Rosner J, Barton M: Effects of a 48-hour fat infusion on insulin secretion and glucose utilization, *Diabetes* 44(10):1239-1242, 1995.
7. Henquin JC: Cell biology of insulin secretion. In Kahn CR, Weir GC (eds): *Joslin's diabetes mellitus,* ed 13, Philadelphia, 1994, Lea & Febiger, pp 56-80.
8. Stryer L: Integration of metabolism. In Stryer L (ed): *Biochemistry,* ed 3, New York, 1988, WH Freeman, pp 627-645.
9. Granner DK: Pituitary and hypothalamic hormones. In Murray RK, Granner DK, Mayes PA, Rodwell VW (eds): *Harper's biochemistry,* ed 25, Stamford, CT, 2000, Appleton & Lange, pp 550-560.
10. Bessey P, Lowe K: Early hormonal changes affect the catabolic response to trauma, *Ann Surg* 218(3):476-491, 1993.
11. Gabay C, Kushner I: Acute-phase proteins and other systemic responses to inflammation, *N Engl J Med* 340(6):448-454, 1999.
12. Schmitz K: Providing the best possible care: an overview of the current understanding of diabetic ketoacidosis, *Australian Crit Care* 13:22-27, 2000.
13. Kitabchi AE, Umpierrez GE, Murphy MB, Barrett EJ, Kreisberg RA, Malone JI, Wall BM: Management of hyperglycemic crises in patients with diabetes, *Diabetes Care* 24(1):131-153, 2001.
14. Ferguson SC, Strachan MWJ, Janes JM, Frier BM: Severe hypoglycemia in patients with type I diabetes and impaired awareness of hypoglycemia: a comparative study of insulin lispro and regular human insulin, *Diab Met Res Rev* 17(4):285-291, 2001.
15. Silverstein JH, Rosenbloom AL: New developments in type I (insulin dependent) diabetes, *Clin Pediatr* 39(5):257-266, 2000.
16. Anderson JH, Brunelle R, Kovisto VA: Reduction of post prandial hyperglycemia and frequency of hypoglycemia in IDDM patients on insulin analog treatment, *Diabetes* 46(2):265-270, 1997.
17. Alberti KGMM: Treating type 2 diabetes—today's targets, tomorrow's goals, *Diabetes Obesity Metab* 3(suppl 1):S3-S10, 2001.
18. Reaven GM, Laws A: Insulin resistance, compensatory hyperinsulinemia and coronary heart disease, *Diabetologia* 37(9):948-952, 1994.
19. Rosenzweig JL: Principles of insulin therapy. In Kahn CR, Weir GC (eds): *Joslin's diabetes mellitus,* ed 13, Philadelphia, 1994, Lea & Febiger, pp 460-487.
20. Christiansen MP, Linfoot PA, Neese RA, Hellerstein MK: Effect of dietary energy restriction on glucose production and substrate utilization in type 2 diabetes, *Diabetes* 49(10):1691-1699, 2000.
21. Heilbronn LK, Noakes M, Clifton PM: Effect of energy restriction, weight loss, and diet composition on plasma lipids and glucose in patients with type II diabetes, *Diabetes Care* 22(6):889-895, 1999.
22. Simonson DC, DelPrato S, Castellino P, et al: Effect of glyburide on glycemic control, insulin requirement, and glucose metabolism in insulin treated diabetic patients, *Diabetes* 36(2):136-146, 1987.
23. Foster D: Diabetes mellitus. In Braunwald E, Isselbacher KJ, Petersdorf RG, et al. (eds): *Harrison's principles of internal medicine,* New York, 1987, McGraw-Hill, pp 1778-1796.

24. Fuhlendorff J, Rorsman P, Kofod H, Brand CL, Rolin B, MacKay P, Shymko R, Carr RD: Stimulation of insulin release by repaglinide and glibenclamide involves both common and distinct processes, *Diabetes* 47(3):345-351, 1998.

25. Jeppesen J, Zhou MY, Chen YD, Reaven GM: Effect of metformin on postprandial lipemia in patients with fairly to poorly controlled NIDDM, *Diabetes Care* 17(10):1093-1099, 1994.

26. Gan SC, Barr J, Arieff AI, Pearl RG: Biguanide-associated lactic acidosis: case report and review of the literature, *Arch Intern Med* 152(11):2333-2336, 1992.

27. Coniff RF, Shapiro JA, Seaton TB, Bray GA: Multicenter, placebo-controlled trial comparing acarbose (BAY g 5421) with placebo, tolbutamide, and tolbutamide-plus-acarbose in non–insulin-dependent diabetes mellitus, *Am J Med* 98(5):443-451, 1995.

28. Porte D: Clinical importance of insulin secretion and its interaction with insulin resistance in the treatment of type II diabetes mellitus and its complications, *Diab Met Res Rev* 17(3):181-188, 2001.

29. Pickavance LC, Buckingham RE, Wilding JPH: Insulin-sensitizing action of rosiglitazone is enhanced by preventing hyperphagia, *Diab Obes Metab* 3(3):171-180, 2001.

30. Lebovitz HE: Oral antidiabetic agents. In Kahn CR, Weir GC (eds): *Joslin's diabetes,* ed 13, Philadelphia, Lea & Febiger, 1994, pp 508-529.

31. DeFronzo RA: Pharmacologic therapy for type 2 diabetes mellitus, *Ann Intern Med* 131(4):281-303, 1999.

32. Quinn L: Diabetes emergencies in the patient with type 2 diabetes, *Nurs Clin North Am* 36(2):341-360, 2001.

33. Bessey P, Watters J, Aoki T, Wilmore D: Combined hormonal infusion stimulates the metabolic response to injury, *Ann Surg* 200(3):264-281, 1984.

34. Shamoon M, Hendler R, Sherwin R: Synergistic interactions among anti-insulin hormones in the pathogenesis of stress hyperglycemia in humans, *J Clin Endocrinol Metab* 52(6):1235-1241, 1981.

35. Shamoon H, Hendler R, Sherwin R: Altered responsiveness to cortisol, epinephrine, and glucagon in insulin-infused juvenile-onset diabetes, *Diabetes* 29(4):284-291, 1980.

36. Horowitz M, Harding PE, Maddox A, et al: Gastric and oesophageal emptying in insulin dependent diabetes mellitus, *J Gastroenterol Hepatol* 1:97-113, 1986.

37. Ireton-Jones CS, Turner WW: Actual or ideal body weight: which should be used to predict energy expenditure? *J Am Diet Assoc* 91(2):193-195, 1991.

38. Maximizing the role of nutrition in diabetes management. In American Diabetes Association, 1994, p 31.

39. Sheard NF, Clark NG: The role of nutrition therapy in the management of diabetes mellitus, *Nutr Clin Care* 3:334-348, 2000.

40. Rezabek KM: Medical nutrition therapy in type 2 diabetes, *Nurs Clin North Am* 36(2):203-216, 2001.

41. Chandalia M, Garg A, Lutjohann D, Von Bergmann K, Grundy SM, Brinkley LJ: Beneficial effects of high dietary fiber intake in patients with type II DM, *N Engl J Med* 342(19):1392-1398, 2000.

42. American Diabetes Association: Nutrition recommendations for people with diabetes mellitus, *Diabetes Care* 22(suppl 1):S42-S45, 1999.

43. Mattson FH, Grundy SM: Comparison of effects of dietary saturated, monounsaturated, and polyunsaturated fatty acids on plasma lipids and lipoproteins in man, *J Lipid Res* 26(2):194-202, 1985.

44. Grundy SM: Comparison of monounsaturated fatty acids and carbohydrates for lowering cholesterol, *N Engl J Med* 314(12):745-748, 1986.

45. Garg A, Bantle JP, Henry RR, et al: Effects of varying carbohydrate content of diet in patients with non-insulin dependent diabetes mellitus, *JAMA* 271(18):1421-1428, 1994.

46. Campbell LV, Marmot PE, Dyer JA, et al: The high monounsaturated fat diet as a practical alternative for NIDDM, *Diabetes Care* 17(3):177-182, 1994.

47. Vessby B: Dietary fat and insulin action in humans, *Br J Nutr* 83(suppl 1):S91-S96, 2000.

48. Barton RG: Nutrition support in critical illness, *Nutr Clin Pract* 9(4):127-139, 1994.

49. Klahr S, Levey AS, Beck GJ, et al: The effects of dietary protein restriction and blood pressure control on the progression of chronic renal disease, *N Engl J Med* 330(13):877-884, 1994.

50. Druml W: Nutritional support in acute renal failure. In Mitch WE, Klahr S (eds): *Nutrition and the kidney,* ed 2, Boston, 1993, Little, Brown, pp 314-345.

51. Henry RR: Protein content of the diabetic diet, *Diabetes Care* 17(12):1502-1513, 1994.

52. Gottschlich MM: Selection of optimal lipid sources in enteral and parenteral nutrition, *Nutr Clin Pract* 7(4):152-165, 1992.

53. Peters AL, Davidson MB, Isaac RM: Lack of glucose elevation after simulated tube feeding with a low-carbohydrate, high fat enteral formula in patients with type 1 diabetes, *Am J Med* 87(2):178-182, 1989.

54. Peters AL, Davidson MB: Effects of various enteral feeding products on postprandial blood glucose response in patients with type I diabetes, *J Parenter Enteral Nutr* 16(1):69-74, 1992.

55. Craig LD, Nicholson S, Silverstone FA, Kennedy RD: Use of a reduced-carbohydrate, modified-fat enteral formula for improving metabolic control and clinical outcomes in long term care residents with type 2 diabetes: results of a pilot study, *Nutrition* 14(6):529-534, 1998.

56. American Diabetes Association: Translation of the diabetes nutrition recommendations for health care institutions, *Diabetes Care* 22(suppl 1):S46-S48, 1999.

57. Jenkins DJA, Leeds AR, Gassull MA, et al: Unabsorbable carbohydrate and diabetes: decreased postprandial hyperglycemia, *Lancet* 2(7978):172-174, 1976.

58. Nuttall FQ: Dietary fiber in the management of diabetes, *Diabetes* 42(4):503-508, 1993.

59. Madar Z: Effect of brown rice and soybean dietary fiber on the control of glucose and lipid metabolism in diabetic rats, *Am J Clin Nutr* 38(3):388-393, 1983.

60. Fukagawa NK, Minaker KL, Hageman G, et al: High-carbohydrate, high-fiber diets increase peripheral insulin sensitivity in healthy young and old adults, *Am J Clin Nutr* 52(3):524-528, 1990.

60. Thomas BL, Laine DC, Goetz FC: Glucose and insulin response in diabetic subjects: acute effect of carbohydrate level and the addition of soy polysaccharide in defined-formula diets, *Am J Clin Nutr* 48:1048-1052, 1988.

61. Silk DBA: Formulation of enteral diets, *Nutrition* 15(7/8):626-632, 1999.

62. Wolfe R, O'Donnell T, Stone M, et al: Investigation of factors determining the optimal glucose infusion rate in total parenteral nutrition, *Metabolism* 29(9):892-900, 1980.

63. McMahon M, Manji N, Driscoll DF, Bistrian BR: Parenteral nutrition in patients with diabetes mellitus: theoretical and practical considerations, *J Parenter Enteral Nutr* 13(5):545-553, 1989.

64. Seidner D, Mascioli E, Istfan NW, et al: Effects of long-chain triglyceride emulsions on reticuloendothelial system function in humans, *J Parenter Enteral Nutr* 13(6):614-619, 1989.

65. Marcuard SP, Dunham B, Hobbs A, Caro JF: Availability of insulin from total parenteral nutrition solutions, *J Parenter Enteral Nutr* 14(3):262-264, 1990.

66. Doglietto GB, Bellantone R, Bossola M, et al: Insulin absorption to 3 liter ethylene vinyl acetate bags during 24 hour infusion, *J Parenter Enteral Nutr* 13(5):539-543, 1989.

67. Hongsermeier T, Bistrian BR: Evaluation of a practical technique for determining insulin requirements in diabetic patients receiving total parenteral nutrition, *J Parenter Enteral Nutr* 17(1):16-19, 1993.

68. Knapke CM, Owens JP, Mirtallo JM: Management of glucose abnormalities in patients receiving total parenteral nutrition, *Clin Pharm* 8(2):136-144, 1989.

69. Pitts DM, Kilo KA, Pontious SL: Nutritional support for the patient with diabetes, *Crit Care Nurs Clin North Am* 5(1):47-56, 1993.

70. American Diabetes Association: Translation of the diabetes nutrition recommendations for health care institutions, *Diabetes Care* 23(suppl 1):S38-S40, 2000.

71. Dudrick SJ, MacFadyen BV, Van Buren CT, et al: Parenteral hyperalimentation: metabolic problems and solutions, *Ann Surg* 176(3):259-264, 1972.

72. Sanderson I, Deitel M: Insulin response in patients receiving concentrated infusions of glucose and casein hydrolysate for complete parenteral nutrition, *Ann Surg* 179(4):387-394, 1974.

73. Wagman LD, Miller KB, Thomas RB, et al: The effect of acute discontinuation of total parenteral nutrition, *Ann Surg* 204(5):524-529, 1986.

74. Krzywda EA, Andris DA, Whipple JK, et al: Glucose response to abrupt initiation and discontinuation of total parenteral nutrition, *J Parenter Enteral Nutr* 17(1):64-67, 1993.

75. Anderson RA, Polansky M, Bryden NA, Canary J: Supplemental chromium effects on glucose, insulin, glucagon, and urinary chromium losses in subjects consuming controlled low chromium diets, *Am J Clin Nutr* 54(5):909-916, 1991.

76. Rayfield EJ, Ault MJ, Keusch GT, et al: Infection and diabetes: the case for glucose control, *Am J Med* 72(3):439-450, 1982.

77. Zerr KJ, Furnary AP, Grunkemeier GL et al: Glucose control lowers the risk of wound infection in diabetics after open heart operations, *Ann Thorac Surg* 63(2):356-361, 1997.

78. Pomposelli JJ, Baxter JK, Babineau TJ, et al: Early postoperative glucose control predicts nosocomial infection rate in diabetic patients, *J Parenter Enteral Nutr* 22(2):77-81, 1998.

79. Golden SH, Peart-Vigilance C, Kao WH, Brancati FL: Perioperative glycemic control and the risk of infectious complications in a cohort of adults with diabetes, *Diabetes Care* 22(9):1408-1414, 1999.

80. Orr ME: Hyperglycemia during nutrition support, *Crit Care Nurs* 12(1):64-70, 1992.

81. Clouse RE, Sandrock M: Intensive nutritional support, *Diabetes Spectrum* 2:329-334, 1989.

82. Nathan DM: Long term complications of diabetes mellitus, *N Engl J Med* 328(23):1676-1685, 1993.

83. The Diabetes Control and Complications Trial Research Group: The effect of intensive treatment of diabetes on the long term complications in insulin dependent diabetes mellitus, *N Engl J Med* 329(14):977-986, 1993.

84. UK Prospective Diabetes Study Group: Intensive blood glucose control with conventional treatment and risk of complications in patients with type 2 diabetes (UKPDS 33), *Lancet* 352(9131):837-853, 1998.

85. Nasr CE, Hoogwerf BJ, Faiman C, Reddy SSK: Effects of glucose and blood pressure control on complications of type 2 diabetes mellitus, *Clev Clin J Med* 66(4):247-253, 1999.

86. Katz LA, Spiro HM: Gastrointestinal manifestations of diabetes, *N Engl J Med* 275(24):1350-1361, 1966.

87. Minami H, McCallum RW: The physiology and pathophysiology of gastric emptying in humans, *Gastroenterology* 86(6):1592-1610, 1984.

88. Iber FL, Parveen S, Vandrunen M, Sood KB, Reza F, Serbovsky R, Reddy S: Relation of symptoms to impaired stomach, small bowel, and colon motility in longstanding diabetes, *Dig Dis Sci* 38(1):45-50, 1993.

89. Kong MF, Horowitz M, Jones KL, Wishart JM, Harding PE: Natural history of diabetic gastroparesis, *Diabetes Care* 22(3):503-507, 1999.

90. Feldman M, Schiller LR: Disorders of gastrointestinal motility associated with diabetes mellitus, *Ann Intern Med* 98(3):378-384, 1983.

91. Nompleggi D, Bell SJ, Blackburn GL, Bistrian BR: Overview of gastrointestinal disorders due to diabetes mellitus: emphasis on nutritional support, *J Parenter Enteral Nutr* 13(1):84-91, 1989.

92. Schade RR, Dugas MC, Lhotsky DM, et al: Effect of metoclopramide on gastric liquid emptying in patients with diabetic gastroparesis, *Dig Dis Sci* 30(1):10-15, 1985.

93. Horowitz M, Harding PE, Chatterton BE, et al: Acute and chronic effects of domperidone on gastric emptying in diabetic autonomic neuropathy, *Dig Dis Sci* 30(1):1-9, 1985.

94. Janssens J, Peeters TL, Vantrappen G, et al: Improvement of gastric emptying in diabetic gastroparesis by erythromycin, *N Engl J Med* 322(15):1028-1031, 1990.

95. Clark CM, Lee DA: Prevention and treatment of the complications of diabetes mellitus, *N Engl J Med* 332(18):1210-1217, 1995.

96. Shimizu H, Shimomura Y, Takahashi M, et al: Enteral hyperalimentation with continuous subcutaneous insulin infusion improved severe diarrhea in poorly controlled diabetic patient, *J Parenter Enteral Nutr* 15(2):181-183, 1991.

97. Anderson AR, Christiansen JS, Anderson JK, et al: Diabetic nephropathy in type I (insulin dependent) diabetes: an epidemiologic study, *Diabetologia* 25:496-501, 1983.

98. Selby JV, Fitzsimmons SC, Newman JM, et al: The natural history and epidemiology of diabetic nephropathy: implications for prevention and control, *JAMA* 263(14):1954-1960, 1990.

99. Jonsson A, Rydberg T, Sterner G, Melander A: Pharmacokinetics of glibenclamide and its metabolites in diabetic patients with impaired renal function, *Eur J Clin Pharmacol* 53(6):429-435, Feb 1998.

100. Harrower AD: Pharmacokinetics of oral antihyperglycemic agents in patients with renal insufficiency, *Clin Parmacokinet* 31(2):111-119, Aug. 1996.

Obesity 38

Jean C. Burge, PhD, RD, CNSD

THE health consequences of obesity are well established. Approximately 325,000 annual deaths are attributable to obesity in the United States.[1] Reduction in the incidence of overweight, defined as a body mass index (BMI) greater than 25 kg/m^2 and obesity as a BMI greater than 30 kg/m^2, among the American population was established as a goal for the *Healthy People 2000: National Health Promotion and Disease Prevention Objectives*.[2] Despite the designation and the inclusion of the goal of reducing the incidence of obesity in the U.S. population, recent observations have revealed that the prevalence of obesity continues to rapidly increase. A recent review by the National Center for Chronic Disease Prevention and Health Promotion reported that the incidence of obesity increased approximately 50% from 1991 to 1998.[3] Current estimates suggest that close to 20% of Americans are obese, approximately 50 million men and women. The incidence of obesity is also increasing rapidly in younger Americans, with a subsequent increase in type 2 diabetes mellitus in children as young as 10.[4] *Healthy People 2010* has again listed reducing the incidence of obesity as one of the top five health initiatives.[5]

The number of overweight hospitalized patients presenting for surgical and/or medical treatment is also reflected in these numbers. In fact, the percentage of the patient population that would be considered overweight should actually be higher than in the normal population because obesity contributes to the etiology and morbidity of many disease processes that frequently require hospitalization. Medical care costs associated with obesity-related morbidity and mortality account for 6.8% of U.S. health care costs[6] or approximately $99 billion annually.[7]

The treatment of the obese hospitalized patient continues to be controversial. Very little research has addressed the appropriate energy and protein requirements for this population, and because these patients appear well nourished, little attention is generally paid to the possibility of malnutrition. Recently, however, it has been shown that obese patients are at high risk for malnutrition,[8,9] and interest in identifying and adjusting treatment protocols based on body weight has increased. Traditionally, in the acute care setting overweight patients were treated just as were their normal weight counterparts. Energy requirements are based on actual or adjusted body weight, and consideration of weight reduction is either delayed or ignored. Although no one would recommend weight loss as a primary objective in the obese trauma patient, delivery of protein and energy necessary to maintain obesity may be associated with additional metabolic stress leading to modifications in estimating energy and protein needs.

In this chapter I define obesity, identify the medical and metabolic complications, and describe current treatment strategies for hospitalized or seriously stressed obese patients.

Defining Overweight

BMI, which is weight in kilograms divided by height in meters squared, is an estimate of adiposity. BMI adjusts for height because 90% of the variation associated with weight at any given height is adipose tissue. Both the National Institute of Health and the World Health Organization have established standards that categorize overweight and obesity based on BMI.[10,11] Table 38-1 provides these standards. BMI should be calculated and included as a vital sign in all patient medical records. See Box 38-1 on determining BMI.

Other indicators of weight status are also available. The Metropolitan Height-Weight Tables provide desirable weights for heights, based on actuarial calculations derived from life insurance data.[12,13] The Metropolitan Height-Weight Tables were revised in 1983 to reflect newer data. The 1983 tables have generated a fair amount of controversy because the normal weights for height are higher than in the previous tables. Recent investigators have suggested that in light of the current trend of weight gain in the general population, the older tables should remain the basis for determining ideal body weight (IBW). Both the original and revised versions of these tables establish weights for adult males and females. The weights obtained are for individuals with light clothes, which may add 1 to 2 pounds to the desirable weight. The height adds 2 inches for women and 1 inch for men to adjust for shoe heel height. Although this data does take into account the individual's height, weight, and frame size, the table must be available for reference. In addition these tables were based on data from primarily middle-income individuals and may not represent norms of specific subpopulations.

Finally, the Hamwi formula,[14] which is 100 pounds for the first 60 inches and 5 pounds for each subsequent inch of height in females and 106 pounds for the first 60 inches and 6 pounds for each subsequent inch of height in males, has been used frequently because of its simplicity. Until the most recent version of the Metropolitan Height-Weight Tables, the Hamwi formula closely approximated the "desirable body weights" published in that table. The advantage of the Hamwi method is that ideal weight can be established quickly. Body build is factored into the formula by adding or subtracting 10% of the derived body weight to the final weight, based on large or small frame size, respectively. Individuals who are greater than 20% above this

TABLE 38-1
Classification of Obesity

Underweight	BMI < 18.5 kg/m^2	Associated health risks low
Normal range	BMI 18.5-24.9 kg/m^2	Associated health risks low
Overweight	BMI 25-29.9 kg/m^2	Associated health risk increased
Class I obesity	BMI 30-34.9 kg/m^2	Associated health risk moderate
Class II obesity	BMI 35-39.9 kg/m^2	Associated health risk severe
Class III obesity	BMI ≥ 40 kg/m^2	Associated health risk very severe

From National Institutes of Health: Clinical guidelines on the identification and treatment of overweight and obesity in adults—the evidence report, *Obes Res* 6:51S-209S, 1998.

BOX 38-1
Determining BMI

Mrs. K is a 40-year-old female with a body weight of 347 pounds. She is 5 foot, 3 inches tall.

$$347 \text{ lb}/2.2 = 157.7 \text{ kg}$$
$$63 \text{ in} \times 0.0254 = 1.6 \text{ m}$$
$$1.6 \times 1.6 = 2.56 \text{ m}^2$$
$$BMI = 157.7 \text{ kg}/2.56 \text{ m}^2 = 61 \text{ kg/m}^2$$

final figure are considered overweight and those who are greater than 40% (or approximately 100 pounds) above this figure are classified as having clinically severe obesity.[15]

Beyond the absolute increase in body weight, the distribution of the excess adiposity also plays a role in determining the risks associated with obesity. Increases in visceral or central fat are associated with a much higher risk of metabolic abnormalities, which in turn increase the risk of comorbid complications such as type 2 diabetes mellitus (DM), cardiovascular disease, and certain types of cancers. Estimation of risk can be assessed through the use of waist to hip ratio. The waist and hip circumference measurements are made in a standing patient. A waist to hip ratio of greater than 0.8 (females) and greater than 1.0 (males) is indicative of central body adiposity and carries an increased health risk.[16]

Comorbid Conditions Associated with Obesity

The significance of obesity as a medical problem derives from the comorbid conditions that are associated with or caused by it. Being overweight is a significant independent risk factor for cardiovascular disease and is associated with an increased risk of hypertension; type 2 DM; hypercholesterolemia; stroke; chronic joint disease; gallstones; gastrointestinal (GI) reflux; urinary stress incontinence; obstructive sleep apnea; and several types of malignancies including breast, endometrial, colon, and prostate cancer.[17-23] A curvilinear relationship between BMI and morbidity and mortality from all causes has been described by a number of investigators.[20] This relationship appears to be a J-shaped curve (Fig. 38-1), with moderate increases in mortality occurring in individuals below a BMI of 20 kg/m^2 and increasing mortality occurring as BMI increases from a normal of 25 kg/m^2.

The Nurses Health Study, a prospective cohort of 115,866 women who were healthy at baseline, reported a strong association between BMI and cardiovascular disease. This association was maintained in women who were only 10% to 20%

above their IBWs.[24] The Lipid Research Clinic Program reported a similar association in males.[25] *Syndrome X* is a term used to describe a cluster of disorders and biochemical abnormalities that are known cardiovascular risk factors. These abnormalities include hypertension, hypertriglyceridemia, and decreased HDL cholesterol. Elevated serum insulin levels and insulin resistance are thought to play a causative role in the development of Syndrome X.[26] Zumoff[27] reported a positive linear relationship between fasting serum insulin levels and BMI. He reported a rise of 1.07 uU/ml of insulin per unit of BMI increase. This relationship held over the entire range of BMIs studied (BMI of 21 to 98 kg/m^2). Although weight loss produced a reduction in the fasting serum insulin levels, there was no correlation between the amount of weight lost and the decrease in insulin levels. Insulin resistance and hyperinsulinemia also appear to be closely associated with the presence of hypertension in this population. The prevalence of hypertension and type 2 DM among obese individuals is three times, and hypercholesterolemia two times, that found in young, normal-weight individuals. Eighty percent of individuals with type 2 DM are overweight. Weight loss not only decreases the severity of type 2 DM but also, in some cases, may result in return to the euglycemic state. The level of insulin resistance may play an important role in determining the amount of parenteral glucose the obese patient is able to tolerate.

Other potentially life-threatening medical problems associated with obesity include the obstructive sleep apnea/obesity hypoventilation syndrome. Sleep apnea is a sleep-related breathing disorder that is characterized by multiple respiratory pauses during sleep. These apneic episodes are defined as complete cessation of airflow for a period of 10 seconds or more.[28] Although sleep apnea is not confined to obese patients, two thirds of patients with this disorder are obese. Two characteristic signs of sleep apnea are daytime somnolence and snoring. Excess adipose tissue results in decreased ventilatory effort as a result of increased body mass interfering with lung expansion or

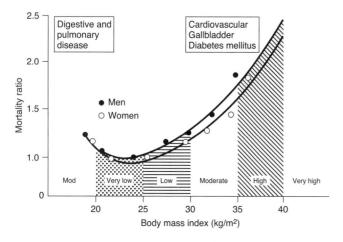

FIGURE 38-1 Mortality risk curve in obesity.[20] Relationship of BMI to risk. The curvilinear plot is based on data adapted from the American Cancer Society study. As BMI increases the excess risk rises. A healthy or good body weight range is between 19 and 25 kg/m². (From Kral JG: Morbid obesity and related health risks, *Ann Intern Med* 103:1043-1047, 1985.

the efficient mechanical functioning of the diaphragm and respiratory accessory muscles. The respiratory status of the obese patient should also be taken into account when determining the ratio of carbohydrate, protein and fats. Efforts should be made to lower the respiratory quotient of the ingested nutrients.

The incidence of GI problems is also significantly increased in the obese population. These include cholelithiasis and gastroesophageal reflux.[29] The association between obesity and gallstones has long been known. Arthritis and degenerative joint disease also occurs with greater frequency among obese patients and may be compounded by the additional weight load on joints.[30] Urinary stress incontinence is another common problem among patients who are obese and frequently improves with weight loss.[31]

Estimating Energy and Protein Needs

Numerous strategies exist for estimating nutrition needs in the obese patient (Box 38-2). Many practitioners believe that the obese patient's energy needs should be the same as the nonobese patient and calculate energy and protein needs on a per kilogram basis adjusted for the perceived degree of stress. Several problems are associated with this approach. Most patients with obesity have some degree of insulin resistance. This underlying metabolic abnormality coupled with the hyperglycemia associated with stress make the delivery of large amounts of carbohydrates difficult. Assuming the patient with obesity has energy needs based on actual body weight does not take into account changes in body composition associated with obesity. It is well known that lean body mass is metabolically active, whereas adipose tissue tends to be metabolically inactive. Body composition does not change in a linear fashion with increasing body weight. As weight increases there is some increase in lean body mass, but overall, there is a disproportionate increase in body fat in the majority of individuals. In addition to changes in body composition and insulin resistance, obesity-induced changes in pulmonary function further com-

---

BOX 38-2

Determining Energy Requirements in the Obese Patient

Mrs. K is a 40-year-old, 63-in, 347-lb female presenting with acute pancreatitis, resulting from obstruction of the common bile duct. She is admitted to the surgical intensive care unit status postcholecystectomy and debridement of the pancreas. Mrs. K is not currently on a ventilator.

Ideal body weight: 115 lb (52 kg)
Adjusted body weight: 202 lb (92 kg)

$$347 \text{ lb} \times 0.25 = 86.75$$
$$86.75 + 115 \text{ lb} = 201.75$$

Harris Benedict: (adjusted) 655.1 + 9.56(92 kg) + 1.85(160 cm) − 4.68(40)
655.1 + 879.52 + 296 − 187.2 = 1643
1643 (activity/stress factors of 1.3) = **2136 kcal**

(Ideal wt) 655.1 + 9.56(52 kg) + 1.85(160 cm) − 4.68(40)
655.1 + 497.12 + 296 − 187.2 = 1261(1.3) = **1639 kcal**

(Actual wt) 655.1 + 9.56(157.7) + 1.85(160) − 4.68(40)
655.1 + 1507.89 + 296 − 187.2 = 2272(1.3) = **2953 kcal**

Ireton-Jones: 629 − (11 × 40) + (25 × 92 kg) − 609 =
629 − 440 + 2300 − 609 = **1880 kcal**

Metabolic cart measurement: REE = 1735 kcal/day, RQ = 0.88
1735 (activity of 1.1) = **1908 kcal**

As this example illustrates, wide variations in the caloric estimation can occur with different methods of determining energy requirements. Although the metabolic cart is the most accurate method of determining energy requirements for the obese patient, the availability, cost, and technical problems associated with its use may make it difficult to obtain in some medical centers. A close approximation can be derived from the Ireton-Jones formula. When the Harris-Benedict equation is used, the adjusted weight should be substituted for the actual or ideal weight.

REE, Resting energy expenditure; *RQ*, respiratory quotient.

---

promise the patient's ability to handle high carbohydrate loads. These variables make it difficult to estimate and fulfill energy needs for obese patients and have resulted in a controversy regarding the best method for determining energy and protein requirements in stress.

There is considerable debate regarding the most appropriate weight to be used when calculating needs.[8] The adjusted body weight formula takes into account the alterations in body composition that occur in obesity and the fact that adipose tissue is metabolically inactive. Adjusted body weight is calculated by determining 25% of the obese patient's actual weight and adding it to the IBW: [adjusted BW = (actual BW × .25) + IBW]. This formula attempts to estimate the increase in lean body mass seen in the obese patient. This value is then substituted into equations such as the Harris-Benedict to predict energy needs. In a recent survey conducted by Ireton-Jones and Francis,[32] 40% of respondents used actual body weight and 40% of respondents used adjusted body weight.

Predictive equations that are based on normal populations, such as the Harris-Benedict equations, have been shown to underestimate the resting energy expenditure (REE) of obese individuals when IBW is used and to overestimate energy expenditure when actual body weight is used in the equations.[33,34] Ireton-Jones developed an equation for estimating energy needs in obese patients[35] and subsequently looked at the use of ideal versus actual body weight in this population[36] (Box 38-3).[37] In a comparison of this formula with the metabolic cart measurement, Ireton-Jones and colleagues found

BOX 38-3

Estimated Energy Expenditure for Obesity

EEE (v) = 1925−10(A) + 5(W) + 281(S) + 292(T) + 851(B), R^2 = 0.43
EEE (s) = 629−11(A) + 25(W)−609(O), R^2 = 0.5

From Ireton-Jones CS, Turner WW, Liepa GU, Baxter CR: Equations for estimation of energy expenditure in patients with burns with special reference to ventilatory status, *J Burn Care Rehabil* 13:330-333, 1992.
EEE, kcal/day; *V,* ventilator dependent; *s,* spontaneously breathing; *A,* age (yr); *W,* wt (kg); *S,* sex (m = 1, f = 0); *T,* trauma; *B,* burn; *O,* obesity (present = 1, absent = 0).

that it more closely approximated the actual energy expenditure in the obese patient.[36] Of interest was the fact that obesity was a significant factor in the nonventilated patient but became less significant in the obese ventilated patient. Ireton-Jones also suggests that actual body weight be used in equations to estimate energy expenditure rather than ideal or adjusted body weight. Although this formula does more closely approximate energy requirements in obese stressed patients, it should be used when indirect calorimetry is unavailable or not feasible.

Measuring Energy and Protein Needs

As previously discussed, as the degree of obesity and the severity of illness increase, it becomes progressively more difficult to estimate energy needs using any formula or theoretic method. In this situation one should consider using indirect calorimetry to obtain a measured resting energy expenditure (MREE). This machine measures O_2 consumption and CO_2 production and from these values energy expenditure in kilocalories per 24 hr can be calculated. In hospitalized patients it is often difficult to meet the conditions needed for a true REE or basal metabolic rate (BMR). Routine care provided, such as baths, physical therapy, dressing changes, respiratory therapy, make it unusual to have patients resting quietly for 30 to 45 minutes after a 2-hour fast, which is required for accurate measurement. Therefore, in hospitalized patients, the level of stress associated with the illness or trauma is incorporated into the measurement and what you obtain is measured energy expenditure (MEE). Consequently, the estimate of 24-hr energy needs from the MEE does not require the use of additional stress factors. Additional energy must be added for activity because activity associated with nursing care increases energy needs. A 10% to 30% increase in caloric intake based on level of activity associated with care is usual. Provision of calories is based on the MEE obtained from the cart, and protein needs are derived separately.

Most institutions, regardless of size, have the capability of measuring urine urea nitrogen (UUN), which allows for estimation of protein requirements. If other clinical conditions permit (i.e., renal and hepatic function are reasonable), nitrogen (protein) is provided to place the patient in +2 to +3 nitrogen balance. The formula frequently used for nitrogen balance is [nitrogen intake − (UUN + 0.2 (UUN) + 2]. The obese patient requires approximately 1.5 to 2 g protein per kilogram of IBW, depending on the energy level of the feedings.

Hypocaloric Nutrition Support

Several investigators have studied the use of hypocaloric feeding in the acutely ill obese patient.[38-44] These studies are based on the premise that reducing the caloric load for the obese patient will lead to improved glucose tolerance and still result in adequate nitrogen balance. Semistarvation diets have been used successfully as treatments for obesity in otherwise healthy obese individuals for some time.[45,46] Adaptive changes during starvation reduce energy requirements and allow fat depots (ketone bodies) to be utilized for energy, while sparing muscle protein from excessive catabolism. In this setting, the administration of adequate amounts of exogenous protein (approximately 1 g/kg IBW) results in nitrogen equilibrium or positive nitrogen balance.

During stress, high insulin levels impede normal adaptive mechanisms. As a result, muscle protein is actively catabolized for energy. Initially it was thought that stressed obese patients may be less able to mobilize fat for energy than stressed nonobese patients.[8,9] However, Dickerson and colleagues in 1986 demonstrated that nitrogen balance could be achieved in mild to moderately stressed obese patients receiving parenteral nutrition (PN) containing approximately 51% of MREE as nonprotein calories.[38] Nonprotein caloric intake averaged 881 kcal/day, and protein intake was 2.13 ± 0.59 g/kg IBW. Serum albumin and total iron-binding capacity improved significantly, and all subjects had complete tissue healing. Hwang and associates in 1993 were also able to show that nitrogen balance could be achieved in patients following multiple traumas if sufficient protein was provided. They also reported improved visceral protein and higher total lymphocyte levels in patients receiving the hypocaloric feedings.[39]

Burge and associates[40] in 1994 completed a prospective, randomized, double-blind trial of hypocaloric nutrition support in hospitalized obese patients. After measuring REE using indirect calorimetry, the formulas were administered at a rate to provide 100% of MEE as nonprotein calories (control) or 50% of MEE as nonprotein calories (hypocaloric). Protein intake was provided based on level of stress and calculated per kilogram actual body weight. The study was limited to 14 days and the main assessment of efficacy was achievement of positive nitrogen balance. There was no difference in the ability of the patient to achieve nitrogen balance based on caloric intake. A subsequent study by Choban and colleagues[43] evaluated the benefit of hypocaloric feedings in stressed obese patients, including those with type 2 DM. Nine patients had glycosuria (5 hypocaloric, 4 control) and one mild ketonuria (hypocaloric) documented during the study. Twelve patients (6 hypocaloric, 6 control) received insulin at some time during the study; 11 of these had an admission diagnosis of DM. Mean insulin dose per day was 36.1 ± 47.1 units in the hypocaloric group compared to 61.1 ± 61.1 units in the control group (NS). An admission diagnosis of DM was present in 13 (43%) patients (4 type I, 9 type 2), 7 patients in the hypocaloric group, and 6 in the control group. There appeared to be a trend toward decreased insulin requirements among the diabetic patients in the hypocaloric group. There was no difference in the number of diabetic patients in each group receiving insulin; however, among the type 2 diabetic patients, the average number of study days in which insulin was required was significantly less in the hypocaloric group (3.2 ± 2.7 days, hypocaloric [*N* = 5], versus 8.0 ± 2.5 days, control [*N* = 4], *p* < .05). Because of large intragroup variability, the differences in average daily serum glucose and the average daily insulin dosage did not reach statistical significance. A second significant finding in both hypocaloric studies was that control patients lost more weight over time than did the hypocaloric patients. The control group also gained more weight initially and subsequently lost this excess gain as they recovered, which probably reflects greater fluctuations in fluid balance in the control group. The objective of hypocaloric feedings should be to achieve optimum nitrogen balance with improved control of glucose status rather than weight loss. The majority of these studies suggest that weight loss in stressed obese patients receiving hypocaloric feedings is minimal.

The results of these studies support the efficacy of hypocaloric feedings in patients who are greater than 130% of IBW and who have normal renal function. The hypocaloric formula is used at a rate that provides 2 g protein per kilogram IBW per day. Successful postoperative hypocaloric nutritional support depends on the provision of adequate protein. For patients with functional GI tracts a similar enteral hypocaloric formula using Promote plus Promod (Ross Laboratories, Columbus, Ohio) can be used. All patients should undergo UUN studies and calculation of nitrogen balance. If the patient is in negative nitrogen balance, the rate of the formula is increased to reach positive nitrogen balance. The primary aim of these studies is to establish safety and to avoid risks inherent in overfeeding, not weight loss.

Although hypocaloric feedings that supply sufficient protein to stressed patients who are mild to moderately obese appear to be capable of producing nitrogen balance in this population, these studies observed a small number of subjects. A recent study in elderly obese, trauma-stressed patients did not support the ability of this group of patients to achieve nitrogen balance with this regimen.[47] Frankenfield and colleagues[44] reported that despite wide variation in energy intake among trauma patients receiving hypocaloric versus eucaloric feedings, there was no attenuation of nitrogen losses in either group. The advantage of this treatment modality seems to include better control of glucose homeostasis, possible improvement of fluid status control, and decreases in weight gain during treatment. Mechanisms resulting in improved fluid and electrolyte status, changes in body composition, differences in length of stay, and other medical outcomes are yet to be studied.

Conclusion

Obesity is a growing public health problem in the United States and is associated with a significant increase in morbidity and mortality in hospitalized patients. Providing appropriate calorie and protein needs for these patients reduces the stress associated with both overfeeding and underfeeding in this population. Further research is needed to identify the appropriate energy and protein requirements of this population of patients at various levels of stress. Hypocaloric feedings appear promising as a therapeutic regimen in obese patients who are mildly to moderately stressed. These feedings protect against the risks of overfeeding on the pulmonary, hepatic, and cardiovascular systems, and it appears they are well tolerated in this group of patients.

REFERENCES

1. Allison DB, Fontaine KR, Manson JE, Stevens J, VanItallie TB: Annual deaths attributable to obesity in the United States, *JAMA* 282(16): 1530-1538, 1999.
2. Public Health Service: *Healthy people 2000: national health promotion and disease prevention objectives,* Publication PHS 90-50212, Washington, DC, 1990, US Department of Health and Human Services.
3. Mokdad AH, Serdula MK, Dietz W, Bowman B, Marks J, Koplan J: The spread of the obesity epidemic in the United States, 1991-1998, *JAMA* 282(16):1519-1522, 1999.
4. Must A, Strauss RS: Risks and consequences of childhood and adolescent obesity, *Int J Obes* 23(suppl 2):S2-S11, 1999.
5. Public Health Service: *Healthy people 2010: conference edition,* Washington, DC, 2000, Office of Disease Prevention and Health Promotion, US Department of Health and Human Services.
6. Wolf AM, Colditz GA: Social and economic effects of body weight in the United States, *Am J Clin Nutr* 63(3 suppl):466S-469S, 1996.
7. Wolf AM, Colditz GA: Current estimates of the economic cost of obesity in the United States, *Obes Res* 6(2):97-106, 1998.
8. Jeevanandam M, Young DH, Schiller WR: Obesity and the metabolic response to severe multiple trauma in man, *J Clin Invest* 87(1):262-269, 1991.
9. Gottschlich MM, Mayes T, Khoury JC, Warden GD: Significance of obesity on nutritional, immunologic, hormonal, and clinical outcome parameters in burns, *J Am Diet Assoc* 193(11):1261-1268, 1993.
10. National Institutes of Health: Clinical guidelines on the identification and treatment of overweight and obesity in adults—the evidence report, *Obes Res* 6(suppl 2):51S-209S, 1998.
11. World Health Organization: Physical status: the use and interpretation of anthropometry. Report of a WHO Expert Committee, *World Health Organ Tech Report Serv* 854:1-452, 1995.
12. Metropolitan Life Insurance Company: *Build and blood pressure study,* vol 1, Chicago IL, 1959, Society of Actuaries.
13. Metropolitan Life Insurance Company: *Statistical Bulletin,* January-June, 1983, pp 64:3-9.
14. Hamwi GJ: Changing dietary concepts. In Donowski TS (ed): *Diabetes mellitus: diagnosis and treatment,* New York, 1964, American Diabetes Association Inc.
15. Simopoulos AP: Body weight reference standards. In VanItallie TB, Simopoulos AP (eds): *Obesity: new directions in assessment and management,* Philadelphia, 1995, Charles Press Publishers.
16. Bouchard C, Bray GA, Hubbard VS: Basic and clinical aspects of regional fat distribution, *Am J Clin Nutr* 52(5):946-950, 1990.
17. Van Itallie TB: Health implications of overweight and obesity in the United States, *Ann Intern Med* 103(6, Pt 2):983-988, 1985.
18. Glass AR: Endocrine aspects of obesity, *Med Clin North Am* 73(1): 139-160, 1989.
19. Bjorntorp P: Abdominal fat distribution and disease: an overview of epidemiological data, *Ann Med* 24(1):15-18, 1992.
20. Bray GA: Complications of obesity, *Ann Intern Med* 103(6 Pt 2): 1052-1062, 1985.)
21. Hubert HB, Feinleib M, McNamara PM, Castelli WP: Obesity as an independent risk factor for cardiovascular disease: a 26 year follow up of participants in the Framingham Heart Study, *Circulation* 67(5):968-977, 1983.
22. Garfinkel L: Overweight and cancer, *Ann Intern Med* 103(6 Pt 2): 1034-1036, 1985.
23. Hershcopf RJ, Bradlow HL: Obesity, diet, endogenous estrogens, and the risk of hormone-sensitive cancer, *Am J Clin Nutr* 45(1 suppl):283-289, 1987.
24. Manson JE, Colditz GA, Stampler MJ, Willett WC, Rosner B, Monson RR, Speizer FE, Hennekens CH: A prospective study of obesity and risk of coronary heart disease in women, *N Engl J Med* 322(13):882-889, 1990.
25. Wilcosky T, Hyde J, Anderson JJB, Bangdiwala S, Duncan B: Obesity and mortality in the lipid research clinics program follow-up study, *J Clin Epidemiol* 43(8):743-752, 1990.
26. Reaven GM: Role of insulin resistance in human disease, *Diabetes* 37(12):1595-1607, 1988.
27. Zumoff B: Hormonal abnormalities in obesity: cause or effect. In VanItallie TB, Simopoulos AP, Gullo SP, Futterweit W (eds): *Obesity: new directions in assessment and management,* Philadelphia, 1995, Charles Press Publishers, pp 40-65.

28. American Sleep Disorders Association: *International classification of sleep disorders,* Rochester, MN, 1990, American Sleep Disorders Association.

29. Bray GA: Complications of obesity, *Ann Intern Med* 103(6 Pt 2): 1052-1062, 1985.

30. Kral JG: Morbid obesity and related health risks, *Ann Intern Med* 103 (6 Pt 2):1043-1047, 1985.

31. National Institutes of Health: Health implications of obesity, *Ann Intern Med* 103(6 Pt 2):1073-1077, 1985.

32. Ireton-Jones CS, Francis C: Obesity: nutrition support practice and application to critical care, *Nutr Clin Pract* 10(4):144-149, 1995.

33. Pavlou KN, Hoefer MA, Blackburn GL: Resting energy expenditure in moderate obesity, *Ann Surg* 203(2):136-141, 1986.

34. Daly JM, Heymsfield SB, Head CA, Harvey LP, Nixon DW, Katzeff H, et al: Human energy requirements: overestimation by widely used prediction equation, *Am J Clin Nutr* 42(6):1170-1174, 1985.

35. Ireton-Jones CS: Evaluation of energy expenditures in obese patients, *Nutr Clin Pract* 4(4):127-129, 1989.

36. Ireton-Jones CS, Turner WW Jr: Actual or ideal body weight: which should be used to predict energy expenditure? *J Am Diet Assoc* 9(2)1: 193-195, 1991.

37. Ireton-Jones CS, Turner WW, Liepa GU, Baxter CR: Equations for estimation of energy expenditure in patients with burns with special reference to ventilatory status, *J Burn Care Rehabil* 13(3):330-333, 1992.

38. Dickerson RN, Rosato EF, Mullen JL: Net protein anabolism with hypocaloric parenteral nutrition in obese stressed patients, *Am J Clin Nutr* 44(6):747-755, 1986.

39. Hwang T, Mou S, Chen M: The importance of a source of sufficient protein in postoperative hypocaloric partial parenteral nutrition support, *J Parenteral Enteral Nutr* 17(3):254-256, 1993.

40. Burge JC, Goon A, Choban PS, Flancbaum L: Efficacy of hypocaloric total parenteral nutrition in hospitalized obese patients: a prospective, double-blind randomized trial, *J Parenter Enteral Nutr* 18(3):203-207, 1994.

41. Pasulka PS, Kohl D: Nutrition support of the stressed obese patient, *Nutr Clin Pract* 4(4):130-132, 1989.

42. Baxter JK, Bistrian BR: Moderate hypocaloric parenteral nutrition in the critically ill, obese patient, *Nutr Clin Pract* 4(4):133-135, 1989.

43. Choban PS, Burge J, Scales D, Flancbaum L: Hypoenergenic nutrition support in hospitalized patients: a simplified method for clinical application, *Am J Clin Nutr* 66(3):546-50, 1997.

44. Frankenfield DC, Smith JS, Cooney RN: Accelerated nitrogen loss after traumatic injury is not attenuated by achievement of energy balance, *J Parenteral Enteral Nutr* 21(6):324-329, 1997.

45. Strang JM, McClugage HB, Evans FA: Further studies in the dietary correction of obesity, *Am J Med Sci* 179:687-694, 1930.

46. Strang JM, McClugage HB, Evans FA: The nitrogen balance during dietary correction of obesity, *Am J Med Sci* 181:336-349, 1931.

47. Liu K, Cho M, Atten M, Panizales E, Walter R, Hawkins D, Donahue P: Hypocaloric parenteral nutrition support in elderly obese patients, *Am Surg* 66(4):394-400, 2000.

Metabolic Stress 39

Gail A. Cresci, MS, RD, CNSD, LD

NUTRITION support is an important supportive treatment in the management of critically ill patients, especially those with prolonged hypercatabolism and hypermetabolism. In such patients, the development of malnutrition is often rapid. This is mainly due to the metabolic alterations that occur in injured and septic patients as opposed to those that occur through starvation (Table 39-1). The metabolic changes that occur during the acute-phase response involve both energy production/use and tissue substrate use.[1] Hypermetabolic patients experience many important nutritional consequences such as decreased tolerance to prolonged fasting, persistent tissue catabolism despite adequate energy and nutrient supply, and a decreased response to anabolic factors.

Metabolic Alterations

The metabolic response to injury and sepsis has been well studied after the pioneering work of Cuthbertson, Selye, Moore, and Kinney.[2] Stressed patients undergo several metabolic phases as a series of ebb and flow states reflecting a patient's response to the severity of the stress (Box 39-1). The earliest, or ebb state, is usually manifested by decreased oxygen consumption, fluid imbalances, inadequate tissue perfusion, and cellular shock. These changes decrease metabolic needs and provide a brief protective environment. The flow state is a hyperdynamic phase in which substrates are mobilized for energy production while increased cellular activity and hormonal stimulation are noted. Subsequently most patients enter a third phase of recovery, or anabolism, which is characterized by normalization of vital signs, increased diuresis, and improved appetite and positive nitrogen balance. Energy expenditure requirements differ for each phase, making the goals of nutrition therapy variable depending on the stage in question. As long as the patient is in a hyperdynamic catabolic state, optimal nutrition support can at best approach zero nitrogen balance in an attempt to minimize further protein wasting. Once the patient enters the anabolic phase, achieving a positive nitrogen balance and repletion of body cell mass through optimal nutrition intervention becomes more realistic. Therefore, early nutrition intervention in critical illness is primarily geared toward sustaining vital organ structure and immune function, ameliorating the catabolic effects of critical illness, and promoting recovery without causing further metabolic derangements.

The high-risk patient usually remains in the catabolic phase for a prolonged period. To meet tissue demands for increased oxygen consumption following acute injury, oxygen delivery increases. This is accomplished by a systemic response that includes an increase in heart rate, minute ventilation, cardiac output, and oxygen consumption and a decrease in peripheral vascular resistance; thus, the cardiac index may exceed 4.5 L/min per meter[2].[2-4] Other systemic responses include hypermetabolism yielding increased proteolysis and nitrogen loss, accelerated gluconeogenesis, hyperglycemia and increased glucose utilization, and retention of salt and water.[1,5] Therefore, critical illness results in a rapid shift from an anabolic state to a catabolic state by mobilizing body stores for energy utilization.[5,6] The mobilization of protein, fat, and glycogen is believed to be mediated through the release of proinflammatory cytokines such as tumor necrosis factor (TNF); interleukins-1, -2 and -6, (IL-1, IL-2, IL-6); and the counterregulatory hormones such as epinephrine, norepinephrine, glucagons, and cortisol.[1-3,7,8] However, Plank and Hill found that prolonged hypermetabolism in septic patients was not reflected in the behavior of circulatory proinflammatory cytokines that were elevated early and then returned to within normal limits within a week or so.[5] It has been suggested that cytokines, compartmentalized within the abdominal cavity, may communicate with the brain via the vagus nerves, accounting for continued catabolism as the result of a neuroendocrine response.[5] Circulating levels of insulin are also elevated in

TABLE 39-1

Metabolic Comparisons Between Starvation and Stress

	Starvation	Stress
Resting energy expenditure	↓	↑↑
Respiratory quotient	↓	↑
Primary fuels	Fat	Mixed
Glucagon	↑	↑
Insulin	↓	↑
Gluconeogenesis	↓	↑↑↑
Plasma glucose	↓	↑
Ketogenesis	↑↑	↓
Plasma lipids	↑	↑↑
Proteolysis	↑	↑↑↑
Hepatic protein synthesis	↑	↑↑
Urinary nitrogen loss	↑	↑↑↑

Data from Barton RG: Nutrition support in critical illness, *Nutr Clin Pract* 10:129, 1994.

Acknowledgment: A special thank you is extended to Judith Fish, MMSc, RD, CNSD, and Janet Friedmann, MS, RD, CNSD, who contributed to the first edition chapter.

most metabolically stressed patients, but the responsiveness of tissues to insulin, especially skeletal muscle, is severely blunted. This relative insulin resistance is believed to be due to the effect of the counterregulatory hormones.[8] The hormonal milieu normalizes only after the injury or metabolic stress has resolved.

Hypermetabolism (resting energy expenditure [REE] and oxygen consumption greater than 115% of basal rate) has been described in critically ill patients, but the degree of hyper-

---

BOX 39-1
Stress Phase Alterations

EBB PHASE

Hormonal
↑ Glucagon
↑ Adrenocorticotropic hormone (ACTH)

Metabolic
Circulatory insufficiency (↑ heart rate, vascular constriction)
↓ Digestive enzyme production
↓ Urine production

Clinical outcomes
Hemodynamic instability

FLOW PHASE

Hormonal and Nonhormonal
↑ Counterregulatory hormones (epinephrine, norepinephrine, glucagon, cortisol)
↑ Insulin
↑ Cytokines (TNF, IL-1,-2, and -6)

Metabolic
Hyperglycemia
↓ Protein synthesis/↑ amino acid efflux
↑ Gluconeogenesis
↑ Glycogenolysis
↑ Lipolysis
↑ Urea nitrogen excretion/net (-) nitrogen balance

Clinical Outcomes
Fluid and electrolyte imbalances
Mild metabolic acidosis
↑ Resting energy expenditure

ANABOLIC PHASE

Hormonal and Nonhormonal
↑ Insulin
↓ Counterregulatory hormones
↓ Cytokines

Metabolic
↑ Protein synthesis
↓ Urea nitrogen excretion/net (+) nitrogen balance
↓ Gluconeogenesis
↓ Lipolysis

Clinical Outcomes
↓ Resting energy expenditure
↑ Lean body mass

IL-1, -2, and -6, Interleukin-1, -2, and -6; *TNF,* tumor necrosis factor.
Data from Seyle H (ed): The physiology and pathology of exposure to stress; a treatise based on concepts of general-adaptation-syndrome and the disease of adaptation. In First Annual Report on Stress, Montreal, Acta, 1951.

---

metabolism reported among studies is variable. For example, reports of REE in trauma patients indicate an elevation of 40% to 60%, whereas the range for patients undergoing major surgery is 10% to 30% and for critically ill medical patients, 35%.[5,9] A recent study found that fever, rather than the marked difference in severity of injury among trauma, surgery, and medical disease, is a more important factor associated with the degree of hypermetabolism in critically ill patients. Frankenfield and colleagues found that the development of fever portends an increase in the hypermetabolic response above that of the injury itself, with energy expenditure being on average 41% above basal across all injury types.[9] Many drugs and supportive treatments influence REE. In normal subjects, the part of REE devoted to the respiratory muscles is limited, amounting to 2% to 3% of total energy expenditure (TEE). In patients with respiratory failure, respiratory work often is increased and the energy expended to breathe is enhanced. The use of mechanical ventilation markedly decreases REE (10% to 30%).[1] Catecholamines are known to exert extensive metabolic activation, including increased glycemia, hepatic glucose production, lipolysis, production of lactic acid, and REE. The importance of catecholamine thermogenesis is dependent on the specific agents, being maximal for epinephrine and minimal for dobutamine. β-blockers have the opposite effect in patients with hyperadrenergic states, such as severe burns and head injury, although they do not abolish the hypermetabolism. Sedatives induce a rapid reduction of energy expenditure, up to less than, or equal to 50%.[1] By contrast, sedation withdrawal induces an elevation of REE in patients with head injury.[1]

The use of alternate fuels to support the hypermetabolic response is reflected in the respiratory quotient (RQ) of critically ill patients. This is exhibited by an elevated RQ of 0.80 to 0.85, reflecting mixed fuel oxidation, as opposed to a nonstressed starved state in which the RQ is in the range of 0.60 to 0.70, reflecting the oxidation of fat as the primary fuel source. Under the influence of the counterregulatory hormones, cytokines, and catecholamines, hepatic glucose production increases through glycogenolysis and gluconeogenesis.[1] The increased endogenous glucose production is poorly suppressed even with exogenous glucose or insulin administration. In stress metabolism, glycogen stores are depleted within 12 to 24 hours of a major catabolic insult, leaving only protein and adipose tissue as potential energy substrates. Gluconeogenic substrates include lactate, alanine, glutamine, glycine, serine, fatty acids, and glycerol. Accompanying the increased glucose production is an increase in flow to and uptake of glucose in the peripheral tissues. Hyperglycemia commonly results from an increased glucagon/insulin ratio and insulin resistance in peripheral tissues (Fig. 39-1).

Alterations in hormone levels also affect lipid metabolism. Elevations of epinephrine, growth hormone, glucagons, and α-adrenergic stimulation induce lipolysis and increase glycerol and free fatty acid (FFA) levels, which are then used as a fuel source.[6,7] Despite elevation in lipolysis, a proportionate increase in lipid oxidation is not observed. This is believed to be due to the elevated insulin levels. Therefore, even though lipid stores are abundant, in most cases they are poorly utilized.[10]

With depleted glycogen stores and diminished ability to utilize fat stores, the body shifts to catabolizing lean body mass

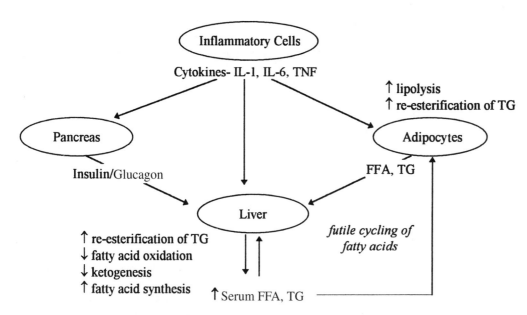

FIGURE 39-1 Fat metabolism in the hypermetabolic patient. *FFA*, free fatty acids; *TG*, triglycerides; *IL*, interleukin; *TNF*, tumor necrosis factor.

as a main energy source and substrate for gluconeogenesis. In addition to gluconeogenesis, amino acids reaching the liver are used for cytokine, immunoglobulin, and hormone synthesis in addition to acute-phase protein synthesis, such as fibrinogen, haptoglobin, C-reactive protein, ceruloplasmin, and α-2 macroglobulin.[7] Alanine is the primary amino acid used for gluconeogenesis, while glutamine transports nitrogen to the kidneys for the synthesis of urea.[4] Although protein synthesis is higher relative to nonstress starvation, its synthesis is significantly reduced from the normal state secondary to the rate of protein catabolism. Nitrogen loss correlates with catabolic rate but not with energy expenditure or energy balance.[11] Accelerated protein breakdown, which is detected by increased urinary nitrogen output, leads to a loss of lean muscle mass, organ failure, and ultimately death. During metabolic stress, ureagenesis and obligatory urinary nitrogen losses may exceed 15 to 20 g/day,[2] resulting in loss of less than or equal to 20% of body protein stores or 2.3 kg body weight over the first 2 weeks,[10] much of which originates from skeletal muscle.[5,12] Furthermore, immobility of patients causes atrophy of skeletal muscle and contributes to a negative nitrogen loss. Spinal cord injury patients have been shown to exhibit an obligatory nitrogen loss for up to 7 weeks of injury.[13] Box 39-2 lists some clinical consequences of protein catabolism.

Metabolic stress deranges normal fluid and electrolyte homeostasis. Electrolyte deficiencies often reflect shifts in concentrations between intravascular and extravascular spaces, rather than total body depletion. With resolution of hemodynamic instability (defined as the time when no further colloid infusion or increasing inotropic support is required) a net accumulation of 5 to 12 L of total body water in trauma and septic patients, respectively, has been found.[14] Resuscitative fluid retention of greater than or equal to 10 L occurs in the extravascular space and results in positive water balance, weight gain, and positive sodium balance.[15] This resuscitative fluid tends to dissipate slowly, 3 weeks in the elderly and 10 days in younger patients.[5,10,16] In addition to inflammatory mediators increasing fluid compartment permeability, altered hydrostatic and colloid oncotic pressures can also result in third-spaced body fluids.

Much of the retained fluid is found in the abdominal cavity, contributing to the common prolonged bowel dysfunction often observed in critically ill patients.[5,16]

Nutrition Assessment

The goals of nutrition intervention during metabolic stress are to minimize loss of body cell mass and support immune function. Nutrient delivery is designed to maintain body cell mass without causing further metabolic complications. Achieving these goals involves accurate and continued nutrition assessment, optimal and timely nutrient delivery, and continuous systematic monitoring of metabolic status. In the absence of carefully designed clinical trials, the rationale for nutrition support is based mostly on clinical judgment. It is not known exactly how long a critically ill patient can tolerate lack of nutrient provision without adverse consequences. Nonetheless, the large nitrogen loss that occurs in catabolic patients suggests that critical depletion of lean tissue may occur after 14 days of starvation.[17] Therefore, nutrition support should be initiated in patients who are not expected to resume oral feeding for 7 to 10 days.[17]

Because critical illness and its treatment can profoundly alter metabolism and significantly increase or decrease energy expenditure, accurate determination of REE is necessary in patients receiving nutrition support to ensure that their energy needs are met and to avoid complications associated with overfeeding or underfeeding.[18] Overfeeding is associated with numerous metabolic complications. It is usually a result of excessive administration of carbohydrate or fat and can result in hepatic steatosis, pulmonary compromise, and hyperglycemia with resultant depressed immune function. Underfeeding leads to poor wound healing, impaired organ function, and altered immunologic status. Unfortunately it is often difficult to achieve estimated energy needs in critically ill patients secondary to delayed return of gastrointestinal (GI) function, decreased renal function, hyperglycemia, and osmolar constraints in patients with brain injury and edema. Typically clinical practice allows for around 60% of TEE to be achieved in trauma patients in the first week and 50% in the

BOX 39-2

Clinical Consequences of Protein Catabolism[12]

Decreased visceral proteins (e.g., albumin, prealbumin)
Increased synthesis of acute phase proteins (e.g., C-reactive protein, fibrinogen)
Decreased coagulation capacity
Impaired immune response
Impaired wound healing
Altered gut function
Intestinal bacterial translocation
Altered parenchymal function
Skeletal muscle wasting
Decreased muscle function (e.g., respiratory muscles)

BOX 39-3

Effect of Injury and Sepsis on Resting Energy Expenditure[1]

Clinical Condition	REE (%)*
Elective uncomplicated surgery	Normal
Major abdominal, thoracic, and vascular surgery	
ICU + mechanical ventilation	105-109 ± 20-28
Cardiac surgery	
ICU + mechanical ventilation	119 ± 21
Multiple injury	
ICU + mechanical ventilation	138 ± 23
Spontaneous ventilation	119 ± 7
Head and multiple injury ICU + mechanical ventilation	150 ± 23
Head injury	
ICU + spontaneous ventilation	126 ± 14
ICU + mechanical ventilation	104 ± 5
Infection	
Sepsis + spontaneous ventilation	121 ± 27
ICU + septic shock + mechanical ventilation	135 ± 28
Sepsis + mechanical ventilation	155 ± 14
Septic shock + mechanical ventilation	102 ± 14
Multiple injury + sepsis + mechanical ventilation + PN	191 ± 38

*Values are percentage of reference value (± standard deviation [SD]).
ICU, Intensive care unit; *REE*, resting energy expenditure; *PN*, parenteral nutrition.

second week, and for septic patients 95% during the first week and 60% during the second week.[19]

Multiple methods for assessing energy requirements in the critically ill are available (see Chapter 6). Although indirect calorimetry remains the "gold standard,"[20] many institutions do not have the technology available and rely upon predictive equations. Predicting energy needs in critical illness can be difficult because of uncertainties about the influence of multiple factors on energy expenditure (Box 39-3). Predictive equations may overestimate energy needs for those mechanically ventilated and sedated because neuromuscular paralysis can decrease energy requirements by as much as 30%.[3] Calculated results are only as accurate as the variables used in the equation. Obesity and resuscitative water weight complicate the use of these equations and lend to a tendency for overfeeding.[21] It is unclear as to whether ideal body weight (IBW) or total body weight should be used in predictive energy equations. It has been reported that obese patients should receive 20 to 30 kcal/kg IBW per day.[22] The use of adjusted body weight, particularly in those whose IBW is greater than 130%, may also be preferable.[21] Predictive equations have been developed to account for obesity; using actual body weight; and trauma, burns, and ventilatory status.[23] Patino and colleagues reported a hypocaloric-hyperproteinic nutrition regimen provided during the first days of the flow phase of the adaptive response to injury, sepsis, and critical illness.[24] The regimen consists of a daily supply of 100 to 200 g of glucose and 1.5 to 2.0 g of protein per kg IBW. Overall, energy requirements for patients with metabolic stress range from 20 to 35 kcal/kg usual body weight per day.[4]

Glucose is the main fuel for the central nervous system (CNS), bone marrow, and injured tissue. A minimum of about 100 g per day is necessary to maintain CNS function as well as drive the citric acid cycle. In the metabolically stressed adult, the maximum rate of glucose oxidation is 4 to 7 mg/kg per minute,[25] roughly equivalent to 400 to 700 g/day in a 70-kg person. Provision of glucose greater than this rate usually results in lipogenesis[4] and hyperglycemia. In the hypermetabolic patient, a portion of the oxidized glucose is derived from endogenous amino acid substrates via gluconeogenesis. In the severely stressed patient, up to 2 mg/kg per minute of glucose may be provided via gluconeogenesis, and this endogenous production is poorly suppressed by exogenous glucose administration.[26] In fact, providing additional glucose in these situations can lead to severe hyperglycemia. Exogenous insulin

delivery tends to be ineffective with increasing cellular glucose uptake in critically ill patients because the rate of glucose oxidation is already maximized and because endogenous insulin concentrations are already elevated. Complications of excess glucose administration include hyperglycemia, hyperosmolar states, excess carbon dioxide production, and hepatic steatosis.[4,26] Therefore it is recommended that glucose be provided at a rate less than or equal to 5 mg/kg per minute or approximately 50% to 60% of total energy requirements in critically ill patients, and that they be monitored closely for metabolic complications.

Protein needs of critically ill patients are significantly increased compared with those patients with simple starvation. In addition to muscle proteolysis during metabolic stress, increased ureagenesis, increased hepatic synthesis of acute phase proteins, increased urinary nitrogen losses, and the increased use of amino acids as oxidative substrate for energy production are also noted. Although the high catabolic rate is not reversed by provision of glucose and protein,[27] the protein synthetic rate is responsive to amino acid infusions, and nitrogen balance is attained through the support of protein synthesis.[28,29] Current recommendations for stressed patients are for 15% to 20% of the total nutrient intake to be provided as protein or 1.5 to 2.0 g/kg per day.[30,31] Excess protein administration has not been shown to be beneficial and, in fact, can cause azotemia; in conjunction with excess calories, this may also increase carbon dioxide production in patients with respiratory compromise.[14,18]

Lipids become an important substrate in critically ill patients because they can facilitate protein sparing, decrease the risk of excess carbohydrate, limit volume delivery by their high caloric density, and provide essential fatty acids. Daily fat can be provided without adverse effect because critically ill patients efficiently metabolize moderate amounts of exogenous lipids.[32] Fat may comprise between 10% to 30% of total energy requirements, with a minimum of 2% to 4% as essential fatty acids to prevent deficiency.[30] Hypermetabolic patients should be monitored for tolerance of lipid delivery, especially if high levels are provided, because it may cause metabolic complications such as hyperlipidemia; coagulopathies; impaired immune function; and hypoxemia, resulting from impaired diffusing capacity and ventilation/perfusion abnormalities.[18] These complications are associated with intravenous infusions and are not only due to the quantity of lipid provided but also result from the rate of delivery. The rate of infusion should not exceed 0.1 g/kg per hour. Infusing lipids continuously over 18 to 24 hours while monitoring serum triglyceride levels and liver function tests to ensure tolerance may minimize complications.[4]

Other therapies provided in the critically ill should be considered for possible energy provision. Examples include lipid-based medications (e.g., propofol) and dextrose (e.g., intravenous fluids, hemofiltration).

Fluid and electrolyte provision can vary greatly in the critically ill. Altered electrolyte levels can impair organ function and are usually manifested by cardiac dysrhythmias, ileus, and impaired mentation. Fluid and electrolytes should be provided to maintain adequate urine output and normal serum electrolytes, with emphasis on the intracellular electrolytes, potassium, phosphorus, and magnesium. These are required for protein synthesis and the attainment of nitrogen balance. Standard fluid requirements are estimated at 35 ml/kg with increased requirements for those with increased losses (e.g., high output fistulas, ostomy) and increased renal solute loads or decreased for those with fluid restrictions (e.g., kidney, liver, heart failure). Once nutrition support is initiated, fluid balance, body weight, and electrolytes should be monitored closely because they may change rapidly once adequate protein and calories have been provided and the patient shifts from catabolism to anabolism.

Currently there are no specific guidelines regarding vitamin and mineral requirements in the critically ill. It is presumed that needs are increased during stress and sepsis because of increased metabolic demands; however, objective data to support supplementation are lacking. The antioxidant vitamins and minerals have received the most recent attention. Oxygen-free radicals and other reactive oxygen metabolites are believed to be generated during critical illness (see Chapter 11). This response is most likely mediated by release of cytokines and initiation of an acute phase response and redistribution of hepatic protein synthesis.[33] Along with increased levels of free radicals, decreased levels of circulating vitamins C and E have been found after surgery, trauma, burns, sepsis, and long-term parenteral nutrition (PN).[4]

Supplementation of large doses of antioxidants in critical illness has not consistently been shown to be beneficial. Studies currently in progress are addressing supplementation at various levels and combinations. Providing more than therapeutic doses of single vitamins or minerals in various metabolic situations may be harmful by potentially upsetting the balance of metabolic pathways.[4] Therefore, current recommendations are to provide the recommended dietary allowance for vitamins and minerals in the critically ill until further research definitely defines optimal dosing.[30] Enteral formulations contain this recommended level when they are provided at specified volumes. If those volumes are not tolerated, patients should be supplemented intravenously.

Nutrition Intervention

The ideal route of nutrition intervention in the critically ill has been well studied. Although PN has been lifesaving and successful in reversing malnutrition in many disease states, it has become more apparent that parenteral formulations currently available in the United States may in fact be systemically immunosuppressive, deliver imbalanced nutrient solutions, and alter nutrient uptake and utilization.[34-37] PN allows for more rapid achievement of nutrient requirements than enteral nutrition (EN), but also allows for increased nitrogen excretion.[38] PN has also been associated with a higher rate of hyperglycemia, adding to patient immunocompromise with decreased neutrophil chemotaxis, phagocytosis, oxidative burst, and superoxide production.[36,39] Prospective clinical trials evaluating perioperative PN have shown that subjects receiving PN had greater postoperative infectious morbidity rates than those receiving no EN or no nutrition intervention.[38-43] PN is also more costly than EN.[44,45] Therefore, PN should be considered in the critically ill only when oral or enteral feeding is not anticipated, achieved, or tolerated within 7 days in previously well-nourished patients, and within 5 to 7 days in malnourished patients.[30,39]

Although research supports providing EN in critically ill patients, it is often difficult to provide full energy requirements because of patient intolerance. The etiology of this intolerance is often multifactorial. One clinically significant factor is low intestinal blood flow. Intestinal ischemia and reperfusion is an important determinant of the subsequent development of the proinflammatory state and multiple organ failure (MOF). Although the gut is able to increase its oxygen extraction up to tenfold in a normal state, it remains extremely vulnerable to ischemic injury during low-flow states. Low flow not only exhibits negative effects on mucosal oxygenation and barrier maintenance,[46-48] but also has adverse effects on motility. It is now known that sepsis, endotoxemia, and low-flow states have significant negative effects on GI tract motility, with the colon being the most affected, followed by the stomach and small intestine, respectively.[49] Low-flow states also cause decreases in nutrient absorption with protein absorption believed to be significantly altered; carbohydrate and lipid absorption are also altered but to a lesser degree.[50] Several investigators using animal models have found enteral nutrient delivery at low rates enhances visceral blood flow during low-flow states.[51-55]

Another common occurrence that prevents full enteral nutrient delivery is that of ileus. After a major metabolic insult, ileus commonly results, lasting 24 to 48 hours in the stomach, 48 to 72 hours in the large intestine, and 12 to 24 hours in the small intestine.[4,49] Several hemodynamic factors can affect ileus such as increased intracranial pressure and hyperglycemia. Generally, if small bowel access is available, then critically ill patients may be fed at a low rate enterally as soon as 8 hours after insult. It has been estimated that only 15% to 30% of caloric requirements delivered enterally is needed to provide immunologic and mucosal protective benefits.[56-58] Attempting to obtain 100% of nutrient requirements in critically ill patients often results in intolerance of early enteral feeding.[59] Therefore, a rational approach to enteral feeding in critically ill populations is to initiate and maintain feedings at a low rate (10 to 20 ml/hr) until tolerance is demonstrated. Signs of intolerance include abdominal distention and pain, hypermotility, significant ileus, pneumatosis intestinalis, significant increase in nasogastric tube output, and uncontrollable diarrhea. Enteral feeding should only be advanced according to patient tolerance and decreased or discontinued if any of the aforementioned symptoms are present. Most critically ill patients will tolerate full enteral feeds within 5 to 7 days. However, if goal tube feedings are not tolerated after 5 to 7 days of injury, then it is appropriate to start PN to either provide the balance of the nutrient requirements or provide full nutrition support as clinically indicated.[4]

Nutrition Pharmacology—New Developments

In the past several years, several nutrients and agents have been investigated to determine if they have a pharmacologic effect on specific metabolic functions. Several amino acids have been investigated because of the hypercatabolism and high nitrogen losses that occur during metabolic stress. Branched-chain amino acids (BCAA) leucine, isoleucine, and valine are essential amino acids required for protein synthetic functions. The properties of the BCAAs as energy substrates, substrates for gluconeogenesis, and modulators of muscle protein metabolism make the use of BCAA-enriched solutions theoretically appropriate for the management of the metabolically stressed patient. Balanced amino acid formulations at a dose of 0.5 to 1.2 g/kg per day of branched chain, can improve nitrogen retention with reduced ureagenesis and increased protein synthetic functions relative to standard amino acid formulations.[30] Bower and colleagues concluded that improved patient outcomes were not seen in septic patients receiving PN with a standard amino acid solution versus two BCAA-enriched solutions,[60] while Garcia-de-Lorenzo and associates found that BCAA-enriched parenteral solutions showed a beneficial effect in septic patients.[61] Therefore, the precise role of BCAA-enriched formulations in improving patient outcomes is still to be determined.

Glutamine is known to be a major fuel source for rapidly dividing cells such as enterocytes, reticulocytes, and lymphocytes. In normal metabolic states, glutamine is a nonessential amino acid. However during times of metabolic stress, glutamine is implicated as being conditionally essential because it has been shown to be needed for maintenance of gut metabolism, structure, and function.[62] Decreased plasma glutamine levels have been reported after severe burns, multiple trauma, or multiple organ failure.[63] Studies have shown beneficial effects with supplemental glutamine, its precursors (ornithine α-ketoglutarate and α-ketoglutarate), or glutamine dipeptides (alanine-glutamine, glycine-glutamine).[62] These studies deliver glutamine in pharmacologic doses of 25% to 35% of the dietary protein. Supplemental glutamine has been shown to have multiple benefits, including increased nitrogen retention and muscle mass, maintenance of the GI mucosa and permeability, preserved immune function and reduced infections, and preserved organ glutathione levels.[62]

Arginine, like glutamine, has gained recent attention in critical care nutrition and is considered a conditionally essential amino acid. Arginine is the specific precursor for nitric oxide production and a potent secretagogue for anabolic hormones such as insulin, prolactin, and growth hormone. Under normal circumstances, arginine is considered a nonessential amino acid because it is adequately synthesized endogenously via the urea cycle. However research suggests that during times of metabolic stress, optimal amounts of arginine are not synthesized to promote tissue regeneration or positive nitrogen balance.[62] Research studies in animals and humans have shown positive outcomes from supplementation to include improved nitrogen balance, wound healing, and immune function, and increased anabolic hormones, insulin, and growth hormone.[62] The outcomes are of special interest in the metabolically stressed patient during the flow phase when enhancement of these processes would yield the greatest advantage.

Although lipids are required in critical illness, excess lipid, particularly long-chain triglycerides, can be detrimental.[18] The long-chain fatty acids (ω-6 and ω-3) share the same enzyme systems because they are elongated and desaturated with each pathway competitive, based on substrate availability (see Chapter 9). Omega-3 fatty acids, eicosapentaenoic acid (EPA), and docosahexaenoic acid (DHA) aid the immune system by competing with arachidonic acid for cyclooxygenase metabolism at the cell membrane. Arachidonic acid is an ω-6 fatty acid that at high levels suppresses the immune functions and promotes inflammation. Modifying the ω-6 to ω-3 content of the cell membranes affects T-cell proliferation, cell-to-cell adhesion, plasma membrane fluidity, and cytokine production.[62] In effect, EPA and DHA prevent T cells from becoming overzealous and overreacting to the inflammatory process.[62] A study of patients with acute respiratory distress syndrome (ARDS) revealed that patients who received an enteral formula with fish oil experienced improvement in laboratory indicators of ventilatory status, less days on the ventilator, and shorter time in the ICU compared with those who received an isonitrogenous, isocaloric control.[64] Therefore the ratio of ω-3 and ω-6 fatty acids in an enteral formula may be important for optimizing immune function in the critically ill.

Enteral formulations containing combinations of nutrients with immune function activity (e.g., glutamine, arginine, ω-3 fatty acids, nucleic acids) have been evaluated as components of a balanced enteral diet for critically ill patients. A consensus panel recently recommended that these formulations either do benefit or should benefit patients with blunt and penetrating torso trauma; severe head injury; burns (≥ 30% total body surface area, third degree); and ventilator-dependent, nonseptic medical and surgical patients at risk of subsequent infectious morbidity.[65] The panel recommended further study of immune-enhancing diets in patients with preexisting sepsis because one study showed an increased mortality rate when patients were fed an immune diet. The expected benefits from delivering these products in the aforementioned populations are decreased ICU length of stay, decreased infectious complications, decreased antibiotic days, decreased ventilator days, and a reduction in multiple organ dysfunction. The panel recommended that the earlier the diet could be started the better (e.g., preoperative for 7 to 10 days or when hemodynamically stable). They also stated that at least 50% of calculated nutrient goals should be provided for at least 5 days postinjury.

Carnitine is a metabolite that is normally present in the diet and increases β-oxidation of long-chain fatty acids by promoting their transport across the mitochondrial membrane. Carnitine has also been associated with improving insulin-mediated glucose utilization in humans and reducing nitrogen loss in septic animals and humans.[11] Hypermetabolic patients exhibit decreased intracellular carnitine concentrations with increased acylcarnitine/free carnitine ratio. It is known that intracellular free carnitine may buffer excessive acyl-CoA production, which in stress conditions frequently derives from accelerated free fatty acid oxidation.[11] Free carnitine may react with acyl-CoA to form acylcarnitine and regenerate free-CoA. Other factors in metabolically stressed patients such as decreased dietary intake and increased urinary output may contribute to low carnitine levels. Whether critically ill patients demonstrate improved outcomes when supplemented with carnitine is yet to be determined.

Selenium is an essential trace element that plays a major role in the intracellular antioxidant system as a structural component of the active center of glutathione peroxidase enzymes (SeGSH-Px).[66] These selenoenzymes catalyze the reduction of hydrogen peroxide and several organic hydroperoxides to less toxic products, and play a unique role in protecting cells against the numerous cytopathologic effects of lipid peroxidation, especially membrane lipid peroxidation induced in conditions of oxidative stress. Selenium also appears to play a role in the regulation of inflammatory processes. Oxidative stress and inflammatory reaction may activate SeGSH-PX synthesis, which may then increase the need for selenium in body tissue.[67] Critically ill ICU patients with systemic inflammatory response syndrome (SIRS) were shown to experience an early 40% decrease in plasma selenium concentration, reaching values observed in deleterious nutritional selenium deficiency.[66] The efficacy of selenium treatment in SIRS patients warrants further investigation.

Resistance to growth hormone (GH) and the decreased production and action of insulin-like growth factor I (IGF-I) may be attributable to the negative nitrogen balance seen in critically ill patients.[68] Positive anabolic effects of GH have been reported in septic, burned, and posttraumatic patients, whereas negative effects have also been demonstrated in such critical illness.[69] High doses of GH were associated with increased morbidity and mortality in critically ill adults receiving prolonged intensive care.[68]

Conclusion

Many metabolic alterations occur during metabolic stress, resulting in hypermetabolism and obligatory negative nitrogen balance. Although nutrition intervention plays a vital role in the medical management of these patients, limited substrate tolerance is often observed. Early initiation of nutrition support in those deemed to require intervention for more than 5 to 7 days is recommended, with enteral preferred over parenteral whenever possible. Careful monitoring and adjusting of the nutrition plan as the patient's medical condition changes is essential to avoid harm and produce optimal patient outcomes. Supplemental nutrients such as glutamine, arginine, and ω-3 fatty acids have shown benefits in this population and should be considered as part of the nutrition plan.

REFERENCES

1. Chiolero R, Revelly JP, Tappy L: Energy metabolism in sepsis and injury, *Nutrition* 13(suppl):45S-51S, 1997.
2. Kinney J: Metabolic responses of the critically ill patient, *Crit Care Clin* 11(3):569, 1995.
3. Barton RG: Nutrition support in critical illness, *Nutr Clin Pract* 10(1):129, 1994.
4. Cresci GA, Martindale RG: Nutrition support in trauma. In Gottschlich M, Fuhrman M, Hammond K, Holcombe B, Seidner D (eds): *The science and practice of nutrition support,* ed 3, Dubuque, IA, 2001, Kendall/Hunt, pp 445-464.
5. Plank LD, Hill GL: Sequential metabolic changes following induction of systemic inflammatory response in patients with severe sepsis or major blunt trauma, *World J Surg* 24(6):630-638, 2000.
6. Wolfe RR, Martini WZ: Changes in intermediary metabolism in severe surgical illness, *World J Surg* 24(6):639-647, 2000.
7. Gabay C, Kushner I: Acute-phase proteins and other systemic responses to inflammation, *N Engl J Med* 340(6):448-454, 1999.
8. Khaodhiar L, McCowen K, Bistrian B: Perioperative hyperglycemia, infection or risk? *Curr Opin Clin Nutr Met Care* 2(1):79-82, 1999.
9. Frankenfield DC, Smith JS, Cooney RN, Blosser SA, Sarson GY: Relative association of fever and injury with hypermetabolism in critically ill patients, *Injury* 28(9-10):617-621, 1997.
10. Monk DN, Plank LD, Franch-Arcas G, Finn P, Streat S, Hill G: Sequential changes in the metabolic response in critically injured patients during the first 25 days after blunt trauma, *Ann Surg* 223(4):395-405, 1996.
11. Frankenfield D, Smith JS, Cooney R: Accelerated nitrogen loss after traumatic injury is not attenuated by achievement of energy balance, *J Parenter Enteral Nutr* 21(6):324-329, 1997.
12. Biolo G, Toigo G, Ciocchi B, Situlin R, Iscra F, Gullo A, Cuarnieri G: Metabolic response to injury and sepsis: changes in protein metabolism, *Nutrition* 13(9 suppl):52S-57S, 1997.
13. Rodriguez DJ, Benzel EC, Clevenger FW: The metabolic response to spinal cord injury, *Spinal Cord* 35(9):599-604, 1997.
14. Hill GL: Implications of critical illness, injury, and sepsis on lean body mass and nutritional needs, *Nutrition* 14(6):557-558, 1998.
15. Streat S, Plank L, Hill G: Overview of modern management of patients with critical injury and severe sepsis, *World J Surg* 24(6):655-663, 2000.
16. Deutsch GS: Medical issues of third-spacing, *Support Line* 23:23, 2001.
17. Klein S, Kinney, Jeejeebhoy K, Alpers D, Hellerstein M, Murray M, Twomey P: Nutrition support in clinical practice: review of published data and recommendations for future research directions, *J Parenter Enteral Nutr* 21(3):133-156, 1997.
18. Klein C, Stanek G, Wiles C: Overfeeding macronutrients to critically ill adults: metabolic complications, *J Am Diet Assoc* 98(7):795-806, 1998.
19. Uehara M, Plank L, Hill G: Components of energy expenditure in patients with severe sepsis and major trauma: a basis for clinical care, *Crit Care Med* 27(7):1295-1302, 1999.
20. Flancbaum L, Choban P, Sambucco S, Verducci J, Burge: Comparison of indirect calorimetry, the Fick method, and prediction equations in estimating the energy requirements of critically ill patients, *Am J Clin Nutr* 69(3):461-466, 1999.
21. Cutts M, Dowdy R, Ellersieck M, Edes T: Predicting energy needs in ventilator-dependent critically ill patients: effect of adjusting weight for edema or adiposity, *Am J Clin Nutr* 66(5):1250-66, 1997.
22. Marik P, Varon J: The obese patient in the ICU, *Chest* 113(2):492-498, 1998.
23. Ireton-Jones CS, Turner WW, Liepa GU, et al: Equations for estimation of energy expenditures in patients with burns with special reference to ventilatory status, *J Burn Care Rehab* 13(3):330-333, 1992.
24. Patino J, Echeverri de Pimiento S, Vergara A, Savino P, Rodriguez M, Escallon J: Hypocaloric support in the critically ill, *World J Surg* 23(6):553-559, 1999.

25. Wolfe R, Allsop J, Burke J: Glucose metabolism in man: responses to intravenous glucose infusion, *Metabolism* 28(3):210-220, 1979.

26. Cerra FB: Hypermetabolism, organ failure and metabolic support, *Surgery* 101(1):1-14, 1987.

27. Elwyn DH: Nutritional requirements of adult surgical patients, *Crit Care Med* 8(1):9-20, 1980.

28. Cerra FB, Siegel JH, Coleman B, et al: Septic autocannibalism, a failure of exogenous nutritional support, *Ann Surg* 192(4):570-580, 1980.

29. Shaw J, Wildbore M, Wolfe R: Whole body protein kinetics in severely septic patients, *Ann Surg* 205(3):288-294, 1987.

30. Cerra F, Benitez M, Blackburn G, Irwin R, Jeejeebhoy, et al: Applied nutrition in ICU patients, *Chest* 111(3):769-778, 1997.

31. ASPEN Board of Directors: Practice guidelines, *J Parenter Enteral Nutr* 17(suppl):20SA-21SA, 1993.

32. Nordenstrom J, Carpentier Y, Askanazi J, et al: Free fatty acid mobilization and oxidation during total parenteral nutrition in trauma and infection, *Ann Surg* 198(6):725-735, 1983.

33. Goode HF, Webster NR: Antioxidants in intensive care medicine, *Clin Intensive Care* 4(3):265-269, 1993.

34. Basu R, Muller D, Papp E, Merryweather I, Eaton S, Klein N, Pierro A: Free radical formation in infants: the effect of critical illness, parenteral nutrition, and enteral feeding, *J Pediatr Surg* 34(7):1091-1095, 1999.

35. McQuiggan M, Marvin R, McKinley B, Moore F: Enteral feeding following major torso trauma: from theory to practice, *New Horizons* 7(2):131-146, 1999.

36. Takagi K, Yamamori H, Toyoda Y, Nakajima N, Tashiro T: Modulating effects of the feeding route on stress response and endotoxin translocation in severely stressed patients receiving thoracic esophagectomy, *Nutrition* 16(5):355-360, 2000.

37. Kennedy B, Hall G: Metabolic support of critically ill patients: parenteral nutrition to immunonutrition, *Br J Anesth* 85(2):185-187, 2000.

38. Moore FA, Feliciano DV, Andrassy RJ, et al: Early enteral feeding, compared with parenteral, reduces postoperative septic complications—the results of a meta-analysis, *Ann Surg* 216(2):62-69, 1992.

39. Napolitano L: Parenteral nutrition in trauma patients: glucose-based, lipid-based, or none? *Crit Care Med* 26(5):813-814, 1998.

40. Veterans Affair Total Parenteral Cooperative Study Group: Perioperative total parenteral nutrition in surgical patients, *N Engl J Med* 325(3):525-532, 1991.

41. Brennan MF, Pisters PWT, Posner M, et al: A prospective randomized trial of total parenteral nutrition after major pancreatic resection for malignancy, *Ann Surg* 220(4):436-444, 1994.

42. Moore FA, Moore EE, Jones TN, et al: TEN versus TPN following major abdominal trauma reduced septic morbidity, *J Trauma* 29(7):916-924, 1989.

43. Kudsk K, Croce M, Fabian T, et al: Enteral vs. parenteral feeding: effects on septic morbidity following blunt and penetrating abdominal trauma, *Ann Surg* 215(5):503-514, 1992.

44. Frost P, Bihari D: The route of nutritional support in the critically ill: physiological and economical considerations, *Nutrition* 13(suppl):58S-63S, 1997.

45. Trice S, Melnik G, Page C: Complications and costs of early postoperative parenteral versus enteral nutrition in trauma patients, *Nutr Clin Pract* 12(1):114-119, 1997.

46. Ohri SK, Somassundaram S, Koak Y, et al: The effect of intestinal hypoperfusion on intestinal absorption and permeability during cardiopulmonary bypass, *Gastroenterology* 106(2):318-323, 1994.

47. Fink MP: Adequacy of gut oxygenation in endotoxemia and sepsis, *Crit Care Med* 21(2 suppl):54-58, 1993.

48. Flynn MP: Gastrointestinal mucosal injury in experimental models of shock, trauma and sepsis, *Crit Care Med* 19(6):627-41, 1991.

49. Singh G, Harkema JM, Mayberry AJ, et al: Severe depression of gut absorptive capacity in patients following trauma or sepsis, *J Trauma* 36(6):803-809, 1994.

50. Gardiner K, Barbul A: Intestinal amino acid absorption during sepsis, *J Parenter Enteral Nutr* 17(3):277-283, 1993.

51. Fiddian-Green RG, Baker S: The predictive value of measurement of pH in the wall of the stomach for complications after cardiac surgery: a comparison with other forms of monitoring, *Crit Care Med* 15(2):153-157, 1987.

52. Gosche J, Garrison R, Harris P, et al: Absorptive hyperemia restores intestinal blood flow during *E. coli* sepsis in rat, *Arch Surg* 125(12):1573-1576, 1990.

53. Flynn W, Gosche J, Garrison R: Intestinal blood flow is restored with glutamine or glucose infusion after hemorrhage, *J Surg Res* 52(5):499-504, 1992.

54. Purcell P, Davis R, Branson R, Johnson D: Continuous duodenal feeding restores gut blood flow and increases gut oxygen utilization during PEEP ventilation for lung injury, *Am J Surg* 165(1):188-194, 1993.

55. Kazamias P, Kotzampass K, Koufogiannis D, et al: Influence of enteral nutrition-induced splanchnic hyperemia on septic origin of splanchnic ischemia, *World J Surg* 22(1):6-11, 1998.

56. Shou J, Lappin J, Minard E, Daly J: Total parenteral nutrition, bacterial translocation, and host immune function, *Am J Surg* 167(1):145-150, 1994.

57. Sax HC, Illig K, Ryan C, et al: Low-dose enteral feeding is beneficial during TPN, *Am J Surg* 171(6):587-590, 1996.

58. Okada Y, Klein N, Vansaene H, et al: Small volumes of enteral feedings normalize immune function in infants receiving parenteral nutrition, *J Pediatr Surg* 33(1):16-19, 1998.

59. Montejo J: Enteral nutrition-related gastrointestinal complications in critically ill patients: a multicenter study, *Crit Care Med* 27(8):1447-1453, 1999.

60. Bower R, Muggia-Sullam M, Vallgren S, et al: Branched chain amino acid-enriched solutions in the septic patient, *Ann Surg* 203(1):13-20, 1986.

61. Garcia-de-Lorenzo A, Ortiz-Leyba C, Planas M, et al: Parenteral administration of different amounts of branch-chain amino acids in septic patients: clinical and metabolic aspects, *Crit Care Med* 25(3):418-424, 1997.

62. Schloerb P: Immune-enhancing diets: products, components, and their rationales, *J Parenter Enteral Nutr* 25(suppl):S3-S7, 2001.

63. De-Souza D, Greene L: Pharmacological nutrition after burn injury, *J Nutr* 128(5):797-803, 1998.

64. Gadek J, DeMichele S, Karlstad M, et al: Effect of enteral feeding with eicosapentaenoic acid, gamma-linolenic acid, and antioxidants in patients with acute respiratory distress syndrome, *Crit Care Med* 27(8):1409-1420, 1999.

65. Kudsk K, Schloerb P, DeLegge M, et al: Consensus recommendations from the U.S. Summit on immune-enhancing enteral therapy, *J Parenter Enteral Nutr* 25(suppl):S61-S62, 2001.

66. Forceville X, Vitoux D, Gauzit R, et al: Selenium, systemic immune response syndrome, sepsis, and outcome in critically ill patients, *Crit Care Med* 26(9):1536-1544, 1998.

67. Crosby AJ, Wahle W, Dughie G: Modulation of glutathione peroxidase activity in human vascular endothelial cells by fatty acids and the cytokine interleukin-1, *Biochim Biophys Acta* 1303(3):187-192, 1996.

68. Takala J, Ruokonen E, Webster N, et al: Increased mortality associated with growth hormone treatment in critically ill adults, *N Engl J Med* 341(11):785-792, 1999.

69. Saito H: Anabolic agents in trauma and sepsis: repleting body mass and function, *Nutrition* 14(6):554-556, 1998.

Solid Organ Transplantation 40

Jeanette M. Hasse, PhD, RD, LD, FADA, CNSD

THE field of organ transplantation is relatively young. Kidney transplantation between identical twins was first successfully accomplished in 1954,[1] and intestinal transplantation joined the ranks of organ transplantation in the 1990s. Solid organ transplantation is an accepted form of treatment for patients with end-stage organ failure who no longer respond to other medical or surgical treatments. Today, transplanted organs include the heart, kidney, liver, lung, pancreas, and small intestine.

Many factors affect the success and outcome of transplantation, and many, including the patient's reaction to a transplanted graft and immunosuppression, are uncontrollable and unpredictable. A patient's nutritional status can be controlled and manipulated by appropriate nutrition therapy both before and after transplantation. Other diseases and medical conditions are improved by nutrition therapy, and it seems likely that the same is true for transplantation. Attention to specific nutritional needs of transplant recipients should improve the outcome and success of organ transplantation.

Pretransplant Phase

Nutritional Status of Transplant Candidates

Nutrition problems plague many transplant patients both before and after transplantation. Appropriate nutrition therapy is vital to the success of transplantation. Before treatment can be applied, an accurate nutrition assessment must be performed. Nutrition assessment is difficult in transplant candidates because organ failure affects many commonly used objective nutrition assessment parameters.[2-7]

OBJECTIVE NUTRITION ASSESSMENT. Objective nutrition assessment parameters include weight, anthropometric measurements, serum protein levels, skin antigen tests, nitrogen balance studies, and other laboratory tests. Body weight, the most widely used assessment parameter, is expressed as a percentage of ideal or usual weight, or as body mass index (BMI). Subjects with organ failure, however, frequently suffer from ascites and edema, which alter body weight and render these measurements unreliable.[2,6-8]

Anthropometry is used to measure somatic fat and muscle stores. Triceps skinfold and midarm muscle circumference measurements have limited usefulness because they are affected by hydration status and age and by the examiner's technique. In addition, they are insensitive measures: small changes over a short period of time are difficult to detect. If arm measurements are used to assess transplant candidates, they must not be performed on an arm where a dialysis shunt is located and they are best used serially over a long time.

Serum concentrations of albumin, transferrin, thyroxine-binding prealbumin, and retinol-binding protein are common measures of visceral protein stores. Again, because hydration status of transplant candidates frequently is altered, these parameters are not useful in fluid-overloaded patients.[6,7] Other factors that affect the interpretation of serum albumin concentrations are liver and renal function, zinc deficiency, administration of albumin or corticosteroids, and losses through the skin, gastrointestinal (GI) tract, wounds, or bleeding. The interpretation of serum transferrin level as a nutrition parameter is affected by liver function, iron status, zinc deficiency, and excessive excretion, as in nephrotic syndrome. Infection and kidney and liver function affect the interpretation of serum prealbumin levels.[6,7] Finally, serum retinol-binding protein is affected by renal failure, vitamin A status, hyperthyroidism, and cystic fibrosis. As nutrition assessment parameters for organ transplant candidates, protein concentrations have limited value.

Some objective assessments of nutritional status are used less frequently than other tests. These methods include skin antigen testing, nitrogen balance, creatinine-height index, 3-methylhistidine excretion, and indirect calorimetry. These tests, too, are of limited value in transplant candidates. Many transplant patients are anergic or will become so when immunosuppressant medications are administered. Therefore, skin antigen tests are not reliable indicators of nutritional status. Nitrogen balance requires an accurate record of nitrogen intake and output. Protein intake may be altered and varies from day to day. Nitrogen output is difficult to measure when poor renal function leads to nitrogen retention, poor liver function prevents conversion of ammonia to urea, or excessive nitrogen loss results from profuse diarrhea or chest tube losses.[6] Age, sex, protein intake, renal function, and infection are all nonnutritional factors that influence 3-methylhistidine excretion.[6] Creatinine-height index also is influenced by renal function, liver function, and protein intake.[2,6] Performed properly, indirect calorimetry accurately measures a transplant candidate's resting energy expenditure (REE). Changes in medical condition, however, such as increased ascites or change in work of breathing, alter the REE, which must be reassessed as the patient's condition changes.

SUBJECTIVE NUTRITION ASSESSMENT. Because the interpretation of objective assessment parameters for organ transplant recipients is fraught with difficulties, a subjective global assessment (SGA) technique is helpful. SGA is a method of nutrition assessment by which a properly trained dietitian can determine nutritional status based on the patient's history, functional capacity, disease state, and physical appearance.[3,7,9,10]

The history portion of the SGA involves questioning the patient and family members about the patient's weight history (considering fluid fluctuations), appetite, factors inhibiting dietary intake, and a diet history. It is important to determine whether the patient is experiencing persistent symptoms that affect nutritional intake, such as bowel irregularity, anorexia, nausea, vomiting, or chewing and swallowing difficulty. A diet history reveals the adequacy of the patient's current diet. The patient's functional status contributes to retention or loss of muscle mass. An understanding of the disease state, intercurrent medical conditions, and medications helps the dietitian determine the degree of nutritional stress these factors cause. Finally, the dietitian must examine the patient for signs of muscle wasting, ascites, edema, and fat depletion. Other information, such as history of diabetes, use of supplements and alcohol, and social history, helps the dietitian devise an individualized nutrition care plan.

Once all of this information is collected, the dietitian makes a final assessment and creates a nutrition care plan. Traditional SGA categories are (1) well-nourished, (2) moderately (or suspected of being) malnourished, and (3) severely malnourished (Table 40-1). Using a combination of valid objective and subjective data seems to be the best approach to assessing transplant candidates.

Malnutrition in Transplant Candidates

PREVALENCE OF PRETRANSPLANT MALNUTRITION. The prevalence of malnutrition among transplant candidates varies with the population assessed and the assessment parameters used to evaluate nutritional status. Table 40-2 summarizes research on nutritional status of solid organ transplant candidates.

EFFECTS OF PRETRANSPLANT MALNUTRITION ON POST-TRANSPLANT OUTCOME. Although many factors affect transplant outcome, nutritional status may be the only reversible one. Malnutrition theoretically contributes to increased posttransplant morbidity because of its effects on immune function, infection, and wound healing. The effect of pretransplant malnutrition on posttransplant outcome has been analyzed among transplant candidates. Frazier and colleagues reported that, among their first 52 heart transplant patients, mortality was higher among poorly nourished patients.[24] Malnutrition, defined by hypoalbuminemia in kidney/pancreas transplant recipients, resulted in an increased rate of cytomegalovirus infection and graft failure, as well as a trend toward reduced survival.[12] Hypoalbuminemia in liver transplant patients corre-

lated with reduced 6-month survival.[25] Lower preoperative handgrip strength and branched-chain amino acid levels were correlated with prolonged intensive care unit stays in patients who had undergone liver transplantation.[15] Malnutrition based on anthropometry and/or body cell mass by bioelectrical impedance correlated with reduced survival in liver transplant recipients.[16,18,20] Two studies of liver transplant patients in which SGA was the nutrition assessment technique suggested that severely malnourished liver transplant patients had reduced survival compared with better nourished patients.[17,19]

CAUSES OF MALNUTRITION. Many factors contribute to malnutrition in patients awaiting organ transplantation. Knowing the cause of malnutrition helps define its treatment. Although each type of organ failure precipitates specific nutrition alterations, some nutrition problems are common to all solid organ transplant candidates. Anorexia and dysgeusia frequently are caused by disease or medication for the disease.[8,24,26] Symptoms of nausea, vomiting, early satiety, and diarrhea result in diminished food intake[26] and drug-nutrient interactions alter nutrient absorption and utilization. Malabsorption secondary to certain disease states results in nutrient loss.[11,24,26] Depression caused by chronic illness often weakens a person's desire to eat. Finally, many symptoms of organ failure are treated with diet restriction, including restriction of protein, carbohydrate, fat, electrolytes, minerals, or fluid. Diet restrictions frequently result in suboptimal intake.

Other causes of malnutrition can be linked to nutrition problems related to specific organ failure. Glucose intolerance, hypertriglyceridemia, protein malnutrition, and abnormalities of calcium, phosphorus, vitamin D, and aluminum are common in patients with end-stage renal disease.[27] Kidney transplant candidates also can suffer from uremia and protein and electrolyte abnormalities. Uremia causes catabolism through impairment of insulin-stimulated protein synthesis and increased muscle protein degradation.[28] Heart transplant candidates often suffer from cardiac cachexia and fluid abnormalities.[8] Cardiac cachexia results from decreased nutrient intake, depressed GI absorptive capacity, increased stool and urine nutrient losses, and hypermetabolism secondary to increased cardiac and pulmonary energy expenditure.[8,11,24] In addition, ascites and early satiety can develop in patients with hepatic congestion due to heart failure,[29] and reduced circulatory function can impair metabolic waste removal and result in poor nutrient delivery to tissues.[30] Patients with hepatic failure may have protein, fluid, and electrolyte abnormalities as well as

TABLE 40-1

Subjective Global Assessment Ratings in Solid Organ Transplant Patients

SGA Rating	Determining Factors
Well-nourished	Stable weight (consider whether ascites or edema masks weight loss) Good appetite, adequate intake No signs of subcutaneous fat loss or muscle wasting
Moderately (or suspected of being) malnourished	Unintentional weight loss (consider whether ascites or edema masks weight loss) Reduction in dietary intake Mild subcutaneous fat loss and muscle wasting
Severely malnourished	Severe, unintentional weight loss (consider whether ascites or edema masks weight loss) Inadequate dietary intake Obvious signs of subcutaneous fat loss and muscle wasting

TABLE 40-2

Nutritional Status of Organ Transplant Candidates

Authors	Transplant Population Studied (No.)	Nutrition Assessment Techniques	Rate of Malnutrition
Grady and Herold[11]	Cardiac transplant patients (65)	Anthropometry, skin-antigen tests	Depressed somatic protein stores (31%) Anergy (32.3%) Pretransplant weight was 102% of ideal and 90% of usual
Becker et al.[12]	Simultaneous kidney-pancreas transplant recipients (232)	Serum albumin level	Pretransplant serum albumin level <3.5 g/dl (44%)
Miller et al.[13]	Kidney transplant patients with diabetes (24) and without (21)	Weighing, anthropometry	Body weight <85% ideal (16/45) Midarm muscle circumference <5th percentile (38%) Midarm muscle circumference >50th percentile (58%)
Akerman et al.[14]	Liver transplant candidates (104)	Weighing, anthropometry, secretory protein levels, 24-hr creatinine and urea nitrogen, immunologic studies	Triceps skinfold <5th percentile (33%) Midarm muscle circumference <5th percentile (43%) Mean serum albumin level 2.5 g/dl Mean nitrogen balance − 0.7 ± 2.5 mM Creatinine height index 69 ± 32% of standard Depressed total lymphoctye count (64%) Anergy (90%)
DiCecco et al.[2]	Liver transplant candidates (74)	Diet history, anthropometry, biochemical and immunocompetence evaluations	Some degree of malnutrition (100%)
Figueiredo et al.[15]	Liver transplant patients (53)	Body cell mass, SGA, anthropometry, handgrip dynamometry, biochemical and amino acid profile, Child's score, dual-energy x-ray absorptiometry	By SGA, mild malnutrition (39.6%) By SGA, moderate to severe malnutrition (45.2%)
Harrison et al.[16]	Liver transplant patients (102)	Anthropometry	Midarm muscle circumference and triceps skinfold thickness ≤25th percentile (79%) <5th percentile (28%)
Hasse et al.[17]	Liver transplant patients (1224)	SGA	Moderate to severe malnutrition (75%)
Lautz et al.[18]	Liver transplant candidates (123)	Anthropometry, 24-hr urinary creatinine excretion, bioelectrical impedance analysis, total body potassium counting, ultrasound examination	Some signs of protein-calorie malnutrition (65%)
Pikul et al.[19]	Liver transplant patients (68)	SGA	Mild to severe malnutrition (79%)
Selberg et al.[20]	Liver transplant patients (150)	Body composition analysis (24-hr urinary creatinine excretion, anthropometry, bioelectrical impedance analysis)	Body cell mass <35% body weight (47%)
Stephenson et al.[21]	Liver transplant patients (109)	SGA	Moderate to severe malnutrition (64%)
Madill et al.[22]	Lung transplant candidates	Diet history, physical examination, anthropometry, biochemical markers, SGA	By SGA, severe (11.4%) or moderate (48.6%) malnutrition Subnormal BMI in patients with emphysema and cystic fibrosis Normal serum albumin and transferrin levels
Williams et al.[23]	Lung transplant patients (220)	Weighing	Weight <90% ideal (38% patients <45 yr, 19% patients >60)

BMI, Body mass index; *SGA*, subjective global assessment.

nutrient malabsorption, esophageal strictures resulting in dysphagia, and mental alterations due to accumulation of toxins in the blood. Ascites leads to early satiety, and liver disease can cause increased intestinal protein losses, impairment of hepatic protein synthesis, altered intermediary metabolism, and elevated energy requirements. Finally, malabsorption occurs in the presence of depressed bile salt levels, dysfunction of the small intestine secondary to portal hypertension or lymph stasis, drug-nutrient interaction, and pancreatic insufficiency.[5] Lung transplant candidates' metabolic rates are often elevated because of increased work of breathing.[22] Hyperinflation in patients with lung disease can cause early satiety.[22] Patients with cystic fibrosis seem to lose weight because of increased energy requirements from chronic lung infection rather than from malabsorption.[22] Long-term diabetes mellitus has nutri-

tional and medical consequences for persons who need a pancreas transplant, including neuropathy, nephropathy, gastroparesis, cardiovascular disease, and blindness. Small-bowel transplant candidates are dependent on parenteral nutrition (PN) and submit to the transplant procedure so they can eat normally. Long-term PN can lead to metabolic bone disease, trace mineral deficiencies, cholestasis, cholelithiasis, hepatic dysfunction, portal hypertension, splenomegaly, and urolithiasis.

Effect of Pretransplant Nutrition Support on Posttransplant Outcome

Pretransplant nutrition is vital to the survival of transplant candidates and plays a major role in their recovery after operation. The waiting period for donor organs continues to increase, and during this time nutritional status can deteriorate. Poor nutritional status at the time of transplantation is associated with increased posttransplant morbidity and mortality.[12,15-20,25] One could hypothesize that improving nutritional status or preventing deterioration during the waiting period should decrease posttransplant morbidity.

In one study of 10 children awaiting liver transplantation, researchers found that enteral nasogastric tube feeding improved pretransplant nutritional status without causing adverse clinical or biochemical effects.[31] Adult liver transplant candidates may also benefit from pretransplant nutrition intervention. In one study, 9 patients received oral diet, 19 received oral diet plus 0.5 g pro/kg per day from a hepatic supplement (Hepatic Aid, B. Braun, Irvine, CA) and 18 received oral diet and 0.5 g pro/kg per day from a casein supplement (Ensure, Ross Products Division, Abbott Laboratories, Columbus, OH).[32] Patients in the supplemented groups consumed more calories and protein than control patients. There were no differences between groups in nutritional status by SGA, anthropometry, encephalopathy, or serum laboratory tests. However, patients drinking the hepatic supplement had fewer hospitalizations per patient (0.2 ± 0.2) versus the casein (1.7 ± 0.2) and control groups (0.8 ± 0.4).

Some studies of patients with organ failure who did not undergo transplantation showed potential improvement with nutrition supplementation. Hirsch and colleagues followed 25 patients with alcoholic cirrhosis (Child-Pugh B or C) for 6 months after initiation of 1000 calories per day of Ensure in addition to diet.[33] Patients drank 85% of prescribed supplement. After 6 months, REE, total body fat, serum albumin levels, and cellular immunity improved. Thirty-one patients with alcoholic liver disease were randomized to receive either a casein-based formula via a feeding tube plus a regular diet or a regular diet alone.[34] Those who were tube fed demonstrated improvement in hepatic encephalopathy, reduced serum bilirubin levels, and shorter antipyrine half-lives than patients who ate only their normal diet. As expected, the tube-fed group received almost twice the calories and protein that the control group received. In a similar study, 35 severely malnourished, cirrhosis patients were randomized to receive either a low-sodium diet or tube feedings.[35] The diet control group had a lower survival rate and lower calorie intakes (1320 versus 2110 calories) than the tube-fed group. In addition, an improvement in serum albumin level and Child's score was seen only in the supplemented patients.

Severe Obesity in Transplant Candidates

Severe obesity in transplant candidates is another concern. Transplant surgeons are reluctant to perform transplantation in extremely obese patients because of technical difficulties and the theoretically increased morbidity rates. For heart transplantation, body weight greater than 110% of ideal body weight (IBW) in a recipient is associated with decreased posttransplant survival.[36]

Obesity has been identified as a factor in delayed graft function in kidney transplant recipients.[37-40] Some researchers have demonstrated that obesity adversely affects kidney and kidney/pancreas graft survival,[38,39,41-44] although this has not been universally shown.[40,45]

Wound infection has been identified as an adverse outcome related to obesity in liver transplant recipients.[46-49] However,

graft function and mortality have not been affected. The conclusion from these studies seems to be that for obese patients, transplantation has some long-term risks, and that, if possible, weight loss should be encouraged before transplantation.

Pretransplant Nutrition Therapy

Until the theory that pretransplant nutrition support improves patient outcome is disproved, the accepted plan of care is to provide nutrition to, at least, prevent further deterioration or, at best, improve nutritional status. Nutrition can be provided orally, by enteral tube feeding, or intravenously.

The most desirable route of nutrition is an oral diet. Many factors affect a transplant candidate's ability to eat. Patients should be instructed to eat small, frequent meals of nutritionally dense foods. Oral nutrition supplements may provide enough additional nutrients to obviate more intensive nutrition support. Many commercial supplements are available to patients in addition to homemade shakes and fortified drinks.

Enteral tube feeding is the alternative feeding method of choice when patients cannot get adequate nutrients from diet and supplements. Even for patients with esophageal varices, small-bore enteral feeding tubes can be used to provide nutrition. Some patients may require only nocturnal feedings to supplement daytime eating. Many standard and disease-specific commercial formulas are available. The chapters on organ failure review the use of disease-specific formulas.

PN sustains life in small-bowel transplant candidates until successful engraftment of a donor intestine is accomplished. In all other organ transplant candidates, PN should be considered only when the gut ceases to function or enteral feeding has failed. PN may actually worsen organ failure in some patients. See Part VI for specific care plans.

PRETRANSPLANT CALORIE AND PROTEIN REQUIREMENTS. The goal of pretransplant nutrition support is to optimize the nutritional status of and maximize the efficiency of medical therapy for patients before transplantation.[7] For well-nourished patients, this means maintaining nutritional status; for obese patients, weight loss with maintenance of protein stores is the goal. For malnourished patients, improving nutritional status is beneficial; however, in the face of organ failure, prevention of further deterioration may be all that can be achieved.[50] Table 40-3 outlines general pretransplant calorie and protein goals.

VITAMIN AND MINERAL REQUIREMENTS. Although specific vitamin and mineral recommendations have not been developed for transplant patients, a daily multivitamin and mineral supplement is recommended for most pretransplant patients unless oral intake is consistently adequate. Vitamin and mineral abnormalities may be due to organ failure or treatment of medical complications. Tables 40-4 and 40-5 outline potential vitamin and mineral abnormalities in transplant candidates.

Posttransplant Phase
Short-Term Posttransplant Nutrition Therapy

The immediate posttransplant period is considered a catabolic phase in which adequate nutrition is vital for patient recovery. The goal of nutrition therapy in this phase is to promote wound healing, deter infection, and replenish depleted nutrient stores.[51]

TABLE 40-3

Pretransplant Calorie and Protein Goals for Solid Organ Transplant Candidates

Nutrition Goal	Calorie Needs
Weight maintenance	1.2-1.3 × basal energy expenditure (by Harris-Benedict equation), depending on activity level 30 kcal/kg
Weight gain	1.5 × basal energy expenditure 35-40 kcal/kg
Weight loss	Deficit of 500 to 1000 kcal/day, depending on current intake, anticipated time until transplant, and ability to exercise

Nutrition Goal	Protein Needs
Maintenance	0.8-1.2 g/kg/day
Repletion	1.3-2.0 g/kg/day
Dialysis	Hemodialysis: 1.2-1.5 g/kg/day Peritoneal: 1.5 g/kg/day
Hepatic encephalopathy	Most hepatic encephalopathy is triggered by conditions such as gastrointestinal bleeding, infection, electrolyte imbalance, sedatives, etc; see requirements for maintenance and repletion; consider branched-chain amino acid supplements

Data from PorayKo MK, DiCecco S, O'Keefe SJ: Impact of malnutrition and its therapy on liver transplantation, *Semin Liver Dis* 11:305-314, 1991; and Poindexter SM: Nutrition support in cardiac transplantation, *Topic Clin Nutr* 7(3):12-16, 1992.

TABLE 40-4

Potential Vitamin Abnormalities in Organ Transplant Candidates

Vitamin	Potential Abnormalities and Causes
A	Deficiency can be caused by steatorrhea, neomycin, cholestyramine, alcoholism, and underproduction of retinol-binding protein by the liver Levels often increase with renal failure
B_6	Alcoholism can cause deficiency
B_{12}	Alcoholism, cholestyramine can cause deficiency
Niacin	Alcoholism can cause deficiency
Thiamine	Alcoholism, high-carbohydrate diet can cause deficiency
C	In renal transplant patients, low plasma and leukocyte levels may result from dietary restriction of fruits and vegetables and dialysis losses
D	Deficiency can result from poor diet, steatorrhea, glucocorticoids, cholestyramine, and inadequate 25-hydroxylation of cholecalciferol and ergocalciferol by a cirrhotic liver Renal transplant candidates may lack the active form of vitamin D
E	Steatorrhea, antibiotics, cholestyramine can cause deficiency
K	Steatorrhea, antibiotics, cholestyramine can cause deficiency
Folate	Alcoholism, antibiotics can cause deficiency May be depressed in dialysis patients

Adapted from Hasse JM, Blue LS, Watkins LA: Solid organ transplantation. In Gottschlich MM, Matarese LE, Shronts EP (eds): Nutrition support dietetics core curriculum, ed 2, Silver Spring, MD, 1993, American Society for Parenteral and Enteral Nutrition, pp 409–422.

TABLE 40-5

Potential Mineral and Electrolyte Abnormalities in Patients Undergoing Organ Transplantation

Mineral/Electrolyte	Potential Abnormalities and Causes
Calcium	Glucocorticoids increase urinary excretion Gastrointestinal loss associated with steatorrhea In renal transplant patients, low serum levels result from abnormal vitamin D, calcium, and phosphorus metabolism
Copper	In liver transplant patients, decreased excretion is associated with biliary obstruction or Wilson's disease
Iron	Chronic bleeding can cause deficiency Decreased erythropoietin and red blood cell production and dialysis losses can cause deficiency in renal transplant patients Liver transplant candidates with hemochromatosis have excess iron stores
Magnesium	Diuretics, alcoholism can cause deficiency Renal failure can cause decreased excretion
Phosphorus	Anabolism, alcoholism, glucocorticoids can cause deficiency Increased levels associated with renal failure
Potassium	Potassium-wasting diuretics, anabolism, insulin use can cause hypokalemia Decreased renal function, potassium-sparing diuretics can cause hyperkalemia
Sodium	Depending on fluid status and blood pressure, sodium restriction may be necessary
Zinc	Diarrhea, diuretics, alcoholism can cause deficiency Renal failure can decrease excretion Low levels may be seen in dialysis patients

vascular complications, pancreatitis, metabolic alterations) can interfere with the provision of nutrition.[51] Delayed organ function, prolonged ventilatory support, infection, impaired mental status, bleeding, or other technical problems can delay oral feedings even longer. Side effects of immunosuppressant drugs also interfere with nutrition.

IMMUNOSUPPRESSANT MEDICATIONS. Immunosuppressant drugs are given to prevent rejection of the transplanted organ. The body recognizes a transplanted organ as "nonself" and mounts an immune response (rejection) if the immune system is not suppressed. The management of immunosuppression is the science and art of transplantation; the goal of immunosuppression is to maintain a balance—to prevent both rejection and infection. Immunosuppressant agents, like many other medications, have food and nutrient interactions. Table 40-6 describes the action of the immunosuppressant, the nutritional side effects, and suggested nutrition therapy.

POSTTRANSPLANT NUTRITION SUPPORT. When patients begin to eat after transplantation, taste changes, anorexia, diarrhea or constipation, and early satiety hamper their ability to eat adequate amounts. Oral nutrition supplementation helps patients achieve adequate nourishment. Monitoring nutrient intake is vital in assessing a patient's progress.

When oral intake is delayed or inadequate, nutrition support, usually tube feeding, is indicated. Four studies have shown that immediate posttransplant tube feedings are possible and may even improve patient outcome. Wicks and coworkers[52]

FACTORS THAT AFFECT ACUTE POSTTRANSPLANT NUTRIENT INTAKE. Patients undergoing renal transplantation usually are able to eat on the day after the transplant; however, heart, lung, pancreas, and liver transplant recipients usually cannot eat before the second or third day.[51] Several obstacles prevent adequate nutrition in the first few days after transplantation. Postoperative complications (including rejection, infection, renal insufficiency, GI complications, abdominal bleeding,

TABLE 40-6

Immunosuppressant Drugs, Nutritional Side Effects, and Interventions

Drug	Activity	Nutritional Side Effects	Suggested Nutrition Therapy
Anti-lymphocyte serum (ATGAM, Thymoglobulin)	Binds with lymphocytes, resulting in phagocytosis Inhibits and destroys lymphocytes	Fever and chills Increased risk of infection, profound leukopenia	Provide nutrient-dense foods patient will eat Ensure patient is receiving adequate protein
Azathioprine (Imuran)	Inhibits purine nucleotide synthesis, blocking T- and B-lymphocyte proliferation	Nausea, vomiting	Try antiemetic medications; if vomiting does not subside, consider tube feeding or PN
		Diarrhea	Review drugs and substitute for those that may be causing diarrhea; make sure that patient is receiving adequate fluid to replace losses
		Sore throat/ mucositis	Provide foods that will not irritate throat
		Altered taste acuity	Offer a variety of foods with different tastes
		Macrocytic anemia	Make sure folate intake is adequate
		Pancreatitis	Initiate PN if pancreatitis is severe
Basiliximab (Simulect)	Acts against the interleukin (IL)-2R-α chain (CD25) on activated T-lymphocytes, and inhibits IL-2-mediated activation of lymphocytes	None reported	
Corticosteroids (methylprednisone, prednisone, prednisolone, Solu-Medrol, Solu-Cortef)	Antiinflammatory properties Inhibits cell-mediated—and, to a lesser degree, humoral—immunity Inhibits lymphocyte proliferation Inhibits lymphokine production	Hyperglycemia	Monitor blood sugar and need for long-term diabetes diet and hypoglycemic agents
		Sodium retention	Avoid high-sodium foods
		Ulcers	Avoid foods that irritate stomach
		Osteoporosis	Ensure adequate calcium and vitamin D intake; consider need for calcitriol, fluoride, or estrogen
		Hyperphagia	Behavior modification to prevent overeating
		Impaired wound healing and increased infection risk	Ensure adequate protein intake; consider need for vitamins A, C, or zinc
		Hypertension	Avoid high-sodium foods, maintain healthy weight
		Pancreatitis	Initiate PN if pancreatitis is severe
Cyclosporine (Neoral, Sandimmune)	Inhibits cell-mediated immunity; inhibits T-cell proliferation Suppresses IL-2 production Prevents γ-interferon release	Hyperkalemia	Restrict high-potassium foods
		Hypomagnesemia	Supplement with high-magnesium foods or supplements
		Hypertension	Avoid high-sodium foods, maintain healthy weight
		Hyperglycemia	Monitor blood sugar and need for long-term diabetes diet and hypoglycemic agents
		Hyperlipidemia	Limit fat intake to <30% calories during long-term phase; maintain healthy weight
Daclizumab (Zenapax)	Inhibits IL-2-dependent human T-lymphocyte activation	None reported	
Muromonab-CD3 (OKT3)	Blocks T3 antigen recognition and T cell effector function Causes T cell lysis	Nausea, vomiting	Try antiemetic medications; if vomiting does not subside, consider tube feeding or PN
		Diarrhea	Review drugs and substitute for those that may be causing diarrhea; make sure that patient is receiving adequate fluid to replace losses
		Anorexia	Offer frequent meals of nutrient-dense foods
Sirolimus (Rapamycin, Rapamune)	Blocks the response of T- and B-cell activation by cytokines, which prevents cell-cycle progression and proliferation	Hyperlipidemia	Limit fat intake to <30% calories during long-term phase; maintain healthy weight
		Gastrointestinal disorders (constipation, diarrhea, nausea/ vomiting, dyspepsia)	Monitor for adequate nutrient intake
Tacrolimus (Prograf, FK506)	Suppresses T cell-mediated immunity and IL-2 production	Nausea, vomiting	Try antiemetic medications; if vomiting does not subside, consider tube feeding or PN
		Hyperkalemia	Avoid high-potassium foods
		Hyperglycemia	Monitor blood sugar and need for long-term diabetes diet and hypoglycemic agents
		Abdominal distress	Monitor oral intake; consider alternate methods of nutrition support if intake is suboptimal
Mycophenolate mofetil (CellCept)	Inhibits DNA synthesis and mixed lymphocyte production Inhibits antibody formation	Diarrhea	Review drugs and substitute for those that may be causing diarrhea; make sure that patient is receiving adequate fluid to replace losses

Data from Hasse J: Role of the dietitian in the nutrition management of adults after liver transplantation, *J Am Diet Assoc* 91(4):473-476, 1991.

randomized 24 liver transplant patients to receive either enteral nutrition (EN) or PN support. Fourteen patients began receiving tube feeding via a nasojejunal tube 18 hours after surgery. PN was started within 24 hours after transplantation in seven patients and up to 60 hours later for the other three. The median number of days for patients to begin eating was similar in both groups. No significant differences were seen between the two groups in anthropometry, intestinal absorptive capacity, or infection rates.

Another transplant group found similar results.[53,54] This group placed jejunostomy tubes at the end of liver transplant surgery in 108 patients and retrospectively reviewed their experience. They concluded that jejunostomy tube feeding was tolerated and reduced postoperative ileus and the need for PN.[54] Complications of the jejunostomy tube occurred in 16 patients, including six kinked tubes, six infections or perforations, two tube displacements, two intestinal obstructions, and two other problems.[54] Surgery was required to correct the complications in seven cases.

Hasse and colleagues[55] prospectively compared immediate posttransplant tube feeding to intravenous hydration and diet in 31 liver transplant recipients. Tube feeding was initiated 12 hours after liver transplant in 14 patients via nasointestinal tube without major complications. All patients began eating on about the third postoperative day. As expected, the tube-fed group had superior nutrient intakes than controls for the first 5 to 6 posttransplant days and better nitrogen balance on posttransplant day 4. Although there were no differences in rejection between the two groups, there was a significant reduction in viral infections and a trend toward fewer bacterial infections and overall numbers of infections in the tube-fed group, as compared with controls.

In a final study, 45 liver transplant patients were assigned to one of three groups.[56] Group 1 underwent selective bowel decontamination for 28 days posttransplant and received fiber-free tube feeding formula. Group 2 received a fiber-containing tube feeding formula and Lactobacillus plantarum 299 twice daily. Group 3 received a fiber-containing tube feeding formula plus Lactobacillus placebo. Tube feeding was administered from day 2 to 12 posttransplant. Group 2 experienced the lowest infection rate.

Selection of the tube-feeding formula depends on a patient's nutritional status, gut absorption, and fluid tolerance.[8] Generally, an isotonic, polymeric, tube-feeding formula can be used for transplant patients. If fluid overload is a problem, a nutrient-dense formula can be used. Small bowel transplant recipients may initially require a semielemental formula.[51]

PN is reserved for patients with no gut function who are expected to need PN for at least 7 days. Infection rates are higher with PN than with tube feeding, and infection in immunosuppressed patients significantly increases their mortality. One study evaluated the benefit of PN in liver transplant patients.[57] Twenty-eight patients were randomly assigned to receive PN with standard amino acids, PN with branched-chain enriched amino acids, or no nutrition support. Both PN groups received 35 kcal/kg per day and 1.5 g of protein per kilogram per day for a total of 7 days. Both PN regimens improved nitrogen balance and shortened intensive care unit stay. However, this study has limited application today because of current

reductions in hospital lengths of stay and preference for EN versus PN.

Candidates for PN include patients who develop severe ileus or, in some cases, pancreatitis. PN solution composition depends on metabolic and medical requirements. Nutrition support for fluid-overloaded patients should begin slowly. When oral feeding is instituted, the diet should advance quickly to solid food. High-protein oral supplements and snacks often are required to help the patient achieve adequate intake. Monitoring intake is crucial to determine if nutrition support should be initiated.

NUTRITION SUPPORT OF SMALL-BOWEL TRANSPLANT PATIENTS. Special nutrition support is necessary for patients who receive small-bowel transplants. All small-bowel transplant patients require PN during the immediate posttransplant period (about 1 to 2 weeks). PN also is required during rejection and infection episodes because the gut becomes "leaky" and loses function. When gut function is established, there will be output via the terminal ileostomy.[58,59] Tube feeding can be initiated when the gut is functional. Feeding tube options for these patients include nasogastric, nasoduodenal, gastric with postpylorus extensions, and jejunostomy tubes.[58,60] Several enteral feeding formulas have been tried in this population—elemental, semi-elemental, and intact protein.[58,60] A small-peptide formula containing glutamine and medium-chain triglycerides may be absorbed best.[61-65]

Oral feeding can begin when the stomach and intestinal tract are functional; however, initially patients must overcome many food aversions. When advancing oral diets, a low-fat diet would be better than a full-liquid diet high in fat and lactose. Fat malabsorption is not uncommon in the early posttransplant period. The lacteals and lymphatics, used for absorption of long-chain fatty acids, are severed during the transplant procedure.[61,66-69] In addition, some carbohydrate enzymes may be deficient in the early posttransplant phase. A lactose- and fat-reduced diet or enteral formula may be tolerated better initially and can decrease ostomy output. Concentrated sweets and hyperosmolar beverages may increase ostomy loss.[70-72]

Other nutrition-related concerns are unique to small bowel transplantation. Intestinal transit time can vary from 30 minutes to 5 hours, so absorption can be variable.[60] Ostomy output can quickly increase and require administration of additional fluid to replace losses. A rehydration solution may be helpful. Metabolic acidosis can occur and is treated with sodium bicarbonate.[60,66] Zinc and other electrolyte losses in ostomy output also must be replaced.

EARLY POSTTRANSPLANT NUTRITIONAL REQUIREMENTS

Calorie requirements. Nutrient needs in the acute posttransplant phase are increased to provide adequate nutrition for repletion of stores and maintenance of organ function. Energy requirements in the initial posttransplant phase are estimated to be 35 kcal/kg or 130% to 150% of basal energy expenditure (BEE) calculated by the Harris-Benedict equation.[8,24,30,73] Some propose that patients receive as much as 175% of the calculated BEE, but several studies that have measured posttransplant energy expenditure by indirect calorimetry do not demonstrate such a rapid metabolic rate (Table 40-7).

Protein requirements. Nitrogen excretion after transplantation is increased because of catabolic effects of corticosteroids

TABLE 40-7

Energy Expenditure After Liver Transplantation as Measured by Indirect Calorimetry

Researchers	Design	Results
Delafosse et al.[74]	REE measured in 8 patients on first 2 posttransplant days	REE was 36%-38% above energy expenditure predicted by Harris-Benedict equation
Shanbhogue et al.[75]	REE measured in 11 posttransplant patients	REE was 7% higher than predicted by Harris-Benedict equation using actual weight
Plevak et al.[76]	REE measured in 28 patients pretransplant and on posttransplant days 1, 3, 5, 14, and 28	REE did not change over time; Harris-Benedict equation (using ideal weight) plus 20% met energy needs for most patients
Hasse et al.[55]	REE measured in 31 patients on posttransplant days 2, 4, 7, and 12	REE rose gradually in first 12 posttransplant days; peak mean REE was 27% above the Harris-Benedict equation using patient's lowest recent weight

and stress of surgery. The amount of nitrogen lost depends on complications after transplantation (infection, bleeding, nitrogen loss through wounds) and corticosteroid doses. Newer immunosuppression protocols use more effective drugs (such as tacrolimus) that decrease the amount of corticosteroids required and, therefore, the amount of nitrogen lost. Traditional therapy for acute cellular rejection is additional doses of corticosteroids. During rejection treatment, protein needs are increased. Protein catabolism can lead to problems with poor wound healing, GI ulceration, osteopenia, myopathy, increased skin fragility, and infection.

Several studies of renal transplant patients have shown that the protein catabolic rate (PCR) parallels corticosteroid doses. Seagraves and associates[77] found this theory to be true in an evaluation of nine renal transplant patients receiving corticosteroids. Hoy and colleagues[78] measured PCR in 50 renal transplant patients who were receiving 60 mg of prednisone per day during their initial hospitalization. Protein catabolic rate rose over the first 3 to 4 posttransplant days and then stabilized. Treating rejection with additional corticosteroids further increased PCR. Neither protein restriction nor protein supplementation affected PCR. The same research group measured PCR in 20 renal transplant patients during posttransplant hospitalizations.[79] Half received 1 mg/kg per day of prednisone, and the other half 3 to 5 mg/kg per day of prednisone, tapering to 1 mg/kg per day by the time of discharge. PCR increased for 3 to 4 days and then stabilized; PCR was greater in the high-steroid dose group. Most patients had negative nitrogen balance, and protein deficits were greater in the high-dose group. This study concluded that the increased PCR caused by steroids is independent of protein intake at levels in the study (1.4 to 1.7 g/kg per day) but that protein balance can be achieved if enough protein is ingested to offset losses.

As previously mentioned, newer immunosuppression protocols use smaller amounts of steroids than these earlier studies. Recommendations for immediate posttransplant protein administration are 1.2 to 2.0 g/kg per day.[51,73,80] Table 40-8 reviews studies that evaluated posttransplant nitrogen loss in liver transplant recipients.

Van Buren and colleagues have suggested that a change in the nucleotide content of a diet can prolong survival of transplant recipients.[82,83] In rat studies, a nucleotide-free diet suppressed cell-mediated immunity, and, in combination with cyclosporine, a nucleotide-free diet prolonged heart transplant survival. The efficacy of this type of diet has not been studied in humans.

Arginine may have beneficial effects on transplantation outcomes. Rats fed 2% or 5% arginine after heart transplant had improved survival rates.[84] Further rat studies showed survival benefits when fish oil, arginine, and RNA were given as Impact diet (Novartis Nutrition, Minneapolis, MN). Graft survival improved when Impact and cyclosporine and sirolimus were given but not in animals who were given tacrolimus.[85] Kidney transplant recipients on cyclosporine-based immunosuppressives receiving arginine (2% of energy) and canola oil (15% of energy for 1800 calories/day) daily experienced reduction in systolic blood pressure and rejection episodes compared with a control group.[86]

Requirements for other nutrients. In the short-term posttransplant recovery phase (approximately 2 to 3 months after transplantation), the nutrition goal is provision of adequate nutrients to promote healing. When nutrition support is administered, carbohydrates should provide 50% to 70% of nonprotein calories. The patient should be monitored for elevated glucose levels because corticosteroids, stress, and organ function can alter glucose metabolism. Generally, 30% of nonprotein calories are provided as fat during the short-term posttransplant phase unless glucose or triglyceride levels are consistently elevated enough to warrant changing the fat component. Electrolyte metabolism is altered during this period. Sodium can be lost via nasogastric tube aspirate, urine, and drains. Cyclosporine, tacrolimus, and some diuretics cause hyperkalemia. Alternatively, other diuretics and aggressive refeeding can lead to hypokalemia. Cyclosporine also enhances loss of magnesium. Small bowel transplant recipients lose bicarbonate through drainage of the allograft organ. Supplementation of bicarbonate usually is required. Although specific vitamin and mineral requirements during this phase are not known, many patients have preexisting deficits secondary to their organ failure, and supplementation to the levels of the recommended dietary allowances (RDAs) is suggested.

Long-Term Posttransplant Nutrition Therapy

COMMON LONG-TERM POSTTRANSPLANT PROBLEMS. While the focus of the acute posttransplant phase is replenishment of lost nutrition stores, the aim of long-term medical nutrition therapy is maintenance of a healthy weight and prevention of nutrition problems. Common, chronic posttransplant nutrition problems include obesity, hyperlipidemia, hypertension, diabetes mellitus, and osteoporosis.

Obesity. Obesity, the most visible posttransplant problem, can contribute to or exacerbate hypertension, hyperlipidemia,

TABLE 40-8

Short-Term Nitrogen Loss After Liver Transplantation

Researchers	Design	Results
Hasse et al.[55]	UUN measured in 17 nontube-fed and 14 tube-fed patients on posttransplant days 2, 4, 7, 11	Daily UUN losses for nontube-fed patients, 9.6 ± 5.1 g to 11.7 ± 6.3 g; for tube-fed patients, 2.9 ± 4.3 g to 15.0 ± 7.7 g
Delafosse et al.[74]	UUN measured in 8 patients on the first 2 posttransplant days	Day 1 UUN, 20.1 g Day 2 UUN, 24.6 g
Shanbhogue et al.[75]	UUN measured in 11 posttransplant patients	Mean UUN excretion, 12.9 ± 4.4 g on day 3
O'Keefe et al.[81]	Evaluated nitrogen losses in 42 transplant patients	Nitrogen state relatively stable on day 4 posttransplant, mean nitrogen loss, 14.4-16 g/day
Plevak et al.[76]	Nitrogen balance measured in 28 patients pretransplant and on posttransplant days 1, 3, 5, 14, and 28	UUN excretion increased after transplant, peaking on day 3; nitrogen losses returned to preoperative level by day 28; despite nutrition support, mean nitrogen balance was negative during study period

and diabetes mellitus and cause strain to joints. Posttransplant obesity also predisposes patients to other medical problems, such as organ dysfunction. In heart transplant patients, BMI is significantly related to luminal narrowing and rejection of the heart.[87] Obesity has been associated with the incidence of hepatic abnormalities in liver transplant recipients.[88]

Several factors contribute to posttransplant obesity. One major determinant of posttransplant obesity may be pretransplant or preillness weight. At least one study suggested that patients with a history of obesity were much more likely to gain weight or remain obese than patients without a history of obesity.[89] Another study in liver transplant patients suggested that underweight patients gained significantly more weight posttransplant than other patients, but patients who were obese at the time of transplantation still had a higher BMI.[90] In heart transplant recipients, history of obesity did not influence the amount of weight gained.[91] Other factors that predispose to excessive weight gain after transplantation include steroid hunger, sedentary lifestyle, elimination of pretransplant diet restrictions, a newfound sense of well-being, and the attitude that patients can eat anything they want without limits.[11,27,91] African-American race, female gender, and young age (18 to 29) were factors found to be strongest predictors of posttransplant weight gain in kidney transplantation.[92] Everhart and colleagues also determined recipient BMI, donor BMI, and being married to be risk factors for increased weight after liver transplantion.[93]

Posttransplant weight gain is also influenced by immunosuppression regimens. Patients maintained on tacrolimus-based immunosuppression have a lower incidence of posttransplant obesity than do patients maintained on cyclosporine.[94,95] It is theorized that reduced corticosteroid doses for patients taking tacrolimus account for the difference.

Some researchers even suggest that neuropeptide Y (a peptide hormone that regulates food intake and energy expenditure) may play a role in posttransplant weight gain. Neuropeptide Y is elevated in renal transplant recipients[96] possibly because of increased synthesis/secretion resulting from increased response to glucocorticoids.[97-99] Increased leptin levels in kidney transplantation have also been correlated with increased BMI and tend to be higher than in healthy subjects with similar BMIs.[100]

Prevention of posttransplant obesity rests on the basic premise of *Eat less, exercise more.* Nutrition education helps

patients learn how to select a healthy diet without excess calories. Behavioral counseling teaches the patients how to deal with hyperphagia caused by steroids and other emotions tied to eating and the transplant. Patients must be taught how to exercise properly and be encouraged to be physically active. Some clinicians have proposed experimentation with appetite suppressants in this population.

Dietary intervention may help reduce posttransplant weight gain. Lopes and colleagues counseled 23 kidney transplant recipients with a BMI greater than 27 on an American Heart Association Step One diet with a moderate energy restriction. After 6 months, mean weight had decreased 3.2 ± 2.9 kg.[101] Patel and associates randomized kidney transplant patients to receive either nutrition counseling for 4 months or no intervention.[102] At 1 year posttransplant, the counseled group had significantly lower weights compared with controls.

Hyperlipidemia. Cardiovascular disease is a leading cause of long-term morbidity in transplant patients.[103] Hyperlipidemia is one of several risk factors for cardiovascular disease.[103,104] Hypercholesterolemia may also be a risk factor for graft loss for specific subgroups of kidney transplant recipients.[105] Alterations in serum triglyceride, cholesterol, high-density lipoprotein (HDL) cholesterol, low-density lipoprotein (LDL) cholesterol, and apolipoprotein concentrations have been observed in liver, kidney, heart, and pancreas recipients.[90, 94, 106-111]

Aside from the cardiovascular disease risks associated with hyperlipidemia, Kobashigawa and Kasiske theorize that hypercholesterolemia increases transplant graft vasculopathy and could manifest as problems such as heart transplant coronary artery disease, chronic renal transplant rejection, or liver transplant vanishing bile duct syndrome.[107] Not all researchers concur with this theory.[112]

The cause of posttransplant hyperlipidemia is multifactorial. Risk factors include obesity, genetic predisposition, diabetes mellitus, high-fat diet, sedentary lifestyle, renal dysfunction, antihypertensive drugs, proteinuria, and immunosuppressive drugs.[107,113] Specifically, cyclosporine-based immunosuppression regimens result in higher long-term lipid levels than tacrolimus-based regimens,[94,95,114-116] and corticosteroid dose is associated with increased posttransplant cholesterol levels.[117] Cyclosporine appears to decrease activity of LDL receptors, inhibit bile acid synthesis, depress lipolipase activity, and stimulate hepatic lipase activity.[107,118] Corticosteroids enhance acetyl Co-A carboxylase and free fatty acid synthesis activity, as well as 3-hydroxy-3-methylglutaryl coenzyme A reductase activity. Corticosteroids may also increase hepatic synthesis of very-low-density lipoprotein cholesterol and downregulate LDL receptor activity.[107,118]

Treatment or prevention of posttransplant hyperlipidemia involves several arms—immunosuppression changes, dietary intervention, drug therapy, and other interventions. Alterations in immunosuppressive drug therapy may improve hyperlipidemias. Patients maintained on tacrolimus-based immunosuppression versus cyclosporine-based immunosuppression tend to have lower total cholesterol and triglyceride levels.[94,95,119,120] Corticosteroid reductions or withdrawals resulted in serum total cholesterol concentration reductions in kidney transplant patients[121,122] and liver transplant patients[123] but not always a reduction in cholesterol to HDL-cholesterol ratio.[121]

Dietary changes may improve posttransplant hyperlipidemia. In some studies, kidney transplant patients adhering to low-fat, low-cholesterol diets experienced lowered cholesterol and LDL-cholesterol levels and unchanged HDL cholesterol levels.[101,124-126] Mediterranean-type diets have also been reported to lower serum total cholesterol and HDL-cholesterol levels in heart transplant patients.[127] However, not all patients experience reductions from diet alone.[124,128,129]

For patients who do not respond to diet therapy, antihyperlipidemic drugs may be necessary. The HMG-CoA reductase inhibitors are usually the drugs of choice for this population. Lovastatin, pravastatin, simvastatin, fluvastatin, atorvastatin, and cerivastatin have been used successfully and safely to lower serum total cholesterol and LDL-cholesterol concentrations in cyclosporine-treated transplant recipients with hyperlipidemia.[124,130-145] Statin drugs may also reduce rejection rates in heart transplant patients.[142] At least one study showed that pravastatin was safe and effective in lowering serum lipid levels in liver transplant patients treated with tacrolimus.[146]

Hyperhomocysteinemia is an additional risk factor for arteriosclerosis among kidney transplant recipients.[147-153] Hyperhomocysteinemia in kidney transplant recipients is correlated with renal function and folate, vitamin B_6, and vitamin B_{12} status.[147,149-154] In at least one study, supplementing with vitamins B_6 and B_{12} and folate effectively lowered postmethionine-loading and fasting plasma total homocysteine levels in renal transplant recipients.[147]

Hypertension. Hypertension occurs in 60% to 80% of transplant recipients maintained on a cyclosporine-based immunosuppression regimen.[110] Conversion from cyclosporine to tacrolimus lowers blood pressure.[120] Factors that lead to posttransplant hypertension include corticosteroids, cyclosporine, renal artery stenosis (kidney recipient), diseased kidneys, rejection, and recurrence of primary renal disease. A moderately sodium-restricted diet (2 to 4 g per day) and antihypertensive drugs are used to control posttransplant hypertension.

Ingestion of fish oil may improve hypertension and other side effects of immunosuppression. Fish oil therapy in renal transplant recipients resulted in lower blood pressure,[155-157] reduced serum triglyceride concentrations and platelet aggregation,[156,157] and improved transplant graft function.[157] Renal hemodynamics were also improved in liver transplant patients receiving fish oil compared with controls receiving corn oil.[158]

Diabetes mellitus. Diabetes mellitus can develop after organ transplantation. Causes of new-onset diabetes mellitus include heredity, renal insufficiency, and drugs—corticosteroids, diuretics, antithymocyte globulin, and tacrolimus. Corticosteroids produce insulin resistance,[159,160] increase gluconeogenesis and glucagon secretion, and antagonize peripheral glucose uptake.[161] Cyclosporine and tacrolimus may inhibit insulin secretion, increase insulin resistance, or exert a direct toxic effect on the beta cell.[160] Tacrolimus may be more diabetogenic than cyclosporine because the onset of diabetes mellitus after transplantation tends to be higher in tacrolimus-treated versus cyclosporine-treated patients despite lower corticosteroid doses.[94,162,163] The treatment of posttransplant diabetes includes a "carbohydrate-controlled diet" and, in some cases, oral hypoglycemic agents or insulin.

Osteoporosis. Solid organ transplant recipients are at risk of accelerated osteoporosis.[164-169] There is a fifteenfold to thirtyfold acceleration in posttransplant bone mineral loss every year.[170] Some transplant patients (e.g., those who had cholestatic liver disease or renal osteodystrophy before transplantation) are at increased risk of bone disease before transplantation.[166,167] Half of patients with cholestatic liver diseases have bone mineral density levels below the fracture threshold before transplantation.[170] After transplantation, there is a significant increase in bone turnover.[166] Corticosteroids accelerate loss of trabecular bone.[171] Corticosteroids also alter sex hormone secretion, depress renal phosphate tubular reabsorption, accelerate synthesis of 1,25 dihydroxy vitamin D, and decrease synthesis of osteocalcin.[166] Secondary hyperparathyroidism may be caused by corticosteroids, resulting in increased osteoblast activity and decreased intestinal absorption of calcium.[166,167] High-turnover osteopenia is caused by cyclosporine via stimulation of bone resorption but may counterbalance the effects of steroids on bone mineral density.[172]

General preventive guidelines for osteoporosis include adequate vitamin D and dietary calcium intake (1000 to 1500 mg calcium per day), avoidance of smoking, weight-bearing exercise, and estrogen replacement for some women. Pamidronate and calcitriol have also been found beneficial in reducing bone loss after kidney transplantation.[173] Treatment with calcitriol, fluoride, and calcium seems to benefit liver transplant patients, especially those with severe osteoporosis.[174] Bone-modulating medications may also reduce osteoporosis and fractures in the organ transplant population.

LONG-TERM POSTTRANSPLANT NUTRITION THERAPY RECOMMENDATIONS. Long-term posttransplant nutrition goals include maintaining healthy weight and preventing other nutrition-related problems. Calories should be adequate to maintain a healthy weight for the patient's activity level (estimated to be 25 to 30 kcal/kg or 1.2 to 1.3 times the BEE). Protein needs are 0.8 to 1.2 g/kg per day. Low-protein diets have been prescribed for patients with chronic renal insufficiency. Whether such a diet would be beneficial long-term for kidney transplant recipients has been questioned. One study evaluated the effect of a low-protein diet (0.6 g/kg per day) in eight stable renal transplant recipients 38 ± 7 months after transplantation.[175] This study concluded that a low-protein diet could maintain nitrogen balance but that it restricted adequate calorie intake and should be used with caution until long-term nutritional consequences have been studied.

Most transplant centers encourage patients to restrict excess simple sugars. A low-fat diet (<30% of calories as fat and <20% as saturated fat) is encouraged to prevent hyperlipidemia. Van der Heide and colleagues have evaluated the effect of fish oil supplementation on renal function and rejection in renal transplant patients receiving cyclosporine-based immunosuppression.[176-178] In all three studies, patients received either 6 g of fish oil or 6 g of coconut oil per day. They concluded that fish oil supplementation did not affect survival of the kidney allograft but when taken for 1 year did reduce the number of rejections and improved mean arterial blood pressure.[177] The same results cannot be inferred from other transplant recipients and with different immunosuppression protocols. Long-term compliance with such a regimen is unknown.

Electrolyte and mineral balance can be altered after transplantation. Restriction of sodium to 2 to 4 g is suggested to help alleviate fluid retention and hypertension. Phosphorus and magnesium frequently are depleted (and may need to be supplemented) and phosphate binders discontinued. Potassium is restricted if serum levels exceed 6 mg/dl. A calcium intake of 1000 to 1500 mg per day is suggested, using calcium supplements if dietary intake is not adequate.

Immunosuppressed transplant recipients should be instructed to take precautions such as cooking meats well, washing all fruits and vegetables, and storing food at proper temperatures to avoid food-borne illness. Herbal supplements should be avoided until effects in transplant patients are known. There is at least one published report in which consumption of St. John's Wort caused the serum cyclosporine level in a liver transplant patient to decrease, resulting in acute rejection.[179]

Conclusion

Nutrition therapy is important during all phases of organ transplantation. Nutrition assessment identifies patients who are nutritionally depleted or are at risk. While a patient awaits transplantation, specific nutrition therapy can be provided to help treat symptoms of organ failure and replenish depleted nutrient stores in preparation for surgery. After a transplant, nutrition support can help recipients recover, minimize infection and wound problems, and diminish nitrogen loss associated with surgery and corticosteroid administration. Long-term nutrition goals for transplant recipients focus on preventing chronic illnesses such as hypertension, hyperlipidemia, and excessive weight gain. Immunosuppressant drugs are key to survival of the transplant but contribute to the development of the chronic illnesses aforementioned. Nutrition interventions can delay or offset some of the drugs' side effects. In conclusion, identification, treatment, and prevention of nutrition problems in transplant recipients are vital in achieving successful outcomes and survival with organ transplantation.

REFERENCES

1. Merrill JP, Murray JE, Harrison JR, Guild WR: Successful homotransplantation of the human kidney between identical twins, *JAMA* 160:277-282, 1956.

2. DiCecco SR, Wieners EJ, Wiesner RH, et al: Assessment of nutritional status of patients with end-stage liver disease undergoing liver transplantation, *Mayo Clin Proc* 64(1):95-102, 1989.

3. Hasse J, Strong S, Gorman MA, Liepa GU: Subjective global assessment: alternative nutritional assessment technique for liver transplant candidates, *Nutrition* 9(4):339-343, 1993.

4. Hasse J: Role of the dietitian in the nutrition management of adults after liver transplantation, *J Am Diet Assoc* 91(4):473-476, 1991.

5. Porayko MK, DiCecco S, O'Keefe SJ: Impact of malnutrition and its therapy on liver transplantation, *Semin Liver Dis* 11(4):305-314, 1991.

6. Shronts EP: Nutritional assessment of adults with end-stage hepatic failure, *Nutr Clin Pract* 3(3):113-119, 1988.

7. Hasse JM: Nutrition assessment and support of organ transplant recipients, *J Parenter Enteral Nutr* 25(3):120-131, 2001.

8. Poindexter SM: Nutrition support in cardiac transplantation, *Top Clin Nutr* 7(3):12-16, 1992.

9. Detsky AS, McLaughlin JR, Baker JP, et al: What is subjective global assessment of nutritional status? *J Parenter Enteral Nutr* 11(1):8-13, 1987.

10. Baker JP, Detsky AS, Wesson DE, et al: Nutritional assessment: a comparison of clinical judgment and objective measurements, *N Engl J Med* 306(16):969-972, 1982.

11. Grady KL, Herold LS: Comparison of nutritional status in patients before and after heart transplantation, *J Heart Transplant* 7(2):123-127, 1988.

12. Becker BN, Becker YT, Heisey DM, et al: The impact of hypoalbuminemia in kidney-pancreas transplant recipients, *Transplantation* 68(1):72-75, 1999.

13. Miller DG, Levine SE, D'Elia JA, Bistrian BR: Nutritional status of diabetic and nondiabetic patients after renal transplantation, *Am J Clin Nutr* 44(1):66-69, 1986.

14. Akerman PA, Jenkins RL, Bistrian R: Preoperative nutrition assessment in liver transplantation, *Nutrition* 9(4):350-356, 1993.

15. Figueiredo F, Dickson ER, Pasha T, et al: Impact of nutritional status on outcomes after liver transplantation, *Transplantation* 70(9):1347-1352, 2000.

16. Harrison J, McKiernan J, Neuberger JM: A prospective study on the effect of recipient nutritional status on outcome in liver transplantation, *Transpl Int* 10(5):369-374, 1997.

17. Hasse JM, Gonwa TA, Jennings LW, et al: Malnutrition affects liver transplant outcomes, *Transplantation* 66(8):S53, 1998 (abstract).

18. Lautz HU, Selberg O, Körber J, Bürger M, Müller MJ: Protein-calorie malnutrition in liver cirrhosis, *Clin Invest* 70(6):478-486, 1992.

19. Pikul J, Sharpe MD, Lowndes R, Ghent CN: Degree of preoperative malnutrition is predictive of postoperative morbidity and mortality in liver transplant recipients, *Transplantation* 57(3):469-472, 1994.

20. Selberg O, Böttcher J, Tusche G, et al: Identification of high- and low-risk patients before liver transplantation: a prospective cohort study of nutritional and metabolic parameters in 150 patients, *Hepatology* 25(3):652-657, 1997.

21. Stephenson GR Jr, Moretti EW, El-Moalem H, Clavien PA, Tuttle-Newhall JE: Malnutrition in liver transplant patients: pre-operative subjective global assessment (SGA) is predictive of outcome following liver transplantation, *J Parenter Enteral Nutr* 24(1):S10-S11, 2000 (abstract).

22. Madill J, Maurer JR, deHoyas A: A comparison of preoperative and postoperative nutritional state of lung transplant recipients, *Transplantation* 56(2):347-350, 1993.

23. Williams J, Kinosian B, Compher C, Kotloff R: Preoperative weight and a percentage of ideal body weight correlates with survival in patients status-post lung transplantation, *J Parenter Enteral Nutr* 24(1):S29-S30, 2000 (abstract).

24. Frazier OH, Van Buren CT, Poindexter SM, Waldenberger F: Nutritional management of the heart transplant recipient, *Heart Transplant* 4(4):450-452, 1985.

25. Shaw BW Jr, Wood RP, Gordon RD, et al: Influence of selected patient variables and operative blood loss on six-month survival following liver transplantation, *Semin Liver Dis* 5(4):385-393, 1985.

26. Hasse JM, Roberts S: Transplantation. In Rombeau JL, Rolandelli RH (eds): *Parenteral nutrition,* ed 3, Philadelphia, 2001, WB Saunders, pp 529-561.

27. Rosenberg ME, Hostetter TH: Nutrition. In Toledo-Pereya LH (ed): *Kidney transplantation,* Philadelphia, 1988, FA Davis, pp 169-186.

28. Mitch WE, May RC, Maroni BJ: Review mechanisms for abnormal protein metabolism in uremia, *J Am Coll Nutr* 8(4):305-309, 1989.

29. Poindexter SM: Nutrition in heart transplantation, *Support Line* 14(1):8-9, 1992.

30. Evans MA, Shronts EP, Fish JA: A case report: nutrition support of a heart-lung transplant recipient, *Support Line* 14(1):1-8, 1992.

31. Charlton CPJ, Buchanan E, Holden CE, et al: Intensive enteral feeding in advanced cirrhosis: Reversal of malnutrition without precipitation of hepatic encephalopathy, *Arch Dis Child* 67(5):603-607, 1992.

32. Hasse JM, Crippin JS, Blue LS, et al: Does nutrition supplementation benefit liver transplant candidates with a history of encephalopathy? *J Parenter Enteral Nutr* 21:S16, 1997 (abstract).

33. Hirsch S, de la Maza MP, Gattás V, et al: Nutritional support in alcoholic cirrhotic patients improves host defenses, *J Am Coll Nutr* 18(5):434-441, 1999.

34. Kearns PJ, Young H, Garcia G, et al: Accelerated improvement of alcoholic liver disease with enteral nutrition, *Gastroenterology* 102(1):200-205, 1992.

35. Cabre E, Gonzalez-Huix G, Abad-Lacruz A, et al: Effect of total enteral nutrition on the short-term outcome of severely malnourished cirrhotics: a randomized controlled trial, *Gastroenterology* 98(3):715-720, 1990.

36. Grady KL, Costanzo MR, Fisher S, Koch D: Preoperative obesity is associated with decreased survival after heart transplantation, *J Heart Lung Transplant* 15(9):863-871, 1996.

37. Moreso F, Serón D, Anunciada AI, et al: Recipient body surface area as a predictor of posttransplant renal allograft evolution, *Transplantation* 65(5):671-676, 1998.

38. Pirsch JD, Armbrust MJ, Knechtle SJ, et al: Obesity as a risk factor following renal transplantation, *Transplantation* 59(4):631-633, 1995.

39. Holley JL, Shapiro R, Lopatin WB, et al: Obesity as a risk factor following cadaveric renal transplantation, *Transplantation* 49(2):387-389, 1990.

40. Drafts HH, Anjum MR, Wynn JJ, Mulloy LL, Bowley JN, Humphries AL: The impact of pre-transplant obesity on renal transplant outcomes, *Clin Transplant* 11 (5 Pt 2):493-496, 1997.

41. Bumgardner GL, Henry ML, Elkhammas E, et al: Obesity as a risk factor after combined pancreas/kidney transplantation, *Transplantation* 60(12):1426-1430, 1995.

42. Gill IS, Hodge EE, Novick AC, et al: Impact of obesity on renal transplantation, *Transplant Proc* 25(1 Pt 2):1047-1048, 1993.

43. Wilson GA, Bumgardner GL, Henry ML, et al: Decreased graft survival rate in obese pancreas/kidney recipients, *Transplant Proc* 27(6):3106-3107, 1995.

44. Halme L, Eklund B, Kyllönen L, Salmela K: Is obesity still a risk factor in renal transplantation? *Transpl Int* 10(4):284-288, 1997.

45. Meier-Kriesche H-U, Vaghela M, Thambuganipalle R, et al: The effect of body mass index on long-term renal allograft survival, *Transplantation* 68(9):1294-1297, 1999.

46. Keeffe EB, Gettys C, Esquivel CO: Liver transplantation in patients with severe obesity, *Transplantation* 57(2):309-311, 1994.

47. Testa G, Hasse JM, Jennings LW, et al: Morbid obesity is not an independent risk factor for liver transplantation, *Transplantation* 66:S53, 1998 (abstract).

48. Braunfeld MYY, Chan S, Pregler J, et al: Liver transplantation in the morbidly obese, *J Clin Anesth* 8(7):585-590, 1996.

49. Sawyer RG, Pelletier SJ, Pruett TL: Increased early morbidity and mortality with acceptable long-term function in severely obese patients undergoing liver transplantation, *Clin Transplant* 13(1 Pt 2):126-130, 1999.

50. Riordan SM, Williams R: Nutrition and liver transplantation, *J Hepatol* 31(5):955-962, 1999.

51. Hasse JM: Recovery after transplantation: the role of nutrition therapy, *Top Clin Nutr* 13(2):15-26, 1998.

52. Wicks C, Somasundaram S, Bjarnason I, et al: Comparison of enteral feeding and total parenteral nutrition after liver transplantation, *Lancet* 344(8926):837-840, 1994.

53. Pescovitz MD, Mehta PL, Leapman SB, et al: Tube jejunostomy in liver transplant recipients, *Surgery* 117(6):642-647, 1995.

54. Mehta PL, Alaka KJ, Filo RS, et al: Nutrition support following liver transplantation: a comparison of jejunal versus parenteral routes, *Clin Transplant* 9(5):364-369, 1995.

55. Hasse JM, Blue LS, Liepa GU, et al: Early enteral nutrition support in patients undergoing liver transplantation, *J Parenter Enteral Nutr* 19(6):437-443, 1995

56. Rayes N, Hansen S, Müller AR, et al: SBD versus fibre-containing enteral nutrition plus lactobacillus or placebo to prevent bacterial infections after liver transplantation, European Transplantation Society Meeting, Oslo, 1999 (abstract).

57. Reilly J, Mehta R, Teperman L, et al: Nutritional support after liver transplantation: a randomized prospective study, *J Parenter Enteral Nutr* 14(4):386-391, 1990.

58. Reyes J, Tzakis AG, Todo S, et al: Post-operative care of small bowel transplant recipients, *Crit Care Ill* 9:193-194, 1993.

59. Todo S, Tzakis A, Abu-Elmagd K, et al: Clinical intestinal transplantation, *Transplant Proc* 25(3):2195-2197, 1993.

60. Reyes J, Tzakis AG, Todo S, et al: Nutritional management of intestinal transplant recipients, *Transplant Proc* 25(1 Pt 2):1200-1201, 1993.

61. Nour B, Reyes J, Tzakis A, et al: Intestinal transplantation with or without other abdominal organs: nutritional and dietary management of 50 patients, *Transplant Proc* 26(3):1432-1433, 1994.

62. Janes S, Beath SV, Jones R, et al: Enteral feeding after intestinal transplantation: the Birmingham experience, *Transplant Proc* 29:1855-1856, 1997.

63. Nemoto A, Krajack A, Suzuki T, et al: Glutamine metabolism of intestine grafts: influence of mucosal injury by prolonged preservation and transplantation, *Transplant Proc* 28(5):2545-2546, 1996.

64. Schroeder P, Schweizer E, Blomer A, et al: Glutamine prevents mucosal injury after small bowel transplantation, *Transplant Proc* 24(3):1104, 1992.

65. Yagi M, Sakamoto K, Inoue T, et al: Effect of a glutamine-enriched elemental diet on regeneration of the small bowel mucosa following isotransplantation of small intestine, *Transplant Proc* 26(4):2297-2298, 1994.

66. Hasse JM, Weseman RA: Solid organ transplant. In Gottschlich MM, Fuhrman MP, Hammond KA, et al. (eds): *The science and practice of nutrition support: a case-based core curriculum*, Silver Spring, MD, 2001, American Society for Parenteral and Enteral *Nutrition*, pp 601-618.

67. Sarr MG: Motility and absorption in the transplanted gut, *Transplant Proc* 28(5):2535-2538, 1996.

68. Pakarinen M, Kuusanmaki P, Halttunen J: Recovery of fat absorption in the transplanted ileum, *Transplant Proc* 26(3):1665-1666, 1994.

69. Schmid TH, Koeroezsi G, Oberhuber G, et al: Lymphatic regeneration after small bowel transplantation, *Transplant Proc* 22(4):2060-2061, 1990.

70. Rovera G, Furudawa H, Reyes J, et al: The use of clonidine for the treatment of high intestinal output following small bowel transplantation, *Transplant Proc* 29(3):1853-1854, 1997.

71. Lykins TC, Stockwell J: Comprehensive modified diet simplifies nutrition management of adults with short-bowel syndrome, *J Am Diet Assoc* 98(3):309-315, 1998.

72. Strohm SL, Koehler AN, Mazariegos GV, et al: Nutrition management in pediatric small bowel transplant, *Nutr Clin Pract* 14:58-63, 1999.

73. Obayashi PAC: Medical nutrition therapy following pancreas transplantation, *Support Line* 22(1):18-22, 2000.

74. Delafosse B, Faure JL, Bouffard Y, et al: Liver transplantation: energy expenditure, nitrogen loss, and substrate oxidation rate in the first two postoperative days, *Transplant Proc* 21(1 Pt 2):2453-2454, 1989.

75. Shanbhogue RLK, Bistrian BR, Jenkins RL, et al: Increased protein catabolism without hypermetabolism after human orthotopic liver transplantation, *Surgery* 101(2):146-149, 1987.

76. Plevak DJ, DiCecco SR, Wiesner RH, et al: Nutritional support for liver transplantation: identifying caloric and protein requirements, *Mayo Clin Proc* 69(3):225-230, 1994.

77. Seagraves A, Moore EE, Moore FA, Weil R: Net protein catabolic rate after kidney transplantation: impact of corticosteroid immunosuppression, *J Parenter Enteral Nutr* 10(5):453-455, 1986.

78. Hoy WE, Sargent JA, Hall D, et al: Protein catabolism during the postoperative course after renal transplantation, *Am J Kidney Dis* 5(3):186-190, 1985.

79. Hoy WE, Sargent JA, Freeman R, et al: The influence of glucocorticoid dose on protein catabolism after renal transplantation, *Am J Med Sci* 291(4):241-247, 1986.

80. Hasse JM: Recovery after transplantation: the role of nutrition therapy, *Top Clin Nutr* 13(2):15-26, 1998.

81. O'Keefe SJ, Williams R, Calne RY: "Catabolic" loss of body protein after human liver transplantation, *Br Med J* 280(6222):1107-1108, 1980.

82. Van Buren CT, Kulkarni AD, Schandle VB, Rudolph FB: The influence of dietary nucleotides on cell-mediated immunity, *Transplantation* 36(3):350-352, 1983.

83. Van Buren CT, Kulkami A, Rudolph FB: Synergistic effect of a nucleotide-free diet and cyclosporine on allograft survival, *Transplant Proc* 15(suppl):2967-2968, 1983.

84. Alexander JW, Levy A, Custer D, et al: Arginine, fish oil, and donor-specific transfusions independently improve cardiac allograft survival in rats given subtherapeutic doses of cyclosporine, *J Parenter Enteral Nutr* 22(3):152-155, 1998.

85. Gibson SW, Valente JF, Alexander JW, et al: Nutritional immunomodulation leads to enhanced allograft survival in combination with cyclosporine A and rapamycin, but not FK506, *Transplantation* 69(10):2034-2038, 2000.

86. Alexander JW: Role of immunonutrition in reducing complications following organ transplantation, *Transplant Proc* 32(3):574-575, 2000.

87. Winters GL, Kendall TJ, Radio SJ, et al: Posttransplant obesity and hyperlipidemia: major predictors of severity of coronary arteriopathy in failed human heart allografts, *J Heart Transplant* 9(4):364-371, 1990.

88. Palmer M, Schaffner F, Thung SN: Excessive weight gain after liver transplantation, *Transplantation* 51:797-800, 1991.

89. Merion RM, Twork AM, Rosenberg L, et al: Obesity and renal transplantation, *Surg Gynecol Obstet* 172(5):367-376, 1991.

90. Hasse JM, Testa G, Gonwa TA, et al: Is pre-liver transplant obesity a risk factor for posttransplant metabolic complications? *Transplantation* 66(8):S53, 1998 (abstract).

91. Baker AM, Levine TB, Goldberg AD, Levine AB: Natural history and predictors of obesity after orthotopic heart transplantation, *J Heart Lung Transplant* 11(6):1156-1159, 1992.

92. Johnson CP, Gallagher-Lepak S, Zhu YR, et al: Factors influencing weight gain after renal transplantation, *Transplantation* 56(4):822-827, 1993.

93. Everhart JE, Lombardero M, Lake JR, Wiesner RK, Zetterman RK, Hoofnagle JH: Weight change and obesity after liver transplantation: incidence and risk factors, *Liver Transplant Surg* 4(4):285-296, 1998.

94. Mor E, Facklam D, Hasse J, et al: Weight gain and lipid profile changes in liver transplant recipients: long-term results of the American FK506 multicenter study, *Transplant Proc* 27(1):1126, 1995.

95. Canzanello VJ, Schwartz L, Taler SJ, et al: Evolution of cardiovascular risk after liver transplantation: a comparison of cyclosporine A and tacrolimus (FK506), *Liver Transplant Surg* 3(1):1-9, 1997.

96. Kokot F, Adamczak M, Wiecek A, Speichowicz U, Mesjasz J: Plasma immunoreactive Leptin and Neuropeptide Y levels in kidney transplant patients, *Am J Nephrol* 19(1):28-33, 1999.

97. Kalra SP, Kalra PS: Is neuropeptide Y a naturally occurring appetite transducer? *Curr Opin Endocrinol Diabetes* 3:157-163, 1996.

98. White BD, Dean RG, Martin RJ: Adrenalectomy decreases neuropeptide and mRNA levels in arcuate nucleus, *Brain Res Bull* 25(5):711-715, 1990.

99. Higuchi H, Yang HY, Sabol SL: Rat neuropeptide Y precursor gene expression, mRNA structure, tissue distribution, and regulation by glucocorticoids, cyclic CNP and phorbol ester, *J Biol Chem* 263(13):6288-6295, 1988.

100. Bączkowska T, Soin J, Soluch L, Lao M, Gaciong Z: The role of leptin in body mass index increase in renal allograft recipients, *Transplant Proc* 32(6):1331-1332, 2000.

101. Lopes IM, Martín M, Errasti P, Martínez JA: Benefits of a dietary intervention on weight loss, body composition, and lipid profile after renal transplantation, *Nutrition* 15(1):7-10, 1999.

102. Patel MG: The effect of dietary intervention on weight gains after renal transplantation, *J Renal Nutr* 8(3):137-141, 1998.

103. Wheeler DC, Steiger J: Evolution and etiology of cardiovascular diseases in renal transplant recipients, *Transplantation* 70(11 suppl):S541-S545, 2000.

104. Lorenzetti M, Giannarelli R, Paleologo G, et al: Risk factors for cardiovascular disease in patients with functioning kidney grafts, *Transplant Proc* 30(5):2047, 1998.

105. Wissing KM, Abramowicz D, Broeders N, Vereerstraeten P: Hypercholesterolemia is associated with increased kidney loss caused by chronic rejection in male patients with previous acute rejection, *Transplantation* 70(3):464-472, 2000.

106. Nyberg G, Fager G, Mjornstedt L, et al: Serum lipids after pancreas and kidney transplantation, *Transplant Proc* 24(3):846-847, 1992.

107. Kobashigawa JA, Kasiske BL: Hyperlipidemia in solid organ transplantation, *Transplantation* 63(3):331-338, 1997.

108. Brann WM, Bennett LE, Keck BM, Hosenpud JD: Morbidity, functional status, an immunosuppressive therapy after heart transplantation: an analysis of the Joint International Society for Heart and Lung Transplantation/United Network for Organ Sharing Thoracic Registry, *J Heart Lung Transplant* 17(4):374-382, 1998.

109. Mathe D, Adam R, Malmendier C, et al: Prevalence of dyslipidemia in liver transplant recipients, *Transplantation* 54(1):167-170, 1992.

110. Munoz SJ, Deems RO, Moritz MJ, et al: Hyperlipidemia and obesity after orthotopic liver transplantation, *Transplant Proc* 23(1 Pt 2):1480-1483, 1991.

111. Stegall MD, Everson G, Schroter G, et al: Metabolic complications after liver transplantation. Diabetes, hypercholesterolemia, and obesity, *Transplantation* 60(9):1057-1060, 1995.

112. Hegeman RL, Hunsicker LG: Chronic rejection in renal allografts: importance of cardiovascular risk factors, *Clin Transplant* 9(2):135-139, 1995.

113. Lye WC, Hughes K, Leong SO, et al: Abnormal lipoprotein (a) and lipid profiles in renal allograft recipients: effects of treatment with pravastatin, *Transplant Proc* 27(1):977-978, 1995.

114. McCune TR, Thacker LR, Peters TG, et al: Effects of tacrolimus on hyperlipidemia after successful renal transplantation, *Transplantation* 65(1):87-92, 1998.

115. Brown JH, Murphy BG, Douglas AF, et al: Influence of immunosuppressive therapy on lipoprotein(a) and other lipoproteins following renal transplantation, *Nephron* 75(3):277-282, 1997.

116. Manu M, Tanabe K, Tokumoto T, et al: Impact of tacrolimus on hyperlipidemia after renal transplantation: a Japanese single center experience, *Transplant Proc* 32(7):1736-1738, 2000.

117. Fernández-Miranda C, de la Calle A, Morales JM, et al: Lipoprotein abnormalities in long-term stable liver and renal transplanted patients. A comparative study, *Clin Transplant* 12(2):136-141, 1998.

118. Perez R: Managing nutrition problems in transplant patients, *Nutr Clin Pract* 8(1):28-32, 1993.

119. Abouljoud MS, Levy MF, Klintmalm GB: Hyperlipidemia after liver transplantation: long-term results of the FK-506/cyclosporine a US multicenter trial, US Multicenter Study Group, *Transplant Proc* 27(1):1121-1123, 1995.

120. Ligtenberg G, Hene RJ, Blankestijn PJ, Koomans HA: Cardiovascular risk factors in renal transplant patients: cyclosporine A versus tacrolimus, *J Am Soc Nephrol* 12(2):368-373, 2001.

121. Hricik DE, Bartucci MR, Mayes JT, Schulak JA: The effects of steroid withdrawal on the lipoprotein profiles of cyclosporine-treated kidney and kidney-pancreas transplant recipients, *Transplantation* 54(5):868-871, 1992.

122. Vanrenterghem Y, Lebranchu Y, Hene R, Oppenheimer F, Ekberg H: Double-blind comparison of two corticosteroid regimens plus mycophenolate mofetil and cyclosporine for prevention of acute renal allograft rejection, *Transplantation* 70(9):1352-1359, 2000.

123. Stegall MD, Everson GT, Schroter G, et al: Prednisone withdrawal late after adult liver transplantation reduces diabetes, hypertension, and hypercholesterolemia without causing graft loss, *Hepatology* 25(1):173-177, 1997.

124. Downey P, Maiz A, Vaccarezza A, Pinto C, Retamal F, Martínez L: Renal transplantation and dyslipidemia: characterization of a population and treatment with diet and low dose lovastatin, *Transplant Proc* 27(2):1803-1805, 1995.

125. Shen SY, Lukens CW, Alongi SV, et al: Patient profile and effect of dietary therapy on post-transplant hyperlipidemia, *Kidney Int* 24(suppl 16):S147-152, 1983.

126. La Rocca E, Ruotolo G, Parlavecchia M, et al: Dietary advice and lipid metabolism in insulin-dependent diabetes mellitus kidney- and pancreas-transplanted patients, *Transplant Proc* 24(3):848-849, 1992.

127. Salen P, de Lorgeril M, Boissonnat P, et al: Effects of a French Mediterranean diet on heart transplant recipients with hypercholesterolemia, *Am J Cardiol* 73(11):825-827, 1994.

128. Moore RA, Callahan MF, Cody M, et al: The effect of the American Heart Association Step One Diet on hyperlipidemia following renal transplantation, *Transplantation* 49(1):60-62, 1990.

129. Tonstad S, Goldaas H, Gørbitz C, Ose L: Is dietary intervention effective in posttransplant hyperlipidaemia? *Nephrol Dial Transplant* 10(1):82-85, 1995.

130. Romero R, Calviño J, Rodriguez J, Sánchez-Guisande D: Short-term effect of atorvastatin in hypercholesterolaemic renal-transplant patients unresponsive to other statins, *Nephrol Dial Transplant* 15(9):1446-1449, 2000.

131. Malyszko JS, Malyszko J, Mysliwiec M: Serum lipids and hemostasis in kidney allograft recipients treated with fluvastatin (Lescol) for 3 months, *Transplant Proc* 32(6):1344-1346, 2000.

132. Caillard S, Leray C, Kunz K, et al: Effects of cerivastatin on lipid profiles, lipid peroxidation and platelet and endothelial activation in renal transplant recipients, *Transplant Proc* 32(8):2787-2788, 2000.

133. Arnadottir M, Eriksson LO, Germershausen JI, et al: Low-dose simvastatin is a well-tolerated and efficacious cholesterol-lowering agent in

ciclosporin-treated kidney transplant recipients: double-blind, randomized, placebo-controlled study in 40 patients, *Nephron* 68(1):57-62, 1994.

134. Martínez-Castelao A, Grinyó JM, Fiol C, et al: Fluvastatin and low-density lipoprotein oxidation in hypercholesterolemic renal transplant patients, *Kid Int* 56(suppl 71):S231-S234, 1999.

135. Barbir M, Rose M, Kushwaha S, et al: Low-dose simvastatin for the treatment of hyperlipidemia in recipients of cardiac transplantation, *Int J Cardiol* 33(2):241-246, 1991.

136. Campana C, Iacona I, Regazzi MB, et al: Efficacy and pharmacokinetics of simvastatin in cardiac transplant recipients treated with cyclosporine, *Ann Pharmacother* 29(2):235-239, 1995.

137. Castelao AM, Grina JM, Gilverner S, et al: HMG-CoA reductase inhibitors lovastatin and simvastatin in the treatment of hyperlipidemia after renal transplantation, *Transplant Proc* 25(1 Pt 2):1043-1046, 1993.

138. Cheung AK, DeVault GA, Gregory MC: A prospective study on treatment of hyperlipidemia with lovastatin in renal transplant patients receiving cyclosporine, *J Am Soc Nephrol* 3(12):1884-1891, 1993.

139. Goldberg RB, Roth D: A preliminary report of the safety and efficacy of fluvastatin for hypercholesterolemia in renal transplant patients receiving cyclosporine, *Am J Cardiol* 76(2):107A-109A, 1995.

140. Holdaas H, Hartmann A, Stenstrom J, et al: Effect of fluvastatin for safely lowering atherogenic lipids in renal transplant patients receiving cyclosporine, *Am J Cardiol* 76(2):102A-106A, 1995.

141. Kasiske BL, Tortorice KL, Heim-Duthoy KL, et al: Lovastatin treatment of hypercholesterolemia in renal transplant recipients, *Transplantation* 49(1):95-100, 1990.

142. Kobashigawa JA, Katznelson S, Laks H, et al: Effect of pravastatin on outcomes after cardiac transplantation, *N Engl J Med* 333(10):621-627, 1995.

143. Vanhaecke J, van Cleemput J, van Lierde J, Daenen W, De Geest H: Safety and efficacy of low dose simvastatin in cardiac transplant recipients treated with cyclosporine, *Transplantation* 58(1):42-45, 1994.

144. Wenke K, Thiery J, Meiser B, Arndtz N, Seidel D, Reichart B: Therapy of hypercholesterolemia after heart transplantation with the HMG-CoA reductase inhibitor simvastatin in long-term follow-up, *Z Kardiol* 84(2):130-136, 1995.

145. Yoshimura N, Oka T, Okamoto M, Ohmori Y: The effects of pravastatin on hyperlipidemia in renal transplant recipients, *Transplantation* 53(1):94-99, 1992.

146. Imagawa DK, Dawson S, Holt CD, et al: Hyperlipidemia after liver transplantation. Natural history and treatment with the hydroxy-methylglutaryl-coenzyme A reductase inhibitor pravastatin, *Transplantation* 62(7):934-942, 1996.

147. Bostom AG, Gohh RY, Beaulieu AJ, et al: Treatment of hyperhomocysteinemia in renal transplant recipients: a randomized placebo-controlled trial, *Ann Intern Med* 127(12):1089-1092, 1997.

148. Bostom AG, Gohh RY, Tsai MY, et al: Excess prevalence of fasting and postmethionine-loading hyperhomocysteinemia in stable renal transplant recipients, *Arteriorscler Thromb Vasc Biol* 17(10):1894-1900, 1997.

149. Arnadottir M, Hultberg B, Vladov V, Nilsson-Ehle P, Thysell H: Hyperhomocysteinemia in cyclosporine-treated renal transplant recipients, *Transplantation* 61(3):509-512, 1996.

150. Arnadottir M, Hultberg B, Wahlberg J, Fellström B, Dimény E: Serum total homocysteine concentration before and after renal transplantation, *Kid Int* 54(4):1380-1384, 1998.

151. Huh W, Kim B, Kim SJ, et al: Changes of fasting plasma total homocysteine in the early phase of renal transplantation, *Transplant Proc* 32(8):2811-2813, 2000.

152. Fonseca I, Queirós JM, Satos JM, et al: Hyperhomocysteinemia in renal transplantation: preliminary results, *Transplant Proc* 32(8):2602-2604, 2000.

153. Kim SI, Yoo TH, Song HY, et al: Hyperhomocysteinemia in renal transplant recipients with cyclosporine, *Transplant Proc* 32(7):1878-1879, 2000.

154. Stein G, Muller A, Busch M, Fleck C, Sperschneider H: Homocysteine, its metabolites, and B-group vitamins in renal transplant patients, *Kidney Int* 59(suppl 78):262-265, 2001.

155. Santos J, Queirós J, Silva F, et al: Effects of fish oil in cyclosporine-treated renal transplant recipients, *Transplant Proc* 32(8):2605-2608, 2000.

156. Donker JM, van der Heide JJ, Bilo HJG, et al: Effect of dietary fish oil on renal function and rejection in cyclosporine-treated recipients of renal transplants, *N Engl J Med* 329(11):769-773, 1993.

157. Sweny P, Wheeler DC, Lui SF, et al: Dietary fish oil supplements preserve renal function in renal transplant recipients with chronic vascular rejection, *Nephrol Dial Transplant* 4(12):1070-1075, 1989.

158. Badalamenti S, Salerno F, Lorenzano E, et al: Renal effects of dietary supplementation with fish oil in cyclosporine-treated liver transplant recipients, *Hepatology* 22(6):1695-1671, 1995.

159. Silva F, Queirós J, Vargas G, Henriques A, Sarmento A, Guimarãs S: Risk factors for posttransplant diabetes mellitus and impact of this complication after renal transplantation, *Transplant Proc* 32(8):2609-2610, 2000.

160. Jindal RM, Sidner RA, Milgrom ML: Post-transplant diabetes mellitus: the role of immunosuppression, *Drug Saf* 16(4):242-257, 1997.

161. Jawad F, Rizvi SAH: Posttransplant diabetes mellitus in live-related renal transplantation, *Transplant Proc* 32(7):1888, 2000.

162. Pirsch JD, Miller J, Deierhoi MJ, et al: A comparison of tacrolimus (FK506) and cyclosporine for immunosuppression after cadaveric renal transplantation, *Transplantation* 63(7):977-983, 1997.

163. Reichenspurner H, Kur F, Treede H, et al: Optimization of the immunosuppressive protocol after lung transplantation, *Transplantation* 86(1):67-71, 1994.

164. Martins L, Queirós J, Ferreira A, et al: Renal osteodistrophy: histologic evaluation after renal transplantation, *Transplant Proc* 32(8):2599-2601, 2000.

165. Keogh JB, Tsalamandris C, Sewell RB, et al: Bone loss at the proximal femur and reduced lean mass following liver transplantation: a longitudinal study, *Nutrition* 15(9):661-664, 1999.

166. Vedi S, Greer S, Skingle SJ, et al: Mechanism of bone loss after liver transplantation: a histomorphometric analysis, *J Bone Miner Res* 14(2):281-287, 1999.

167. Trautwein C, Possienke M, Schlitt H-J, et al: Bone density and metabolism in patients with viral hepatitis and cholestatic liver diseases before and after liver transplantation, *Am J Gastroenterol* 95(9):2343-2351, 2000.

168. Leidig-Bruckner G, Hosch S, Dodidou P, et al: Frequency and predictors of osteoporotic fractures after cardiac or liver transplantation: a follow-up study, *Lancet* 357(9253):342-347, 2001.

169. Nisbeth Ulf, Lindh E, Ljunghall S, Backman U, Fellström B: Increased fracture rate in diabetes mellitus and females after renal transplantation, *Transplantation* 67(9):1218-1222, 1999.

170. Porayko MK, Wiesner RH, Hay JE, et al: Bone disease in liver transplant recipients: Incidence, timing, and risk factors, *Transplant Proc* 23(1 Pt 2):1462-1465, 1991.

171. Katz IA, Epstein S: Posttransplantation bone disease, *J Bone Miner Res* 7(2):123-126, 1992.

172. Westeel FP, Mazouz K, Ezaitouni F, et al: Cyclosporine bone remodeling effect prevents steroid osteopenia after kidney transplantation, *Kid Int* 58(4):1788-1796, 2000.

173. Nam JH, Moon JI, Chung SS, et al: Pamidronate and calcitriol trial for the prevention of early bone loss after renal transplantation, *Transplant Proc* 32(7):1870, 2000.

174. Neuhaus R, Lohmann R, Platz KP, et al: Treatment of osteoporosis after liver transplantation, *Transplant Proc* 27(1):1226-1227, 1995.

175. Windus DW, Lacson S, Delmez JA: The short-term effects of a low-protein diet in stable renal transplant recipients, *Am J Kidney Dis* 17(6):693-699, 1991.

176. van der Heide JJ, Bilo HJ, Donker AJ, et al: Dietary supplemention with fish oil modifies renal reserve filtration capacity in postoperative, cyclosporin A-treated renal transplant recipients, *Transplant Int* 3:171-175, 1990.

177. van der Heide JJ, Bilo HJ, Donker JM, et al: Effect of dietary fish oil on renal function and rejection in cyclosporine-treated recipients of renal transplants, *N Engl J Med* 329(11):769-773, 1993.

178. van der Heide JJ, Bilo HJ, Donker AJ, et al: The effects of dietary supplementation with fish oil on renal function and the course of early postoperative rejection episodes in cyclosporine-treated renal transplant recipients, *Transplantation* 54(2):257-263, 1992.

179. Karliova M, Treichel Ulrich, Malagò M, Frilling, A, Gerken G, Broelsch CE: Interaction of hypericum perforatum (St. John's wort) with cyclosporin A metabolism in a patient after liver transplantation, *J Hepatol* 33(5):853-855, 2000.

Hematopoietic Cell Transplantation 41

Polly Lenssen, MS, RD, CD, FADA

HEMATOPOIETIC cell transplantation (HCT) is the infusion of stem cells collected from the bone marrow, peripheral blood, or placental cord blood to treat blood and other cancers, bone marrow–related diseases, and a variety of immunologic and genetic disorders. Stem cells may be harvested from the patient (autologous HCT) or a family member or volunteer donor (allogeneic HCT). It is the therapeutic standard for many hematologic malignancies. Its effectiveness in solid tumors, including breast, ovarian, testicular, and other solid tumors, is yet to be firmly established. To prepare the patient for the new stem cells requires intensive chemotherapy and often radiation, which are associated with significant infectious morbidity; major organ dysfunction; lengthy hospitalization; and often, long-term health problems. Hematopoietic cell transplantation is a complex and challenging area of practice, continuously evolving as the latest advances in immunology, molecular biology, and cancer basic science are applied in the clinical setting. Our understanding of how nutrients and nutrition therapy interface with the anticancer therapy, prolonged period of immunosuppression, and the recovery process lags behind. Nonetheless, nutrition assessment, diet therapy, patient education and counseling, and specialized nutrition support are key components in the medical care of patients undergoing HCT.

Historical Overview

The Early Years, the 1970s

The first successful HCT was achieved in the late 1960s in patients with severe combined immunodeficiency and advanced leukemia who received bone marrow from a sibling.[1] The ability to match tissue types via human leukocyte antigens (HLA) was a necessary precursor to the development of HCT. In the absence of HLA compatibility between the patient and donor, a fatal reaction occurred in which the donor marrow attacked key organs of the patient. Even with compatible HLA typing, the grafted marrow could initiate life-threatening graft-versus-host disease (GVHD). Few patients were candidates for transplant because a patient had only one chance in four of having the same HLA antigens as any sibling. Typically, patients were protected against infections in ultraisolation environments, sometimes for months. Patients undergoing HCT were among the first beneficiaries of central venous catheters and parenteral nutrition (PN) in the early 1970s.[2]

Expansion of Treatment, 1980s

By the 1980s HCT emerged as standard therapy for aplastic anemia, chronic myelogenous leukemia, and many types of acute leukemia. Progress in the understanding of the HLA system allowed successful transplants from family members whose HLA antigens did not fully match those of the patient. The establishment of several international registries of volunteer donors further expanded the pool of eligible patients who had no family members to donate.[3] Treatment-related mortality decreased with improved therapies to prevent and treat infections and GVHD. Whereas in the early years only young patients were believed able to tolerate the rigors of HCT, throughout the 1980s the average age of patients gradually grew older.[4]

Investigations expanded to the area of autologous HCT for both hematologic malignancies and solid tumors. In autologous transplant for leukemia, the patient's own marrow was extracted during disease remission and reinfused, often after processing to remove residual tumor cells, or frozen until the patient relapsed. For patients with solid tumors that did not involve the bone marrow, such as breast, neuroblastoma, testicular, and ovarian cancers, autologous transplant was a promising modality. By the end of the 1980s it was estimated that more patients underwent autologous than allogeneic transplantation.[3]

Increased Heterogeneity in Patients and Approaches, 1990s

In the 1990s the technology and application of HCT expanded further. Peripheral blood replaced bone marrow as the source for autologous stem cells because of the reduced surgical risk and expense and earlier hematopoietic recovery compared with bone marrow.[5] Recent studies suggest peripheral blood stem cells may be the superior source in allogeneic patients as well.[6,7] Transplantation of placental cord blood also developed as an alternative donor source.[8]

Oncologists explored new chemotherapy combinations in order to lower the disease relapse after HCT, especially among autologous patients. Recipients of autologous and syngeneic (identical twin) transplants do not benefit from the antitumor immunity that donor immune cells induce in allogeneic transplantation. This immunity, termed the graft-versus-leukemia (GVL) or graft-versus-tumor effect, leads to significantly lower relapse rates after allogeneic compared with autologous HCT.[9,10] Trials of immunotherapy in combination with HCT were conducted to boost the patient's immunity against tumor cells in a fashion similar to GVL.[11] In the same vein, discontinuation of GVHD medications and infusions of donor T lymphocytes were found successful in treating relapse after allogeneic HCT.[12]

Experimentation with diseases that had an autoimmune origin, such as multiple sclerosis and systemic sclerosis, began.[13] Patients as old as 70+ years were undergoing HCT. By the end of the decade nearly 50,000 transplants were performed annually.

Current Status and Trends

The field of HCT continues to take new directions. Mixed-chimera grafts, in which donor and host cells coexist, are being investigated with the goal to reduce mortality yet retain the GVL effect. By using less intensive treatment regimens, this approach expands HCT to older patients and to those with wide ranging immune-mediated or genetic diseases.[14,15] Novel immunologic strategies to overcome the histocompatibility barrier will expand transplantation to all patients, not just the 60% to 70% whose HLA antigens match with a family member or volunteer donor. Box 41-1 describes diseases for which HCT has been utilized.

Overview of the Phases of Transplantation

Transplantation can be conceptualized into five phases, each distinguished by key events (Fig. 41-1).

Preparation Phase

TREATMENT PLAN. Establishment of an accurate diagnosis, staging of tumor for cancer diagnoses, and identification of the donor and the histocompatibility between patient and donor are critical before HCT to ensure patients receive optimal treatment to eradicate the cancer and create marrow space for the new graft. Patients are frequently part of research protocols that aim for cure with an acceptable rate of treatment-related toxicity. In general, patients with resistant tumor types, advanced stage disease, or HLA-incompatible or unrelated donors receive more intensive treatment. Any organ dysfunction or infectious complications that might alter the treatment plan are also thoroughly investigated.

STEM CELL MOBILIZATION. Patients undergoing autologous HCT receive a short course of chemotherapy, usually as outpatients, with or without hematopoietic growth factors, to mobilize large numbers of stem cells from their bone marrow into their peripheral blood. Stem cells are then collected and cryopreserved (frozen) until ready for reinfusion. Stem cells are typically purged of residual tumor cells by cytotoxic or physical methods. Patients often develop neutropenia after chemotherapy mobilization; an interval of time appears necessary between chemotherapy mobilization and the transplant treatment to reduce toxicities.

Cytoreduction Phase and Stem Cell or Marrow Infusion

For most transplants, patients require high-dose chemotherapy with or without radiation to ablate the patient's immune system, allowing engraftment of donated stem cells and, in the case of cancers, to eradicate the tumor. Lower dose regimens are used when there is limited immunity to ablate, such as with immune deficiency disorders, or when the goal is to establish a mixed chimera graft.

The use of chemotherapy-only regimens has increased over the years to reduce the toxicities of radiation.[4] Patients under-

---

BOX 41-1

Diseases Treated by Hematopoietic Cell Transplantation

HEMATOLOGIC MALIGNANCIES
Acute leukemias, myelogenous and lymphoblastic
Chronic myelogenous leukemia
Lymphomas, non-Hodgkin and Hodgkin
Myelodysplastic and myeloproliferative disorders
Multiple myeloma

SOLID TUMORS
Breast cancer (metastatic or high-risk primary disease)
Neuroblastoma
Ovarian cancer
Sarcoma
Testicular cancer
Small-cell lung cancer
Brain tumors
Renal carcinoma

GENETIC DISORDERS
Thalassemia
Sickle cell disease
Immunodeficiency disorders (severe combined immunodeficiency disorder, combined immunodeficiency, Wiskott-Aldrich syndrome)
Fanconi's anemia
Osteopetrosis
Enzyme deficiency diseases*

OTHER NONMALIGNANT DISEASES
Severe aplastic anemia
Paroxysmal nocturnal hemoglobinuria
Acquired immunodeficiency disease
Autoimmune disorders (multiple sclerosis, systemic sclerosis, systemic lupus erythematosus, rheumatoid arthritis)

*Maroteaux-Lamy syndrome, metachromatic leukodystrophy, globoid cell leukodystrophy, adrenoleukodystrophy, Hurler's syndrome, Hunter's syndrome.

---

going total body irradiation (TBI) experience more severe mucositis,[16] acute and chronic pulmonary complications,[17] and other serious late complications, including secondary malignancies,[18-20] leukoencephalopathy, impaired cognitive function, and endocrine abnormalities (hypothyroidism, infertility, and delayed growth and development).[21-23] However, for some cancers, such as acute lymphoblastic leukemia in children, TBI remains the most effective regimen for a cure.[24] Other forms of radiation that shield vital organs or that target only lymphoid tissue or bone marrow may be utilized to reduce toxicity.

Chemotherapy drugs commonly used for cytoreduction and their major nutrition-related toxicities are described in Table 41-1. All these agents can induce some degree of nausea and vomiting, necessitating antiemetic premedication. Many cytoreductive regimens can safely be administered on an outpatient basis.

Neutropenia Phase

INFECTION CONTROL. High doses of cytoreduction therapy lead to profound neutropenia, thrombocytopenia, and anemia. Frequent transfusions of platelets and red blood cells are usually required. Circulating neutrophils may be negligible up

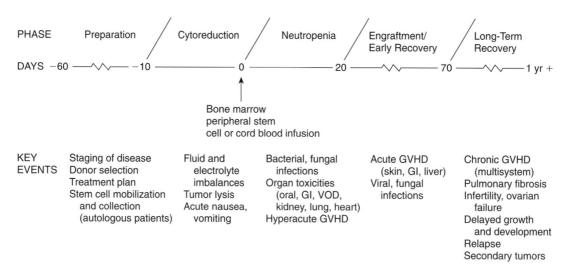

FIGURE 41-1 Hematopoietic cell transplantation can be characterized by events that occur in five general phases or time periods. The day of transplant is referred to as day 0. *GI,* Gastrointestinal; *GVHD,* graft-versus-host disease; *VOD,* venoocclusive disease.

until 2 weeks after stem cell, 3 weeks after marrow, and 4 weeks after cord blood infusion. To prevent bacterial and fungal infections, intravenous antimicrobials are administered and special protective environments, high-efficiency particulate air filtration systems, gut decontamination with oral nonabsorbable antibiotics, or low-microbial diets may be utilized. Patients may receive an antiviral agent to prevent reactivation of herpes simplex virus, which causes painful oral and esophageal lesions. If a patient becomes febrile or develops an infection, additional antibiotics are added that often contribute to organ toxicity (see Table 41-1).

REGIMEN-RELATED TOXICITIES. It is during the early posttransplant phase of neutropenia that the most serious toxicities associated with cytoreduction therapy occur. Most conditioning regimens disrupt the gastrointestinal (GI) tract, resulting in painful mucositis and esophagitis, gastritis with prolonged nausea and vomiting, and diarrhea (see Table 41-1); those containing TBI and alkylating agents are especially toxic to the gut.[25,26] With allogeneic grafts, GI toxicity is aggravated by posttransplant administration of methotrexate to minimize acute GVHD.[27]

Hepatic venoocclusive disease (VOD), renal failure, and pulmonary and cardiac damage are potential morbid events in the early posttransplant period. VOD is the clinical syndrome that results from cytoreductive damage to terminal hepatic venules and hepatocytes.[28] Severe disease is characterized by 15% or greater weight gain and elevation of serum bilirubin over 20 mg/L within the first 20 days after transplant,[29] although some chemotherapies are associated with a more delayed onset.[30] Ascites, renal insufficiency, and cardiopulmonary failure are common sequelae of severe VOD. A higher incidence is observed among patients with previous liver damage as well as those receiving cytoreduction regimens containing large doses of TBI or busulfan.[31] No effective medical treatment has been established for severe VOD.

Other causes of liver dysfunction in the early posttransplant period include medications, sepsis, hemolysis, and biliary sludge syndrome.[32] Renal insufficiency is multifactorial and is associated with TBI; chemotherapy; nephrotoxic antimicro-

bials; anti-GVHD drugs; sepsis; and especially, liver toxicity. Among patients with no liver toxicity, renal dysfunction occurs in approximately 10% of patients, whereas more than 80% of patients with severe liver toxicity may expect to develop renal dysfunction.[33] Congestive cardiomyopathy syndromes occur in as many as 5% of patients receiving TBI, cyclophosphamide, or anthracycline-containing regimens. Patients are also at risk for pulmonary edema, both infectious and idiopathic pneumonia, pulmonary hemorrhage, sepsis, adult respiratory distress syndrome, and multiorgan failure during this phase. The requirement for mechanical ventilation carries a poor prognosis, especially if complicated by other organ dysfunction or hypotension.[34]

ENGRAFTMENT AND EARLY RECOVERY PHASE. As white cell engraftment occurs (usually defined as a neutrophil count > 500 per cm³), infection precautions are still necessary. Patients require medications to prevent *Pneumocystis carinii* pneumonia and cytomegalovirus infections of the lung or GI tract.

Unless they have developed organ toxicities, autologous graft patients can expect rapid improvement in physical status with recovery of neutrophil and platelet counts. Allogeneic patients, however, may develop GVHD, which can significantly prolong recovery.

GRAFT-VERSUS-HOST DISEASE. With engraftment, allogeneic graft recipients enter the risk period for GVHD. GVHD is initiated when immunocompetent donor T cells orchestrate damage to host (patient) target tissues, especially the skin, liver, and GI tract.[35] GVHD can occur as early as the first week after transplant but more typically appears after there is evidence of donor cell engraftment in the peripheral blood. Approximately 30% of patients with HLA-identical sibling donors develop clinically significant GVHD.[36] Both the incidence and severity are higher for older patients, for patients with unrelated or mismatched family donors, and for patients who fail to tolerate sufficient immunosuppressive drug therapy.[37]

Pharmacologic immunosuppression to prevent GVHD is started at the time the marrow or peripheral stem cells are

TABLE 41-1
Nutritional Implications of Drugs Used During Hematopoietic Transplantation

Medication	Classification	Nutritional Implications
CHEMOTHERAPY AGENTS		
Busulfan	Alkylating agent	Mild nausea, vomiting, anorexia, mucositis; hepatotoxic; absorption impaired by food (take on empty stomach); delayed growth in children
Carmustine (BCNU)	Alkylating agent	Moderate to severe nausea, vomiting, anorexia; mucositis, esophagitis; hepatotoxic; nephrotoxic
Cisplatin	Heavy metal	Severe nausea, vomiting; diarrhea; nephrotoxicity; magnesium, potassium and zinc wasting; metallic aftertaste
Cyclophosphamide	Alkylating agent	Moderate to severe nausea, vomiting, mucositis, esophagitis; nephrotoxicity; may cause inappropriate ADH-like syndrome with total body water excess; cardiotoxicity
Cytosine arabinoside (ARA-C)	Antimetabolite	Severe nausea, vomiting, anorexia, diarrhea, mucositis, esophagitis; nephrotoxicity; hepatotoxicity
Etoposide (VP-16)	Plant alkaloid	Mild to moderate nausea, vomiting, mucositis, diarrhea
Fludarabine	Purine analog	Mild to moderate nausea, vomiting; peripheral edema
Fluorouracil (5-FU)	Antimetabolite	Severe mucositis, esophagitis; diarrhea; hepatotoxicity
Ifosfamide	Alkylating agent	Mild to moderate nausea, vomiting; electrolyte wasting; nephrotoxicity
Melphalan	Alkylating agent	Mild to moderate nausea, vomiting
Thiotepa	Alkylating agent	Moderate nausea, vomiting; mucositis
IMMUNOTHERAPY AND BIOLOGIC RESPONSE MODIFIERS		
Granulocyte colony-stimulating factor, granulocyte-macrophage colony-stimulating factor	Growth maturation factors	Mild nausea, vomiting, anorexia, diarrhea
Interferons	Cytokine	Mild to moderate nausea, vomiting, anorexia, diarrhea; hepatotoxicity
Interleukin-1	Cytokine	Mild to moderate nausea, vomiting, anorexia; hepatotoxicity; capillary leak (fluid retention)
ANTIMICROBIALS		
Acyclovir, gancyclovir, valacyclovir	Antiviral	Renal tubular damage; synergy with other nephrotoxins
Amphotericin	Broad-spectrum antifungal	Nephrotoxicity, hypokalemia, hypomagnesemia, anorexia, nausea and vomiting; lipid complex form of drug less nephrotoxic
Ceftazidime	Cephalosporin antibacterial	Nausea, vomiting, diarrhea; hepatotoxicity
Ciprofloxacin	Fluoroquinolone	Nausea, vomiting, diarrhea; nephrotoxicity
Fluconazole	Triazole antifungal	Nausea and vomiting, diarrhea, nephrotoxicity, hepatotoxicity
Foscarnet	Antiviral	Nephrotoxicity; calcium, phosphorus, magnesium, and potassium wasting
Gentamicin	Aminoglycoside antibacterial	Nephrotoxicity, hepatotoxicity
Tobramycin	Aminoglycoside antibacterial	Nephrotoxicity, hepatotoxicity
Trimethoprim/sulfamethoxazole or Cotrimazole	Broad-spectrum sulfonamide antibacterial	Anorexia, nausea, vomiting, nephrotoxicity, hepatotoxicity
Vancomycin	Glycopeptide antibacterial (gram-positive organisms, including *Staphylococcus*)	Nausea
GVHD PROPHYLAXIS AND TREATMENT		
Antithymocyte globulin (ATG)	Immunosuppressant	Requires large-volume normal saline that may affect fluid and electrolyte status
Azathioprine	Immunosuppressant	Uncommon: nausea and vomiting, anorexia, diarrhea
Beclomethasone dipropionate	Oral nonabsorbable synthetic glucocorticoid	Xerostomia, dysgeusia, adrenal insufficiency, nausea
Corticosteroids	Synthetic glucocorticoid	Sodium and fluid retention, hyperphagia and weight gain, hyperglycemia, muscle wasting, gastritis, esophageal reflux, hypokalemia, osteoporosis, growth retardation, hyperlipidemia
Cyclosporine	Immunosuppressive macrolide	Nephrotoxicity, hepatotoxicity, hypomagnesemia, hyperkalemia, hyperlipidemia; should not be taken with grapefruit, pineapple, or papaya juice or carbonated beverages
Humanized Anti-Tac and other murine or human anti-IL-2 receptor antibodies	Monoclonal antibodies that bind to IL-2 receptor on T and B cells	Mild nausea, vomiting; mucositis; diarrhea
Methotrexate	Antimetabolite	Anorexia, mucositis, esophagitis, nausea, vomiting, nephrotoxicity, hepatotoxicity; trimetrexate an experimental alternative
Mycophenolate mofetil (MMF)	Enzyme inhibitor; blocks purine synthesis in T and B cells	Diarrhea, vomiting, viral activation
Psoralen and ultraviolet radiation (PUVA)	Photosensitizer and light therapy to treat skin GVHD	Nausea, hepatotoxicity
Rapamycin	Immunosuppressive macrolide	Hypertriglyceridemia; intravenous lipid emulsions contraindicated
Tacrolimus (FK-506)	Immunosuppressive macrolide	Nephrotoxicity, hypomagnesemia, hyperkalemia, glucose intolerance
Thalidomide	Glutamic acid derivative	Constipation, nausea, sedation
Ursodeoxycholic acid (UDCA)	Synthetic bile acid to displace toxic bile acids in liver disease	Nausea, vomiting, diarrhea, dyspepsia

GVHD, Graft-versus-host disease; *Il-2,* interleukin-2.

infused and continues usually for a minimum of 6 months after transplant. Common regimens are methotrexate and cyclosporine[38] or tacrolimus.[39] New strategies are under continual investigation, most of them targeted for the specific T cells that initiate GVHD. Removal of donor T cells has been very effective in preventing GVHD but unfortunately has led to increased graft rejection and recurrent leukemia.[40] T-cell depletion is most effective in patients with little risk of graft rejection and with nonmalignant diseases (see Box 41-1).

Additional immunosuppression is necessary to treat established GVHD, which adds to the risk for bacterial, fungal, and viral infections. In turn, infections can stimulate or cause a "flare" of GVHD, leading to a downward spiral in which the immune system becomes profoundly impaired and life-threatening infections occur. The nutrition-related side effects of GVHD drugs are described in Table 41-1. GVHD occasionally occurs with autologous HCT and usually responds to a short course of immunosuppression.

Long-Term Recovery Phase

With gradual recovery of immunocompetence over the next several months, the risk of infection diminishes. Autologous grafts carry little risk of late infections, as do allogeneic ones in the absence of GVHD. Patients with chronic GVHD require prolonged immunosuppression and are susceptible to recurrent bacterial and fungal infections.

CHRONIC GRAFT-VERSUS-HOST DISEASE. Chronic GVHD develops 70 to 400 days (or more) after allogeneic HCT in 30% of patients with HLA-identical sibling donors and in as many as 70% of patients with unrelated donors.[36] It is viewed not simply as a chronic form of the acute disease but as a separate immune-mediated phenomenon. In contrast to the cell destruction observed in acute GVHD, the pathophysiology is more similar to that of autoimmune disorders such as systemic lupus erythematosus and primary biliary cirrhosis. The pathologic findings are characterized principally by increased collagen deposition and fibrosis due to autoreactive T lymphocytes.

Chronic GVHD can present as *progressive* disease evolving from the acute form, which is associated with the poorest prognosis. Approximately 20% of patients will present *de novo* with no history of acute GVHD. Patients undergo diagnostic screening studies approximately 2 to 3 months after transplant to monitor disease activity.[40] If there is clinical evidence of extensive disease, immunosuppression is indicated for at least 6 months to 1 year after the graft, at which time disease activity can be reevaluated. Patients with subclinical or limited disease are not treated unless the GVHD progresses because treatment may increase the risk of relapse, presumably because of abrogation of the GVL or graft-versus-tumor effect.

DISEASE RELAPSE. The risk of disease recurrence varies widely and depends on the type of malignancy and the stage of disease at the time of HCT. For some patients who relapse, further treatment options may be available (e.g., a second transplant)[41] or with allogeneic grafts, stimulation of GVL with discontinuation of immunosuppression and/or infusion of donor T cells.[12,42,43]

OTHER LONG-TERM COMPLICATIONS. Some of the complications patients experience as a long-term consequence of the transplant are poor engraftment with associated immunodeficiency, restrictive and obstructive lung disease, cataracts, osteoporosis and aseptic bone necrosis, retarded growth, gonadal and ovarian failure, tooth decay, and hemosiderosis.[21-23, 43-45] Fatigue and the deconditioning associated with HCT persist for many months in most patients, and psychosocial adjustment is often difficult.[46] Patients with transplant-related problems may be disabled for years.[47] For those patients without chronic GVHD or other serious complications, normal activities resume within 6 months to 2 years posttransplant. Eventually even patients with chronic GVHD appear to have disease stabilization and abatement of symptoms as time passes; the vast majority of patients surveyed an average of 10 years after the transplant report leading productive, meaningful lives.[48]

The Role of Nutrition Intervention

Pretransplantation Nutrition Assessment

EARLY SCREENING FOR NUTRITIONAL RISK. All patients undergoing HCT may be considered at nutritional risk because of the anticipated toxicities that affect ability to sustain adequate oral intake for a minimum of 3 to 4 weeks.[49] The majority of patients have adequate nutritional status at the time of transplant.[50,51] For patients who are underweight, prognosis is less favorable. In one large series of 1662 adults and 576 children undergoing either allogeneic or autologous HCT, nonrelapse mortality was significantly higher in patients whose ideal body weight (IBW) was less than 95%.[51] Other studies have confirmed the association of malnutrition and increased mortality in both autologous and allogeneic patients.[52,53] Thus, the earlier candidates for HCT are screened for nutritional risk, the earlier nutrition intervention can begin to reverse weight loss and minimize this risk factor. The risk of obesity on outcome is less clear.[51,52,54]

Assessment of nutritional status is similar to a thorough assessment appropriate to any complex medical condition. Table 41-2 suggests measures and clinically significant indicators of nutritional status before and subsequent to transplant. Some special considerations of pretransplant nutrition assessment are discussed next.

ANTHROPOMETRIC STATUS. Weight history, including preillness weight, is important in determining IBW because of the fluctuations that may occur with previous treatment and often over an extended period of time. Splenomegaly can add weight, and some attempt should be made to estimate the weight of the spleen and correct for its effect on IBW. Patients with multiple myeloma may become shorter as a result of vertebral compression, although their lean body mass is not significantly altered; thus, it may be appropriate to use their premorbid height to evaluate IBW status.

For chemotherapy that is dosed by body weight, doses may be adjusted downward for obese patients.[52] Adjusted body weight is often used (see Table 41-2), which accounts for the increased lean tissue needed to support excess fat stores.[55] Upper arm anthropometry helps distinguish overfat persons from very muscular ones. In the latter cases, adjusted body weight may be inappropriate and drug dosing may best be based on actual weight. In the other extreme, patients who recently took corticosteroid therapy may weigh more because

TABLE 41-2

Nutrition Assessment and Monitoring in Hematopoietic Cell Transplantation

Measure	Interval	Significant Indicators	Intervention/Comments
ANTHROPOMETRY			
Ideal body weight	Pretransplant; continuous monitoring	Adults: <95% IBW Children: <10th %tile weight for length or body mass index for age	Intervene early with nutrition support if unable to eat adequate kcal for weight gain. In cytoreduction and neutropenia phases and during severe complications, provide kcal to maintain weight (at risk for substrate intolerance and fluid overload). In early recovery phase and if medically stable, increase kcal for weight gain to >95% IBW.
		>125% IBW	Standardize method for adjusted IBW for cyclophosphamide, busulfan, cyclosporine, and other drug dosing* If indirect calorimetry inaccessible, adjusted IBW may be used for calculation of energy and protein needs.
Body weight	Daily during cytoreduction, neutropenia, and periods of hospitalization Weekly (minimum) during early and long-term recovery through first posttransplant year	>5% gain in 7-10 days associated with capillary leak syndrome (due to cytoreduction, early acute GVHD, or sepsis), VOD ascites, congestive heart failure, acute severe skin GVHD, corticosteroid use, decreased urine output	Restrict fluid in PN, IV fluid, and diet as needed; if urine sodium excretion <10 mEq, restrict all sources of sodium.
		>5% loss in 7-10 days associated with fluid mobilization in resolving VOD or capillary leak syndrome, dehydration (due to inadequate input or excessive output such as diarrhea, glycosuria, or diuretic use), hypermetabolism or hypercatabolism	Assess volume status and provide adequate fluid support as indicated; correct glucose abnormalities. If volume status and glucose abnormalities are ruled out, measure metabolic rate.
Upper arm muscle and fat areas	Pretransplant, day 50-100, 1 yr posttransplant	<5th %tile	For low muscle mass, initiate physical therapy consult and monitor activity levels. For low fat, at risk for more weight loss during periods of hypermetabolism because of hydrated muscle tissue loss.
Height	Pretransplant Adults and postpubertal adolescents: Yearly posttransplant if on corticosteroids Children: Every 3 mo posttransplant; plot growth rate annually	Adults and postpubertal adolescents: Serial decrements (a sign of vertebral compression and osteoporosis) associated with corticosteroids, ovarian failure Children: <5th %tile associated with chronic disease, prior chemoradiotherapy, corticosteroids, chronic malnutrition Growth velocity[†] <10th %tile associated with chemoradiotherapy before HCT cytoreduction with TBI or busulfan, chronic GVHD, corticosteroids, malnutrition	Identify and correct any contributory nutritional deficiencies (energy, protein, zinc, vitamin D, calcium, and vitamin A). Evaluate bone absorptiometry, 25(OH) vitamin D status, and/or initiate endocrinology consult for osteoporosis therapy
SERUM PROTEIN STATUS			
Albumin	Pretransplant	<3.3 mg/dl	If other signs of inadequate nutrition status, intervene early with nutrition counseling and/or support.
	Weekly (to correct serum calcium status)	<2.5 mg/dl associated with intravascular volume overload, capillary leak syndrome, diarrhea, hepatic disease	Occurs independent of adequate nutrition support; exogenous infusions considered not helpful for maintenance of oncotic pressure but sometimes used with diuretic to promote diuresis.
Prealbumin	As clinically indicated	Adults: <20 mg/dl Children: <10 mg/dl associated with neutropenia, infection, inflammation, hepatic disease	As sign of metabolic stress, may help determine need for nutrition intervention. Not helpful to determine adequacy of nutrition support in early posttransplant period.
SUBSTRATE UTILIZATION			
Indirect calorimetry	Pretransplant if body composition altered (obesity, high muscle mass, malnutrition) Posttransplant if at high risk for adverse consequences or overfeeding or	Measured resting energy expenditure + activity factor differs from current intake by >10%	Adjust nutrition support or counsel patient to target kcal intake according to measured energy expenditure. Consider whether respiratory quotient is consistent with overfeeding (>1.0) or underfeeding (<0.7).

Continued.

TABLE 41-2

Nutrition Assessment and Monitoring in Hematopoietic Cell Transplantation—cont'd

Measure	Interval	Significant Indicators	Intervention/Comments
	underfeeding (critically ill, on PN >1mo, liver disease, chronic GVHD) or if significant weight and muscle mass loss make energy estimations difficult		
Serum glucose	Daily until stable if on nutrition support then once or twice weekly Twice weekly (minimum) with large doses of steroids Once or twice weekly in ambulatory care	>180 mg/dl (random draw) >140 mg/dl (fasting; minimum 4 hours off PN or overnight if on oral diet) associated with PN, sepsis, corticosteroids, tacrolimus, preexisting diabetes, pancreatitis	If on PN: Provide kcal appropriate to clinical status, daily IV lipids to reduce dextrose load, insulin to maintain serum glucose <180 mg/dl. If high insulin requirements (>0.3-0.4 m/g dextrose), restrict dextrose to 2-3 mg/kg/min in adults and adolescents and increase lipids to maximum 50-60% of total kcal; insulin drip may allow for better glucose control. If on IVF: Provide dextrose-free solution. If on oral diet (including transitioning off PN): Determine if SC insulin required (fasting >160-180 mg/dl or symptomatic with osmotic diuresis); provide NPH and Regular insulin based on preprandial blood glucose; monitor fasting blood glucose frequently to determine NPH dose, especially if escalating insulin doses or tapering corticosteroids. Teach home blood glucose monitoring to ambulatory patients. Restrict total kcal and/or carbohydrate intake if excessive. Assess for signs and symptoms of dehydration (osmotic diuresis) or hypoglycemia.
Serum triglyceride	Pretransplant Weekly if on PN and >350 mg/dl pretransplant, on dialysis, or with hepatic dysfunction, persistent sepsis, pancreatitis	>400-500 mg/dl associated with preexisting hypertriglyceridemia, glucose intolerance, pancreatitis, hepatic dysfunction, sepsis, corticosteroid or cyclosporine use	If on PN: Provide IV lipids at 4-8% of total kcal for essential fatty acids. If >1000 mg/dl or if serum lipemic, hold IV lipids. If on oral diet (normal serum lipids pretransplant): Reassess when off all lipid-raising drugs. If on oral diet (elevated serum lipids pretransplant): Assess for other risk factors for heart disease and provide or refer for counseling as indicated.
Nitrogen balance	As clinically indicated in patients able to separate urine and stool, not on diuretics, and with stable renal function (otherwise correct for urea pool‡)	Loss of >5 g/day associated with protein intakes less than twice normal requirements, corticosteroids, preexisting large muscle mass, persistent fevers and sepsis	Increase protein support.
Plasma amino acid profile	In patients with encephalopathy due to liver disease	Plasma phenylalanine >twice normal	Consider trial of reduced-phenylalanine solution (PN or enteral); efficacy not established.§

SERUM ELECTROLYTES AND TRACE ELEMENTS

Measure	Interval	Significant Indicators	Intervention/Comments
Potassium	Daily if potassium wasting or significant renal insufficiency 2-3 times weekly during neutropenia, early recovery or if on PN	<3.5 mEq/dl associated with amphotericin, thiazide diuretics, gastrointestinal losses, corticosteroids, aminoglycosides, foscarnet, anabolism >5.5 mEq/dl associated with renal failure, cyclosporine, tacrolimus, aldactone	Supplement in PN, hydration or separate infusion up to maximum 20 mEq/hr (0.3 mEq/kg/hr in children) without a cardiac monitor; maximum 10-15 mEq/hr in ambulatory care). If GI symptoms absent, provide oral supplement and high-potassium diet. Delete all supplemental potassium; rarely a moderate restriction of dietary potassium may be indicated.
Magnesium	Twice weekly if magnesium wasting Once weekly if on PN, cyclosporine, or tacrolimus	<1.5 mEq/dl associated with cyclosporine, tacrolimus, amphotericin, aminoglycosides, gastrointestinal losses	If on PN: Initial supplement 16 mEq/L; may reach up to 48 mEq/L. If off PN/IVF but on magnesium-wasting medication: Maintain level >1.3 mEq/L with oral magnesium ± MgSO₄ boluses; maximum tolerated oral dose varies (protein complex form usually better tolerated).

Continued.

Nutrition Assessment and Monitoring in Hematopoietic Cell Transplantation—cont'd

Measure	Interval	Significant Indicators	Intervention/Comments
Calcium	Once twice weekly if on PN	>10 mg/dl (corrected for hypoalbuminemia); associated with tumor lysis, renal failure, multiple myeloma, metastatic breast cancer	If on PN: Delete calcium. If on oral diet: Restrict if sources (diet, antacids, supplements) far exceed RDA.
		<8.5 mg/dl (corrected for hypoalbuminemia or obtain ionized serum calcium); associated with corticosteroids, foscarnet, high calcium needs in children	If on PN: Maximize calcium intake within calcium/phosphorus solubility limitations; occasionally IV calcium gluconate must be provided as separate infusate. If on oral diet: Provide 1.5 times DRI of calcium via diet and supplements (maximum single dose 500 mg, citrate form if on gastric acid blockers).
Phosphorus	Twice weekly inpatient Once weekly in ambulatory care if on PN or steroids	Adults: <2.5 mEq/dl Children: <4.0 mEq/dl associated with anabolism (refeeding syndrome), cyclophosphamide, renal acidosis, steatorrhea, diabetes, mineralocorticoid deficiency	If on PN: Increase phosphate salts (sodium or potassium). If on oral diet: Oral phosphate replacement.
		Adults: >4.5 mEq/dl Children: >6.0 mEq/dl associated with renal failure, multiple myeloma, tumor lysis syndrome	If on PN: Delete phosphate salts. If on oral diet: Provide phosphate binder (calcium carbonate).
Zinc	Posttransplant if excessive diarrhea >1 wk or severe skin GVHD	<60-80 µg/dl associated with gastrointestinal losses, increased needs for healing	Serum levels do not reflect tissue stores so only crudely guide replacement therapy (see Table 41-3).
Copper	If on PN when chronic liver disease or diarrhea present	<70-90 µg/dl associated with gastrointestinal losses >200 µg/dl associated with lymphoma, liver disease	Serum levels do not reflect tissue stores so only crudely guide replacement therapy.

*Adjusted body weight = ideal weight + 0.25 (actual weight − ideal weight). Renal Dietitians Practice Group: Adjustment in body weight for obese patients (Appendix B). In *Suggested guidelines for nutrition care of renal patients*, Chicago, 1990, American Dietetic Association, p. 34.

+Tanner JM: *North American growth and development longitudinal standards. Height: distance and velocity for girls and boys*, Castlemead Publications, Swains Mill, 4A Crane Mead, Ware, Herts. SG129PY, England. 1985.

‡{[0.6 × wt in kg + (previous day fluid input − output in ml$_{previous\ day}$/1000 ml)] × BUN$_{previous\ day}$ × 10]} − {[0.6 × wt in kg + (fluid input − output in ml/1000 ml)] × BUN × 10]} where BUN = Blood urea nitrogen in mg/dl.

§Lenssen P, Spencer GD, McDonald GB: A randomized trial of FreAmine vs. HepatAmine vs. placebo in acute hepatic coma, *Gastroenterology* 92:1749, 1987 (abstract).

DRI, dietary reference intakes; *GVHD*, graft-versus-host disease; *IBW*, ideal body weight; *IV*, intravenous; *IVF*, intravenous fluids; *PN*, parenteral nutrition, *RDA*, recommended dietary allowance; *SC*, subcutaneous; *TBI*, total body irradiation; *VOD*, venoocclusive disease; *HCT*, hematopoietic cell transplantation.

of fluid retention or fat deposition without gaining any lean body mass. The dietitian can bring these aspects of nutrition assessment to the attention of the medical team.

Arm anthropometry and other techniques that estimate muscle mass and function, such as bioelectric impedance or hand dynamometry, are also useful in establishing baseline values and monitoring serial changes, especially in allogeneic grafts that carry a higher risk of long-term complications and cumulative muscle protein losses.[56]

LABORATORY AND MEDICAL EVALUATION. Major renal or hepatic dysfunction is almost always a contraindication to transplantation. The pretransplant serum creatinine value serves as a benchmark for evaluating posttransplant renal insufficiency. Metabolic problems such as diabetes and hyperlipidemia can influence nutrition support strategies.

DIET HISTORY. During the pretransplant patient interview, any active problems that interfere with the ability to meet nutrient needs and sustain weight should be evaluated and a care plan instituted. Some patients may follow diets that limit food variety such as very low fat or other special diets; fitting these individuals' diet preferences into posttransplant care plans can be a special challenge. Large-dose vitamin supplementation and use of herbals are common practices, some of which carry risks, such as fungal or bacterial contamination[57] or organ toxicity, and it may be prudent to restrict consumption. Our knowledge in these areas is, unfortunately, very rudimentary, and common sense must substitute for scientifically based recommendations.

PEDIATRIC ISSUES. Accurate measurements of height and length on a vertical and a recumbent stadiometer, respectively, provide critical baseline data for posttransplant growth assessment. Delayed feeding development should be identified in infants and young children so that intervention with occupational therapy specialists can be initiated as early as possible in the transplant process. Breast feeding is controversial; some institutions may not allow it for allogeneic graft patients, whereas others have succeeded without immune sequelae when breast milk is irradiated.[58]

Cytoreduction and Neutropenia
NUTRIENT NEEDS

Energy. Few data on the energy and protein needs of HCT patients are available. Data on the measured resting energy expenditure of approximately 100 adult patients, derived from both abstracts and published papers during the cytoreduction and neutropenia phases, suggest large interindividual variability but average energy needs of 25 to 35 kcal/kg (assuming bed rest or a 10% activity factor) or approximately 1.3 to 1.5 times basal energy needs.[59-65] No studies with children have been reported, but 1.6 times basal energy needs is a safe starting point.

Taveroff and colleagues reported that energy intake of 25 kcal/kg in adults (as compared with 35 kcal/kg) resulted in less pronounced derangements in serum sodium, potassium, and albumin without adverse effects on nitrogen balance.[66] However, in this small, nonrandomized trial the groups were not balanced for important variables, such as types of transplants, administration of medications that affect electrolyte status, and body weight status. On the contrary, underfeeding allogeneic graft patients during the early posttransplant period may result in significant weight loss before onset of acute and chronic GVHD when metabolic needs appear higher and may be more difficult to achieve.[67] In autologous graft patients, who may generally be expected to recover earlier, potential underfeeding in the neutropenic period should be weighed against a variety of factors, including initial nutritional status, the severity of regimen-related toxicities and projected length of recovery, and whether further treatment is planned, such as immunotherapy or consolidation with local irradiation.

Protein. Negative nitrogen balance despite PN has been described in several studies.[68-70] In adult patients undergoing allogeneic HCT, median daily nitrogen losses exceed 5 g during the first month after transplant when protein support is targeted at 1.5 g/kg.[69] Cumulative protein losses during this period are associated with a loss of approximately 5% of body cell mass that is not reflected in weight loss owing to expansion of extracellular water.[68] The magnitude of protein loss is greater in men[71] and is markedly accelerated with the administration of corticosteroids.[60, 70] Based on these data, protein needs are estimated at twice normal requirements, probably for all age groups, although nitrogen balance studies have not included children younger than 12 years. Individual requirements may be estimated with serial nitrogen balance studies, but these are labor intensive and frequently inaccurate outside the research setting because of incomplete collections or mixing of stool and urine.

Fluid and electrolytes. Fluid needs during cytoreduction are based on individual drug regimens and may range from 1.0 to 2.0 times maintenance needs. Maintenance fluid needs are calculated as:

100 ml/kg up to 10 kg
1000 ml + 50 ml/kg for 10-20 kg
1500 ml + 20 ml/kg for 20-40 kg
1500 ml per square meter of body surface area for weights greater than 40 kg in which body surface area is calculated by the square root of (ht in cm × wt in kg) divided by 60.

$$\sqrt{\frac{\text{height (cm)} \times \text{weight (kg)}}{60}}$$

During cytoreduction and neutropenia, daily input and output records and weights are assessed to detect fluid overload or deficits (see Table 41-2). Fluid input from blood product support, PN, oral intake, and intravenous medications typically exceeds maintenance needs. Patients with signs and symptoms of pulmonary edema, heart failure, ascites, or other serious consequences of fluid overload require restriction of fluid and usually of sodium. Fluid replacement greater than maintenance needs is usually necessary for patients whose stool volume is greater than 500 ml, which is often observed after cytoreduction and with intestinal GVHD (Table 41-3).

Electrolytes may be provided in PN or hydration solution, as separate infusions, or as a combination of these means, depending on institutional practice and cost considerations. Some practitioners find that separate electrolyte supplementation avoids frequent reformulation of PN, but others find it more cost-effective to supplement in the PN formula. In the early posttransplant period, patients frequently excrete little sodium and, unless diarrhea is voluminous, may require minimal sodium repletion. Patients should be instructed not to swallow saline rinses used for oral hygiene. Some amino acid solutions contain moderate amounts of sodium and need to be factored into total sodium delivery, as, of course, should hydration solutions with saline (see Chapter 19).

Potassium, in contrast, may be required in very large amounts. Potassium losses with amphotericin, especially in conjunction with other potassium-wasting drugs such as furosemide, can surpass 500 to 700 mEq per day, far exceeding maximal infusion rates without a cardiac monitor (see Table 41-2). Replacement therapy must be carefully planned to avoid concurrent infusions of potassium piggybacks or drips with potassium-containing hydration or PN. Adding 200 to 250 mEq/L of potassium in PN or hydration solution to provide a continuous infusion may be safer than trying to juggle multiple potassium infusates. During the period of escalating or deescalating requirements, patients may require twice daily monitoring of serum potassium. Potassium wasting can persist for many weeks after discontinuation of amphotericin, challenging professionals to maintain potassium homeostasis safely for ambulatory patients. A combination of oral and intravenous replacement may be necessary as well as medical supervision in a clinic when potassium supplementation exceeds 15 mEq per hour (or 0.3 mEq/kg/hr in children). Oral supplementation generally is not tolerated well if GI symptoms are present.

Magnesium supplementation is required with many nephrotoxins, in particular amphotericin, cyclosporine, tacrolimus, and foscarnet.[72] Oral supplementation is poorly tolerated in the early posttransplant period and should not be attempted until stools are formed (see Table 41-2).

Vitamins and minerals. The data on vitamin and mineral requirements are negligible; intervention related to complications is largely driven by clinical judgment. A few reports on micronutrients in patients receiving PN are described later.

Vitamin K status has generated interest because dietary intake is low and the administration of broad-spectrum antibiotics may predispose patients to more thrombolytic events associated with vitamin K–dependent anticoagulant protein functions.[73] A study in HCT patients comparing intravenous vitamin K supplementation of 10 mg per week or 5 mg per day found that daily dosing produced more anticoagulant protein in its fully functional form.[74] The clinical significance of these findings has yet to be determined.

TABLE 41-3

Nutrition Care Plans for Management of Posttransplant Organ Toxicity

Organ Dysfunction	Evaluation	Intervention	Desired Nutritional Outcome
Liver disease secondary to VOD, acute or chronic GVHD; drugs (cyclosporine, Bactrim, interferon, methotrexate); PN; infection (fungal, viral, sepsis associated multiorgan failure); hemochromatosis	*Patients on PN:* Assess energy support to minimize risk of overfeeding and ensure good glucose control	Maintain dextrose load in adults <5 mg/kg/min; in adolescents and school age children <7-10 mg/kg/min; in infants and toddlers <15/kg/min; if on PN >3 wk, measure metabolite rate to target energy needs	Minimize component of PN-induced damage
	Screen for serum turbidity; if bilirubin >10 mg/d, assess serum triglyceride	If serum turbid or triglycerides >400-500 mg/dl, discontinue lipids until turbidity resolves and then provide at 4%-8% total kcal to prevent essential fatty acid deficiency	
	If hyperbilirubinemia persists >7-10 days, assess risk for toxicity of biliary-excreted trace metals	Delete manganese and copper from PN (rule out hypocupremia first if diarrhea present)	
	Assess appropriateness of transition to oral or tube feeding (i.e., absence of significant GI symptoms)	Maximize oral intake; nasogastric/intestinal feeding, or, if prolonged tube feeding anticipated, percutaneous endoscopic gastrostomy placement; and/or trial off PN	Maximize use of GI tract
	Patients on enteral intake/oral diet: If signs/symptoms of fat malabsorption, obtain quantitative fecal fat and vitamin assays	If decreased fat absorption, low-fat diet, supplementcalcium and fat-soluble vitamins with water-miscible form, MCT-based supplements	Weight stabilization, correction of nutritional deficiencies
	If iron overload, assess for excessive iron or vitamin C intake (vitamin C acts as pro-oxidant in presence of iron)	Discontinue supplements with iron or large doses of vitamin C	Minimize iron-induced organ damage
	For patients with ascites or excessive third-spacing of fluids: Monitor fluid and sodium intake	Decrease IV and oral sodium and fluid. If on PN, provide reduced-volume solutions	Minimize rate of fluid accumulation
Renal insufficiency secondary to: Hepatorenal syndrome (most common with VOD) Drugs (cyclosporine, tacrolimus amphotericin, aminoglycosides, Bactrim, foscarnet)	If serum creatinine >50% baseline, assess if maintenance fluid needs met; further volume status assessment often necessary (fluid output, weight, postural blood pressure, presence of edema)	If volume depleted, increase oral and/or IVF If fluid restriction indicated (weight gain and decreased urine output), maximize nutrient intake within fluid restriction	Optimize renal perfusion to minimize drug toxicity Maintain nutritional status
	If calculated GFR is <30 ml/min[1] assess protein support	Protein at 1.0 g/kg in adults (1.25 RDA for age)	Decrease rate of BUN rise Maintain nutritional status
Sepsis Intravascular volume depletion Hemolytic syndromes	If dialysis required and on PN, assess serum triglyceride weekly, provide renal-dose vitamins, replace protein losses	If triglyceride >400-500 mg/dl, see section on Liver Disease; provide folate and reduce MVI dose by 50%; provide protein at 2.0 RDA for age	Maintain vitamin status; avoid vitamin A toxicity and excessive hyperlipidemia
Tumor lysis syndrome	If renal function changing rapidly, monitor serum potassium daily and calcium, phosphorus, and magnesium frequently	Adjust IV or PN electrolytes accordingly	Electrolyte homeostasis
Pulmonary compromise secondary to: Pneumonia Pulmonary edema Acute respiratory distress syndrome Bronchiolitis obliterans	Assess volume status	If pulmonary edema, restrict IV and oral fluids and sodium; maximize nutrient intake within fluid restriction	Maintain nutritional status
	Assess energy support to avoid overfeeding if ventilated and underfeeding if increased work of breathing	Measure metabolic rate; if unavailable, patients with chronic disease (bronchiolitis obliterans) may need >1.7 × basal kcal	
Skin toxicities secondary to: Severe skin GVHD Conditioning therapy Bed sores	Assess nutrient support	Measure metabolic rate; if unavailable, provide 1.7 × basal kcal (or greater dependent on % skin involved); protein at 2.0 RDA for age; 1000 mg vitamin C daily; supplemental zinc if low serum zinc	Provide adequate substrate for tissue repair
	Assess volume status (at risk for fluid shifts to extravascular space and for high insensible losses, especially if on air bed)	If intravascular depletion, increase IV fluid	Maintain intravascular volume status
Neurologic deficits secondary to: Sepsis Oversedation Hypoxia Uremia	If liver disease, obtain plasma amino acid profile	If phenylalanine or methionine >twice normal, consider trial of reduced aromatic amino acid solution	Correct abnormal plasma amino acids
	If BUN >100 mg/dl in absence of corticosteroids, assess protein support	Trial of decreased protein 0.6-0.7 RDA for age	Decrease in rate of blood urea nitrogen rise

Continued.

TABLE 41-3

Nutrition Care Plans for Management of Posttransplant Organ Toxicity—cont'd

Organ Dysfunction	Evaluation	Intervention	Desired Nutritional Outcome
Liver failure Drugs (corticosteroids, cyclosporine, interferon) Metabolic imbalances (sodium, glucose, manganese)			
GASTROINTESTINAL DISORDERS			
Mucositits secondary to: Conditioning therapy Oral infection (fungal, viral)	Monitor adequacy of nutrient intake	Oral supplements, cold clear liquids, soft, bland foods. If oral supplementation unsuccessful, provide PN (or if chronic GVHD, tube feeding)	Maintain weight
Methotrexate Acute or chronic GVHD	Assess oral hygiene measures	Encourage good oral hygiene; if persists after engraftment, obtain cultures and treat infections as indicated	Symptom control and improved food tolerance
Dysphagia/esophagitis secondary to: Conditioning therapy	Monitor adequacy of nutrient intake	Oral supplements, soft bland foods. If oral supplementation unsuccessful, provide PN (or if chronic GVHD, tube feeding)	Maintain weight
Gastric reflux (corticosteroids, GVHD, stress)	If gagging present and/or high aspiration risk, obtain swallowing evaluation	Altered food consistency as indicated	Minimize aspiration risk
Esophageal infection (fungal, viral, bacterial) Chronic GVHD Prolonged intubation	Assess antireflux regimen	Antireflux measures (upright position postprandially, elevate head of bed); routine use of antacids and gastric acid inhibitors	Symptom control and improved food tolerance
Nausea/vomiting secondary to: Conditioning therapy	Determine frequency and volume of emesis, relationship to oral intake	Clear cold liquids, small frequent meals, low fat	Maintain weight
GVHD, gastrointestinal, liver Drugs (cyclosporine, clotrimazole,amphotericin)	Assess antiemetic regimen Monitor adequacy of nutrient intake	Scheduled antiemetics, including gastric motility agents and gastric acid inhibitors If interventions unsuccessful, provide PN	Symptom control and improved food tolerance
Gastrointestinal or systemic infections Liver disease Gastric reflux or ulcers Thick salivary secretions		If symptoms persist after engraftment, endoscopic evaluation to rule out treatable infection or GVHD If gastrointestinal workup negative, psychology referral for behavior modification and food desensitization	
Pancreatitis Food aversions		Provide additional fluids as appropriate	Maintain hydration status
Anticipatory vomiting	Assess volume status		
Anorexia and/or early satiety secondary to: Hypomotility of GI tract (conditioning therapy, prolonged NPO, GVHD)	Monitor adequacy of nutrient intake	Oral supplements, small frequent meals, low fat meals, food experimentation Trial of gastric motility agent	Maintain weight
Drugs (cyclosporine, narcotics, antibiotics) Upper gastrointestinal GVHD Liver disease		If on PN, cycle overnight; if nutritionally and medically stable, trial off PN and/or transition to tube feeding	
Anxiety or depression Adrenal insufficiency Food aversions History of prior eating disorder		If depression or history of eating disorder, psychology consult	
Diarrhea secondary to: Conditioning therapy	Assess volume, frequency, other characteristics of stool output (color, odor, consistency), relation to oral intake or dietary components (lactose, fiber, fat), other signs or symptoms of gastrointestinal dysfunction (abdominal cramping, presence of blood in stool, moderate to severe nausea and vomiting)	If steatorrhea: see section on Liver disease; if chronic, trial of pancreatics enzymes	Minimize stool volumes Symptom control
Intestinal infection (viral, fungal, bacterial overgrowth) Gastrointestinal GVHD Drugs (magnesium salts, gastric motility agents, antibiotics)		If mild: trial of antidiarrheals (contraindicated with GVHD and infectious causes) and empiric use of lactase-treated milk and lactase tablets with other dairy products	
Pseudomembranous colitis *(Clostridium difficile)* Typhlitis (other Clostridium species)		If secretory (large volume with minimal oral stimulation) and/or presence of other symptoms: Gut rest and PN until stool <4-5 ml/kg Extra zinc 1 mg/100 ml stool Extra copper 1 mg/d (adult dose) if hypocupremia	Maintain weight and provide substrate to repair tissues

Continued.

TABLE 41-3

Nutrition Care Plans for Management of Posttransplant Organ Toxicity—cont'd

Organ Dysfunction	Evaluation	Intervention	Desired Nutritional Outcome
Lactose intolerance		Refeed in moderate to severe GVHD with slow diet progression (low in lactose, insoluble fiber, fat, gastric irritants and motility stimulants); one new food at a time	
Past medical history of gastrointestinal pathology	Review medications	Discontinue medications not otherwise medically necessary; if magnesium related, may respond to decrease in dose	
Liver or pancreatic disease (usually steatorrhea)	Assess volume status	Replace losses cc/cc with D5 1/4-1/2 NS (100-130 mEq sodium/L with GVHD)	Maintain hydration status

Modified with permission from Nutrition Care Criteria, Seattle Cancer Care Alliance, Seattle, Washington, 98104, 2002.
BUN, Blood urea nitrogen; *GFR*, glomerular filtration rate; *GI*, gastrointestinal; *GVHD*, graft-versus-host disease; *IV*, intravenous, *IVF*, intravenous fluids; *MCT*, medium-chain triglycerides; *NPO*, nil per os (nothing by mouth); *PN*, parenteral nutrition, *RDA*, recommended dietary allowance; *VOD*, venoocclusive disease.

Acute folic acid deficiency, even with oral or intravenous supplementation, has been described following bone marrow transplantation (BMT).[75] Poor oral intake, inadequate absorption, drug therapy (especially methotrexate and trimethoprim sulfamethoxazole), and possibly increased requirements may contribute to folic acid deficiency. No data have been published to suggest what dose is required to prevent deficiency.

Several reports describe low levels of α-tocopherol or vitamin E when given standard PN multivitamins, especially among those receiving daily intravenous lipids.[76-78] Low levels of α-tocopherol occur after transplant even when patients are preloaded with 825 mg α-tocopherol for three weeks before high-dose chemotherapy and TBI.[79] One study, however, did not support this decline in vitamin E.[80] Supplementation of vitamin C at 500 to 700 mg/day appears to maintain plasma levels in the normal range.[77, 80] Although some investigators advocate antioxidant supplementation to prevent lipid preoxidation and attendant regimen-related toxicity, this approach is controversial because of the potential to interfere with the oxidative damage targeted by radiation and some chemotherapy toward oxygen rich tumors, such as leukemia.[81]

For all patients not receiving PN it is prudent to provide an oral multivitamin and mineral supplement because of the restricted intake of a normal diet, often for an extended period. Iron usually is not required because of red cell transfusions; each unit of red blood cells contains 200 to 250 mg of iron. In fact, patients who have received multiple transfusions, either before or after transplantation, have a grossly elevated serum ferritin value and are at risk for iron overload and attendant organ damage.[82] Iron supplements are absolutely contraindicated for these patients.

Oral Dietary Management

GASTROINTESTINAL TOXICITIES. Care plans for nutrition management associated with the common GI toxicities are detailed in Table 41-3. Nausea and vomiting are most acute during administration of cytoreduction therapy, but mild symptoms persist for 3 to 6 weeks.[83] Mucositis peaks at 10 to 14 days posttransplant,[16] and the associated pain and swelling are the principal deterrents to eating during the neutropenic phase. Intravenous narcotic analgesics to control mucositis pain are required for the majority of patients and can lead to gastric stasis and intestinal ileus.[84] Crampy abdominal pain and

diarrhea secondary to mucosal crypt aberrations, epithelial flattening, cell degeneration, and increased bowel permeability peak 1 to 2 weeks after the start of conditioning and return to normal by 3 to 4 weeks after the transplant.[84,85]

Figure 41-2 illustrates the decline in oral energy intake during cytoreduction to minimal levels during the neutropenic period. For patients still in the hospital 1 month after transplant, oral intake remains far below estimated needs. While individual patients may be able to consume enough calories to maintain acceptable nutritional status, most patients experience one or more regimen-related GI toxicities that dramatically impair eating and drinking.

The use of pharmacologic doses of oral glutamine to reduce the severity of oral mucositis following cytoreduction has been explored by several investigators (Table 41-4).[86-91] Only one study reported a favorable result among autologous patients but paradoxically found that glutamine made mucositis worse, as measured by opiate use, in allogeneic patients with matched sibling donors.[89]

"Low-Microbial" Diets. The protective benefit of low-microbial diets against infection has never been established.[92] Nonetheless, such diets are often fed to patients with neutropenia to minimize acquisition of organisms from food sources and food handlers.[93] The high production costs, lack of scientific data, empiric nature of most diets, and shift of treatment toward ambulatory care have caused some transplant centers to switch from very restrictive diets that are sterile[94] or of known microbial content[92] to less stringent diets that patients can also follow at home. Educating patients and their caregivers in the basics of food safety takes priority over extensive diet restrictions. Table 41-5 describes one set of diet restrictions for HCT patients undergoing treatment both in the hospital and at home. Autologous graft recipients are advised to follow the diet for 3 months after chemotherapy and allogeneic graft patients until 1 year after transplant, or longer if they are still taking immunosuppressants for GVHD.

Special Food Service Needs. Traditional hospital food services with set mealtimes, limited food choices, and advance menu selection may fail to meet the dietary needs of the majority of HCT patients. Ways of providing more flexible food service have been reviewed by Stern and Lenssen.[95] Key points include sufficient trained personnel to help with meal selection,

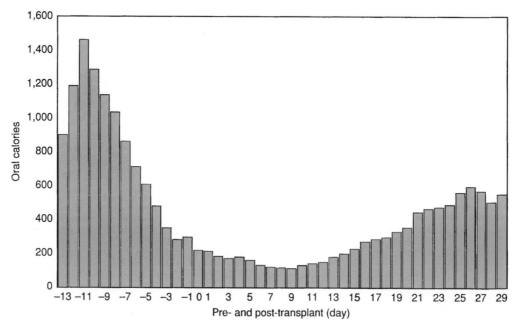

FIGURE 41-2 Average daily oral calorie intake in 295 adult marrow transplant recipients. (From Aker SN, Lenssen P: Nutrition support of patients with hematologic malignancies. In Hoffman P, Benz EJ, et al [eds]: *Hematology: basic principles and practices,* ed 3, Philadelphia, 2000, WB Saunders.)

a satellite kitchen on the HCT or oncology unit, availability of foods and beverages typically requested (e.g., a special menu for HCT and oncology patients),[96] and a way of accurately assessing daily oral intake.

Enteral and Parenteral Nutrition

Clinicians must determine when to intervene with nutrition support and with what strategies. There are limited published studies on the use of enteral feeding in the early posttransplant period.[97-100] Several reports have attempted to determine if safe enteral access could be established via endoscopically placed gastrostomy tubes several weeks prior to transplant[99] or nasal jejunal (NJ) tubes placed immediately prior to high-dose conditioning therapy and the onset of mucositis.[99,100] The risk of infection after a gastrostomy tube limits this approach to those patients with good neutrophil counts and for whom a potential delay in transplant would not be medically contraindicated, or in the case of an unrelated donor, logistically difficult. Nasal tubes are frequently vomited; however, 8 of 15 allograft patients were able to maintain a Bengmark self-propelling NJ tube until engraftment.[100] The use of enteral nutrients to improve mucosal integrity and recovery, reduce infections, and alter incidence and severity of GVHD are intriguing hypotheses but as yet unproven.

The standard of care since the 1970s has been to institute PN early. Evidence suggests that among allogeneic patients implementation of PN during cytoreduction improves long-term survival and reduces relapse rates.[101] Similar results have not been demonstrated for autologous patients with hematologic malignancies,[101] but large trials with sufficient statistical power to detect differences in outcome have not been conducted in autologous graft patients who have hematologic malignancies or solid tumors. Iestra and colleagues applied standard criteria used in cancer patients as indications for PN to a retrospective

cohort of 86 HCT patients treated for acute myelogenous leukemia or lymphoma.[50] Among patients undergoing autologous grafting, PN was indicated in only 37% and 50% of patients prepared without and with TBI, respectively. In allogeneic patients, who all received TBI, PN was indicated for 58% with HLA-matched donors and 92% with HLA-mismatched donors. These data are consistent with the increased oral and gut toxicity observed with TBI-based regimens and the use of methotrexate to prevent GVHD. PN does not appear to affect short-term outcomes, such as engraftment or duration of hospitalization and, in fact, appears be associated with more bacteremia.[97,101,102]

LIPIDS. The optimal substrate distribution and lipid composition for HCT patients are unknown. The effect of lipids on immunity has been a cause for concern, but a large randomized trial in autologous and allogeneic patients with hematologic malignancies failed to show an association between a moderate dose (25% to 35% of total energy) and a low dose (6% to 8% of total energy) linoleic-based lipid emulsion and bacterial and fungal infections.[103] One novel approach used very high dose lipids (80% of energy) in an attempt to modulate or dampen cytokine activation that is associated with GVHD.[104] Although these investigators reported less mortality in those patients with severe GVHD who received high dose versus no lipids, the study size was very small. Because biochemical evidence of essential fatty acid deficiency may occur within 1 week of starting PN in HCT patients,[105,106] there is no reason to withhold intravenous lipids except in the presence of severe hypertriglyceridemia.

AMINO ACIDS. Attenuation of negative nitrogen balance has been a goal of several studies utilizing branched chain amino acids, high doses of protein, or glutamine. Lenssen and coworkers found no difference in nitrogen balance with a branched chain-enriched amino acid solution compared with

TABLE 41-4

Summary of Randomized Glutamine Trials in Hematopoietic Cell Transplantation

Study	No. of Autograft Patients	No. of Allograft Patients	Conditioning Regimen (No. Patients)	Mucositis	Days of PN	Infection	GVHD	Relapse	Long-Term Survival
			IV Glutamine						
Ziegler, et al., 1992[90]	45		Cy/TBI/ARA-C (40) Bu/Cy (3)	ND	ND	+ (see text)	ND	?	?
Schloerb, et al., 1993[91]	14	15	Cy/VP-16/BCNU (2) Cy/TBI/ARA-C (26) Bu/Cy (3)	ND	ND	ND	?	?	?
			Oral Glutamine						
Jebb, et al., 1995[86]	24		BCNU/VP-16/ melphalan (24)	ND	ND	?	Not applicable	ND at 6 mo	?
Anderson, et al., 1998[89]	87	55 sibling 51 URD	Only TBI specified (54 auto, 45 sibling, 42 URD)	+ auto – sibling ND URD	ND	ND	ND	?	ND*
Schloerb and Skikne, 1999[87]	48	18	Cy + TBI or Bu (19) Cy/VP-16/BCNU (19) Cy/thiotepa (23) Unknown (3)	ND	ND	ND	ND	?	ND†
Couglin Dickson, et al., 2000[88]	34	24	Only TBI specified (33 auto, 23 allo)	ND	ND	?	?	ND	ND

Reprinted with permission from Lenssen P, Bruemmer B, Aker SN, McDonald GB: Nutrient support in hematopoietic cell transplantation, *J Parenteral Enteral Nutr* 25:4, 2001.
ARA-C, cytosine arabinoside; *BCNU*, carmustine; *Bu*, busulfan; *Cy*, cyclophosphamide; *ND*, no difference between glutamine and placebo; *TBI*, total body irradiation; *URD*, unrelated donor; *VP-16*, etoposide; +, benefit of glutamine over placebo; –, benefit of placebo control over glutamine; ?, not reported.
*Day 28 survival significantly better for glutamine group but no difference at day 100.
†Nonsignificant positive trend for autograft and allograft patients with hematologic malignancy.

TABLE 41-5

Diet for Immunosuppressed Patients

Food Groups	Allowed	Not Allowed
Dairy	All *pasteurized*, grade A milk and milk products; commercially packaged cheese and cheese products made with pasteurized milk (e.g., mild and medium cheddar, mozzarella, Parmesan, Swiss); *pasteurized* yogurt; dry, refrigerated, and frozen *pasteurized* whipped topping; ice cream, frozen yogurt, sherbet, ice cream bars, homemade milkshakes; commercial nutritional supplements and baby formulas (liquid and powdered)	*Unpasteurized* or *raw* milk, cheese, yogurt, and other milk products; cheeses from delicatessens; cheeses containing chili peppers or other uncooked vegetables; cheeses with molds (e.g., Blue, Stilton, Roquefort, Gorgonzola); sharp cheddar, Brie, Camembert, feta, farmer's cheese
Meat and meat substitutes	All *well-cooked* or *canned meats* (beef, pork, lamb, poultry, fish, shellfish, game, ham, bacon, sausage, hot dogs); well-cooked eggs (white cooked firm with thickened yolk is acceptable); *pasteurized* egg substitutes (e.g., Egg Beaters); *commercially packaged* salami, bologna, and other luncheon meats; canned and commercially packaged *hard smoked* fish; refrigerated after opening; cooked tofu (cut into 1-in or smaller cubes, boiled a minimum of 5 minutes in water or broth before eating or using in recipes)	Raw or *undercooked* meat, poultry, fish, game, tofu; meats and cold cuts from delicatessens; hard cured salami in natural wrap; cold smoked salmon (fish); lox; pickled fish; tempeh
Entrees, soups	All cooked entrees and soups	All miso products (e.g., miso soup)
Fruit and nuts	Canned and frozen fruit and fruit juices; *well-washed* raw fruit; foods containing well-washed raw fruits, dried fruits; canned or bottled roasted nuts; nuts in baked products; commercially packaged peanut butter	*Unwashed* raw fruits; unroasted raw nuts; roasted nuts in the shell; unpasteurized fruit juice
Vegetables	All cooked frozen, canned, or fresh vegetables and potatoes; *well-washed* raw vegetables; fresh, *well-washed* herbs and dried herbs and spices (added to raw or cooked foods)	*Unwashed* raw vegetables or herbs; salads from delicatessens; commercial salsas stored in refrigerated case
Bread, grain, and cereal products	All breads, bagels, rolls, muffins, pancakes, sweet rolls, waffles, French toast; potato chips, corn chips, tortilla chips, pretzels, popcorn; cooked pasta, rice, and other grains; all cereals, cooked and ready to eat	Raw grain products
Beverages	Tap water, commercial bottled distilled, spring, and natural water; all canned, bottled, powdered beverages; instant and brewed coffee, tea; cold tea brewed with boiling water, brewed herbal teas using commercially packaged tea bags; commercial nutritional supplements, liquid and powdered	Well water (unless tested yearly and found safe); cold-brewed tea made with warm or cold water; unpasteurized fruit and vegetable juices
Desserts	Refrigerated commercial and homemade cakes, pies, pastries, and pudding; refrigerated, cream-filled pastries; homemade and commercial cookies; shelf-stable* cream-filled cupcakes (e.g., Twinkies, Ding Dongs), fruit pies (e.g., Poptarts, Hostess fruit pies), and canned pudding; ices, popsicle-like products	*Unrefrigerated*, cream-filled pastry products (not shelf stable*)
Fats	Oil, shortening; refrigerated lard, margarine, butter; commercial, shelf-stable* mayonnaise and salad dressings (including cheese-based salad dressings; refrigerated after opening); cooked gravy and sauces	Fresh salad dressings containing aged cheese (e.g., Blue, Roquefort) or raw eggs, stored in refrigerated case
Other	Salt, granulated sugar, brown sugar; jam, jelly, syrups, (refrigerated after opening); commercially packaged (pasteurized) honey (may not say "pasteurized" on label); catsup, mustard, BBQ sauce, soy sauce, other condiments (refrigerated after opening); pickles, pickle relish, olives (refrigerated after opening); candy, gum	Raw or unpasteurized honey; herbal and nontraditional (health food store) nutrient supplements, Chinese herbs; brewer's yeast if eaten uncooked

Courtesy Seattle Cancer Care Alliance, Seattle, Washington, 98104.
Shelf-stable refers to unopened canned, bottled, or packaged food products that can be stored before opening at room temperature; container may require refrigeration after opening.

standard amino acid solution during the first month after allogeneic grafting in a randomized trial of 40 patients.[69] Geibig and colleagues showed an arithmetic, but not statistically significant, improvement in nitrogen balance assessed intermittently during the first 2 weeks after transplant by increasing protein to 2.25 g/kg.[60] Improved nitrogen balance has been reported with glutamine.[105] In allogeneic graft recipients studied between posttransplant days 4 and 11, daily nitrogen balance was -1.4 ± 0.5 g in patients receiving 0.57 g/kg body weight per day of glutamine as compared with -4.2 ± 1.2 g for patients receiving glutamine-free PN.

Concentrated solutions of amino acids are usually required to achieve protein needs in most adults and older children, especially for fluid-restricted patients. However, caution should be urged in using solutions with relatively higher phenylalanine

content because HCT patients demonstrate elevated circulating levels of plasma phenylalanine.[107]

Low plasma taurine has been described following HCT, possibly because of taurine release from white cells and platelets following cytoreduction.[108] The clinical significance of the deficiency is not known, but the ability of taurine to conjugate bile acids toxic to the liver offers an intriguing direction for research. The only commercially available taurine-supplemented solutions are for infants. Consideration should be given to routine use of pediatric amino acid solutions for the very youngest transplant patients, given the evidence of relative taurine deficiency after transplant.

GLUTAMINE. The role of intravenous glutamine has been examined in several studies, with conflicting results (see Table 41-4). Ziegler and colleagues reported fewer clinical infections among allogeneic graft patients who received gluta-mine-supplemented PN,[90] whereas Schloerb and coworkers failed to confirm these findings in a study that included autolo-gous and allogeneic grafts.[91] Both groups of investigators reported shorter hospital stays but failed to provide objective criteria for hospital discharge that would assist in the interpre-tation of their findings.

Additional reports derived from the Ziegler trial found improvement in mood,[109] decreased hospital costs,[110] and less expansion of extracellular water and fluid retention[111] in patients supplemented with intravenous glutamine. Multiple end points in a small study raise serious questions about statis-tical validity, and additional trials are needed to validate the efficacy of glutamine in these desirable clinical end points.

ELECTROLYTES AND MICRONUTRIENTS. Electrolyte management is discussed in a previous section and in Table 41-2. Several studies have been undertaken to characterize micronutrient status. In a retrospective study of allogeneic graft patients, normal serum levels of copper and zinc were maintained during the first 3 weeks after HCT in more than 90% of the patients by daily supplementation of 1 mg of copper and 4 mg of zinc.[112] Serum levels are of questionable value as an index of zinc status because of the frequent finding of hypo-albuminemia and an acute-phase response. In zinc and copper balance studies performed between days 7 and 20 posttransplant, Mulder and colleagues found that daily excretion was approxi-mately 2 mg of copper and 10 mg of zinc in autologous patients who were treated with cyclophosphamide and etoposide or mitoxantrone for solid tumors.[98] Papadopoulou and coworkers suggest that in children undergoing HCT, a decrease in plasma alkaline phosphatase activity predicts zinc depletion.[113]

Manganese toxicity that manifested as a Parkinson's-like syndrome with brain magnetic resonance imaging (MRI) sug-gestive of manganese accumulation has been described in a patient with cholestatic liver disease who was supplemented with 0.3 mg per day of manganese during 2 months of PN.[114] These investigators found elevated serum manganese levels in eight other HCT patients with liver disease, suggesting the need to restrict manganese for patients with cholestasis.[114]

Engraftment and Early Recovery

Transition to Oral Feeding

Delayed toxicities from cytoreduction present challenges for patients trying to resume adequate dietary intake. Xerostomia and blunted taste may be pronounced in the first few months after transplant, especially among adult patients receiving TBI,[115,116] and may persist longer than a year.[56,117] Abdominal pain and nausea on eating are common and may be associated with biliary stasis and gallbladder sludge. As many as 70% of allogeneic patients exhibit ultrasound evidence of gallbladder sludge by the second week after transplant.[84]

Some clinicians advocate lactose restriction for up to a year after transplant,[118] but no data conclusively demonstrate lactose intolerance in these patients. In the absence of diarrhea, feeding milk products can be attempted.

PN has been associated with delayed resumption of ade-quate oral energy intake after hospital discharge.[119] In a large,

randomized, double-blind trial that included both autologous and allogeneic patients greater than 2 years old who were not able to consume at least 70% of estimated energy needs (130% of basal energy) at hospital discharge, Charuhas and coworkers provided PN or hydration.[119] Patients who received hydration were able to meet calorie goals earlier. No adverse conse-quences, such as increased readmissions or clinically significant weight loss, were found when PN was withheld for up to a month. Unless a clinical condition, such as malnutrition, malabsorption, or significant GI toxicity, warrants otherwise, PN can be safely discontinued in patients whose oral intake is as little as 20% to 25% of total needs.

Nutrition Management of Graft-Versus-Host Disease

The nutritional consequences of GVHD can be profound. Patients have increased nutrient requirements because of hypermetabolism and tissue regeneration. Corticosteroids have remained the mainstay of treatment for over three decades, intensifying the muscle and lean body mass loss and often leading to insulin resistance and hypertriglyceridemia. Anorexia is common, and tolerance to oral feedings may be poor, especially if the GI tract is involved.

SKIN DISEASE. Acute GVHD usually presents initially as a skin rash, and when it exceeds 25% to 50% of body surface area it requires treatment. Severe skin disease leads to ulcera-tions and bullae, mimicking a total body burn and evoking similar increased nutritional requirements (see Table 41-3).

Skin involvement affects 70% to 90% of patients with chronic GVHD. The primary nutrition concern is maintenance of bone health by ensuring an adequate source of vitamin D. Sun-blocking agents and clothing that cover exposed skin and protect against photoactivation or exacerbation of skin disease also block photosynthesis of vitamin D in the epidermis and dermis. Multivitamin supplementation is recommended for all allogeneic graft patients during the risk period for skin GVHD ($\geq$1 year). Severe chronic skin involvement, which today is less common than it once was thanks to developments in immuno-suppressant therapy, is characterized by hidebound skin, hypopigmentation, contractures, ulceration, pain, and dimin-ished physical activity. Rigorous physical therapy is necessary to maintain mobility and attenuate muscle loss. If ulcers are present, adequate energy, protein, vitamin C, and zinc must be supplied to promote healing.

Psoralen plus ultraviolet A (PUVA) radiation is an adjunctive therapy for skin GVHD. Beta-carotene is protective against ultraviolet radiation;[120] thus, it seems prudent to discourage the intake of supplemental beta-carotene during PUVA therapy.

GASTROINTESTINAL DISEASE. In its most severe form, acute GI GVHD causes profuse, watery diarrhea, abdominal cramping and pain due to bowel wall edema, and extensive intestinal protein loss.[84,121] The secretory diarrhea is independent of oral intake and may progress to frank GI bleeding and total cell necrosis mediated by cytotoxic T cells. The total volume is roughly correlated with the degree of mucosal damage.[122] GI disease is usually diagnosed when it presents in the setting of skin GVHD. In the absence of skin disease, diagnosis by the histologic findings of crypt cell necrosis and apoptosis in mucosal biopsies of the stomach or colon is recommended before initiating treatment. Other causes of diarrhea must always be ruled out because enteric pathogens and late-onset conditioning toxicities can have signs and symptoms similar to those of acute GVHD.[123]

Fluid and electrolyte management and debilitation secondary to frequent bowel movements are problems for patients with high-volume diarrhea (more than 2.5 to 3.0 L per day). Antidiarrheal agents, such as opiate derivatives and anticholinergics, are generally contraindicated because of the risk of ileus and abdominal distention and their masking of the response to immunosuppressant therapy. The use of octreotide acetate, the synthetic analog of somatostatin, has been reported to control diarrhea with variable success.[124-126] In one report, patients who failed to respond to octreotide acetate also failed immunosuppressant therapy for the underlying disease.[125] As adjunctive therapy for symptom management in acute GI GVHD, it is not totally benign because it can lower the serum level of cyclosporine.[125]

The decision to rest the gut and support exclusively with PN depends on the severity of the diarrhea and abdominal pain; frequently patients voluntarily restrict their intake. When stool volumes exceed 8 to 10 ml/kg per day, fluid and electrolyte management is easier if oral challenges are restricted until stool volume subsides. Gauvreau and colleagues originally described a diet progression that follows gut rest, beginning with limited volumes of isotonic beverages.[127] A similar diet has been recommended by Vickers.[128] If stool volume and abdominal symptoms do not increase, foods that are low in lactose, insoluble fiber, acidity, and fat are introduced incrementally until a regular diet is tolerated. Patients with severe ileal involvement may have to restrict fat intake more. The potential of food as a vector for pathogens merits emphasis during acute GI GVHD because GI tract immunocompetence is seriously impaired by the mucosal damage and diminished secretory immunoglobulins.[129] Energy needs have been predicted during acute GVHD to be 45 to 50 kcal/kg in adults and 65 kcal/kg in children.[67] No balance studies have been conducted to establish protein and other nutrient needs; thus, clinical judgment must serve as a guide (see Table 41-3).

A more moderate form of upper GI GVHD has been identified that presents as anorexia, nausea, and vomiting and is associated with edematous stomach epithelium on esophagogastroduodenoscopy (EGD).[130] In one series of 76 patients with persistent nausea and vomiting and poor oral intake after day 20 posttransplant, 86% had histologic evidence of GVHD on EGD.[131] Often smaller doses of corticosteroids are sufficient to treat upper GI GVHD effectively in conjunction with gastric acid inhibitors and antiemetics for symptom management; prolonged nutrition support may thus be avoided. Strategies for diet management are based on the particular GI symptoms (as described in Table 43-3) that the patient is experiencing.

Chronic involvement of the intestinal tract is less common; when it occurs, management strategies are similar to those of acute GI GVHD. In patients with chronic diarrhea, which either fails to respond to immunosuppressive therapy or is not associated with histologic evidence of GVHD on biopsy, a malabsorption workup, specifically a quantitative fecal fat study, is recommended. Usually a stool pattern consistent with steatorrhea can be elicited from the patient. It is my experience and

that of others[132] that diarrhea may resolve with pancreatic enzyme replacement. The etiology of pancreatic insufficiency is unknown, but prior pancreatic damage, drug therapy (cyclosporine, corticosteroids) and even pancreatic GVHD have all been hypothesized as contributing factors.[132,133]

ORAL DISEASE. Erythema and lichenoid changes in the oral mucosa are typical of oral GVHD and are difficult to differentiate from conditioning-associated mucositis until approximately 3 weeks after transplant.[134] Topical oral steroids and local analgesics may provide some relief. Management can be a frustrating problem because GVHD cannot be expected to resolve within a given interval, as can conditioning-related mucositis, and it can evolve into the chronic form. With prolonged use of oral supplements and bland foods patients can develop taste fatigue and weight loss, thus requiring nutrition support.

Oral GVHD occurs in as many as 70% of patients with chronic GVHD, presenting as frank mucositis in its more severe forms and persisting for years. Microbiologic cultures should be obtained in symptomatic patients to rule out or detect concurrent infections. Approximately 30% of patients with oral symptoms complain of severe xerostomia.[56] Patients should be encouraged to undergo routine evaluation by a dental professional and to practice vigorous daily oral hygiene. If significant weight loss occurs, percutaneous endoscopic gastrostomy feeding may be indicated.

LIVER DISEASE. Liver GVHD is characterized by moderate to marked elevations of serum alkaline phosphatase and bilirubin levels; jaundice; hepatomegaly; and, in severe cases of acute disease, ascites and encephalopathy.[84] The acute disease is usually diagnosed in the setting of skin or GI GVHD, but in their absence it may depend on biopsy because of the high prevalence of other liver diseases after transplantation. Hepatic synthesis and enterohepatic circulation of bile salts may diminish with resultant steatorrhea. Nutrition management is similar to that for other liver complications (see Table 41-3).

Liver involvement affects 50% to 85% of patients with chronic GVHD. It is primarily cholestatic and may progress to cholestasis. Liver disease responds more slowly to immunosuppressant therapy than other organ involvement. Adjunctive therapy may include ursodeoxycholic acid, a less toxic bile acid than native bile acids in models of cholestatic liver injury.[135]

When weight loss occurs in chronic liver GVHD, the relative contributions of deficient energy intake and malabsorption need to be determined. Patients are often anorexic, but some may have a good appetite and diet intake but significant stool nutrient losses. If malabsorption is clinically evident, other treatable causes such as bacterial overgrowth should be investigated. A workup may include quantitative stool fat collection, Sudan stain for stool fat, serum carotene, serum D-xylose or Schilling test, or serum vitamin D. In patients with malabsorption, moderate fat restriction generally controls symptoms and allows weight gain, especially if dietary fat intake has been excessive to compensate for weight loss. Vitamin D status is a special concern because it is likely that hepatic hydroxylation to the active metabolite is inadequate. Some patients with malabsorption may respond to pancreatic enzymes (see preceding discussion on pancreatic insufficiency in Gastrointestinal Disease).

For patients who fail to gain weight, nutrition support is often indicated. PN should be avoided when possible. If chronic liver GVHD is of progressive onset, it is likely that PN exposure is already lengthy. Percutaneous endoscopic gastrostomy feeding should be seriously considered given the slow resolution of the disease.

Long-Term Recovery

SPECIAL CONSIDERATIONS IN CHRONIC GRAFT-VERSUS-HOST DISEASE. Allogeneic transplant patients are at risk of developing chronic GVHD at any time during the first posttransplant year and beyond as they are "tapered off" prophylactic or therapeutic immunosuppressants. While the skin, mouth, and liver are most often the target organs for chronic GVHD, involvement elsewhere (esophagus and lung) or long-term immunosuppression (steroids in particular) can adversely affect nutrition status.

CHRONIC ESOPHAGEAL DISEASE. Esophageal complications occur in fewer than 5% of patients with chronic GVHD but are usually associated with multiple nutrient deficiencies. If dysphagia and retrosternal pain develop, esophageal GVHD should be suspected. Pathologic lesions include generalized desquamation of the epithelium of the upper and middle esophagus and esophageal webbing and stricture formation.[136] Webs and strictures require periodic dilation and systemic immunosuppression. Weight loss may be profound and may best be managed by gastrostomy for delivery of food and medications.

PULMONARY DISEASE. Approximately 10% of patients develop obstructive lung disease or bronchiolitis obliterans after allogeneic HCT.[137] Nutrition-related signs and symptoms are characterized by weight loss and anorexia. Even if the appetite is good, eating sufficient calories for weight maintenance is difficult, as it is for patients with chronic obstructive lung disease. Patients with lung disease have significant muscle wasting because of limited exercise tolerance and corticosteroid therapy. It is important to incorporate some physical activity into their care plan to prevent further muscle loss.

OSTEOPOROSIS. Loss of bone mineral density 6 months and longer after allogeneic HCT has been chronicled by several investigators.[138 139] Bone loss correlates with cumulative corticosteroid dose, 4% per 10 g prednisolone at the lumbar spine and 9% per 10 g prednisolone at the femoral neck.[139] Women undergoing autologous HCT are also at risk of osteoporosis, especially if they have received corticosteroid therapy before HCT.[139] Patients with additional risk factors include sedentary ones, women who have not taken estrogen replacement, children with higher bone turnover rates, and patients who have malabsorption or consume little calcium and vitamin D.

Osteoporosis may not become clinically evident until several years posttransplant, at which point, the patient with vertebral fractures suffers chronic, debilitating pain. Prevention includes routine supplementation of calcium and vitamin D according to standards established for other populations on long-term corticosteroids, with periodic monitoring of bone mineral density.[140] Treatment of established osteoporosis is recommended under the guidance of an endocrinologist or other expert on osteoporosis.

Pediatric Growth and Development

Children who receive a transplant during puberty attain adult heights that are (on average) comparable to U.S. standards; those who receive a transplant at or before age 10 will be shorter than average as adults without hormonal intervention.[22] Reduction of linear growth is multifactorial. Endocrine imbalances that contribute to poor growth are hypothyroidism (which occurs in approximately 10% of children receiving fractionated doses of TBI), reduced growth hormone production after TBI or prior central nervous irradiation, and deficiency of sex hormones during puberty.[22] Chronic GVHD and corticosteroid therapy further impair growth. Treatment with growth hormone is recommended during the prepubertal period and before the growth rate drops below the third percentile to optimize growth potential.[22] Stature should be measured every 3 months after HCT to detect growth failure early.

Nutritional status and intake have not been investigated as factors in growth failure. Annual nutritional evaluation for deficiencies is appropriate. Children with chronic GVHD are a special challenge because they have the same risk for weight loss and depleted muscle mass as do adults with chronic GVHD.[56] Frequent nutritional follow-up is recommended, with intervention as required to maintain length-for-height or body mass index-for-age at or above the 25th percentile.

Community-Based Care

Many HCT patients are treated in general oncology and hematology units without benefit of the day-to-day expertise that specialty transplant centers accumulate. The nutritional aspects of care are particularly underappreciated. Many oncologists and hematologists have limited access to or underutilize available nutrition resources. The nutrition resources available in the community may not include practitioners with expertise in HCT, especially its chronic complications. Home-care companies likewise may not have experienced clinicians available for transplant clients with nutrition-related complications. Even transplant centers may not offer ambulatory patients routine nutrition services.

A system for ongoing screening for correctable nutrition problems after discharge from the hospital or transplant center is strongly recommended. Formal nutrition summaries to patients' primary medical providers with patient-specific diet and nutrition support recommendations help the providers incorporate nutritional concerns into follow-up care. It is important for patients to understand that they are their own best advocates; allogeneic graft recipients in particular should be instructed on potential nutrition-related signs and symptoms that could occur in the long-term recovery period. Symptoms that they should report to their physicians include increased oral sensitivity or dryness, difficulty swallowing pills or food, weight loss, persistent nausea or vomiting, and frequent, loose bowel movements or diarrhea. Recovery of normal dietary intake and nutrition status can be a long, slow process measured in years, not the few short months the patients originally anticipate.

Conclusion

HCT is an intense and often prolonged medical therapy that presents a wide range of nutritional challenges. The clinical nutrition practitioner must be skilled in (1) PN and tube feeding management; (2) both the critical and ambulatory care settings;

(3) the management of multiple drug-nutrient interactions; (4) patient education and counseling; and (5) the development of short-term and more global, long-term nutrition goals and care plans. A basic understanding of immunology, especially the unique aspects of allogeneic grafting, is essential to competent dietetics practice in this setting. The relationship of impaired immunity and all modes of feeding—oral, tube, and parenteral—must be continuously reviewed as therapies change and related nutrition research is published.

REFERENCES

1. Thomas ED, Storb R: The development of the scientific foundation of hematopoietic cell transplantation based on animal and human studies. In Thomas ED, Blume KG, Forman SJ (eds): *Hematopoietic cell transplantation,* ed 2, Malden, MA, 1999, Blackwell Science, pp 1-11.
2. Hickman RO, Buckner CD, Clift RA, Sanders JE, Stewart P, Thomas ED: A modified right atrial catheter for access to the venous system in marrow transplant recipients, *Surg Gynecol Obstet* 148(6):871-875, 1979.
3. Bortin MM, Horowitz MM, Rimm AA: Increasing utilization of allogeneic bone marrow transplantation. Results of the 1988-1990 survey, *Ann Intern Med* 116(6):505-512, 1992.
4. Bortin MM, Horowitz MM, Gale RP, et al: Changing trends in allogeneic bone marrow transplantation for leukemia in the 1980's, *JAMA* 268(5):607-612, 1992.
5. King CR: Peripheral stem cell transplantation: past, present and future. In Buchsel PC, Whedon MB (eds): *Bone marrow transplantation: clinical and administrative strategies,* Boston, 1995, Jones and Bartlett, pp 187-211.
6. Powles R, Mehta J, Kulkarni S et al: Allogeneic blood and bone marrow stem-cell transplantation in haematological malignant diseases: a randomised trial, *Lancet* 355(92II):1231-1237, 2000.
7. Bensinger WI, Martin PJ, Storer B et al: Transplantation of bone marrow as compared with peripheral-blood cells from HLA-identical relatives in patients with hematologic cancers, *N Engl J Med* 344(3):175-181, 2001.
8. Laughlin MJ: Umbilical cord blood for allogeneic transplantation in children and adults, *Bone Marrow Transplant* 27(1):1-6, 2001.
9. Gale RP, Horowitz MM, Ash RC, et al: Identical-twin bone marrow transplants for leukemia, *Ann Intern Med* 120(8):646-652, 1994.
10. Horowitz MM, Gale RP, Sondel PM, et al: Graft-versus-leukemia reactions after bone marrow transplantation, *Blood* 75(3):555-562, 1990.
11. Fefer A: Graft-versus-tumor responses. In Thomas Ed, Blume KG, Forman SJ (eds): *Hematopoietic cell transplantation,* ed 2, Malden, MA, 1999, Blackwell Science, pp 316-326.
12. Porter DL, Roth MS, McGarigle C, et al: Induction of graft-versus-host disease as immunotherapy for relapsed chronic myeloid leukemia, *N Engl J Med* 330(2):100-106, 1994.
13. Tyndall A: Haematological stem cell transplantation in the treatment of severe autoimmune diseases: first experiences from an international project, *Rheumatology* 38(8):774-776, 1999.
14. Storb R, Yu C, McSweeney P: Mixed chimerism after transplantation of allogeneic hematopoietic cells. In Thomas ED, Blume KG, Forman SJ (eds): *Hematopoietic cell transplantation,* ed 2, Malden, MA, 1999, Blackwell Science, pp 287-295.
15. Exner BG, Domenick MA, Bergheim M, et al: Clinical applications of mixed chimerism, *Ann NY Acad Sci* 872:377-386, 1999.
16. Schubert MM, Williams BE, Lloid ME, et al: Clinical assessment scale for the rating of oral mucosal changes associated with bone marrow transplantation, *Cancer* 69(10):2469-2477, 1992.
17. Keane TJ, Van Dyk J, Rider WD: Idiopathic interstitial pneumonia following bone marrow transplantation: the relationship with total body irradiation, *Int J Radiat Oncol Biol Phys* 7(10):1365-1370, 1981.
18. Curtis RE, Rowlings PA, Deeg HJ, et al: Solid cancers after bone marrow transplantation, *N Engl J Med* 336(13):897-904, 1997.
19. Socie G, Curtis RE, Deeg HJ, et al: New malignant diseases after allogeneic marrow transplantation for childhood acute leukemia, *J Clin Oncol* 18(2):348-357, 2000.
20. Bhatia S, Louie AD, Bhatia R, et al: Solid cancers after bone marrow transplantation, *J Clin Oncol* 19(2):464-471, 2001.

21. Deeg HJ: Delayed complications after hematopoietic cell transplantation. In Thomas ED, Blume KG, Forman SJ (eds): *Hematopoietic cell transplantation,* Malden, MA, 1999, Blackwell Science, pp 776-789.
22. Sanders JE: Growth and development after hematopoietic cell transplantation. In Thomas ED, Blume KG, Forman SJ (eds): *Hematopoietic cell transplantation,* Malden, MA, 1999, Blackwell Science, pp 764-765.
23. Giri N, Vowels MR, Davis EA: Long-term complications following bone marrow transplantation in children, *J Paediatr Child Health* 29(3):201-205, 1993.
24. Davies SM, Ramsay NKC, Klein JP, et al: Comparison of preparative regimens in transplants for children with acute lymphoblastic leukemia, *J Clin Oncol* 18(2):340-347, 2000.
25. Bearman SI, Appelbaum FR, Buckner CD, et al: Regimen-related toxicity in patients undergoing bone marrow transplantation, *J Clin Oncol* 6(10):1562-1568, 1988.
26. Bensinger WI, Buckner CD: Preparative regimens. In Thomas ED, Blume KG, Forman SJ (eds): *Hematopoietic cell transplantation,* Malden, MA, 1999, Blackwell Science, pp 123-134.
27. Storb R, Deeg HJ, Thomas ED, et al: Marrow transplantation for chronic myelocytic leukemia: a controlled trial of cyclosporine versus methotrexate for prophylaxis of graft-versus-host disease, *Blood* 66(3):698-702, 1985.
28. Shulman HM, McDonald GB, Matthews D, et al: An analysis of hepatic venoocclusive disease and centrilobular hepatic degeneration following bone marrow transplantation, *Gastroenterology* 79(6):1178-1191, 1980.
29. McDonald GB, Hinds MS, Fisher LD, et al: Veno-occlusive disease of the liver and multiorgan failure after bone marrow transplantation: a cohort study of 355 patients, *Ann Intern Med* 118(4):255-267, 1993.
30. Lee JL, Gooley T, Bensinger W, Schiffman K, McDonald GB: Veno-occlusive disease of the liver after busulfan, melphalan, and thiotepa conditioning therapy: incidence, risk factors, and outcome, *Biol Blood Marrow Transplant* 5(5):306-315, 1999.
31. Shulman HM, Hinterberger W: Hepatic veno-occlusive disease: liver toxicity syndrome after bone marrow transplantation, *Bone Marrow Transplant* 10(3):197-214, 1992.
32. Strasser SI, Shulman HM, McDonald GB: Cholestasis after hematopoietic cell transplantation, *Clin Liver Dis* 3(3):651-667, 1999.
33. Zager RA, O'Quigley J, Zager BK, et al: Acute renal failure following bone marrow transplantation: a retrospective study of 272 patients, *Am J Kidney Dis* 13(3):210-216, 1989.
34. Rubenfeld GD, Crawford SW: Withdrawing life-support for mechanically-ventilated bone marrow transplant patients: a case for evidence-based guidelines, *Ann Intern Med* 125(8):625-633, 1996.
35. Ferrara JLM, Antin JH: The pathophysiology of graft-versus-host disease. In Thomas ED, Blume KG, Forman SJ (eds): *Hematopoietic cell transplantation,* Malden, MA, 1999, Blackwell Science, pp 305-315.
36. Sullivan KM: Graft-versus-host disease. In Thomas ED, Blume KG, Forman SJ (eds): *Hematopoietic cell transplantation,* Malden, MA, 1999, Blackwell Science, pp 515-536.
37. Anasetti C, Beatty PG, Storb R, et al: Effect of HLA incompatibility on graft-versus-host disease, relapse and survival after marrow transplantation for patients with leukemia or lymphoma, *Hum Immunol* 289(2):79-91, 1990.
38. Storb R, Deeg HJ, Whitehead J, et al: Methotrexate and cyclosporine compared to cyclosporine alone for prophylaxis of acute graft-versus-host disease after marrow transplantation for leukemia, *N Engl J Med* 314(12):729-735, 1986.
39. Nash RA, Antin JH, Karanes C, et al: Phase 3 study comparing methotrexate and tacrolimus with methotrexate and cyclosporine for prophylaxis of acute graft-versus-host disease after marrow transplantation from unrelated donors, *Blood* 96(6):2062-2068, 2000.
40. Vogelsang GB: How I treat chronic graft-versus-host disease, *Blood* 97(5):1196-1201, 2001.
41. Radich JP, Sanders JE, Buckner CD, et al: Second allogeneic marrow transplantation for patients with recurrent leukemia after initial transplant with total-body irradiation–containing regimens, *J Clin Oncol* 11(2):304-313, 1993.
42. Kolb HJ: Management of relapse after hematopoietic cell transplantation. The pathophysiology of graft-versus-host disease. In Thomas ED, Blume KG, Forman SJ (eds): *Hematopoietic cell transplantation,* Malden, MA, 1999, Blackwell Science, pp 929-937.
43. Collins RH Jr, Shpilberg O, Drobyski WR, et al: Donor leukocyte infusions in 140 patients with relapsed malignancy after allogeneic bone marrow transplantation, *J Clin Oncol* 15(2):433-444, 1997.

44. Socie G, Cahn JY, Carmelo J, et al: Avascular necrosis of bone after allogeneic bone marrow transplantation: analysis of risk factors for 4388 patients by the Societe Francaise de Greffe de Moelle (SFGM), *Br J Hematol* 97(4):865-870, 1997.
45. Mahendra P, Hood IM, Bass G, et al: Severe hemosiderosis post allogeneic bone marrow transplantation, *Hematol Oncol* 14(1):33-35, 1996.
46. Nims JW: Survivorship and rehabilitation. In Whedon MB (ed): *Bone marrow transplantation, principles, practices and nursing insights,* Boston,1991, Jones and Bartlett, pp 334-345.
47. Molassiotis A, van den Akker OBA, Milligan DW, et al: Quality of life in long-term survivors of marrow transplantation: comparison with a matched group receiving maintenance chemotherapy, *Bone Marrow Transplant* 17(2):249-258, 1996.
48. Bush NE, Haberman M, Donaldson G, Sullivan KM: Quality of life of 125 adults surviving 6-18 years after bone marrow transplantation, *Soc Sci Med* 40(4):479-490, 1995.
49. Aker SN: Bone marrow transplantation: nutrition support and monitoring. In Bloch AS (ed): *Nutrition management of the cancer patient,* Rockville, MD, 1990, Aspen Publishing, pp 199-225.
50. Iestra JA, Fibbe WE, Zwinderman AH, et al: Parenteral nutrition following intensive cytotoxic therapy: an exploratory study on the need for parenteral nutrition after various treatment approaches for haematological malignancies, *Bone Marrow Transplant* 23(9):933-939, 1999.
51. Deeg HJ, Seidel K, Bruemmer B, et al: Impact of patient weight on non-relapse mortality after marrow transplantation, *Bone Marrow Transplant* 15(3):461-468, 1995.
52. Dickson TM: Kusnierz-Glaz CR, Blume KG, et al: Impact of admission body weight and chemotherapy dose adjustment on the outcome of autologous bone marrow transplantation, *Biol Blood Marrow Transplant* 5(5):299-305, 1999.
53. Morton AJ, Gooley T, Hansen JA, et al: Association between pretransplant interferon-alpha and outcome after unrelated donor marrow transplantation for chronic myelogenous leukemia in chronic phase, *Blood* 92(2):394-401, 1998.
54. Fleming DR, Rayens MK, Garrison J: Impact of obesity on allogeneic stem cell transplant patients: a matched case-controlled study, *Am J Med* 102(3):265-268, 1997.
55. Forbes GB, Welle SL: Lean body mass in obesity, *Int J Obesity* 7(2):99-107, 1983.
56. Lenssen P, Sherry ME, Cheney CL, et al: Prevalence of nutrition-related problems among long-term survivors of allogeneic marrow transplantation, *J Am Diet Assoc* 90(6):835-842, 1990.
57. Oliver MR, Van Voorhis WC, Boeckh M, et al: Hepatic mucormycosis in a bone marrow transplant recipient who ingested naturopathic medicine, *Clin Infect Dis* 22(3):521-524, 1996.
58. Myre S, McCorkle N, Kumar M: Management of the breastfed infant during bone marrow transplantation program (abstract). In *Program of the 19th Clinical Congress,* Miami Beach, FL, 1995, American Society of Parenteral and Enteral Nutrition, p 598.
59. Annis K, Henslee-Downey J, DeWitt P, McClain C: Measured energy expenditure in bone marrow transplant patients, *J Parenter Enteral Nutr* 15(1):34S, 1991 (abstract).
60. Geibig CB, Owens JP, Mirtallo JM, et al: Parenteral nutrition for marrow transplant recipients: Evaluation of an increased nitrogen dose, *J Parenter Enteral Nutr* 15(2):184-188, 1991.
61. Hutchinson ML, Clemans GW, Springmeyer SC, Flournoy N: Energy expenditure estimation in recipients of marrow transplant, *Cancer* 54(8):1734-1738, 1984.
62. Stravolich A, Porter C: Energy expenditure of bone marrrow transplant patients, *J Parenter Enteral Nutr* 15(1):36S, 1991 (abstract).
63. Peters E, Beck J, Lemaistre C: Changes in resting energy expenditure (REE) during bone marrow transplantation, *Am J Clin Nutr* 51:521, 1990 (abstract).
64. Cogoluenhes VC, Chambrier C, Michallet M, et al: Energy expenditure during allogeneic and autologous bone marrow transplantation, *Clin Nutr* 17(6):253-257, 1998.
65. Tomalis L, Kennedy MJ, Caballero B: Resting energy expenditure in patients undergoing autologous bone marrow transplant, *J Parenter Enteral Nutr* 18(1):27S, 1994 (abstract).
66. Taveroff A, McArdle AH, Rybka WB: Reducing parenteral energy and protein intake improves metabolic homeostasis after bone marrow transplantation, *Am J Clin Nutr* 54(6):1087-1092, 1991.
67. Szeluga DJ, Stuart RK, Brookmeyer R, et al: Energy requirements of parenterally fed bone marrow transplant recipients, *J Parenter Enteral Nutr* 9(2):139-143, 1985.
68. Cheney CL, Abson KM, Aker SN, et al: Body composition changes in marrow transplant recipients receiving total parenteral nutrition, *Cancer* 58(8):1515-1519, 1987.
69. Lenssen P, Cheney CL, Aker SN, et al: Intravenous branched chain amino acid trial in marrow transplant recipients, *J Parenter Enteral Nutr* 11(2):112-118, 1987.
70. Keller U, Kraenzlin ME, Gratwohl A, et al: Protein metabolism assessed by 1-^{13}C leucine infusions in patients undergoing bone marrow transplantation, *J Parenter Enteral Nutr* 14(5):480-484, 1990.
71. Cheney CL, Lenssen P, Aker SN, et al: Sex differences in nitrogen balance following marrow grafting for leukemia, *J Am Coll Nutr* 6(3):223-230, 1987.
72. Matarese LE, Speerhas R, Seidner DL, Steiger E: Foscarnet-induced electrolyte abnormalities in a bone marrow transplant patient receiving parenteral nutrition, *J Parenter Enteral Nutr* 24(3):170-173, 2000.
73. Gordon BG, Haire WD, Patton DF, et al: Thrombotic complications of BMT: association with protein C deficiency, *Bone Marrow Transplant* 11(1):61-65, 1993.
74. Gordon BG, Haire WD, Stephens LC, et al: Protein C deficiency following hematopoietic stem cell transplantation: optimization of intravenous vitamin K dose, *Bone Marrow Transplant* 12(1):73-76, 1993.
75. Link H, Blaurock M, Wernet P, et al: Acute folic acid deficiency after bone marrow transplantation, *Klin Wochenschr* 64(9):423-432, 1986.
76. Clemens MR, Ladner C, Ehninger G, et al: Plasma vitamin E and β-carotene concentrations during radiochemotherapy preceding bone marrow transplantation, *Am J Clin Nutr* 51(2):216-219, 1990.
77. Jonas CR, Puckett AB, Jones DP, et al: Plasma antioxidant status after high-dose chemotherapy: a randomized trial of parenteral nutrition in bone marrow transplantation patients, *Am J Clin Nutr* 72(1):181-189, 2000.
78. Hunnisett A, Davies S, McLaren-Howard J, et al: Lipoperoxides as an index of free radical activity in bone marrow transplant recipients, *Biol Trace Element Res* 47(1-3):125-132, 1995.
79. Clemens MR, Waladkhani AR, Bublitz K, et al: Supplementation with antioxidants prior to bone marrow transplantation, *Vien Klin Wochenschr* 109(19):771-776, 1997.
80. Dürken M, Agbenu J, Finckh B, et al: Deteriorating free radical-trapping capacity and antioxidant status in plasma during bone marrow transplantation, *Bone Marrow Transplant* 15(5):757-762, 1995.
81. Labriola D, Livingston R: Possible interactions between dietary antioxidants and chemotherapy, *Oncology* 13(7):1003-1008, 1999.
82. McKay PJ, Murphy JA, Cameron S, et al: Iron overload and liver dysfunction after allogeneic or autologous bone marrow transplantation, *Bone Marrow Transplant* 17(1):63-66, 1996.
83. Chapko MK, Syrjala KL, Schilter I, et al: Chemoradiotherapy toxicity during bone marrow transplantation: Time course and variation in pain and nausea, *Bone Marrow Transplant* 4(2):181-186, 1989.
84. Strasser SI, McDonald GB: Gastrointestinal and hepatic complications. In Thomas ED, Blume KG, Forman SJ (eds): *Hematopoietic cell transplantation,* Malden, MA, 1999, Blackwell Science, pp 627-658.
85. Fegan C, Poynton CH, Whittaker JA: The gut mucosal barrier in bone marrow transplantation, *Bone Marrow Transplant* 5(6):373-377, 1990.
86. Jebb SA, Marcus R, Elia M: A pilot study of oral glutamine supplementation in patients receiving bone marrow transplants, *Clin Nutr* 14:162-165, 1995.
87. Schloerb PR, Skikne BS: Oral and parenteral glutamine in bone marrow transplantation: a randomized, double-blind study, *J Parenter Enteral Nutr* 23(3):117-122, 1999.
88. Coghlin Dickson TM, Wong RM, Offrin RS, et al: Effect of oral glutamine supplementation during bone marrow transplantation, *J Parenter Enteral Nutr* 24(2):61-66, 2000.
89. Anderson PM, Ramsay NKC, Shu XO, et al: Effect of low-dose oral glutamine on painful stomatitis during bone marrow transplantation, *Bone Marrow Transplant* 22(4):339-344, 1998.
90. Ziegler TR, Young LS, Benfell K, et al: Clinical and metabolic efficacy of glutamine-supplemented parenteral nutrition after bone marrow transplantation. A randomized, double-blind, controlled study, *Ann Intern Med* 116(10):821-828, 1992.
91. Schloerb PR, Amare M: Total parenteral nutrition with glutamine in bone marrow transplantation and other clinical applications (a randomized, double-blind study), *J Parenter Enteral Nutr* 17(5):407-413, 1993.

92. Moe G: Enteral feeding and infection in the immunocompromised patient, *Nutr Clin Pract* 6(2):55-64, 1991.
93. Dezenhall A, Curry-Bartley K, Blackburn SA, et al: Food and nutrition services in bone marrow transplant centers, *J Am Diet Assoc* 87(10):1351-1353, 1987.
94. Aker SN, Cheney CL: The use of sterile and low microbial diets in ultraisolation environments, *J Parenter Enteral Nutr* 7(4):390-397, 1983.
95. Stern JM, Lenssen P: Food and nutrition services for the BMT patient. In Buchsel PC, Whedon MB (eds): *Bone marrow transplantation: clinical and administrative strategies,* Boston, 1995, Jones and Bartlett, pp 113-136.
96. Gauvreau-Stern JM, Cheney CL, Aker SN, et al: Food intake patterns and foodservice requirements on a marrow transplant unit, *J Am Diet Assoc* 89(3):367-372, 1989.
97. Szeluga DJ, Stuart RK, Brookmeyer R, et al: Nutritional support of bone marrow transplant recipients: a prospective randomized clinical trial comparing total parenteral nutrition to an enteral feeding program, *Cancer Res* 47(12):3309-3316, 1987.
98. Mulder POM, Bouman JG, Gietema JA, et al: Hyperalimentation in autologous bone marrow transplantation for solid tumors, *Cancer* 64(10):2045-2052, 1989.
99. Lenssen P, Bruemmer B, Aker SN, McDonald GB: Nutrient support in hematopoietic cell transplantation, *J Parenter Enteral Nutr* 25(4):219-228, 2001 (in press).
100. Sefcick A, Anderton A, Byrne JL, et al: Naso-jejunal feeding in allogeneic bone marrow transplant recipients: results of a pilot study, *Bone Marrow Transplant* 28(12):1135-1139, 2001.
101. Weisdorf SA, Lysne J, Wind D, et al: Positive effect of prophylactic total parenteral nutrition on long-term outcome of bone marrow transplantation, *Transplantation* 43(6):833-838, 1987.
102. Lough M, Watkins R, Campbell M, et al: Parenteral nutrition in bone marrow transplantation, *Clin Nutr* 9(2):97-101, 1990.
103. Lenssen P, Bruemmer BA, Bowden RA, et al: Intravenous lipid dose and incidence of bacteremia and fungemia in patients undergoing bone marrow transplantation, *Am J Clin Nutr* 67(5):927-933, 1998.
104. Muscaritoli M, Conversano L, Torelli GF, et al: Clinical and metabolic effects of different parenteral nutrition regimens in patients undergoing allogeneic bone marrow transplantation, *Transplantation* 66(5):610-616, 1998.
105. Clemans G, Yamanaka W, Flournoy N, et al: Plasma fatty acid patterns of bone marrow transplant patients primarily supported by fat-free parenteral nutrition, *J Parenter Enteral Nutr* 5(3):221-225, 1981.
106. Yamanaka WK, Tilmont G, Aker SN: Plasma fatty acids of marrow transplant recipients on fat-supplemented parenteral nutrition, *Am J Clin Nutr* 39(4):607-611, 1984.
107. Hutchinson ML, Clemans GW, Detter F: Abnormal plasma amino acid profiles in patients undergoing bone marrow transplant, *Clin Nutr* 3:133-139, 1984.
108. Desai TK, Maliakkal J, Kinzie JL, et al: Taurine deficiency after intensive chemotherapy and/or radiation, *Am J Clin Nutr* 55(3):708-711, 1992.
109. Young LS, Bye R, Scheltinga M, et al: Patients receiving glutamine-supplemented intravenous feedings report an improvement in mood, *J Parenter Enteral Nutr* 17(5):422-427, 1993.
110. MacBurney M, Young LS, Ziegler TR, Wilmore DW: A cost-evaluation of glutamine-supplemented parenteral nutrition in adult bone marrow transplant patients, *J Am Diet Assoc* 94(11):1263-1266, 1994.
111. Scheltinga MR, Young LS, Benfell K, et al: Glutamine-enriched intravenous feedings attenuate extracellular fluid expansion after a standard stress, *Ann Surg* 214(4):385-395, 1991.
112. Antila HM, Salo MS, Kirvela O, et al: Serum trace element concentrations and iron metabolism in allogeneic bone marrow transplant recipients, *Ann Med* 24(1):55-59, 1992.
113. Papadopoulou A, Nathavitharana K, Williams MD, et al: Diagnosis and clinical applications of zinc depletion following bone marrow transplantation, *Arch Dis Child* 74(4):328-331, 1996.
114. Fredstrom S, Rogosheske, Gupta P, Burns LJ: Extrapyramidal symptoms in a BMT recipient with hyperintense basal ganglia and elevated manganese, *Bone Marrow Transplant* 15(6):989-999, 1995.
115. Boock CA, Reddick JE: Taste alterations in bone marrow transplant patients, *J Am Diet Assoc* 91(9):1121-1122, 1991.
116. Okada JE: Identification of primary taste thresholds in adults with leukemia undergoing marrow transplantation, master's thesis, University of Washington, Seattle, 1984.
117. Mattsson T, Arvidson K, Heimdahl A, et al: Alterations in taste acuity associated with allogeneic bone marrow transplantation, *J Oral Pathol Med* 21(1):33-37, 1992.
118. Weisdorf SA, Schwarzenberg SJ: Nutritional support of hematopoietic stem cell recipients. In Thomas ED, Blume KG, Forman SJ (eds): *Hematopoietic cell transplantation,* Malden, MA, 1999, Blackwell Science, pp 723-732.
119. Charuhas PM, Fosberg KL, Bruemmer B, et al: A double-blind randomized trial comparing outpatient parenteral nutrition with intravenous hydration: effect on resumption of oral intake after marrow transplantation, *J Parenter Enteral Nutr* 21(3):157-161, 1997.
120. Fuller CJ, Faulkner H, Bendich A, et al: Effect of beta-carotene supplementation on photosuppression of delayed-type hypersensitivity in normal young men, *Am J Clin Nutr* 56(4):684-690, 1992.
121. Weisdorf SA, Salati LM, Longsdorf JA, et al: Graft-versus-host disease of the intestine: a protein losing enteropathy characterized by fecal alpha 1-antitrypsin, *Gastroenterology* 85(5):1076-1081, 1985.
122. Sale GE, Shulman HM, McDonald GB, Thomas ED: Gastrointestinal graft-versus-host disease in man. A clinicopathologic study of the rectal biopsy, *Am J Surg Pathol* 3(4):291-299, 1979.
123. Cox GJ, Matsui M, Lo RS, et al: Etiology and outcome of diarrhea after marrow transplantation: a prospective study, *Gastroenterology* 107(5):1398-1407, 1994.
124. Bianco JA, Higano C, Singer J, et al: The somatostatin analog octreotide in the management of the secretory diarrhea of the acute intestinal graft-versus-host disease in a patient after bone marrow transplantation, *Transplantation* 49(6):1194-1195, 1990.
125. Ely P, Dunitz J, Rogosheske J, Weisdorf D: Use of a somatostatin analogue, octreotide acetate, in the management of acute gastrointestinal graft-versus-host disease, *Am J Med* 90(6):707-710, 1991.
126. Morton AJ, Durrant ST: Efficacy of octreotide in controlling refractory diarrhea following bone marrow transplantation, *Clin Transplant* 9(3 Pt 1):205-208, 1995.
127. Gauvreau JM, Lenssen P, Cheney C, et al: Nutrition management of patients with intestinal graft-versus-host disease, *J Am Diet Assoc* 79(6):673-677, 1981.
128. Vickers CR: Gastrointestinal complications. In Atkinson K (ed): *Clinical bone marrow transplantation,* Cambridge, 1994, Cambridge University Press, pp 435-443.
129. Beschorner WE, Yardley JH, Tutschka PJ, Santos GW: Deficiency of intestinal immunity with graft-vs-host disease in humans, *J Infect Dis* 144(1):38-46, 1981.
130. Weisdorf DJ, Snover DC, Haake R, et al: Acute upper gastrointestinal graft-versus-host disease: clinical significance and response to immunosuppressive therapy, *Blood* 76(3):624-629, 1990.
131. Wu D, Hockenberry DM, Brentnall TA, et al: Persistent nausea and anorexia after marrow transplantation, *Transplantation* 66(10):1319-1324, 1998.
132. Akpek G, Valladares JL, Lee L et al: Pancreatic insufficiency in patients with chronic graft-versus-host disease, *Bone Marrow Transplant* 27(2):163-166, 2001.
133. Maringhini A, Gertz MA, DiMagno EP: Exocrine pancreatic insufficiency after allogeneic bone marrow transplantation, *Int J Pancreatol* 17(3):243-247, 1995.
134. Schubert MM, Sullivan KM: Recognition, incidence and management of oral graft-versus-host disease, *NCI Monogr* 9:135-143, 1990.
135. Fried RH, Murakami CS, Fisher LD, et al: Ursodeoxycholic acid treatment of refractory chronic graft-versus-host disease of the liver, *Ann Intern Med* 116(8):624-629, 1992.
136. McDonald GB, Sullivan KM, Plumley TF: Radiographic features of esophageal involvement in chronic graft-versus-host disease, *Am J Roentgenol* 142(3):501-506, 1984.
137. Clark JG, Schwartz DA, Flournoy N, et al: Risk factors for airflow obstruction in recipients of bone marrow transplants, *Ann Intern Med* 107(5):648-656, 1987.
138. Stern JM, Sullivan KM, Ott SM, et al: Bone density loss after allogeneic hematopoietic stem cell transplantation: a prospective study, *Biol Blood Marrow Transplant* 7(5):257-264, 2001.
139. Ebeling PR, Thomas DM, Erbas B, et al: Mechanisms of bone loss following allogeneic and autologous hemopoietic stem cell transplantation, *J Bone Miner Res* 14(3):342-350, 1999.
140. American College of Rheumatology Task Force on Osteoporosis Guidelines: Recommendations for the prevention and treatment of glucocorticoid-induced osteoporosis, *Arthritis Rheum* 39(11):1791-1801, 1996.

Burns and Wound Healing 42

Theresa Mayes, RD, LD

Michele M. Gottschlich, PhD, RD, LD, CNSD

WOUND healing involves an elaborate sequence of events that is affected by postinjury alterations in the hormonal environment, immune system, metabolic processes, and the circulatory and thermoregulatory systems. These physiologic aberrations are more prominent after extensive burn than following any other kind of trauma. Nutritional status is affected by the deranged atmosphere, and demands for energy, protein, cofactors, and coenzymes are increased. An aggressive nutrition support program is indicated to provide ideal conditions for wound healing. However, decisions on optimal nutrient composition and provision are complex. In this chapter, we review wound classifications and events of normal wound healing, pathophysiologic responses to injury, and current knowledge of the implications for nutrition support and assessment of its efficacy.

Pathophysiology of Wound Healing

Physical Destruction of Skin

Pressure ulcers, burns, necrotizing fasciitis, toxic epidermal necrolysis, and frostbite are examples of diagnoses associated with open wounds. Of these etiologies, pressure sores and burns are the most common. A pressure sore results from unrelieved pressure most often to bony prominences causing anoxic necrosis of surrounding tissues. Multiple factors contribute to the development of pressure sores. These include pressure due to body position, friction and/or appliance use, infection, moisture, malnutrition, and immobility.

The extent and depth of a wound are crucial to the determination of a treatment plan. The rule of nines is a convenient tool used in burns to estimate the extent of total body surface area (TBSA) involved in the injury.[1] This method divides the body into sections that represent 9%, or a multiple of 9%, of total surface area. Each upper extremity counts as 9%, each lower extremity 18%, the anterior trunk 18%, the posterior trunk 18%, and the head 9% of the total surface area.

Wounds are also classified by the depth of skin injury. A first-degree burn or stage I pressure ulcer affects the epidermal layers of the skin only. A second-degree (partial-thickness) burn or stage II pressure ulcer involves the epidermis and some of the dermis. A third-degree (full-thickness) burn or stage III pressure ulcer destroys all epithelial components of the skin. A fourth degree burn or stage IV pressure ulcer is characterized by extensive tissue necrosis extending to, thus

exposing, muscle, fascia, tendons, and ultimately bone/joints (Fig. 42-1). Such massive devastation of the skin barrier permits loss of heat, fluids, and most water-soluble compounds through the open wound and admits pathogens into subcutaneous tissue. Furthermore, major alterations occur in metabolism, in proportion to the depth and severity of the wound.

Phases of Wound Repair

Wound healing is a multifaceted sequence of events. The process is composed of three phases: inflammation, proliferation, and maturation.

The inflammatory phase typically lasts 3 to 10 days and is characterized initially by clot formation and lymphocyte attraction. The primary leukocyte during this stage is the neutrophil, which phagocytizes bacteria and other foreign bodies. Monocytes are also present in the inflammatory stage. The monocyte population steadily increases so that by the third to fifth day, these cells are actively working with neutrophils to debride the wound by phagocytosis. Monocytes secrete cytokines. Some of the key cytokines released at this time are tumor necrosis factor (TNF), interleukin-1 (IL-1), and interleukin-6 (IL-6). These local mediators fight invading organisms, attract other inflammatory cells to the wound, and stimulate their proliferation, thus easing into the second phase of wound healing.

This proliferative phase generally lasts for the next 2 weeks. As cytokines propagate, fibroblasts are attracted to the wound to release and deposit connective tissue proteins, most notably collagen. Collagen strengthens the integrity of the wound. This new connective tissue matrix replaces the lost dermis and is termed *reepithelialization.* Angiogenesis from the intact vasculature surrounding the dermis occurs during this phase as well. The new vasculature supports the nutritional/energy requirements for the synthesis and deposition of scar tissue. Wounds also gain resistance to infection in proportion to the rate of angiogenesis.[2-4] When local perfusion is diminished, delivery of oxygen, leukocytes, and other mediators of wound healing is decreased, and the risk for infection is increased.[5]

Remodeling of collagen, a process that continues over months to years, occurs in the final, maturation phase of wound healing. This stage is characterized by a state of balance between collagen production and degradation. The remodeling process occurs under a newly epithelialized surface, as is present following second degree/partial-thickness wound closure and beneath the skin graft that accompanies a third

Acknowledgment: A special thank you is extended to Debbie Lown, MS, RD, CNSD, who contributed to the first edition chapter on wound healing.

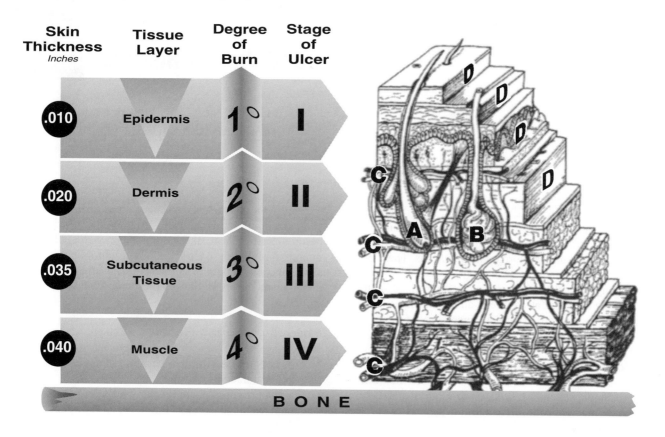

FIGURE 42-1 Interpretation of wound classification based on damage to the integument.

degree/full-thickness injury. This phase is further characterized by a reduction in fibroblast density, a process known as *apoptosis,* whereby fibroblast death is programmed without invoking an inflammatory response. Over time, the blood flow/nutritional needs of the scar diminish, leading to reduced vasculature. Collagen fiber bundles organize and increase in thickness affording the wound tensile strength.

Metabolic Response to Injury

Cuthbertson and Tilstone[6] described the metabolic response to trauma in two specific phases, the ebb and the flow response. Each is distinguished by peculiar phenomena. Burn injury in particular provides the most obvious manifestation of the categorized responses. The ebb phase is fairly transient: usually it lasts 3 to 5 days after injury, but in some patients, only hours. The ebb response is identified by loss of plasma volume, shock, and low plasma insulin levels. Decreased oxygen consumption, energy expenditure, blood pressure, cardiac output, and body temperature are other features (Table 42-1).

The transition to the flow phase is dominated by alterations in the hormonal environment that play an important role in mediating the metabolic response. An increase in catabolic hormones such as the catecholamines (epinephrine, norepinephrine, and their metabolites), glucocorticoids, and glucagon is observed during the flow response. These hormones counteract the anabolic effects of insulin that would normally force glucose and amino acids into cells for tissue and protein anabolism. Instead, the formidable effects of the catabolic hormones drive ureagenesis via accelerated protein breakdown, gluconeogenesis, and mobilization of fat reserves.[7]

Hormonal Alterations

The catecholamines, glucocorticoids, and glucagon have synergistic effects on metabolism after burn trauma. Shamoon and colleagues[8] infused the three hormones into normal subjects until concentrations were similar to those observed after mild to moderate injury. Triple-hormone infusion induced hypermetabolism, negative nitrogen balance, sodium retention, glucose intolerance, hyperinsulinemia, insulin resistance, and

TABLE 42-1

Metabolic Alterations Produced by Burns

	Ebb Response	Flow Response	
		Acute Phase	**Adaptive Phase**
Dominant factors	Loss of plasma volume Poor tissue perfusion Shock Low plasma insulin levels	Heightened total body blood flow Elevated catecholamines Elevated glucagon Elevated glucocorticoids Normal or elevated serum insulin High glucagon-insulin ratio	Stress hormone response subsiding Convalescence
Metabolic and clinical characteristics	Decreased oxygen consumption Depressed resting energy expenditure Decreased blood pressure Cardiac output below normal Decreased body temperature	Catabolism Hyperglycemia Increased respiratory rate Increased oxygen consumption and hypermetabolism Increased carbon dioxide production Increased body temperature Redistribution of polyvalent cations such as zinc and iron Increased urinary excretion of nitrogen, sulfur, magnesium, phosphorus, potassium, and creatinine Accelerated gluconeogenesis Fat mobilization Increased use of amino acids as oxidative fuels	Anabolism Normoglycemia Energy expenditure diminished Nutrient requirements approaching preinjury needs

Adapted from Gottschlich MM, Alexander JW, Bower RH: Enteral nutrition in patients with burns or trauma. In Rombeau JL, Caldwell MD (eds): *Enteral and tube feeding,* vol 1, Philadelphia, 1990, WB Saunders, p 307.

altered fuel metabolism. Others provide evidence to support the role of catecholamines, cortisol, and glucagon in catabolism.[9-12]

Many studies have been directed at the metabolic effects of the catecholamines, specifically in response to stress or trauma.[9,12-19] Studies from the 1960s through the 1980s suggested that the postburn surge of catecholamines had a significant effect on resting energy expenditure (REE). In addition, increased catecholamine concentration greatly affects the nervous, cardiovascular, and thermoregulatory systems and smooth muscle. Gottschlich and colleagues, however, recently evaluated the interrelationship between catecholamines and metabolic rate. Their data do not support the contention that epinephrine is the primary sustained mediator of postburn hypermetabolism.[19]

Serum insulin levels may be within normal limits after burn injury but are disproportionate to the rise in glucagon. As the glucagon to insulin ratio and tissue insulin resistance increase, the body attempts to provide a glucose source for wound repair by stimulating glycogenolysis and gluconeogenesis. In less than 24 hours, glycogen reserves are exhausted.[7] It is at this time that gluconeogenesis secondary to skeletal muscle breakdown begins.

Circulatory and Immunologic Considerations

After wounding, cardiac output increases to dissipate the glucose generated by glycogenolysis and gluconeogenesis. Disbursement of elevated amounts of blood to the wound provides an energy source directly at the affected site. As a result, loss of plasma volume through the open wound increases. Ongoing fluid and electrolyte resuscitation for large burns/wounds helps restore that lost through the open area. Adequate

fluid provision maintains homeostatic equilibrium by restoring acid-base balance; reestablishing cardiovascular, pulmonary, and renal hemodynamics; and supporting the transport of oxygen and nutrients to the wound.

Immunologic functions are abnormal, specifically following a large burn injury. Damage sustained to the protective skin barrier, coupled with massive nutrient loss via the open wound, predisposes the patient to an invasion of microorganisms. Infectious episodes contribute to hypermetabolism and hypercatabolism. Infection may precipitate or exacerbate malnutrition, placing the patient at even higher risk of morbidity and mortality.

Physiology of Burn Hypermetabolism

Many metabolic derangements following burn injury cause energy needs to surpass those associated with any other form of trauma. Energy needs peak approximately at postburn day 12 and typically return slowly to normal as the percentage of open wound decreases with reepithelialization or skin grafting. If, however, an infectious episode or multisystem organ failure develops, the hypermetabolic response is revived. Debate among clinicians persists, but a single agent does not appear to be responsible for the dramatic rise in metabolic needs during the flow phase of burn injury. Rather, the causes of hypermetabolism appear to be multiple.

Increased evaporative water loss from the burn wound has been implicated as a cause of the hypermetabolic response. Burned skin is no longer a barrier to water loss, and evaporative heat loss occurs through the open wound. The increase in heat production and elevation of core and skin temperatures produced by skin loss appear to enhance metabolic sequelae that normally maintain body temperature.[20,21] Debate over the implications of evaporative heat loss on hypermetabolism continues: many investigators support the theory at least in part,[13,20,22-27] whereas others refute the cause-effect relationship.[28,29] Most would agree that controlling ambient room temperature appears to reduce the metabolic rate, but it does not completely abolish the hypermetabolism associated with burn injury.

Neuroendocrine changes may contribute to the development of hypermetabolism. Epinephrine is secreted from the adrenal medulla. Studies that used pharmacologic adrenergic blockade demonstrated a significant decrease in metabolic rate;[16,30] however, adrenergic blockade did not completely avert the hypermetabolic response. This implies that other processes are involved.

Prevention of infection and wound closure are the principal means of reducing energy expenditure, although caregivers are in control of certain stress factors that can also help reduce the metabolic rate. Supporting the patient in a warm environment with wounds covered helps decrease energy needs. Wallace and colleagues recommend interviewing the patient to determine their subjective level of thermal comfort.[31] Maintaining an environmental temperature at the upper level of the established zone of thermal preference decreases calorie needs. In addition, adequate pain medication reduces anxiety and relieves suffering, both decreasing energy expenditure. As an aside, it should be noted that minor fevers are normal in patients with large burns and do not require treatment. Burn patients have lost the insulating function of the skin, and until the wounds are healed core temperature remains slightly elevated.

Other factors thought to be responsible for the hypermetabolic response to burn injury have been investigated. Early enteral feeding of burn patients has been implicated as a means of reducing energy needs.[32-34] In addition, Gottschlich and colleagues document significant sleep pattern disturbances with burns and suggest that sleep deprivation may be an extraneous component of the postburn course that promotes hypermetabolism.[35] Furthermore, research has attempted to discern the role of nonhormonal factors such as cytokines (IL-1, TNF) and prostaglandins on hypermetabolism after physiologic stress.[36-39] Rapidly emerging evidence supports the role of cytokines and prostaglandins in substrate utilization.[32-41] In addition, the cytokines appear to be responsible for stimulation of neuromediators that activate endocrine organs to release increased concentrations of catecholamines, cortisol, and glucagon, thus indirectly affecting REE. These investigations provide promising insights into the hypermetabolic response to injury and will be the focus of future research.

Nutritional Factors in Wound Repair

To combat the metabolic complications of injury, nutrition support is a critical component of the treatment plan to promote wound healing. The elicited hypermetabolism, hypercatabolism, and elevated nutrient loss via urine and open wound predispose persons with a burn injury or chronic wound to heightened nutritional requirements. Calories, protein, vitamins A and C, and zinc are essential constituents of the nutrition care plan.[42,43] The positive effects of nutritional repletion include promotion of wound healing, reduced risk of infection, perpetuation of body stores, and repletion of visceral and somatic proteins.

The multiple hormonal, biochemical, circulatory, and immune-mediated changes that transpire in the postinjury period have profound effects on nutritional requirements. The patient with a large open wound, as is present following thermal injury in particular, must overcome the devastating metabolic milieu of the flow phase of injury to progress to anabolism, and ultimately to survive. An adequate nutrition support regimen is essential to facilitating this transition. Although the following sections discuss nutrients separately to emphasize individual roles in wound healing, all are interrelated, and collective consideration is recommended for the most effective nutrition assessment and treatment plan.

Energy

Wound healing requires energy for synthesis of collagen, millions of new cells, new blood vessels, serum hepatic transport proteins, and more. Poor wound closure is present in patients who lack nutritional reserves to support healing and resist infection. Therefore, the energy requirement for wound repair is a dominant factor in healing.

The energy requirements of burn patients may be either estimated from predictive equations or measured by indirect calorimetry. At least 25 mathematical equations have been devised for estimating the daily energy requirements of burn patients. Table 42-2 lists several of the more commonly referenced ones. The various equations use different demographic variables to estimate calorie needs. There is no consensus on the use of body weight, body surface area, surface area of burn, or basal metabolic rate in such formulas. An initial nutrition care plan for a patient with decubitus ulcer should consist of 30 to 35 calories per kilogram per day.[63]

The reliability of some of the equations has been questioned by several investigators,[56,64-67] whereas other methods are criticized for not validating results with direct or indirect calorimetry.[52,59,61] In addition, many confounding factors (Box 42-1) are not accounted for in any equation. Body weight (affected by edema), burn dressings, and amputations can be sources of error when incorporated into an equation. Furthermore, several of these equations were developed more than 20 years ago. In the interim, improvements in wound management, early enteral feeding, and pain and infection control have reduced postburn hypermetabolism, thus, perhaps, decreasing the applicability of certain equations to today's burned population. Finally, the postburn metabolic ceiling described by Wilmore further complicates the use of an equation to estimate energy needs because most burn formulas incorporate total percent burn.[62]

The imprecision of the various burn formulas and the lack of evidence supporting a calculation specifically for wound healing justify the use of indirect calorimetry as a guide for determining energy requirements. Indirect calorimetry is the best tool for determination of REE because it accounts for differences in wound size, weight, body surface area, sex, infectious episodes, and other extraneous variables and is thus a more individualized representation of calorie needs. A factor of 20% to 30% should be added to REE to account for

TABLE 42-2

Formulas for Calculating Energy and Protein Requirements of Burn Patients

Reference	Age	% BSAB	Calories per Day	Protein per Day
Alexander[44]	Child	Any		22%-25% of kcal
Curreri[45–47]	0–1 yr	<50	Basal + (15 × % burn)	
	1–3 yr	<50	Basal + (25 × % burn)	
	4–15 yr	<50	Basal + (25 × % burn)	
	16–59 yr	Any	(25 × W) + (40 × % burn)	3 g/kg
	>60 yr	Any	Basal + (65 × % burn)	
Davies and Lilijdahl[48]	Adult	Any	20/kg + 70% BSAB	1 g/kg + 3 g/% BSAB
	Child	Any	60/kg + 35/% BSAB	3 g/kg + 1 g/% BSAB
Long[49,50] modification of the Harris-Benedict[51] equation	Male	Any	(66.47 + 13.7W + 5.0H − 6.76A) × (activity factor) × (injury factor)	
	Female	Any	(655.1 + 9.56W + 1.85H − 6.68A) × (activity factor) × (injury factor)	
Hildreth[52–54]	<15 yr	>30	(1800/m² BSA) + (2200/m² burn)	
Hildreth[55]	<12 yr		(1800/m² BSA) + 1300/m² burn	
Mayes[56]	<3 yr	10–50	108 + 68W + 3.9 × % BSAB	
	5–10 yr	10–50	818 + 37.4W + 9.3 × % BSAB	
Molnar[57]	Adult	Any	2 × BMR	2.5 g/kg
Parks[1]	Adult	Any	(1800/m² BSA) + (2200 kcal/m² BSAB)	
Pruitt[58]	Adult	Any	2000-2200/m² BSA	
Soroff[59]	Adult	Any	3500/m² BSA	
Sutherland[60]	Adult	Any	(20 × W) + (70 × % BSAB)	
Troell and Wretlind[61]	Adult	Any	40-60/kg	
Wilmore[62]	Any	Adult	2000/m² BSA	

Adapted from Kagan RJ, Gottschlich MM, Jenkins ME: Nutritional support in the burn patient. In Robin AP (ed): *Problems in general surgery*, vol 8, Philadelphia, 1991, JB Lippincott, p 65.
BMR, Basal metabolic rate; *BSA*, body surface area; *BSAB*, body surface area burned; *W*, weight in kg; *A*, age in years; *H*, height in cm.
Activity factor:
(a) confined to bed, use 1.2
(b) out of bed, use 1.3
Injury factor:
(a) severe burn, use 2.0

increased energy demands from physical therapy, dressing changes, temperature spikes, and other circumstances that elevate energy needs not accounted for by indirect calorimetry.[65,68,69] Optimally, metabolic testing is repeated two or three times per week postburn because transient alterations in calorie needs persist into the rehabilitation phase of recovery. The nutrition support regimen should be routinely adjusted to coincide with the results of indirect calorimetry.

Underfeeding is known to impair wound healing and immunocompetence and to increase the risk of morbidity and mortality. Overfeeding, on the other hand, can cause hyperglycemia, fatty liver, and elevated carbon dioxide production. Increased carbon dioxide levels can lead to respiratory insufficiency and difficulties with ventilator weaning. Thus, another advantage to utilizing indirect calorimetry is the concurrent disclosure of the respiratory quotient. Respiratory quotient indicates substrate utilization (Table 42-3) and may be an effective tool for avoiding underfeeding or overfeeding. For example, a respiratory quotient exceeding 1.00 necessitates a reduction in total calorie intake or the carbohydrate-lipid ratio. If the respiratory quotient is less than 0.80, the patient is experiencing an energy deficit and must increase calorie intake.

Indirect calorimetry is optimal for determining calorie goals for patients with acute or chronic wounds because the nutrition regimen can be tailored to meet individual needs. Because this tool is not available to all clinicians, using a reliable formula for caloric projection is a reasonable alternative. (See Table 42-2 for severe burns or 30 to 35 calories per kilogram body weight per day as an initial calorie goal for adults with

BOX 42-1

Factors Known to Affect Metabolic Rate

Activity
Age
Ambient temperature and humidity
Anxiety
Body surface area
Convalescence
Dressing changes
Drugs and anesthesia
Evaporative heat loss
Lean body gender
Metabolic cost of various nutrients when digested and absorbed
Pain
Physical therapy
Sepsis
Sleep deprivation
Surgery
Treatments rendered
Type and severity of injury
Weight

Adapted from Gottschlich MM, Alexander JW, Bower RH: Enteral nutrition in patients with burns or trauma. In Rombeau JL, Caldwell MD (eds): *Enteral and tube feeding*, vol 1, Philadelphia, 1990, WB Saunders, p 309.

minor wounds.) In either circumstance, the nutrition support program should be reevaluated regularly and modifications implemented in accordance with nutrition assessment parameters.

Increasing evidence suggests that energy demands are lower than those previously proposed for pediatric burn patients.[55,56]

TABLE 42-3

Implications of Respiratory Quotient (RQ)

RQ	Significance
<0.70	Oxidation of alcohol
	Oxidation of ketones
	Carbohydrate synthesis
	Measurement problem
0.70–0.75	Mostly lipid oxidation
	Possible starvation
0.85–0.95	Mixed substrate oxidation
	Calories adequate
>1.00	Lipogenesis
	Primarily carbohydrate oxidation
	Hyperventilation
	Measurement problem

Study results from the Shriners Hospitals for Children in Cincinnati and Galveston have resulted in the implementation of regimens that provide fewer calories than were previously recommended. Both hospitals theorize that early excision and grafting techniques that allow prompt closure of the open wound affect energy needs.

CUMULATIVE CALORIE BALANCE. It is recommended that the diet order for supplemental nutrition meet the daily energy goal by ±10%. Cumulative balance is a means of assessing and monitoring the adequacy of the diet order. Cumulative balance determination (current 24-hour energy intake minus the caloric goal added to the cumulative balance from the previous day) is a useful clinical indicator or monitor of nutritional adequacy. Over the hospital course, achieving a cumulative balance within ±7000 calories is considered within acceptable limits for the indicator. If the ±7000 cumulative balance goal is not achieved, an explanation for noncompliance is documented in the performance improvement report along with an action plan for preventing a similar incident in the future.

Carbohydrate

Glucose is the primary energy source for leukocytes, cell proliferation, phagocytic activity, and fibroblast function. An inadequate supply of carbohydrate results in decreased accumulation of collagen and thus diminished wound strength and ultimately, poor wound healing.

Hyperglycemia is a recognized consequence of severe thermal insult. The postburn phase appears to determine the mechanism of elevated blood glucose concentration. In the shock phase, elevated glucose levels principally result from a lack of insulin in relation to glucose concentration.[70,71] Glucose intolerance persists into the flow phase of injury but at this time is predominantly caused by increased peripheral tissue insulin resistance[71,72] and increased gluconeogenesis[70] rather than decreased utilization.[73] This glucose intolerance has been referred to as *stress diabetes* or *diabetes of injury.*[74,75] The use of the term *diabetes* is somewhat misleading because sufficient insulin is being produced in the flow phase and would, under normal conditions, effectively counteract the increases in blood sugar concentration.

Two gluconeogenic mechanisms that promote a rise in serum glucose concentration after burn injury, even in the fasting state, have been identified. First, the postburn hormonal environment with the increased glucagon-insulin ratio is known to activate gluconeogenesis. Secondly, alanine and other amino acids are increasingly cycled into the gluconeogenic pathway after burns.[70,76] These amino acids are rendered unavailable to build proteins. Instead, progressive depletion of body protein stores is augmented in this manner.

There is little evidence of impaired glucose oxidation following an injury whereby an open wound is created. In fact, wounds appear to metabolize large quantities of glucose. Glucose uptake by an injured extremity can be at least ten times that of an uninjured extremity.[77] The wound satisfies its energy requirements by enhancing circulation to the affected area. Given the fact that glucose metabolism is accelerated after a burn plus studies that describe the immunosuppressant consequences of fat delivery,[73,78-81] carbohydrate has become a vital energy-yielding nutrient. In severely hypermetabolic patients receiving constant doses of amino acids, carbohydrate decreased nitrogen excretion while equicaloric doses of fat failed to have a similar effect.[82] In addition, carbohydrate intake stimulates production of insulin, which is known for its anabolic properties. Dietary intake of carbohydrate approaching 60% to 65% total calories is recommended in patients with extensive burns to preserve muscle and liver glycogen stores in efforts to spare protein.[83,84]

Abundant carbohydrate facilitates the use of nitrogen for wound healing,[82,85] while suppressing gluconeogenesis. However, it should be noted that excessive administration has potentially damaging side effects.[86-92] Excessive enteral or parenteral carbohydrate provision can be associated with osmotic diuresis, resulting in dehydration and hypovolemia,[86,88-90] hyperglycemia, hyperosmolality, and increased lipogenesis, fatty liver, and carbon dioxide retention,[90-92] resulting in increased respiratory effort preventing ventilatory wean. All severely burned patients should be monitored for hyperglycemia and glycosuria. Provision of exogenous insulin is often necessary to improve serum glucose levels and maximize glucose uptake. From a practical point of view, the provision of 60% to 65% of calories as carbohydrate is a reasonable guideline, assuming that the amount does not exceed the reported 5 mg/kg per minute[88,93,94] maximum oxidation rate.

Protein

Chronic protein deficiency impairs angiogenesis and decreases fibroblast proliferation, thus diminishing reparative collagen synthesis, accumulation, and remodeling necessary for wound healing. Adequate protein supports the immune response specifically through antibody formation and phagocytosis. Normal protein synthesis and cell multiplication cannot occur without an adequate supply of protein. It has been suggested that prolonged hypoalbuminemia, whether from the acute phase of injury or prolonged protein deprivation can result in increased oncotic pressure and resultant tissue edema that slows oxygen diffusion, causing further insult to tissue and preventing repair.[95,96] Greenhalgh and associates randomized pediatric burn patients to either receive supplemental albumin to maintain levels between 2.5 to 3.5 g/dl or to give exogenous albumin only if levels dropped below 1.5g/dl following burn resuscitation. No differences in morbidity or mortality were noted between groups.[97] Therefore our institution provides exogenous albumin to patients with large burns only when the serum level falls below 1.5 g/dl or when edema is clinically noted.

Protein metabolism is drastically altered following thermal insult. If calorie needs are not met, nutritional status is compromised because amino acids become a principal energy source in the acute phase of injury. Alanine and glutamine are the primary amino acids released from structural and functional protein. These amino acids are transported to the liver and enter the gluconeogenesis pathway. The magnitude of amino acid liberation in this manner is dictated by the extent of the burn.[98,99] In addition to increased degradation, protein status is further compromised by extensive nitrogen losses through wound exudate and urine, impairment of the liver to form protein and, finally, inadequate nutrition therapy. Amino acids provide the fundamental building blocks for wound healing and nitrogen for growth in children. To reduce progressive somatic degradation, combat accelerated nitrogen losses, and prevent a syndrome of protein malnutrition, aggressive nutrition support is obligatory.

The effect of increased protein intake in critical care has been extensively studied.[100-102] These studies support enteral protein fortification as a means of improving hepatic transport protein synthesis, promoting positive nitrogen balance, enhancing host defense mechanisms, and supporting wound healing. Perhaps the most insightful study in burns has been conducted by Alexander and colleagues, who demonstrate that supplementation of protein as approximately 23% of total calories improves survival, opsonic index, serum total protein, retinol-binding protein, prealbumin, transferrin, C3, immunoglobulin G, and nitrogen balance and decreases incidence of infection in severely burned children.[44] Therefore, a recommendation of 23% to 25% of calories from protein is appropriate in serious burns.[44,103] This provision translates to an inherently low calorie-nitrogen ratio of approximately 80:1 or 2.5 to 4.0 g of protein per kilogram of body weight. A goal of 1.25 to 1.5 g of protein per kilogram of body weight per day usually supports anabolism in patients with an open area (<20% total body surface), including pressure sores. Administration of such high quantity of protein requires continuous monitoring of fluid status, blood urea nitrogen, and serum creatinine, especially in patients with severe injury, because of the high renal solute load.

In addition to the amount of protein provided, the quality of the protein is important. The use of high-biologic value protein such as whey or casein is preferred over soy for nutrition therapy in burn patients.[44,103] Furthermore, whey is endorsed over casein for multiple reasons, including improvement in tube feeding tolerance,[98-104] enhanced solubility in gastric acid,[98] greater digestibility (over casein),[105,106] association with unidentified growth factors, and nitrogen retention effects. Moreover, Alexander and associates conclude that animals fed intact whey protein have statistically significant increases in body weight; cumulative nitrogen balance; liver, gut, and gastrocnemius weights; and serum albumin, transferrin, and C3 levels than animals fed free amino acids in a whey protein pattern.[44,107,108]

BRANCHED-CHAIN AMINO ACIDS. Branched-chain amino acids (BCAAs) are known to regulate protein synthesis, suggesting potential beneficial effects in catabolic states. As a result, fortification of enteral feedings with BCAAs in the presence of skin destruction has been investigated.[109-113] Positive outcomes with BCAA supplementation in the burn population have not been demonstrated. Mochizuki and colleagues compared a BCAA-supplemented formula to a nonsupplemented formula in 71 guinea pigs with burns over more than 30% of body surface.[109] The BCAA group did not exhibit superior results in body weight, carcass weight, gastrocnemius muscle weight, gut mucosal mass, nitrogen content of muscle, serum albumin, or transferrin. In addition, cumulative nitrogen balance and mortality were significantly increased in the BCAA-supplemented group. In a study conducted by McCauley and colleagues, no improvement in wound healing was demonstrated by supplementing BCAA formulations.[113] For these reasons, BCAA fortification is not recommended as a part of the nutrition support program following skin and soft tissue injury.

ARGININE. Under normal circumstances, arginine is classified as a dispensable amino acid;[114-116] however, increasing research suggests that endogenous arginine synthesis via the urea cycle, sufficient under normal conditions, may be inadequate to support tissue regeneration or positive nitrogen balance following trauma or stress.[117-119] Arginine is a precursor of proline and hydroxyproline, essential components of collagen. Animals receiving supplemental arginine demonstrated increased wound tensile strength and deposition of hydroxyproline in subcutaneously implanted sponges.[120]

Following burn injury, dietary arginine supplementation improves nitrogen retention,[117,121] wound healing,[122-125] immune function,[126-131] and increases the anabolic hormones insulin and human growth hormone.[118,132-134] These outcomes are especially noteworthy in the acute postburn phase, when enhancement of these processes would be beneficial. A summary of the effects of supplemental arginine is listed in Box 42-2.

To determine the amount of supplemental arginine needed to promote its beneficial effects in burns, Saito and colleagues[127] designed a study whereby four groups of burned guinea pigs received varying amounts of arginine. The total number of calories as protein remained constant at 22%. The best cell-mediated immune response and the lowest mortality rate were noted in the group that received 20% of calories as whey protein and an additional 2% of calories as arginine. Therefore, a 2% provision of calories as arginine is the present postburn recommendation, an amount that was subsequently tested clinically.[73]

GLUTAMINE. It is becoming increasingly evident that the gut plays a key role as a regulator of amino acid metabolism after surgery and in other states of catabolic stress.[154-158] Glutamine is regarded as a conditionally indispensable amino acid important for maintenance of gut metabolism, structure, and function. The elevated glutamine requirement after injury is the result of increased utilization by small bowel epithelium. Following critical illness, glutamine is the principal fuel for the small bowel and is responsible for maintenance of the mucosal barrier. To date, most research has concentrated on the positive effects of glutamine fortification on intestinal mucosa. Glutamine supplementation after trauma is associated with improved villus height, restoration of intestinal mucosa,

BOX 42-2

Effects of Supplemental Arginine

1. Decreased protein catabolism and enhanced nitrogen retention after injury[117-120,135]
2. Corrected some cases of hyperammonemia[136-138]
3. Increased insulin and human growth hormone secretion[118,132-134]
4. Accelerated wound healing[122-125,139,140]
5. Enhanced immune response[126-131,140]
6. Increased thymic size and number of thymic lymphocytes[124,127-129,141-144]
7. Lessened the decrease in thymic weight and lymphocyte content that ordinarily follows injury[118,122-124]
8. Decreased body weight loss after injury[119,122,123,125]
9. Suppressed tumor growth[131,145-147]
10. Improved fat absorption and weight gain in cystic fibrosis[134]
11. Decreased incidence of sepsis and reduced length of hospital stay[73,148]
12. Necessary for maximal rate of recovery from protein-calorie malnutrition[149]
13. Required in the presence of excessive lysine (an antagonist) in foods, such as a high-casein diet[150]
14. Increased albumin and liver protein synthesis during sepsis[151]
15. Reduced intestinal protein turnover following enterectomy[152]
16. Improved survival in gut-derived sepsis and peritonitis by modulating bacterial clearance[153]

Adapted from Gottschlich M, Alexander JW, Bower RH: Enteral nutrition in patients with burns or trauma. In Rombeau JL, Caldwell MD (eds): *Enteral and tube feeding,* vol 1, Philadelphia, 1990, WB Saunders, p 312.

BOX 42-3

Benefits of Glutamine Supplementation After Injury

1. Maintains gut barrier function[160,163]
2. Improves villus height[162,163]
3. Regenerates intestinal mucosa[160-162]
4. Improves mucosal cellularity[159,160,163]
5. Maintains tissue glutathione concentration, an important oxygen radical scavenger
6. Improves weight status[158]
7. Reduces severity of intestinal mucosal injury secondary to chemotherapy,[160,166] radiation therapy,[164,167,168] and intestinal resection[162,169]
8. Regulates nitrogen metabolism in normal and catabolic states,[155,158,170] improving nitrogen balance[171,172]
9. Improves survival[171-173]

prevention of intestinal bacterial translocation, and improved mucosal cellularity.[159-165] Additional benefits of glutamine supplementation are noted in Box 42-3.

Given the anabolic properties of glutamine, preliminarily it appears that fortification with this nutrient might benefit burn patients. Tenenhaus and associates demonstrated a decrease in bacterial translocation in burned mice receiving glutamine-supplemented enteral feeds as compared with a nonsupplemented group.[163] In addition, Parry-Billings and colleagues concluded that a decrease in plasma glutamine concentration after a major burn insult may contribute to an already suppressed immune response.[174] Safe and efficacious administration of glutamine for burns is an area of promising future nutrition research.

ORNITHINE α-KETOGLUTARATE Many studies have evaluated the efficacy of ornithine α-ketoglutarate (OKG) supplementation postburn.[175-179] OKG combats postburn catabolism through its potent secretagogic effects on the production of insulin and growth hormone. In addition, the biotransformation of OKG to its metabolites glutamine and arginine supports immune enhancement. These beneficial effects strongly favor OKG supplementation following thermal injury, although further studies are necessary to determine if the metabolic and immunologic effects of OKG administration offer benefit over direct exogenous supplementation of arginine and glutamine.[180]

Fat

Enteral provision of lipid contributes calories and theoretically minimizes catabolism of endogenous protein by helping to fulfill energy requirements. Lipid is an essential component of cell membranes and acts as a carrier of the fat-soluble vitamins. An estimated 15 to 25 g of fat per day is necessary to meet vitamin demands. Finally, dietary lipid is imperative to satisfy essential fatty acid (EFA) requirements. Hulsey and coworkers showed delayed burn wound healing with EFA deficiency.[181]

As integral a component of the dietary regimen that fat may play in burns and wound healing, complications of excessive fat intake have been described.[73,78-81,182] Large amounts of dietary lipid are associated with accumulation of fat in the blood and liver and impaired clotting ability.[182] Of particular importance are studies of the effects of enteral lipids on depression of the immune response.[73,78-81,182,183] Liver damage, changes in prostaglandin metabolism, reduced antibody formation, inhibited neutrophil chemotaxis, impaired phagocytosis, and depressed function of the reticuloendothelial system are proposed mechanisms by which fat negatively affects the immune system. Furthermore, fat does not stimulate the secretion of the anabolic hormone insulin, nor does it share the nitrogen-sparing effects of carbohydrate.[80,182,184] For these reasons, enteral nutrition (EN) support containing high levels of fat may be detrimental to wound healing and ultimately, the survival of patients with large open wounds.

In an effort to define the optimal percentage of calories from fat, Mochizuki and colleagues studied 5 groups of guinea pigs, each with a 30% body surface area full-thickness burn.[80] Each group received equal calories, protein, vitamins, and minerals by continuous gastrostomy tube feeding; however, each group received a different amount (range 0 to 50%) of nonprotein calories in a lipid emulsion with a high concentration of linoleic acid. Results indicate significant differences among the varying groups in body weight, muscle mass, cumulative nitrogen balance, serum albumin level, and total fat in the liver. Based on these findings, diets containing between 5% and 15% of nonprotein calories as fat are considered optimal for nutrition support following burn injury.

OMEGA-6 VERSUS OMEGA-3 FATTY ACIDS. Linoleic acid, an ω-6, long-chain fatty acid, is the precursor of arachidonic acid. Arachidonic acid further metabolizes to the 1 and 2 series of prostaglandins (PGE_1 and PGE_2), thromboxane, prostacyclin, and series 4 leukotrienes.[185-188] Inflammation, increased immunosuppression,[81,189-191] and enhanced muscle breakdown are associated with these arachidonic acid metabolites.[80,192,193] Series 4 leukotrienes are known bronchorestrictors and stimulate mucous secretion.[194] For these reasons, diets high in linoleic acid are contraindicated for critically ill persons.

The ω-3 fatty acids, particularly eicosapentaenoic acid (EPA) and its parent α-linolenic acid, and docosahexanoic acid (DHA) are precursors of the triene prostaglandins (PGE_3) and series 5 leukotrienes.[185,195] The biologic activities of these metabolites differ immensely from those derived from the ω-6 fatty acids because PGE$_3$ and series 5 leukotrienes are proven antiinflammatory and immune-enhancing agents.[196-197] Furthermore, PGE$_3$ is a potent vasodilator.[198] In addition, numerous studies reveal that ω-3 fatty acids have competitive and inhibitory effects on the conversion of linoleic acid to PGE$_1$ and PGE$_2$.[199-204]

Because of the noted positive effects, a dietary supplement that is high in ω-3 fatty acids appears favorable for burn patients. With knowledge of the ω-3 versus ω-6 fatty acid controversy, Alexander and associates followed up the previously noted study, which determined the optimal percentage of calories from fat in the burn diet, with two trials that attempted to discern the importance of lipid type for burns. In the first study,[81] three groups of burned guinea pigs were randomly assigned to receive one of three enteral formulas that differed only in lipid source. Animals in group 1 received safflower oil as the sole lipid; those in group 2 received oleic acid; and those in group 3 received fish oil. Safflower oil contains 74% linoleic acid and fish oil contains only 2%. Both of these lipid solutions have similar oleic acid content, 15% and 13%, respectively. Fish oil, however, contains the ω-3 fatty acids EPA (18%) and DHA (17%). The group that received the fish oil experienced less weight loss, improved skeletal muscle mass, lower resting metabolic rate, enhanced cell-mediated immunity, better opsonic index, higher spleen weight, and improved serum transferrin.

Second, Alexander and colleagues further evaluated the use of fish oil, inherently high in ω-3 fatty acids, in their search for optimal lipid provision for burn patients.[189] Thirty-seven burned guinea pigs were fed enteral diets containing between 5% and 50% of nonprotein calories as fish oil. Increased weight loss and decreased carcass and liver weights were noted in animals receiving 30% to 50% fish oil, confirming that high lipid doses negatively affect outcome variables. In addition, high levels of fish oil did not compromise immunity. The authors postulate that, unlike high linoleic acid provision, known for its immunosuppressant precursor, PGE$_2$,[189-191] the ω-3 fatty acids present in fish oil might enhance the immune response to burns.

PRINCIPLES OF FAT DELIVERY IN BURNS. The principles of recommended fat delivery documented in the animal laboratory were investigated in a clinical trial conducted by Gottschlich and colleagues.[73] Three groups of burn patients were randomized to receive one of three enteral feedings. Two groups received commercial products widely used for nutrition management of burn patients. These formulas provided moderate to large doses of fat and linoleic acid. The third group was given a modular tube feeding (Table 42-4) used in the previously cited guinea pig model. This formula was low in fat, restricted in linoleic acid, and supplemented with ω-3 fatty acids. The provision of the modular tube feeding was associated with a significantly decreased incidence of wound infection and reduced length of stay. Trends in data also supported a relationship between the modular group and decreased incidence of diarrhea, improved glucose tolerance, and enhanced maintenance of muscle mass. Furthermore, 70% of deaths occurred in the group receiving the diet highest in fat and linoleic acid

content. This study supports an enteral diet that is low in fat and linoleic acid with ω-3 fatty acid fortification because this regimen appears to offer immunity-enhancing properties and other positive outcomes in burns.

Because of the many documented detrimental effects of arachidonic acid metabolites,[80,81,189-195] the continued use of large amounts of ω-6 fatty acids in enteral and parenteral formulas should be reevaluated. Recognizing 12% to 15% of calories from fat as the recommended amount for burn patients and that consumption of 1% to 3% of total calories as linoleic acid is sufficient to prevent EFA deficiency in humans,[200,201] it is clear that the majority of commercial enteral tube feeding products remain considerably high in fat content. Although improved in the past few years, most available enteral products are also practically devoid of ω-3 fatty acids. For these reasons, many of the currently available enteral products may not maximize the nutrition support of burn patients. Modular modification or careful scrutiny of commercially available products can help eliminate the "nutrition injustices" suffered by burn patients in the past.

STRUCTURED LIPIDS. Structured lipids are formed by the transesterification of medium-chain with long-chain triglycerides. Having both kinds on the same glycerol backbone may offer distinct advantages over a simple mixture of medium-chain and long-chain triglycerides. For example, structured lipids that combine medium-chain triglycerides and fish oils have been shown to optimize whole-body protein synthesis and serum albumin levels in burn injury and cancer animal models.[205] Structured lipids of this type have also been shown to decrease infection and increase survival as compared with traditional triglycerides because they provide fewer inflammatory and immunosuppressant fatty acids than conventional lipid emulsions.[186,206-213] Hayashi and colleagues recently concluded that supplementation of only 1% of total calories from a structured lipid containing EPA and DHA improved protein metabolism in burned rats receiving parenteral nutrition (PN).[214] The clinical relevance of structured lipid provision in burns and critical care remains to be determined.

Micronutrients

Micronutrients function as coenzymes and cofactors necessary for physiologic reactions at the cellular level, enabling protein and energy to be efficiently utilized. Given the increased energy and protein demands of burns and wound healing, it seems logical that vitamin and mineral needs increase as well. In addition to the roles of coenzymes and cofactors, vitamins and minerals are important for wound healing, immunocompetence, and other biologic functions. Enhanced losses through the open wound and changes in metabolism, absorption, excretion, and utilization, support supplementation of certain micronutrients beyond the recommended dietary allowance (RDA)[215]/dietary reference intake (DRI)[216] guidelines. The RDAs/DRIs are based on healthy persons and, thus, do not seem applicable to patients with an acute or chronic wound.

Table 42-5 characterizes the most prominent micronutrients associated with wound healing. The function of each nutrient in wound healing, food sources, deficiency symptoms, and the recommended test to determine micronutrient status are detailed. Deficiencies of any one or number of these

TABLE 42-4

Modular Tube Feeding Recipe*

Ingredients	1000	2000	3000	4000	5000	Method
			Amount			
Sterile water	750 ml	1500 ml	2250 ml	3000 ml	3750 ml	1. Measure sterile water and pour into blender.
MaxEpa (fish oil)	6 ml	13 ml	19 ml	25 ml	31 ml	2. Measure MaxEpa using a graduated cylinder. Add to blender.
Selenium-copper mixture	2 ml	4 ml	6 ml	8 ml	10 ml	3. Add selenium-copper mixture to blender.
Centrum Liquid	30 ml	60 ml	90 ml	120 ml	150 ml	4. Measure Centrum Liquid using graduated cylinder. Add to blender.
Microlipid	9 ml	18 ml	25 ml	34 ml	43 ml	5. Shake Microlipid preparation very well. Open and measure using a pipette. Refrigerate and date leftover Microlipid. Discard within 5 days.
Promix	62 g	125 g	187 g	249 g	311 g	6. Weigh Promix. Add to liquids in blender.
Polycose	165 g	330 g	495 g	650 g	825 g	7. Weigh Polycose. Add to liquids in blender.
Arginine HCl	5 g	10 g	15 g	20 g	25 g	8. Weigh arginine HCl. Add to liquids in blender.
Histidine	1 g	2 g	3 g	4 g	5 g	9. Weigh histidine. Add to liquids in blender.
Cysteine	1 g	2 g	3 g	4 g	5 g	10. Weigh cysteine. Add to liquids in blender.
Vitamin A	0.1 ml	0.2 ml	0.3 ml	0.4 ml	0.5 ml	11. Add vitamin A preparation.
						12. Mix all ingredients in blender on low for 30 seconds. Pour into proper container. Refrigerate immediately.

*Patent pending.

vitamins/minerals potentially impairs immunity and wound healing capacity. For these reasons, a daily multivitamin should be routinely administered to patients with an open wound. Further enrichment of vitamins A and C and zinc is indicated in large burns.[42,43] Dose recommendations for these nutrients for burn patients who weigh more than 40 pounds are vitamin A, 5000 IU per 1000 calories of EN; vitamin C, 1 g per day (usually administered as 500 mg twice daily); and zinc, 220 mg of zinc sulfate (or another compound providing approximately 46 mg of elemental zinc) daily. Children who weigh less than 40 pounds should have their doses of vitamin C and zinc reduced by half.[42] In addition, supplementation of the trace minerals copper and selenium (as well as zinc) above that of the standard may be warranted in burns, given a recent investigation by Berger and associates.[218] Supplementation of these minerals postburn was associated with a decrease in bronchopneumonial infections and shortened length of stay.[218]

Precise vitamin and mineral requirements for patients with an acute or chronic open wound are not known. Therefore, supplementing specific nutrients above that of the standard multivitamin may not be warranted (except for acute burns in excess of 20% TBSA) unless there are clinical signs of deficiency.

Nonnutritional Factors in Wound Repair

In addition to nutritional status, multiple factors affect wound healing. Boxes 42-4 and 42-5 list positive and negative influences. A number of these factors prevent or promote the supply of oxygen to the wound, thus inhibiting or supporting wound healing by this means. Chemotherapy, radiation, age, infection, adrenocortical steroids and immunosuppressant drugs are known to reduce the immune response and thus negatively impact healing, while certain therapies attenuate the hypermetabolic, hypercatabolic postinjury response. Modulation of cytokines[219] and prostaglandins[219,220] have been shown to enhance immunity and thus promote wound healing. Exogenous insulin stimulates muscle protein synthesis supporting anabolism, thus wound healing.[221-223] Pharmacologic agents such as anabolic steroids,[224-227] recombinant growth hormone,[228-232] and growth factors[228] reportedly improve wound healing although controversy regarding the effects of recombinant growth hormone on morbidity and mortality in critical care and burns is evident.[231,232]

Nutrition Assessment

Patients presenting with acute or chronic wounds should be screened upon admission and in the outpatient setting. A detailed nutrition assessment of these patients should follow in those patients identified at nutritional risk in order to determine the most appropriate approach to nutrition support. Details of nutrition support recommendations are discussed in the Enteral and Parenteral Nutrition sections of this chapter.

The goals of nutrition therapy should be to provide adequate nutrients to support wound healing, immune competence, and resultant hypermetabolism, thereby preventing malnutrition. This section reviews various monitors used to determine the effectiveness of the nutrition care plan's promotion of the above stated goals. Determination of calorie and protein intake is an important component of the ongoing nutrition evaluation. As applicable, tolerance of the nutrition support regimen along with calorie and protein intake from all sources including tube feedings, dextrose, albumin, and immunoglobulin G infusions should be recorded daily. Follow-up appraisals of nutritional status should include monitoring of body weight, body composition, and biochemical parameters that measure hepatic transport and somatic protein stores, and immune status. In general, regular assessment of nutrition intervention should continue until the patient has achieved closure of at least 95% of the wound.

Anthropometric Data

BODY WEIGHT. Fluctuations in body weight can be an important indicator of the adequacy of nutrition support; however, for the victim of a large burn injury, the interpretation of weight must consider factors known to affect body mass. For example, weight gain from fluid resuscitation in the first 24 to 48 hours after a burn is typical. Edema may continue well into the second or third postburn week, or even longer in some patients. In addition, fluid shifts, bulky dressings, amputations, escharotomies, other attached equipment, and supportive devices alter body weight dramatically.

It is important to obtain a "dry weight" on admission before measurement is skewed by edema. If the patient has been resuscitated at a referring hospital or was not promptly weighed on admission, preinjury weight should be used as a baseline. Biweekly body weights are recommended. It is helpful to designate particular days for weighing. For example, if Mondays and Thursdays are routinely known as *weight days,* the likelihood of procurement is increased. Weight measurements are optimally acquired in conjunction with scheduled hydrotherapy or dressing changes to avoid erroneous errors contributed by splints, bulky dressings, elastic bandages, clothes, and shoes. Determination of current weight as a percentage of the dry/preinjury weight is a useful assessment parameter. A goal of 90% to 110% of dry/preinjury weight indicates optimal nutrition intervention. Furthermore, this standard may be incorporated into a quality improvement program as an indicator of the success of diet therapy.

TRICEPS SKINFOLD THICKNESS AND MIDARM MUSCLE CIRCUMFERENCE. Triceps skinfold thickness and midarm muscle circumference are inexpensive measures of changes in body composition because fat and somatic stores can be rapidly depleted after a burn. These tests may be performed only on uninjured skin because eschar, swelling, fresh grafts, dressings, splints, and pressure garments can confound readings or render them inaccurate. Initial readings should be obtained on admission and repeated weekly thereafter.

Biochemical Parameters

ALBUMIN. Serum albumin decreases within a few days of wounding. The rapid decline is due to increased loss of albumin as plasma leaks from microvasculature to the burned area. Adequate nutrition support is necessary to replenish serum albumin levels. Albumin is increasingly effective as an assessment tool as the size of the open wound diminishes; however, because of its long half-life and insensitivity to rapid changes in nutritional status, trends in albumin values are monitored rather than assessing a single determination. In addition,

TABLE 42-5

Micronutrient Summary Pertinent to Wound Healing

Micronutrient	Function in Wound Healing	Food Sources	Deficiency Symptoms	Test to Determine Deficiency State[217]
Vitamin A	Enhances tissue regeneration by aiding in glycoprotein synthesis; cofactor for collagen synthesis and cross-linkage	Liver; fish liver oils; enriched dairy products; egg yolk; carrots; sweet potatoes; squash; apricots; peaches; and dark green, leafy vegetables	Xerophthalmia (night blindness, conjunctival xerosis, Bitot's spots), respiratory ailments (pneumonia, bronchopulmonary dysplasia), affects epithelial tissues of the gut	Serum vitamin A
Vitamin E	Antioxidant properties promote cell membrane integrity	Wheat germ; rice germ; vegetable oil; dark green, leafy vegetables; nuts; legumes	Increased platelet aggregation, decreased red blood cell survival, hemolytic anemia, neurologic abnormalities, decreased serum creatinine levels, excessive creatinuria	Serum vitamin E
Vitamin D	Regulates the synthesis of several structural proteins, including collagen type I	Eggs, liver, fatty fish, butter, margarine, fortified dairy products	Rickets in children, osteomalacia in adults	Serum 25-hydroxy vitamin D
Vitamin K	Essential for coagulation—a prerequisite for wound healing	Green, leafy vegetables; dairy products; meat; eggs; cereals; fruits	Hemorrhage	Plasma vitamin K, prothrombin time
Thiamine (B_1)	Cofactor in collagen cross-linking	Brewer's yeast, unrefined cereal, grains, organ meats, pork, legumes, nuts, seeds	Beriberi, anorexia, fatigue, peripheral neuropathy, foot and wrist drop, cardiomegaly, hyperlactatemia	Serum or 24–hour urinary thiamine
Riboflavin (B_2)	Cofactor in collagen cross-linking	Broccoli, spinach, asparagus, turnip greens, meat, poultry, fish, yeast, egg whites, dairy products, milk, fortified grain products	Cheilosis, angular stomatitis, glossitis, scrotal dermatitis, cessation of growth, photophobia	Serum erythrocyte glutathione reductase
Pyridoxine (B_6)	Coenzyme that activates protein synthesis	Chicken, fish, kidney, liver, pork, bananas, eggs, soy beans, oats, whole wheat products, peanuts, walnuts	Irritability, depression, stomatitis, glossitis, cheilosis, seborrhea of the nasal labial folds, normochromic, microcytic, or sideroblastic anemia	Serum erythrocytic glutamic-oxaloacetic transaminase (EGOT) and serum erythrocytic glutamic-pyruvic transaminase (EGPT)
Cobalamin (B_{12})	Coenzyme for protein and DNA synthesis	Meat and meat products, fish, shellfish, poultry, eggs	Megaloblastic anemia, loss of appetite, weight loss, fatigue, glossitis, leukopenia, thrombocytopenia, achlorhydria	Serum cobalamin
Vitamin C	Necessary for hydroxylation of lysine and proline in collagen formation and cross-linking; protects tissue from superoxide damage; enhances tissue regeneration	Citrus fruits, green vegetables, potatoes	Fatigue; anorexia; muscular pain; scurvy characterized by anemia, hemorrhagic disorders, weakening of collagenous structures in bone cartilage, teeth, and connective tissue, degeneration of muscle, gingivitis, capillary weakness, and rheumatic leg pain	Serum vitamin C
Magnesium	Cofactor for enzymes involved in protein and collagen synthesis	Nuts, legumes, unmilled grains, green vegetables, bananas	Nausea, muscle weakness, irritability, mental derangement	Serum magnesium
Calcium	Both the remodeling process and the degradation of collagen are accomplished through the action of various collagenases, all of which require calcium	Dairy products, sardines, oysters, kale, greens, tofu	Osteoporosis	Serum calcium
Copper	Promotes the cross-linking reactions of collagen and elastin synthesis; scavenges free radicals	Whole grain breads and cereals; shellfish, especially oysters; organ meats; poultry; dried peas and beans; dark green, leafy vegetables	Skeletal demineralization, impaired glucose tolerance, anemia, neutropenia, leukopenia, changes in hair and skin pigmentation	Serum copper or ceruloplasmin
Iron	Necessary for hydroxylation of lysine and proline in collagen synthesis and transportation of oxygen to the wound bed	Egg yolk; red meats; dark green, leafy vegetables; enriched breads and cereals; legumes; dried fruits	Anemia, cheilosis, glossitis, atrophy of the tongue, hair loss, brittle fingernails, koilonychia, pallor, tissue hypoxia, exertional dyspnea, heart enlargement	Serum ferritin, hemoglobin, hematocrit

Continued.

TABLE 42-5

Micronutrient Summary Pertinent to Wound Healing—cont'd

Micronutrient	Function in Wound Healing	Food Sources	Deficiency Symptoms	Test to Determine Deficiency State[217]
Selenium	Reduces intracellular hydroperoxides, thereby protecting membrane lipids from oxidant damage	Seafood, kidney, liver, meats, grains	Growth retardation, muscle pain and weakness, myopathy, cardiomyopathy	Serum or plasma selenium
Zinc	Cofactor in over 100 different enzyme systems that promote protein synthesis, cellular replication, and collagen formation	Oysters, dark meat turkey, liver, lima beans, pork	Hair loss, dermatitis, growth retardation, delayed sexual maturation, testicular atrophy, decreased appetite, depressed smell and taste acuity, depression, diarrhea, decreased dark adaptation	Serum or plasma zinc

Adapted with permission from Mayes T, Gottschlich MM: Burns and wound healing. In Gottschlich MM (ed): *American Society for Parenteral and Enteral Nutrition: The science and practice of nutrition support,* Dubuque, 2001, Kendall/Hunt Publishing, pp 391–392.

BOX 42-4

Nonnutritional Factors That Promote Wound Healing

- Anabolic agents
  - Anabolic steroids
  - Growth factors
  - Recombinant growth hormone
- Massage
- Perioperative prophylactic antibiotics
- Proper positioning/frequent position changes
- Prostaglandin/cytokine modulation
- Surgical debridement of eschar
- Topical antibiotics

BOX 42-5

Nonnutritional Factors That Attenuate Wound Healing

- Chemotherapy
- Increased age
- Infection
- Immunosuppressant drugs
- Radiation
- Smoking
- Underlying medical condition
  - Atheroslerosis
  - Cancer
  - Coagulation disorders
  - Congestive heart failure
  - Diabetes/hyperglycemia
  - Edema
  - Immunologic deficiencies
  - Ischemia
  - Obesity
  - Uremia

---

nonnutritional effects on variations in albumin concentration should be evaluated for proper interpretation. Dehydration, redistribution of total body water as in third-spacing, or exogenous albumin infusions raise the measured serum level. Overhydration, edema, surgery, blood loss, and sepsis are associated with hypoalbuminemia.

Transferrin

Serum transferrin is a more useful tool in defining malnutrition than albumin because its half-life (8 days) is shorter. The transferrin value of a burn victim obtained within hours of injury may be normal or nearly so, but as plasma is lost through the open wound the level declines dramatically over the next 1 to 3 days. Although the burn injury is responsible for the dramatic decrease in serum levels, it is nutrition support that will expedite the repletion of stores. Apart from dietary factors, decreased values are associated with fluid overload, iron overload, chronic infection, catabolic stress, nephrotic syndrome, and antibiotic therapy (particularly aminoglycosides, tetracycline, and cephalosporins). Serum levels may increase with hepatitis, pregnancy, iron-deficiency anemia, chronic blood loss, and dehydration. A weekly measurement of serum transferrin is recommended for long-term monitoring of nutritional status in burns.

Thyroxine-Binding Prealbumin

Prealbumin, like transferrin and albumin, is an indicator of hepatic transport protein synthesis. It is an extremely sensitive measure, given the small total body pool and half-life of 2 days. In addition, prealbumin is a more useful gauge of malnutrition

than albumin because it is not affected by exogenous albumin administration.

Because of its classification as an acute-phase reactant, prealbumin levels may have limited clinical relevance during the early stages of burn injury. Fluid shifts, wound exudate, transfusions, and infections affect serum concentration. Because prealbumin is degraded in the kidneys, increased levels are also observed during renal failure. The measure is more useful in evaluating the appropriateness of diet therapy during the convalescent stage of recovery when the effectors of serum concentrations are at a minimum. A weekly serum prealbumin level is recommended throughout the postburn phase and would be helpful in the assessment of the nutritional status of the patient with a chronic open wound.

NITROGEN BALANCE. Nitrogen balance calculations, with proper interpretation, may be used to verify the adequacy of the nutrition support program. The standard formula used to estimate the degree of anabolism or catabolism accounts for nonurinary, insensible losses; however, a primary additional source of nitrogen loss is the open wound. Formulas for estimating the amount of nitrogen wasted through burn exudate have been useful (Box 42-6).[233] A precise determination of nitrogen intake and a complete 24-hour urine collection are essential for accurate calculation of nitrogen balance. A

BOX 42-6

Formula for Calculating Nitrogen Balance in Burn Patients

Nitrogen intake – (24-hr urine urea nitrogen + fecal nitrogen loss g/24 hr + wound nitrogen loss g/24 hr)

Wound Nitrogen Loss:

≤ 10% open wound	= 0.02 g N/kg/day
11% to 30% open wound	= 0.05 g N/kg/day
≥31% open wound	= 0.12 g N/kg/day

See reference 233 for formula contained in box.

---

nutrition regimen that favors nitrogen balance determinations exceeding +5 for adults and children older than 3 years of age with burns in excess of 25% TBSA and a nitrogen balance greater than +2 in children less than 3 years is optimal for wound healing and anabolism. Nitrogen balance determinations in patients with chronic open wounds would be helpful in the assessment of the adequacy of calorie and protein intake/needs. The discretion of the clinician is needed to ensure that a full 24-hour urine sample as well as nutritional intake can be obtained.

CREATININE-HEIGHT INDEX. Creatinine is an excreted end product of somatic protein breakdown. Creatinine-height index (CHI), derived from the urinary creatinine value, is a useful assessment tool for monitoring lean body mass and nutritional status. Evaluations may be used when upper-arm anthropometry cannot be obtained or may be used in conjunction with anthropometry to verify results. CHI is depressed with malnutrition and poor muscle mass nutriture. Results of less than 40% of the standard suggest severe nutritional depletion. Some 40% to 60% of the standard signifies a marginal nutritional deficiency, and over 60% of the standard is evidence of adequate nutrition support.

If nitrogen balance studies requiring a 24-hour urine collection are ordered, urinary nitrogen loss and urinary creatinine concentration may be reported simultaneously. The availability of urinary creatinine values in this manner facilitates the calculation and evaluation of CHI. It is important to note that reliable CHI computations depend on normal renal function.

TOTAL LYMPHOCYTE COUNT. Malnutrition depresses immunocompetence and lowers lymphocyte counts. Total lymphocyte count (TLC) instead of white blood cell differential is a sensitive nutrition index. A TLC above 1200 per cubic millimeter suggests no depletion, 800 to 1200 per cubic millimeter suggests moderate depletion, and less than 800 per cubic millimeter may represent severe nutritional depletion.

Effectors of white cell count must be considered before TLC can be used as a nutrition assessment tool. These include the presence of a large wound, which could result in temporary depletion of peripheral lymphocytes because of tissue migration, causing a transient depression in the TLC calculation; an elevated white cell count, common with infection, causing a false rise in TLC; and suppression of leukocyte count by drugs and topical agents frequently used in treating burns and open wounds, such as silver sulfadiazine, cimetidine, penicillin,

furosemide, and sulfonamides. Because of these multiple factors, trends in TLC are most useful as a nutrition assessment tool during the convalescent stage of recovery, or for a patient with a smaller wound whose TLC value is not confounded by any of the aforementioned variables.

SKIN TESTS. Malnutrition has a profound effect on host defense mechanisms. The extent of immune compromise has been assessed in burn patients using cell-mediated immunity techniques. As malnutrition advances, the ability of an individual to react to common skin test antigens is impaired. Antigens are injected intradermally, usually on the forearm, circled and numbered to facilitate identification. The induration at the site of the antigen injection is measured after 24 to 72 hours. A positive response is defined as an induration of 5 mm or larger. Anergy, or failure of the host to produce a delayed hypersensitivity reaction to any one of the four skin tests, has been associated with host resistance, sepsis, morbidity, and mortality.[234,235] Additional factors implicated in anergy are age older than 80 years, cancer, sepsis, shock, major trauma,[236] malnutrition, technical errors in administration, and no previous exposure to the antigen.[233,237]

Because immunocompetence may be jeopardized by a number of factors other than malnutrition, one must exercise caution in using skin tests to assess the nutritional status of the critically ill burn patients. Skin test reactivity can be used for nutrition assessment if other factors in the development of anergy are eliminated.

PROGNOSTIC INFLAMMATORY AND NUTRITIONAL INDEX. The typical nutrition assessment parameters applied in burns are likely to be abnormal, particularly during the acute phase of injury. To strengthen the predictive value of individual assessment variables, multiparameter nutrition risk indices have been devised.[238-240] One such guide, prognostic inflammatory and nutritional index (PINI), combines positive and negative acute-phase reactants capturing inflammatory and nutrition-dependent rapid turnover proteins.[238] PINI incorporates albumin (Alb) and prealbumin (Palb) (negative acute-phase proteins) that characteristically decrease after thermal injury,[241-244] with C-reactive protein (CRP), and α_1-acid glycoprotein (AAG) (positive acute-phase proteins), which markedly increase.[245-248] Changes in these positive and negative reactants depend on the extent of injury.[241]

$$PINI = [AAG \times CRP] \div [Alb \times Palb]$$

A PINI value of 175 or more is considered abnormal and appears to be an important indicator of morbidity and mortality for patients with burns.[240]

Gottschlich and coworkers have reported a less costly model that incorporates CRP and Palb only.[240] The differences between the standard four-variable PINI and the two-tier CRP/Palb were negligible in predicting outcome. Therefore, the authors assert that the CRP/Palb index is more practical in burns.

Nutrition Support Guidelines

Oral Versus Tube Feeding

Adequate oral intake can usually be achieved in a well-nourished individual when the wound involves less than 20% of

TBSA (minor burns, minimal surgical wound/trauma or decubitus ulcer). A combination of food preference provision, oral supplementation of high-calorie, high-protein products, and concealing carbohydrate and protein modules in foods and beverages is helpful in increasing nutrient intake. These same guidelines can be applied to patients nearing discontinuation of enteral feeds to ensure that adequate oral nutriture exists before termination of tube feeding. Attempts to raise calories by supplying more food are discouraged. This practice often leads to poor oral intake because the patient is overwhelmed by the food presented at mealtimes and having to consume large amounts of food may drastically alter eating patterns. The overeating could become a habit and might predispose the patient to unnecessary weight gain. If the patient is determined to be undernourished, the factors contributing to the malnutrition should be examined and nutrition support initiated.

Enteral Nutrition Support

Enteral support offers specific advantages over parenteral administration and is the preferred route of nutrient provision for wound healing.[249-252] Kiyama and associates demonstrated significantly enhanced early wound breaking strength and wound collagen accumulation in enterally fed, wounded rats versus those parenterally sustained.[250] Increased intestinal blood flow, preserved gastrointestinal function, decreased mucosal atrophy,[253-256] and reduced bacterial translocation from the gastrointestinal tract[253,256-258] have been proven with enteral alimentation. In addition, enteral alimentation is much less expensive than PN. Finally, risks such as pneumothorax, bleeding, infection, air embolism, pulmonary or hepatic dysfunction, and decreased utilization of nutrients, associated with PN, are not issues with enteral feeding.

Supplemental enteral calories and protein are usually necessary for patients with greater than 20% TBSA burns, those who are unable to eat because of prolonged ventilator dependence, patients with preexisting malnutrition, individuals with oral facial/injury, or patients with poor intake over a period of 2 to 3 days. Although the stomach may be affected by posttraumatic ileus, the small intestine is a viable means of nutrition provision because its functional and absorptive capacities are maintained postburn.[259,260] Consequently, the absence of bowel sounds does not preclude the provision of tube feeding. Nasoduodenal feeding tubes may be placed under fluoroscopy, with radiographic confirmation, into the third portion of the duodenum, just beyond the ligament of Treitz. Simultaneous decompression of stomach acids by a nasogastric tube is necessary until gastric motility is established. Administration of antacid medications through the nasogastric tube is essential to prevent Curling's ulcer. Once gastric function is confirmed, if the feeding tube remains in the small bowel and the patient is receiving nothing by mouth, the nasogastric tube should remain in place. If the patient is able to accept oral foodstuff, the recommendations noted under the Oral versus Tube Feeding section of this chapter should be implemented. Furthermore, because of the minimal aspiration risk associated with feeding tubes in the small bowel, interruption of the enteral regimen for various postburn procedures is obviated.

Early Enteral Intervention in Burns

Because a delay in EN is associated with reduced concentration and activity of intestinal enzymes and gastric hormones that are necessary for digestion and optimal nutrient usage, the institution of EN after a burn should be a priority. In addition, structural and functional intestinal atrophy is also recognized with delayed or absent enteral feeds[255] (see Chapter 21). Mochizuki and colleagues[32] and Dominioni's group[33] have demonstrated that immediate enteral feeding postburn prevented the hypermetabolic response observed in control animals not fed for 24 to 72 hours after injury. Furthermore, animals fed early lost less weight, had positive nitrogen balance, and had a lower prevalence of diarrhea.

Jenkins and associates further evaluated early enteral feeding by applying the principle in the clinical setting.[34] In support of the previous study, the group fed early (less than 24 hours after the burn) did not exhibit as much of a hypermetabolic response as the group fed 72 hours after the burn. Trends toward improved hepatic transport protein store measures and decreased infectious complications (thus reducing systemic antibiotic therapy) were also observed in the group fed early. Early enteral feeding in burns is also associated with a reduction in infectious episodes and decreased length of stay.[261]

It is essential that EN be a priority for burn patients because the practice appears to have multiple anabolic effects. Decreased energy requirement is a surprising yet welcome feature of immediate small bowel feeds. Further studies are necessary to confirm the existence of lower energy needs in patients fed early and to elucidate the mechanisms.

Guidelines for Enteral Nutrition Administration

There is no need to delay enteral alimentation until after the burn resuscitation period. The tube feeding rate should be run above total hourly fluid requirements until the shock phase has ended. Once resuscitation is complete, the amount of tube feeding per hour is included in the overall hourly fluid rate. Delivery of full-strength product is usually tolerated well and is essential for meeting nutrient requirements. The initial hourly infusion rate should begin at half of the final desired volume and be advanced by 5 ml per hour for children younger than 3 years and 10 to 20 ml per hour for older children and adults.

Most pharmaceutical companies market high-protein enteral formulas, but the majority of commercial products continue to provide insufficient ω-3 fatty acids, coenzymes, cofactors, and other substances the body needs after a significant thermal injury. The addition of one or more dietary modules such as whey protein or extra vitamins and minerals, or amino acid supplementation may enhance its nutritional quality greatly. Maldigestion is rarely a concern with burns and wound healing, so an elemental product is seldom indicated.[262] Elemental formulas should be considered only in the unusual cases of gut trauma or severe malabsorption. When predigested enteral formulas are necessary, a peptide protein source should be used based on research showing that, in comparison to free amino acids, peptides are more rapidly absorbed in the small intestine and have a stimulatory effect on water and electrolyte absorption.[263,264]

Perioperative Enteral Feeding

Studies support the definitive relationship between malnutrition and poor postoperative wound healing, suggesting that adequate nutrition in the perioperative period is warranted.[265-271] Further discussion of perioperative enteral feeding is included in Chapter 21.

It is common to allow patients nothing by mouth for hours before and after surgical procedures. At our institution, grafting of the burn wound takes place following an overnight period of stabilization after the wound excision. In the past, patients would receive negligible nutrition support during this 2-day period. The minimal alimentation may have abolished the reduction in hypermetabolism realized from immediate enteral feeding. In addition, this protocol of reduced nutrition support does not promote the immune enhancement or wound healing benefits all burn victims deserve.

Successful demonstration of continued enteral feedings throughout excision and grafting procedures has been documented without complications.[265,266,272] Jenkins and coworkers compared two sets of patients with burns of equal size, one set fed through surgery and the other not fed through surgery. Results indicate significantly reduced calorie deficits and less albumin requirements to maintain adequate serum levels in patients fed through surgery.[265] Although strong support is provided for feeding through surgical procedures at our institution, it is important to recognize that strict safety protocols are in place. These standards ensure that diligent monitoring of feeding tube position and gastric reflux occur throughout the operation.

Parenteral Nutrition Support

Because of the association of PN with increased prevalence of blood-borne infections, lower helper-suppressor T-cell ratios, and impaired neutrophil function as compared with enteral feeding,[273,274] instituting parenteral alimentation as a matter of standard protocol for an individual with an intact gastrointestinal system, like a burn patient, is unjustified. To avert the morbidity and mortality associated with malnutrition, intravenous feedings should be reserved for patients who cannot meet calorie requirements by enteral feeding for an expected protracted time. Indications for parenteral feeds are limited: concurrent abdominal trauma; persistent intestinal ileus; severe diarrhea, most often due to sepsis or prolonged antibiotic therapy; stress ulceration of the stomach or duodenum;[275] pancreatitis;[276] pseudo-obstruction of the colon;[277] and superior mesenteric artery syndrome.[278-280]

In the rare case when PN is implemented, the standards of gut stimulation and low fat provision should be maintained. Whenever possible, simultaneous trophic enteral feedings are recommended for parenterally supported patients to promote small bowel function. Advances in tube feeding rate are accompanied by respective decreases in parenteral solution administration. Conservative provision of intravenous fat is encouraged because of its hyperlipidemic and immunosuppressant effects. If enteral trophic feeds provide 1% to 2% of total calorie requirements as linoleic acid and 1% to 2% of calories derive from an ω-3 fatty acid source, naturally rich in α-linolenate, then additional lipid in the parenteral solution is not necessary. When parenteral alimentation is the sole source of nutrition support, 500 ml of a 10% lipid emulsion two times per week is adequate for adults. Less fat would be necessary for children.

Conclusion

Because an open wound induces many pathophysiologic derangements that ultimately affect nutritional status and, thus, healing, ongoing assessment of clinical course with appropriate nutrition intervention should be a priority of care in the inpatient and outpatient settings. Research continues to discern the proper amounts of carbohydrate, protein, fat, and micronutrients necessary to compensate for the deleterious effects of extensive injuries such as burns. Current knowledge supports a high-protein, high-carbohydrate, low-fat, low-linoleic acid diet for severely burned patients. Supplementation of vitamins and minerals, particularly vitamins A and C and zinc, is also necessary for healing of a large burn wound. The current supplementation recommendation for healing a nonburn wound is increased calories and protein. Micronutrient fortification of a patient with a nonburn-induced wound is supported only upon suspected or documented deficiency. Enteral feeding is the superior mode of nutrition because it has specific advantages over intravenous management. Exciting advances have been made in the past decade with respect to the nutrients involved in wound healing. Research must now focus on whether manipulation of specific nutrients can accelerate wound healing, enhance immune response, and minimize negative metabolic sequelae, thus improving clinical outcomes.

REFERENCES

1. Parks DH, Carvajal HF, Larson DL: Management of burns, *Surg Clin North Am* 57(5):875-894, 1977.
2. Allen DB, Maquire JJ, Mani M, et al: Wound hypoxia and acidosis limit neutrophil bacterial killing mechanisms, *Arch Surg* 132(9):991-996, 1997.
3. Gibson JJ, Angeles A, Hunt TK: Increased oxygen tension potentiates angiogenesis, *Surg Forum* 48:696-699, 1997.
4. Hopf HW, Hunt TK, West JM, et al: Wound tissue oxygen tension predicts the risk of wound infection in surgical patients, *Arch Surg* 132(9):997-1004, 1997.
5. Hartmann M, Jonsson K, Zederfeldt B: Effect of tissue perfusion and oxygenation on accumulation of collagen in healing wounds. Randomized study in patients after major abdominal operations, *Eur J Surg* 158(10):521-526, 1992.
6. Cuthbertson D, Tilstone WJ: Metabolism during the postinjury period, *Adv Clin Chem* 12:1-55, 1969.
7. Clowes GHA: Metabolic responses to injury. Part I: The production of energy, *J Trauma* 3:149-195, 1963.
8. Shamoon HM, Hendler R, Sherwin RS: Synergistic interactions among anti-insulin hormones in the pathogenesis of stress hyperglycemia in humans, *J Clin Endocrinol Metab* 52(6):1235-1241, 1981.
9. Bessey PQ, Walters JM, Aoki TT, Wilmore DW: Combined hormonal infusion simulates the metabolic response to injury, *Ann Surg* 200(3):264-281, 1984.
10. Simmons PS, Miles JM, Gerich JE, Haymond MW: Increased proteolysis: an effect of increases in plasma cortisol within the physiologic range, *J Clin Invest* 73(2):412-420, 1984.
11. Darmaun D, Matthews DE, Bier DM: Physiological hypercortisolemia increases proteolysis, glutamine and alanine production, *Am J Physiol* 255(3 Pt 1):E366-E373, 1988.
12. Gelfand RA, Matthews DE, Bier DM, Sherwin RS: Role of counterregulatory hormones in the catabolic response to stress, *J Clin Invest* 74(6):2238-2248, 1984.

13. Aikawa N, Caulfield JB, Thomas RJS, Burke JF: Postburn hypermetabolism: relation to evaporative heat loss and catecholamine level, *Surg Forum* 26:74-76, 1975.

14. Matthews DE, Pesola G, Cambell RG: Effect of epinephrine upon amino acid and energy metabolism in humans, *Am J Physiol* 258(6 Pt 1):E948-E956, 1990.

15. Stalen MA, Matthews DE, Cryer PE, Bier DM: Physiologic increments in epinephrine stimulate metabolic rate in humans, *Am J Physiol* 253(3 Pt 1):E322-E330, 1987.

16. Wilmore DW, Long JM, Mason AD, et al: Catecholamines: mediator of the hypermetabolic response to thermal injury, *Ann Surg* 180(4):653-669, 1974.

17. Aprille JR, Horn JA, Rulfs J: Liver and skeletal muscle mitochondrial function following burn injury, *J Trauma* 17(4):279-288, 1977.

18. Harrison TS, Seton JF, Feller I: Relationship of increased oxygen consumption to catecholamine excretion in thermal burns, *Ann Surg* 165(2):169-172, 1967.

19. Gottschlich MM, James JH, Mayes T, et al: Interrelationship between catecholamines, metabolic rate and burn severity: the concept revisited, *Proc Am Burn Assn* 33, 2001.

20. Birke G, Carlson LA, vonEuler VS, et al: Lipid metabolism, catecholamine excretion, basal metabolic rate, and water loss during treatment of burns with warm dry air, *Acta Chir Scand* 138(4):321-333, 1972.

21. Harrison HN, Moncrief JA, Durkett JW, Mason AD: The relationship between energy metabolism and water loss from vaporization in severely burned patients, *Surgery* 56:203-211, 1964.

22. Caldwell FT, Bowser GH, Crabtree JH: The effect of occlusive dressings on the energy metabolism of severely burned children, *Ann Surg* 193(5):579-591, 1981.

23. Barr PO, Birke G, Liljedahl SO, Planting LO: Oxygen consumption and water loss during treatment of burns with warm, dry air, *Lancet* 1:164-168, 1968.

24. Roe CF, Kinney JM, Blair C: Water and heat exchange in third-degree burns, *Surgery* 56:212-220, 1964.

25. Lieberman ZH, Lansche JM: Effects of thermal injury on metabolic rate and insensible water loss in the rat, *Surg Forum* 7:83-88, 1957

26. Neely WA, Petro AB, Holloman GH, et al: Researches on the cause of burn hypermetabolism, *Ann Surg* 179(3):291-294, 1974.

27. Caldwell FT: Energy metabolism following thermal burns, *Arch Surg* 111:181-185, 1976.

28. Zawacki BE, Spitzer KW, Mason AD, et al: Does increased evaporative water loss cause hypermetabolism in burn patients? *Ann Surg* 171(2):236-240, 1970.

29. Wilmore DW, Mason AD, Johnson DW, Pruitt BA: Effect of ambient temperature on heat production and heat loss in burn patients, *J Appl Physiol* 38(4):593-597, 1975.

30. Wilmore DW: Hormonal responses and their effect on metabolism, *Surg Clin North Am* 56(5):999-1018, 1976.

31. Wallace BH, Caldwell FT, Cone JB: The interrelationships between wound management, thermal stress, energy metabolism and temperature profiles of patients with burns, *J Burn Care Rehabil* 15(6):499-508, 1994.

32. Mochizuki H, Trocki O, Dominioni L, et al: Mechanisms of prevention of postburn hypermetabolism and catabolism by early enteral feeding, *Ann Surg* 200(3):297-310, 1984.

33. Dominioni L, Trocki O, Mochizuki H, Fang CH: Prevention of severe postburn hypermetabolism and catabolism by immediate intragastric feeding, *J Burn Care Rehabil* 5(2):106-112, 1984.

34. Jenkins M, Gottschlich M, Alexander JW, Warden GD: An evaluation of the effect of immediate enteral feeding on the hypermetabolic response following severe burn injury, *J Burn Care Rehabil* 15(2):199-205, 1994.

35. Gottschlich MM, Jenkins ME, Mayes T, et al: A prospective clinical study of the polysomnographic stages of sleep following burn injury, *J Burn Care Rehabil* 15(6):486-492, 1994.

36. Cerami A: Inflammatory cytokines, *Clin Immunopathol* 62(1):S3-S10, 1992.

37. Tracey KJ: TNF and other cytokines in the metabolism of septic shock and cachexia, *Clin Nutr* 11:1-11, 1992.

38. Deitch EA: Multiple organ failure: pathophysiology and potential future therapy, *Ann Surg* 216(2):117-134, 1992.

39. Tredgett EE, Yu YM, Zhong S, et al: Role of interleukin-1 and tumor necrosis factor on energy metabolism in rabbits, *Am J Physiol* 255(6 Pt 1):E760-E768, 1988.

40. Dinarello CA: Overview: interleukin-1 and tumor necrosis factor in inflammatory disease and the effect of dietary fatty acids on their production. In Kinney JM, Tucker HN (eds): *Organ metabolism and nutritional ideas for future critical care,* New York, 1994, Raven Press, pp 181-195.

41. Warren RS, Starnes HF, Gabrilove JL: The acute metabolic effects of tumor necrosis factor administration, *Arch Surg* 122(12):1396-1400, 1987.

42. Gottschlich MM, Warden GD: Vitamin supplementation in the patient with burns, *J Burn Care Rehabil* 11(3):275-279, 1990.

43. Gamliel Z, DeBiasse MA, Demling RH: Essential microminerals and their response to burn injury, *J Burn Care Rehabil* 17(3):264-272, 1996.

44. Alexander JW, MacMillan BG, Stinnett JP, et al: Beneficial effects of aggressive protein feeding in severely burned children, *Ann Surg* 192(4):505-517, 1980.

45. Curreri PW, Richmond D, Marvin J, Baxter CR: Dietary requirements of patients with major burns, *J Am Diet Assoc* 65(4):415-417, 1974

46. Day T, Dean P, Adams MC, et al: Nutritional requirements of the burned child: the Curreri junior formula, *Proc Am Burn Assoc* 18:86, 1986 (abstract).

47. Adams MR, Kelley CH, Luterman A, Curreri PW: Nutritional requirements of the burned senior citizen: the Curreri senior formula, *Proc Am Burn Assoc* 19:83, 1987 (abstract).

48. Davies JWL, Liljedahl SL: Metabolic consequences of an extensive burn. In Polk HC, Stone HH (eds): *Contemporary burn management,* Boston, 1971, Little, Brown, pp 151-169.

49. Long CL: Energy expenditure of major burns, *J Trauma* 19(11 suppl):904-906, 1979.

50. Long CL, Schaffel N, Geiger JW, et al: Metabolic response to injury and illness: estimation of energy and protein needs from indirect calorimetry and nitrogen balance, *J Parenter Enteral Nutr* 3(6):452-456, 1979.

51. Harris JA, Benedict FS: *Biometric studies of basal metabolism in man,* Carnegie Institute of Washington, Pub. No. 279, 1919.

52. Hildreth M, Carvajal HF: Caloric requirements in burned children: a simple formula to estimate daily caloric requirements, *J Burn Care Rehabil* 3:78-80, 1982.

53. Hildreth MA, Herndon DN, Desai MH, Duke MA: Calorie needs of adolescent patients with burns, *J Burn Care Rehabil* 10(6):523-526, 1989.

54. Hildreth MA, Herndon DN, Parks DH, et al: Evaluation of a caloric requirement formula in burned children treated with early excision, *J Trauma* 27(2):188-189, 1987.

55. Hildreth MA, Herndon DN, Desai MH, Broemeling LD: Current treatment reduces calories required to maintain weight in pediatric patients with burns, *J Burn Care Rehabil* 11(5):405-409, 1990.

56. Mayes TM, Gottschlich MM, Khoury J, Warden GD: An evaluation of predicted and measured energy requirements in burned children, *J Am Diet Assoc* 96(1):24-29, 1996.

57. Molnar JA, Bell SS, Goodenough RD, Burke JF: Enteral nutrition in patients with burns or trauma. In Rombeau JL, Caldwell FT (eds): *Enteral and tube feeding,* vol 1, Philadelphia, 1984, WB Saunders, pp 412-433.

58. Pruitt BA: Metabolic changes and nutrition in burn patients, *Ann Chir Plast* 24(1):21-25, 1979.

59. Soroff HS, Pearson E, Artz CP: An estimation of nitrogen requirements for equilibrium in burned patients, *Surg Gynecol Obstet* 112:159-172, 1961.

60. Sutherland AB: Nitrogen balance and nutritional requirements in the burn patient: a reappraisal, *Burns* 2:238-244, 1976.

61. Troell L, Wretlind A: Protein and caloric requirements in burns, *Acta Chir Scand* 122:15-20, 1961.

62. Wilmore DW: Nutrition and metabolism following thermal injury, *Clin Plast Surg* 1(4):603-619, 1974.

63. Panel for the Prediction of Pressure Ulcers in Adults: Treatment of pressure ulcers. *Clinical Practice Guideline,* No15, AHCPR Publication No 92-0047, Rockville, MD, Dec 1994, Agency for Health Care Policy and Research, Public Health Service, US Department of Health and Human Services, pp 29-30.

64. Ireton CS, Hunt JL, Liepa GU, Liepa GO: Evaluation of energy requirements in thermally injured patients, *J Am Diet Assoc* 86(3):331-333, 1986.

65. Saffle JR, Medina E, Raymond J, et al: Use of indirect calorimetry in the nutritional management of burned patients, *J Trauma* 25(1):32-39, 1985.

66. Turner WW, Ireton CS, Hunt JL, Baxter CR: Predicting energy expenditures in burned patients, *J Trauma* 25(1):11-16, 1985.

67. Gottschlich MM, Ireton-Jones CS: The Curreri formula: a landmark process for estimating the caloric needs of burn patients, *Nutr Clin Pract* 16(3):172-173, 2001.
68. Goran MI, Peters EJ, Herndon DN, Wolfe RR: Total energy expenditure in burned children using the doubly labeled water technique, *Am J Physiol* 259(4 Pt 1):E576-E585, 1990.
69. Kagan RJ, Gottschlich MM, Mayes T, Warden GD: Estimation of calorie needs in the thermally injured child, *Proc Am Burn Assoc* 27:283, 1995 (abstract).
70. Wolfe RR: Glucose metabolism in burn injury: a review, *J Burn Care Rehabil* 6(5):408-418, 1985.
71. Allison SP, Hinton P, Chamberlain MJ: Intravenous glucose-tolerance, insulin and free fatty acid levels in burned patients, *Lancet* 2(7578):1113-1116, 1968.
72. Wolfe RR, Durkot MJ, Allsop JR, Burke JF: Glucose metabolism in severely burned patients, *Metabolism* 28(10):1031-1039, 1979.
73. Gottschlich MM, Jenkins M, Warden GD, et al: Differential effects of three enteral dietary regimens on selected outcome variables in burn patients, *J Parenter Enteral Nutr* 14(3):225-236, 1990.
74. Bingham HG, Spellacy W, Linquist J, Powell M: Burn diabetes: a review, *J Burn Care Rehabil* 3(3):179-182, 1982.
75. Arney GK, Pearson E, Sutherland AB: Burn stress pseudodiabetes, *Ann Surg* 152(1):77-90, 1960.
76. Wilmore DW, Goodwin CW, Aulick CH, et al: Effect of injury and infection on visceral metabolism and circulation, *Ann Surg* 192(4):491-504, 1980.
77. Wilmore DW, Aulick LH, Mason AD, Pruitt BA: Influence of the burn wound on local and systemic responses to injury, *Ann Surg* 186(4):444-458, 1977.
78. Beisil WR, Edelman R, Nauss K, Suskind R: Single-nutrient effects on immunologic functions, *JAMA* 245(1):53-58, 1981.
79. Fiser RH, Rollins JB, Beisel WR: Decreased resistance against infectious canine hepatitis in dogs fed high-fat ration, *Am J Vet Res* 33(4):713-719, 1972.
80. Mochizuki H, Trocki O, Dominioni L, Alexander JW: Optimal lipid content for enteral diets following thermal injury, *J Parenter Enteral Nutr* 8(6):638-646, 1984.
81. Alexander JW, Saito H, Trocki O, Ogle CK: The importance of lipid type in the diet after burn injury, *Ann Surg* 204(1):1-8, 1986.
82. Long JM, Wilmore DW, Mason AD, Pruitt BA: Effect of carbohydrate and fat intake on nitrogen excretion during total intravenous feeding, *Ann Surg* 185(4):417-422, 1977.
83. Pearson E, Soroff HS: Burns. In Schneider HA, Anderson CE, Coursin DB (eds): *Nutritional support of medical practice,* New York, 1977, Harper & Row, pp 222-235.
84. Wilmore DW: Glucose metabolism following severe injury, *J Trauma* 21(8 suppl):705-707, 1981.
85. Cuthbertson DP, Tilstone WJ: Nutrition of the injured, *Am J Clin Nutr* 21(9):911-922, 1968.
86. Barrocas A, Webb GL, Webb WR, St. Romain CM: Nutritional considerations in the critically ill, *South Med J* 75(7):848-851, 1982.
87. Barrocas A, Tretola R, Alonso A: Nutrition and the critically ill pulmonary patient, *Respir Care* 28(1):50-59, 1983.
88. Burke JF, Wolfe RR, Mullany CS, et al: Glucose requirements following the burn injury: parameters of optimal glucose infusion and possible hepatic and respiratory abnormalities following excessive glucose intake, *Ann Surg* 190(3):274-283, 1979.
89. Gottschlich MM: Nutritional strategies for burn patients, *RD* 8:6-8, 1988.
90. Askanazi J, Rosenbaum SH, Hyman AI, et al: Respiratory changes induced by large glucose loads of total parenteral nutrition, *JAMA* 243(14):1444-1447, 1980.
91. Covelli HD, Black JW, Olsen MS, Beekman JF: Respiratory failure precipitated by high carbohydrate loads, *Ann Intern Med* 95(5):579-581, 1981.
92. Hunker FO, Bruton CW, Hunker EM, et al: Metabolic and nutritional evaluation of patients supported with mechanical ventilation, *Crit Care Med* 8(11):628-632, 1980.
93. Elwyn DH, Kinney JM, Jeevanandam M, et al: Influence of increasing carbohydrate intake on glucose kinetics in injured patients, *Ann Surg* 190(1):117-127, 1979.
94. Sheridan RL, Yu YM, Prelack K, et al: Maximal parenteral glucose oxidation in hypermetabolic young children: a stable isotope, *J Parenteral Enteral Nutr* 22(4):212-216, 1998.
95. Winkler MF, Mandry MK: Nutrition and wound healing, *Support Line* 14(3):1-4, 1992.
96. Roberts P: Nutrition and wound healing. In Zaloga GP, (ed): *Nutrition in critical care,* St Louis, Mosby, 1994, pp 525-544.
97. Greenhalgh DG, Housinger TA, Kagan RJ, et al: Maintenance of serum albumin levels in pediatric burn patients: a prospective, randomized trial, *J Trauma* 39(1):67-74, 1995.
98. Batstone GF, Alberti KG, Hinks L: Metabolic studies in subjects following thermal injury, *Burns* 2:207-225, 1975.
99. Cynober L, Nguyen Dinh F, Saizy R, et al: Plasma amino acid levels in the first few days and their predictive value, *Intensive Care Med* 9(6):325-331, 1983.
100. Cerra FB: Branched chain amino acids. I. Stress nutrition, *Nutr Support Serv* 5:8-40, 1985.
101. Dominioni L, Trocki O, Fang CH, Alexander JW: Nitrogen balance and liver changes in burned guinea pigs undergoing prolonged high-protein enteral feeding, *Surg Forum* 34:99-101, 1983.
102. Dominioni L, Trocki O, Fang CH, et al: Enteral feeding in burn hypermetabolism: Nutritional and metabolic effects of different levels of calorie and protein intake, *J Parenter Enteral Nutr* 9(3):269-279, 1985.
103. Young VR, Motel KJ, Burke JF: Energy and protein metabolism in relation to requirements of the burned pediatric patient. In Suskind RM (ed): *Textbook of pediatric nutrition,* New York, 1981, Raven Press, pp 309-340.
104. Prokop-Oliet M, Trocki O, Alexander JW, MacMillen BG: Whey protein supplementation of complete tube feeding in the nutritional support of thermally injured patients, *Proc Am Burn Assoc* 15:45, 1983.
105. Newport MJ, Henschel MJ: Evaluation of the neonatal pig as a model for infant nutrition. Effects of different proportion of casein and whey protein in milk on nitrogen metabolism and composition of digesta in the stomach, *Pediatr Res* 18(7):658-662, 1984.
106. O'Leary MJ: Nourishing the premature and low birthweight infant. In Pipes PL (ed): *Nutrition in infancy and childhood,* St Louis, 1989, Mosby, pp 301-360.
107. Trocki O, Mochizuki H, Dominioni L, Alexander JW: Intact protein versus free amino acids in the nutritional support of thermally injured animals, *J Parenter Enteral Nutr* 10(2):139-145, 1986.
108. Stinnett JD, Ogle CK, Alexander JW, et al: Alterations of immunologic function in experimental animals following severe thermal injury, *J Burn Care Rehabil* 2(3):150-157, 1981.
109. Mochizuki H, Trocki O, Dominioni L, Alexander JW: Effect of a diet rich in branched chain amino acids on severely burned guinea pigs, *J Trauma* 26(12):1077-1085, 1986.
110. Aussel C, Cynober L, Lioret N, et al: Plasma branched chain keto-acids in burn patients, *Am J Clin Nutr* 44(6):825-831, 1986.
111. Young E, Raymond J, Kravitz M, et al: A randomized trial of branched chain amino acid-enriched feedings in thermally injured patients, *Proc Am Burn Assn* 18,1986, p 83 (abstract).
112. Snelling CFT, Woolf LI, Groves AC, et al: Amino acid metabolism in patients with severe burns, *Surgery* 91(4):474-481, 1982.
113. McCauley C, Platell C, Hall J, et al: Influence of branched chain amino acid solutions on wound healing, *Aust NZ J Surg* 60(6):471-473, 1990.
114. Holt LE, Snyderman SE: The amino acid requirements in infants, *JAMA* 175(2):100-103, 1961.
115. Rose WC: The amino acid requirements of adult man, *Nutr Abstr Rev* 27:631-647, 1957.
116. Leverton RM: Amino acid requirements of young adults. In Albanese AA (ed): *Protein and amino acid nutrition,* New York, 1959, Academic Press, pp 477-506.
117. Sitren HS, Fischer H: Nitrogen retention in rats fed diets enriched with arginine and glycine, *Br J Nutr* 37(2):195-208, 1977.
118. Barbul A, Sisto DA, Wasserkrug HL, et al: Nitrogen sparing and immune mechanisms of arginine: Differential dose-dependent responses during post injury intravenous hyperalimentation, *Curr Surg* 40:114-116, 1963.
119. Pui YML, Fischer H: Factorial supplementation with arginine and glycine on nitrogen retention and body weight gain in the traumatized rat, *J Nutr* 109(2):240-246, 1979.
120. Barbul A, Lazarow SA, Efrom DT, et al: Arginine enhances wound healing and lymphocyte immune responses in humans, *Surgery* 108(2):331-337, 1990.
121. Minuskin ML, Lavine ME, Ulman EA, Fisher H: Nitrogen retention, muscle creatinine and orotic acid excretion in traumatized rats fed arginine and glycine enriched diets, *J Nutr* 111(7):1265-1274, 1981.
122. Barbul A, Rettura G, Levenson SM, Seifter E: Wound healing and thymotrophic effects of arginine: a pituitary mechanism of action, *Am J Clin Nutr* 37(5):786-794, 1983.

123. Barbul A, Rettura G, Levenson SM, Seifter E: Arginine: a thymotrophic and wound healing promoting agent, *Surg Forum* 28: 101-103, 1977.

124. Barbul A, Fishel RS, Shimazu S, et al: Intravenous hyperalimentation with high arginine levels improves wound healing and immune function, *J Surg Res* 38(4):328-334, 1985.

125. Seifter E, Terrura G, Barbul A, Levenson SM: Arginine: an essential amino acid for injured rats, *Surgery* 84(2):224-230, 1978.

126. Daly JM, Reynolds J, Thom A, et al: Immune and metabolic effects of arginine in the surgical patient, *Ann Surg* 208(4):512-521, 1988.

127. Saito H, Trocki O, Wang S, et al: Metabolic and immune effects of dietary arginine supplementation after burn, *Arch Surg* 122(7):784-789, 1987.

128. Barbul A, Rettura G, Levenson SM, Seifter E: Thymotrophic actions of arginine, ornithine and growth hormone, *Fed Proc* 37:264, 1978.

129. Barbul A, Wasserkrug HL, Sisto DA, et al: Thymic stimulatory actions of arginine, *J Parenter Enteral Nutr* 4(5):446-449, 1980.

130. Barbul A, Sisto DA, Wasserkrug HL, Efron G: Arginine stimulates lymphocyte immune response in healthy human beings, *Surgery* 90(2):244-251, 1981.

131. Tachibana K, Mukai K, Hiraoka I, et al: Evaluation of the effect of arginine-enriched amino acid solution on tumor growth, *J Parenter Enteral Nutr* 9(4):428-434, 1985.

132. Merimee TJ, Lillicrop DA, Rabinowitz D: Effect of arginine on serum levels of human growth hormone, *Lancet* 2(7414):668-670, 1965.

133. Mulloy AL, Kari FW, Visek WJ: Dietary arginine, insulin secretion, glucose tolerance and liver lipids during repletion of protein-depleted rats, *Horm Metab Res* 14(9):471-475, 1982.

134. Solomons CC, Cotton EK, Dubois R, Pinney M: The use of buffered L-arginine in the treatment of cystic fibrosis, *Pediatrics* 47(2):384-390, 1971.

135. Jeevanandam M, Ali MR, Holaday NJ, et al: Relative nutritional efficacy of arginine and ornithine salts of alpha-ketoisocaproic acid in traumatized rats, *Am J Clin Nutr* 57(6):889-896, 1993.

136. Batshaw ML, Wachtel RC, Thomas GH, et al: Arginine-responsive asymptomatic hyperammonemia in the premature infant, *J Pediatr* 105(1):86-91, 1984.

137. Heird WC, Nicholson JF, Driscoll JM, et al: Hyperammonemia resulting from intravenous alimentation using a mixture of synthetic L-amino acids: a preliminary report, *J Pediatr* 81(1):162-165, 1972.

138. Najarian JS, Harper HA: A clinical study of the effect of arginine on blood ammonia, *Am J Med* 21:832-842, 1956.

139. Barbul A, Lazarow SA, Efron DT, et al: Arginine enhances wound healing and lymphocyte immune responses in humans, *Surgery* 108: 331-336, 1980.

140. Nirgiotis JG, Hennessey PJ, Andrassy RJ: The effects of an arginine-free enteral diet on wound healing and immune function in the post-surgical rat, *J Pediatr Surg* 26(8):936-941, 1991.

141. Barbul A, Wasserkrug HL, Seifter E, et al: Immunostimulatory effects of arginine in normal and injured rats, *J Surg Res* 29(3):228-235, 1980.

142. Barbul A, Wasserkrug HL, Penberthy LT, et al: Optimal levels of arginine in maintenance intravenous hyperalimentation, *J Parenter Enteral Nutr* 8(3):281-284, 1984.

143. Rettura G, Barbul A, Levenson SM, Seifter E: Citrulline does not share the thymotrophic properties of arginine and ornithine, *Fed Proc* 38:289, 1979.

144. Kirk S, Regan MC, Wasserkrug HL, et al: Arginine enhances T-cell responses in athymic nude mice, *J Parenter Enteral Nutr* 16(5):429-432, 1992.

145. Reynolds JV, Daly JM, Show J, et al: Immunologic effects of arginine supplementation of tumor-bearing and non–tumor-bearing hosts, *Ann Surg* 211(2):202-210, 1990.

146. Reynolds JV, Thom AK, Zhang SM, et al: Arginine, protein malnutrition and cancer, *J Surg Res* 45(6):513-522, 1988.

147. Oka T, Dhwada K, Nagao M, Kitazato K: Effect of arginine-enriched total parenteral nutrition on the host-tumor interaction in cancer-bearing rats, *J Parenter Enteral Nutr* 17(4):375-383, 1993.

148. Gottschlich MM, Stone M, Havens P, et al: Therapeutic effects of a modular tube feeding recipe in pediatric burn patients, *Proc Am Burn Assn* 84, 1986.

149. Kari FW, Ulman EA, Mulloy AL, Visek WJ: Arginine requirement of mature protein-malnourished rats for maximal rate of repletion, *J Nutr* 111(8):1489-1493, 1981.

150. Jones JD, Walters R, Burnett PC: Lysine-arginine electrolyte relationship in the rat, *J Nutr* 89(2):171-188, 1966.

151. Leon P, Redmond HP, Stein TP, et al: Arginine supplementation improves histone and acute-phase protein synthesis during gram negative sepsis in rats, *J Parenter Enteral Nutr* 15(5):503-508, 1991.

152. Welters CFM, Deutz NEP, Dejong CHC, Heineman E: Arginine supplementation reduces intestinal protein turnover in rats with short bowel syndrome, *Clin Nutr* 13:4S, 1994.

153. Gianotti L, Alexander JW, Pyles T, Fukushima R: Arginine-supplemented diets improve survival in gut-derived sepsis and peritonitis by modulating bacterial clearance: the role of nitric oxide, *Ann Surg* 217(6):644-654, 1993.

154. Souba WW, Smith RJ, Wilmore DW: Glutamine metabolism by the intestinal tract, *J Parenter Enteral Nutr* 9(5):608-617, 1985.

155. Souba WW, Smith RJ, Wilmore DW: Effect of glucocorticoids on glutamine metabolism in visceral organs, *Metabolism* 34(5):450-456, 1985.

156. Souba WW, Roughneen PT, Goldwater DL, et al: Postoperative alterations in interorgan glutamine exchange in enterectomized dogs, *J Surg Res* 42(2):117-125, 1987.

157. Souba WW, Wilmore DW: Gut-liver interaction during accelerated gluconeogenesis, *Arch Surg* 120(1):66-70, 1985.

158. Souba WW, Wilmore DW: Postoperative alteration of arteriovenous exchange of amino acids across the gastrointestinal tract, *Surgery* 94(2):342-350, 1983.

159. O'Dwyer ST, Smith RJ, Hwang TL, Wilmore DW: Maintenance of small bowel mucosa with glutamine-enriched parenteral nutrition, *J Parenter Enteral Nutr* 13(6):579-585, 1989.

160. O'Dwyer ST, Scott T, Smith RJ, Wilmore DW: 5 fluorouracil toxicity on small intestinal mucosa but not white blood cells is decreased by glutamine, *Clin Res* 35(3):369a, 1987 (abstract).

161. Smith RJ, Wilmore DW: Glutamine nutrition and requirements, *J Parenter Enteral Nutr* 14(4 suppl):94S-99S, 1990.

162. Smith RJ, O'Dwyer ST, Wang XD, Wilmore DW: Glutamine nutrition and the gastrointestinal tract. In *The gastrointestinal response to injury, starvation and enteral nutrition: report of the Eighth Ross Conference on Medical Research,* Columbus, OH, 1988, Ross Laboratories, pp 76-78.

163. Tenenhaus M, Hansbrough JF, Zapata-Sirvent RL, et al: Supplementation of an elemental enteral diet with alanyl-glutamine decreases bacterial translocation in burned mice, *Burns* 20(3):220-225, 1994.

164. Souba WW, Klimberg VS, Hautamaki RD, et al: Oral glutamine reduces bacterial translocation following abdominal radiation, *J Surg Res* 48(1):1-5, 1990.

165. Burke D, Alverdy JC, Aoys E, Moss GS: Glutamine supplemented TPN improves gut immune function, *Arch Surg* 124(12):1396-1399, 1989.

166. Jacobs DO, Evans A, O'Dwyer ST, et al: Disparate effects of 5-fluorouracil on the ileum and colon of enterally fed rats with protection by dietary glutamine, *Surg Forum* 38:45-47, 1987.

167. Klimberg VS, Souba WW, Dolson DJ, Copeland EM: Oral glutamine supports crypt cell turnover and accelerates intestinal healing following abdominal radiation, *J Parenter Enteral Nutr* 13:11(suppl 1) , 1989.

168. Klimberg VS, Souba WW, Dolson DJ, et al: Prophylactic glutamine protects the intestinal mucosa from radiation therapy, *Cancer* 66(1): 62-68, 1990.

169. Wang XD, Jacobs DO, O'Dwyer ST, et al: Glutamine-enriched parenteral nutrition prevents mucosal atrophy following massive bowel resection, *Surg Forum* 39:44-46, 1988.

170. Grant J: Use of L-glutamine in total parenteral nutrition, *J Surg Res* 44(5):506-513, 1988.

171. Hammarqvist F, Wernerman J, Ali R, et al: Addition of glutamine to total parenteral nutrition after elective abdominal surgery spares free glutamine in muscle, counteracts the fall in muscle protein synthesis and improves nitrogen balance, *Ann Surg* 209(4):455-461, 1989.

172. Ziegler TR, Benfell K, Smith RJ, et al: Safety and metabolic effects of L-glutamine administration in humans, *J Parenter Enteral Nutr* 14(suppl 4):137S-146S, 1990.

173. Stehle P, Zander J, Mertes N, et al: Effect of parenteral glutamine peptide supplements on muscle glutamine loss and nitrogen balance after major surgery, *Lancet* 8632:231-233, 1989.

174. Parry-Billings M, Evans J, Calder PC, Newsholme EA: Does glutamine contribute to immunosuppression after major burns? *Lancet* 336(8714):523-525, 1990.

175. Vaubourdolle M, Coudray-Lucas C, Jardel A, et al: Action of enterally administered ornithine alpha ketoglutarate on protein breakdown in skeletal muscle and liver of the burned rat, *J Parenter Enteral Nutr* 15(5):517-520, 1991.

176. Donati L, Ziegler F, Pongelli G, Signorini MS: Nutritional and clinical efficacy of ornithine alpha ketoglutarate in severe burn patients, *Clin Nutr* 18(5):307-311, 1999.

177. LeBoucher J, Eurengbiol, Farges MC, et al: Modulation of immune response with ornithine alpha ketoglutarate in burn injury: an arginine or glutamine dependency? *Nutrition* 15(10):773-777, 1999.

178. Cynober L, Liolet N, Coudray-Lucas C, et al: Action of ornithine alpha ketoglutarate on protein metabolism in burn patients, *Nutrition* 3:187-191, 1987.

179. Cynober L, Saizy R, Nguyen Dinh F, et al: Effect of enterally administered ornithine alpha ketoglutarate on plasma and urinary amino acid levels after burn injury, *J Trauma* 24(7):590-596, 1984.

180. Jeevanandam M: Immune modulation with OKG supplementation in burn injury, editorial comment, *Nutrition* 15(11-12):952-953, 1999.

181. Hulsey TK, Burnham SJ, Neblett WW, et al: Delayed burn wound healing in essential fatty acid deficiency, *Surg Forum* 28:31-32, 1977.

182. Moore FD: Energy and maintenance of the body cell mass, *J Parenter Enteral Nutr* 4(3):228-260, 1980.

183. Penturf ME, McGlone JJ, Griswold JA: Modulation of immune response in thermal injury by essential fatty acid-deficient diet, *J Burn Care Rehabil* 17(5):465-470, 1996.

184. Wolfe BM, Culebras AJ, Sim MR, et al: Substrate interaction in intravenous feeding, *Ann Surg* 186(4):518-538, 1977.

185. Gottschlich MM: Selection of optimal lipid sources in enteral and parenteral nutrition, *Nutr Clin Pract* 7(4):152-165, 1992.

186. Bell SJ, Mascioli EA, Bistrian BR, et al: Alternative lipid sources for enteral and parenteral nutrition. Long- and medium-chain triglycerides, structured triglycerides and fish oils, *J Am Diet Assoc* 91(1):74-78, 1991.

187. Haw MP, Bell SJ, Blackburn GL: Potential of parenteral and enteral nutrition in inflammation and immune dysfunction: a new challenge for dietitians, *J Am Diet Assoc* 91(6):701-709, 1991.

188. Sardesai VM: The essential fatty acids, *Nutr Clin Pract* 7(4):179-186, 1992.

189. Trocki O, Heyd TJ, Waymack JP, Alexander JW: Effects of fish oil on postburn metabolism and immunity, *J Parenter Enteral Nutr* 11(6):521-528, 1987.

190. Arturson MG: Arachidonic acid metabolism and prostaglandin activity following burn injury. In Ninnemann JL (ed): *Traumatic injury: infection and other immunologic sequela*, Baltimore, 1983, University Press, pp 57-78.

191. Ellner JJ: Suppressor cells of man, *Clin Immunol Rev* 1(1):119-123, 1981.

192. Barrocas A, Rodemann HP, Dinarello CA, Goldberg AL: Stimulation of muscle protein degradation and prostaglandin E_2 release by leukocyte pyrogen (interleukin 1) a mechanism for the increased degradation of muscle proteins during fever, *N Engl J Med* 308(10):553-558, 1983.

193. Rodeman HP, Goldberg AL: Arachidonic acid, prostaglandin E_2 and F_2-alpha influence rates of protein turnover in skeletal and cardiac muscle, *J Biol Chem* 257(4):1632-1638, 1982.

194. Wan JF, Teo TC, Babayan VK, and Blackburn GL: Invited comment: lipids and the development of immune dysfunction and infection, *J Parenter Enteral Nutr* 12(6):43S-48S, 1988.

195. Mayes PA: Lipids of physiologic significance. In Mournay RK, Ganner DK, Mayes PA, Rodwell VW (eds): *Harper's biochemistry*, ed 22, Norwalk, CT, 1990, Appleton & Lange, pp 218-225.

196. Merlin J: Omega-6 and omega-3 polyunsaturates and the immune system, *Br J Clin Pract* 38(5)suppl 31:111-114, 1984.

197. Ninneman JL, Stockland AE: Participation of prostaglandin E in immunosuppression following thermal injury, *J Trauma* 24(3):201-207, 1984.

198. Moncada S: Biology and therapeutic potential of prostaglandin, *Stroke* 14(2):157-168, 1983.

199. Steinberg G, Slayton WH, Howton DR, Mead JF: Metabolism of essential fatty acids. IV. Incorporation of lineolate into arachidonic acid, *J Biol Chem* 220(1):257-264, 1956.

200. Holman RT: Nutritional and metabolic interrelationships between fatty acids, *Proc FASEB* 23:1062-1067, 1964.

201. Holman RT: Essential fatty acid deficiency, *Prog Chem Fats Lipids* 9:275-348, 1970.

202. Hwang DH, Carroll AE: Decreased formation of prostaglandins derived from arachidonic acid by dietary linolenate in rats, *Am J Clin Nutr* 33(3):590-597, 1980.

203. Marshall LA, Szczesnwski A, Johnston PV: Dietary alpha-linolenic acid and prostaglandins synthesis. A time course study, *Am J Clin Nutr* 38(6):895-900, 1983.

204. Meng HC: Fat emulsions in parenteral nutrition. In Fischer JE (ed): *Total parenteral nutrition*, Boston, 1976, Little, Brown, pp 305-334.

205. Gallaher CJ, Fechner K, Karlstad M: The effect of increasing levels of fish oil containing structured triglycerides on protein metabolism in parenterally fed rats stressed by burn plus endotoxin, *J Parenter Enteral Nutr* 17(3):247-253, 1993.

206. Sorbrado J, Moldawer LL, Pomposelli J, et al: Lipid emulsions and reticuloendothelium system function in healthy and burned guinea pigs, *Am J Clin Nutr* 42(5):855-863, 1985.

207. Mascioli EA, Bistrian BR, Babayan VK, Blackburn GL: Medium chain triglycerides and structured lipids as unique non glucose energy sources in hyperalimentation, *Lipids* 22(6):421-423, 1987.

208. Bach AC, Babayan VK: Medium chain triglycerides: an update, *Am J Clin Nutr* 36(5):950-962, 1982.

209. Yamazaki K, Maiz A, Sobrado J, et al: Hypocaloric lipid emulsions and amino acid metabolism in injured rats, *J Parenter Enteral Nutr* 8(4):361-366, 1984.

210. Maiz A, Yamazaki K, Sobrado J, et al: Protein metabolism during total parenteral nutrition (TPN) in injured rats using medium-chain triglycerides, *Metabolism* 33(10):901-909, 1984.

211. Mok KT, Maiz A, Yamazaki K, et al: Structured medium-chain and long-chain triglyceride emulsions are superior to physical mixtures in sparing body protein in the burned rat, *Metabolism* 33(10):910-915, 1984.

212. DeMichele SJ, Karlstad MD, Babayan VK, et al: Enhanced skeletal muscle and liver protein synthesis with structured lipid in enterally fed burned rats, *Metabolism* 37(8):787-795, 1988.

213. Ling PR, Istfan NW, Lopes SM, et al: Structured lipid made from fish oil and medium-chain triglycerides alters tumor and host metabolism in Yoshida-sarcoma-bearing rats, *Am J Clin Nutr* 53(5):1177-1184, 1991.

214. Hyashi N, Tashiro T, Yamamori H, et al: Effects of intravenous omega-3 and omega-6 fat emulsion on cytokine production and delayed hypersensitivity in burned rats receiving total parenteral nutrition, *J Parenter Enteral Nutr* 22(6):363-367, 1998.

215. Food and Nutrition Board and National Research Council: *Recommended dietary allowances*, ed 9, Washington, DC, 1980, National Academy of Sciences.

216. Food and Nutrition Board: *Dietary reference intakes for thiamin, riboflavin, niacin, vitamin B_6, folate, vitamin B_{12}, pantothenic acid, biotin and choline*, Washington, DC, 1998, National Academy of Sciences, National Academy Press.

217. Sauberlich Howerde E: Laboratory tests for the assessment of nutritional status, ed 2, New York, 1999, CRC Press, pp 1-486.

218. Berger MM, Spertini F, Shenkin A, et al: Trace element supplementation modulates pulmonary infection rates after major burns: a double-blind, placebo-controlled trial, *Clin Nutr* 68:365-371, 1998.

219. Nirgiotis JG, Hennessey PJ, Black CT, et al: Low-fat, high carbohydrate diets improve wound healing and increase protein levels in surgically stressed rats, *J Pediatr Surg* 26(8):925-929, 1991.

220. Linz DN, Garcia VF, Arya G, Ziegler MM: Prostaglandin and tumor necrosis factor levels in early wound inflammatory fluid. Effect of parenteral omega-3 and omega-6 fatty acid administration, *J Pediatr Surg* 29(8):1065-1070, 1994.

221. Sakurai Y, Aarsland A, Herndon DN, et al: Stimulation of muscle protein synthesis by long term insulin infusion in severely burned patients, *Ann Surg* 222(3):283-297, 1995.

222. Pierre EJ, Barrow RE, Hawkins HK, et al: Effects of insulin on wound healing, *J Trauma* 44(2):342-345, 1998.

223. Ferrando AA, Chinkes DL, Wolf SE, et al: A submaximal dose of insulin promotes net skeletal muscle protein synthesis in patients with severe burns, *Ann Surg* 229(1):11-18, 1999.

224. Demling RH, Desante L: Oxandrolone, an anabolic steroid, significantly increases the rate of weight gain in the recovery phase after major burns, *J Trauma* 43(1):47-51, 1997.

225. Demling RH: Comparison of the anabolic effects and complications of human growth hormone and the testosterone analog, oxandrolone, after severe burn injury, *Burns* 25(3):215-221, 1999.

226. Demling RH, Desante L: Involuntary weight loss and the nonhealing wound: the role of anabolic agents, *Adv Wound Care* 12(suppl 1):1-14, 1999.

227. Hart DW, Wolf SE, Ramzy PI, et al: Anabolic effects of oxandrolone after severe burn, *Ann Surg* 233(4):556-564, 2001.

228. Gilpin DA, Barrow RE, Rutan RL, et al: Recombinant human growth hormone accelerates wound healing in children with large cutaneous burns, *Ann Surg* 220(1):19-24, 1994.

229. Mueller RV, Lee C, Jacobovicz J: The effect of insulin-like growth factor on wound healing variables and macrophages in rats, *Arch Surg* 129(3):262-265, 1994.

230. Ziegler TR, Young LS, Manson JM, Wilmore DW: Metabolic effects of recombinant human growth hormone in patients receiving parenteral nutrition, *Ann Surg* 208(1):6-16, 1988.

231. Gottschlich MM, Mayes T, Jenkins M, et al: An examination of the clinical effectiveness of growth hormone in pediatric burns, *Proc Am Burn Assn* 18:S197, 1997.

232. Takala J, Ruokonen E, Webster NR, et al: Increased mortality associated with growth hormone treatment in critically ill adults, *N Engl J Med* 341(11):785-792, 1999.

233. Kien CL, Young VR, Rohrbaugh DK, Burke JF: Increased rates of whole body protein synthesis and breakdown in children recovering from burns, *Ann Surg* 187(4):383-391, 1978.

234. Meakins JL, Pietsch JB, Bubenick O: Delayed hypersensitivity: indicator of acquired failure of host defenses in sepsis and trauma, *Ann Surg* 186(3):241-250, 1977.

235. Eilber FR, Morton DL: Impaired immunologic reactivity and recurrence following cancer surgery, *Cancer* 24(2):362-367, 1970.

236. Meakins JL, McLean APH, Kelly R, et al: Delayed hypersensitivity and neutrophil chemotaxis: effect of trauma, *J Trauma* 18(4):240-247, 1978.

237. Pietsch JB, Meakins JL, MacLean LD: Delayed hypersensitivity response: application in clinical surgery, *Surgery* 82(3):349-355, 1977.

238. Inglenbleek Y, Carpentier YA: A prognostic inflammatory and nutritional index scoring critically ill patients, *Int J Vitam Nutr* 55:91-101, 1985.

239. Mullen JL, Buzby GP, Waldman MT, et al: Prediction of operative morbidity and mortality by preoperative nutritional assessment, *Surg Forum* 30(2):80-82, 1979.

240. Gottschlich MM, Baumer T, Jenkins M, Warden GD: The prognostic value of nutritional and inflammatory indices in patients with burns, *J Burn Care Rehabil* 13(1):105-113, 1992.

241. Batstone GF, Levick PL, Spurr E, et al: Changes in acute phase reactants and disturbances in metabolism after burn injury, *Burns* 9(4):234-239, 1982.

242. Birke G, Liljedahl SO, Plantin LO, Reizenstein P: Studies on burns. Part IX. The distribution and losses through the wound of 131-I-albumin measured by whole-body counting, *Acta Chir Scand* 134(1):27-36, 1968.

243. Daniels JC, Larson DL, Abston S, Ritzmann SE: Serum protein profiles in thermal burns. Part I. Serum electrophoretic patterns immunoglobulins and transport proteins, *J Trauma* 14(2):137-152, 1974.

244. Moody BJ: Changes in serum concentrations of thyroxine-binding prealbumin and retinol-binding protein following burn injury, *Clin Chim Acta* 118(1):87-92, 1982.

245. Daniels JC, Larson DL, Abston S, Ritzmann SE: Serum protein profiles in thermal burns. Part II. Protease inhibitors, complement factors and C-reactive protein, *J Trauma* 14(2):153-162, 1974.

246. Faymonville ME, Michels J, Bodson L, et al: Biochemical investigations after burning injury: Complement system, protease-anti-protease balance and acute-phase reactants, *Burns* 13(1):26-33, 1987.

247. Shenkin A, Neuhauser M, Bergstrom J, et al: Biochemical changes associated with severe trauma, *Am J Clin Nutr* 33(10):2119-2127, 1980.

248. Zeireh RA, Kukral JC: The turnover rate of orosomucoid in burn patients, *J Trauma* 10(6):493-498, 1970.

249. Trice S, Melnik G, Page CP: Complications and costs of early postoperative parenteral versus enteral nutrition in trauma patients, *Nutr Clin Pract* 12(3):114-119, 1997.

250. Kiyama T, Witte MB, Thornton FJ, Barbul A: The route of nutrition support affects the early phase of wound healing, *J Parenter Enteral Nutr* 22(5):276-279, 1998.

251. Gottschlich MM: Burns. In *Guidelines for the use of parenteral and enteral nutrition,* Silver Spring, MD (in press).

252. Mayes T, Gottschlich MM, Warden GD: Nutrition protocols for continuous quality improvements in the outcomes of patients with burns, *J Burn Care Rehab* 18(4):365-368, 1997.

253. Alexander JW: Recent advances in burn injuries. *Proceedings of International Society of Burn Injuries,* Istanbul, Turkey 48, 1988 (abstract).

254. Levine GM, Deren JJ, Steiger E, Zinno R: Role of oral intake in maintenance of gut mass and disaccharide activity, *Gastroenterology* 67(5):975-982, 1974.

255. Saito H, Trocki O, Alexander JW: Comparison of immediate postburn enteral vs parenteral nutrition, *J Parenter Enteral Nutr* 9(1):115, 1985.

256. Saito H, Trocki O, Alexander JW, et al: The effect of route of nutrient administration on the nutritional state, catabolic hormone secretion, and gut mucosal integrity after burn injury, *J Parenter Enteral Nutr* 11(1):1-7, 1987.

257. Deitch EA, Maejima K, Berg R: Effect of oral antibiotics and bacterial overgrowth on the translocation of the gastrointestinal tract microflora in burned rats, *J Trauma* 25(5):385-392, 1985.

258. Moore EE, Jones TW: Benefits of immediate jejunostomy feedings after major abdominal trauma—a prospective randomized study, *J Trauma* 26(10):874-881, 1986.

259. Glucksman DL, Halser MA, Warren WD: Small intestinal absorption in the immediate postoperative period, *Surgery* 60(5):1020-1025, 1966.

260. Moore EE, Jones TN: Nutritional assessment and preliminary report on early support of the trauma patient, *J Am Coll Nutr* 2(1):45-54, 1983.

261. Taylor SJ: Early enhanced enteral nutrition in burned patients is associated with fewer infective complications and shorter hospital stay, *J Hum Nutr Diet* 12:85-91, 1999.

262. Fairfull-Smith R, Abunassar R, Freeman JB, Maroun JA: Rational use of elemental and nonelemental diets in hospitalized patients, *Ann Surg* 192(5):600-603, 1980.

263. Silk DBA, Fairclough PD, Clark ML, et al: Use of peptide rather than free amino acid nitrogen source in chemically defined "elemental" diets, *J Parenter Enteral Nutr* 4(6):548-553, 1980.

264. Matthews DM, Adibi SA: Peptide absorption, *Gastroenterology* 71(1):151-161, 1976.

265. Jenkins ME, Gottschlich MM, Warden GD: Enteral feeding during operative procedures in thermal injuries, *J Burn Care Rehabil* 15(2):199-205, 1994.

266. Buescher TM, Cioffi WG, Becker WK, et al: Perioperative enteral feedings, *Proc Am Burn Assoc* 22:162, 1990.

267. Haydock DA, Hill GL: Impaired wound healing in surgical patients with varying degrees of malnutrition, *J Parenter Enteral Nutr* 10(6):550-554, 1986.

268. Kay SP, Moreland JR, Schmitter E. Nutritional status and wound healing in lower extremity amputations, *Clin Orthop* 217(Apr):253-256, 1987.

269. Casey J, Flinn WR, Yao JST, et al: Correlation of immune and nutritional status with wound complications in patients undergoing vascular operations, *Surgery* 93(6):822-827, 1983.

270. Haydock DA, Hill GL: Improved wound healing response in surgical patients receiving intravenous nutrition, *Br J Surg* 74(4):320-323, 1987.

271. Schroeder D, Gillanders L, Mahr K, Hill G: Effects of immediate postoperative enteral nutrition on body composition, muscle function, and wound healing, *J Parenter Enteral Nutr* 15(4):376-383, 1991.

272. Pearson KS, From RJP, Symreng T, Kealey GP: Continuous enteral feeding and short fasting periods enhances perioperative nutrition in patients with burns, *J Burn Care Rehabil* 13(4):477-481, 1992.

273. Herndon DN, Stein MD, Rutan TC, et al: Failure of TPN supplementation to improve liver function, immunity and mortality in thermally injured patients, *J Trauma* 27(2):195-204, 1987.

274. Lennard ES, Alexander JW, Craycroft T, MacMillan BG: Association in burn patients of improved antibacterial defense with nutritional supplementation by the oral route, *Burns* 1:98-107, 1974.

275. Czaja AJ, McAlhany JD, Pruitt BA: Gastric acid secretion and acute gastroduodenal disease after burns, *Arch Surg* 111(3):243-245, 1976.

276. Goodwin CW, Pruitt BA: Increased incidence of pancreatitis in thermally injured patients: a prospective study, *Proc Am Assoc Surg Trauma* 13:106, 1981.

277. Lescher TJ, Teejarden DK, Pruitt BA: Acute pseudo-obstruction of the colon in thermally injured patients, *Dis Colon Rectum* 21(8):618-622, 1978.

278. Lescher TJ, Sirinek KR, Pruitt BA: Superior mesenteric artery syndrome in thermally injured patients, *J Trauma* 19(8):567-571, 1979.

279. Reckler JM, Brucke HM, Munster AM, et al: Superior mesenteric artery syndrome as a consequence of burn injury, *J Trauma* 12(11):979-985, 1972.

280. Popp MB, Law EJ, MacMillan BG: Parenteral nutrition in the burned child: a study of twenty-six patients, *Ann Surg* 179(2):219-225, 1974.

Quality and Performance Improvement 43

Marion F. Winkler, MS, RD, LDN, CNSD
Ann-Marie Hedberg, DrPh, RD, LD

What Is Quality Care?

Quality is an infinitely subjective concept. It reflects judgments made by consumers, patients, purchasers, and providers about products or services and how well their needs (stated or implied) are satisfied. Quality, as it relates to health care, has been defined as "the optimal achievable result for each patient, the avoidance of iatrogenic complications, and the attention to patient and family needs in a manner that is cost-effective and reasonably documented."[1] The Joint Commission on Accreditation of Healthcare Organizations (JCAHO) defines quality of care as the degree to which health services for individuals and populations increase the likelihood of desired health outcomes and are consistent with current professional knowledge.[2] The dimensions of performance include patient perspective issues, safety of the care environment, and accessibility, appropriateness, continuity, effectiveness, efficacy, efficiency, and timeliness of care.[2] In February 1997, JCAHO implemented the ORYX initiative, which serves as the critical link between accreditation and the outcomes of patient care. This initiative provides a mechanism for review of data trends and patterns that organizations can use to improve patient care.

In this chapter we review the regulatory aspects of health care quality, the role of JCAHO, performance measurement, and involvement of other professional organizations in the development of standards and practice guidelines. Recommendations for establishing a performance improvement program for nutrition support and examples of a nutrition care quality monitor flow sheet are provided (Fig. 43-1).

Historical Perspective

The quality of patient care has always been important. The measurement tools have changed, and there has been a shift from self-regulation to external regulation, but quality continues to be emphasized. Establishment of patient care standards and statistical monitoring of patient admissions, recoveries, and discharges were proposed in the late nineteenth century by Florence Nightingale.[1] In 1914, Dr. Ernest A. Codman established a method of reviewing patient outcomes 1 year after surgery.[3] He raised several quality care issues that eventually led to the initiation of the American College of Surgeons' Hospital Standardization Program in 1918. These programs addressed licensure, certification, accreditation, severity of disease or illness, comorbidity, patient behavior, and economics; these issues are still important in the twenty-first century.

The establishment of JCAHO in 1952 occurred because of the growth of nonsurgical specialties after World War II and the need for hospitals and the entire medical field to have uniformly high standards of care in all areas, including medicine, nursing, pharmacy, and radiology.[1]

Role of Regulatory Agencies

Federal regulation of health care increased in the 1960s with the enactment of Medicare and Medicaid as part of the Social Security Amendment in 1965. In the 1970s, Professional Standards Review Organizations (PSRO) were created to safeguard federal monies paid through the Social Security Act by identifying services that were not considered medically appropriate. The utilization review functions, still in existence today, were mandated by federal legislation in 1983. As consumers were beginning to hold health care professionals and institutions more accountable for quality, emphasis was placed on a patient-oriented approach to health care. The establishment of diagnostic related groups (DRGs) in 1983, providing hospital reimbursement under a prospective payment system, prompted health care administrators to scrutinize operational costs more closely, to produce revenue, and to increase marketing of programs and services. Health care costs became a major focus.

The Transition from Quality Assurance to Continuous Quality Improvement to Performance Improvement

JCAHO is synonymous with quality assurance (QA), quality improvement (QI), and performance improvement (PI). In the 1970s, accreditation manuals for hospitals focused on retrospective process and outcome-oriented audits. In the 1980s standards of care and departmental monitoring of quality and appropriateness of care were emphasized. The agenda for change in the 1990s resulted in standards that emphasize continuous quality improvement (CQI) and evaluation of quality from the patient's perspective, outcome assessment, and an interdisciplinary approach to patient care.[4] The focus in the twenty-first century is performance measurement. The ORYX initiative provides a basis for continuously monitoring actual performance and for guiding and stimulating continuous improvement in health care organizations. JCAHO plans to identify standardized core performance measures allowing health care organizations to begin collecting core measure data in 2002.[5]

The transition from QA to CQI required a philosophic shift in how we viewed quality patient care and how we monitored

Unit _____

ST. LUKE'S
EPISCOPAL HOSPITAL

**Nutrition Care
Quality Monitor**

Addressograph _____

Chart monitor by: _____

Date: _____

RD Documentation by: _____

#	JCAHO Standard	Specifics	YES	NO	N/A	Comments
PE.1.2 *Intent* of PE.1.2-3	"Nutritional status is assessed when warranted by the patient's needs or condition." "The hospital refers such patients to a dietitian for further assessment."	Initiation of nutrition consult documented as soon as possible (no more than 24 hours, based on prioritized need) after referral from: • Patient database referral on admit • PN report • TF report • Ventilator dependency report • NPO, clear and/or full liquid > 7 days report • Lab results - pathology report • Multidisciplinary team rounds				
TX.4 *Intent of* TX.4	"Each patient's nutrition care is **planned."** "Based on results of the nutrition screen and, when appropriate, nutrition assessment and reassessment, the nutrition therapy plan is **implemented** for all patients determined to be at nutritional risk."	Nutrition documentation for patients identified at nutrition 1 risk addressed: • Evaluation based on age, culture, food-drug interactions, physical examination, patient interview, diet education needs, and subjective global assessment • Monitoring of mechanical, gastrointestinal, metabolic and infectious complications • Adequacy of intake and appropriateness of diet/nutrition support • **Specific** recommendations				
TX.4.5 *Intent* TX.4.5 *Intent* TX.4.1	"Each patient's response to nutrition care is monitored." "Nutrition care monitoring is a **collaborative** process..." "The plan identified **measur goals and actions** to achieve them."	Monitoring (follow-up) documentation for patients identified at risk addressed: • Monitoring based on change in clinical status, critical pathways, outcomes management team protocols • **Adequacy** and appropriateness of nutrition support • Monitoring of mechanical, gastrointestinal, metabolic, and infectious complications • **Specific** recommendations				
PE.2	"Each patient is reassessed at points designated in hospital policy."	Reassessment for patients identified at risk documented based on: • Change in clinical status • Critical pathways • Outcomes management team protocols				
PF.3.1 Implementation	"Before discharge a multidisciplinary team approach is used to teach patients about drug-food interaction."	Food-drug interaction education documented (including objective assessment of comprehension) on Patient and Family Education Documentation form				☐ Warfarin (Coumadin) ☐ Grapefruit ☐ MAOI ☐ Isoniazide ☐ _____
PF.3.2	"The patient is educated about nutrition interventions, modified diets, or oral health when applicable."	Nutrition/diet education documented (including objective assessment of comprehension) on Patient and Family Education Documentation form				

Please attach copy of Nutrition note if problem identified.

FIGURE 43-1 Nutrition care quality monitor chart (Courtesy St. Luke's Episcopal Hospital, TX.)

or measured it. The American Dietetic Association (ADA) in 1986 defined QA as a process that certifies continuous, optimal, effective, and efficient health and nutrition care.[6] Quality assurance was implemented as a design or plan to attain a predetermined level of quality. Continuous quality improvement was an approach to quality management that built on traditional QA methods by emphasizing the organization and systems (rather than individuals), the need for objective data with which to analyze and improve processes, and the ideal that systems and performance can always improve even when high standards appear to have been met. Whereas QA focused principally on clinical aspects of care, CQI focused on the relationship of governance, managerial support, and clinical processes that affect patient outcomes. QA programs were compartmentalized with activities conducted by departments. CQI organized activities around the flow of patient care. Audits were used to identify deficiencies retrospectively, whereas CQI used tools such as cause-and-effect diagrams, flow charts, and interdisciplinary teams to track how well systems or processes were performing. Individual performance or problem performance were cornerstones to QA. Action was initiated only when a problem was identified. CQI programs focused on how processes could be improved and acknowledged that there were always better ways.

Today, surveyors assess how health care organizations have integrated and used ORYX performance measurement data in their performance improvement activities. During the performance improvement interview, health care organizations are asked for the rationale used to select institution-specific measures, how the data have been incorporated into institution performance improvement activities, and the results of these activities. The ORYX program moves toward the development of specific performance measures focusing on clinical performance, patient perception of care, health status, and administrative or financial measures. The initial core measure sets for hospitals include: acute myocardial infarction including coronary artery disease, congestive heart failure, pneumonia, surgical procedures and complications, and pregnancy and related conditions.[5] These core measures are based on disease prevalence, high-volume, high-risk or problem-prone areas, or areas known to have significant variations in patterns of care. For example, dietitians at St. Luke's Episcopal Hospital in Texas have collaborated with speech pathologists to assess risk for aspiration and are immediately changing a patient's diet order to the appropriate consistency or NPO until further evaluation is completed. This ties in with the institution's current ORYX measures of "aspiration pneumonia rate." It is clear that each of the five identified core measures have nutritional implications, and dietetic professionals and nutrition support practitioners should identify how nutrition-related activities and outcomes can be incorporated into the institution's performance improvement plan.

The American Medical Association, JCAHO, and the National Committee for Quality Assurance recently released "Coordinated Performance Measurement for the Management of Adult Diabetes."[7] This measurement set addresses the following aspects of the outpatient care of adult patients for which performance measurement is warranted and feasible: HbA$_{1c}$ management, lipid management, urine protein testing, eye examination, foot examination, influenza immunization, blood pressure management, and office visits. The core measurement set includes information on importance for patient care and treatment goals, clinical recommendations, standardized data elements, performance measures, aggregate data element values, and the rationale for each aspect of care.

Nutrition Care Standards—Hospitals

JCAHO manuals are now organized into chapters of functions or required activities[5] (Box 43-1). Because of the emphasis on interdisciplinary processes and coordinated activities, standards related to nutrition care and nutrition support have been integrated into the Assessment of Patients (PE), Care of Patients (TX), Education of Patients (PF), and Continuum of Care (CC) functional chapters (Table 43-1).

The nutrition care process, defined in the JCAHO accreditation manual includes: screening, assessment, reassessment, development of a plan for nutrition therapy, prescribing or ordering, preparing, distributing, administering, and patient monitoring.[5] When screening criteria identify a patient who is at high nutritional risk, an assessment with the following elements should be conducted: adequacy of nutrient intake; anthropometric measurements including weight and weight history; nutritional implications of selected laboratory tests; physical examination for manifestations of nutrient deficiency or excess; medications that may affect nutritional status; conditions that may affect ingestion, digestion, absorption, or use of nutrients; food intolerances or allergies; religious, cultural, ethnic, and personal food preferences; and diet prescription or number of days of nothing by mouth. The assessment process for an infant, child, or adolescent must be individualized, and other age-related issues must be considered. Examples include guidelines for handling human breast milk, infant formulary, and pediatric parenteral nutrition (PN) forms with age-weight appropriate ordering instructions.

BOX 43-1

JCAHO 2001 Patient-Focused and Organization-Focused Functions[5]

PATIENT-FOCUSED FUNCTIONS
Patient Rights and Organization Ethics
Assessment of Patients
Care of Patients
Education
Continuum of Care

ORGANIZATION-FOCUSED FUNCTIONS
Improving Organization Performance
Leadership
Management of the Environment of Care
Management of Human Resources
Management of Information
Surveillance, Prevention, and Control of Infection

Joint Commission: Automated Comprehensive Accreditation Manual for Hospitals, Joint Commission on Accreditation of Healthcare Organizations, Oakbrook Terrace, IL, 2001. Reprinted with permission.

TABLE 43-1

JCAHO (2001) Standards Applicable to Nutrition Services

Standard		Intent/Comment
Assessment of Patients (PE)		
PE.1.2	Nutritional status is assessed when warranted by the patient's needs or condition.	Nutrition screening is conducted to determine the patient's need for a comprehensive nutrition assessment. Approved policies define the content of nutrition screening. When indicated by results of the nutrition screen, a nutrition assessment is completed and updated at specified intervals. A written prescription or order for nutrition assessment is not required.
PE 1.5	Diagnostic testing necessary for determining the patient's health care needs is performed.	
PE 1.7	Each admitted patient's initial assessment is conducted within a time frame specified by hospital policy.	
PE 2.1	Reassessment occurs at regular intervals in the course of care.	
PE 2.2	Reassessment determines a patient's response to care.	
PE. 2.3	Significant change in a patient's condition or diagnosis results in reassessment.	
PE. 4.1	The hospital defines the scope of assessment performed by each discipline.	
PE 5	The assessment process for an infant, child, or adolescent patient is individualized.	
Care of Patients (TX)		
TX.4	Each patient's nutrition care is planned.	Based on the results of the nutrition screen and, when appropriate, nutrition assessment and reassessment, the nutrition therapy plan is implemented for all patients determined to be at nutritional risk. Patients at nutritional risk include: patients with actual or potential malnutrition; on altered diets or diet schedules; with inadequate nutrition; lactating and pregnant women; and geriatric surgical patients. All patients, regardless of their nutritional status or need, receive a prescription or order for food or other nutrients. The food or other nutrients ordered can range from nothing by mouth (NPO orders), to regular diets, to parenteral or enteral tube nutrition.
TX.4.1	An interdisciplinary nutrition therapy plan is developed and periodically updated for patients at nutritional risk.	A more intensive plan for nutrition therapy may be indicated for patients at high nutritional risk. The patient's physician, the registered dietitian, nursing, and pharmaceutical services staff participate in developing the plan, and their roles in implementation are clearly defined.
TX.4.1.1	When appropriate to the patient groups served by a unit, meals and snacks support program goals.	
TX.4.2	Authorized individuals prescribe or order food and nutrition products in a timely manner.	Food and nutrition products are administered only when prescribed or ordered by medical staff, authorized house staff, or other individuals with appropriate clinical privileges. Verbal prescriptions or orders for food and nutrition products are accepted by designated personnel.
TX.4.3	Responsibilities are assigned for all activities involved in safe and accurate provision of food and nutrition products.	The organization used the HACCP process to manage food and enteral tube feeding safety. Staff responsibilities for preparation, storage, distribution, and administration of food and nutrition products are clearly defined to ensure safety and accuracy.
TX.4.4	Food and nutrition products are distributed and administered in a safe, accurate, timely, and acceptable manner.	Food is distributed in a timely manner to preserve nutrient value and serving temperature and provide nutrition that is appetizing and palatable. There is documentation of HACCP for food and enteral nutrition.
TX.4.5	Each patient's response to nutrition care is monitored.	Ongoing patient monitoring is essential to effective, appropriate, and continuous nutrition care. Nutrition care monitoring is a collaborative process that may involve a formal nutrition care team; representatives from multiple disciplines conducting patient care rounds; communication among the various disciplines; or integration of nutrition care with the patient care team.
TX.4.6	The nutrition care service meets patients' needs for special diets and accommodates altered diet schedules.	Food and nutrition services include processes for meeting special diet or diet schedule needs; providing food or nutrition products at times other than the regular delivery schedule; accommodating personal dietary requests; and storing, handling, and controlling food or nutrition products obtained from outside sources. (Documentation of HACCP for food and enteral tube feeding.)
TX.4.7	Nutrition care practices are standardized throughout the organization.	Standardized approaches to nutrition care are developed and maintained. Approaches are communicated and used throughout the organization. A nutrition care manual reflects the standards for nutrition care, RDA, the basis for all prescriptions or orders for food and nutrition products including enteral and parenteral nutrition, and incorporates HACCP into hospital policies.
TX.5	The medical staff defines the scope of assessment for operative and other procedures.	Preoperative nutrition assessment is an example of implementation.

Continued.

TABLE 43-1

JCAHO (2001) Standards Applicable to Nutrition Services—cont'd

Standard		Intent/Comment
Management of Information (IM)		
IM.7.7	Verbal orders of authorized individuals are accepted and transcribed by qualified personnel who are identified by title or category in the medical staff rules and regulations.	
Education (PF)		
PF.2	The patient education process is coordinated among appropriate staff or disciplines who are providing care or services.	
PF.3	The patient receives education and training specific to the patient's assessed needs, abilities, learning preferences, and readiness to learn as appropriate to the care and services provided by the hospital.	Patient and family education, discharge planning, and continuity of care are interrelated. Discharge planning helps develop and implement a workable postdischarge care plan. Such planning involves teaching the patient and family about when and how to obtain further care or treatment after discharge; specific treatment procedures; self-care; how to manage continuing care, whether it is carried out at home (with or without home health care services) or at another organization.
PF 3.1	Based on assessed needs, the patient is educated about how to safely and effectively use medications, according to law and regulation, and the hospital's scope of services, as appropriate.	Drug-food interactions are listed as one of the components for which hospitals have a responsibility for educating patients.
PF.3.2	The patient is educated about nutrition. Interventions, modified diets, or oral health, when applicable.	The hospital is responsible for educating patients and families about issues related to nutrition.
PF 3.3	The hospital assures that the patient is educated about how to safely and effectively use medical equipment or supplies, as appropriate.	Patients and families are instructed how to safely use medical equipment and supplies. This has application to enteral and parenteral feeding supplies and pumps.
PF.3.9	Discharge instructions are given to the patient and those responsible for providing continuing care.	Instructions should include how to make lifestyle choices and changes.
Control of Infection (IC)		
IC.4	The hospital takes action to prevent or reduce the risk of nosocomial infections in patients, employees, and visitors.	Policies and procedures address infection prevention issues in the process of food and nutrition product preparation and distribution.
Improving Organization Performance (PI)		
PI 3.1	The organization collects data to monitor its performance.	Included among the data that the organization should monitor are patient safety needs (adverse drug events), perceptions of risks to patients, outcomes of processes or services, infection control surveillance and reporting, and effectiveness of pain management.

Joint Commission: Automated Comprehensive Accreditation Manual for Hospitals, Joint Commission on Accreditation of Healthcare Organizations, Oakbrook Terrace, IL, 2001. Reprinted with permission.

To meet these standards, the organization must have policies and procedures that address nutrition screening and nutrition assessment, including criteria for identifying patients at nutrition risk. In changing the orientation away from process, professionals might look at the outcome of nutrition screening in terms of identifying patients at high nutritional risk and providing timely nutrition intervention. Most institutions have incorporated nutrition screening criteria into the initial patient assessment and database that is completed upon admission. This system minimizes duplication of efforts in data collection and emphasizes interdisciplinary care. Referrals to appropriate health care professionals are automatically obtained when admission screening indicates high risk. Surveyors want to see a system or tool implemented that can identify high nutrition risk patients on admission through a referral process. Standard PE 1.7.1 specifies that the patient's history and physical examination, nursing assessment, and other screening assessments as needed, be completed within 24 hours of inpatient admission.[5] The intent is for these elements to be performed and documented by all hospitals and for all patients within 24 hours even on weekends and holidays. "Other screening assessments" is not defined; however, dietetic professionals and even surveyors, have interpreted this as including nutrition screening. A hospital may, according to the intent statement, establish different time frames for the initial assessment in different areas or services.

A plan of care is based on data gathered during patient assessment that identifies the patient's care needs, lists the strategy for providing services to meet those needs, documents treat-

BOX 43-2

HACCP Critical Steps Applied to Enteral Feeding: An Example from St. Luke's Episcopal Hospital, TX

1. PURCHASING:	All tube feeding formulas are purchased in liter ready-to-hang sterile containers with at least a 6-month expiration date.
2. RECEIVING:	The containers are inspected to ensure the protective cover is intact.
3. STORAGE:	Normal storage is in a cool dry area off the floor as with other similar shelf-stable products.
4. PREPARATION:	No formula will be mixed either in the Food Service Department or on the patient care units. Any additional water, electrolytes, medications, dyes, or modular caloric enhancers are delivered via the Y-port on a scheduled basis.
5. HOLDING:	Any unused formula should be covered, labeled, dated, and stored in the refrigerator until needed again.
6. DELIVERY TO UNITS:	All formula has an intact original label including expiration date. Cans are wiped before opening.
7. ADMINISTRATION:	Ready-to-hang formulas must be dated when hung and may be hung for 24 hours per hospital policy. Tubing must be changed every 24 hours and dated and timed. If a canned product is poured into a feeding bag, only 4 hours of formula should be poured and documented. The remaining formula should be covered, dated, and labeled when refrigerated. All opened formula is discarded after 24 hours.

Used with permission from St. Luke's Episcopal Hospital, Houston, Texas.

ment goals and objectives, outlines the criteria for terminating specified interventions, and documents the individual's progress in meeting specified goals and objectives. Nutrition care plans should show evidence of an interdisciplinary approach and include measurable goals and plans to achieve such goals. Practitioners are encouraged to document any discussions pertaining to the nutrition care plan, treatment, and interventions that occur during one-on-one conversations with other disciplines, interdisciplinary care conferences, and/or clinical rounds. A nutrition care model developed by the Health Services Research task force of the ADA is a framework for which a standard set of core nutrition measures could be developed.[8] The nutrition care process has the following five steps:

- Assess
- Establish goals and determine nutrition plan
- Implement intervention
- Document and communicate
- Evaluate and reassess

Patient-centered outcomes, direct nutrition outcomes, clinical outcomes, and health care utilization/cost savings outcomes can be documented using this model. Measures must be routinely implemented; accurately documented; and tracked for each patient, institution, and health system.

Nutrition care policies and procedures must show compliance with Hazard Analysis Critical Control Point (HACCP)[9] guidelines for handling of food and nutrition products. Federal and State Health Departments have gradually begun requiring implementation of these guidelines in the food production industry since 1993. Although these plans have not specifically included enteral tube feeding formulas provided to patients in hospitals and other health care facilities, it makes sense that dietetics professionals include nutritional formulas in this process. Each step in the process of food production must be evaluated to determine if there are critical control points for temperature control during which the food or nutrition product is susceptible to bacterial growth. The critical points include purchasing, receiving, storage, preparation, holding delivery to the nursing care unit, and administration. An example of how one institution has addressed each of these critical steps in shown in Box 43-2. Many manufacturers now provide information and continuing education on preventing microbial contamination in enteral nutrition (EN) products and delivery systems.

Education of patients and families is an important function of health care organizations. Instruction on potential drug-food

interactions and counseling on medical nutrition therapy as well as instruction in proper breast-feeding technique and proper nutrition while lactating are examples of interdisciplinary education responsibilities. Surveyors have placed much focus on drug-nutrient interaction education. Institutions should have a clearly defined policy with updated drug lists and explicit delineation of which health care practitioner is responsible for teaching about each drug.[10] For example, when a patient is taking one or more chemotherapeutic drugs, the physician may provide the primary education. In situations in which the drugs taken by a patient limit the patient's food choices, the dietitian may be the educator. The pharmacy department plays an important role in tracking drug-drug and drug-food interactions and in notifying nurses of these interactions. In some hospitals the pharmacy prints a list of patients on preselected medications for the dietetics staff to review. Although JCAHO leaves it up to individual facilities to select the drugs to be targeted for education, the decision should involve consideration of degree or risk associated with a drug and frequency of use at the institution.[10] During a recent survey at St. Luke's Episcopal Hospital, surveyors advised the dietitians to pick three or four high-usage drugs to begin with and really do an excellent job educating patients on them. Many institutions have incorporated systems that dispense drug-nutrient education materials at the same time medication is dispensed from a unit. The health care professional responsible for completing the instruction and assessing understanding of each drug must be designated in the institutional policy; for example, the pharmacist may have primary responsibility for Coumadin, while dietitians may provide education for monoamine oxidase inhibitors (MAOI).

Any discharge instructions given to the patient or his or her family must be provided to the organization or person responsible for the patient's continuing care. The role of the nutrition support team in providing patient education and ensuring continuity of care as it relates to tube feeding, care and maintenance of vascular access devices and feeding tubes, equipment, aseptic technique, and transitional feeding are examples of areas in which interdisciplinary teaching occurs and responsibilities should be clearly delineated. Similarly, the Comprehensive Accreditation Manual for Hospitals (CAMH) chapter on Continuum of Care specifies that the discharge process provides for continuing care based on the patient's assessed needs at the time of discharge. The role of nutrition support practitioners in arranging for home care services, EN or PN support equipment, supplies and formulations, and follow-up teaching or counseling on nutrition-related issues should also be addressed. Emphasizing the importance of continuity of care, surveyors conduct individual centered evaluations. They begin at an entry point in the hospital (e.g., the emergency department) and identify a patient on admission whom they follow for the entire survey week to prospectively determine if care and documentation reflect continuity of care.

The decision to forego or withdraw nutrition support is pertinent to the standards that deal with patient rights and organization ethics.[5] A discussion of the patient's preferences, goals, and values, and the potential benefits or burdens of nutrition support is in order.[8] Consideration of the appropriateness of nutrition support therapy, as well as benefit and risk, is a typical discussion on daily nutrition support rounds. The nutrition support team's role in patient rights and organizational ethics should be defined or communicated as part of the institution's overall performance improvement plan. Nutrition support practitioners should also participate in medical staff committees that discuss and provide guidance for ethical issues and advanced directives. Practitioners should review the organization-focused chapters, including Improving Organizational Performance (PI), Leadership (LD), Management of the Environment of Care (EC), Management of Human Resources (HR), Management of Information (IM), and Surveillance, Prevention, and Control of Infection (IC) to identify standards applicable to nutrition care. The Management of Information chapter includes standards that pharmacists and nutrition support specialists need to specifically review. They specify that a hospital formulary or drug list be readily available to the staff who use it. EN formularies are fairly commonplace, and, whether coordinated by pharmacy or food and nutrition services, the information should be made available to physicians and other health care staff. This is particularly necessary when generic tube feeding order forms are used to accommodate formulary changes imposed by annual contract bidding.

Similarly, the standards related to surveillance, prevention, and infection control are very important to nutrition support practice. The CAMH states that an organization uses a coordinated process to reduce the risks of endemic and epidemic nosocomial infections in patients and health care workers.[5] The hospital's infection control program must address issues defined by the hospital to be epidemiologically important. Examples of implementation in the CAMH that are relevant to nutrition support teams include addressing device-related infections (especially those associated with intravascular devices) and tube feeding.[5] Responsibility for this monitoring typically is assigned to infectious disease services; however, many nutrition support teams monitor similar data as they relate to PN catheter sepsis, hospital-acquired pneumonia in patients receiving PN, and aspiration pneumonia in tube-fed patients.[11] Demonstration of the role of nutrition in patient outcome, particularly as it relates to infection, should also be emphasized. Insurers and third-party payers frequently use infection rates to compare health care institutions and providers because of the associated costs. Nutrition support teams can collaborate with the infection control department to evaluate data and document decreased infection in patients receiving nutrition therapy. Dietitians at St. Luke's Episcopal Hospital receive a daily list of all patients with positive cultures as a screening referral in addition to more traditional screens such as low prealbumin levels and number of days a patient is NPO. They have been able to document decreased nosocomial infections with early EN in patients undergoing bowel resection.[12,13]

A major emphasis in current JCAHO Standards is pain. Standards for pain appear in most of the patient-focused function chapters. While much of the focus is on assessment, treatment, and monitoring of pain in patients, hospitals must also educate staff about pain assessment and treatment. Because patient care is interdisciplinary, dietetics professionals and nutrition support practitioners need to consider how pain influences nutrition care. Consider how pain affects intake of food (e.g., Does the medication induce drowsiness, causing the patient to sleep through a meal?) and how food intake affects pain (e.g., Does acidic food worsen oral pain related to severe mucositis in an immunosuppressed patient?).[14] This information should be incorporated into a set of policies, procedures, measurements, and plans for improvement of services.

Nutrition Care Standards—Home and Long-Term Care

Nutrition care standards for home and long-term care are similar to those for hospitals.[15,16] All patients admitted for home care services should undergo nutrition screening. It is suggested that nutrition screening be conducted for patients on medically prescribed diets; patients with nutrition-related problems or open wounds; elderly patients who live alone and depend on others for meal preparation, grocery shopping, and feeding; and for patients whose need for enteral product suddenly increases or decreases.[17] Likewise, the standards for nutrition care in long-term care are similar to those for hospital and home care, but they also define standards specific to that setting.[18] For example, emphasis is placed on menu cycles, resident access to dining facilities, nutrition and hydration needs, and oral health assessment as well as intervention. The manual includes certain certification requirements mandating that the facility ensure that a resident maintain acceptable parameters of nutritional status, such as body weight and protein levels, unless the resident's clinical condition demonstrates that this is not possible. Residents fed by nasogastric or gastrostomy tubes must also receive appropriate treatment and services to prevent aspiration pneumonia, diarrhea, vomiting, dehydration, metabolic abnormalities, and nasopharyngeal ulcers, and to restore, if possible, normal feeding function. An example of a collaborative or interdisciplinary performance improvement process may include tracking the cause for an increased incidence of pressure ulcers or unintentional weight loss and comparing the findings with those of other facilities, regionally and nationally.[19]

Professional Standards and Practice Guidelines

Professional organizations offer many guidelines for quality performance improvement programs. These documents provide an important framework for performance measurement and other monitoring tools. The American Society for Parenteral and Enteral Nutrition (ASPEN) Standards for Nutrition Support: Hospitalized Patients include several standards related to quality and performance improvement.[20]

Examples of standards from professional organizations are useful to nutrition support practitioners who are implementing performance improvement programs. The American Society for Hospital Pharmacists (ASHP) published Guidelines on the Pharmacist's Role in Home Care.[21] Similar to ASPEN's standards of practice for dietitians, nurses, physicians, and pharmacists,[22-25] ASHP's standards outline in detail professional responsibilities as they relate to patient assessment, patient education, training and counseling, product selection, drug preparation and administration, care plan development, clinical monitoring, communication, universal precautions, documentation and reporting mechanisms, QI, policies and procedures, licensure and accreditation, and continuing education. ASPEN also published "Interdisciplinary Nutrition Support Core Competencies" to aid in the required documentation of professional competence assessment.[26] The core competency statements are examples of critical aspects of job performance, which supervisors or managers may use or adapt for performance appraisal of nutrition support practitioners, while meeting the accreditation standards.

Practice guidelines describe how to do an activity or intervention.[27,28] They specify a recommended course of action. Protocols, algorithms, care maps, critical pathways, and flow diagrams are all examples of practice guidelines that help illustrate the process of providing nutrition support. Typically, guidelines combine scientific evidence and practitioner experience. Dietitians in Nutrition Support (DNS), a dietetic practice group of the ADA, has validated practice guidelines for EN and PN, home nutrition support, and diseases or conditions, including acquired immunodeficiency syndrome (AIDS), burns, diabetes, geriatrics, multiple system organ failure, cancer, pulmonary dysfunction, renal failure, short-gut syndrome, and solid organ and bone marrow transplantation.[29] A recent study conducted by Mueller also validates several of the DNS guidelines.[30] He found that adequate feeding and absence of gastrointestinal complications were associated with increased body weight in residents of long-term care facilities requiring EN.[30] Excellent resources, including a tool kit for developing and validating evidence-based guides for practice and medical nutrition therapy protocols for EN and PN, are also available from the ADA.[31,32]

When nutrition support care is delivered according to established protocols or practice guidelines, specific end results or outcomes should be achieved and documented. Failure to achieve the desired goals or deviation from the protocol triggers an extensive review as part of the performance improvement process. Any problems, strengths, weaknesses, or inconsistencies in the process of delivering care are identified. Review of the scientific literature and clinical applications, and corrective action such as protocol revision, procedural change, retraining, and professional education are then directed at improving the process and outcomes.

Establishing a Performance Improvement Program

Fundamental to the establishment of any departmental performance improvement program are defined objectives that have a clear connection to the organization's mission and vision. There are many ways to approach performance improvement, but each plan should include the following essential processes: process design, performance measurement, performance assessment, and performance improvement.[5] A *performance measure* is a standard or indicator used to assess the performance of a function or process. An *indicator* is a tool or measure used over time to determine the performance of an organization's functions, processes, and outcomes. Indicators measure three types of events:

- Structure—measures whether or not enough resources are in place to deliver health care
- Process—measures a care activity and is linked to clients' outcomes
- Outcome—what happens or does not happen after an intervention is provided

There are two types of indicators. A *comparative rate indicator* is an instrument that monitors a patient care event over a period of time within an institution or organization.[33] Trends within an organization over varying time periods can be evaluated or significant variations between organizations or similar institutions may warrant further assessment. A *sentinel event indicator* measures a serious, undesirable, and often avoidable process or outcome.[33] JCAHO's sentinel event policy is designed to help organizations identify sentinel events and take action to prevent their recurrence. JCAHO defines a sentinel event as an unexpected occurrence involving death or serious physical or psychologic injury, or the risk thereof.[5] Any time a sentinel event occurs, the organization is expected to complete a root cause analysis, implement improvements to reduce risk, and monitor the effectiveness of those improvements. Examples of adverse events include medication errors, wrong-site surgery, restraint-related deaths, blood transfusion errors, inpatient suicides, infant abductions, fatal falls, and operative/postoperative complications. A collaboration of nutrition organizations has published indicators that have application to nutrition support practice.[34] Another performance improvement tool used by practitioners and health care organizations is clinical benchmarking. Clinical benchmarks serve as a standard of best practice against which other similar practices can be measured.[35]

The purpose of a nutrition support team's performance improvement plan is to provide a systematic process for monitoring and evaluating the quality and appropriateness of nutrition support therapy and nutritional care outcomes, and to identify and resolve problems related to provision of care. Objectives for a nutrition support team CQI or PI plan might include these:

- Provision of quality patient care based on professional standards of care and practice for nutrition support
- Identification of opportunities for improvement and resolution of patient care or practitioner problems that inhibit quality care
- Interdisciplinary involvement and communication with other departments involved in the provision of nutrition support
- Establishment of responsibility for ongoing monitoring of quality care by all nutrition support team members

Data Collection and Evaluation

To achieve its full potential, the medical record should function as a database for performance improvement activities.[36] Patient information, including goals and outcomes, should be systematically documented. Figure 43-1 shows an example of a nutrition care quality monitor tool that can be used to evaluate whether standards are being met. Performance improvement should be an integral part of the daily workload of all nutrition support practitioners. Outcomes of quality nutrition care should be shared with the profession through presentation and publication. Similar to the database organized by JCAHO, professional organizations could establish a central data bank where practitioners compare experiences, and patients, clients, consumers, insurers, and providers evaluate efficiency and effectiveness of care. Aggregate data could be used to compare different treatments, to describe the typical course of nutrition therapy for certain diseases, and to evaluate variations in outcome when similar standards of care or practice guidelines are followed.

Preparing for an Audit or Survey

The best way to prepare for a JCAHO survey is to always be ready. Familiarize yourself with the standards that apply to nutrition care and nutrition support services. Set up a system that allows you to monitor compliance on a regular basis.[14] Evaluate opportunities for improved performance in all aspects of departmental activities. Network with colleagues and attend performance improvement sessions at professional meetings and workshops. Conduct "mock" surveys on a regular basis and share results and findings with others in your institution.

Conclusion

Quality nutrition care is a dynamic, expanding target that requires continuous performance evaluation and improvement to achieve. Nutrition professionals and other health care providers must stay abreast of current research, regulatory changes, and industry standards of practice. We must be the ones to define excellence in nutritional care that is the right of each patient.

REFERENCES

1. Graham NO: *Quality assurance in hospitals,* Rockville, MD, 1990, Aspen Publishers, pp 3-13.
2. Joint Commission on Accreditation of Healthcare Organizations (JCAHO): *2002 Automated Accreditation manual for hospitals,* Oakbrook Terrace, IL, 2002, JCAHO; www.jcaho.org
3. Codman E: The product of a hospital, *Surg Gynecol Obstet* 18:491-496, 1914.
4. O'Leary DS: Agenda for change fosters CQI concepts, *Joint Commission Perspectives* 12:2-3, 1992.
5. Joint Commission on Accreditation of Healthcare Organizations (JCAHO): *2001 Automated comprehensive accreditation manual for hospitals,* Oakbrook Terrace, IL, 2001, JCAHO, 2001; www.jcaho.org.
6. American Dietetic Association: *Standards of practice: a practitioner's guide to implementation,* Chicago, 1986, American Dietetic Association, p 13.
7. American Medical Association, the Joint Commission on Accreditation of Healthcare Organizations, and the National Committee for Quality Assurance: Coordinated performance measurement for the management of adult diabetes: a consensus statement, April 2001. Retrieved from http://www.ama-assn.org/ama/pub/category/3798.html.
8. Splett P, Meyers EF: A proposed model for effective nutrition care, *J Am Diet Assoc* 101:357-363, 2001.
9. *The complete HACCP manual for institutional food service operations,* Dunkirk, NY, 1995, Food Services Associates.
10. Jackson R: Food-drug interactions, *Food & Nutrition Focus* 14:1-5, 1998.
11. Dougherty D, Bankhead R, Kushner R, et al: Nutrition care given new importance in JCAHO standards, *Nutr Clin Pract* 10:26-31, 1995.
12. Hedberg AM, Lairson DR, Aday LA, Chow J, Suki R, Cole L, Wolf JA: Effectiveness of an early postoperative enteral feeding protocol, *J Clin Outcomes Management* 5:21-28, 1998.
13. Hedberg AM, Lairson DR, Aday LA, Chow J, Suki R, Cole L, Wolf JA: Implications of an early postoperative enteral feeding protocol, *J Am Diet Assoc* 99:802-807, 1999.
14. Clairmont MA: Are you audit ready? *Today's Dietitian* 3(5):39-40, May, 2001.
15. Mirtallo JM: JCAHO nutrition care standards adopted for home care, *Nutr Clin Pract* 10(2 suppl):63S-65S, 1995.
16. Joint Commission on Accreditation of Healthcare Organizations (JCAHO): *Comprehensive accreditation manual for home care,* Oakbrook Terrace, IL, 2001, JCAHO.
17. Westbrook NH: Applying the 1995 JCAHO standards to dietetics practice in home care, *J Am Diet Assoc* 96:404-406, 1996.
18. Joint Commission on Accreditation of Healthcare Organizations (JCAHO): *Accreditation manual for long term care,* Oakbrook Terrace, IL, 2001, JCAHO.
19. Robinson GE: Applying the 1996 JCAHO nutrition care standards in a long-term care setting, *J Am Diet Assoc* 96:400-403, 1996.
20. Standards for nutrition support: hospitalized patients, *Nutr Clin Pract* 10:208-219, 1995.
21. ASHP guidelines on the pharmacist's role in home care, *Am J Hosp Pharm* 50:1940-1944, 1993.
22. Standards of practice for the nutrition support dietitian, *Nutr Clin Pract* 15:53-59, 2000.
23. Standards of practice: nutrition support nurse, *Nutr Clin Pract* 56-62, 2001.
24. Standards of practice: nutrition support physician, *Nutr Clin Pract* 11:235-240, 1996.
25. Standards of practice: nutrition support pharmacist, *Nutr Clin Pract* 14:275-281, 1999.
26. Board of Directors, American Society for Parenteral and Enteral Nutrition: Interdisciplinary nutrition support core competencies, *Nutr Clin Pract* 14:331-333, 1999; www.nutritioncare.org
27. Gottlieb LK, Margoles CA, Schoenbaum SC: Clinical practice guidelines at an HMO: development and implementation in a quality improvement model, *Qual Rev Bull* 16:80-86, 1990.
28. Leape LL: Practice guidelines and standards. An overview, *Qual Rev Bull* 16:42-49, 1990.
29. Winkler MF, Lysen LK: *Suggested guidelines for the nutrition and metabolic management of adults receiving nutrition support,* Chicago, 1994, American Dietetic Association.
30. Mueller CM: Enteral nutrition and selected health care outcomes among elderly residents of long-term care facilities. Submitted in partial fulfillment of the requirements for the degree of Doctor of Philosophy in the School of Education, New York University, 2001 (personal communication).
31. Splett PL: *Developing and validating evidence-based guides for practice: a tool kit for dietetics professionals,* Chicago, IL, 2000, American Dietetic Association.
32. *Medical nutrition therapy across the continuum of care,* ed 2, Chicago, IL, 1998, American Dietetic Association and Morrison Health Care.
33. Council on Practice Quality Management Task Force: Learning the language of quality care, *J Am Diet Assoc* 93:531-532, 1993.
34. Kushner RF, Ayello EA, Beyer PL, et al: National Coordinating Committee clinical indicators of nutrition care, *J Am Diet Assoc* 94:1168-1177, 1994.
35. Weissman NW, Allison JJ, Kiefe C, et al: Achievable benchmarks of care: the ABCs of benchmarking, *J Eval Clin Pract* 3:269-281, 1999.
36. Davies AR, Doyle MAT, Lansky D, et al: Outcomes assessment in clinical settings: a consensus statement on principles and best practices in project management, *J Qual Improve* 20:6-16, 1994.

Julie O'Sullivan Maillet, PhD, RD, FADA

WHEN health professionals think about ethical and legal issues in nutrition support, two aspects are often considered: the issue of autonomy and self-determination, and legalities surrounding artificial nutrition as a medical therapy. A variety of principles, values, and beliefs create the dilemmas in individual cases. The purpose of this chapter is

- To provide readers with the knowledge and skills they need to participate effectively in ethical decision making
- To provide ethical guidelines for dietitians and other practitioners who engage in ethical decision making
- To offer guidelines or references to facilitate decision making in specific cases
- To provide an overview of common ethical dilemmas
- To help readers clarify their personal values and ethical bases for decision making
- To present different points of view that must be considered in ethical decision making

Ethical Issues Surrounding Feeding

Nourishment is essential for life. From conception to death, nourishment is required to sustain life, and proper nutrition helps to sustain health. The typical human can survive 7 to 10 days without fluids and will die of starvation after being deprived of food for 50 to 70 days. Throughout life, people are encouraged to eat for growth, healing, and well-being. On a community basis, agencies are established to reduce hunger and malnutrition. Providing nutrition is basic, humane care.

Food has many symbolic, psychologic, cultural, and religious connotations that must be considered in patient care. Various cultures have beliefs about what foods to eat or avoid when ill, foods tied to special occasions, and food-based rituals. And, of course, food selection guidelines vary with medical conditions and therapies. Food is essential from a psychologic perspective as well as a physiologic one. Feeding is associated with affection, and withholding food may be tied to punishment.

Ethical dilemmas surrounding oral feeding include the following:

- What rights do persons have to select the foods they eat, especially in institutional settings?
- Can a diet be liberalized if doing so is detrimental to care?
- Can an individual refuse to eat?
- Does a health professional ever have an obligation to force feed someone or control what an individual eats? If so, under what circumstances?

When oral feeding is insufficient, tube feeding or parenteral nutrition may be a possibility. From an ethical standpoint, is there a difference between the two? Often in literature on termination of feeding, they are lumped together as *artificial feeding*. When is there an ethical obligation for a health professional to start or stop artificial feeding? Providing oral intake is basic care; is artificial feeding basic care or not? Can individuals refuse artificial feeding initially or discontinue it later? How aggressive should the health care provider be in recommending artificial feeding to patients? Can health professionals stop feeding if it is futile? Can health professionals refuse to administer particular feedings, such as refusing to administer parenteral feeding when enteral feeding is acceptable? Can parenteral feeding be recommended as palliative care?

There are no definitive rules, because each individual situation must be reviewed. The basic premise remains: When in doubt, feed. Enteral and parenteral feeding should not be withheld unless feeding is medically harmful or conflicts with the client's informed choice. Guidelines for providing or withholding feeding, and the court decisions regarding food and fluids, have been written for terminally ill persons and those in persistent vegetative states. Feeding critically ill or comatose patients who have not been declared permanently unconscious is an essential part of care for that person. Several recent articles[1,2] question the premise of feeding, based on the question of whether nutrition has been proven to improve the patient's prognosis or health, thus questioning the futility of nutrition.

The difference between withholding and withdrawing feeding affects health care providers on a practical and ethical level. In 1982 The President's Commission for the Study of Ethical Problems in Medicine and Biomedical and Behavioral Research[3] stated that withdrawing of feeding, after determining it to be futile, was more ethical than withholding feeding without knowing its futility; however, some make a moral distinction between withholding and withdrawing feeding, often on religious grounds, and in practice many patients and families support withholding versus withdrawing feeding.

Definition of Terms

The definitions for terminal illness and permanent unconsciousness (also called *persistent vegetative state* [PVS]) continue to evolve. Some current definitions are provided here.

Terminal illness has been defined as "the end or final stage of a specific, progressive, normally irreversible lethal disease when physicians have 'determined, through objective medical validation, that medical treatment of that disease is futile' and the disease will cause the patient's death in the foreseeable future."[4]

The PVS patient is defined by The American Academy of Neurology as a patient who "at no time is aware of himself or his environment," and has a "total loss of cerebral functioning."[5] Persons in a PVS have lost the function of their cerebral cortex and thalamus, although the brain stem is relatively intact.[6] Thus, after trauma, "the patient will begin to breathe spontaneously, the eyes will open and 'wander' and respond normally to light, and periods of sleep will occur. The protective gag, cough, and swallow reflexes are usually normal and hand-feeding is possible by placing food at the back of the throat, thus activating the involuntary swallow reflex. All voluntary reactions or behavioral responses reflecting consciousness, volition, or emotion at the cerebral cortical level are absent."[7] Absence of progressive improvement for a prolonged time is essential to the diagnosis. The Multi-Society Task Force on PVS[5] defines PVS as "a vegetative state present one month after acute traumatic or nontraumatic brain injury or lasting for at least one month in patients with degenerative or metabolic disorders or developmental malformations." In the Task Force's judgment, PVS is only one form of permanent unconsciousness. Alternatively, Freeman suggests categorizing "a person as in *prolonged coma* between 2 weeks and 3 months after trauma, *vegetative state* from 3 to 12 months, and *persistent vegetative state* after 12 months."[8]

The diagnosis of PVS is determined through clinical judgment. The results of imaging and laboratory studies do not confirm the diagnosis. The Multi-Society Task Force Report provides a thorough review of the status of diagnostic tests and cautions making the diagnosis when there is any "degree of sustained visual pursuit, consistent and reproducible visual fixation, or response to threatening gestures."[5]

Medical futility is still being defined.[9] Nelson suggests this working definition: "A treatment is medically futile when the magnitude of the benefit, however it contributes to the patient's treatment goals, is disproportionately small in relation to the magnitude of the risks of violating the patient's integrity, worsening the patient's condition, or when compared to the magnitude of the effort needed to achieve the benefit."[10]

Guidelines from Health Professional Associations

Guidelines on the ethical considerations of foregoing or discontinuing hydration and nutrition support have been written by numerous organizations, including The American Dietetic Association (ADA),[11] The American Medical Society (AMA),[12] The American Nurses Association (ANA),[13] and the Hastings Center.[14] Aimed at their particular specialty, each promotes the rights of self-determination for competent patients and incompetent patients when there is evidence of a patient's living will or advance directive. The multidisciplinary association, the American Society for Parenteral and Enteral Nutrition (ASPEN), provides guidelines on the use of enteral nutrition (EN) and parenteral nutrition (PN), and promotes use of advance directives, the patient's desires, and a team to assist surrogate decision makers.[15]

Specifically for dietitians, the joint ADA-Commission on Dietetic Registration's Code of Ethics[16] requires that the dietitian respect the unique needs and values of the individual, provide sufficient information to enable clients to make their own informed decisions, and interpret controversial information without personal bias. In addition, the ADA has its position on ethical and legal issues in feeding:

> "It is the position of The American Dietetic Association that the development of clinical and ethical criteria for the nutrition and hydration of persons through the lifespan should be established by members of the health care team. Registered dietitians should work collaboratively to make nutrition, hydration and feeding recommendations in individual cases." [14]

In 2002, the two positions have been combined into one position. The paper can be found at http://www.eatright. org/adar0502.html.The AMA states that the physician cannot act intentionally to cause death but has a responsibility to sustain life, relieve suffering, and respect patient dignity and patient choice. Without a proxy, the physician acts in the best interest of the patient.[12] Statements from other associations mirror these statements.

The American Thoracic Society has published a position on futility of care: "A physician has no ethical obligation to provide a life-sustaining intervention that is judged futile as defined previously, even if the intervention is requested by the patient or surrogate decision maker. To force physicians to provide medical interventions that are clearly futile would undermine the ethical integrity of the medical profession."[17]

Ethical Issues

Health care professionals have an inherent ethical duty to respect the sanctity of life and to relieve suffering. The moral principles of autonomy, beneficence, nonmaleficence, and justice govern the behavior of health care professionals. The principle of *autonomy* promotes the individual's right to self-determination and independent decision making. *Beneficence* means to do well, to act charitably toward another. For health care providers, this is the helping principle. *Nonmaleficence* is the principle of not doing harm to the patient. *Justice* is the process of being fair and equitable. When all of these principles can be followed simultaneously, there is no dilemma. Ethical dilemmas most often occur when autonomy conflicts with nonmaleficence or beneficence, the conflict between individual rights (autonomy) and societal duty (nonmaleficence or beneficence) (Fig. 44-1).

When conflict occurs, the question is, What is in the best interest of the individual, and who determines this? The decisions include determining which moral principle takes precedence in what situation. For example, a patient terminally ill with esophageal cancer has refused a tube feeding. The moral principle of respecting self-determination conflicts with the obligation of health professionals to beneficence and nonmaleficence. The dilemma is determining which moral principle takes precedence. Figure 44-1 illustrates a matrix for identifying the ethical dilemmas of feeding. The health care professional has an obligation of responsibility to maintain life and value the sanctity of life; however, the dilemma arises

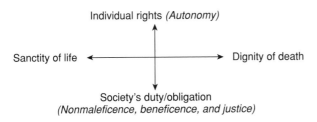

FIGURE 44-1 Dimensions of decision making.

because the health care professional must also respect the values of the individual and allow patients to die in a dignified manner. Legally, the courts have given precedence to self-determination and individual rights.

The dilemma on the horizontal axis of Fig. 44-1 is predominantly related to technologic advances over the past quarter century, especially in the area of nutrition support. Technologic advances have created the ability to feed almost any patient in any situation. In addition, technology can keep persons alive who 10 or 20 years ago would have died. Because nutrition support is possible, the question arises, "Because we have the technology to feed, do we as professionals have to feed?" In a broader statement, does the ability to act imply the need to act? While the question is open to debate, the general response is that people control technology and should act in the best interests of the individual. Thus, the ability to act does not cause the need to act. Although artificial feeding is not required, the professional obligation to protect the sanctity of life may interfere with the individual's decision of what is death with dignity. The issue of assisted suicide is part of this dilemma.

Since the days of Hippocrates and Plato, physicians have been encouraged to understand when medical care has reached its level of usefulness.[18] Health care professionals have a duty to attempt to restore health, not to prolong life at any cost. Without more information on a patient with esophageal cancer, the balance between prolonging life and prolonging death, and the individual's right to self-determination versus society's obligation to feed cannot be determined. Box 44-1 identifies four key questions to address in making care decisions. The first question prompts determination of which moral principles are in conflict or which dimension of decision making from Fig. 44-1 is causing the dilemma. Question 2 seeks information about the current health/nutritional status of the individual. Question 3 identifies the decisions that must be made. Finally, question 4 urges a consideration of the consequences of any action.

Patient Ethics

Two diverse ethical theories, the utilitarian or consequentialist view and the formalist or deontological view, influence attitudes toward provision of health care interventions. The ethical theory espoused by the patient affects discussions about options for nutrition support. The utilitarian viewpoint[19] approaches ethical decisions by seeking to balance the individual's needs with those of the society as a whole. The utilitarian approach holds as appropriate that which produces the greatest positive balance of value over negative value for all persons affected. The utilitarian approach emphasizes examination of

the entire set of consequences to determine feeding options. Referring back to Fig. 44-1, the principle of justice could influence society's duty. The deontological approach to ethics[20] posits that acts or decisions are inherently wrong or right, independent of their consequences for the individual or society. The deontological viewpoint provides a firm statement of the appropriateness of withholding or withdrawing feeding that is much more independent of the situation. The vertical dimension in Fig. 44-1 does not exist in the deontological viewpoint.

As a society, Americans are tolerant of conflicting moral and ethical values. We value the right of the individual to control or govern himself or herself according to his or her own reason and ethical values. Guidelines for feeding the terminally ill and permanently unconscious support the individual's right to self-determination as the overriding principle. Within American society, the individual's right to self-determination takes precedence over the beliefs or wishes of health care providers. "Each patient approaches that universal, common end called death with different religious, philosophic, and personal attitudes and values. For some, every moment of life, no matter how painful and limited in quality, is of inestimable value. On the other hand, because of their circumstances and values, competent, informed patients may seek to forego various medical procedures, which may include nutrition support."[4]

The preferences of those deemed legally "incompetent" are more perplexing; however, the Supreme Court's ruling in the Cruzan case[21] states that, when "clear and convincing evidence" of the wishes of the incompetent person is known, those wishes are sufficient for action. The questions are, what constitutes clear and convincing evidence and what happens if none is available. The methods of determining an incompetent person's wishes include "living wills" or "durable power of attorney for health care" or family discussions, depending on the laws of the state. A 1992 conference brought together families involved in "right to die" cases. All of them "stressed the abysmal quality of life of their loved ones, how 'personal' such a decision is, and how they would support another's decision not to terminate treatment under the very same circumstances that caused them to do so."[22]

Cultural and religious beliefs affect an individual's attitudes toward feeding. Because every person is unique, health professionals must use cultural and religious values as a platform for assessing a patient's opinion on feeding, but realize that the individual's viewpoint may not necessarily reflect their culture or religion. For example, in the traditional Jewish faith, life support once initiated would not be discontinued; however, the Jewish faith has a variety of denominations whose beliefs about life support differ, and many persons of Jewish heritage believe that discontinuation of life support is an appropriate action at certain times.

Religious Viewpoints

The four most prevalent religions in the United States split on their guidelines regarding life support including artificial nutrition. Catholic[23] and Protestant[24] authorities do not distinguish between initiation and discontinuation of feeding, whereas the Jewish[25] and Islamic faiths[26] do. Each believes in the sanctity of life; however, the Catholic and Protestant faiths have stated that there are instances when prolonging death is not necessary.

The Archbishop of Canterbury stated in 1977 that it is "misleading to extend the term *euthanasia* to cover decisions not to preserve life by artificial means when it would be better for the patient to be allowed to die."[24] However, for those who believe that the PVS is a God-mandated fate, life-prolonging treatment is a benefit rather than a burden.[22]

The Catholic press[23] released a paper in 1992 that opposed all willful suicides but stated that Catholics are not obliged to use extraordinary or disproportionate means when there is no hope and only a burden. Catholic theologians agree that unconscious patients must be treated with value and dignity but disagree on care for the permanently unconscious. The debate centers on moral obligation and whether any procedure can be obligatory if it offers no benefit. The argument continues that a decision can be made to omit nonobligatory care to avoid a burden. While expressing a need for continued reflection concerning permanently unconscious patients, the Catholic statement concludes, "We are concerned that withdrawal of all life support, including nutrition and hydration, not be viewed as appropriate or automatically indicated for the entire class of PVS patients simply because of a judgment that they are beyond the reach of medical treatment that would restore consciousness…Recognizing that judgments about the benefits and burdens of medically assisted nutrition and hydration in individual cases have a subjective element and are generally best made by the patient directly involved, we also affirm a legitimate role for families' love and guidance, health care professionals' ethical concerns, and society's interest in preserving life and protecting the helpless."[23]

Jewish ethical perspective[25] contends that man should not intervene in the process of death because the principle of sanctity of life means that every moment of life is invaluable. Schostak's has attempted to develop artificial feeding guidelines that are "medically viable, Halachically-sensitive, and compatible with state and federal law."[25] He states that some Halachic authorities maintain "that providing proper nutrition is imperative, even in situations where intravenous feeding might only prolong a life of pain," while others maintain that artificial nutrition is a medical procedure that may be refused. Some Halachic authorities suggest that patients may refuse extraordinary treatment, especially those associated with pain. Jewish law distinguishes between commission and omission in regard to treatment. The Islamic faith mirrors the Jewish faith. It adds the belief that the physician "should avoid predicting whether the patient will live or die, should treat the strong and the weak, the rich and the poor, the wise and the illiterate."[26] The belief is that, while removing care is wrong, not initiating care is acceptable.

The religious viewpoint of an individual must be considered before initiating artificial feeding. For those who believe that withdrawing feeding is acceptable, it may be initiated early in the care process. For those who will not withdraw feeding, more deliberation is needed on when to initiate it. The outer limits of acceptability for nutritional well-being may be used as the point to initiate nutrition support rather than earlier implementation of feeding.

Key Legal Decisions

Within the past two decades landmark judicial decisions addressing the withdrawal of life-sustaining medical procedures have been made. The question of whether nutrition and hydration constitute a medical procedure has been debated. The determination of the wishes of the patient and the role of surrogate decision makers continues to evolve. The Nancy Cruzan case[21] constitutes the current U.S. legal framework for care of the PVS patient. Five U.S. Supreme Court Justices wrote opinions on the case.

The Cruzan family requested removal of their adult daughter's feeding tube after the daughter had been in a PVS for 5 years. The hospital staff refused to honor the request without a court order. The Missouri trial court found that Nancy had a fundamental right to "refuse or direct the withdrawal of 'death-prolonging procedures,'"[21] however, the Supreme Court of Missouri reversed the lower court's ruling, skeptical that the right to refuse treatment applied in this case. It upheld the State's right to preserve life, and ruled that there was insufficient evidence to support the parents' claim of Nancy's wishes. The U.S. Supreme Court agreed to "consider the question of whether Cruzan has a right under the United States Constitution which would require the hospital to withdraw life-sustaining treatment from her under these circumstances."[21] The U.S. Supreme Court's 1990, five-four decision affirmed the state's right to determine its level "for clear and convincing evidence" in "proceedings where a guardian seeks to discontinue nutrition and hydration of a person diagnosed to be in a persistent vegetative state."[21] The definition of "clear and convincing evidence" is decided upon by each state, and ranges from oral substitute judgment to written statements. The Supreme Court also affirmed that artificial nutrition was medical treatment and thus could be refused, as can all other medical treatments. The health care community has generally endorsed this concept that artificial nutrition is a medical treatment. However, there is still a minority viewpoint that there is limited difference between tube feeding and oral nutrition and that "food provided is not transformed into an exotic medical substance by pouring it into a tube."[27]

In its opinion, the U.S. Supreme Court states, "[the] principle that a competent person has a constitutionally protected liberty interest in refusing unwanted medical treatment may be inferred from our prior decisions," and later says, "we assume that the United States Constitution would grant a competent person a constitution protected right to refuse lifesaving hydration and nutrition."[21] The deeply personal decision of life or death is mentioned in the various opinions.

Six months after the U.S. Supreme Court decision, after three new witnesses testified to Nancy's desire not to continue life-sustaining medical treatment, the court case was dropped and court permission was granted for the feeding tube to be removed. The decision of the Court emphasizes the need for written directives and the use of health care proxies.

For 25 years, decisions on medical treatment have favored personal autonomy and the patient's beliefs as taking precedence over the professional's belief. These cases focused on the right to stop medical treatment. In the mid-1990s a growing number of cases and articles focused on the issue of futility of care. A foundation in ethics and a review of key cases is necessary to provide a basis for ethical considerations in nutrition support.

The issue of futility of care was raised in the Helga Wanglie case shortly after the Cruzan case was settled.[28] Mrs. Wanglie, an 86-year-old woman, suffered severe brain damage after a stroke in a nursing home and was diagnosed as permanently unconscious, after rehospitalization. Her physicians stated that her respirator and feeding tube were of no benefit to her in restoring consciousness. The physician described her care as nonbeneficial and medically inappropriate. The family argued the intrinsic value of life to Mrs. Wanglie. The Minnesota District Court decided the best decision maker was her husband because she had no advance directive. Wanglie died with the respirator and feeding tube in place. "Because the Wanglie case ended as it did, no court has yet ruled whether, in the presence of clear and convincing evidence that a PVS patient wants life-sustaining treatment, physicians may nonetheless withhold or withdraw treatment on the grounds that it is medically inappropriate or nonbeneficial."[28] Nelson, at the National Center for Clinical Ethics, states that a patient's request for care does not "obligate a physician or other health provider to provide that treatment."[10] However, medical futility does not preclude care, and compassionate care includes extending life for a few days based on the wishes of the patient. The issue of futility of care is discussed further under Ethical Considerations.

In February 1993, the British House of Lords determined that the withdrawal of medical treatment and support, including hydration and nutrition, from Anthony Bland, a PVS patient, was lawful. Using the Bolam principle, a principle based on a responsible body of medical opinion, the House of Lords stated that health professionals can act on what they believe is in the best interest of the patient and thus may start treatment considered appropriate or curtail treatment considered inappropriate.[29]

Back in the United States, a case in the Massachusetts courts in spring 1995[30] involved a daughter who was suing the doctors and hospital for mental anguish caused by their refusing to take extraordinary steps to keep her comatose mother alive. The needed balance is trust that any physician or health care provider will give the best care while not being required to give futile care.

In an institutional setting, the right of the patient to have feeding withdrawn is in direct conflict with society's obligation to preserve life. The courts have decided numerous cases. In general, the patient's interests take precedence over the State's interest when the patient has an incurable condition and the burden outweighs the benefit. In a long-term care facility in New York State an 85-year-old man was allowed to fast. He died after 45 days.[31] In cases in which the patient's interests are not known, the family's judgment predominates if there is agreement within the family. In 1998, the right of a wife to stop the feeding of her permanently unconscious husband was challenged by the Governor of Virginia; the courts ruled in favor of the wife.[32]

Assisted Suicide

While withholding or withdrawing life-sustaining treatments has become well accepted, euthanasia remains illegal. A study of physician-assisted suicide and euthanasia in Washington State[33] found that 26% of physicians in the State had received explicit requests from patients for assistance. Patients with cancer, acquired immunodeficiency syndrome (AIDS), and neurologic disorders most frequently made the request. Physicians granted the request for 24% of the patients; the physician's decision often related to the extent of physical symptoms. In a similar study[34] of critical care nurses across the United States, 17% reported receiving requests for euthanasia or assisted suicide from a patient or the family. Approximately 19% of the nurses had complied with the request at least once. The reasons given by the nurses "include concern about the overuse of life-sustaining technology, a profound sense of responsibility for the patient's welfare, a desire to relieve suffering, and a desire to overcome the perceived unresponsiveness of physicians toward that suffering"[11] The ANA's position statements hold that nurses should not participate in these activities.[35]

In 1994, Oregon approved a law supporting physician-assisted suicide for terminally ill patients.[36] In Oregon, the physician must be willing to participate and must determine if the patient meets the provisions of the law. The Oregon Act sets forth specific procedures for the patient and the physician to attempt to prevent coercion or impaired judgment. The Law states that a physician cannot assist with the death, except through writing the drug prescription. The Alper and Momeyer articles provide good discussion of these complex issues.[36,37] In 1996, the State of Oregon voted to approve assisted suicide. At least 70 people have taken their lives with medication prescribed by their doctors since the law took effect in 1997. The constitutionality of the new law is now being questioned. In November 2001, the U.S. Attorney General authorized federal agents to take action against physicians who prescribe medication that would hasten death.[38] The State of Oregon ruled in April 2002 that the federal government could not interfere with Oregon. In May 2002, the U.S. Department of Justice appealed this decision.[39]

The debate on assisted suicide is intensifying. In March 1996, a Federal appeals court for the nine western states struck down a Washington State law that made assisted suicide a felony.[40] This increases the odds that the Oregon law may be upheld. Eight other states are actively considering laws allowing assisted suicide. In April 1996, The Federal Court of Appeals covering New York struck down a law prohibiting doctors from assisting in suicides.[41] The debate is one of personal liberty on the *pro* side, and fear of mistakes and abuse, especially during this period of cost containment in health care, on the *con* side.

The American College of Physicians-American Society of Internal Medicine published a position paper in 2000 recommending terminal sedation and voluntary withholding of food and fluids as an alternative to physician-assisted suicide for patients with intolerable pain.[42] The purpose of the sedation is to alleviate suffering, not cause death. A decision to cease consuming food is a patient's choice that the health care team should respect, forcing feeding in this situation could be considered assault. This is only suggested if the patient has decision-making capacity and the suffering cannot be relieved. Miller[43] points out that dehydration is preferred over assisted suicide because of its voluntary nature and because it cannot be accomplished on impulse.

Self-Determination

The Patient Self-Determination Act took effect on December 1, 1991.[44] It requires all Medicare/Medicaid health care providers to inform patients of their right to prepare advance directives and to refuse treatment.[45] Advance directives may take the form of a living will, a proxy appointment, or a durable power of attorney for health care. They were designed to give patients a means of influencing their medical care when they do not have the capacity to do so.[46] The living will legally states what treatments patients wish or do not wish if they become incompetent to express an opinion. Any adult may change their advance directives at any time. The advance directive may include the designation of someone to make proxy health care decisions in the event that the person cannot make these decisions himself or herself.

Only a capable adult may write advance directives. A distinction is made between being capable of handling a medical treatment decision and being *competent*.[47] A patient may be incompetent to handle money but have the *capability* to make an informed decision using reasonable judgment. The determination of whether the *incompetent* patient has made a reasonable judgment can be based on whether the decision is "internally consistent with the patient's other expressed beliefs."[41] Each state has regulations on advance directives, do-not-resuscitate orders, and declaration of death. These are found in the state register. For example, in New Jersey,[48] *decision-making capacity* means "a patient's ability to understand and appreciate the nature and consequences of health care decisions, including the benefits and risks of each, and alternatives to any proposed health care, and to reach an informed decision. A patient's decision-making capacity is evaluated relative to the demands of a particular health care decision." In New Jersey, fluids and nutrition are also listed as life-sustaining treatment.

The Patient Self-Determination Act places the patient as the decision maker regarding medical treatment. It is important to note that many persons of Asian, Spanish, or Russian descent believe that "it is harmful for physicians to tell patients about serious diagnoses and that the family should monitor what is told to the patient and should make the decisions about treatment."[49] Again, the balance of the individual's preference and the rule should go to an ethics committee and to legal counsel. Pantilat[49] suggests health care providers may want to discuss the issue of preference in knowing the results of any diagnostic tests before initiating testing. Table 44-1 suggests a framework for cultural sensitivity.[50]

A study published in *JAMA* in November 1995[46] explored communication of advance directives from outpatient to inpatient in a geriatric population. To achieve their purpose, such

TABLE 44-1

A Framework for Cultural Sensitivity in Discussions of Advance Directives

Goals of Discussion	Cultural Considerations
Providing information	Identify language problems
	Determine comprehension
	Recognize power and status differences
	Include culturally relevant persons (e.g., family members, spiritual advisors, traditional healers, community or tribal leaders)
Eliciting patient values	Recognize beliefs about illness and disease; role of family, spiritual advisors, healers; care of the dying; treatment of the dead; organ donation
Determining patient wishes	Identify appropriate decision maker
	Avoid cultural stereotyping
	Do not make assumptions
Acting on patient wishes	Respect cultural differences
	Recognize own cultural prejudices and biases
Reviewing patient wishes	Recognize potential for change in views

From Marshall PA: Issues of ethnic, racial, and cultural diversity. In *Advance directives: the role of health care professionals*. Report of the Sixteenth Ross Roundtable on Medical Issues, Columbus, OH, 1996, Ross Products Division, Abbott Laboratories, pp 25–30.

documents must be "available, recognized, and honored under clinical circumstances when they should be invoked."[46] The study indicated that only 25% of the advance directives were recognized but, when recognized, were used correctly.

For the nutritionist, the two major ethical responsibilities are to ensure that the patient makes the decision about nutrition treatments and that the patient has sufficient information to determine whether artificial nutrition is desirable for their well-being. Patients, often not understanding what tube feedings are, indicate that they do not want *artificial nutrition*. The dietitian has the responsibility to be sensitive to the values and other preferences of the patient and to seek clarification of the desire for artificial feeding when a discrepancy is noted. The organizational structure of the institution often dictates whether the dietitian has this discussion or whether another member of the team talks with the patient. Boxes 44-2 and 44-3 provide considerations for examining the efficacy of foregoing or providing aggressive nutrition support.

Futility of Care

Since the beginnings of medicine, physicians have been encouraged to limit useless care. The problem has been to determine when care is futile and what to do when there is disagreement on the futility of care. The question of benefit enters in when futility is discussed. The question of whether care is obligatory or optional surfaces. A common method of distinguishing between obligatory and optional is to consider the effects or the outcome, the benefits, and burdens. The question goes back to the issue of whether nutrition is medical treatment or basic care. Nutrition can be effective in that it maintains life, but it cannot prevent death from a terminal illness or restore consciousness. In such cases nutrition may be considered futile as a medical treatment "because the ultimate goal of any

Considerations for Examining the Efficacy of Forgoing or Discontinuing Aggressive Nutrition Support

I. Questions that can help determine the potential burdens include:
   A. What is the level of risk for potential medical and metabolic complications from each available nutrition alternative?
   B. Will the administration of tube feeding or parenteral nutrition at home or in a health care facility be contraindicated because of staffing, monitoring ability, or financial constraints?
   C. Will the nutritional benefits of the insertion of an enteral or parenteral feeding tube during hospitalization create feelings of abandonment if tube feeding is unavailable upon discharge?
II. Forgoing or discontinuing enteral or parenteral nutrition support may be considered when some or all of the following are present:
   A. Death is imminent, within hours or a few days.
   B. Enteral or parenteral feeding will probably worsen the condition, symptoms, or pain, such as during shock, when pulmonary edema or diarrhea, vomiting, or aspiration would cause further complications.
   C. A competent patient has expressed an informed preference not to receive aggressive nutrition support that would be ineffective in improving the quality of life and/or which may be perceived by the patient as undignified, degrading, and physically or emotionally unacceptable.
   D. If available and legally recognized, written advanced directives such as the "living will" or "durable power of attorney for medical care" may indicate the preference of an incompetent patient. Otherwise, the next of kin or patient appointed surrogate of an incompetent patient should be consulted about the patient's probable preference for the level of nutrition intervention, as well as state law.
III. Written ethical guidelines for assessing and implementing these considerations should be established through the facility's ethics committee, if available, and in accordance with legal guidance.
IV. Legal precedents and regulations or statutes establishing feeding parameters within local and state jurisdiction should be considered when deciding to require or forgo nutrition support. The facility's written protocol and legal counsel should also be consulted.

From The American Dietetic Association Position Paper. Issues in feeding the terminally ill adult, *J Am Diet Assoc* 92:996-1005, 1992.

medical intervention should be improvement of the patient's prognosis, comfort, well-being, or general state of health."[7] Conversely, one may be reluctant to withdraw feeding, thinking it is morally obligatory, because the withdrawal of nutrition may hasten death.[7]

If the decision is that there is an obligation to feed the terminally ill or permanently unconscious patient, is there ever a time when the obligation stops? Can it be overridden when we are certain that the condition is irreversible for the permanently unconscious or increases pain for the terminally ill? Does moral obligation change to moral option?

For the unconscious patient, does a time frame suggesting permanency, whether that be 1, 12, or more months, shift the moral duty to a moral option? If the patient cannot feel the burden of pain and suffering it cannot be a physical burden. Can it, however, be an emotional or financial one? For the terminally ill person, can the burden or pain and suffering make feeding a moral option? Can it be medically futile but emotionally beneficial? To argue that feeding is a benefit because of sanctity of life, can be countered with the "dignity of death" arguments. The singular goal of prolonging life as a patient goal is not an independent, but rather a dependent, goal accord-

ing to Tong.[22] The physician's responsibility is "restoring and correcting." There is general agreement that patients have the right to refuse treatment and decide for themselves if a treatment is a moral obligation or option, based on physical, emotional, and financial burdens.

The next debatable question is, because the patient has a right to refuse care, does that also mean that the patient has the right to demand care? Does the patient have the right to set treatment decisions or are those decisions in the hands of the doctors or the insurance carriers? If a patient were to demand parenteral feeding when it was unwarranted, should it be given? The consensus of nutrition support providers is that as health professionals our stewardship responsibility requires that we not waste health dollar resources. Thus, if enteral feeding is the best therapy, its cost should be covered; if the patient wanted PN, the patient should pay the difference. Thorny issues such as this should be addressed in policies formulated by an institutional committee, possibly the ethics committee. The dietitian's role is to explain options and present them. The discussion should encompass the unique needs and values of the individual. These include culturally diverse attitudes and the patient's personal attitudes toward feeding.

Regarding enteral feeding, the Wanglie case started to examine whether patients have the right to demand treatment if it is not beneficial or is medically inappropriate. There is as yet "no official consensus among physicians that it is inappropriate to aggressively treat PVS patients or that prolonging life is not an 'independent' and 'overriding' goal of medicine, and such a consensus may be long in coming,"[22] and may not be desirable. A survey conducted of 1000 members of the American College of Physicians after the Cruzan case generally "favored either withholding tube feeding from the severely demented patient or withdrawing tube feeding from the patient in a persistent vegetative state."[51] Even if physicians agreed, society might be foolish to give over to the health care provider unilateral say on what is better for the patient.[52] The debate on futility is in the early stages. Public values and standards of care for PVS patients will evolve. Angell reminds health care providers, "any solution must be a principled one that applies generally and is established by consensus, in the same way that death was redefined as brain death."[52]

The question of the definition of death and the need to redefine the death is surfacing. One argument is that some "potential for cognitive function is necessary for personhood, and that, when this is absent in cases of anencephaly and persistent vegetative state, the individual should be considered dead."[53] Lizza believes that the definition of death is a philosophic one of whether cognitive function is essential to be a person.[53] Tong suggests that legislative or social changes may be the solution.[22] The definition of *death* could change to include when higher brain function ceases. This would then include the PVS. Such changes would have society rather than the physicians decide, but the lack of diagnostic certainty complicates this approach.[22]

Justice and Scarce Resources

The cost of health care confronts health care providers daily. The question of whether cost should be a factor in clinical

BOX 44-3

Suggested Ethical Deliberations about Nutrition and Hydration

1. The patient's expressed desire for extent of medical care is a primary guide for determining the level of nutrition intervention.
2. The decision to forgo hydration or nutrition should be weighed carefully because such a decision may be difficult or impossible to reverse with a period of days or weeks.
3. The expected benefits, in contrast to the potential burdens, of nonoral feeding must be evaluated by the health care team and discussed with the patient. The focus of care should include the patient's physical and psychological comfort.
4. Food and hydration are considered medical interventions.
5. Consider whether or not nutrition, either oral or artificial, will improve the patient's quality of life during the final stages of life.
6. Consider whether or not nutrient support, either oral or artificial, can be expected to provide the patient with emotional comfort, decreased anxiety about disease cachexia, improved self-esteem with cosmetic benefits, improved interpersonal relationships, or relief from fear of abandonment.
7. If death is imminent and feeding will not alter condition consider whether or not nutrient support will be burdensome.
8. When oral intake is appropriate:
   a. Oral feeding should be advocated whenever possible. Food and control of food intake may give comfort, pleasure and sense of autonomy and dignity. The most important priority is to provide food according to the individual patient's wishes.
   b. Efforts should be made to enhance the patient's physical and emotional enjoyment of food by encouraging staff and family assistance in feeding the patient.
   c. Nutrition supplements, including commercial products and other alternatives, should be used to encourage intake and ameliorate symptoms associated with hunger, thirst, or malnutrition.
   d. The therapeutic rationale of previous diet prescriptions for an individual patient should be reevaluated. Many dietary restrictions can be liberalized. Coordination of medication or medication schedules with the diet should be discussed with the physician, with the objective of maximizing food choice and intake by the patient.
   e. The patient's right to self-determination must be considered in determining whether to allow the patient to consume foods that are not generally permitted within the diet prescription.
   f. Suboptimal oral feedings may be more appropriate than burdensome tube or parenteral feeding.
9. When tube feeding or parenteral feeding is being considered:
   a. The patient's informed preference for the level of nutrition intervention is primary. The patient or substitute decision maker should be advised on how to accomplish whatever feeding the patient desires.
   b. When palliative care is the agreed goal nutritional support must be part of the palliative plan. A palliative care plan does not automatically preclude aggressive nutrition support. The decision to forgo "heroic" medical treatment does not preclude baseline nutrition support. All options for nutritional support can be considered.
   c. Feeding may not be desirable if death is expected within hours or a few days and the effects of partial dehydration or the withdrawal of nutrition support will not adversely alter patient comfort.
   d. Facilities should provide and distribute written protocols for the provision of and termination of tube feedings and parenteral feedings. The protocols should be reviewed periodically, and revised if necessary, by the health care team. Legal and ethical counsel should be routinely sought during the development and interpretation of the guidelines. The institution's ethics committee, if available, should assist in establishing and implementing defined, written guidelines for nutrition support protocol. The registered dietitian should be a contributing member of or consultant to such a committee.
   e. Conflict within the family or among stakeholders can be resolved by referring to an ethics committee or consultant if available within the institution.
   f. The potential benefits vs. burdens of tube feeding or parenteral feeding should be weighed on the basis of specific facts concerning the patient's medical and mental status, as well as on the facility's options and limitations.
   g. Facility options and limitations—one should consider the following:
      (1) lack of staffing—no one to manage or monitor feeding
      (2) too costly without financial help
      (3) if a feeding strategy is started in one site it will have to be stopped when the patient is transferred to another site, which can lead to a sense of abandonment.
10. Either short- or long-term parenteral nutrition should be considered only when other routes are impossible or inadequate to meet the comfort needs of the patient.
11. The physician's written diet order in the medical chart documents the decision to administer or forgo nutrition support.
    a. The registered dietitian should participate in the decision.
    b. If a decision is made that the registered dietitian does not agree with, appeal to the facility's ethics mechanism (committee or consultant) is appropriate.
    c. If the court has ordered feeding or no feeding and you do not agree with the court's decision, appealing to the facility's ethics mechanism is appropriate.

From the American Dietetic Association Position Paper: Ethical and legal issues in nutrition, hydration, and feeding, *J Am Diet Assoc* 102:716-726, 2002.

---

ethical decision making is intensifying as resources become scarcer. What constitutes just and fair allocation of scarce resources?[7] Because it is widely accepted that medical treatment may be withdrawn when the burden outweighs the benefit, and because the PVS patient is said to experience nothing, the "benefits and burdens" question changes. The issue is thus *futility*. To date, the principle of justice has not been applied as the sole ethical consideration in individual patient care decisions.

The issue of justice for the PVS patient may intensify within society and the medical community because of economics. For PVS patients, Tong and Angell offer some interesting points to consider. For example, it could be required, as a principle of justice, that people who want to live in a PVS purchase insurance for the care and feeding or pay out-of-pocket.[22, 52] Angell suggests that the presumption be that the PVS patient would not want to be alive permanently unconscious. The health care team would then need to establish guidelines for when to stop artificial feeding, based on when irreversibility is virtually certain. Families could then object and document the patient's earlier wishes.[52]

The cost of enteral feeding for terminally ill persons should not be an issue, because of the minimal expense. The broader ethical issues of end-of-life decisions; and the process of prolonging death; and pain, for those dying in acute care, will be addressed in the coming decade. Miller and Fins[54] suggest remodeling hospital care for dying patients to take the form of an alternative-care unit that focuses on comfort care rather than aggressive care and that allows more patient and family participation in treatment planning. They conclude, "To integrate life-sustaining treatment and palliative care, it is important to address the idea that many clinicians, patients, and family members continue to hold: that forgoing life-sustaining treatment means 'giving up' and 'doing nothing' for the patient.

BOX 44-4

Dietary Management of Common Symptoms in Terminally Ill Patients

BELCHING

- Try to determine which foods cause the belching, especially the gas producers: carbonated drinks, beer and alcohol, dairy products, other high-fat foods, and legumes and vegetables high in fiber. Let the patient make all final choices about what to and what not to eat.
- Have the patient eat solids at mealtime and take fluids between meals, not with solid foods.
- Have the patient eat slowly and relax before, during, and after eating. The patient should not, however, recline just after eating.
- The patient should, to the degree possible, keep his or her mouth closed when chewing or swallowing, not chew gum, and not suck through straws.

CONSTIPATION

- If adequate fluid intake can be maintained, the patient should eat high fiber foods—whole grains, nuts, vegetables and fruits such as pineapple, prunes, and raisins. If severe constipation, dehydration, or obstruction become problems high-fiber foods should be avoided.
- If they contribute to constipation, discontinue calcium and iron supplements, and limit cheeses and rich desserts.
- Have the patient increase his or her fluid intake to maximum tolerable levels. This is especially important if bulk-forming laxatives are being used. Offer cider, fruit juices, and prune juice. An effective, low cost laxative: 1–2 ounces with the evening meal of a mixture of two cups applesauce, two cups unprocessed bran, and one cup 100% prune juice.

DIARRHEA

- If they are contributing to the diarrhea, urge the limitation of foods such as milk and ice cream; whole grain products; nuts and legumes; greens, raw and gas-forming vegetables; fruits with seeds and skins; fresh pineapple and raisins; alcohol and caffeine-containing beverages.
- Urge the patient to eat bananas, applesauce, peeled apples, tapioca, rice, peanut butter, refined grains, crackers, pasta, cream of wheat, oatmeal, and cooked vegetables.
- Encourage eating the meal without liquids. Offer fluids, especially those containing sugar and electrolytes, an hour after eating.
- Have the patient relax before, during, and after a meal.
- If dehydration accompanies the diarrhea, offer foods high in potassium.
- With AIDS patients, enteral and/or parenteral nutrition support may be appropriate. In such cases the diet formula should be high in calories and protein, and low in fiber.

HYPERCALCEMIA

- Do not discourage foods with a high calcium content, such as ice cream, if the patient wants them; but caution against the use of calcium and vitamin D supplements.
- Encourage fluids as tolerated, particularly carbonated drinks containing phosphoric acid.

MENTAL DISORDERS

- Urge the patient to discontinue alcohol and foods and beverages high in caffeine—coffee, tea, chocolate—if they contribute to anxiety, sleep deprivation, or depression.
- With the *drowsy or apathetic* patient help the family to assume the responsibility for feeding him or her. Urge them to prepare the patient's favorite foods in bite sizes and/or soft forms if the patient can be helped to spoon feed him- or herself. Help the family protect the patient and others from possible harm that might be inflicted by the patient by shutting off stoves or removing knobs, removing matches, and locking doors to cupboards that contain alcohol, medications, or poisons. Unplug microwave ovens and put away small electrical appliances.

- Urge the family to be cautious when hand feeding the *agitated or confused* patient: feed with a spoon and do not allow patient to handle utensils. Use reality orientation by reminding the patient what time of day it is, what meal is being served, and that the foods being served are his or her favorites. While trying to make mealtime pleasant by reminiscing about the past, minimize conversation if the patient appears frightened or confused. Urge the family to care fully consider the pros and cons of waking the patient if he or she is asleep at mealtime.
- In the case of the *stuporous or comatose* patient, remind the family that semi-starvation and dehydration are not painful to the patient and, if they ask about it, explore with them the pros and cons of enteral and parenteral nutrition support.

MOUTH PROBLEMS

- When foods taste *bitter* to the patient—instead of the foods usually associated with bitter tastes: red meats, sour juices, tomatoes, coffee, and tea, chocolate—suggest that he or she try poultry, fish, dairy products, and eggs. Do not serve foods in metallic containers or use metallic utensils. Use herbs and spices as seasoning and encourage sweet fruit drinks, ice lollipops, and carbonated beverages.
- When foods taste *too sweet* to the patient, encourage the drinking of sour juices; cooking with lemon juice, vinegar, spices, herbs, and mint; add pickles when appropriate.
- When foods have *no taste* for the patient suggest marination, if appropriate; the serving of highly seasoned foods; the addition of sugar; and serving foods at room temperature.
- When the patient has *difficulty swallowing* urge frequent small meals of soft or pureed foods; caution against foods that might irritate the mouth or esophagus, such as acidic fruits or juices; foods that are spicy or very hot or cold, alcohol, and carbonated beverages.
- When the patient has *mouth sores* urge cold and blenderized foods, cream soups and gravies, eggnog, milkshakes, cheesecake and cream pies, and macaroni and cheese. Have the patient avoid alcohol, and acidic, spicy, rough, hot, and highly salted foods.
- When the patient has a *dry mouth* urge frequent sips of water, juice, ice chips, ice lollipops, ice cream, fruitades, or slushy-frozen baby foods mixed with fruit juices. Suggest sucking on hard candies to stimulate saliva production. Solid foods should be moist, pureed if necessary, and not too tart, too hot, or too cold.

NAUSEA AND VOMITING

- Suggest that the patient not eat.
- If the patient wants to and can tolerate eating, encourage small meals of cool, odor-free foods. Avoid fatty or greasy and fried foods; avoid high bulk foods; do not mix hot and cold foods at the same meal. Discourage the intake of alcohol, and sweet and/or spicy foods.
- Urge the patient to eat slowly and avoid overeating, to relax before and after meals, and to avoid physical activity or lying flat for 2 hours after eating.
- Recommend that the patient not prepare his or her own food.

INTESTINAL OBSTRUCTION

- If oral intake is not contraindicated, encourage the patient to eat small meals of blenderized or strained foods that are low in fiber and residue. Offer the biggest meal early in the day. Many patients eat large portions of their favorite foods and then vomit. A gastric tube open to straight or intermittent drainage may relieve this need for frequent vomiting. With vomiting, foods high in potassium should be encouraged.
- In the case of "squashed stomach syndrome" have the patient eat frequent small meals, avoid nausea- and gas-producing foods, avoid high-fat or fried foods and foods that have strong odors. Limit fluid with meals, offering them 45 minutes before and after the meal.

From Maillet JO, King D: Nutritional care of the terminally ill, *The Hospice Journal* 9(2/3):37–54, 1993; adapted from Gallagher-Allred C: *Nutritional care of the terminally ill,* Rockville, MD, Aspen Publishers, Inc., 1989; pp 151-195.

Coordination of the ICU with the alternative-care unit should help dispel this misconception by demonstrating that when aggressive life support stops, there remains the challenging and rewarding task of helping patients manage the process of dying with comfort and dignity." [54]

The Dietitian's Role

Dietitians have the expertise in EN and PN and should study and keep up with debates on the ethical, social, and legal principles of feeding patients and should participate with the health care team and society in the debate and development of these principles and standards of care. The dietitian's special professional responsibility is in achieving the goal of informed nutrition care decision making by the patient, for the patient's physical and emotional comfort. Dietitians should provide patients, their families, and the health care team with the best options for oral nutrition, EN, and PN.

Box 44-4 suggests some ways of helping terminally ill persons eat when they can eat orally but have common symptoms associated with terminal illness.[55,56] The dietitian should encourage oral intake when possible and set the stage to make eating a pleasurable experience. The common and unique needs of each patient, including organ dysfunction, symptoms, and caregiver issues, will have to be addressed. Patients' apprehension about feeding decisions range from the fear of being coerced and force fed, at one extreme, to the fear of being starved by "passive neglect," at the other. Developing ethical, humane feeding guidelines that seek a delicate balance between too much and too little requires wise deliberation. By weighing all crucial factors, it is possible to provide appropriate care for each patient in the context of changing physical and environmental conditions. This requires that the practitioner listens well, clarifies options, sets forth pros and cons, and supports the patient's or family's choices.[57] Patients should have the opportunity to continue to discuss the ramifications of their choices and the opportunity to change their mind. Clarification of what EN and PN involve and their benefits and risks are an important part of the patient's informed consent. The pros and cons of initiating EN or PN should be presented, incorporating the patient's beliefs concerning withdrawal of feeding into the discussion. An example follows: A terminally ill patient who practices Orthodox Judaism tells you that he does not want a tubefeeding. Since maximizing life is the norm for that religion, the dietitian should explain what enteral feeding entails to ensure that the patient is making an informed decision without placing a value on the final decision. The dietitian may also be called upon to explain the natural process of dying when a family is struggling that the patient has stopped eating and drinking.

Conclusion

The health care team members, including the dietitian, must set treatment goals that are patient centered and tailored to the patient's personal values. The patient's expressed desire is the touchstone for determining the extent of nutrition and hydration. Good communication is essential to ensure informed consent. Consistent stances the patient takes over time support

their authenticity. The health care team and the family should share in decision making when the patient's preference is not stated and the family agrees with the legal parameters of the state. The health care team should discuss with the family, when necessary, ethics, values, religious guidelines, and referral for pastoral counseling.

If the patient's choice is feeding, the dietitian should ensure that the composition of the meals or feeding promotes nutritional health. If the patient's choice is cessation of feeding, the dietitian should explain what is known about the interval between cessation and death. Sensitivity to the family's needs and questions is imperative in both scenarios.

When the benefits of the treatment are in dispute the situation requires "clarification, further discussion and, perhaps, negotiation and mediation."[10] Patients and families daily request that "everything possible be done," while health professionals face the futility of some treatments. "Do everything possible" might simply be a request for comfort and dignity. A shift from aggressive care to a caring ethic is encouraged.[58] This may require a shift in the perception of what medicine can do, and moving from a technology-driven approach to caring, humane patient care.

Institutional ethics committees should participate in establishing and implementing written guidelines for withholding or withdrawing feeding. A dietitian should be a member of (or a consultant to) any such committee and should have an integral role in institutional policy development. The dietitian should educate others in nutrition and hydration issues, advocate for the patient, and participate in legal and ethical considerations regarding feeding.

REFERENCES

1. Winter S: Terminal nutrition: framing the debate for withdrawal of nutrition support in terminally ill patients, *Am J Med* 109:723-726, 2000.
2. Callahan C, Haag K, Buchanan N, Nisi R: Decision-making for percutaneous endoscopic gastrostomy among older adults in a community setting, *J Am Geriatr Soc* 47(9):1105-1109, 1999.
3. President's Commission for the Study of Ethical Problems in Medicine and Biomedical and Behavioral Research. Making Health Care Decisions: *The ethical and legal implications of informed consent in the patient/practitioner relationship*, vol 1-3, No 82:6000637, Washington, DC, 1982, US Government Printing Office.
4. American Dietetic Association: Position of the American Dietetic Association: issues in feeding the terminally ill adult, *J Am Diet Assoc* 92:996-1005, 1992.
5. American Academy of Neurology: Position on certain aspects of the care and management of the persistent vegetative state patient, *Neurology* 39:125-126, 1989.
6. Kinney HC, Korein J, Panigraphy A, et al: Neuropathological findings in the brain of Karen Ann Quinlan, *N Engl J Med* 330(21):1469-1474, 1994.
7. Mitchell K, Kerridge I, Lovat T: Medical futility, treatment withdrawal and the persistent vegetative state, *J Med Ethics* 19:71-76, 1973.
8. Freeman EA: Protocols for vegetative patients, *Med J Aust* 159:428, 1993.
9. AMA Report of the Council on Ethical and Judicial Affairs. Medical futility and end-of-life care, *JAMA* 281(10):937-941, 1999.
10. Nelson W, Durnan JR, Spritz N, et al: Futility: the concept and its use, *Trends Health Care Law Ethics* 9(3):19-26, 1994.
11. American Dietetic Association: Position of the American Dietetic Association: Ethical and legal issues in nutrition, hydration, and feeding, *J Am Diet Assoc* 102(5):716-726, 2002.
12. Council on Scientific Affairs and Council on Ethical and Judicial Affairs: Persistent vegetative state and the decision to withdraw or withhold life support, *JAMA* 263(3):426-430, 1990.

13. American Nurses Association: Guidelines on withdrawing or withholding food and fluids. Ethics in nursing: position statements and guidelines, Kansas City, MO, 1988, American Nurses Association, 1988.

14. *Guidelines on the termination of life-sustaining treatment and the care of the dying. A report by the Hastings Center,* Briarcliff Manor, NY, 1987, The Hastings Center, 1987.

15. ASPEN Board of Directors: Guidelines for the use of parenteral and enteral nutrition in adult and pediatric patients, *J Parenter Enteral Nutr* 17(Suppl):505A-525A, 1993.

16. Code of Ethics for the Profession of Dietetics, *J Am Diet Assoc* 99:109-113, 1999.

17. American Thoracic Society: Withholding and withdrawing life-sustaining therapy, *Am Rev Respir Dis* 144:726-731, 1991.

18. Rappaport M, Dougherty A, Kelting DL: Evaluation of coma and vegetative states, *Arch Phys Med Rehabil* 73:628-634, 1992.

19. Mill JS: *On liberty,* New York, 1975, WW Norton.

20. Kant I: *The Philosophy of Kant: Immanuel Kant's moral and political writings,* NewYork, 1977, The Modern Library.

21. Nancy Beth Cruzan, by her parents and Co-Guardians, Lester L. Cruzan, et al., Petitioners v. Director, Missouri Department of Health, et al. Supreme Court Docket Number 88-15503. Argued: December 6, 1989; Decided: June 25, 1990.

22. Tong R: An exercise in futility: are we bidden to "treat" the untreatable?" *N Car Med J* 54(8):386-391, 1993.

23. Committee for Prolife Activities: *National Conference of Catholic Bishops. Nutrition and hydration: moral and pastoral reflections,* Washington, DC, 1992, US Catholic Conference Offices of Publishing and Promotion Services, pp 18-20.

24. Coggan F: On dying and dying well: spiritual and moral aspects, *Proc R Soc Med* 70:75-81, 1977.

25. Schostak RZ: Jewish ethical guidelines for resuscitation and artificial nutrition and hydration of the dying elderly, *J Med Ethics* 20:93-100, 1994.

26. Nanji AA: Medical ethics and the Islamic tradition, *J Med Phil* 13:257-275, 1988.

27. Rosner F: Why nutrition and hydration should not be withheld from patients, *Chest* 104(6):1892-1896, 1993.

28. In re Helga Wanglie, Fourth Judicial District (Dist. Ct. Div.) PX-91-283, Minnesota, Hennepin County.

29. Brahams D: Persistent vegetative state, *Lancet* 341:428, 1993.

30. Kolata G: Withholding care from patients: Boston case asks, who decides, *The New York Times,* April 3, 1995, pp A1, B8.

31. In the Matter of the Application of Plaza Health and Rehabilitation Center. (New York Supreme Court, Syracuse, February 6, 1984, Miller, J.)

32. James S. Gilmore, III, Governor of the Commonwealth of Virginia, et al v. Michele P. Finn; Michele P. Finn v. James S. Gilmore, III et al. Record No. 990796. Supreme Court of Virginia 259 Va.448;527 S.E. 2d 426;2000 Va.

33. Back AL, Wallace JI, Starks HE, Pearlman RA: Physician-assisted suicide and euthanasia in Washington State: patient requests and physician responses, *JAMA* 275(12):919-925, 1996.

34. Asch DA: The role of critical care nurses in euthanasia and assisted suicide, *N Engl J Med* 334(21):1374-1379, 1996.

35. Scanlon C: Euthanasia and nursing practice: right question, wrong answer, *N Engl J Med* 334(21):1401-1402, 1996.

36. Alpers A, Lo B: Physician-assisted suicide in Oregon, *JAMA* 274(6): 483-487, 1995.

37. Momeyer R: Does physician assisted suicide violate the integrity of medicine? *J Med Phil* 20:13-24, 1995.

38. Verhoveh SH: Federal agents are directed to stop physicians who assist suicides, *The New York Times,* Nov 7, 2001, p.A20.

39. The Health Care Advisory Board, 5/29/02. Accessed at http://www.advisory.com/members.

40. Lewin T: Ruling sharpens assisted-suicide debate: court, backing idea of personal liberty, brings issue to new level, *The New York Times,* March 8, 1996, p A14.

41. Fein E: Court overturns ban in New York on aided suicides: for doctors, an anxiety is removed, *The New York Times,* April 3, 1996, p 1, B5.

42. Quill T, Byock I: Responding to intractable terminal suffering: the role of terminal sedation and voluntary refusal of food and fluids, *Ann Intern Med* 132(5):408-414, 2000.

43. Miller FG, Meier D: Voluntary death: a comparison of terminal dehydration and physician-assisted suicide, *Ann Intern Med* 128:559-562, 1998.

44. La Puma J, Orentilicher D, Moss RJ: Advanced directives on admission. Clinical implications and analysis of the patient self-determination act of 1990, *JAMA* 266:402-405, 1991.

45. White M, Fletcher J: The patient self-determination act, *JAMA* 266(3):410B-412B, 1991.

46. Morrison RS, Olson E, Mertz K, Meier DE: The inaccessibility of advance directive on transfer from ambulatory to acute care settings, *JAMA* 274(6):478-482, 1995.

47. Goldstein MK, Fuller JD: Intensity of treatment in malnutrition: the ethical considerations, *Nutr Old Age* 21(1):191, 1994.

48. Advance directives to make health care decisions, do not resuscitate orders (DNR orders), and declaration of death, *N J Register* Jan 3, 1994, p 26NJR222.

49. Pantilat SZ: Patient-physician communication: respect for culture, religion, and autonomy, *JAMA* 275(2):107, 1996.

50. Marshall PA: Issues of ethnic, racial, and cultural diversity. In *Advanced directives: the role of health care professionals: report of the Sixteenth Ross Roundtable on Medical Issues,* Columbus, OH, 1996, Ross Products Division, Abbott Laboratories, pp 125-130.

51. Hodges M, Tolle SW, Stocking C, Cassel CK: Tube feeding. Internists' attitudes regarding ethical obligations, *Arch Intern Med* 154:1013-1020, 1994.

52. Angell M: After Quinlan: The dilemma of the persistent vegetative state, *N Engl J Med* 330(21):1524-1525, 1994.

53. Lizza JP: Persons and death: what's metaphysically wrong with our current statutory definition of death? *J Med Phil* 18:351-374, 1993.

54. Miller FG, Fins JJ: A proposal to restructure hospital care for dying patients, *N Engl J Med* 334(26):1740-1742, 1996.

55. Maillet JO, King D: Nutritional care of the terminally ill adult, *Hospice J* 9:37-54, 1993.

56. Gallagher-Allred C: *Nutritional care of the terminally ill,* Rockville, MD, 1989, Aspen Publishers, pp 151-195.

57. Gallagher-Allred CR: Managing ethical issues in nutrition support of terminally ill patients, *Nutr Clin Pract* 6:113-116, 1991.

58. Jecker NS, Schneiderman LJ: When families request that 'everything possible' be done, *J Med Phil* 20:145-163, 1995.

Economics of Nutrition Support 45

Charlene W. Compher, PhD, RD, FADA, CNSD
Jennifer Kay Nelson, MS, RD, LD, CNSD

THE economic issues around provision of parenteral nutrition (PN) and enteral nutrition (EN) to patients who need it are a complex and constantly changing force, with vital importance to nutrition professionals involved in the care of these patients. The purpose of this chapter is to elucidate the historic and current regulations pertaining to the economics of nutrition support provided in the hospital and at home.

Health Care Costs

U.S. health care economics have been the focus of much attention from consumers, employers, legislators, and health care providers. In the most recent year of data, the Health Care Financing Administration (HCFA) reported total health care costs of $1210.7 billion, 13% of the gross domestic product (GDP), and a reduction from the 13.4% spent in 1993. [1]

The Office of the Actuary at HCFA makes annual projections of future health expenditures, based on historical data interpreted with an actuarial, econometric, and judgment model. [1] In March, 2001, projections were made for 2000-2010, based on 1999 data. U.S. health expenditures are projected to total $2.6 trillion and reach 15.9% of the GDP by 2010. [1] This projection in part reflects faster health spending growth, in a setting of somewhat slower GDP growth.

The pattern of type of expenditure is also expected to change (Table 45-1). [1] A rapid increase in spending for prescription drugs is an important factor in the projected increase in total spending. Drug costs are impacted by low-cost copays for drug insurance coverage, direct advertising to consumers, and higher-cost medications. [1] Hospitalization costs are steadily being reduced as a portion of the total health care spending bill, to 27% in 2010. A final factor with significant impact on health care spending is the expansion of the elderly population from 34.7 million in 1999 to 39.3 million in 2010, thus increasing the total dollars needed for Medicare beneficiary coverage. [1]

These cost estimates generally underestimate actual health care expenditures. Direct medical costs do not include lost productivity in the workplace by patients or their family members. The time and cost of patient training, telephone support by medical professionals, and troubleshooting for home-delivered therapies are not included. The costs of home nutrition support, in particular, reflect only the supplies and equipment used, and thus grossly underestimate true cost.

Cost Containment

Government efforts to control costs historically have included the Balanced Budget Act (BBA) of the Prospective Payment System (PPS) in 1997, which reduced payments to health care providers. [2] After 3000 home health agencies closed, nursing homes sought bankruptcy protection, and many hospitals closed, the BBA Refinement legislation was enacted in 1999 to soften some of the 1997 budget cuts. [2]

Health care providers have also implemented measures to contain costs. To keep patient care decisions in the domain of physicians, primary gatekeeper arrangements have been created to respond to case-management strategies implemented by third-party carriers. A host of other efforts are under way to improve efficiency: development of practice guidelines, quality improvement initiatives, critical pathways, and clinical indicators. Efforts to assess and eliminate procedures and services that have no clearly demonstrable benefit include cost studies (cost minimization, cost benefit, cost effectiveness, cost utility) and outcomes management.

Expensive therapies such as nutrition support have been affected by efforts aimed at controlling reimbursement and costs, and these trends will continue. The effectiveness of nutrition support in relation to both cost and outcome will also determine its future course and utilization in the health care arena. These issues and future reimbursement trends of importance to nutrition support are discussed here.

TABLE 45-1

Health Care Expenditures in the United States: HCFA Data, Percentage Total Cost[1]

Year	Hospitalization	Professional Services	Nursing Home/Home Health	Prescription Drugs	Age > 65 yr*
1993	36%	32%	10%	5.7%	12.6%
1999	32%	33%	10%	8%	12.5%
2010[†]	27%	32%	10%	13.8%	13%

*Percentage of total population.
[†]Projected costs.

The Third-Party System

The term *third-party system* describes the current method of payment for health care services. Three parties are involved: the patient (first party), the provider of care (second party), and the insurer who manages the payment for the care (third party). Insurance companies exist to spread the costs of health care across many subscribers, rather than requiring any one patient to pay the entire cost.

Under the traditional third-party payer system, policy guidelines for coverage vary, so reimbursement can vary. All services may be reimbursed, or only selected ones, and the amount of reimbursement can also vary to cover only a portion of or the entire cost of the service. In most instances the patient is responsible for paying a limited portion of the provider's bill, in addition to the annual premium paid to the insurer. Medical services may also be covered as a benefit of employment.

The traditional third-party system evolved as health care costs began to escalate in the mid-1970s. Insurers placed greater limitations in their policies for inpatient services. To encourage health care providers to control costs, policies reimbursed a predetermined amount of money for a service (regardless of actual cost). This encouraged health care providers to control costs. An example of this is the PPS introduced by Medicare (see below).[3] Many private insurers have adopted a similar scheme. In the outpatient setting, managed care plans such as those of health maintenance organizations (HMOs) have been established. Insurers have also begun to reimburse care at alternative sites (such as skilled nursing facilities, or in the home), where therapies can be delivered at reduced cost.

Economics of Hospital-Based Nutrition Support

Simply stated, the system required to deliver nutrition support in the hospital includes the patient, the product (enteral or PN system), and the health care providers (physician, nurse, dietitian, pharmacist). It is difficult to establish a price for nutrition support because there are direct costs for the product and equipment and indirect costs for the facilities and personnel who administer it. In addition, the response of patients to nutrition support varies, and the response affects the type and duration of therapy and, in turn, costs.

Table 45-2 lists the average daily wholesale prices for PN and EN solutions and sets in the year 2000.[4] The actual costs to a hospital vary because of differences in purchasing power, type of product, manufacturer, and wholesaler. In most cases the patient charge is adjusted to offset labor and other indirect costs. Although hospitals may itemize these charges, their actual payment for these fees varies because of the terms of insurer payment agreements.

The ways in which hospital services are reimbursed vary considerably and depend on type of insurance. Insurance policies reimburse in any number of ways: as a percentage of gross charges, as a capitated rate, under *per diem* arrangements, or according to prospective payment schemes. Hospital accounting departments collect information on the types of reimbursement received and refer to it as a *payer mix*. This mix determines the amount of monies received by the hospital for services rendered. Because it is difficult to control payer mix, it is in the best

TABLE 45-2

Average 2000 Wholesale Prices for Parenteral and Enteral Nutrition Products[4]

	Parenteral	Enteral
Solution/formula*	$235	$18
Sets (each)	$30	$11
Total	$265	$29

*Parenteral solution: 500 ml of 50% dextrose in water with 500 ml of 10% amino acids, 500 ml of 10% intravenous fat, standard electrolytes, vitamins, and trace elements. Enteral formula: 1500 ml of 1 kcal/cc, isotonic formula.

financial interests of the hospital to control costs for services provided while maintaining maximum reimbursement.

The Prospective Payment System

The Prospective Payment System (PPS) was initiated by Medicare in 1983.[3] Many state Medicaid programs and Blue Cross plans also use this type of payment plan for inpatient services. Under this system, the hospital receives a set amount of money based on the specific diagnosis-related group (DRG) assigned to the patient's condition upon discharge. Payments are determined by the average cost of caring for patients in each DRG. There are a finite number of DRGs for which average costs for care (or reimbursement levels) have been established. There is also a base rate for payment that is determined by the characteristics of the hospital (e.g., urban or rural, a training hospital).

The PPS is intended to provide hospitals with incentive to control costs. A hospital receives the same amount of money for a patient who stays a short time and requires few services as for a patient with the same diagnosis who stays longer and requires many expensive services. As a result, this system for reimbursement encourages cost containment, increased efficiency, and improved outcome.

Although reimbursement is determined by the base rate and the DRG assignment, the presence of complications or comorbid conditions (CCs) can affect length of stay, number of treatment services, and cost.[3] CCs, when properly documented, can also increase the reimbursement.[5] The current DRG system is designed so that the presence of one or more CCs triggers a predetermined adjustment to reimbursement. Although only one CC is needed to increase reimbursement, it is important that all relevant diagnostic information be clearly documented in the medical record. In preparing DRG coding documents, hospital accounting departments compare all possible combinations of primary diagnoses and relevant CCs, to choose the combination that best describes the patient's condition while maximizing reimbursement. Most hospitals list five or more CCs on the DRG coding document.

Nutrition support is not directly reimbursed under the PPS. However, clearly documenting the presence of malnutrition or a nutrition-related diagnosis as a primary diagnosis or as a CC can affect reimbursement, as shown in Table 45-3.[6] In this scenario, a patient with gastrointestinal obstruction and no CC would be classified as DRG 181. The assigned relative weight for this diagnosis is 0.4979. Multiplying this by the base rate assigned to the hospital results in a payment of $1990 for this admission. A patient who has documented CCs (e.g.,

---

TABLE 45-3

Prospective Payment With and Without Complication or Comorbid Conditions[6]

Diagnosis	DRG	Relative Weight	Reimbursement*
Gastrointestinal obstruction, no comorbid condition	181	0.4979	$1990
Gastrointestinal obstruction, with comorbid condition	180	0.9139	$3655

*Calculated with average hospital Medicare base rate of $4000. Relative weight × base rate = amount reimbursed (figures rounded).

---

malnutrition) would be reclassified into DRG 180. The relative weight is increased to 0.9139, and the hospital would receive $3655 for this patient for this admission. The difference is $1665 that the hospital would either receive or forgo, depending on the patient's diagnosis and the CC.

Diagnosis coding for malnutrition has been shown to enhance hospital reimbursement, especially in hospitals with large patient populations covered under the PPS. Studies published in the late 1980s[7-12] indicated that some hospitals were able to increase revenue substantially, by $100,000 to $300,000 annually, by clearly coding malnutrition as a CC. On the other hand, hospitals with higher risk, more complicated, high acuity level patients may not be able to increase revenues because in all cases malnutrition was among many CCs and thus did not affect final reimbursement.[12]

Current payment is not the only reason to code all malnutrition or nutrition-related CCs that apply to a given case. New CCs may be considered in future revisions to the DRG system; likewise, some existing CCs may be eliminated because of infrequent use.[11] Prospective payment systems may vary from state to state, and all recorded CCs for a patient may be used to make annual adjustments to base DRG rates.[12] In addition, some hospitals may use CCs to track utilization rates for therapies and to signify the importance of a service, level of staffing, and need for additional resources.[12] In addition to ensuring that revenues for nutrition support are provided, nutrition support practitioners must also focus on cost containment and justify nutrition support results with positive outcomes.

Cost Containment and Outcomes in Hospital Nutrition Support

Malnutrition is common in hospitalized patients. As many as 40% to 50% are at risk for malnutrition;[13] up to 12% of them may be severely malnourished.[14] Patients with malnutrition are two to three times more likely to experience morbid complications than the well-nourished, and they are more likely to die.[15-17] Malnourished patients have significantly longer hospital stays, extended by as much as 90%.[18,19] In 1985, among malnourished hospitalized adults, costs per stay were estimated to be 35% and 75% higher than for well-nourished surgical and medical patients, respectively.[18,19] These data strongly suggest that malnutrition is associated with negative health outcomes, greater utilization of resources, and increased costs.[20]

Nutrition support is expensive, and efforts must be made to utilize it appropriately, effectively, and efficiently. A review of comparative trials[21-24] examining the influence of nutrition support teams on the provision of PN and EN found that teams produced significant benefits in the application of these therapies, largely through the development of protocols and standardization of practices. These resulted in reductions in sepsis,

mechanical complications, and metabolic abnormalities. Although savings have been accomplished, the cost effectiveness of nutrition support and of the teams who administer it remains controversial. By one report, the loss of a nutrition support nurse was associated with increased cost, inappropriate PN use, and catheter sepsis events.[25] Nutrition support team consultation was associated with reduced inappropriate PN starts and less hyperglycemia.[26] Few prospective studies have described fully the financial impact of personnel, supplies, solutions, monitoring activities, therapy-related complications, malnutrition-related complications, and patient outcomes.[23]

The challenge to nutrition support providers in the hospital setting includes justification of the use of nutrition support modalities and employment of the persons who oversee it. Continued efforts to reduce costs and improve patient outcomes are needed.

Economics of Home Nutrition Support

The events described thus far have dramatically affected the growth of home nutrition support. Implementation of Medicare's PPS in 1983 provided financial incentives for hospitals to discharge patients earlier. Also in the early 1980s, Medicare (and other insurers) acknowledged home nutrition support and began to cover it as a benefit. At that time nutrition support technology was available to sustain patients who did not require sophisticated medical monitoring in the hospital.

Home infusion therapy, which includes home nutrition support, is one of the most expensive and fastest-growing components of home health care.[27] In the most recent available data, at least 192,000 patients receive home nutrition support, 20% of the PN and 50% of home tube-feeding patients paid by Medicare.[28] The home infusion therapy industry represents a significant part of the total $33.1 billion home care costs in 1999.[1] From the early 1980s into the early 1990s, the number of providers of home infusion therapy had grown from a handful to more than 4500, but was reduced again after the BBA in 1997.[2]

It is difficult to establish a price for home nutrition support because direct costs for product and equipment and indirect costs for the support system needed to execute the therapy are intertwined. The current cost of 1 year of home PN has been estimated at $150,000 to $250,000, only 25% to 50% of the hospital-based cost.[29] When costs per patient were based on Medicare charges, the annual cost per patient for parenteral solutions was $55,193 ± 30,596, and for enteral solutions was $9605 ± 9327.[30] Annual hospitalizations were 0.52 to 1.1 for parenteral and 0 to 0.5 for the enteral group, costing $0 to $149,220 for the parenteral and $0 to $39,204 for the enteral group.[30]

TABLE 45-4

Prevailing Medicare Fees for Home Nutrition Support in Year 2000[31]

	Parenteral ($)	Enteral ($)
Solution/formula	248	9
20% Lipid, 3/wk	95	
Pump	22	11
Gravity set		7
Syringe set		6
IV pole	1	1
Pump	109	4
Supply kit	7	7
NG tube (1/mo)		1
Daily Total Fee	482	Syringe 16
		Gravity 25
		Pump 31
Medicare Reimbursement (80%)	396	Syringe 13
		Gravity 20
		Pump 25

BOX 45-1

2001 Medicare Criteria for Home Nutrition Support[31,32]

- Covered under Part B Prosthetic Device Benefit
- Inoperative body organ or function
- Parenteral: nonfunctioning gastrointestinal tract with malabsorption
- Enteral: nonfunctioning structure that permits food to reach small bowel
- Permanence: 90 or more consecutive days
- Sole source of nutrition: 20 to 35 kcal/kg body weight/day
- Subject to 80-20 split of allowed costs
- Certification of need

ADDITIONAL DOCUMENTATION REQUIRED

- Home parenteral nutrition
  - Kilocalories < 20 or > 35 kcal/kg body weight/day
  - Dextrose concentration < 10%
  - Protein < 1.0 or > 1.5 g/kg body weight/day
  - Lipid 500 ml units > 12/mo
  - "Special" nutrient sources
  - Less than daily infusion
- Home enteral nutrition
  - Kilocalories < 20 or > 35 kcal/kg body weight/day
  - Blended, elemental, disease-specific formulas
  - Pump-assisted feedings

As with hospital nutrition support, the response to the therapy can vary, and that affects the type, duration, and cost of care. Owing in part to these variations, little is known about the actual costs of home nutrition support. However, data that reflect the prevailing reimbursement fees paid by Medicare to primary suppliers of home nutrition support are available (Table 45-4).[31] It is important to note that these fees are set at 25% of arrayed customary charges received from providers. Individual charges can vary substantially. It can be seen from these data that the financial burden for home nutrition support is significant.

The rapid growth in both the utilization and cost of home nutrition support has led government and private insurers to scrutinize this treatment modality. Legislation has been developed to control access to services and to govern the sharing of costs by patient, supplier, and insurer. The regulations described below were developed by HCFA, which administers the Medicare program. Medicare regulations have also been incorporated into the reimbursement policies of many private insurers. Reimbursement regulations for home nutrition support govern who can be reimbursed, what is reimbursable, a capitation on how much is reimbursed, and how reimbursement programs are administered. Medicare and private insurers practice tight utilization review and case management to ensure that the cost of home nutrition support is distributed fairly among patient, supplier, and third-party payer. Familiarity with the regulations and compliance with them are important.

Medicare

In 1965, Congress enacted Title XVII of the Social Security Act, creating the Medicare program. This legislation established health insurance for individuals over age 65 years, regardless of income, and for disabled persons, regardless of age and income. The Medicare program is divided into two parts. Part A addresses reimbursement for inpatient hospital care, skilled nursing care, home health care, hospice care, and care provided through an HMO. Part B is voluntary, and the enrollment premium is paid by the individual. It provides coverage for physician services and includes provisions for durable medical equipment, prosthetic devices, clinic services, therapy, and rehabilitation services. HCFA administers the Medicare program and contracts with private insurance carriers to implement and oversee payments on a claim-by-claim basis.

In 1981, the Medicare program was amended to acknowledge coverage for home nutrition support. Home PN and EN therapies are covered under Medicare Part B as a "prosthetic device." HCFA identified nutrition support as the prosthetic device that replaces all or part of an inoperative body organ or function (a malfunctioning gastrointestinal tract) that is permanent (in practice, > 90 days). The benefit includes not only the access catheter and ancillary equipment for administering the therapy but also the nutrients or solutions that make the entire system effective. Services associated with the execution and monitoring of home nutrition support are not covered, other than those provided by a physician during an office visit or incident to his professional services.

Box 45-1 summarizes selected aspects of the prevailing Medicare guidelines for home nutrition support.[30,31] The physician must document that the patient has a permanent (at least 90 days' duration) gastrointestinal dysfunction that justifies home PN support, such as short bowel syndrome or severe malabsorption. For home EN there must be nonfunctional swallowing or motility of the upper gastrointestinal tract that prevents food from safely reaching the stomach for digestion, and the patient must be NPO. "Cognitive diagnoses" are not covered: for example, a patient who has unexplained anorexia or has lost the "will to eat" is not eligible for coverage.

Coverage is intended for those who require total sustenance; supplemental nutrition is not covered. The Medicare claims for nutrition support treatment plans that provide between 20 and 35 kcal/kg of body weight per day are generally accepted.

Claims outside this range require additional documentation justifying the patient's particular needs. In addition, for PN to be approved, the ordering physician must provide justification for protein orders less than 1.0 or greater than 1.5 g/kg per day; dextrose concentrations less than 10%; lipid use greater than 12 units (500 ml/unit) per month, and infusions on a less-than-daily basis.

The types of solutions and formulas are also scrutinized. Products are grouped according to their common compositions and the reimbursement rate is set at 25% of the arrayed customary charges for the group of products. Parenteral and enteral products that are designed to meet disease-specific or "special" needs of patients (e.g., renal, hepatic, or trauma products) are costly, and Medicare requires additional medical justification of the patient's need.

Coverage for equipment and supplies needed to administer home PN and EN is "capped"; that is, the amount of reimbursement is fixed, regardless of the actual cost of a particular brand of equipment or supplies. In addition, for EN the need for a feeding pump must be documented as medically necessary. The request is approved when there has been documented (or there is great risk for) aspiration, unresolved severe diarrhea or dumping syndrome, blood glucose fluctuations, circulatory overload, or the need to control infusion rates at less than 100 ml per hour.

Certificates of Medical Necessity (CMN) (Figs. 45-1 and 45-2)[1] have been developed by HCFA to facilitate standardization of documentation for claims and to facilitate processing by its carriers. These forms are required on initiation of therapy. If the patient is to continue to receive coverage for home nutrition support, the medical need must be recertified periodically. For stable patients, recertification is required after 3, 9, and 24 months of therapy. After 2 years, the need for further recertification is determined case by case.

It is required that the patient be monitored throughout the course of therapy. The physician signing the certificate of medical necessity is expected to see the patient at the time of initial certification and within 30 days of recertification. If the physician is unable to see the patient within this time frame, the reason must be documented and other monitoring methods used to evaluate the patient's nutrition needs described. The physician signing the certificate authorizes the medical necessity of the therapy and certifies that the information is accurate and truthful. The certificate is a legal document.

Documentation is ordinarily sent to the supplier, who then forwards the claim to one of the designated Medicare carriers. The claim is reviewed, and, if approved, Medicare will reimburse 80% of the established prevailing fee for the needed supplies. The patient (or supplemental insurance) pays the remainder.

Medical Nutrition Therapy

Medical nutrition therapies (MNT), which are necessary to treat illness or injury, include assessment of the nutritional status of a patient, review and analysis of the medical and nutritional histories, laboratory values, anthropometric measurements, and nutrition-focused physical assessment. The MNT provided can range from modification of diet to administration of PN.[33]

In 2002, coverage of MNT services by dietitians will be provided to Medicare patients with diabetes or renal disease. The Institute of Medicine recommended MNT coverage for dietitians' services for these patients because clinical outcomes showed improvement in quality of life, reduced hospital stays, and medication costs for patients who received MNT for these diseases.[32] As positive outcomes and cost effectiveness for nutrition support become available, it is possible that reimbursement will be expanded to cover MNT services provided by dietitians for other patients. To stay in touch with this developing issue, the American Dietetic Association maintains an updated website.[33]

At the current time, however, dietitians cannot bill Medicare for their services directly. Hospital, skilled nursing facility (SNF), home health, and hospice services provided by a dietitian are included with the total "per diem" cost of care and not reimbursable as a separate charge. However, under Medicare Part B coverage, practitioners who are not authorized to bill Medicare directly (including dietitians) may be covered for their services if they are furnished "incident to" a physician's professional services. The dietitian must generally be employed and supervised by the physician or his medical practice.[32]

Table 45-5 represents a series of recognized procedure codes used to describe these MNT services when making charges to Medicare.[33] The 99200 series is for physician charges, but the new 97800 series was specifically designed to reflect MNT services performed by a dietitian. These latter codes are published in the *American Medical Association's Current Procedural Terminology 2001* book, although the charges associated with these codes are yet to be established.

Medicaid

Besides Medicare, Medicaid programs also cover home nutrition support. Unlike Medicare, Medicaid programs are run by each state and are designed to reimburse medical care for the indigent. Although state programs must comply with general federal guidelines, each state formulates its own program. Because of this, broad generalizations about coverage for home nutrition support are difficult to make because each state determines the extent of coverage and reimbursement. States have considerable discretion in judging the need for services and have freedom to control their utilization. Many states require

TABLE 45-5

Current Procedural Terminology (CPT) Codes for Nutrition Services[33]

Code Number	Description of Care Provided	Provider
99200	Nutrition office visit	MD*
99230	Subsequent nutrition office visit	MD*
99240	Outpatient nutrition assessment	MD*
97802	Individual initial nutrition assessment and intervention, q 15min	RD
97803	Individual nutrition reassessment and intervention, q 15min	RD
97804	Group session, q 30min	RD

*These services may be billed incident to physician professional services by a registered dietitian who works for, is supervised by the physician, and whose practice bills Medicare directly.

U.S. DEPARTMENT OF HEALTH & HUMAN SERVICES
HEALTH CARE FINANCING ADMINISTRATION

FORM APPROVED
OMB NO. 0938-0679

CERTIFICATE OF MEDICAL NECESSITY

DMERC 10.02B

ENTERAL NUTRITION

SECTION A   Certification Type/Date: INITIAL __/__/__   REVISED __/__/__   RECERTIFICATION __/__/__

PATIENT NAME, ADDRESS, TELEPHONE and HIC NUMBER

(__ __ __) __ __ __ - __ __ __ __   HICN _____

SUPPLIER NAME, ADDRESS, TELEPHONE and NSC NUMBER

(__ __ __) __ __ __ - __ __ __ __   NSC# _____

PLACE OF SERVICE _____

NAME and ADDRESS of FACILITY if applicable (See Reverse)

HCPCS CODE
_____
_____
_____
_____

PT DOB ___/___/___;   Sex ___ (M/F);   HT. _____ (in.);   WT. _____ (lbs.)

PHYSICIAN NAME, ADDRESS (Printed or Typed)

PHYSICIAN'S UPIN: _____

PHYSICIAN'S TELEPHONE #: (__ __ __) __ __ __ - __ __ __ __

SECTION B   Information in this Section May Not Be Completed by the Supplier of the Items/Supplies.

EST. LENGTH OF NEED (# OF MONTHS): _____ 1-99 (99=LIFETIME)   DIAGNOSIS CODES (ICD-9): _____ _____ _____ _____

ANSWERS	ANSWER QUESTIONS 7, 8, AND 10 - 15 FOR ENTERAL NUTRITION (Circle **Y** for Yes, **N** for No, **D** for Does Not Apply, Unless Otherwise Noted)
	Question 1 - 6, and 9, reserved for other or future use.
Y N	7. Does the patient have permanent non-function or disease of the structures that normally permit food to reach or be absorbed from the small bowel?
Y N	8. Does the patient require tube feedings to provide sufficient nutrients to maintain weight and strength commensurate with the patient's overall health status?
A) _____ B) _____	10. <u>Print</u> product name(s).
A) _____ B) _____	11. Calories per day for each product?
_____	12. Days per week administered? (Enter 1 - 7)
1 2 3 4	13. Circle the number for method of administration. 1 - Syringe 2 - Gravity 3 - Pump 4 - Does not apply
Y N D	14. Does the patient have a documented allergy or intolerance to semi-synthetic nutrients?
	15. Additional information when required by policy:

NAME OF PERSON ANSWERING SECTION B QUESTIONS, IF OTHER THAN PHYSICIAN (Please Print):
NAME: _____   TITLE: _____   EMPLOYER: _____

SECTION C   Narrative Description Of Equipment And Cost

(1) <u>Narrative</u> description of all items, accessories and options ordered; (2) Supplier's charge; and (3) Medicare Fee Schedule Allowance for <u>each</u> item, accessory, and option. (See Instructions On Back)

SECTION D   Physician Attestation and Signature/Date

I certify that I am the physician identified in Section A of this form. I have received Section A, B and C of the Certificate of Medical Necessity (including charges for items ordered). Any statement on my letterhead attached hereto, has been reviewed and signed by me. I certify that the medical necessity information in Section B is true, accurate and complete, to the best of my knowledge, and I understand that any falsification, omission, or concealment of material fact in that section may subject me to civil or criminal liability.

PHYSICIAN'S SIGNATURE_____   DATE __/__/__   (SIGNATURE AND DATE STAMPS ARE NOT ACCEPTABLE)

FORM HCFA 853 (4/96)

FIGURE 45-1 Certificate of medical necessity for enteral nutrition.[1] (From the US Department of Health and Human Services, Health Care Financing Administration.)

U.S. DEPARTMENT OF HEALTH & HUMAN SERVICES
HEALTH CARE FINANCING ADMINISTRATION

FORM APPROVED
OMB NO. 0938-0679

CERTIFICATE OF MEDICAL NECESSITY

DMERC 10.02A

PARENTERAL NUTRITION

SECTION A   Certification Type/Date: INITIAL __ / __ / __   REVISED __ / __ / __   RECERTIFICATION __ / __ / __

PATIENT NAME, ADDRESS, TELEPHONE and HIC NUMBER	SUPPLIER NAME, ADDRESS, TELEPHONE and NSC NUMBER
(__ __ __) __ __ __ - __ __ __ __ HICN _____	(__ __ __) __ __ __ - __ __ __ __ NSC# _____

| PLACE OF SERVICE _____

NAME and ADDRESS of FACILITY if applicable
(See Reverse) | HCPCS CODE

_____
_____
_____
_____ | PT DOB ___ / ___ / ___;   Sex ___ (M/F);   HT. _____ (in.);   WT. _____ (lbs.)

PHYSICIAN NAME, ADDRESS (Printed or Typed)

PHYSICIAN'S UPIN: _____

PHYSICIAN'S TELEPHONE #: (__ __ __) __ __ __ - __ __ __ __ |

SECTION B   **Information in this Section May Not Be Completed by the Supplier of the Items/Supplies**

EST. LENGTH OF NEED (# OF MONTHS): _____ 1-99 (99=LIFETIME)   **DIAGNOSIS CODES (ICD-9):** _____ _____ _____ _____

ANSWERS	ANSWER QUESTIONS 1, AND 3 - 5 FOR PARENTERAL NUTRITION (Circle **Y** for Yes, **N** for No, **D** for Does Not Apply, Unless Otherwise Noted)
	Question 2 reserved for other or future use.
Y N	1. Does the patient have severe permanent disease of the gastrointestinal tract causing malabsorption severe enough to prevent maintenance of weight and strength commensurate with the patient's overall health status?
_____	3. Days per week infused? (Enter 1 - 7)

	4. Formula components:
	
	        Amino Acid _____ (ml/day) _____ concentration % _____ gms protein/day
	
	        Dextrose _____ (ml/day) _____ concentration %
	
	        Lipids _____ (ml/day) _____ days/week _____ concentration %

1 3 7	5. Circle the number for the route of administration. 2, 4, 5, 6 - Reserved for other or future use. 1 - Central Line; 3 - Hemodialysis Access Line; 7 - Peripherally Inserted Catheter (PIC)

NAME OF PERSON ANSWERING SECTION B QUESTIONS, IF OTHER THAN PHYSICIAN (Please Print):
NAME: _____   TITLE: _____   EMPLOYER: _____

SECTION C   **Narrative Description Of Equipment And Cost**

(1) <u>Narrative</u> description of all items, accessories and options ordered; (2) Supplier's charge; and (3) Medicare Fee Schedule Allowance for <u>each</u> item, accessory, and option. (See Instructions On Back)

SECTION D   **Physician Attestation and Signature/Date**

I certify that I am the physician identified in Section A of this form. I have received Sections A, B and C of the Certificate of Medical Necessity (including charges for items ordered). Any statement on my letterhead attached hereto, has been reviewed and signed by me. I certify that the medical necessity information in Section B is true, accurate and complete, to the best of my knowledge, and I understand that any falsification, omission, or concealment of material fact in that section may subject me to civil or criminal liability.

PHYSICIAN'S SIGNATURE_____   DATE ___ / ___ / ___   (SIGNATURE AND DATE STAMPS ARE NOT ACCEPTABLE)

FORM HCFA 852 (4/96)

FIGURE 45-2 Certificate of medical necessity for parenteral nutrition.[1] (From the US Department of Health and Human Services, Health Care Financing Administration.)

preauthorization as a condition for coverage. Each case is subject to individual review by a state board. Each state may also have an established contract with a supplier for the products. Because Medicaid is a joint federal-state program, it is especially sensitive to budgetary concerns at both levels. As availability of health care dollars decreases, this program may be particularly affected.

Private Insurers

Private insurers vary greatly in the way they reimburse for home nutrition support. In addition, individual policies within a single company can vary in their coverage for this therapy. Thus, generalizations about reimbursement practices by private insurers are also difficult. Many carriers have adopted Medicare's system and approach to reimbursement. On the other hand, a few treat home nutrition support as a basic benefit and cover it fully. The services that are needed to manage and monitor the home program may or may not be covered by some private insurers.

Most private insurers are aggressively pursuing cost containment with strategies such as approval before initiation of therapy, case management, and capitation of reimbursement (per diem or lifetime maximum). The future of coverage for home nutrition support by private insurers will likely be dictated by the economics of the overall health care environment.

The Uninsured

A further issue impacting the health care system in the United States is the 43 million Americans who lack health insurance, and thus have limited access to health care.[34] Of these, 50% to 60% either work full-time or are dependents of full-time workers.

A viable plan is needed to provide coverage to this vulnerable group. It has been suggested that the portion of the federal budget surplus that was gleaned from Medicare and Medicaid cuts, might be redirected to insuring these individuals.[35] In the year 2000, Medicare and Medicaid costs were $104 billion less than projected.[35] This important issue, however, will require extensive discussion in the political arena before it can be resolved.

Cost Containment and Outcomes in Home Nutrition Support

Expenditures for home health care have been increasing dramatically. Increased expenditures can be attributed to the increased utilization of home care as a viable alternative to hospitalization; however, the method of charging that is used by the home care industry for products and services has also been viewed as inflationary. A 1990 study by the U.S. General Accounting Office found that the fees charged to Medicare carriers for selected equipment items varied by as much as 100% to 600%.[36] Others have found weak relationships between costs to the company and charges to the consumer.[37,38] The current freedoms in home care to bundle services, negotiate prices, and manipulate patient and payer mix further cloud true cost.

Regulatory agencies and insurers are taking steps to exercise more control over reimbursement for costly home therapies, including nutrition support.[39] These efforts have focused mainly on cost containment by regulating access to coverage (i.e., controlling what medical conditions qualify for reimbursement) and by placing limits on what is reimbursed (absolute dollars).

However, establishing true product costs is difficult, in part, because of the number of suppliers. Indirect costs are even more difficult to establish and control. It is conceivable that the total costs associated with home care, including equipment, products, and cost for health care personnel needed to execute and monitor home nutrition support, may be greater than hospital treatment. The lost earning power of home caregivers and the emotional cost to household members of caring for the patient must also be considered.

In addition to ensuring that costs are contained, regulatory agencies have become increasingly interested in the clinical appropriateness of home therapies. It has been pointed out that therapies that do not improve health outcomes are inefficient, a waste of resources, and that such therapies should be cut.[39] Only a few studies have addressed outcomes of home nutrition support.

One longitudinal study[40] of 1594 home PN support patients concluded that clinical outcomes justified such therapy for people with serious, long-term, chronic illness. Utilization and appropriateness of home PN were questioned for end-stage diseases such as cancer and the acquired immunodeficiency syndrome (AIDS), where expected survival was relatively short and additional therapy was unlikely to alter the outcome.

Another follow-up study[41] looked specifically at home PN outcomes for cancer patients. It was found that home PN was justified in patients with "cured" cancer and severe radiation enteritis. However, justification for home PN for patients with "active" cancer was less conclusive because of variability in outcomes. For those with "slowly growing tumors" or "potentially curable disease," home nutrition support appeared justified. On the other hand, for patients with "aggressive disease" or a life expectancy of less than 6 to 9 months, the appropriateness of home nutrition support was not confirmed. For this population, further study was recommended. Questions to be addressed included these: Does simple hydration with fluid and electrolytes produce the same medical outcome and quality of life as home PN? Would simple hydration for such a patient be cost effective if it avoided a terminal hospital stay? (Note: Medicare Part B does not currently reimburse for simple hydration.) Do current reimbursement policies increase use of home PN or expensive hospitalizations?

A more recent report[28] of patients receiving home nutrition support contained outcome profiles for a variety of diseases. Clinical outcomes were positive for home parenterally nourished patients with gastrointestinal diseases (Crohn's, ischemic bowel disease, motility disorders, congenital bowel defects), hyperemesis gravidarum, chronic pancreatitis, and radiation enteritis. Clinical outcomes were poor for patients with a poor prognosis such as those who had AIDS or an aggressive neoplasm. A subgroup of patients with neuromuscular swallowing disorders receiving home EN was also assessed. Older subjects were found to experience minimal rehabilitation, whereas younger subjects had much better survival and rehabilitation. The appropriateness of home EN as standard practice for older patients was questioned.

These studies focused on traditional outcomes measurements such as morbidity and mortality. More outcome studies are needed, particularly for the home nutrition support population. In keeping with today's broad definitions of health, newer outcomes measures to explore in this population should include functional status, performance, quality of life, and satisfaction with the therapy.

Conclusion

The economics of health care reform will continue to be debated. Because health care expenditures consume a large portion of the national budget, pressures will mount to control costs and to eliminate services whose benefits are not clearly demonstrable. Expensive therapies, such as nutrition support, will be scrutinized and subject to legislation governing reimbursement. Nutrition support professionals must be keenly aware of the existing regulations governing reimbursement, to ensure appropriate coverage for this therapy.

Nutrition professionals must lead the effort to control costs. Identification and implementation of less expensive, but effective interventions should be a part of each patient's care plan. It is important to identify all costs for therapy, including personnel, supplies, solutions, and complications and their effects (both therapy related and nutrition related).

In addition, nutrition professionals must document outcomes of nutrition support interventions or the withholding thereof. Health care reforms aimed at controlling health expenditures present a threat to nutrition services in the absence of outcomes data. Cost containment, by itself, is insufficient. Whatever the cost of a therapy, if it does not accomplish its goal or is inappropriate, it yields no benefit and is not needed. The challenge for nutrition professionals is to document the effectiveness of nutrition support, using not only cost and biochemical end points but also length of stay, complications, hospital readmission rates, functional status, and quality of life parameters. The effectiveness of nutrition support in relation to both cost and outcome will determine future utilization and course in health care.

REFERENCES

1. *National health care expenditures projections: 2000-2010.* Retrieved from http://www.hcfa.gov/stats. Office of the Actuary of the Health Care Financing Administration.
2. Parver A: *Medicare PEN issues 2000: voice your concerns.* Retrieved 10/07/01 from http://www.oley.org/lifeline/99-023.html.
3. Bowers CR, Stafford KE, Johnson C (eds): *St. Anthony's DRG guidebook 1995,* Reston, VA, 1994, St. Anthony's Publishing, p xvi.
4. Finkel AS, Hammond JM, Karlin DS, et al: (eds): *2000 drug topics Red Book Pharmacy's fundamental reference,* Montvale, NJ, 2000, Medical Economics.
5. Ridge M: DRG coding for malnutrition may improve reimbursement status, *Clin Manage* 4:41-44, 1988.
6. Myers M, Landye ST: Malnutrition in the hospital: impact on costs, DRG coding for nutrition reimbursement, *J Am Diet Assoc* 89(6):764, 1989 (letter).
7. Rowan ML: The impact of malnutrition as a comorbidity on final DRG and reimbursement, *J Am Diet Assoc* 89(suppl):A-77, 1989 (abstract).
8. Funk KL, Ayton CM: Improving malnutrition documentation enhances reimbursement, *J Am Diet Assoc* 95(4):468-475, 1995.
9. Delhey DM, Anderson EJ, Laramee SH: Implications of malnutrition and diagnosis-related groups (DRGs), *J Am Diet Assoc* 89(10):1448-1451, 1989.
10. Cicenas DD: Increasing Medicare reimbursement through improved DRG coding. In Fox MK (ed): *Reimbursement and insurance coverage for nutrition services,* Chicago, 1991, The American Dietetic Association, pp 51-55.
11. Trimble JM: Reimbursement enhancement in a New Jersey hospital: coding for malnutrition in prospective payment systems, *J Am Diet Assoc* 92(6):737-738, 1992.
12. McCulley JA, Myers EF: Dietitians take the lead in diagnosis-related group coding, *J Am Diet Assoc* 94(6):650-651, 1994.
13. Bistrian BR, Blackburn GL, Vitale J, et al: Prevalence of malnutrition in general medical patients, *JAMA* 235(15):1567-1570, 1976.
14. Detsky AS, Baker JP, O'Rourke K, Goel V: Perioperative parenteral nutrition: a meta-analysis, *Ann Intern Med* 107(2):195-203, 1987.
15. Buzby GP, Mullen JL, Matthews DC, et al: Prognostic nutritional index in gastrointestinal surgery, *Am J Surg* 139(1):160-167, 1980.
16. Hickman DM, Miller RA, Rombeau JL, et al: Serum albumin and body weight as predictors of postoperative course in colorectal cancer, *J Parenter Enteral Nutr* 4(3):314-316, 1980.
17. Klidjian AM, Archer TJ, Foster KJ, Karran SJ: Detection of dangerous malnutrition, *J Parenter Enteral Nutr* 6(2):119-121, 1982.
18. Epstein AM, Read JL, Hoefer M: The relation of body weight to length of stay and charges for hospital services for patients undergoing elective surgery: a study of two procedures, *Am J Public Health* 77(8):993-997, 1987.
19. Robinson G, Goldstein M, Levine GM: Impact of nutrition status on DRG length of stay, *J Parenter Enteral Nutr* 11(1):49-51, 1987.
20. Reilly JJ, Hull SF, Albert N, et al: Economic impact of malnutrition: a model system for hospitalized patients, *J Parenter Enteral Nutr* 12(4):371-376, 1988.
21. Gales BJ, Gales MJ: Nutritional support teams: a review of comparative trials, *Ann Pharmacother* 28(2):227-235, 1994.
22. Hassell JT, Games AD, Shaffer B, Harkins LE: Nutrition support team management of enterally fed patients in a community hospital is cost beneficial, *J Am Diet Assoc* 94(9):993-998, 1994.
23. Baumgartner TG: More cost-containment literature needed, *J Parenter Enteral Nutr* 11(3):330-331, 1987.
24. McCamish MA: Malnutrition and nutrition support interventions: cost, benefits and outcomes, *Nutrition* 9(6):556-557, 1993.
25. Goldstein M, Braitman LE, Levine GM: The medical and financial cost associated with termination of a nutrition support nurse, *J Parenter Enteral Nutr* 24(6):323-327, 2000.
26. Trujillo EB, Young LS, Chertow GM, Randall S, Clemons T, Jacobs DO, Robinson MK: Metabolic and monetary costs of avoidable parenteral nutrition use, *J Parenter Enteral Nutr* 23(2):109-113, 1999.
27. Webb LC: Home infusion therapy services, Robert W. Baird and Co., Inc.'s., Health Care Research, May 1992.
28. The Oley Foundation: *North American home parenteral and enteral nutrition patient registry. Annual report with outcome profiles: 1985-1992,* Albany, 1994, The Oley Foundation.
29. Pontis JW: The economics of home parenteral nutrition, *Nutrition* 14(10):809-812, 1998.
30. Reddy P, Malone M: Cost and outcome analysis of home parenteral and enteral nutrition, *J Parenter Enteral Nutr* 22(5):302-310, 1998.
31. Region A DMERC: *Medicare supplier manual,* February 2001.
32. Sheils JF, Rubin R, Stapleton DC: The estimated costs and savings of medical nutrition therapy: the Medicare population, *J Am Diet Assoc* 99(4):428-435, 1999.
33. Retrieved 4/2/01 from http://www.eatright.org/gov/mntindex.html. The Campaign for Coverage of Medical Nutrition Therapy.
34. Dalen J: A bold proposal to achieve near-universal health care coverage in the United States, *Arch Int Med* 160(22):3354-3355, Dec 2000.
35. Davis K, Schoen C, Schoenbaum SC: A 2020 vision for American health care, *Arch Int Med* 160(22):3357-3362, Dec 2000.
36. Medicare program: payment for home intravenous drug therapy services, *Federal Register* Nov 11, 1989.
37. Margolis RE: The home infusion industry: patients' angel or their ruthless plunderer? *HealthSpan* 10(6):18-20, 1993.
38. Curtiss FR: Recent developments in federal reimbursement for home health care services and products, *Am J Hosp Pharm* 45(8):1682-1690, 1988.
39. Donabedian A: Quality and cost: choices and responsibilities, *Inquirer* 25:90-99, 1988.
40. Howard L, Heaphey L, Fleming CR, et al: Four years of North American registry home parenteral nutrition outcome data and their implications for patient management, *J Parenter Enteral Nutr* 15(4):384-393, 1991.
41. Howard L: Home parenteral and enteral nutrition in cancer patients, *Cancer (Suppl)* 72(11):3531-3541, 1993.

Understanding and Conducting Clinical Research

46

Elaine R. Monsen, PhD, RD
Ann M. Coulston, MS, RD

Developing a Research Environment

The results of research form the backbone of scientific, medical, or clinical knowledge, and dietetics is no exception. Research is a *process,* not a product. It is a careful and thorough search, a studious inquiry or examination, or thorough testing or exploration of ideas. It is this type of exploration and study that leads to the discovery of new knowledge. Research produces concepts not known before or never before applied in a particular context.[1] "Never in the history of nutrition has the need for science been greater than it is today. Dietitians should strive... to (be) open to new ideas but based on scientific evidence."[2]

Many readers of this book may not think of themselves as researchers, yet all participate (knowingly or unknowingly) in research activities every day. Not all research is performed in the laboratory; much new information is generated by research conducted in clinical settings where nutrition therapy is applied to patients. Appreciating how every practicing dietitian is positioned to contribute actively to research is the major focus of this chapter.

Evaluating the Literature

Research can be defined in many different ways. It can be defined broadly as the *studious and critical inquiry and examination of information aimed at the discovery and interpretation of new knowledge.* The research process involves problem solving and decision making. Health care professionals perform research functions daily, whether they work in a clinical, management, or research setting. For most nutrition practitioners, daily research activity is evaluation of the scientific literature, not exhaustive review of all available studies in a specific area, but reading current journals and considering the value of new findings. With the recent multiplication of information resources available through computer on-line services, dietetics professionals with access to a computer and modem can quickly scan a great deal of information. Government health and regulatory agencies, the National Library of Medicine, health care research journals, and professional societies carry late-breaking research findings updated at least daily. For many, on-line searches and the use of e-journals are the preferred way of staying current with the literature in their field.

A key skill in the practice of nutrition support is the ability to critically appraise the scientific value of findings. Guidelines can assist in this activity, and periodic practice can sharpen skills of identification of information appropriate to a given setting and of interpretation for use in nutrition care. Not everyone reads research with a critical eye. Some questions to guide the reading of research articles are discussed in the following sections.[3] As you read, ask yourself these questions.

WHAT TYPE OF STUDY IS THIS? Is it a preliminary study? Has it been reviewed by other scientists before publication (i.e., has it been *refereed*)? How do the findings fit into the cumulative evidence in the area? For example, a study published in a peer-review journal has had more scrutiny and review than research presented for the first time at a scientific meeting or directly to the media.

WAS THE RESEARCH DESIGN APPROPRIATE? Epidemiologic research, for example, is very different from clinical research. Epidemiologic research is observational and does not prove cause and effect. Rather, it identifies only relationships between a factor in the diet and an outcome in the population. This is a valuable first step in the research process, which can lead to controlled, intervention studies. Walter Willett has provided a comprehensive review of nutritional epidemiology.[4]

For clinical trials that contain an intervention, the appropriateness of the control group is an important consideration. Critical readers look for documentation of similarities between study groups and for comments about biases that might influence the direction of the results. For example, was a control group used to provide a point of comparison, and was dietary intake assessed consistently and with appropriate methods throughout the study period? It is good to know what methods were used for data gathering. For example, self-reported diet data tend to underestimate portion size, calories, and alcohol.[5] Were the subjects randomly selected and assigned to treatment groups? Randomized studies minimize bias.

The critical decision in study design is what variable should be measured to reflect the outcome. If the end point measurement is not a good reflection of the outcome, the conclusions may be weak. For example, if the end point is total fat intake, does the study address changes in other calorie-containing nutrients that might alter the measured outcome?

ARE ALL RELEVANT HEALTH OUTCOMES REPORTED? Does the paper report morbidity and mortality and quality of life? The reader should check the validity, objectivity, and reproducibility of the measurements and whether the investigators were blinded to the outcome assessment. Who were the study population? What were the eligibility criteria and inclusion criteria? Was the intervention feasible? What were the intervention strategy and compliance measurements? Cointervention contamination should be sought, such as subjects who were in multiple studies or had been in studies that had lingering impact. Were all subjects who entered the study accounted for at its conclusion? The investigators should account for dropouts, noncompliant subjects, and potential study crossovers.

WERE THE STATISTICAL CRITERIA APPROPRIATE? Both statistical significance and clinical differences are important. Significant statistical differences tell you whether the difference in end points (measurements) between two groups is real and not just an effect of chance; however, statistical significance can be questioned if the sample size is extremely large or small. In some cases the clinical difference, in practical terms, is impressive even when statistical significance is not achieved because of small sample size.

Critical readers are skeptics: big breakthroughs in nutrition science are few. Remember, science is *evolutionary* not *revolutionary*! Numbers and statistics can be misleading and can be manipulated. Results should be expressed in meaningful, practical terms. For example, research reports may indicate that there are statistical differences in levels of blood cholesterol, blood glucose, or body weight, when all reported plasma concentrations or body weights are within the normal range. Some clinical scientists describe such findings as *statistically* significant results that have no *clinical* significance. Not everyone agrees on what is clinically significant, but results that fall within normal laboratory ranges certainly should not be considered clinically significant. Perspective comes from discussing recent findings with other nutrition scientists.

In addition to our own reading of the literature, critical literature review can be formalized in the setting of what is called a *journal club,* in which one member is assigned to choose a research article, review it, and discuss the research question, research design and methods, and results. Usually, all members have read the article and contribute to the discussion. This activity is useful not only for acquiring new clinical knowledge but also for improving research skills or your approach to research questions.

Critical appraisal of the scientific literature helps the practitioner confront daily clinical problems. Busy clinicians who think this critical method is too time consuming must keep in mind that critical appraisal skills develop rapidly when used regularly. These skills enable one to optimize reading time and enhance ventures into clinical research. The benefits—to clinicians and to their patients—will quickly bring rewards.

Developing Research Teams
Benefits of Collaboration

By nature, research is a collaborative effort. Members of the research team include the investigator(s); research subjects; laboratory technicians; statisticians or consultants; and frequently, scientific collaborators. Each participant brings unique expertise. Collaboration guards against pitfalls and unidentified weaknesses in the research project that could invalidate the results. Because research activity is a resource-intensive effort in terms of dollars and professional time the best possible project should be the goal. One research team member in the clinical nutrition setting is the dietitian, who initiates the

project, outlines the research question, and serves as the principal investigator. Frequently, a physician is needed for expertise in medicine or surgery or to perform some of the clinical measurements in data collection. If the study involves the determination of substances in blood or urine, the laboratory technician is important. At most major hospitals and medical centers, statisticians are available to help with research design and data analysis. Although data analysis might seem to occur later in the research project, it is extremely important to enlist the advice of the statistician early, so that the data can be collected to coordinate with the most appropriate statistical analysis design. Finally, the subjects are important members of the research team. The investigator needs the full cooperation of the subjects once they have agreed to participate. Compliance-with-protocol problems are greatly reduced when subjects understand the research and feel part of it.

Internal Colleagues in the Investigator's Institution

As a research project begins to develop or while the research question is being formulated, new and seasoned investigators find it useful to discuss ideas with institutional colleagues and department members in the same field (i.e., nutrition) or in related ones such as surgery, medicine, or nursing. The value of input from colleagues early in the planning and development stages of research must not be overlooked.

External Colleagues at Other Institutions

Frequently, it is necessary to discuss research ideas with others who have conducted research in your area of interest. Often these scientists are located elsewhere, but they can help to "fine tune" a research design because they are familiar with projects in the same area. Investigators get to know others through meeting contacts, literature review, and introductions from colleagues. When a research area is quite narrow and sample size to reach statistical significance becomes an issue, colleagues from other institutions that treat similar patient populations may contribute subjects to the study. Many important clinical intervention studies have been conducted in this manner.

Conceiving Research
Research Question

One of the most challenging tasks of a research project is developing the research question. It seems straightforward: This is, after all, the statement that drives the entire project. Albert Einstein said, "The formulation of a problem is far more often essential than its solution, which may be merely a matter of mathematical or experimental skill. To raise new questions, new possibilities, to regard old problems from a new angle requires creative imagination and marks real advance in science."[6]

For most clinicians, research ideas are born of daily experience, observations, and questions that come up in the course of patient care. When a question arises and a search of the literature reveals no answers, that question can be the basic topic for research. Clinical research is a very rewarding endeavor. The knowledge gained through careful evaluation of a research topic provides objective support for practice-based observations and furthers the knowledge base of dietetics. How often we read a research report or a journal article and say to ourselves, I could have done that. It is just these types of experiences that trigger research ideas and prompt investigators to pursue them. The American Dietetic Association (ADA) recognizes the value of research, but members find it difficult to envision how to plan and conduct research in the clinical setting.[7] They should ask themselves not, Can I do this research project? but, How can I do this research project? The information in this chapter is designed to help practitioners become comfortable with research.

Most studies in clinical nutrition are clinical research studies. The practice setting is an excellent place to identify research issues that have clinical applications. Let us look at the process of identifying a project. All research questions evolve from an area of the researcher's interest. Questions may arise from ideas for improving patient care, suggestions for increasing effectiveness of services and products, untested concepts published in the literature, and unsolved clinical problems.

A research project should address needs of the investigator's own practice area. Being most familiar with the related literature, the researcher already possesses knowledge about what has been studied and what needs to be. A word of caution is warranted here. It is generally good to stay within one's area of expertise.

Conception of a research project and development of a research question begins with the writing of a one- or two-paragraph vignette, an idea or observation that includes the area of possible study.[8] Rereading the vignette, the researcher underlines the word or phrase that represents the essence of what she wants to study. This word or phrase is the topic, and eventually becomes the *dependent* (or *outcome*) *variable*. Words and phrases such as *length of stay, nitrogen balance, body weight,* and *calorie or nutrient intake* are examples of a quantity or aspect of something tangible whose change or difference it is necessary to understand, explain, or predict.

The *independent variables* in the vignette are the words or concepts that cause a change in the outcome or dependent variable you are trying to understand. A study may have several independent variables. It is generally a good idea to keep the independent variables to a minimum by carefully defining the study criteria.

To define the dependent and independent variables, the investigator writes a series of questions—Who? What? When? Where? and Why?—to help narrow the definition of variables. The variables to be controlled or measured must be defined in quantifiable terms. Appropriate ones can be seen, felt, heard, or measured objectively in some way (e.g., days of hospitalization, bacterial count of *E. coli* 0157:H7 in selected food samples, or μmol cholesterol/L serum).

Once research variables have been defined, it is time to write specific questions that will become the research question or topic: relationship (or descriptive) questions or cause-and-effect ("if, then") questions. These questions are reformulated into the research hypothesis.

Another technique for better understanding the development of a research question and of dependent and independent variables is to examine published papers with the aforementioned guidelines in mind. The last sentence of the introduction in a journal research article should be the research question or hypothesis. The methods section demonstrates how other authors have defined terms. The most interesting and easily understood articles closely follow the guidelines described in this chapter. Clarity of a research paper is not the result of its scientific content alone.

When the research question is clearly stated, the research project can be designed and implemented more easily. When researchers follow this process, more than one relevant or related question may emerge. It is best, however, to plan to study one concept at a time and to build on existing data. The results from the first research project can shape the plan for a second project, and so forth.

Research Design

Information about nutrition can be derived from a variety of study types. Each design has a different purpose, which must be understood (Table 46-1). For example, epidemiologic studies are observational and identify some relationship between a factor in the diet and an outcome in the population. They are *directional,* not *conclusive. Case-control studies* compare different groups of people who have a given condition but different treatments to determine differences between the effects of the two treatments. Clinical trials determine if making a specific change will affect a health outcome, usually a measure related to the disease, such as blood cholesterol concentration. Basic research studies originate in the laboratory and use animals to test scientific hypotheses that often are generated by observational or epidemiologic studies.

Research may be broadly classified, according to purpose, as *descriptive* or *analytic.* Descriptive studies include qualitative research, case studies, and survey research. Descriptive research is used to describe a situation or area of interest factually and accurately. For example, a descriptive study might describe the nutrition status of patients who require ventilation assistance for more than 7 days. The design is flexible so that the investigator can discover ideas, gain insight, and formulate a research question for further investigation. Subjects are selected according to their compatibility with the topic under investigation. Research subjects in descriptive studies have special characteristics and are not considered typical or representative of the population.

Case studies (or survey research) fall into this category. The background, current status, and environmental interactions of a given unit (i.e., individual, group, institution, or community) are studied intensively. Reports of observations may be on one or more subjects. The purpose is to describe the experience of a series of cases of a common disease or condition. The information gathered can provide evidence of an association between the disease or condition and a suspected etiologic or therapeutic factor. The data collected usually cover a broad range of factors in detail, producing a detailed description of the case. A case description of a rare illness with a related nutrition component or of the nutrient intake of a section of the population taken from a national database such as the Health and Nutrition Examination Survey (HANES) are examples.

Analytic research studies include some type of intervention. It is this experimental design that most identify as *research.* Experimental or analytic studies in which

TABLE 46-1

Basic Research Methods

Method	Purpose	Example
Descriptive	To describe systematically a group of patients, a situation or area of interest factually and accurately	Nutritional status of patients who present for total parenteral nutrition
Epidemiologic	To identify relationships between something and an outcome in the population	Vitamin E intake of a population with cardiovascular disease before the age of 65
Case-control	To compare different groups of patients who have the same diagnosis but different therapies	Mortality statistics of breast cancer patients who received nutritional support during radiation treatment versus those who did not
True experimental	To study cause and effect relationships by applying an intervention to one group and not to another	Differences in length of hospitalization as a function of nutrition support program
Quasi experimental	To investigate an intervention when a control group cannot be utilized	Determination of need for rehospitalization of patients who received nutritional support during treatment of thermal injury
Clinical trials	To determine a specific intervention for a disease or condition will result in a change in health outcome	Supplementation with vitamin C of patients with lung cancer will decrease mortality

interventions are devised by the investigator provide evidence for cause and effect. This research design investigates cause-and-effect relationships by exposing one or more experimental groups to one or more treatment conditions and compares the results with one or more control groups not receiving the treatment. Random assignment to treatment or control group is essential. For example, a study to investigate whether enterally fed surgical and medical patients given a formula enriched with partially hydrolyzed guar have less diarrhea than patients fed a standard formula containing no soluble fibers falls into this category.[9] Other types of analytic methods of research include causal comparative or *ex post facto studies*. In this design, observing existing consequences and searching back through the data produce plausible cause-and-effect relationships. An example of this research method is a study to determine the effects of nutrition intervention on weight in a group of adult, HIV-positive outpatients in New York City.[10] Partially controlled (or quasiexperimental) designs are less rigorous than true experimental methods but are appropriate when a setting does not afford control or manipulation of all relevant variables. An example of this type of study is an investigation of a treatment method when random assignment of subjects is not possible.

With the current pressure on health care resources and the perceived needs for health care reform, *outcomes research* is becoming popular in the clinical setting. In health care, an *outcome* is defined as what is accomplished for, or what happens to, a patient. The following are different types of outcomes: (1) *Clinical outcomes* are changes in laboratory parameters, rehospitalization, and drug utilization. (2) *Functional outcomes* are measures of physical capability; social, mental, or emotional well-being; patient satisfaction measures; or how well health care meets customer expectations. (3) *Economic outcomes* are the actual costs of a service.

Outcomes research collects data to quantify the results of an intervention on overall patient care, be it a medication, product, or process. The goal is to maximize quality of care when quality meets standards of clinicians, patients, and costs to the system are considered. The logical first step in outcomes research is to develop or describe a model for nutrition care.[11] Figure 46-1 describes a generic nutrition care model that can be adapted to fit the nutrition care setting under study.

The underlying assumption of outcomes research is that consumer, provider, and payer need access to information that helps them weigh care options according to how much they will cost and what the effects are likely to be. In summary, outcomes research is conducted to measure the effects of services and interventions provided to patients. It measures the quantifiable change in patients' health status between two or more points in time.

It is not always possible to classify the research design or method used to conduct a study, but understanding the basic research methods allows the investigator to imagine the variety of methods that can be used to approach a research question. The choice of research design depends on the research question, the setting of the study, and available resources. Frequently, a descriptive study might antedate an experimental study so that information gained from the descriptive study can be used to optimize the experimental study design.

Statistical Analysis

Many important aspects of selecting a research design and determining the scope of the project can be answered only with statistical consultation. Frequently investigators enlist a biostatistician to answer the following concerns:

Which statistical analyses are most appropriate for the proposed study sample?

How many subjects must be studied to be able to detect a true difference?

To benefit from consultation with a statistician, the investigator must be familiar with the fundamentals of statistics. Most practicing dietitians, especially those with postgraduate education, have studied basic statistics. Statistical awareness is also enhanced by consideration of data analysis methods utilized in the literature. The dietitian is not expected to be an expert in statistics, just as the statistician is not an expert in nutrition. Each brings special talents. Together, they determine which statistical analysis methods are best for the research in question and how large the sample must be in order to determine that a difference cannot be accounted for by chance. A useful reference for statistical considerations is *Research: Successful Approaches*.[12]

This section reviews the fundamentals of statistics and provides examples from nutrition research. Basically, four

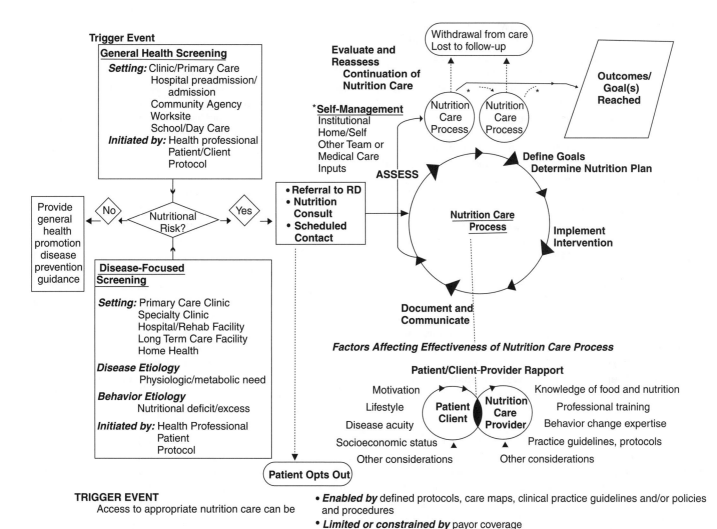

FIGURE 46-1 A nutrition care model (From Splett P, Meyers EF: A proposed model for effective nutrition care, *J Am Diet Assoc* 101:357-363, 2001.)

elements of study design guide the selection of appropriate statistical analysis: the research question, descriptive or analytical; the scale of measurement in which the data are collected or the type of data, whether discrete or continuous; the relationship among samples; and the number of samples to be evaluated. These four elements are discussed briefly in the following section or in other sections of this chapter.

SCALE OF MEASUREMENT. The measurements collected in research are called *variables*. Discrete variables are not necessarily numbers (i.e., gender, race, or clinical stage of disease). Continuous variables, however, have numerical meaning (i.e., blood glucose levels, blood pressure, body weight, or weight changes).

RELATIONSHIP AMONG SAMPLES. These can be independent, meaning that the data points in one sample are unrelated to the data points in the second sample, for example, insulin receptors and blood pressure. Dependent measurements are inherently correlated, such as crossover studies, serial measures, or replicate measures.

NUMBER OF SAMPLES AND ANALYSIS METHODS TO COMPARE THEM. This area of statistical design becomes more complex with the addition of samples. Statistical tests are designed to compare one sample, two samples, or more than two samples.

When the number of groups increases, the number of pair-wise comparisons increases. The chances of finding spuriously significant results increase as the number of tests applied to a single set of data increases.

SAMPLE SIZE DETERMINATION. Keep in mind that statistics allows the investigator to estimate the unknown. Characteristics of a population are estimated from observations of a sample drawn from that population. The size of the sample largely determines how accurate or precise the estimates will be. To be able to conclude that there are differences as a result of the study intervention, a large enough sample size must be drawn from the population, so that the end point will be the result of the intervention and not of chance. The information needed to calculate sample size is the main end point of the study and how it is to be measured. Four estimates must be made. First, how much of a difference is expected between treatment groups? Second, what is the estimated variability in that measurement (i.e., the standard deviation)? This can be obtained from the literature or, better yet, from data collected in a pilot study. Third, the maximum acceptable risk of a false-positive conclusion (or α error) is determined. Most studies base sample calculations on a probability estimate of 0.05. Fourth, the maximum acceptable risk of a false-negative conclusion (or β error) is determined. Most studies select 0.8 to 0.9 for power, which is equivalent to false-negative probabilities of 0.1 to 0.2. Computer software programs are available to assist with sample size (power) calculations.

Preliminary sample size requirements must be reconciled with your estimates of the number of available subjects. A clear picture of the number of willing subjects who meet the inclusion criteria (considering the exclusion criteria as well) and are likely to complete the study and not be lost to follow-up is essential before embarking on the study. If the number of available subjects is insufficient you may want to consider expanding the inclusion criteria (i.e., widening the acceptable age range), eliminating uncritical exclusion criteria, lengthening the time for subject recruitment and enrollment, seeking additional sources for subjects, devising more precise measurements, or considering a different research design that requires fewer subjects.

If the sample size is fixed, as in a retrospective study or a follow-up study, you can estimate the potential power of the study to detect a given effect or the size of the effect that the study can detect at a given power. In general, a study should have a power of 80% or higher. If the sample size is too small, the result of the study may be negative merely because the power is inadequate. In these cases, the study needs to be redesigned and estimates reevaluated.

Financial Support

The amount of financial support needed for a research project depends on the extent of the data collection, the research setting, the number of subjects studied, and the time and effort involved in data analysis. The necessary resources must not be underestimated. Financial support for research is not generally incorporated into the salary of a clinical or nutrition support dietitian. Thus, part of designing a research project is to estimate the needed resources and then to identify a funding source. A chapter by Schiller and Burge in *Research: Successful Approaches* presents many useful suggestions.[12] Funding of clinical research can come from a variety of sources. Sometimes there is money in the budget of an institution to support in-house studies, but usually relatively little. Generally, the scope and nature of the research proposal determine appropriate sources to approach for financial support. Research colleagues can help identify appropriate funding sources. Although the details of this area are beyond the scope of this chapter, the following groups can be considered as potential funding sources: local, state, and national professional associations such as the ADA, American Heart Association, and American Diabetes Association; pharmaceutical companies such as Bristol-Meyers Squibb, Abbott Laboratories, or Novartis; foundations such as the Kaiser Family Foundation or National Kidney Foundation; and federal funding agencies such as the National Institutes of Health, National Science Foundation, or U.S. Department of Agriculture. University grants and contracts offices have lists of potential sources and can help you in making applications.

In any case, the research idea must be developed into a proposal so that it can be evaluated for consideration for funding. Potential funding sources often have specific proposal formats that must be followed. Although most applications contain

similar sections, each potential source has specific guidelines. Paying close attention to the specific guidelines hastens funding.

Networking, both inside and outside the potential funding source, is a good way to position a proposal for maximum success. Before writing a proposal, a personal conversation with the designated staff person in charge of receiving proposals is recommended and welcomed by the granting agency. Information thus gained can help the researcher present the proposal in a light that best suits the funding source.

Scheduling Time for Research

A major concern of clinicians is planning sufficient time to conduct research. Research activities do take time, and frequently the total amount is not easily predicted. It is not unusual for a scientist to discover that one part of a study requires much less time than anticipated and another part, considerably more. While we think our workday is completely filled, when interesting opportunities are presented, time can usually be found. Generally, the amount of time to conduct a research project should be estimated. This is not impossible, if the project is approached in segments. The investigator may be willing to do some of the proposal writing on personal time. For the data collection phase, how long will it take to perform the protocol activities for each subject? How many subjects will be expected over a given period, and how many will be enrolled in the study? Once the samples have been collected and the results from each subject are in hand, the data analysis begins. Again, like proposal writing, this part of the research activity can be accomplished in "off hours" and on personal time. For the sample collection activity, the time investigators deal directly with the research subjects, a research assistant might be useful and must be included in the research budget. The clinical setting offers several alternatives: dietetics students or interns, graduate students looking for opportunities in research as they prepare to conduct their own, dietitian colleagues in the department, or dietetic technicians.

Although research assistants can save some of the researcher's time, such "helpers" have to be trained in the techniques of data collection and measurement. Enough assistants are needed to comfortably conduct the project, but not so many as to produce interobserver variation. The lead investigator blocks out time to supervise the research. This can be a few hours each day or parts of days or a block of days. Arrangements will have to be made with the supervisor for clinical coverage. The nature of the study and the type and timing of the samples (data) to be collected will help determine how to manage time.

Data Maintenance

Extreme care must be taken to protect collected data. Data collection forms should be tested in a pilot study or on several patients before they are finalized. Frequently, data are collected in writing during the course of observations and then later entered into a more permanent record. Data are entered into a computer database for storage and analytic manipulation.

Data must be recorded meticulously. For example, the year is always part of the date. Sufficient identification information on the subject consists of full name, record number, and study number. Many subjects have similar names or initials, and what once seemed easy to remember can be impossible to recall later. Workers must write clearly and double-check numbers, decimal points, and units of measure. All written records are kept in a notebook throughout the study and retained for several years afterward. This notebook should be kept in a safe place and should not leave the research environment. When data are entered from the written record into the computer program, an independent observer must verify the entries. That is, data entered by one assistant have to be verified by a second person for accuracy. Computer records also must be carefully protected. Backup disks or tapes (depending on the system) should be made whenever new data are entered and the copies protected from destruction. Data collection and maintenance of files are not matters to be taken lightly. Most research data cannot easily be retrieved if they are lost or unintelligible.

Confidentiality of Data

Any human subject research requires confidentiality of data. When data are originally collected they can be readily associated with the individual, but as they are transferred into the permanent data file on the computer the name is replaced with an identifying number. In a separate file, identifying numbers and subject names can be recorded. Once the data become available for a variety of assistants or reviewers to examine, there can be no obvious track to the subject. When research results are presented in public forums, whether orally, in poster format, or in print, no personal identification with the human subject is present.

Ethics of Research Design, Conduct, and Presentation

Throughout the course of planning, conducting, and reporting research, ethical practices are involved. Ethical practice is an issue in three areas of the research process. First, the research idea must be investigator initiated. It is not ethical to co-opt a research idea from an idea generated by another investigator or one that might have been gleaned from the peer review process. There are certainly variations on a theme, but anyone in a position to review others' grants for funding must hold their ideas in confidence and not adopt them.[13]

During the planning phase, ethical issues in provision of nutrition services must be considered. To use or withhold special products that have not been demonstrated effective in specific cases, such as parenteral nutrition, must be carefully designed to ensure that accepted therapies are not withheld. Second, equal access to dietetics services for all potential research subjects is an ethical consideration. Equal access to care may be important when research involves clinical practice data. For example, in the study of nutrition support, investigators must not discriminate against some who need it but do not receive it because of reimbursement issues or the policies of the care setting. When possible or appropriate for the analysis of results, these ethical issues should be identified and discussed.

Ethics in study design for clinical research must foremost consider the welfare and health of subjects.[14] In the conduct of human studies all investigators are responsible for the welfare of participants. To protect the well-being of study subjects,

three factors should be taken into consideration: invasiveness of procedures; promoting malaise in the subjects as a result of the summation of procedures; and burdening subjects with too many measurements, activities, or restrictions.

All of these proscriptions are reviewed by the Institutional Review Board for the protection of human subjects involved in research. The foundation of ethical conduct of human studies is a full and truthful description of all study details to enable subjects to give informed consent.[15] This includes helping the subject understand the ramifications of study requirements, which may include time and money to come to the study site daily or family and social contact. A full discussion of these and similar issues helps prevent study dropouts.

In addition, each study has a set of inclusion and exclusion criteria that must be followed carefully to avoid selection bias. Other safety issues must be considered, such as pregnancy tests for women of child-bearing age and whether it is ethical to screen for infectious conditions such as human immunodeficiency virus (HIV), hepatitis, and tuberculosis.

Payment for study participation recognizes subjects' time and effort in participating in studies that do not relate to their disease. The ethical considerations of paying participants generally are guided by the Institutional Review Board criteria. Such payment should be modest, so that subjects do not remain in a study solely for the remuneration.

After data are collected, ethics are important in their analysis and reporting. The relationships that are appropriate to analyze and report are those outlined in the research design. The investigator should fully disclose research data and the methods by which they were collected and analyzed. Scientific proof must be rigorous and without bias. Selective reporting of findings is unethical. Such behavior is driven by efforts to support the research hypothesis. An investigator may be tempted to conceal data, present only favorable data, or in some way "massage" the data to make the results compatible with the hypothesis. In this vein, data analysis must account for all subjects enrolled in the study. Dropouts must be dealt with in the research report and frequently must be included in the analysis under the heading of *intention to treat.*

Ethical considerations also inform presentation of findings. Oral presentation of original research is properly permitted at one national meeting. Similarly, written research reports are submitted and accepted for publication in only one professional journal. It is not appropriate to submit the same data set and analysis for oral presentation to the American Heart Association one month and to the ADA the next. Likewise, articles submitted for publication in the *Journal of the American Dietetic Association* cannot also be considered for the *Journal of the American Medical Association.* After data have been published, written review articles or review presentations must give attribution when data from another laboratory and investigator are cited. An author cannot lead the audience to believe that data presented in review format are the author's own.

Pilot Studies

Pilot studies are critical to solid research for three reasons: (1) to ensure the appropriateness and adequacy of the methods to be used, (2) to increase the effectiveness and efficiency of data collection, and (3) to develop preliminary data. It is critical, in any study, that valid, reliable methods be used. Issues such as accuracy, precision, sensitivity, and specificity must be carefully considered.

Appropriateness and Adequacy of Methods

If you have selected methods that have been tested and validated previously by others or for another purpose, then your goal is to see that the methods are valid and reliable in your hands and for the purposes of your study. On the other hand, if you have devised new methods (e.g., made modifications to established methods), then it falls on your shoulders to validate those new methods. Such validation is a necessity when methods are modified or questionnaires changed, as when a technique used for one population is applied to a different age, gender, socioeconomic, or ethnic group.

To ensure that the methods are reliable and reproducible, it is customary to compare them to "a gold standard," but making assumptions about what is *gold* can be fraught with danger. A great deal of alchemy has been employed over the years with regard to the quality of the gold. Just because a method is commonly used, unless you can find where in the scientific literature it has been acceptably validated, you should make the appropriate comparisons so that you are sure that the method is indeed giving you the data that you seek.

Methods for estimating protein balance are examples of multiple assumptions. The ratio of urinary urea nitrogen to creatinine serves as a substitute for 24-hour total urinary nitrogen, which in turn is a substitute for protein balance. The gold standard is protein intake and protein output. Intake is based on the protein content of foods and may be assessed in the laboratory by proximate analyses. Such analyses show that food protein, on average, is 16% nitrogen. Thus, on average, 1 g of dietary nitrogen is equivalent to 6.25 g of protein. Because the predominant source of dietary nitrogen is protein, it is customary to assume that dietary nitrogen reflects dietary protein and to ignore the relatively small amount of nonprotein nitrogen. This is a close approximation, but not relatively precise for every food (i.e., for most seeds and nuts, 1 g of nitrogen is equivalent to 5.30 g protein, whereas milk has 6.38 g of protein to 1 g of nitrogen).

Protein output is observed in the loss of protein and its metabolic products in feces, skin, nails, and hair, but principally in urine. Generally, it is estimated by measuring urinary nitrogen, but measuring only that ignores extrarenal losses. Nitrogen losses from skin (including hair and nails) and feces have been estimated to be about 2 g per day nitrogen (or 12.5 g of protein per day). Such adjustment is acceptable if the patient is in nitrogen balance, but there can be large individual variations in fecal nitrogen excretion. For example, dietary intake of either protein or fiber affects fecal nitrogen losses. Exercise also affects nitrogen loss, and the accelerated protein catabolism seen in sepsis and burns further exaggerates potential errors. Subjects who have malabsorption or diarrhea lose more protein and nitrogen in feces than those subjects without these protein-wasting conditions.

In addition to the problems of not knowing what the fecal losses are, there is a major problem in assessing the completeness of a 24-hour urine collection. To make such estimates, creatinine excretion in 24 hours has been used as an indicator of the completeness of the urine collection. Because creatinine excretion reflects an individual's muscle mass, it is fairly consistent over 24 hours, and thus should be consistent from day to day in complete 24-hour urine collections. Yet, creatinine excretion is not constant, and coefficients of variation as high as 25% have been estimated. Many factors affect circadian and day-to-day variations in creatinine excretion. Factors such as dietary intake of creatine and creatinine from meat; the extent of strenuous exercise; menstruation; age; infection; fever; trauma; and, of course, chronic renal failure can markedly alter creatinine excretion. To assess urinary nitrogen excretion it would be ideal to make eight 24-hour urine collections per subject, to account for intrasubject variation. If only group means are desired, a single 24-hour collection from each person may suffice.

A substitute measure for 24-hour total urinary nitrogen, urinary urea nitrogen, was selected as a yardstick because urea is the predominant form of nitrogen in urine. Urea nitrogen, however, misses the nitrogen in creatinine, ammonia, and uric acid, all of which are normally excreted in the urine. It is thus customary to add 2 g of nitrogen per day for urinary nonurea nitrogen in addition to the 2 g of nitrogen per day added to adjust for assessing only urinary losses. These two adjustments are equivalent to 25 g of protein per day. The ratio includes creatinine to estimate 24-hour excretion from a single urine sample. The test may be improved if the analyses are made on the first or second voided fasting urine sample. The estimate appears to be acceptable for normal, average persons; however, with low protein intake, urinary urea nitrogen underestimates protein intake. Correspondingly, urea synthesis increases when parenteral and enteral solutions with high levels of arginine and glutamine are administered. An additional caution to note is that metabolic acidosis increases urinary ammonia, whereas metabolic alkalosis reduces it.

Thus, when using a surrogate method, such as the urinary urea nitrogen-creatinine ratio, recognize that the method is based on many assumptions (i.e., that urine urea represents urinary total nitrogen, creatinine represents an estimate of solute concentration for 24 hours, urinary nitrogen represents total nitrogen loss, and nitrogen represents protein). Making the estimate further assumes that skin, hair, and fecal losses are within normal ranges. If they are not, methods must be chosen that will provide accurate data.

Effective and Efficient Data Collection

The effectiveness and efficiency of a large long-term study can be much enhanced by first securing several pilot subjects and working through the planned procedures. The experience gained in explaining the purpose of the study to the pilot subjects and securing their informed consent will make an investigator more effective with the subjects in the full-scale study, as in allaying fears and evaluating the procedures, the sequence, and forms that have been devised and making useful improvements. Of obvious benefit is that the researcher can assess how much time will be needed to secure samples or data from the subjects.

Securing Preliminary Data

Pilot studies allow collection of preliminary data from a small cohort of subjects.[16] The protocol can mimic that of the larger study. The early data may be extremely useful in securing funding, if they lend support to the hypothesis to be tested. In addition, retrospective studies are often a good source of useful data and can serve as a springboard from which to devise prospective studies.[17] Preliminary data may come also from descriptive studies.[18] From rigorous retrospective or descriptive studies, investigators can move on to prospective studies, where analytic designs are paramount.[19]

Refinement of the Research Design

In most pilot studies, at some point it becomes apparent that the test forms can be improved and that certain steps in the procedures can be restructured to be more effective and more efficient. At this time, it is appropriate to refine the research design. For example, it may become apparent that the time needed to secure urine and blood samples from a subject is 20 minutes rather than the 30 minutes the research team had estimated. If this is the case, three subjects can be scheduled in an hour rather than two.

It is wise, while designing the research and planning the pilot study, to be alert for variables that may need to be controlled by establishing well-defined procedures. For example, when subjects are to be enrolled in a study where each will be randomly assigned to one of three parenteral formulas of different glutamine content, it is important to minimize or control other variables, such as total energy and percentage of energy from carbohydrate, protein, and fat. If several dietitians are involved in the study, practitioner variability must be minimized. One way to accomplish this is to devise, ahead of time, precise calculations for assessing nutrition needs so that each practitioner is using the same formulas. For example, formulas to calculate basal energy requirements can be based on the subject's age, gender, height, weight, ideal body weight, and medications (e.g., prednisone); from these calculations, basal energy expenditures, fluid requirements, and the amounts of protein, fat, and carbohydrate to be supplied may be generated and used initially as the subjects are enrolled. Using the equations consistently ensures that the subjects are handled similarly, regardless of which practitioner is interacting with them.

Conducting Research

Having completed the pilot study and being sure that the methods are appropriate for the purpose, test forms and procedures are revised appropriately, and practitioner variability is minimized, the researcher is ready to launch the project. We have discussed the importance of the research teams and colleagues in conducting research. Some dietitians work in rural settings or in less populated areas where access to colleagues with research interests is limited. With the information explosion via computer communication, anyone can participate in research via the Internet, as by collecting data from subjects they work with. You may also be able to conduct secondary analyses of data from larger studies that can be accessed through the Internet.

We have already discussed the importance of data maintenance and appropriate computer backup; the importance of maintaining confidentiality of data; the need to secure approval

from the Institutional Review Board; and the obligation ethically to design, conduct, and present research.[20] These four issues are requisite components of the research process.

Conducting research must be done on a clear schedule. It is necessary to be objective and to maintain the research protocol. Minimum and maximum time limits need to be established by the research team. It is important when conducting research that you are firm in securing the data in such a manner that the protocol is followed within the limits that you as a research team have established. For example, if an experimental procedure is to start at 0800 it must start precisely at 8:00 o'clock, to eliminate possible deviations that reflect circadian rhythms or length of fasting. If fasting data are to be assessed, the research team needs to make a scientific decision about whether fasting data from blood drawn at 1100 are equivalent to fasting blood samples drawn at 0800. If the protocol states that the fasting blood sample is to be taken between 0800 and 0900 and the pilot study determined that 20 minutes be allowed to take the sample, the subject must be there between 0740 and 0840 and not 0930 or later. Guidelines must be clearly defined with the research team and with subjects. The use of a 24-hour clock or "military" time avoids confusion with AM and PM. Guidelines thoughtfully established by the research team are considered sacrosanct. Any leeway given to the subjects must be within guidelines agreed upon beforehand by the entire research team. To do otherwise would lead to chaos and endanger interpretation of the data.

Instructions need to be clearly given; the protocol on instruction sheets needs to be reaffirmed. Instructions given verbally can be very helpful, whether or not they are followed up with written ones. All written instructions should be based on the reading skills level appropriate for the subjects. Subjects should not be expected to understand what researchers are thinking. They need clear verbal instructions and written ones to read later. People differ in their learning styles: some learn aurally, others visually. Thus, it is wise to consider both learning styles and to develop both oral and written instructions. The language and cultural challenge of various subjects need to be recognized in such materials. Repetition of key points is prudent and saves time in the long run.

For data to be useful they must be thoughtfully collected, clearly recorded, and handled consistently. Protocols must be clear and detailed. Rather than saying, Draw a blood sample, the task should state where in the clinic the blood is to be drawn, by whom, how much, and into which tubes; how the sample is to be handled, stored, and transported; and what analyses are to be performed. The chain of responsibility must be clearly established. To that end it is wise to devise flow sheets for the research team that clearly indicate who is to do what and within what time limits, how the samples and data are to be followed from one point to another, and who is responsible. Flow sheets can follow each subject as they proceed through the protocol. Spaces can be provided for the investigators to initial each step.

Data Evaluation

Once data are collected it is wise to graph or plot them. This affords an opportunity to *see* how each data point relates to the others. Such graphs are extremely useful in collating the various pieces of data and in understanding them as a whole. To avoid skewing the visual impact of the data, it is helpful to use the same grid when plotting similar data. For example, when plotting serum cholesterol or serum triglyceride levels against different diets, employ the same grid used for cholesterol, even if the range of cholesterol values is greater than for serum triglycerides. Thus, the effects of the variables may be seen more clearly than if the grid for serum cholesterol were magnified for serum triglycerides to make the differences seem greater than they are. Frequently, the graphs are not used in formal presentations, but they have served their purpose well when such global assessment enhances the opportunity to use the data wisely and with clarity.

It is important to avoid overgeneralization of data. Thoughtful choice of the study population and, within that population, careful selection of test subjects and enrollment of a sufficient number of subjects to meet the goal as determined by power calculations for sample size, will allow investigators to use the data that represent that group. To extend beyond that group, however, must be done with great caution and care. For example, serum transferrin levels for a group of college students in a nutrition class cannot be considered representative of all students on campus, or of all college students in the nation, or all 18- to 22-year-olds, or all the people in the nation, and they definitely would not be representative of persons with hepatic or renal disease. Avoiding overgeneralization is a primary concern. It is a temptation that needs to be resisted.

In evaluating and interpreting data, researchers must remain cognizant of the original data and their precision. If the original serum transferrin levels collected from five subjects are 3.94, 2.76, 1.87, 4.07, and 2.45 g/L, the mean should be reported with the same number of significant figures (i.e., 3.02 g/L, not 3.018 g/L, which implies more precision than the original data could generate).

It is an act of balance to neither underinterpret nor overinterpret data. Perhaps that is one reason why so many reports of data end with the comment, "Additional studies are necessary." If the subjects are selected well and the design generated thoughtfully, the research should be able to answer the question. This will allow future research to answer other questions, rather than addressing the original question again and again.

Disseminating Research Results

There is a great deal of pleasure and responsibility in sharing research data. Pleasure comes from many directions: good feelings from the successful completion of a major creative project, the sense that you have added to the scientific knowledge base of your discipline, the assurance that the data will be useful in problem solving and decision making, and the opportunity to hear the comments and critique of peers. Likewise, responsibility has many sources: the obligation to present data clearly, accurately, and without bias, and ethical with interpretation. Presenting data is exciting and challenging. Fortunately, there are many ways to share research, within an institution, to the scientific community, and to the public, at many times and in many ways. Internal discussion and presentation are extremely helpful in evaluating and refining ideas. Initial presentations

should remain internal and be considered "confidential" unless the researcher plans to forego formal routes of presentation. It is important to remember that data may be published only once in the scientific literature as "original." Before that original publication, oral or poster presentation at scientific meetings, or both, is appropriate and anticipated. Subsequent to the original publication, oral or secondary written publications are both desirable and appropriate as long as acknowledgment is made to the original publication. Information on preparing data for presentation in a variety of settings is available in the ADA publication *Communicating as Professionals*.[21]

Communicating Internally

The value of internal presentation should not be underestimated. Presenting data at departmental meetings is extremely good for letting colleagues know what one is doing. The feedback can really be useful. Interested colleagues may come forward to offer assistance and professional breadth. Pilot studies are very appropriate to present internally.

It is good to show colleagues data as they are being gathered and plotted. Colleagues' feedback can help clarify the final presentation. Internal presentations may take the form of showing a colleague a proposed table or figure, giving a full oral presentation, giving a presentation to an internal group before presenting the data elsewhere, or making internal poster presentations. It is wise to remember that a poster presentation posted within the institution makes the work known and encourages collaboration.

Internal presentations also allow colleagues to see manuscripts in preparation. But such sharing of manuscripts should make clear that they are in draft form and must remain confidential, lest the researcher lose control of the data.

Reporting to the Professional and Scientific Communities

External reports can be very beneficial to both researcher and institution. External oral and poster presentations may be given at subject matter meetings and at regional and national ones. External reports also include manuscript preparation and publication. External presentations make research data available to be added to the body of science.

The public are keenly interested in research that affects them or their families. Researchers have an obligation to inform the public of such information in a way that avoids bias and misinterpretation. Critical to proper application is to avoid overgeneralization. Simple and direct explanations are best. When the media are involved, it is all too easy to mislead (and to be misled by) overinterpreting data, as when data from experimental animal models are extrapolated to humans. Clear and effective presentation is the goal whether the audience is staff, colleagues, the broader professional community, clients, or the public.

Clear and Effective Data Presentation

There are several ways to present research data: written reports, oral presentations, and visual presentation such as posters. Most researchers use tables and figures. Specific formatting depends on the specific use—written or oral—and the audience—research team, a group of practitioners, or readers of the scientific literature.

Tables and Figures

Tables and figures are worthless and ineffective if they are not simple and straightforward. Readers' interest is lost if the tables or figures are too complicated. Tables and figures differ depending on whether they are developed for an oral presentation, a poster, or a manuscript. In general, illustrations (slides) for oral presentations must be simpler and less dense than those for posters or manuscripts.

Tables and figures should be intelligible by themselves, so that readers and viewers can understand material from viewing an individual table or figure. Unusual acronyms and jargon must be avoided and informative category labels should be used. For example, when comparing two groups receiving low and high levels of glutamine, respectively, it is clearer for the reader and viewer if the groups are designated as *Low-Glutamine* and *High-Glutamine* than as *Group 1* and *Group 2*.

The data presentation should be logical; for example, with data ranked from highest to lowest values, or vice versa, or as appropriate or alternatively, chronologically. It is tempting to present data in the order in which they were generated because the researcher is familiar with this. Someone unfamiliar with the data might perceive it as a visual jumble. The investigator should consider several forms of presentation and select the one that seems most effective.

Oral or Written Presentations

The text for the oral presentation must be developed clearly and logically. With oral presentation, it is helpful to give people a map at the beginning to review what will be discussed. Frequent recaps along the way help listeners know where they have been. Repetition supports your comments and confirms listeners' understanding, but repetition can be overdone. Good summaries are useful, either at the beginning, as an abstract, or at the end, as a conclusion or summary. To repeat frequently in written formats is unnecessary and irritates many readers. Readers, at their own discretion, can look back in a printed text.

The text should consist of *clear* sentences that *inform*. Be as active in voice as the content allows. For example, "The subjects were 25 to 50 years of old," a clear statement in the active voice, is preferable to, "It was noted that the subjects were 25 to 50 years old."

Subheads can be an excellent guide to listener or readers. Subheads are "signs" of upcoming material. They serve as an outline for the reader, showing the organization of large components and the parts within each one. Because the goal is to transmit information, a title should be informative, for example, "Glutamine Enhances Cost-Effectiveness of Parenteral Nutrition," rather than "Impact of Glutamine on Cost-Effectiveness of Parenteral Nutrition."

Abstracts

The abstract is one of the most useful components of any presentation, be it an oral summary, abstract summary in a poster, or the abstract in a manuscript. An abstract that is fully informative and is intelligible by itself is one that readers greatly respect. Structured abstracts are now obligatory for many research publications. Information presented under descriptive headings, as in structured abstracts, provides an organized overview of the research design and outcomes. Further, readers can quickly and easily compare similarly organized abstracts of several research reports.

For analytic research such as an intervention that compares two different enteral formulas, a structured abstract with the following descriptive headings would be appropriate: Objective, Design, Subjects/Setting, Intervention (unless presented adequately under Design), Main Outcome Measures (unless presented adequately under Design), Statistical Analyses, Results, and Applications/Conclusions. For a descriptive research project such as a comparison of two equations to predict energy expenditure in children with cystic fibrosis, the structured abstract would have the following descriptive headings: Objective, Design, Subjects/Setting, Statistical Analyses, Results, and Applications/Conclusions.

Slides for Oral Presentations

Presentation of data and other information in slides and overheads is a pleasure in effective oral presentations. Slides should (1) have no more than 45 characters per line; (2) be no more than six lines long, and (3) have no large spaces between the lines. This "45 character–6 line rule" counts blank spaces and punctuation.

In general, tables of data appropriate for publication have to be revised for slide presentation by formatting the data into two or more slides. It is a good idea to project the slide in a room similar to the presentation room and periodically to go to the back of the room to see how readable the slides are. If a slide is too challenging, it may have to be simplified or made into two slides. Appropriate line spacing of text or data improves viewer readability and visibility of the slide to the viewer. Line spacing variation can be by 0.1 increments with the use of PowerPoint software.

Posters

Poster sessions are increasingly popular for sharing new findings or innovative practice techniques at professional meetings. Poster presentations are a combination of written and oral reports, of formal and informal presentations, at professional meetings. Data are presented in formal tables and graphs with written statements of research design, statistical analysis, and conclusions in an environment of informal discussions and question/answer sessions as interest is generated around the poster.[21]

There are several considerations to bear in mind when devising an effective poster presentation.[22] The poster should be divided into specific segments, usually Abstract, Introduction, Methods, Results, Summary, and Conclusions. Brevity; focused, detailed information; and superior visual interest are important components of the presentation. Several people will likely be looking at it at one time, and if the presentation is very successful there may be a small crowd around the display board.

The text and graphics should be bold, interspersing the two to avoid monotonous blocks of "gray material." Color photographs and graphics also lend visual interest. Within text sections, an outline form with bullets can be visually effective. Use this technique to highlight important points and present the logic of your research design and conclusions. It is wise in a poster presentation to place the most important aspect of the research—the results—in an upper and central space where it will receive the most attention. One large sheet of bold text, followed by supporting graphics illustrating research results, should be placed at eye level and central. This part of your presentation must be positioned so that it can be viewed over the heads of people standing in front of others.

Poster sessions are valuable opportunities for a "first run" of a research project in the professional community before findings are submitted to the rigors of a peer-reviewed publication.

Conclusion

The practice of dietetics is based on science. Thus, it behooves dietitians to maintain a research orientation in practice. Documentation of and the outcome of practice is a good beginning for research. Only through documentation and research reporting is it possible to enhance the effectiveness of medical nutrition therapy and to justify costs in a time of cost consciousness. This is the challenge and the opportunity of today.

REFERENCES

1. Sims LS: Nutrition education research: reaching toward the leading edge, *J Am Diet Assoc* 87(9 suppl):S10-S18, 1987.
2. Glore S: Show me the science, *J Am Diet Assoc* 101(2):186, 2001.
3. Labrecque M: Critical appraisal of medical literature: practical update, *Can Fam Phys* 35:786-789, 1989.
4. Willett W: *Nutritional epidemiology,* ed 2, New York, 1998, Oxford University Press.
5. Stallone DD, Brunner EJ, Bingham SA, Marmot MG: Dietary assessment in Whitehall II: the influence of reporting bias on apparent socioeconomic variation in nutrient intakes, *Eur J Clin Nutr* 51(12):815-825, 1997.
6. Einstein A, Infeld L: *The evolution of physics,* New York, 1938, Simon and Schuster.
7. Smitherman AL, Wyse BW: President's page: the backbone of our profession, *J Am Diet Assoc* 87(10):1394, 1987.
8. Coulston AM: Developing the research question, *Cutting Edge* 11(6):7-8, 1990.
9. Homann HH, Kemen M, Fuessenich C, et al: Reduction in diarrhea incidence by soluble fiber in patients receiving total or supplemental enteral nutrition, *J Parenter Enteral Nutr* 18(6):486-490, 1994.
10. McKinley MJ, Goodman-Block J, Lesser ML, Salbe AD: Improved body weight status as a result of nutrition intervention in adult, HIV-positive outpatients, *J Am Diet Assoc* 94(9):1014-1017, 1994.
11. Splett P, Meyers EF: A proposed model for effective nutrition care, *J Am Diet Assoc* 101(3):357-363, 2001.
12. Monsen ER (ed): *Research: successful approaches,* ed 2, Chicago, 2002, The American Dietetic Association (in press).
13. Monsen ER, Vanderpool HY, Halsted CH, et al: Ethics: responsible scientific conduct, *Am J Clin Nutr* 54(1):1-6, 1991.
14. Kahn JP, Mastroianni AC: Moving from compliance to conscience: why we can and should improve on the ethics of clinical research, *Arch Intern Med* 161(7):925-928, 2001.
15. Moreno J, Caplan AL, Wolpe PR: Updating protections for human subjects involved in research: Project on Informed Consent, Human Research Ethics Group, *JAMA* 280(22):1951-1958, 1998.
16. Weddle DO, Tu NS, Guzik CJ, Ramakrishnan V: Positive association between dietetics recommendations and achievement of enteral nutrition outcomes of care, *J Am Diet Assoc* 95(3):753-764, 1995.
17. MacBurney M, Young LS, Ziegler TR, Wilmore DW: A cost-evaluation of glutamine-supplemented parenteral nutrition in adult bone marrow transplant patients, *J Am Diet Assoc* 94(11):1263-1266, 1994.
18. Goldstein DJ, Frederico CB: The effect of urea kinetic modeling on the nutrition management of hemodialysis patients, *J Am Diet Assoc* 87(4):474-479, 1987.
19. Gottschlich MM, Mayes T, Khoury JC, Warden GD: Significance of obesity on nutritional, immunologic, hormonal, and clinical outcome parameters in burns, *J Am Diet Assoc* 93(11):1261-1268, 1993.
20. Committee on Science, Engineering, and Public Policy (COSEPUP) of the National Academy of Sciences: *On being a scientist: responsible conduct in research,* Washington, DC, 1995, National Academy Press.
21. Chernoff R (ed): *Communicating as professionals,* ed 2, Chicago, 1994, American Dietetic Association, pp 3-42.
22. Coulston AM, Stivers M: A poster is worth a thousand words, *J Am Diet Assoc* 93(8):865-866, 1993.

Future Directions 47

Tina Colaizzo-Anas, PhD, RD, CDN
Laura E. Matarese, MS, RD, LD, FADA, CNSD

THE future is elusive and unpredictable. Several areas of nutrition support are ripe for research and development. In this chapter, we present some of the new and emerging technologies. It is a starting point. Perhaps we can direct the future of nutrition support by infusing these technologies into dietetics practice.

Nutrition and Genetics

The impetus for including a discussion on nutrition and genetics is the Human Genome Project, an international research program designed to determine the complete nucleotide sequence of human deoxyribonucleic acid (DNA) and to localize the 30,000 to 40,000 genes within its structure.[1] By definition, *human genome* is all the DNA contained in human cells, which includes the DNA comprising chromosomes within the nucleus, and the DNA in mitochondria. On June 26, 2000 the Human Genome Project announced the completion of a working draft of the sequence of the human genome.[2] This sequence information has been released continuously to the world as it has become available. The significance of this monumental scientific achievement will become celebrated as it revolutionizes the practice of medicine in the twenty-first century. Knowing the sequence of human DNA makes it easier and speedier to identify gene mutations associated with disease. Knowing the sequence of human DNA facilitates the application of microarrays that show how thousands of genes are turned on or off in different types of cells in response to different stimuli (e.g., nutrients). This likely will also facilitate the identification of more precise estimates of nutrient requirements.

It is believed that virtually all diseases have a genetic component.[3] Some diseases are primarily genetic, whereas others have strong genetic and environmental influences. Genetically, humans are 99.9% the same and 0.1% different. The differences are often in the form of single nucleotide polymorphisms (SNPs), which occur 1 in 1000 nucleotides. The identification of SNPs will help scientists pinpoint genetic differences that predispose some to disease and affect individual response to treatment.

Because environment can influence the expression of the genetic predisposition to disease, it is advantageous to know ones genotype in order to decrease disease risk by modifying the environment (e.g., nutrition).[3] In order to prepare for genomic medicine, some have encouraged all health professions to think genetically. This means knowing when genetics may play a role, how to take and use a family history, how to protect genetic privacy, how and when to refer patients for genetic counseling, and how to use genetics to individualize care. This knowledge will be important for dietitians who expand their scope of practice to include genetic nutrition. The discussion that follows highlights the potential influence the Human Genome Project will have on the practice of dietetics and nutrition support.

The New Genetics

Dr. Alan E. Guttmacher, Senior Clinical Advisor, National Human Genome Research Institute, NIH, has offered the perspective that the Human Genome Project provides the tool to deal with what is now termed *genomic medicine (genomics)*.[4] *Genomics* is the study of the structure and function of genes and the roles genes play in health and disease.[5] Genomics takes into consideration the interaction of multiple genes and their interaction with the environment. The old genetics focused primarily on conditions involving a whole or part of a chromosome (e.g., Down syndrome) or mutations in single genes (e.g., cystic fibrosis or phenylketonuria). These conditions, while devastating for families, are relatively rare. Conditions addressed by the new genetics include nine of the top ten causes of death in the United States. These conditions have a high frequency and include heart disease, cancer, stroke, chronic obstructive pulmonary disease (COPD), pneumonia, diabetes, renal disease, and chronic liver disease.[4]

The new genetics addresses conditions that may be only partly caused by genetic mutations. Examples include colon cancer, breast cancer, atherosclerosis, inflammatory bowel disease, Alzheimer's disease, mood disorders, and many others. The diseases/conditions that are encompassed by the new genetics have a high incidence. However, there is a shortage of health professionals who are trained to address genetic issues related to these diseases. Currently, there are only 3300 genetics specialists in the country. What this means is that genetic issues will increasingly need to be addressed by primary care providers.[6]

It is often the primary care provider that identifies genetically related problems. For this reason, it is beneficial when primary care providers can offer patients knowledge of their individual genetic predisposition to disease and individualized schedules for screening. Furthermore, counseling regarding nutrition and lifestyle choices to reduce risk and presymptomatic therapy (e.g., antihypertensive medication and diet to reduce risk of hypertension) may be offered to patients in a seamless fashion. In order to help health professionals prepare for the new genetics, the National Coalition for Health Professional Education in Genetics (NCHPEG) has developed core competencies in genetics. These competencies may be found on the NCHPEG website (http://www.nchpeg.org). Currently there is an initiative to include some of these competencies in dietetics standards of education.

More responsibility for the use and interpretation of genetic tests and information is falling on physicians, nurses, dietitians, speech pathologists, social workers, psychologists, occupational and physical therapists, and other health professionals who may not be formally trained in genetics. A recent survey of members of health-related professions indicated that 80% heard little or nothing about the Human Genome Project.[6] Consequently, integrating genetics education into the curricula of allied health disciplines and its content into credentialing examinations has become a pressing priority. Recently, funding was granted by the U.S. Department of Health and Human Services to develop discipline-specific competencies in genetics. An example of a core competency that may apply to all allied health professions is knowledge of the ethical, legal, and social issues related to genetic testing and recording of genetic information (e.g., the potential for genetic discrimination in health insurance and employment).

A potential competency specific to the profession of dietetics is knowledge of the influence of genetic variation associated with ethnoculture on response to medical nutrition therapy. An example is in predicting the response to a low-cholesterol diet related to variation of the apolipoprotein E (Apo E4) gene. Apo E4 is a genetic variant found in 15% of whites, 35% of African and Asian populations, 22.7% of Finns, 20.3 % of Swedes, and 9.4% of Italians. Men with ApoE4 genotype show improvement in their serum lipids on a low-fat diet but realize no benefit when consuming oat bran.[7] A brief summary of known and hypothesized diet-gene interactions is outlined in Table 47-1. Dietetics professionals need to be adept at: (1) distinguishing between genetic and environmental influences on disease when applying medical nutrition therapy; (2) understanding how genetic heritage influences food and nutrient requirements and response to medical nutrition therapy;[8] and (3) collaborating with genetics specialists.[8,9]

Despite the fact that few dietetic practitioners have had formal training in genetics, 68% have reported that they discussed the genetic component of a problem with at least a few of their patients.[6] Likewise, 24% reported that they provided counseling about genetic concerns to at least a few of their clients. Only 10% reported high confidence in their ability to provide guidance to clients with genetic disorders about the impact of the genetic condition in the future.

The new genetics likely will require dietitians to gain skills in genetic counseling. In general, the goals of genetics counseling include the following components:
1. Patient education
2. Risk assessment
3. Facilitation of decision-making and coping strategies

The process of genetics counseling includes taking a family history (pedigree), obtaining a medical history, performing risk assessment, and making appropriate referrals to health professionals and support groups. Patient education may include many topics related to genetic testing such as eligibility criteria, purpose of testing, sensitivity and specificity of genetic tests, and patients' rights related to genetic testing.[5] Patient education may also be directed toward 'helping the patient understand that in certain situations, genes may determine susceptibility to disease and that disease may not manifest itself under proper environmental influences such as nutrition. The goal here would be to provide patients with information about potential risks, benefits, and limitations of genetic testing. Risks may include insurance or employment discrimination. Limitations may include lack of sensitivity or specificity of genetic tests. Risk assessment may include explaining concepts of probability and disease susceptibility related to genotype. Appropriate referrals may include psychosocial counseling related to genetic diagnoses, referrals for genetic testing, and genetic counseling. Written reports may be forwarded to the physician. Through the process of genetic counseling, the patient will recognize that genotype is permanent and that it has implications for other family members and for reproductive decision-making and choice of partner.[10,11]

A set of competencies for a medical school core curriculum in genetics has been developed.[12] These competencies include targeted knowledge, skills, and attitudes. More recently, a set of clinical objectives in medical genetics for undergraduate medical students was developed.[13] A set of genetics competencies for undergraduate dietetic curriculum has been proposed. These competencies were based on those developed by the NCHPEG.

From its start, the Human Genome Project has earmarked funds for consideration of the related ethical, legal, and social implications (ELSI) of genomic research. It has included the largest funding ever devoted to bioethics. ELSI issues may address many questions. Examples include: What should people know before choosing to have a genetic test? Who should have access to the information stored in our DNA? What is genetic discrimination? How can it be prevented?[14] The ELSI program of the National Human Genome Research Institute (NHGRI) focuses on the following four areas:
1. The use and interpretation of genetic information
2. Clinical integration of genetic technologies
3. Issues surrounding genetics research
4. Public and professional education and training about these issues

As new data become available, physicians and genetic counselors will increasingly refer patients with susceptible genotypes to dietitians for medical nutrition therapy. Accordingly, dietary advice will need to be presented in terms of probabilities for reducing risk of disease.[15]

Genomics and Nutrition Support

The last decade has been marked by the introduction of many disease-specific or functional foodlike nutritional products on the clinical nutrition market. The goals with these products have expanded from simply the prevention of malnutrition and its associated complications to optimization of clinical response via metabolic enhancers. In addition to immune-enhancing formulas, we now have formulas designed to attenuate the stress response, limit the inflammation associated with inflammatory bowel disease, decrease CO_2 production in COPD patients, and prevent hepatic encephalopathy and control blood sugar. Many manufacturers are towing their weight by generating data that demonstrate beneficial effects of these products in terms of patient outcome with regard to hospital stay and rates of common complications. But is this enough? As practitioners, are we using an evidence-based approach to clinical-decision making? When we review the literature related to these products, are we asking whether the authors evaluated all possible outcomes?

In the future, in order to ascertain whether all possible outcomes have been evaluated, we will need to ask what the molecular effects of functional formulas are. If additives are modulating the expression of one gene, what are their effects on other genes that are regulated by the same or similar pathways? These questions are particularly relevant when formulas are designed to modulate the immune response. If formulas are designed to modify the expression/activity of specific cytokines, are we always obtaining a desired effect? Cytokines at various levels have different effects, some desirable and some undesirable.

To ask and answer these questions, it will be helpful to target the competencies that have been proposed by NCHPEG as areas for professional development. These include obtaining knowledge of basic human genetics terminology and knowledge of how the identification of disease-associated genetic variation facilitates development of prevention, diagnosis, and treatment options. Additionally, it will be helpful to gain an understanding of the techniques used in genetics research to critically evaluate the scientific literature. Boxes 47-1 and 47-2 have been constructed to guide the reader in planning personal professional development in the areas of nutrition, genetics, and gene expression.

Knowledge of individual genotypes will enhance the physician's ability to diagnose, treat, prevent, and predict the course of disease. Likewise, knowing an individual's genetic profile will increasingly be helpful to nutrition support dietitians in weighing the risks and benefits of different nutrition support strategies.

Impact of Nutrition Support on Gene Expression

Nutrient gene interactions extend beyond considerations of the genetic predisposition to disease. Numerous components of food are known to affect gene expression and the body's ability to respond to oxidative stress.[18] Some nutrients, metabolites of vitamins A and D, fatty acids, and zinc, directly regulate gene transcription.[19] Other food components, such as dietary fiber and oxidized fatty acid (eicosanoid), may affect gene expression by altering membrane signals to the nucleus.[19] Furthermore, some dietary constituents may regulate mRNA stability and posttranscriptional modification of mRNA.[20] Phytochemicals such as genistein may decrease prostate and liver cancer by modifying gene expression.[21] A variety of enteral formulas are supplemented with many of these additives. Unfortunately, a paucity of data describes their influence on gene expression. Future research should be directed towards delineating the molecular effects of medical foods.

Impact of Nutrition Support on Oxidative Stress, Associated Gene Expression, and Genomic Stability

Antioxidants are frequent additives to enteral formulas. Dietary antioxidants influence gene expression and apoptosis (programmed cell death). Apoptosis can occur normally in development, as in the resorption of a tadpole tail, or it can be initiated when DNA damage exceeds the capacity of normal cellular DNA repair mechanisms.[22] Additionally, antioxidants prevent free radical damage to DNA and lipid membranes. Many clinical manifestations are associated with uncontrolled oxidative stress, including cancer resulting from DNA damage and atherosclerosis due to the damaging action of oxidized low-density lipoprotein (LDL).

TABLE 47-1
Examples of Diet-Gene Interactions

Polymorphism (genotype)	Gene Product Function	Environmental Exposure(s)	Associated Condition/Disease
KNOWN DIET-GENE INTERACTIONS			
Glucose-6-phosphate dehydrogenase	Metabolism	Fava bean consumption	Hemolytic anemia
Phenylketonuria	Metabolism of phenylalanine	Dietary phenylalanine	Phenylketonuria
HFE gene	Iron absorption	Dietary iron	Hemochromatosis
HYPOTHESIZED DIET-GENE INTERACTIONS			
Glutathione S-transferase mu 1	Detoxification	Smoking combined with diet low in antioxidants	Lung cancer
Epoxide hydrolase glutathione S-transferase mu 1	Detoxification	Aflatoxin (fungal contaminant, especially of peanuts)	Liver cancer
Apolipoprotein E, apolipoprotein AIV, apolipoprotein B	Lipoprotein metabolism	Dietary cholesterol and fat	Responsiveness to dietary cholesterol and fat intake
Methylenetetrahydrofolate reductase	Metabolism of folate affecting plasma homocysteine levels	Low folate intake	Coronary artery disease, stroke, colon cancer, and neural tube defects

Adapted from Patterson, Eaton DL, Potter JD: The genetic revolution: change and challenge for the dietetics profession, *J Am Diet Assoc* 99:1412-1420, 1999.

The redox state of a cell may exert its effects on gene expression via activation of the transcription factors NF-kß or AP-1. NF-kß regulates the expression of many genes that may be involved in nutrition support practice. Among them are cytokines, cytokine receptors, and acute phase proteins.[23] AP-1 regulates the expression of many genes that are involved in cell proliferation and differentiation. The transcription of genes regulated by the binding of the AP-1 protein complex to DNA is inhibited under conditions of oxidative stress.[24] Because nutrients or food components can alter the cellular redox state, it is conceivable that nutritional intervention may some day offer targeted modulation of NF-kß and AP-1 activity to affect cytokine expression, acute phase protein synthesis, and cell proliferation and differentiation. Perhaps one day it will be demonstrated that alterations in the activities in these transcription factors will affect the cell proliferation associated with wound healing or the immune response.

A proposed listing of continuing education topics for dietitians endeavoring to position themselves to apply genetics to nutrition support practice is presented in Table 47-2. Additional opportunities for professional development may be found by visiting the websites listed in Table 47-3.

BOX 47-1
Molecular Biology of the Cell: Review Topics

STRUCTURE OF DNA
Replication
Transcription
RNA processing and posttranscriptional control
Translation
Mutations
  Sporadic
  Inherited
  Types
    Point mutations
    Insertions
    Deletions
    Single nucleotide polymorphisms (SNPs)
  Effects of mutations
    Silent
    Missense
    Nonsense
    Frameshift
Regulation of gene expression
Chromosome structure
Cell cycle
Signal transduction
Meiosis
The *immune* system
  Nonspecific internal defenses
    Macrophages
    Natural killer cells
  Inflammatory responses
    Local injury
    Systemic infection
  Specific defense mechanisms
    Humoral-antibodies
    Cell-mediated
    B and T lymphocytes
    T-cell receptors
    Recombinant DNA technology

Intestinal Rehabilitation and Multivisceral Transplantation

Many patients suffer from severe gastrointestinal (GI) dysfunction and irreversible intestinal failure secondary to advanced Crohn's disease, ulcerative colitis, ischemic bowel disease, motility disorders, and radiation enteritis. Currently, three main therapies are available to these patients: long-term parenteral nutrition (PN), intestinal rehabilitation, and isolated intestinal or multivisceral transplantation. At the time of this writing, the latter two therapies are still considered to be in the refinement stages, but rapid progress is being made. Long-term PN, whether in the home or alternate site, is now considered a safe and standard therapy. Without this technology, these patients would have been destined to a life of institutionalization for provision of fluid and nutrients or would have succumbed to malnutrition and dehydration.

There has been a great deal of interest in transplanting small intestine and creative restorative surgeries to make the GI tract continuous. Small bowel transplantation has become a lifesaving procedure for patients with irreversible intestinal failure who can no longer be maintained on PN. Reports of intestinal and multiple abdominal viscera began to appear in the late 1980s.[43-48] Many of these early cyclosporine-based immunosuppression cases, were complicated by rejection, host-versus-graft disease, and infection. However, with the development of new immunosuppressive agents, specifically tacrolimus, and surgical techniques, bone marrow augmentation, allograft irradiation, and the use of daclizumab, outcomes have been improving.[49-52] Survival rates have been reported to be as high as 78% at 1 year and 63% at 5 years.[53]

BOX 47-2
Review Topics in Genetics

Mendelian principles and their application
Genotype/Phenotype
Inheritance
  Autosomal dominant
  Autosomal recessive
  X-linked
  Mitochondrial disorders
Genetics and common diseases
  Hypertension
  Vascular disease
  Diabetes
Gene/environment interactions/genetic markers
Chromosomal abnormalities and cytogenics
Pedigree analysis[16]
The genetics of cancer
  Carcinogenesis and the multiple hit hypothesis
  Proto-oncogenes/oncogenes
  Tumor suppressor genes/loss of function
  Loss of heterozygosity
  Chromosomal rearrangements
  Mechanisms of cancer chemoprevention
Genome projects
Population genetics
Single nucleotide polymorphisms (SNPs)
Genetic testing ¾ indications, interpretation, limitations, risks
Genetic counseling
Ethical, social, and legal issues involved in genetic testing[15,17]

TABLE 47-2

Topics for Continuing Education in Genetics and Nutrition with Resources

Topic	Resources
Genetics and nutrition: general	25, 26
Use of transgenic animals in nutrition research	27, 28
Nutrient effects on gene expression	19, 29, 30
Genetics of nutrition and cancer	31-33
Molecular techniques for studying nutrient effects on gene expression	34
Nutrient effects on posttranscriptional modification	20
Diet-gene interactions in obesity	35
Nutrition and oxidative stress	36,37
Genetic variation and nutrition	38
Genetic risk assessment	39
Cytogenetics	40
Genetic counseling	39-40
Genetic variation, polymorphism, and mutation	40
Genetic variants in apolipoprotein E and cardiovascular risk	7, 41-42

The type of transplant graft depends on the clinical condition and severity of the disease of the recipient. Isolated intestinal transplant is generally recommended for patients with irreversible intestinal failure who can no longer be safely maintained on PN because of repeated bouts of life-threatening sepsis or lack of vascular access. Intestinal transplantation has also been used in patients with complicated desmoid tumors associated with familial adenomatous polyposis.[54] Combined liver-intestinal transplantation is the procedure of choice for patients with irreversible failure of both organs. Multivisceral transplants involving stomach, intestine, liver, pancreas and/or kidney is performed when three or more of these organs have failed. Survival, functional outcome, and quality of life for these patients have improved over the years. But a great deal of work still needs to be done. On April 1, 2001, the Health Care Financing Administration authorized Medicare coverage for intestinal transplantation as a treatment for children and adults with irreversible intestinal failure.

Developing and implementing protocols for gut adaptation and nutritional rehabilitation is another option for patients with severe GI tract dysfunction. It is well known that luminal nutrition plays a role in bowel adaptation. Several nutrients and substrates such as glutamine, zinc, short-chain fatty acids, and dietary fiber have been shown to be gut-tropic. Interest has been renewed in modifying the diet and providing oral rehydration as well as pharmaceutical agents to stimulate bowel growth and adaptation. A variety of growth factors, such as growth hormone, insulin-like growth factor-I, keratinocyte growth factor, epidermal growth factor, and glucagon-like peptide-2 (GLP-2), have been shown to stimulate intestinal growth and repair primarily in animal models with some limited data in humans. ALX-0600 is a 33 amino acid analog of the naturally occurring GLP-2, an intestinotropic hormone that promotes regeneration and repair of the intestinal epithelium.[55-58] It is primarily secreted from the intestinal mucosa of the terminal ileum and colon after food ingestion. Treatment with GLP-2 has been shown to increase the height of the villi of the intestine, thus enhancing its absorptive capacity.[59] It has also been shown to reduce intestinal permeability.[60] Administration of GLP-2 to patients receiving PN has been shown to reduce mucosal atrophy.[61] It has also been demonstrated that the adaptive growth response to major intestinal resections can be augmented by GLP-2 treatment.[62] Treatment with GLP-2 has been shown to improve intestinal absorption and nutritional status, including lean body mass in short-bowel patients.[63] It is possible that with careful dietary modification; close monitoring of fluid, electrolyte, and nutritional status; and the use of agents such as GLP-2, many patients who were dependent on PN will be able to become free of PN.

Although long-term PN has been safely used for about three decades, intestinal transplantation and intestinal rehabilitation each for a decade, the concept of offering patients all three therapies in one center is new.[64] In this decade we will see the emergence of intestinal rehabilitation centers and digestive disease centers that will offer patients evaluation and several treatment options in order to restore nutritional status through

TABLE 47-3

Genetic Information Web Sites*

National Human Genome Research Institute (NHGRI)	http://www.nhgri.nih.gov
Genetic Education Materials database	http://www.dnai.com
Virtual Hospital Clinical Genetics: A Self Study for Health Care Provider	http://www.vh.org
Genetics Education Center	
University of Kansas Medical Center	http://kumc.edu/gec
DNA Learning Center Cold Spring Harbor	http://vector.cshl.org
Genetic Science Learning Center	
University of Utah	http://gslc.genetics.utah.edu
The New Genetics: A Resource for Teachers and Students UMDNJ	http://arginine.umdnj.edu
National Coalition of Health Professionals for Education in Genetics (NCHPEG)	http://www.nchpeg.org
Department of Energy/Human Genome Program Information	http://www.ornl.gov/hgmis
Genetic Organizations:	http://www.faseb.org/genetics
American Society of Human Genetics	
American College of Medical Genetics	
Association of Professors of Human and Medical Genetics	
Lists of genetics services	http://www.genetests.org

*Data from Joann Boughman: Oral presentation. Human Genetics for Health Professions Curricula Project Meeting, Oct 2000, Washington, DC.

the safest, most physiologic techniques compatible with the patient's lifestyle.

Future Practice Roles

Preparing for the future is not easy. As outlined in earlier chapters, the health care environment is changing rapidly and will continue to change. These changes will undoubtedly affect dietetic practice. Increased health care costs, downsizing, and outsourcing trends are changing health care today. Dietetics will continue to undergo change in response to budget constraints, advances in knowledge and technology, and the demands of the marketplace. Nontraditional roles will become the norm. Not only is health care moving from the intensive care unit into the home, but health care professionals are being asked to do more with less. Given our current economic environment, this trend is likely to continue. Our goal is to provide the best possible care for our patients at the lowest cost and in the most efficient manner.

We are already beginning to see the role of the dietitian changing. Dietitians will continue to function at higher levels and with more clinical privileges. And with increased privilege comes increased responsibility and accountability. The need for specialization and subspecialties will continue, and these specialists will have to provide care across the continuum of care from hospital to home. Cross-training to expand the dietitian's skills will increase, allowing for greater job flexibility. The goal is not to replace or "water down" nutrition expertise but rather to expand it. We will see more generalists with advanced skill sets. But expanding skills means more than learning new technical skills such as taking blood pressures or performing a physical examination. Successful dietitians of the future will broaden their horizons, think globally, and learn to be responsive to the marketplace. Successful dietitians of the future will be more creative with the types of services they provide and the way they provide them. For example, dietitians are already obtaining employment in departments in hospitals other than traditional food and nutrition services. Dietitians are acting as entrepreneurs and making their services indispensable.

Dietitians of the future are likely to have increased managerial responsibilities and will manage multiple departments within a facility or like departments in multiple facilities. Dietitians will continue to develop business and communication skills. Good leadership skills will be essential. It will no longer be enough to be clinically competent.

Research will continue to be an area of growing practice for dietitians (see Chapter 46). The future of health care and the profession of dietetics depend on it. We have a tremendous obligation to the patients we serve to advance nutrition knowledge and practice. We must generate data to demonstrate the clinical efficacy and cost-effectiveness of nutrition support.

But in each of these arenas, there will be barriers to overcome. There will be financial issues to contend with, including lack of reimbursement and the overall high cost of health care. Dietitians will face credentialing and licensure issues. Will there be adequate training sites to obtain new skill sets? And, there will always be those who doubt the ability of the registered dietitian to practice in many of these nontraditional roles. So, dietitians will have to learn how to effectively market their skills and expertise.

In his book, *Future Edge*, Joel Barker states, "You can and should shape your own future. Because if you don't someone else surely will."[65] The future is ours to create. We must embrace the many challenges before us. Dietetic practice in the coming years will be very different. Dietitians are in a unique position to take on new roles with broadened scope and added responsibilities as we attempt to balance cost and volume measures with quality and service. But this must be done with a solid knowledge base and a high level of competency. It is the hope of all the dietitians who participated in writing this book that you will be able to use the information contained within it to enhance patient care, advance the practice of dietetics, and create the future.

Conclusion

In this chapter we described some of the areas related to nutrition support that seem to show the greatest potential to alter dietetic practice and hold the greatest promise for future research. The details must be elucidated. DNA technology will continue to have an enormous impact on the practice of medicine. It is possible that in the future, the true potential of this technology will be harnessed and utilized as therapy in clinical nutrition and metabolism. For those patients with compromised GI function, aggressive intestinal rehabilitation with diet modification, oral rehydration, medication, gut-trophic substances, and restorative surgery hold promise for complete nutritional autonomy. The development and refinement of intestinal and multivisceral transplantation offer yet another option for those patients with irreversible organ failure. This concept of offering several interrelated options to patients with GI dysfunction is applicable to other areas of medicine and nutrition practice. The developments in technology will drive dietetic practice, and dietetic practice will drive advancement.

REFERENCES

1. The Human Genome Project, February 9, 2000, Retrieved from http://www.nhgri.nih.gov/HGP.
2. National Human Genome Research Institute in the news (press release), International Human Genome Sequencing Consortium Announces "Working Draft" of Human Genome, 2000, Retrieved from http://www.nhrgi.nih.gov/NEWS/sequencing consortium.html.
3. Mansoura M: Oral presentation. Human Genetics for Health Professions Curricula Project Meeting, Oct 2000, Washington, DC.
4. Guttmacher AE: Oral presentation. Human Genetics for Health Professions Curricula Project Meeting, March 2001, Washington, DC.
5. Gilbride JA: Finding and using genetic resources, *Top Clin Nutr* 14:51-57, 1999.
6. Lapham EV, Kozma C, Weiss JO, et al: The gap between practice and genetics education of health professionals: HuGEM survey results, *Gen Med* 2(4):226-231, 2000.
7. Simopoulos AP: Genetic variation and nutrition, *Nutr Rev* 57(S5 Pt 2):S10-19, 1999.
8. Simopoulos AP: Genetic variants, diet, and physical activity, *J Am Diet Assoc* 101(3):819-820, 2001.
9. White JV, Gilbride J: President's page, *J Am Diet Assoc* 100(9):996, 2000.
10. Scanlon C, Fibison W: *Managing genetic information: implications for nursing practice,* 1995, Washington, DC, American Nurses Association.

11. Lapham EV, Kozma C, Weiss JO: Genetic discrimination: perspectives of consumers, *Science* 274(5287):621-623, 1996.

12. ASHG Information and Education Committee: Report from the ASHG information and education committee: medical school core curriculum in genetics, *Am J Hum Genet* 56:535-537, 1995.

13. Association of Professors of Human or Medical Genetics: Clinical objectives in medical genetics for undergraduate medical students, June 1998. Retrieved from http://www.faseb.org/genetics/aphmg/aphmg12.htm.

14. National Human Genome Research Institute: *Ethical legal and social implications of the human genome project: fact sheet,* Bethesda, MD.

15. Patterson RE, Eaton DL, Potter JD: The genetic revolution: change and challenge for the dietetics profession, *J Am Diet Assoc* 99(11):1412-1420, 1999.

16. Bennett RL, Steinhaus KA, Uhrich SB, O'Sullivan CK, Resta RG, Lochner-Doyle D, Markel DS, Vincent V, Hamanishi J: Recommendations for standardized human pedigree nomenclature, *Am J Hum Genet* 56:745-752, 1996.

17. Board of Directors of the American Society of Human Genetics: ASHG statement: eugenics and the misuse of genetic information to restrict reproductive freedom, *Am J Hum Genet* 64:335-338, 1999.

18. Berdanier CD: Mitochondrial gene expression in diabetes: effect of nutrition, *Nutr Rev* 59(3 Pt 1):61-70, 2001.

19. Cousins RJ: Nutritional regulation gene expression, *Am J Med* 106(1A):20S-23S, 1999.

20. Hesketh JE, Vasconcelos MH, Bermano G: Regulatory signals in messenger RNA: determinants of nutrient-gene interaction and metabolic compartmentation, *Br J Nutr* 80(4):305-306, 1998.

21. Davis JN, Kucuk O, Sarkar FH: Genistein inhibits NF-kappa B activation in prostate cancer cells, *Nutr Cancer* 35(3):167-174, 1999.

22. Sen CK, Packer L: Antioxidant and redox regulation of gene transcription, *FASEB J* 10(7):709-720, 1996.

23. Pinkus R, Weiner LM, Daniel V: Role of oxidants and antioxidants in the induction of AP-1, NF-kß, and glutathione s-transferase gene expression, *J Biol Chem* 23(271):13422-13429, 1996.

24. Gomez del Arco P, Martinez-Martinez S, Calvo V, Armesilla AL, Redondo JM: Antioxidants and AP-1 activation: a brief overview, *Immunobiology* 198(1-3):273-278, 1997.

25. DeBusk RM: Genetics and nutrition: the future is now, *Nutr Comp Care Newsletter* 3:17-21, 2000.

26. Simopoulos AP, Herbert V, Jacobson B: *Genetic nutrition: designing a diet based on your family medical history,* New York, 1993, Macmillan Publishing Company.

27. Knapp JR, Kopchick JJ: The use of transgenic mice in nutrition research, *J Nutr* 124(4):461-468, 1994.

28. McMillen T: The importance of transgenic mouse models for nutrition research, *Support Line* 22(3):7-12, 2000.

29. Clarke SD: Nutrient regulation of gene expression: a methodological strategy, *Miner Electrolyte Metab* 23(3-6):130-134, 1997.

30. Moustaid-Moussa N, Berdanier CD: *Nutrient-gene interactions in health and disease,* Boca Raton, FL, 2001, CRC Press.

31. Rock CL, Lampe JW, Patterson RE: Nutrition, genetics and risks of cancer, *Ann Rev Public Health* 21:47-64, 2000.

32. Heber D, Blackburn GL, Go VLW (eds): *Nutritional oncology,* San Diego, 1999, Academic Press.

33. Greenwald P, Clifford CK, Milner JA: Diet and Cancer Prevention, *Eur J Cancer* 37(8):948-965, 2001.

34. Hirschi KD, Kreps JA, Hirschi KK: Molecular approaches to studying nutrient metabolism and function: an array of possibilities, *J Nutr* 131(5):1605S-1609S, 2001.

35. Perusse L, Bouchard C: Gene-diet interactions in obesity, *Am J Clin Nutr* 72(5 Suppl):1285S-1290S, 2000.

36. Lof S, Poulsen HE: Antioxidant intervention studies related to DNA damage, DNA repair, and gene expression, *Free Radic Res* 33S:S67-83, 2000.

37. Oldham KM: Oxidative stress and gene expression, *Support Line* 22(3):24-27, 2000.

38. Simopoulos AP: Genetic variation: nutrients, physical activity, and gene expression, *World Rev Nutr Diet* 81:61-71, 1997.

39. Wilson GN: *Clinical genetics,* New York, 2000, John Wiley & Sons.

40. Nussbaum RL, Mclnnes RR, Willard HF: *Thompson & Thompson genetics in medicine,* ed 6, Phildelphia, 2001, WB Saunders Co.

41. Cobb MM, Teitlebaum H, Risch N, et al: Influence of dietary fat, apolipoprotein E, phenotype, and sex on plasma lipoprotein levels, *Circulation* 8(3):849-857, 1992.

42. Uusitupa MI J, Ruuskanen E, Makinen E, et al: A controlled study on the effect of beta-glucan-rich oat bran on serum lipids in hypercholesterolemic subjects: relation to apolipoprotein E phenotype, *J Am Coll Nutr* 11(6):65-659, 1992.

43. Starzl TE, Rowe MI, Todo S, et al: Transplantation of multiple abdominal viscera, *JAMA* 261(10):1449-1457, 1989.

44. Deltz E, Schroeder P, Gebhardt H, et al: Successful clinical small bowel transplantation: report of a case, *Clin Transplantation* 3:89-91, 1989.

45. Grant D, Wall W, Mimeault R, et al: Successful small-bowel/liver transplantation, *Lancet* 335(8683):181-184, 1990.

46. Margreiter R, Konigsrainer A, Schmidt T, et al: Successful multivisceral transplantation, *Transplant Proc* 24(3):1226-1227, 1992.

47. Goulet O, Revillon Y, Brousse N, et al: Successful small bowel transplantation in an infant, *Transplantation* 53(4):940-943, 1992.

48. Starzl TE, Todo S, Tzakis A, et al: The many faces of multivisceral transplantation, *Surg Gynecol Obstet* 172(5):335-344, 1991.

49. Starzl TE, Todo S, Fung J, et al: FK506 for human liver, kidney and pancreas transplantation, *Lancet* 2(8670):1000-1004, 1989.

50. Todo S, Fung J, Starzl TE, et al: Liver, kidney, and thoracic organ transplantation under FK506, *Ann Surg* 212(3):295-305, 1990.

51. Vincenti F, Kirkman R, Light S, Blumgardner G, Pescovitz M, Halloran P, et al: Interleukin-2-receptor blockade with daclizumab to prevent acute rejection in renal transplantation, *N Engl J Med* 338(3):161-165, 1998.

52. Kato T, O'Brien CB, Nishida S, Hope H, Gusser M, Berho M, et al: The first case report of the use of a zoom video endoscope for evaluation of small bowel graft mucosa in a human after intestinal transplantation, *Gastrointest Endosc* 50(2):257-261, 1999.

53. Abu-Elmagd K, Reyes J, Bond G, et al: Clinical intestinal transplantation: a decade of a single center experience, *Ann Surg* 234(3):404-417, 2001.

54. Chatzipetrou M, Tzakis A, Pinna A, et al: Intestinal transplantation for the treatment of desmoid rumors associated with familial adenomatous polyposis, *Surgery* 129(3):277-281, 2000.

55. Lovshin J, Drucker DJ: New frontiers in the biology of GLP-2, *Regulatory Peptides* 90(1-3):27-32, 2000.

56. Drucker DJ, Boushey RP, Wang F, Hill M, Brubaker P, Yusta B: Biologic properties and therapeutic potential of glucagon-like peptide-2, *J Parenteral Enteral Nutr* 23(5):S98-S100, 1999.

57. Tsai C-H, Hill M, Asa SL, Brubaker PL, Drucker DJ: Intestinal growth-promoting properties of glucagon-like peptide-2 in mice, *Am J Physiol* 273(1 Pt 1);E77-E84, 1997.

58. Drucker DJ, Ehrlich P, Asa SL, Brubaker PL: Induction of intestinal epithelial proliferation by glucagon-like peptide 2, *Proc Natl Acad Sci USA* 23:93(15):7911-7916, 1996.

59. Kato Y, et al: Glucagon like peptide-2 enhances small intestinal absorptive function and mucosal mass in vivo, *J Pediatr Surg* 34(1):18-21, 1999.

60. Benjamin MA, McKay DM, Yang P-C, Cameron H, Perdue MH: Glucagon-like peptide-2 enhances intestinal epithelial barrier function of both transcellular and paracellular pathways in the mouse, *Gut* 47(1):112-119, 2000.

61. Chance WT, Foley-Nelson T, Thomas I, Balasubramaniam A: Prevention of parenteral nutrition-induced gut hypoplasia by coinfusion of glucagon-like peptide-2, *Am J Physiol* 273(2 Pt 1):G559-563, 1997.

62. Scott RB, Kirk D, MacNaughton WK, Meddings JB: GLP-2 augments the adaptive response to massive intestinal resection in rat, *Am J Physiol* 275(5 Pt 1):G911-G921,1998.

63. Jeppesen PB, Hartmann B, Thulesen J, Graff J, Lohmann J, Hansen BS, Tofteng F, Poulsen SS, Madsen JL, Hoist JJ, Mortensen PB: Glucagon-like peptide 2 improves nutrient absorption and nutritional status in short-bowel patients with no colon, *Gastroenterology* 120(4):806-815, 2001.

64. Matarese LE: Establishment of an intestinal rehabilitation program in an international tertiary care center, *Nutrition* 18(9), 2002.

65. Barker J: *Future edge: discovering the new paradigms of success,* New York, 1992, William Morrow & Company.

Means, Standard Deviations, and Percentiles of Weight (kg) by Height (cm) for Males of 2 to 74 Years

| Height (cm) | N | Mean | SD | Percentiles | | | | | | | | |
				5	10	15	25	50	75	85	90	95
BOYS: 2 TO 11 YR												
84-086	75	12.1	1.1	10.7	10.9	11.1	11.3	11.9	12.8	13.1	13.5	14.3
87-089	170	12.8	1.1	11.2	11.4	11.7	12.0	12.7	13.4	13.8	14.2	14.6
90-092	207	13.5	1.0	11.9	12.1	12.5	12.8	13.6	14.2	14.6	14.9	15.2
93-095	278	14.4	1.2	12.7	13.0	13.4	13.6	14.3	15.1	15.5	15.8	16.3
96-098	310	15.0	1.3	13.3	13.6	13.8	14.2	15.0	15.6	16.1	16.4	17.0
99-101	300	16.0	1.3	13.9	14.4	14.7	15.1	15.9	16.7	17.2	17.6	18.3
102-104	290	16.9	1.4	15.1	15.4	15.6	15.9	16.8	17.7	18.0	18.5	19.3
105-107	291	17.6	1.6	15.4	15.9	16.2	16.6	17.5	18.4	19.0	19.4	19.8
108-110	298	18.7	1.7	16.7	17.0	17.1	17.6	18.5	19.6	20.1	20.5	21.3
111-113	274	20.0	2.2	17.0	17.8	18.1	18.7	19.6	21.0	21.7	22.4	23.4
114-116	223	20.9	2.2	18.6	19.0	19.2	19.6	20.5	21.7	22.3	22.7	23.6
117-119	199	21.9	2.3	19.0	19.6	20.2	20.5	21.5	23.0	23.8	24.3	26.0
120-122	177	23.3	2.4	19.8	20.8	21.2	21.9	23.1	24.5	25.4	26.0	27.3
123-125	174	25.0	2.8	21.5	22.0	22.7	23.4	24.5	26.2	27.0	28.2	30.0
126-128	185	26.5	3.8	22.6	23.1	23.8	24.3	25.9	27.8	29.4	30.6	32.0
129-131	174	27.6	3.1	23.5	24.4	24.7	25.6	27.3	28.9	30.0	31.0	32.9
132-134	180	29.3	3.5	25.1	25.7	25.8	26.8	28.5	31.0	33.0	34.4	35.4
135-137	175	31.4	4.6	26.2	27.1	27.6	28.5	30.4	33.0	34.9	37.4	41.5
138-140	150	33.5	4.7	28.2	28.9	29.4	30.5	32.3	35.1	37.8	39.9	42.0
141-143	153	36.1	5.0	30.4	31.3	31.8	33.0	34.9	38.2	40.5	43.3	45.4
144-146	114	38.9	6.6	31.6	32.7	33.1	35.1	37.6	41.2	43.9	46.3	50.7
147-149	87	40.9	6.8	33.6	34.3	35.3	35.9	39.2	43.8	47.3	51.5	56.7
BOYS: 12 TO 17 YR												
144-146	59	38.1	5.5	31.1	32.4	33.6	34.6	36.5	40.3	42.1	46.1	53.0
147-149	77	40.9	7.1	33.6	34.0	34.7	36.5	38.3	43.8	47.4	49.4	59.8
150-152	103	43.4	6.6	36.3	37.2	38.0	38.7	41.4	46.5	51.5	54.7	56.7
153-155	106	45.9	7.9	36.5	38.1	39.1	40.6	43.7	49.7	51.9	55.2	60.9
156-158	113	48.5	9.2	39.9	40.7	41.3	42.5	45.8	50.0	57.9	62.0	67.3
159-161	146	51.1	9.2	40.8	42.9	43.9	45.6	48.6	53.6	60.9	65.4	68.4
162-164	177	54.8	8.9	44.7	45.9	46.9	49.1	53.2	58.4	61.8	64.3	69.1
165-167	197	57.3	9.2	47.1	48.8	49.9	51.3	55.3	61.0	64.8	68.6	73.3
168-170	235	61.4	10.4	49.2	51.4	52.4	55.0	59.9	65.5	69.6	72.5	79.1
171-173	233	62.8	8.8	51.4	53.4	54.8	56.9	61.3	66.1	71.2	73.7	78.2
174-176	202	66.7	10.9	52.3	55.7	57.4	60.0	64.8	71.2	75.5	81.4	89.9
177-179	166	68.8	12.0	55.8	58.7	59.6	61.6	66.3	72.3	75.5	79.6	88.0
180-182	103	71.8	9.7	60.2	60.9	62.1	64.0	70.1	79.5	82.2	85.2	88.7
183-185	64	73.5	9.1	62.4	63.6	65.4	67.8	72.1	77.3	79.4	89.9	91.1

Continued.

Means, Standard Deviations, and Percentiles of Weight (kg) by Height (cm) for Males of 2 to 74 Years—cont'd

Height (cm)	N	Mean	SD	Percentiles								
				5	10	15	25	50	75	85	90	95
MALES: 18 TO 74 YR												
153-155	56	64.6	13.0	48.6	51.3	54.5	57.1	62.0	66.8	76.8	80.6	83.5
156-158	140	65.5	11.2	48.3	51.4	54.0	57.4	64.9	72.0	77.3	79.3	86.0
159-161	292	66.2	10.8	49.1	53.8	56.4	59.2	66.0	71.2	76.9	80.2	84.3
162-164	643	68.0	10.5	52.2	55.2	57.0	60.4	67.3	74.5	79.1	81.6	86.9
165-167	1147	70.8	11.6	53.0	56.6	59.6	62.7	70.3	77.6	82.3	85.2	90.1
168-170	1582	73.5	12.0	55.9	58.6	61.3	65.9	72.7	80.2	84.5	87.9	93.4
171-173	2047	76.1	12.5	58.2	61.3	63.6	67.6	75.1	83.2	88.1	92.0	97.8
174-176	2053	78.3	12.7	60.0	63.8	66.1	69.5	77.3	84.9	90.1	93.8	99.7
177-179	1750	80.3	12.8	61.9	65.1	67.5	71.4	79.4	87.3	92.6	96.5	102.6
180-182	1252	82.6	13.6	63.4	67.3	69.6	72.9	81.4	90.1	95.0	99.4	105.7
183-185	833	85.2	13.9	65.1	69.2	71.5	75.3	83.3	93.4	99.1	103.2	110.4
186-188	398	88.0	13.3	68.9	72.3	74.8	79.4	85.6	95.1	100.4	103.5	109.8
189-191	161	92.0	16.0	71.3	75.3	77.8	80.7	89.9	99.4	105.0	110.8	123.7
192-194	66	95.9	15.8	71.8	78.6	80.2	84.8	94.2	105.2	109.1	111.8	123.8

From Frisancho AR: *Anthropometric standards for the assessment of growth and nutritional status,* Ann Arbor, 1990, The University of Michigan Press, p 41.

Means, Standard Deviations, and Percentiles of Weight (kg) by Height (cm) for Females of 2 to 74 Years

Height (cm)	N	Mean	SD	Percentiles								
				5	10	15	25	50	75	85	90	95
GIRLS: 2 TO 10 YR												
81-083	36	11.2	.8	10.1	10.2	10.3	10.4	11.0	11.7	12.1	12.6	12.6
84-086	118	11.9	.9	10.5	10.8	11.0	11.3	12.0	12.5	12.7	13.0	13.6
87-089	156	12.5	1.2	11.0	11.3	11.6	11.8	12.4	13.0	13.6	13.8	14.6
90-092	229	13.2	1.2	11.6	11.8	12.0	12.3	13.0	13.8	14.3	14.6	15.2
93-095	259	13.9	1.2	12.0	12.6	12.8	13.1	13.8	14.6	15.1	15.5	16.1
96-098	275	15.0	1.3	13.1	13.5	13.7	14.1	14.9	15.6	16.3	16.7	17.2
99-101	272	15.8	1.6	13.8	14.1	14.3	14.6	15.5	16.6	17.2	17.6	18.4
102-104	278	16.6	2.0	14.2	14.6	15.0	15.5	16.4	17.3	18.0	18.5	19.4
105-107	270	17.6	1.6	15.3	15.8	16.1	16.6	17.3	18.4	19.2	19.4	20.1
108-110	275	18.3	1.6	15.9	16.6	16.8	17.2	18.1	19.2	20.0	20.4	21.1
111-113	251	19.4	1.9	16.6	17.1	17.3	17.9	19.4	20.4	21.2	21.8	22.8
114-116	215	20.7	2.5	17.5	18.3	18.6	19.0	20.2	21.8	22.9	23.9	25.7
117-119	191	21.9	2.6	19.0	19.4	19.5	20.2	21.4	23.0	24.0	24.8	26.6
120-122	181	23.1	2.5	20.1	20.4	20.9	21.5	22.6	24.0	25.3	26.2	27.7
123-125	162	24.5	2.5	21.2	21.8	22.3	22.8	24.0	25.9	26.5	27.2	29.0
126-128	172	26.2	3.1	22.6	23.0	23.4	23.9	25.6	27.7	29.4	30.0	31.5
129-131	157	28.0	3.8	23.6	24.3	24.8	25.6	27.3	29.4	31.1	33.4	36.6
132-134	148	30.3	4.4	25.1	25.8	26.2	27.0	29.4	32.3	34.5	37.2	39.9
135-137	135	32.1	5.4	25.6	27.2	27.7	28.3	30.8	33.9	35.8	41.6	44.1
138-140	124	34.6	7.3	27.6	28.8	29.1	30.6	32.5	35.5	40.9	43.5	47.5
141-143	97	36.0	6.3	28.8	29.8	30.7	32.2	34.8	37.9	41.3	45.6	49.9
144-146	65	39.2	7.0	31.0	31.9	32.9	34.5	37.6	42.9	45.3	48.4	51.8
147-149	45	40.0	7.3	30.7	32.3	34.0	35.0	38.3	44.2	48.0	50.8	54.8
GIRLS: 11 TO 17 YR												
141-143	54	37.1	7.8	28.9	29.8	31.1	32.2	34.9	38.6	42.4	45.7	59.5
144-146	67	38.5	6.8	30.4	30.8	31.6	32.9	38.4	41.4	44.1	46.5	52.4
147-149	127	43.4	10.0	32.7	34.3	35.4	37.0	40.7	46.7	51.3	56.4	61.2
150-152	180	45.8	9.1	34.7	36.3	37.4	39.5	44.1	49.9	54.3	56.1	61.9
153-155	235	48.8	8.9	38.0	39.5	40.6	43.1	46.7	53.6	56.5	60.0	66.3
156-158	352	52.3	10.4	39.7	41.7	43.1	45.1	49.9	57.5	62.5	66.0	72.3
159-161	372	55.1	11.0	42.2	44.3	46.0	48.3	52.8	59.2	62.9	68.4	77.6
162-164	344	56.6	9.9	44.9	46.6	47.5	50.2	54.4	60.6	65.3	68.6	73.8
165-167	243	60.0	12.5	46.3	48.8	50.1	52.8	57.6	62.7	69.4	74.7	84.7
168-170	124	61.2	10.8	48.9	49.2	51.1	53.5	59.0	65.7	73.4	75.1	82.4
171-173	74	67.5	15.0	53.0	54.3	54.9	57.7	62.1	72.3	80.1	89.1	104.2

Continued.

Means, Standard Deviations, and Percentiles of Weight (kg) by Height (cm) for Females of
2 to 74 Years—cont'd

Height (cm)	N	Mean	SD	Percentiles								
				5	10	15	25	50	75	85	90	95
FEMALES: 18 TO 74 YR												
141-143	64	55.9	10.2	39.2	41.3	43.9	49.0	56.5	63.3	64.9	67.7	76.6
144-146	178	57.1	14.2	38.7	42.0	44.3	48.1	54.3	64.4	71.3	74.6	82.0
147-149	430	59.4	13.2	41.5	44.6	46.8	50.1	56.9	66.9	71.9	76.1	84.8
150-152	928	61.1	13.2	43.1	46.5	48.1	51.5	59.0	68.3	74.3	78.4	86.2
153-155	1685	63.0	13.7	45.3	47.5	49.8	53.2	60.7	70.2	77.3	81.6	88.6
156-158	2670	63.8	14.6	46.6	49.1	50.8	53.5	60.7	70.9	77.1	82.3	90.0
159-161	3041	65.3	14.5	47.7	50.2	52.0	55.2	62.3	72.6	79.4	84.6	92.9
162-164	2849	66.9	14.6	49.4	51.5	53.4	56.6	63.5	74.2	81.4	86.0	94.9
165-167	2327	68.2	15.3	50.3	52.8	54.9	57.8	64.5	74.7	82.4	88.6	98.2
168-170	1327	69.5	15.1	52.5	54.7	56.5	59.2	65.4	76.1	83.5	90.1	99.4
171-173	685	71.8	15.8	54.1	55.9	57.9	60.5	67.6	78.9	86.1	93.9	105.0
174-176	334	72.9	17.3	56.1	57.9	59.6	62.3	68.4	77.6	85.7	93.1	106.9
177-179	97	75.3	16.5	57.6	59.9	60.7	64.4	71.2	81.8	89.6	102.1	112.8

From Frisancho AR: *Anthropometric standards for the assessment of growth and nutritional status,* Ann Arbor, 1990, The University of Michigan Press, p 42.

Means, Standard Deviations, and Percentiles of Weight (kg) by Age for Adult Females of Small, Medium, and Large Frames

| Age (yr) | N | Mean | SD | Percentiles | | | | | | | | |
				5	10	15	25	50	75	85	90	95
FEMALES WITH SMALL FRAMES												
28.0-24.9	652	56.2	8.7	44.0	46.1	48.0	50.3	55.1	60.9	64.4	66.9	71.5
25.0-29.9	487	56.9	9.5	44.1	47.3	48.6	50.9	55.6	61.1	64.5	67.6	72.6
30.0-34.9	413	59.1	10.0	45.7	48.2	50.0	52.7	57.6	63.4	68.1	71.8	77.7
35.0-39.9	369	61.1	11.4	45.8	48.2	50.8	53.4	59.5	66.7	71.9	76.0	79.5
40.0-44.9	353	60.6	9.4	48.1	50.3	51.8	54.5	59.1	66.1	70.0	73.6	80.3
45.0-49.9	244	61.4	11.1	46.3	47.8	50.8	53.6	60.3	67.3	71.4	75.1	80.8
50.0-54.9	257	61.3	10.8	46.3	49.1	51.7	54.5	60.3	66.9	71.0	73.1	78.4
55.0-59.9	224	61.3	11.1	47.3	49.5	52.2	54.7	59.9	65.3	70.2	73.6	81.5
60.0-64.9	351	61.9	11.0	46.4	48.9	50.6	54.2	60.9	68.5	71.7	74.0	82.2
65.0-69.9	491	61.1	10.7	44.9	48.4	50.7	53.6	60.2	67.4	71.7	74.0	79.3
70.0-74.9	369	60.6	12.1	42.6	45.9	48.5	51.6	60.2	67.0	72.3	75.4	81.0
FEMALES WITH MEDIUM FRAMES												
18.0-24.9	1297	59.5	10.4	46.0	48.4	50.0	52.5	58.1	64.4	69.5	72.8	78.4
25.0-29.9	967	60.9	11.5	46.9	49.1	50.6	53.0	58.6	66.3	72.2	76.9	83.0
30.0-34.9	815	63.5	13.4	47.2	50.0	51.7	54.3	60.7	69.3	76.7	80.6	87.2
35.0-39.9	730	64.1	12.1	49.2	51.7	53.0	56.1	61.8	69.8	74.7	79.4	87.9
40.0-44.9	700	65.6	13.3	48.8	51.3	53.6	57.0	62.8	71.8	77.3	82.4	92.1
45.0-49.9	484	65.8	13.4	48.3	51.4	53.3	56.4	63.4	72.2	77.8	83.1	91.6
50.0-54.9	504	66.4	12.2	48.9	52.0	54.4	57.7	64.4	73.1	79.3	82.8	89.7
55.0-59.9	444	68.0	15.3	48.2	51.1	54.3	58.1	66.3	74.8	81.0	86.2	92.1
60.0-64.9	695	66.2	12.4	49.1	52.3	54.0	57.5	64.5	73.5	78.1	82.2	89.0
65.0-69.9	973	66.2	12.7	48.1	51.4	53.6	57.1	64.9	73.1	78.7	82.4	88.8
70.0-74.9	731	64.3	11.9	46.8	50.5	52.5	56.8	62.9	70.8	76.9	80.2	84.7
FEMALES WITH LARGE FRAMES												
18.0-24.9	642	68.0	17.2	48.9	51.3	53.1	56.3	62.9	76.2	83.8	89.0	102.7
25.0-29.9	480	72.6	17.7	49.9	53.4	55.6	59.3	68.7	82.9	90.9	98.8	105.0
30.0-34.9	402	76.4	19.7	51.1	54.9	57.7	61.1	72.7	88.4	97.3	102.8	111.9
35.0-39.9	361	79.1	19.5	52.8	56.1	59.1	64.5	76.7	90.4	98.1	106.0	117.9
40.0-44.9	346	79.7	19.8	53.4	57.3	60.7	65.7	77.1	91.3	99.2	104.9	114.2
45.0-49.9	240	80.1	19.6	54.5	60.1	63.2	66.7	76.8	86.6	97.6	105.0	116.9
50.0-54.9	250	79.4	16.9	55.6	60.0	63.0	67.8	77.7	88.8	97.1	103.3	112.1
55.0-59.9	218	79.8	17.5	56.4	60.2	62.5	67.6	77.6	89.9	97.0	101.6	111.3
60.0-64.9	346	77.8	15.6	56.0	59.4	62.8	66.8	76.8	85.7	92.8	100.0	104.8
65.0-69.9	484	76.6	15.4	55.3	59.4	62.0	65.8	74.5	84.6	91.7	97.8	105.0
70.0-74.9	363	74.9	14.0	53.5	57.9	60.9	65.8	74.5	82.7	87.9	91.3	99.1

From Frisancho AR: *Anthropometric standards for the assessment of growth and nutritional status*, Ann Arbor, 1990, The University of Michigan Press, p 61.

Means, Standard Deviations, and Percentiles of Weight (kg) by Age for Adult Males of Small, Medium, and Large Frames

| Age (yr) | N | Mean | SD | Percentiles | | | | | | | | |
				5	10	15	25	50	75	85	90	95
MALES WITH SMALL FRAMES												
18.0-24.9	444	69.9	11.5	54.5	57.4	59.0	62.3	68.3	76.1	80.5	83.8	89.8
25.0-29.9	318	73.4	12.0	56.7	60.3	61.9	65.1	71.8	79.4	84.7	87.5	97.9
30.0-34.9	239	75.7	12.5	57.9	61.6	63.2	67.0	74.6	83.1	87.8	92.9	98.0
35.0-39.9	212	75.5	12.0	56.0	59.9	62.1	66.6	75.9	83.5	87.8	91.4	96.0
40.0-44.9	210	78.3	12.4	58.8	62.8	65.4	70.3	76.1	86.3	92.3	94.8	101.0
45.0-49.9	220	76.3	11.7	57.7	60.9	63.2	67.6	76.2	83.6	89.0	92.1	95.8
50.0-54.9	225	75.4	11.9	57.3	60.2	64.5	67.1	74.7	82.8	88.2	90.5	99.3
55.0-59.9	204	74.5	12.0	54.7	58.2	61.5	66.7	74.8	81.9	87.2	90.6	94.7
60.0-64.9	318	74.0	12.3	54.2	59.2	62.5	65.9	73.4	80.7	85.7	88.4	93.8
65.0-69.9	446	70.7	12.1	50.8	55.4	57.8	61.9	70.3	79.0	83.3	86.8	92.4
70.0-74.9	315	70.5	12.5	49.9	54.4	57.3	61.9	70.1	78.4	83.0	85.5	92.8
MALES WITH MEDIUM FRAMES												
18.0-24.9	877	74.0	12.7	57.5	60.6	62.3	65.3	71.5	80.3	86.0	91.6	99.6
25.0-29.9	627	77.0	13.2	58.5	61.8	64.5	68.4	75.9	84.1	88.3	92.4	100.4
30.0-34.9	473	78.5	12.9	59.8	63.0	65.9	69.5	77.8	85.8	91.1	93.8	98.8
35.0-39.9	419	80.5	12.8	58.7	64.8	68.4	72.9	80.4	87.4	91.5	95.9	102.5
40.0-44.9	414	80.1	12.4	60.8	64.2	67.9	71.9	79.3	88.1	92.4	96.8	102.6
45.0-49.9	436	80.7	13.0	60.3	65.1	67.1	71.9	79.8	88.7	93.3	96.7	101.3
50.0-54.9	441	79.0	13.7	58.4	62.5	65.8	70.0	78.3	86.3	91.7	96.6	103.1
55.0-59.9	404	78.8	12.7	59.9	64.5	66.7	70.5	77.9	85.3	91.1	95.4	102.2
60.0-64.9	629	76.7	11.9	58.3	61.5	64.5	68.7	76.3	84.4	88.4	91.6	97.8
65.0-69.9	886	75.0	12.2	56.1	59.5	62.5	66.9	74.5	82.9	86.9	90.8	97.2
70.0-74.9	627	73.6	12.2	54.3	58.3	61.1	65.5	72.6	81.0	86.1	89.8	93.9
MALES WITH LARGE FRAMES												
18.0-24.9	433	77.5	15.4	58.2	61.3	62.6	67.4	74.7	85.0	91.2	95.0	104.9
25.0-29.9	310	84.3	17.4	61.2	66.0	68.4	72.6	82.2	91.6	99.8	102.8	115.2
30.0-34.9	233	86.5	16.6	65.5	68.4	70.2	75.2	85.4	94.0	101.6	106.7	116.7
35.0-39.9	206	85.0	15.0	59.6	67.4	71.8	75.4	84.1	93.1	98.9	104.1	113.3
40.0-44.9	205	85.8	16.4	63.7	67.7	68.8	74.3	84.9	94.5	100.3	107.4	113.3
45.0-49.9	215	85.5	16.5	62.7	67.0	69.4	74.0	84.0	94.0	101.3	105.9	119.2
50.0-54.9	216	84.7	14.7	64.4	66.9	68.8	73.3	83.1	94.3	101.7	103.6	108.4
55.0-59.9	199	85.7	15.7	64.5	67.1	70.3	74.8	84.5	93.5	100.5	103.5	121.1
60.0-64.9	313	82.1	14.6	61.5	66.6	69.3	73.1	80.7	89.4	94.5	98.9	107.7
65.0-69.9	440	79.5	13.8	57.0	61.5	64.9	70.4	78.9	87.8	93.0	96.3	104.0
70.0-74.9	310	77.1	13.8	55.3	59.9	63.6	67.9	76.7	84.1	90.5	95.8	101.4

From Frisancho AR: *Anthropometric standards for the assessment of growth and nutritional status*, Ann Arbor, 1990, The University of Michigan Press, p 60.

Means, Standard Deviations, and Percentiles of Triceps Skinfold Thickness (mm) by Age for Males and Females of 1 to 74 Years

| Age (yr) | N | Mean | SD | Percentiles | | | | | | | | |
				5	10	15	25	50	75	85	90	95
MALES												
1.0-1.9	681	10.4	2.9	6.5	7.0	7.5	8.0	10.0	12.0	13.0	14.0	15.5
2.0-2.9	677	10.0	2.9	6.0	6.5	7.0	8.0	10.0	12.0	13.0	14.0	15.0
3.0-3.9	717	9.9	2.7	6.0	7.0	7.0	8.0	9.5	11.5	12.5	13.5	15.0
4.0-4.9	708	9.2	2.7	5.5	6.5	7.0	7.5	9.0	11.0	12.0	12.5	14.0
5.0-5.9	677	8.9	3.1	5.0	6.0	6.0	7.0	8.0	10.0	11.5	13.0	14.5
6.0-6.9	298	8.9	3.8	5.0	5.5	6.0	6.5	8.0	10.0	12.0	13.0	16.0
7.0-7.9	312	9.0	4.0	4.5	5.0	6.0	6.0	8.0	10.5	12.5	14.0	16.0
8.0-8.9	296	9.6	4.4	5.0	5.5	6.0	7.0	8.5	11.0	13.0	16.0	19.0
9.0-9.9	322	10.2	5.1	5.0	5.5	6.0	6.5	9.0	12.5	15.5	17.0	20.0
10.0-10.9	334	11.5	5.7	5.0	6.0	6.0	7.5	10.0	14.0	17.0	20.0	24.0
11.0-11.9	324	12.5	7.0	5.0	6.0	6.5	7.5	10.0	16.0	19.5	23.0	27.0
12.0-12.9	348	12.2	6.8	4.5	6.0	6.0	7.5	10.5	14.5	18.0	22.5	27.5
13.0-13.9	350	11.0	6.7	4.5	5.0	5.5	7.0	9.0	13.0	17.0	20.5	25.0
14.0-14.9	358	10.4	6.5	4.0	5.0	5.0	6.0	8.5	12.5	15.0	18.0	23.5
15.0-15.9	356	9.8	6.5	5.0	5.0	5.0	6.0	7.5	11.0	15.0	18.0	23.5
16.0-16.9	350	10.0	5.9	4.0	5.0	5.1	6.0	8.0	12.0	14.0	17.0	23.0
17.0-17.9	337	9.1	5.3	4.0	5.0	5.0	6.0	7.0	11.0	13.5	16.0	19.5
18.0-24.9	1752	11.3	6.4	4.0	5.0	5.5	6.5	10.0	14.5	17.5	20.0	23.5
25.0-29.9	1251	12.2	6.7	4.0	5.0	6.0	7.0	11.0	15.5	19.0	21.5	25.0
30.0-34.9	941	13.1	6.7	4.5	6.0	6.5	8.0	12.0	16.5	20.0	22.0	25.0
35.0-39.9	832	12.9	6.2	4.5	6.0	7.0	8.5	12.0	16.0	18.5	20.5	24.5
40.0-44.9	828	13.0	6.6	5.0	6.0	6.9	8.0	12.0	16.0	19.0	21.5	26.0
45.0-49.9	867	12.9	6.4	5.0	6.0	7.0	8.0	12.0	16.0	19.0	21.0	25.0
50.0-54.9	879	12.6	6.1	5.0	6.0	7.0	8.0	11.5	15.0	18.5	20.8	25.0
55.0-59.9	807	12.4	6.0	5.0	6.0	6.5	8.0	11.5	15.0	18.0	20.5	25.0
60.0-64.9	1259	12.5	6.0	5.0	6.0	7.0	8.0	11.5	15.5	18.5	20.5	24.0
65.0-69.9	1774	12.1	5.9	4.5	5.0	6.5	8.0	11.0	15.0	18.0	20.0	23.5
70.0-74.9	1251	12.0	5.8	4.5	6.0	6.5	8.0	11.0	15.0	17.0	19.0	23.0
FEMALES												
1.0-1.9	622	10.4	3.1	6.0	7.0	7.0	8.0	10.0	12.0	13.0	14.0	16.0
2.0-2.9	614	10.5	2.9	6.0	7.0	7.5	8.5	10.0	12.0	13.5	14.5	16.0
3.0-3.9	652	10.4	2.9	6.0	7.0	7.5	8.5	10.0	12.0	13.0	14.0	16.0
4.0-4.9	681	10.3	3.0	6.0	7.0	7.5	8.0	10.0	12.0	13.0	14.0	15.5
5.0-5.9	673	10.4	3.5	5.5	7.0	7.0	8.0	10.0	12.0	13.5	15.0	17.0
6.0-6.9	296	10.4	3.7	6.0	6.5	7.0	8.0	10.0	12.0	13.0	15.0	17.0
7.0-7.9	330	11.1	4.2	6.0	7.0	7.0	8.0	10.5	12.5	15.0	16.0	19.0
8.0-8.9	276	12.1	5.4	6.0	7.0	7.5	8.5	11.0	14.5	17.0	18.0	22.5
9.0-9.9	322	13.4	5.9	6.5	7.0	8.0	9.0	12.0	16.0	19.0	21.0	25.0
10.0-10.9	329	13.9	6.1	7.0	8.0	8.0	9.0	12.5	17.5	20.0	22.5	27.0
11.0-11.9	302	15.0	6.8	7.0	8.0	8.5	10.0	13.0	18.0	21.5	24.0	29.0
12.0-12.9	323	15.1	6.3	7.0	8.0	9.0	11.0	14.0	18.5	21.5	24.0	27.5
13.0-13.9	360	16.4	7.4	7.0	8.0	9.0	11.0	15.0	20.0	24.0	25.0	30.0
14.0-14.9	370	17.1	7.3	8.0	9.0	10.0	11.5	16.0	21.0	23.5	26.5	32.0
15.0-15.9	309	17.3	7.4	8.0	9.5	10.5	12.0	16.5	20.5	23.0	26.0	32.5
16.0-16.9	343	19.2	7.0	10.5	11.5	12.0	14.0	18.0	23.0	26.0	29.0	32.5
17.0-17.9	291	19.1	8.0	9.0	10.0	12.0	13.0	18.0	24.0	26.5	29.0	34.5

Continued.

Means, Standard Deviations, and Percentiles of Triceps Skinfold Thickness (mm) by Age for Males and Females of 1 to 74 Years—cont'd

Age (yr)	N	Mean	SD	Percentiles								
				5	10	15	25	50	75	85	90	95
FEMALES												
18.0-24.9	2588	20.0	8.2	9.0	11.0	12.0	14.0	18.5	24.5	28.5	31.0	36.0
25.0-29.9	1921	21.7	8.8	10.0	12.0	13.0	15.0	20.0	26.5	31.0	34.0	38.0
30.0-34.9	1619	23.7	9.2	10.5	13.0	15.0	17.0	22.5	29.5	33.0	35.5	41.5
35.0-39.9	1453	24.7	9.3	11.0	13.0	15.5	18.0	23.5	30.0	35.0	37.0	41.0
40.0-44.9	1391	25.1	9.0	12.0	14.0	16.0	19.0	24.5	30.5	35.0	37.0	41.0
45.0-49.9	962	26.1	9.3	12.0	14.5	16.5	19.5	25.5	32.0	35.5	38.0	42.5
50.0-54.9	1006	26.5	9.0	12.0	15.0	17.5	20.5	25.5	32.0	36.0	38.5	42.0
55.0-59.9	880	26.6	9.4	12.0	15.0	17.0	20.5	26.0	32.0	36.0	39.0	42.5
60.0-64.9	1389	26.6	8.8	12.5	16.0	17.5	20.5	26.0	32.0	35.5	38.0	42.5
65.0-69.9	1946	25.1	8.5	12.0	14.5	16.0	19.0	25.0	30.0	33.5	36.0	40.0
70.0-74.9	1463	24.0	8.5	11.0	13.5	15.5	18.0	24.0	29.5	32.0	35.0	38.5

From Frisancho AR: *Anthropometric standards for the assessment of growth and nutritional status,* Ann Arbor, 1990, The University of Michigan Press, p 54.

Means, Standard Deviations, and Percentiles of Upper Arm Muscle Area (cm²) by Height (cm) for Boys and Girls of 2 to 17 Years

Height (cm)	N	Mean	SD	5	10	15	25	50	75	85	90	95
BOYS: 2 TO 11 YR												
87-092	94	12.9	2.2	9.3	10.4	10.6	11.2	12.9	14.2	15.0	15.8	16.5
93-098	373	13.7	2.4	10.2	10.9	11.2	12.1	13.5	15.3	15.9	16.5	17.0
99-104	587	14.6	3.1	10.9	11.7	12.2	13.0	14.5	15.9	16.5	17.1	18.4
105-110	587	15.7	3.1	12.0	12.8	13.3	14.1	15.4	17.0	17.8	18.6	19.8
111-116	588	16.7	2.9	12.6	13.6	14.3	15.0	16.6	18.1	18.9	19.6	20.7
117-122	496	18.1	3.5	14.1	14.5	15.0	16.1	17.7	19.7	20.7	21.6	23.4
123-128	376	19.5	3.6	15.0	15.9	16.3	17.4	19.2	21.2	22.3	23.2	24.2
129-134	359	21.6	4.3	16.1	17.3	18.4	19.3	21.1	23.2	24.7	25.3	27.9
135-140	354	22.9	4.2	17.2	18.1	18.9	20.4	22.6	24.9	26.1	27.2	30.2
141-146	325	25.1	5.2	19.3	20.1	20.8	21.9	24.0	27.2	29.0	30.5	34.0
147-152	266	27.5	4.8	21.2	22.4	23.2	24.8	27.0	29.8	31.8	32.9	34.4
153-158	150	29.8	7.2	22.3	23.2	24.3	25.4	28.4	32.2	34.8	36.9	40.1
159-164	65	32.5	6.5	23.7	24.5	25.3	27.5	31.9	35.6	39.7	41.4	44.5
BOYS: 12 TO 17 YR												
141-146	31	26.8	4.7	20.7	21.4	22.7	24.1	25.6	30.3	32.8	33.9	36.3
147-152	90	28.2	4.1	22.4	23.4	24.1	25.6	27.5	30.2	33.1	34.2	36.1
153-158	181	31.4	6.4	22.7	24.9	26.1	27.5	30.4	34.1	36.4	39.1	41.5
159-164	218	35.0	7.7	23.7	26.7	27.8	30.2	34.1	38.6	41.5	44.3	48.4
165-170	323	40.8	9.3	28.1	29.7	31.5	34.2	40.0	45.6	49.0	52.9	58.9
171-176	431	46.6	9.9	32.8	35.2	36.6	39.5	45.8	52.6	56.0	59.1	66.0
177-182	431	50.3	9.3	36.1	38.7	40.8	43.4	49.5	56.4	59.4	62.6	65.9
183-188	269	53.4	11.2	38.3	41.3	42.8	46.1	52.6	57.8	63.0	67.5	74.3
189-194	99	55.4	9.9	41.4	44.2	45.7	48.9	53.9	60.3	65.0	68.5	74.0
GIRLS: 2 TO 10 YR												
87-092	154	12.6	2.1	9.5	10.1	10.5	11.0	12.6	14.2	14.8	15.5	16.2
93-098	384	13.2	2.1	10.1	10.7	11.0	11.8	13.2	14.4	15.3	15.8	16.9
99-104	533	14.1	2.3	10.6	11.2	11.7	12.5	14.0	15.5	16.4	16.9	18.0
105-110	550	14.8	2.4	11.3	11.9	12.4	13.2	14.6	16.3	17.3	17.9	18.9
111-116	543	15.9	2.8	12.3	13.0	13.5	14.2	15.7	17.4	18.4	19.1	20.3
117-122	465	17.0	2.8	13.0	13.9	14.4	15.2	16.7	18.5	19.6	20.3	21.4
123-128	372	18.2	2.8	14.2	15.0	15.5	16.2	17.9	19.6	20.8	21.6	22.9
129-134	333	20.1	4.6	15.3	16.1	16.8	17.6	19.7	21.7	22.9	23.8	25.4
135-140	303	21.6	4.2	16.1	17.4	18.1	19.2	21.1	23.8	24.8	26.3	27.9
141-146	258	23.3	4.0	17.6	18.5	19.5	20.5	23.0	25.8	27.9	28.8	30.6
147-152	161	25.2	5.2	18.5	20.0	20.7	21.7	24.4	27.8	30.0	31.2	32.9
153-158	66	26.7	6.7	19.4	20.1	22.4	23.0	25.4	29.2	31.8	34.0	38.2
GIRLS: 11 TO 17 YR												
141-146	53	23.8	4.4	17.1	19.3	19.5	21.0	23.4	25.5	27.9	28.6	33.4
147-152	119	25.2	4.6	18.5	19.7	20.9	22.0	24.3	28.0	29.8	30.3	34.4
153-158	305	29.1	6.4	20.8	22.0	23.0	24.7	28.3	32.9	35.0	37.5	39.2
159-164	587	32.2	7.1	23.3	24.8	26.0	27.7	31.2	35.7	38.0	40.1	43.5
165-170	715	34.2	7.4	25.0	26.6	27.8	29.5	33.2	37.6	40.2	42.8	46.9
171-176	367	34.9	8.0	25.9	27.1	28.0	29.9	33.7	38.0	41.2	43.5	47.6
177-182	113	37.8	8.4	28.6	29.5	30.5	31.7	35.9	41.1	45.9	47.8	58.2

From Frisancho AR: *Anthropometric standards for the assessment of growth and nutritional status*, Ann Arbor, 1990, The University of Michigan Press, p 51.

Appendix 7

Means, Standard Deviations, and Percentiles of Muscle Area (cm²) by Age for Adult Females of Small, Medium, and Large Frames

Age (yr)	N	Mean	SD	5	10	15	25	50	75	85	90	95
FEMALES WITH SMALL FRAMES												
18.0-24.9	651	26.2	6.0	18.2	19.6	20.7	22.5	25.5	29.2	31.2	32.8	36.2
25.0-29.9	486	27.8	7.4	19.5	20.6	21.6	23.2	26.9	30.8	33.3	35.2	38.1
30.0-34.9	413	28.6	7.8	19.1	21.6	22.4	24.5	27.8	31.4	33.7	36.2	38.8
35.0-39.9	368	20.6	10.1	19.7	21.4	22.9	24.4	28.8	32.5	35.4	37.5	42.2
40.0-44.9	350	29.8	6.6	20.9	22.1	23.4	25.7	28.9	33.2	36.0	37.9	41.8
45.0-49.9	241	29.2	7.4	19.1	21.5	22.6	24.3	28.3	33.3	36.1	38.7	41.2
50.0-54.9	256	30.3	7.3	20.8	22.1	23.9	25.5	29.1	33.4	36.7	38.5	41.3
55.0-59.9	223	30.9	7.6	20.4	22.3	23.6	25.8	30.2	34.8	37.6	41.3	45.1
60.0-64.9	351	31.9	8.7	20.9	22.4	23.6	25.8	31.2	36.4	39.1	41.1	46.2
65.0-69.9	491	31.3	8.1	19.4	22.1	23.7	25.7	30.6	35.4	39.8	41.8	45.7
70.0-74.9	367	32.0	9.9	20.3	22.5	24.1	25.9	30.3	36.1	39.8	42.6	47.3
FEMALES WITH MEDIUM FRAMES												
18.0-24.9	1296	29.3	7.0	19.8	21.9	23.2	24.9	28.4	32.8	35.2	37.2	40.7
25.0-29.9	964	30.0	7.2	20.7	22.1	23.3	25.0	29.0	33.9	36.8	39.0	43.3
30.0-34.9	814	32.0	9.1	21.4	23.1	24.2	26.3	30.8	36.1	39.4	41.8	46.4
35.0-39.9	728	32.7	8.4	21.4	23.6	24.9	27.3	31.4	37.3	40.8	43.0	47.0
40.0-44.9	696	33.7	12.1	21.2	23.2	25.1	27.2	31.6	37.7	43.1	47.1	52.3
45.0-49.9	484	33.8	8.8	22.2	23.6	25.5	27.9	32.2	37.9	42.5	45.4	49.6
50.0-54.9	502	35.0	9.7	22.8	25.2	26.2	28.5	33.7	40.0	43.5	46.7	51.4
55.0-59.9	442	36.3	11.5	23.7	25.3	26.6	28.7	34.5	41.5	44.9	49.2	53.4
60.0-64.9	695	35.1	9.1	23.0	25.3	26.5	29.2	33.9	39.9	43.7	46.1	49.4
65.0-69.9	971	35.7	10.0	22.4	24.8	26.4	29.1	34.6	40.7	44.5	48.1	51.9
70.0-74.9	731	35.3	9.7	22.2	24.3	26.1	28.9	34.0	40.0	44.4	46.7	51.3
FEMALES WITH LARGE FRAMES												
18.0-24.9	641	34.4	10.7	21.9	23.8	25.3	27.3	31.9	38.7	43.9	47.5	55.8
25.0-29.9	471	36.7	11.5	22.2	25.4	26.8	29.3	34.5	42.0	46.8	50.3	60.1
30.0-34.9	392	38.8	12.3	24.0	25.8	27.3	30.1	36.3	45.1	50.7	55.1	61.2
35.0-39.9	357	41.6	14.4	23.9	27.4	29.1	32.2	39.1	47.2	53.7	61.0	72.1
40.0-44.9	344	43.5	16.6	26.2	28.8	30.5	32.9	40.3	49.5	54.4	58.7	71.6
45.0-49.9	236	43.0	15.8	25.0	28.0	29.4	32.5	39.7	49.0	58.3	62.8	69.9
50.0-54.9	246	42.4	13.1	25.1	28.4	30.1	33.4	39.6	49.5	54.8	59.7	68.4
55.0-59.9	213	45.2	16.9	27.0	30.0	32.4	35.8	42.0	51.0	58.5	62.2	65.7
60.0-64.9	341	43.1	14.2	26.6	29.1	31.2	33.9	40.7	49.8	54.8	57.5	67.6
65.0-69.9	482	42.5	13.4	26.4	28.4	30.6	33.5	40.0	48.7	55.3	58.7	66.5
70.0-74.9	363	41.5	11.6	25.7	28.8	30.2	32.8	40.1	48.7	51.4	54.8	60.3

From Frisancho AR: *Anthropometric standards for the assessment of growth and nutritional status*, Ann Arbor, 1990, The University of Michigan Press, p. 63.
Note: Values for females aged 18 years and older have been adjusted for bone area by subtracting 6.5 cm² from the calculated mid upper arm muscle area.

Means, Standard Deviations, and Percentiles of Muscle Area (cm²) by Age for Adult Males of Small, Medium, and Large Frames

| Age (yr) | N | Mean | SD | Percentiles | | | | | | | | |
				5	10	15	25	50	75	85	90	95
MALES WITH SMALL FRAMES												
18.0-24.9	443	45.6	10.6	30.8	33.8	35.8	38.7	44.6	51.3	55.2	58.1	63.2
25.0-29.9	318	48.2	9.8	33.5	36.8	39.2	41.8	47.6	53.5	57.7	61.2	63.7
30.0-34.9	237	49.6	10.2	35.0	37.5	38.9	42.0	48.8	56.4	60.0	62.7	66.9
35.0-39.9	212	51.2	10.4	34.7	38.7	40.9	44.1	50.7	57.5	61.7	63.8	70.0
40.0-44.9	210	51.5	10.1	34.9	38.1	40.6	44.2	51.6	58.2	61.6	64.5	66.9
45.0-49.9	220	49.7	10.8	32.8	36.5	38.9	42.9	49.1	55.7	59.5	63.3	68.8
50.0-54.9	225	49.1	11.2	33.8	36.0	38.2	41.5	47.6	55.5	60.7	63.8	69.3
55.0-59.9	204	47.9	10.1	31.2	35.4	37.8	41.7	47.8	54.3	58.8	61.4	64.2
60.0-64.9	318	48.7	11.2	32.5	36.3	38.7	41.4	48.0	54.6	59.6	62.2	68.0
64.0-69.9	446	45.1	10.7	26.7	31.5	34.7	37.6	44.7	52.5	56.1	58.5	62.7
70.0-74.9	314	43.5	10.3	27.7	30.8	32.9	36.1	43.4	49.6	53.4	56.6	59.9
MALES WITH MEDIUM FRAMES												
18.0-24.9	875	50.5	10.5	35.5	38.2	40.8	43.6	49.5	56.5	60.8	63.2	69.3
25.0-29.9	626	54.0	11.3	37.0	40.1	42.9	46.8	53.2	60.9	65.6	67.7	73.0
30.0-34.9	472	55.0	10.4	38.5	42.2	44.8	48.0	54.3	61.8	65.7	68.6	72.7
35.0-39.9	416	56.7	11.7	39.9	43.1	45.2	48.8	55.9	64.0	69.0	71.6	75.6
40.0-44.9	413	56.7	11.0	39.2	42.6	45.8	49.2	56.3	64.0	68.0	71.1	74.4
45.0-49.9	433	56.6	11.2	39.0	42.6	45.6	49.4	55.9	63.7	69.6	72.8	76.2
50.0-54.9	440	55.3	11.7	37.6	41.8	44.5	47.7	54.2	62.5	65.9	69.6	74.1
55.0-59.9	403	55.4	10.8	39.2	42.5	44.4	48.5	54.8	62.2	66.7	69.5	75.0
60.0-64.9	627	52.3	10.8	34.5	38.3	41.6	45.0	52.1	59.2	63.3	66.3	70.4
65.0-69.9	886	49.8	10.5	33.4	37.2	39.6	43.0	49.2	56.7	60.1	62.4	68.1
70.0-74.9	626	47.8	10.8	30.8	34.6	36.9	40.6	47.5	54.4	59.1	62.0	66.8
MALES WITH LARGE FRAMES												
18.0-24.9	431	55.7	12.2	37.6	40.8	43.0	47.3	54.6	63.5	67.0	71.6	76.7
25.0-29.9	305	60.3	12.0	42.6	45.7	48.4	52.6	60.4	67.3	72.8	75.8	81.2
30.0-34.9	230	62.8	13.4	44.2	46.9	49.2	53.3	62.6	70.6	75.3	78.8	84.0
35.0-39.9	203	61.6	13.3	43.2	46.0	48.9	51.8	59.9	70.3	76.6	79.4	82.8
40.0-44.9	204	61.8	12.3	44.9	47.4	49.6	53.2	60.0	69.8	74.4	79.4	83.7
45.0-49.9	214	61.1	13.0	42.9	46.3	48.1	52.4	59.6	67.5	71.1	74.9	86.4
50.0-54.9	214	60.5	12.8	41.8	46.0	47.8	51.6	59.4	67.6	72.5	77.6	85.4
55.0-59.9	198	60.2	12.0	42.3	45.0	47.9	52.9	59.8	66.9	71.8	75.3	83.8
60.0-64.9	311	57.9	12.1	38.9	43.9	46.8	50.1	57.5	65.8	69.0	71.8	77.4
65.0-69.9	439	54.5	12.7	35.6	39.4	41.7	46.0	53.7	62.7	66.9	70.7	75.6
70.0-74.9	310	52.0	12.4	33.2	38.3	40.3	43.6	51.6	59.0	63.8	67.2	72.2

From Frisancho AR: *Anthropometric standards for the assessment of growth and nutritional status*, Ann Arbor, 1990, The University of Michigan Press, p 62.
Note: Values for males aged 18 years and older have been adjusted for bone area by subtracting 10.0 cm² from the calculated mid upper arm muscle area.

Means, Standard Deviations, and Percentiles of Upper Arm Fat Area (cm²) by Age for Males and Females 1 to 74 Years

Age (yr)	N	Mean	SD	Percentiles								
				5	10	15	25	50	75	85	90	95
MALES												
1.0-1.9	681	7.5	2.2	4.5	4.9	5.3	5.9	7.4	8.9	9.6	10.3	11.7
2.0-2.9	672	7.4	2.3	4.2	4.8	5.1	5.8	7.3	8.6	9.7	10.6	11.6
3.0-3.9	715	7.6	2.4	4.5	5.0	5.4	5.9	7.2	8.8	9.8	10.6	11.8
4.0-4.9	707	7.3	2.5	4.1	4.7	5.2	5.7	6.9	8.5	9.3	10.0	11.4
5.0-5.9	676	7.4	3.1	4.0	4.5	4.9	5.5	6.7	8.3	9.8	10.9	12.7
6.0-6.9	298	7.7	4.1	3.7	4.3	4.6	5.2	6.7	8.6	10.3	11.2	15.2
7.0-7.9	312	8.1	4.2	3.8	4.3	4.7	5.4	7.1	9.6	11.6	12.8	15.5
8.0-8.9	296	8.9	5.0	4.1	4.8	5.1	5.8	7.6	10.4	12.4	15.6	18.6
9.0-9.9	322	10.1	6.2	4.2	4.8	5.4	6.1	8.3	11.8	15.8	18.2	21.7
10.0-10.9	333	12.0	7.3	4.7	5.3	5.7	6.9	9.8	14.7	18.3	21.5	27.0
11.0-11.9	324	13.6	9.4	4.9	5.5	6.2	7.3	10.4	16.9	22.3	26.0	32.5
12.0-12.9	348	13.9	9.6	4.7	5.6	6.3	7.6	11.3	15.8	21.1	27.3	35.0
13.0-13.9	350	13.0	9.2	4.7	5.7	6.3	7.6	10.1	14.9	21.2	25.4	32.1
14.0-14.9	358	13.3	10.2	4.6	5.6	6.3	7.4	10.1	15.9	19.5	25.5	31.8
15.0-15.9	356	12.8	9.0	5.6	6.1	6.5	7.3	9.6	14.6	20.2	24.5	31.3
16.0-16.9	350	13.9	9.5	5.6	6.1	6.9	8.3	10.5	16.6	20.6	24.8	33.5
17.0-17.9	337	12.9	8.9	5.4	6.1	6.7	7.4	9.9	15.6	19.7	23.7	28.9
18.0-24.9	1752	16.9	10.8	5.5	6.9	7.7	9.2	13.9	21.5	26.8	30.7	37.2
25.0-29.9	1250	18.8	11.6	6.0	7.3	8.4	10.2	16.3	23.9	29.7	33.3	40.4
30.0-34.9	940	20.4	11.4	6.2	8.4	9.7	11.9	18.4	25.6	31.6	34.8	41.9
35.0-39.9	832	20.1	10.5	6.5	8.1	9.6	12.8	18.8	25.2	29.6	33.4	39.4
40.0-44.9	828	20.4	11.2	7.1	8.7	9.9	12.4	18.0	25.3	30.1	35.3	42.1
45.0-49.9	867	20.1	11.0	7.4	9.0	10.2	12.3	18.1	24.9	29.7	33.7	40.4
50.0-54.9	879	19.4	10.3	7.0	8.6	10.1	12.3	17.3	23.9	29.0	32.4	40.0
55.0-59.9	807	19.2	10.2	6.4	8.2	9.7	12.3	17.4	23.8	28.4	33.3	39.1
60.0-64.9	1259	19.1	10.2	6.9	8.7	9.9	12.1	17.0	23.5	28.3	31.8	38.7
65.0-69.9	1773	18.0	9.8	5.8	7.4	8.5	10.9	16.5	22.8	27.2	30.7	36.3
70.0-74.9	1250	17.5	9.4	6.0	7.5	8.9	11.0	15.9	22.0	25.7	29.1	34.9
FEMALES												
1.0-1.9	622	7.3	2.3	4.1	4.6	5.0	5.6	7.1	8.6	9.5	10.4	11.7
2.0-2.9	614	7.7	2.3	4.4	5.0	5.4	6.1	7.5	9.0	10.0	10.8	12.0
3.0-3.9	651	7.8	2.5	4.3	5.0	5.4	6.1	7.6	9.2	10.2	10.8	12.2
4.0-4.9	680	8.0	2.6	4.3	4.9	5.4	6.2	7.7	9.3	10.4	11.3	12.8
5.0-5.9	672	8.5	3.4	4.4	5.0	5.4	6.3	7.8	9.8	11.3	12.5	14.5
6.0-6.9	296	8.7	3.9	4.5	5.0	5.6	6.2	8.1	10.0	11.2	13.3	16.5
7.0-7.9	329	9.8	4.5	4.8	5.5	6.0	7.0	8.8	11.0	13.2	14.7	19.0
8.0-8.9	275	11.3	6.5	5.2	5.7	6.4	7.2	9.8	13.3	15.8	18.0	23.7
9.0-9.9	321	13.1	7.3	5.4	6.2	6.8	8.1	11.5	15.6	18.8	22.0	27.5
10.0-10.9	329	14.1	7.7	6.1	6.9	7.2	8.4	11.9	18.0	21.5	25.3	29.9
11.0-11.9	302	16.3	9.7	6.6	7.5	8.2	9.8	13.1	19.9	24.4	28.2	36.8
12.0-12.9	323	16.9	8.9	6.7	8.0	8.8	10.8	14.8	20.8	24.8	29.4	34.0
13.0-13.9	360	19.1	11.0	6.7	7.7	9.4	11.6	16.5	23.7	28.7	32.7	40.8
14.0-14.9	370	20.4	11.0	8.3	9.6	10.9	12.4	17.7	25.1	29.5	34.6	41.2
15.0-15.9	309	20.7	11.4	8.6	10.0	11.4	12.8	18.2	24.4	29.2	32.9	44.3
16.0-16.9	343	23.5	10.9	11.3	12.8	13.7	15.9	20.5	28.0	32.7	37.0	46.0
17.0-17.9	291	23.9	13.0	9.5	11.7	13.0	14.6	21.0	29.5	33.5	38.0	51.6

Continued.

Means, Standard Deviations, and Percentiles of Upper Arm Fat Area (cm²) by Age for Males and Females 1 to 74 Years—cont'd

Age (yr)	N	Mean	SD	5	10	15	25	50	75	85	90	95
FEMALES												
18.0-24.9	2588	25.2	13.4	10.0	12.0	13.5	16.1	21.9	30.6	37.2	42.0	51.6
25.0-29.9	1921	28.1	14.7	11.0	13.3	15.1	17.7	24.5	34.8	42.1	47.1	57.5
30.0-34.9	1619	31.6	16.1	12.2	14.8	17.2	20.4	28.2	39.0	46.8	52.3	64.5
35.0-39.9	1453	33.6	16.8	13.0	15.8	18.0	21.8	29.7	41.7	49.2	55.5	64.9
40.0-44.9	1390	34.3	16.2	13.8	16.7	19.2	23.0	31.3	42.6	51.0	56.3	64.5
45.0-49.9	961	36.0	17.2	13.6	17.1	19.8	24.3	33.0	44.4	52.3	58.4	68.8
50.0-54.9	1004	36.7	15.9	14.3	18.3	21.4	25.7	34.1	45.6	53.9	57.7	65.7
55.0-59.9	879	37.6	17.7	13.7	18.2	20.7	26.0	34.5	46.4	53.9	59.1	69.7
60.0-64.9	1389	37.1	16.0	15.3	19.1	21.9	26.0	34.8	45.7	51.7	58.3	68.3
65.0-69.9	1946	34.7	15.1	13.9	17.6	20.0	24.1	32.7	42.7	49.2	53.6	62.4
70.0-74.9	1463	32.9	14.6	13.0	16.2	18.8	22.7	31.2	41.0	46.4	51.4	57.7

From Frisancho AR: *Anthropometric standards for the assessment of growth and nutritional status,* Ann Arbor, 1990, The University of Michigan Press, p 52.

INDEX

Page references followed by *f, b, n* or *t* indicate figures, boxes, notes, or tables, respectively.

Feeding tubes *(Continued)*
  gastrostomy, 206, 207*f*
  length of, 202
  materials, 204-205, 205*t*
  medication delivery via, 329, 329*b*
  nasal, 208
  nasoenteral, 202, 203*t*-204*t*
    insertion of, 206-207
  nasogastric, 206, 206*f*
  obstruction of, 217
    in combined feeding, 294
    preventing, 217, 218*b*
  placement of
    bedside methods to verify, 215
    initial, 215-217
  ports, 206, 206*f*
  selection of, 202, 202*b*
  surgically and endoscopically inserted, 207-208
  tips, 206
  weights of, 205
Females
  adult
    creatinine excretion, 50, 51*t*
    muscle area, 673*t*
    weight, 668*t*
  basal energy expenditures, 83-84, 84*t*, 87-88, 88*t*
  height or stature, 38
  triceps skinfold thickness, 670*t*-671*t*
  upper arm fat area, 675*t*-676*t*
  weight, 666*t*-667*t*
Fentanyl, 317*t*
Feosol elixir, 319*t*
Ferricytochrome c reduction, 64, 64*t*
Ferrous Sulfate liquid, 325*t*
Fiber
  added, 174
  in adult enteral formulas, 197, 197*t*
  categories of, 174
  crude, 174
  dietary, 173-180
  in enteral formulas, 177, 194-198, 197*t*
  intake, 174
  optimal formulations, 285
  sources of, 174
  total, 174
Fiber-containing enteral formulas
  bowel function with, 177-179
Fibersource, 197*t*
Fibersource HN, 195*t*
Fibersource Std., 195*t*
Fiber-supplemented enteral formulas, 179
Fibronectin, 46*t*, 48-49
  serial changes in, 49, 50*f*
Fick equation, 81-82
  points of measurement for, 79*f*
Field methods, 34-41
Figures, 655
Filters, 334
Filtration, 123
Financial support, 650
FIO₂. *See* Inspired oxygen
FIO₂. *See* Fractional inspired oxygen concentration
Fish oils
  cancer benefit vs harm, 503*t*
  for inflammatory bowel disease, 423
  modular tube feeding recipe for burn patients, 603, 604*t*
FK-506. *See* Tacrolimus
Flagyl. *See* Metronidazole
Flaxseed oil, 503*t*
Fleet Phosphosoda, 319*t*
Flexiflo Companion Clearstar enteral nutrition pump, 212*t*-213*t*

Flexiflo Companion enteral nutrition pump, 211*f*, 212*t*-213*t*
Flexiflo enteral feeding tube, 205*f*
Flexiflo gastrostomy tube, 207, 207*f*
Flexiflo III enteral infusion pump, 212*t*-213*t*
Flexiflo Stomate, 207, 207*f*
Flexitainer enteral feeding containers, 209*f*
Flow cytofluorometry, 69
Flow cytometry, 65*t*, 69-70
Flow microfluorometry, 69
Flow-through stylets, 205
Floxuridine (FUDR), 491*t*
Fluconazole, 317*t*, 577*t*
Fludarabine, 491*t*, 577*t*
  nutritional implications of, 577*t*
Fluid(s)
  body, 122-128
  complications of parenteral nutrition, 254
  excess, 23*t*
  malabsorption of, 425
  movement between compartments, 123-124
  regulation of, 125-126
  requirements for, 125, 582
    in acute renal failure, 464-465
    in cytoreduction and neutropenia, 582
    determination of, 125, 125*b*, 498
    in infants and children, 363, 364*t*
    in older adults, 380, 380*t*
    in pulmonary failure, 405
Fluid balance, 124-126
  with parenteral nutrition, 254
  regulation of, 461
Fluid compartments, 123-124
Fluid deficiency, 22*t*
Fluid gains, 124, 124*b*
Fluid limitations, 318
Fluid losses, 124-125, 124*b*
Fluid management
  for acute renal failure, 465-466, 466*t*
  for chronic renal failure, 468, 468*t*
  for neonates, 349
  after traumatic brain injury, 386
Fluoride supplementation, daily, 365, 365*t*
Fluorochrome-release assay, 64*t*, 67-68
Fluorosis, 23*t*
5-Fluorouracil (5-FU), 490*t*, 491*t*, 494*t*, 577*t*
Fluphenazine hydrochloride elixir, 325*t*
FN. *See* Fibronectin
Folacin, 233-234, 234*t*
Folic acid toxicity, 154-155
Folic acid/folate, 154-155
  enteral, for neonates, 345*t*
  intake recommendations, 145, 145*t*
  for malabsorption, 427*t*
  in organ transplant candidates, 563, 564*t*
  parenteral multivitamin injection guidelines for, 351, 351*t*
  requirements for, 145*t*, 155
    in older adults, 380, 380*t*
    in pregnancy, 339-340, 340*t*
Folic acid/folate deficiency
  causes of, 57, 58*b*
  megaloblastic anemia caused by, 57-58
  signs and symptoms of, 22*t*, 23*t*, 154
Follow-up formulas, 347
Food(s)
  and cancer, 489, 502-503, 503*t*, 504*f*-505*f*
  carbohydrate functions as, 105
  and gastric emptying, 416, 417*t*
  medical, 263
  patient-reported intake, 476
Food intake
  adequate, 145

Preterm infant formulas, 346-347
 enteral, 366*t*
Preterm infants
 enteral nutrient guidelines for, 345, 345*t*
 gut priming for, 347-348
 nutrient requirements for, 345
 parenteral guidelines for, 345, 345*t*
 parenteral multivitamin injection guidelines for, 351, 351*t*
Primaxin. *See* Imipenem-cilastatin
Primidone suspension, 325*t*
Private insurers, 643
ProBalance, 191*t*, 196*t*, 197*t*
Probiotics, 424
ProCalAmine, 110
Procarbazine, 490*t*, 494*t*
Procarboxypeptidase, 413*t*
Prochlorperazine (Compazine), 319, 497, 498*t*
Prochlorperazine syrup, 325*t*
Product 80056, 366*t*
Professional challenges, 10-11
Professional staff, 6
Professional standards, 622-623
Professional Standards Review Organizations (PSROs), 616
Prognostic inflammatory and nutritional index, 608
Prograf. *See* Tacrolimus
Proliferation assays, 64*t*, 70
Proline, 94*t*
Promethazine (Phenergan), 319
Promethazine hydrochloride syrup, 325*t*
Promix, 603, 604*t*
Pro-Mix RDP, 366*t*
ProMod, 366*t*, 478*t*
Promote, 190*t*, 196*t*
Promote with Fiber, 196*t*, 197*t*
Propac, 366*t*
PRO-Peptide, 191*t*
PRO-Peptide for Kids, 189*t*
PRO-Peptide VHN, 191*t*
Pro-Phree, 366*t*
Propofol, 317*t*, 371
Prosobee, 365, 366*t*, 368*t*
Prospective payment system, 2-3, 637-638
 with comorbid conditions, 637, 639*t*
Prostaglandin, 115, 116*f*
Prostate cancer, 487, 503*t*
Protease inhibitors, 523, 523*t*
Protein(s), 94-104. *See also specific proteins*
 for acute renal failure, 465-466, 466*t*
 biologic value of, 95
 in breast milk substitutes, 365
 chemical score, 95
 dietary, for inflammatory bowel disease, 424
 enteral, for neonates, 345*t*
 in enteral formulas, 101-102, 188, 189*t*, 190-193, 191*t*
 heat release and gas exchange constants for, 78, 78*t*
 hepatic synthesis of, 447
 hepatic transport of, 45-49, 46*t*
 in home parenteral nutrition solutions, 309
 and immune function, 97
 metabolism of, in cancer, 492-493
 parenteral, 101-102, 230-231
  daily amounts for maintenance solutions, 364*t*
  for neonates, 350
 in pediatric enteral formulas, 366*t*
 requirements for
  in acute pancreatitis, 434-435
  in acute renal failure, 464
  in burn patients, 598, 599*t*, 600-602
  in cancer, 498
  in chronic renal failure, 471-472
  in cytoreduction and neutropenia, 582

Protein(s) *(Continued)*
 requirements for
  determination of, 498
  in diabetes mellitus, 539
  early posttransplantation, 566-567
  estimation of, 52-54
  in obesity, 548-549
  in older adults, 380, 380*t*
  in pregnancy, 339
  pretransplant, 563
  in pulmonary failure, 403
  in solid organ transplant candidates, 563, 564*t*
 serum levels
  in acute renal failure, 463
  in dialysis patients, 474
  in hematopoietic cell transplantation, 579*t*
 turnover of, 95-96
 underfeeding and, 222
 visceral
  serial changes in, 49, 50*f*
Protein assessment
 with hepatic transport proteins, 45-49
 methods for, 95
 somatic, 49-52
 after traumatic brain injury, 386
Protein (amino acid) balance, 101
Protein catabolic rate, 53
Protein catabolism, 554, 555*b*
Protein deficiency, 22*t*, 23*t*
Protein malabsorption, 425
Protein XL, 196*t*, 197*t*
Protein-calorie malnutrition, 366*t*
Protein-energy malnutrition, 66
Protestant faith, 628
Prothrombin time, 451, 452*t*
Proton pump inhibitors, 417*t*
PRSL. *See* Potential renal solute load
Pseudohyponatremia, 130
Pseudo-obstruction, 373
Psoralen and ultraviolet radiation, 577*t*
PSROs. *See* Professional Standards Review Organizations
Publication
 ethics of, 651
 internal communication, 654
 oral or written presentations, 655
 posters, 655-656
 reporting to professional and scientific communities, 654
 slides for oral presentations, 655
Pulmocare, 194*t*, 196*t*, 323*t*, 478*t*
Pulmonary complications, postoperative, 399-400
Pulmonary compromise
 nutritional assessment of, 402-403
 posttransplant, 583*t*
Pulmonary disease
 long-term posttransplant, 591
 specialized formulas for, 266-267
Pulmonary failure, 396-411
 enteral nutrition in, 406
 malnutrition role in, 400-401
 medications for, 399
 nutrition support in, 405-407
 oral nutrition therapy in, 405
 parenteral nutrition in, 406
 types of, 396-397
Pulmonary function
 nutrient requirements and substrate impact on, 403-404
 refeeding and, 405
Pulmonary surfactant deficit, 401
Pumps
 considerations for selection of, 210*b*
 enteral feeding, 210-211